A TEXTBOOK OF
Children's and Young People's Nursing

3RD EDITION

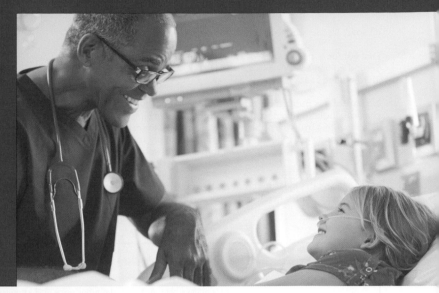

A TEXTBOOK OF
Children's and Young People's Nursing
THIRD EDITION

Edited by

Edward Alan Glasper, PhD
Emeritus Professor of Nursing Studies,
The School of Health Sciences, The University of Southampton
Southampton, UK

Jim Richardson, BA, PhD
Formerly Senior Lecturer (Children's and Young People's Nursing),
School of Nursing, Kingston University/St George's University of London,
London, UK

Duncan C. Randall, BSc(Hons), PGCert, PhD
Senior Lecturer,
Children's Nursing,
Bournemouth University,
Bournemouth, UK

Foreword by
Bernie Carter, PhD, PGCE, BSc, SRN, RSCN
Professor of Children's Nursing; Faculty of Health, Social Care and Medicine,
Edge Hill University,
Ormskirk, UK and Alder Hey Children's NHSFT, Liverpool, UK

London New York Oxford Philadelphia St Louis Sydney 2021

ELSEVIER

First edition 2006
Second edition 2010
Third edition 2021

Notices

ISBN: 978-0-7020-6232-2

Senior Content Strategist: Alison Taylor
Senior Content Development Specialist: Helen Leng
Intake Coordinator: Deanna Sorenson
Project Manager: Andrew Riley
Design: Brian Salisbury
Illustration Manager: Muthukumaran Thangaraj
Marketing Manager: Deborah Watkins

Printed in Scotland

Last digit is the print number: 9 8 7 6 5 4 3 2 1

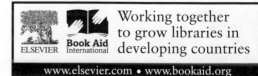

CONTENTS

Nursing children and young people makes one a privileged part of their life stories. The way we nurse inevitably influences their experiences and memories, shapes the way they make sense of things that happen to them whilst they are ill, in need of support and within our care. The way we nurse also shapes and frames the way we grow as nurses.

Nursing children and young people is an act of connection, and an act of commitment to understanding not only what needs to be done in a technical sense, but also understanding what matters to each child as an individual. Our care becomes expert when we can apply and tailor our skills and knowledge to each individual child's context and needs.

Nursing children and young people is skilled, challenging, rewarding and complex. We affect the lives of children and young people every time we are with them, no matter how short or prolonged that contact.

Becoming a children's and young people's nurse requires learning from people who have authentic knowledge, genuine skills and real-life experience. The editors and contributors of this book bring an impressive depth and breadth of experience and expertise to guide the readers to develop their knowledge and appreciation of nursing children and young people. Recognised leaders within the fields of practice, education, management and research, the editors and contributors are shaping the way that we think about and care for child and young people and the way that we ensure that they are able to participate in their own health care. Every chapter in this contemporary textbook addresses an essential element of nursing children and young people; together these 43 chapters reveal and inform reader of the wonderful and complex world of children's and young people's nursing.

Professor Bernie Carter
Edge Hill University and Alder Hey Children's NHSFT

PREFACE

The very fact that this third edition of the *Textbook of Children's and Young People's Nursing* has been published, highlights how useful children's nurses have found this text over the last 19 years. With this in mind, the key characteristics of the original editions have been retained as tried and tested features which readers will know, find accessible and are likely to use in day-to-day clinical practice. In addition, the content of the textbook has been comprehensively reviewed and brought up to date not only with respect to rapidly dynamic clinical knowledge and practice, but also to reflect the issues affecting modern childhood and society's views of the priorities to ensure the health and well-being of today's children and young people. The new edition content has been mapped to the 2018 Standards for Nurse Education from the Nursing Midwifery Council both at registration level and for nursing associates.

The textbook has been edited to ensure that clinical experts have been engaged to produce authoritative explorations of the children's nursing considerations in their particular field of practice. Care has also been taken to ensure that the content is comprehensive and addresses all aspects of modern children's and young people's nursing. The most up-to-date clinical evidence and current clinical guidelines are integrated throughout the text. This will help nurses to ensure their practice with children and their families is evidence based.

We know from reader feedback that the *Textbook of Children's and Young People's Nursing* has been found to be useful by students and newly qualified practitioners of children's and young people's nursing, as well as serving as a useful reference text for more experienced nurses. Our objective has been to try to ensure that this textbook will also be available to assist nurses and other professionals working with children and young people in areas, which are not specifically dedicated to children's services.

The modern professional practitioner is committed to providing evidence-based practice to ensure the safety and effectiveness of that care. This textbook will help these practitioners to access knowledge and understanding of each individual topic. This can be used as the basis for care, which is supplemented by use of the most recent evidence being highlighted in evidence-based journals and guidelines.

We hope that this new edition of the *Textbook of Children's and Young People's Nursing* will provide help and insight as a basis for real world children's and young people's nursing.

E. Alan Glasper
Jim Richardson
Duncan C. Randall

The editor(s) would like to acknowledge and offer grateful thanks for the input of all previous editions' contributors, without whom this new edition would not have been possible.

Kathryn Bailey, MSc, PGCE, BSc Hons, DipHE
Lecturer
School of Nursing and Health Sciences
University of Dundee
Dundee, UK

Virginia Bennett, DPhil, MA, BSc, RGN/RSCN
Lecturer in Children and Young People's
    Nursing
University of Manchester
Manchester, UK

Lesley Bloomfield, BSc
Senior Lead Nurse
W&C Care Group
Portsmouth Hospitals Trust
Portsmouth, UK

Sonya Clarke, MSc, PGCHET, PGCert, BSc Hons, RGN, RN
Senior Lecturer
School of Nursing and Midwifery
Queen's University Belfast
UK

Jane Coad, BA, BSc, PG Dip, PhD, RGN/RSCN
Professor
Faculty of Health and Life Sciences
Coventry University
Coventry, UK

Rachel Cooke, RSCN
Bereavement Service Manager and Joint
    National Child Death Helpline Manager
Great Ormond Street Hospital for Children
    NHS Foundation Trust
London, UK

Rebecca Cooke, BSc, RN, IIHH
Safeguarding Nurse Practitioner
Birmingham Women's & Children's
    Hospital NHS Foundation Trust
Birmingham, UK

Amanda Daniels, RSCN, RGN, MSc Advanced Practice
Associate Lecturer
Three Counties School of Nursing
University of Worcester
Worcester, UK

Philip Davey, MSc Advanced Practice, BN, PG Dip, PGCE
Senior Lecturer in Children's Nursing
London South Bank University
London, UK

Kath Evans, RGN, RSCN, MSc (Nursing), PG Dip (Education), PG Dipl (Management) BSc
Director of Children's Nursing/Chair of the
    Children's Board
Child Health
Barts Health; Nursing and Academic Fellow
School of Health Sciences
City University
London, UK

Susan Fairclough, MBA, PGDip (Management Studies), NNEB, Health Play Specialist Education Trust (Registered)
Therapeutic and Specialised Play Service
    Manager/Events Lead
Royal Manchester Children's Hospital
Manchester University NHS Foundation
    Trust
Manchester, UK

Debbie Fallon, BSc, MA, PhD
Senior Lecturer
Division of Nursing
Midwifery and Social Work
University of Manchester
Manchester, UK

Celeste Foster, RMN, BSc(Hons), PGCE, MA
Mental Health Nursing
University of Salford
Salford, UK

Kerry Louise Gaskin, PhD, MSc, BSc
Department of Post Qualifying Courses
School of Nursing and Midwifery
University of Worcester
Worcester, UK

Alan Glasper, PhD, RSCN
Emeritus Professor of Children and Young
    Peoples' Nursing
University of Southampton School of
    Nursing and Midwifery
Southampton, UK

Liz Gormley-Fleming, RHN, RSCN, RNT, MA, PGDip, PG Cert, SFHEA, BSc(Hons)
Centre for Academic Quality Assurance
University of Hertfordshire
Hatfield, UK

Louise Hair, BSc(Hons), PGDip, RN
Clinical Nurse Specialist for Paediatric Liver
King's College Hospital NHS Foundation
    Trust
London, UK

Anna Haviland, BSc(Hons), Cert Ed
Former Practice Development Nurse
Child and Young People's Nursing
London, UK

Sarah Adrienne Hughes, MA, BA(Hons) Community Health
Senior Teaching Fellow
Nursing
Southampton University
Southampton, UK

Janet Kelsey, MSC, BSc(Hons), MSc, PGDip, PGCEA, RN, RSCN, RNT
Associate Professor Child Health Nursing
    (Education)
Associate Head of School
    (Internationalisation)
Faculty of Health and Human Sciences
University of Plymouth
Plymouth, UK

Kate Khair, PhD, MSC, MCGI, RSCN, RN
Consultant Nurse
Haemophilia Centre
Great Ormond Street Hospital for Children
London, UK

Joann Kiernan, BSc Health Studies, MSc Profound and Multiple Learning Disability and Multi-Sensory Impairment, PhD
Senior Lecturer
Faculty of Health Social Care and Medicine
Edge Hill University
Ormskirk, West Lancashire;
Consultant Learning Disability Nurse
Community and Mental Health Division
Alder Hey Children's Hospital in the Park
Liverpool, UK

Maggie Kirk, PhD, BSc(Hons), DipNurs, Cert. Counselling, SFHEA, FRCN
Emeritus Professor, Genomics Policy Unit,
Faculty of Life Sciences and Education,
    University of
South Wales, Pontypridd, Wales, UK

Hannah Liversedge, PhD, BN(Hons), RN
Senior Teaching Fellow in Children's
    Nursing
University of Southampton
Southampton, UK

Joseph C. Manning, RN, MNursSci(Hons), PGCert, PhD
NIHR ICA Clinical Lecturer;
Clinical Associate Professor in Children,
    Young People and Families Nursing;
Charge Nurse
Paediatric Critical Care Outreach
Nottingham Children's Hospital
Nottingham University Hospitals NHS
    Trust
Nottingham, UK

Catherine Martin, BSc(Hons) RN, V300
Clinical Nurse Specialist
Martin House Children's Hospice
Boston Spa
Wetherby, UK

Deborah Martin, MSc, BSc
Health and Social Care
University of Hertfordshire
Hatfield, UK

Lisa McCann, PhD, MSc, BSc(Hons)
Senior Lecturer in Digital Health & Care
Computer and Information Sciences
University of Strathclyde
Glasgow, UK

Marisa McFarlane, RGN RSCN BSc (Hons)
Paediatric Macmillan Nurse, Royal Belfast
Hospital for Children, Belfast, Northern
Ireland, UK

Wendy Margaret McInally, MSc, BSc(Hons), RSCN
Macmillan Lecturer in Child and Cancer
    Nursing
School of Health and Social Care
Edinburgh Napier University
Edinburgh, UK

Peter McNee, MSc (Nursing), BA(Hons)
Professional Head and Lecturer in Children
    and Young People's Nursing
School of Healthcare Sciences
Cardiff University
Cardiff, UK

Nicholas Medforth
School of Nursing and Allied Health
Faculty of Education, Health and
    Community
Liverpool John Moores University
    Liverpool, UK

Alison Mosenthal, MSc, Diploma Nurse Education, RGN, RSCN
Senior Lecturer Children's Nursing
University of Hertfordshire
Hatfield, UK

Alex Murray MB BS, FRCP
Consultant Clinical Geneticist & Clinical
    Lead
All Wales Medical Genomics Service
University Hospital of Wales, Heath Park
Cardiff, Wales, UK

Arija Parker, BA(Hons), MA
Faculty of Nursing
Midwifery and Social Work
University of Manchester
Manchester, UK

Jackie Parkes PhD BNurs (Hons) RSCN RGN NONCert
Senior Lecturer, School of Nursing and
Midwifery, Queen's University Belfast,
Belfast, Northern Ireland

Elizabeth Podesta, BNurs Adult Nursing
Clinical Skills Tutor
School of Health Sciences
University of Manchester
Manchester, UK

Jayne Price MSc BSc (Hons) PGDipEd RGN RN (Child)
Senior Teaching Fellow, School of Nursing
and Midwifery, Queen's University Belfast,
Belfast, Northern Ireland, UK

Duncan Christopher Randall, BSc(Hons), PGCert, PhD
Principal Teaching Fellow
School of Health Sciences
University of Southampton
Southampton, UK

Sarah Reed, MSc, BN
Lecturer in Children's and Young Peoples'
    Nursing
Outreach Lead With Children and Young
    People
School of Health Sciences
University of Southampton
Southampton, UK

Jim Richardson, BA, PhD
Senior Lecturer (Children's Nursing)
School of Nursing
Kingston University/St George's University of
    London
London, UK

Jean Robinson, SRN, RSCN, CCN, BSc, MA
Clinical Nurse Specialist
Paediatric Dermatology
Paediatrics
The Royal London Hospital Barts Health
    NHS Trust
London, UK

Lee-Anne Rylatt, BSc, PGCert, PGCAP, MAEd
Lecturer
Faculty of Health and Human Sciences
Plymouth University
Plymouth, UK

Rebecca Saul, RGN, RSCN, PgCE, Graduate Certificate Non-Medical Prescribing, MSc
Children's Advanced Nurse Practitioner
Clinical Nurse Specialist
Pain Control Service
Great Ormond Street Hospital for Children
    NHS Foundation Trust
London, UK

Brian Silverwood
Head of Nursing for Surgery and Critical
    Care
Sheffield Children's Hospital
Sheffield, UK

Joanna Smith, PhD, MSc(Hons), BSc(Hons), RNT, RSCN, RGN
Associate Professor Children's Nursing
School of Healthcare
Faculty of Medicine and Health
University of Leeds
Leeds, UK

Kaye Spence, AM, RN, BEd(N), MN(Research)
Adjunct Associate Professor/Clinical Nurse
    Consultant
Grace Centre for Newborn Intensive Care
The Children's Hospital at Westmead
    School of Nursing and Midwifery
Western Sydney University
NSW, Australia

Jennifer Stinson, RN, PhD
Senior Scientist
Child Health Evaluative Sciences
Hospital for Sick Children
Toronto, ON, Canada

Julie Taylor, PhD, MSc, RN, BSc(Hons), RNT, FRCN
Professor of Child Protection
University of Birmingham
Birmingham, UK

Louise M. Terry, PhD, SHFEA, PGCertEd, LLB(Hons), FIBMS
Associate Professor
Department of Adult Nursing and
    Midwifery
London South Bank University
London, UK

Emma Tonkin, PhD, BSc(Hons)
Associate Professor (Genomics Healthcare)
Genomics Policy Unit
Faculty of Life Sciences and Education
University of South Wales
Pontypridd, Wales, UK

Karen Tosh, MSc, Specialist Cert., BSc Hons, DipHE
Lecturer
School of Nursing and Health Sciences
University of Dundee
Dundee, UK

Alison Twycross, PhD, DMS, MSc
Senior Lecturer in Children and Young
    People's Nursing
Open University

Annette Williamson, PGDip, BSc(Hons), RGN, RM, RHV, CPT
Named Nurse for Safeguarding
Birmingham Women's & Children's Hospital
    NHS Foundation Trust
Birmingham, UK

Julia Winter, MSc, BSc(Hons), RN
Head of Quality and Validation
Faculty of Health and Life Sciences
Oxford Brookes University
Oxford, UK

This book is dedicated to the memory of Michael Clift, a highly regarded and respected children's nurse.

We dedicate this book to our esteemed colleague in children's nursing, Michael Clift, following his early and untimely death in 2018. Michael was a revered and valued children's nurse who worked at London's Royal Free Hospital as the lead for clinical practice education in nursing across children's services. He consistently endeavoured, almost as a vocation, to support the student nurses within the children's wards at the hospital, and was passionate about their education and welfare within clinical practice. In his clinical role he was especially interested in providing optimum care for young people with mental health problems.

It is for this reason that we honour Michael's memory and his dedication in providing optimum education and support to tomorrow's registered children's nurses. We know he would be proud of this book and its aspirations to give student nurse readers access to high quality, clinically viable and credible information.

Alan, Jim and Duncan on behalf of all the contributors to this text book, who have unanimously endorsed this dedication to a truly inspirational children nurse.

Context of Children's Nursing Theories and Practices

Historical Perspectives of Children's Nursing

E. Alan Glasper, Sonya E. Clarke

LEARNING OUTCOMES

- Consider the origins of children's nursing in the context of the changing concepts of childhood.
- Understand the fight for registration and the subsequent evolution of children's nursing.

- Explore the developments in nurse education designed to ensure that children's nurses are fit for practice and purpose.
- Examine some of the key challenges facing child health nurses in the 21st century.

INTRODUCTION

Children in our present society are given 'rights' that were not accorded to children in previous generations. In Victorian times it was often said that children should be 'seen but not heard'. In today's society, children have rights under the United Nations Convention on the Rights of the Child (United Nations General Assembly 1989). This sets out the basic human rights that all children are entitled to without discrimination. The Convention is underpinned by four guiding principles, which are those of non-discrimination (Article 2), the best interests of the child (Article 3), survival and development (Article 6) and participation (Article 12). The British government ratified the document in 1991 and, by so doing, committed itself to protecting and ensuring children's rights and agreed to hold itself accountable before the international community. Although in itself it is not a legal statute, the United Nations Convention on the Rights of the Child can be used to support the rights of children. Legislation, which builds on the Articles contained in the Convention on the Rights of the Child, seeks to offer further protection to one of the most vulnerable groups within our society.

The Children Act (1989), which applies in England and Wales, is based on the principle that the child's welfare is the paramount consideration and that effective interventions should be in place to ensure the safety and well-being of children who are at risk of harm. It states that children should, wherever possible, be brought up and cared for within their own family, with both parents playing a full part in their lives, without resorting to legal proceedings. Only in situations where there is fundamental disagreement between parents, or concerns about the child's welfare, will the Courts make orders about a child's place of residence and contact arrangements. The Act emphasises the rights of children to be kept informed about issues that affect them.

The Children (Scotland) Act (1995), which applies in Scotland, is based on the following key principles:
- Each child has a right to be treated as an individual.
- Each child who can form his or her views on matters affecting him or her has the right to express those views if he or she wishes.
- Parents should normally be responsible for the upbringing of their children and should share that responsibility.
- Each child has the right to the protection from all forms of abuse, neglect or exploitation.
- In decisions relating to the protection of a child, every effort should be made to keep the child in the family home.
- Any intervention by a public authority in the life of a child should be properly supported by services from all relevant agencies working in collaboration.

Within Northern Ireland (NI) the Children's (NI) Order of 1995 continues to be the principal statute governing the care, upbringing and protection of children. It affects all those who work and care for children, whether parents, paid carers or volunteers. The NI Order changed the philosophy and practice of the law in relation to children as it reformed, and brought together, most of the 'public' and 'private' law relating to children in a single coherent statutory framework similar to the Children Act (1989) in England and Wales.

WWW

Check out the UN convention on:
- http://www.unicef.org/crc/fulltext.htm

With the introduction of the Human Rights Act (DoH, 1998) some of the rights set out in the European Convention for the Protection of Human Rights and Fundamental Freedoms (1950) became part of British law. Many rights are set out in the Act but of particular relevance to children's nurses, and indeed to all health professionals, are:

- the right to life: Article 2
- the right not to be subjected to degrading treatment: Article 3
- the right to a fair hearing: Article 5
- the right to respect for private and family life: Article 6
- the right not to suffer discrimination in relation to any of the other basic rights: Article 14.

The Human Rights Act, which is central to the right to self-determination by children and young people (CYP), includes their right to consent to or refuse treatment (Lowden, 2002). However, the Children Act (1989) and the Children (Scotland) Act (1995), although providing legislation that relates to the care of children and their upbringing and protection from harm, do not go beyond establishing their right to be involved in decision making about their welfare. The Human Rights Act enables action to be taken if it is proved that children's rights have been infringed (Power 2002).

 POWERPOINT

Access the companion PowerPoint presentation and look up the following web pages and consider the extent of the material on children's rights:
- http://www.unhchr.ch/html/menu3/b/k2crc.htm
- http://www.hmso.gov.uk/acts/acts1998/19980042.htm

ACTIVITY

Access, read and reflect upon a child centred approach and the child as a rights holder:
- Soderback, M., Coyne, I., Harder, M., 2011. The importance of including both a child perspective and the child's perspective within health care settings to provide truly child-centred care. J Child Health Care 15 (2), 99–106.
- http://chc.sagepub.com/content/15/2/99.full.pdf+html

Children in our society are without a political voice and, until recently, played no significant role in the political processes that impact and influence their lives.

The recent appointment of Children's Commissioners in Wales, Northern Ireland and Scotland is a response to the need to address the rights of children. England delayed the appointment of a children's commissioner after lengthy discussions about the proposed role and powers. The role was felt to fall short of the United Nations international guidelines. In the interim, Margaret Hodge, the Minister for Children in England, held responsibility for children's services, childcare and the protection of the under-fives as part of her portfolio. Al Aynsley-Green was appointed Commissioner for Children in England in March 2005. The appointment of Peter Clarke in Wales, Nigel Williams in Northern Ireland and Kathleen Marshall in Scotland did ensure the children in these countries had an advocate in all matters that affect them, either

directly or indirectly. All four countries continue to appoint a children's commissioner. Part of the role of the Commissioner is to monitor all proposed legislation to ensure that the needs and best interests of children are met. They will also have a remit in relation to the safe guarding of children and young people (see Chapter 19). Undertaking and commissioning research is another strand of their work. This activity should contribute to the body of knowledge on which sound decisions can be made on matters affecting children.

 WWW

Look up the following web pages and read about the role and remit of the recently appointed Children's Commissioners:
- http://www.crights.org.uk/commissioner/commissioner.html
- http://www.niccy.org
- http://www.childcom.org.uk/english/index.html
- http://www.scottish.parliament.uk/news/news-04/pa04-008.htm

With rights come societal responsibilities and subsequently new challenges for nurses caring for children and their families in hospital and community. In the past, children were considered as individuals with needs, whereas in contemporary society they are considered to be individuals with rights. The two standpoints are not mutually exclusive. However, the task facing children's nurses today is very different from the task faced by those caring for children at the time of the inception of children's nursing in 1852.

THE CHANGING CONCEPTS OF CHILDHOOD

The material that follows traces the origins of children's nursing in the UK in the context of changing concepts of childhood. Consideration will be given to the fight for registration for sick children's nurses and the evolution of children's nursing in response to greater understanding of the needs of children and their families. Consideration will be given to the educational provision that seeks to ensure that the children's nurses of tomorrow are equipped to provide high standards of care for children and families. Finally, an overview will be given of some of the challenges currently facing children's nurses in the UK.

Children's nursing has undergone a number of fundamental changes since its inception in the mid-18th century. The changes reflect developments within the nursing profession but also changes in societal views towards children themselves and to the needs of children and families. Reference to the sociological analysis of childhood provides substantial evidence of the ambivalent attitude of the British towards children (Scraton, 1997). Indeed, this began to change in the time of the European Enlightenment when, rather than looking at children as poor and weak, whose survival was little valued, society increasingly recognised that children were its future and that their healthy survival was essential for the continuation of society (Seidler, 1990). However, there is continued evidence of a lack of respect for children and their specific needs within society in general, and this attitude is even more evident in the NHS than in the general population.

It is generally agreed that the perspective from which they are considered influences perceptions about children and childhood. Writers on the subject rarely reach a consensus. Thomas, cited by Avery and Briggs (1989), highlights the difficulties of unravelling the concept of childhood by suggesting that historians and modern writers continue to write the history of adults' attitudes towards children rather than the history of childhood. This can still be seen in society today, when debates about what constitutes the best interests of children often centre on what adults define as 'best interests'.

One of the most influential writers on the subject of childhood is Aries (1962), a French historian. He and de Mause (1995) are referred to in many childcare texts. Aries' (1962) views are often misrepresented, as he did not consider the absence of a concept of childhood as detrimental to children. He noted that children in the Middle Ages mingled with adults and spent considerable time in their presence, working and playing. In his opinion the separation of adults from children occurred in the 17th century, with the start of education dominated by religion-based morality. Not all historians agree with this view and, in his writings, de Mause makes the dramatic statement:

The historical record points to childhood being a nightmare from which we have only begun to awaken. The further back in history one goes, the lower the levels of childcare, the more likely children are to be killed, abandoned, beaten, terrorised and sexually abused

(de Mause, 1982)

During the 18th century the needs of children were increasingly recognised and by the 19th century children were considered valuable and therefore in need of protection (Stone, 1977). It was this change in attitude that led to the establishment of foundling hospitals and dispensaries for children. In the 20th century the individuality of the child has become more evident. Family life has become increasingly important. The status of the child has increased significantly with the introduction of the European Convention on the Rights of the Child in 1989 and the Human Rights Act (1998). In our society today children have the right to expect protection from harm and a right to self-determination. This is in stark contrast to the Victorian view of children, whom they considered should be seen and not heard. It has been suggested that changing perceptions of childhood over the years can be analysed by studying the themes of play, art and literature (Watt and Mitchell, 1995).

Children throughout history and in all cultures engage in some form of play through which they learn to make sense of the world of which they are part. They use imitation and experimentation to learn and experience essential social roles and values. Before the 17th century, little evidence exists for children's play, although in the 4th century BC Aristotle – a proponent of play as a prerequisite to health – advocated that children under the age of 5 years should not work. He considered that to do so would be detrimental to their health and well-being. Singer (1973) suggests

that it is likely that children did play but, as it was not considered an important activity, adults did not comment upon it.

According to Aries (1962) there were few attempts to portray childhood in art before the 12th century. This reflected society at that time and the place of children within it. In some of the early artwork images children were depicted as miniature adults. It was not until the 15th and 16th centuries that it became popular to portray children in a social context. The Dutch artist Rembrandt achieved popular acclaim for his work, which included portraits of individual children.

> ### 👤 ACTIVITY
>
> In your learning group explore how art and childhood have been portrayed.

There is limited evidence of children's literature prior to the 18th century. *Orbis Sensualism Pictus* by Comenius, which was printed in 1658, is said to be the earliest illustrated book specifically designed for children. Much of the early children's literature was written to appeal to adults and often contained moral messages. Der Struwwelpeter is a good example of this. Heinrich Hoffman (1809–1894), a German psychiatrist, wrote and illustrated it in 1845 for his son (Hoffman, 1845).

> ### 👤 ACTIVITY
>
> Look at the following extract from Der Struwwelpeter and compare it with an extract from a contemporary children's storybook. Consider what messages the books convey to young readers.
>
> **The story of little suck-a-thumb**
> *One day, Mamma said, 'Conrad dear,*
> *I must go out and leave you here.*
> *But mind now, Conrad, what I say,*
> *Don't suck your thumb while I'm away.*
> *The great tall tailor always comes*
> *To little boys who suck their thumbs:*
> *And ere they dream what he's about,*
> *He takes his great sharp scissors out*
> *And cuts their thumbs off, and then,*
> *You know, they never grow again.'*
> *Mamma had scarcely turn'd her back,*
> *The thumb was in, Alack! Alack!*
> *The door flew open, in he ran,*
> *The great, long, red-legged scissor-man.*
> *Oh! Children, see! The tailor's come*
> *And caught out little Suck-a-Thumb.*
> *Snip! Snap! Snip! the scissors go;*
> *And Conrad cries out - Oh! Oh! Oh!*
> *Snip! Snap! Snip! They go so fast*
> *That both his thumbs are off at last.*
> *Mamma comes home; there Conrad stands*
> *And looks quite sad and shows his hands*
> *'Ah!' said Mamma, 'I knew he'd come*
> *To naughty little Suck-a-Thumb.'*
> Look up the following website and read more about some of the early children's books:
> • http://www.sc.edu/library/spcoll/kidlit/kidlit/kidlit.html
> The following website contains details of the original illustrations which Dr Hoffman included in the original version of Der Struwwelpeter.
> • http://www.fln.vcu.edu/struwwel/struwwel.html

DR CHARLES WEST – FATHER OF CHILDREN'S NURSING

Dr Charles West, widely regarded as the father of paediatrics and, some would argue, children's nursing, was born more than 200 years ago on August 8, 1816, in a period of history in which the care of sick children was elementary and poorly understood. This era of health care for children is perhaps best appreciated through the eyes of the painter Sir Luke Fildes (1843–1927), a well-known English artist who painted 'The Doctor' in 1890. Although somewhat later than West's own birth, this painting perhaps symbolises the lack of knowledge about illness in childhood in the early part of the 19th century. This painting hangs in London's Tate Gallery and was inspired by Fildes own personal tragedy, when in 1877 his first son, Philip, died in infancy. A close examination of the painting shows a puzzled doctor visiting a sick child in a country hovel, looking at, and wondering how he can help. The child is lying across two cushioned kitchen chairs which make up his sick bed and is obviously in extremis. In the foreground is the father, standing stoically and silently wishing for the doctor to be able to cure his child, whilst the mother is slumped over the kitchen table crying inconsolably. This may not have been her first loss of a child, as infant mortality throughout the 19th century remained high with an average of 149 deaths per 1000 (Dyhouse, 1978). Although knowledge about the care of sick children was elementary throughout much of the 19th century, infectious disease exacerbated by poor diet was a prime cause of both morbidity and mortality.

It was into a London society where childhood death from disease was not uncommon that Charles West was born on August 8, 1816, just over a year after the famous battle of Waterloo in Belgium where the later British prime minster the Duke of Wellington defeated the French army of Napoleon Bonaparte. The end of the war with France led to almost four decades of international peace in Europe and another major war did not begin until the 1853 Crimean war, which saw the beginnings of modern nursing under the influence of Florence Nightingale.

In 1956, a young teacher named R.A. Clavering was able to access a range of archive documents and literature pertinent to the life at Charles West. Much of this homage to the legacy of West is derived from this unpublished manuscript (Clavering 1956) and West's own obituary (unknown BMJ, 1898).

West's Early Life

Charles West's father was a former toy shop keeper in London before he accepted a position as a Baptist lay preacher in a village in the county of Hertfordshire in 1821. West's father combined his ecclesiastical duties with the keeping of a local boy's school which he managed. West later attended the school to receive his early education (BMJ, 1898). In 1831, at the age of 15, West displayed an early fascination with medicine and went on to be apprenticed to a Mr Gray, a general practitioner who was also a pharmacist in the adjacent county of Buckinghamshire. He applied to study medicine at Oxford but because of his Baptist beliefs was barred from undertaking further studies. Religious aspects of his life continued to influence his future career even after he later converted to Catholicism. West found this an interesting period of his life as he was able to formulate and dispense medicines, something which he would later find useful when he later worked at a dispensary for children. West stayed with Mr Gray as his apprentice until 1833 when at the age of 17, he obtained a place to study medicine at London's Saint Bartholomew's Hospital. After 2 years West transferred to the University of Bonn for a year and additionally spent a year in Paris before completing his MD in Berlin in 1837. After completing his medical degree West returned to London where he embarked on a failed mission to develop a private practice. Having but few private patients he commenced work within the medical wards at Saint Bartholomew's Hospital as a junior doctor under the patronage of a certain Dr Latham, where he gained enormous experience in caring for the victims of a typhus fever epidemic during the winter season of 1837–1838. Most of the deaths from fever in London were attributed to typhus, and new cases averaged about 16000 in England in each of the subsequent 4 years. This disease of poverty, poor sanitation and close human contact was then, and is still today, caused by the bites from infected body lice (The Victorian Web, n.d.).

This experience of working with typhus fever patients also kindled within West the scholar and academic leading to the publication of a scientific paper in the Edinburgh Medical and Surgical Journal (West, 1838). Later in 1838, West travelled to Dublin where he studied at the Rotunda Lying-in Hospital for women. During his time in Dublin West visited the Institute for Sick Children which had been founded in 1821. Later called the National Children's Hospital, it was the first children's hospital in Ireland which was then part of Great Britain and the second oldest children's hospital in Europe. West lamented that a capital city the size and importance of London should not have the facilities to treat inpatient children. Likewise, during his stay in Paris, West had visited the Hospital des Enfants Malades, opened in June 1802, which was the first paediatric hospital in Europe. On his return from Ireland in 1839, West once again sought work at Saint Bartholomew's Hospital where he began to exploit his scholarly acumen in publishing a range of books and papers, becoming a well-known Victorian medical academic. It was also during this time that West first began to take a serious interest in the illnesses of children, although he maintained a corresponding interest in obstetrics. It was the study of childhood illness for which he will be most remembered some two hundred years after his birth (Dunn, 1991). He commenced these studies of childhood illness at the Infirmary for Children in Waterloo Road, London. The Infirmary had no inpatient beds and was primarily a dispensary but in modern medical nomenclature functioned as an ambulatory care unit, outpatient department and paediatric assessment unit. West was offered a medical position at the Infirmary in 1842 where his background as an apprentice pharmacist was to stand him in good stead.

By 1849, West had ambitions to convert the Waterloo Dispensary into an inpatient children's hospital but his aspiration failed after he was unable to secure the support of local physicians, something which was to plague him for the rest of his career. Of interest in this context is the legacy of George Armstrong, now known as the father of ambulatory care, who opened the first recorded dispensary for poor children in London in 1769. It was Armstrong who famously quoted that children and their parents should not be separated and this may have hindered the opening of the first children's inpatient hospital. Furthermore, Armstrong did not believe that parents would be able to look after their sick children in hospital because of economic pressures and the need to work (Glasper and Lowson, 1998). West's ability to communicate with children is in no doubt but his interpersonal relationships with his colleagues were perceived to be less than optimum and he is said to have been of an acerbic character. Perhaps his Baptist background made it difficult for him to really succeed in the world of adult medicine at that period of history and Clavering (1956) reports that he felt aggrieved when men younger than himself and with less experience were gaining more prestigious salaried positions than he.

Charles West's Quest to Open a Children's Hospital

In 1849 and despite these setbacks, West set about investigating which hospitals in London were offering inpatient beds to sick children. He also corresponded with the continental children's hospitals to gather data to help his cause, many of which had developed after the founding of the children's hospital in Paris (Lomax, 1996). Although not a common occurrence some hospitals did admit sick children prior to the advent of the paediatric hospitals and Williams (2007) gives examples of children admitted to the English Northampton Infirmary in the period 1744–1745. It was patronage that West needed in an era where his religious background was a disadvantage, leading to overt discrimination and fortuitously he was befriended by Dr Bence Jones, a well-known and admired physician who was interested in West's ambitions to open a children's hospital. He helped introduce West to well-known philanthropists of the time, including Lord Shaftesbury, who helped reform the hours that children worked in factories, and Edwin Chadwick, famous for his sanitary reforms which led to a decline in cholera. Notes written by West himself and held in the archives of Great Ormond Street Hospital show that Dr Bence Jones loaned his house to Charles West to hold a meeting of a provisional committee for the founding of a children's hospital. In these notes written for posterity, West acknowledges that Bence Jones's social influence was much greater than his own and that through his influence, many people cooperated with his plan to open a children's hospital.

By 1850 West had located premises suitable for conversion in Upper Gloucester Street, Marylebone Road, London, and he set about drawing up plans for the alterations but before these were completed he found another, and in his opinion, more suitable premises, located at 49 Great Ormond Street. In May 1851, West called a meeting which was held at the Hannover Square Rooms to bring the project of the Hospital before the public. To help in the quest, West as always needed data and in July and August 1851, he travelled through France and Germany, visiting hospitals for children in order to learn all that he could about their constitutions, equipment, and organisations to help equip him with the knowledge to

supervise and direct the alterations of the premises in Great Ormond Street. This 'new hospital' was actually a large palatial house and garden which had formerly been the home of a well-known London royal court physician, Dr Meade, in the early part of the 18th century. In the intervening century, the area of London which housed the premises in Great Ormond Street in the now fashionable borough of Bloomsbury had fallen into decline and was situated near the famous and squalid 'Rookeries' so vividly described by the English author Charles Dickens in novels such as Oliver Twist. The alterations and the furnishing were undertaken by West and his wife, the daughter of a certain Mr Cartwright of Stroud in Gloustershire, by whom he later had a son and a daughter.

Kosky and Lunnon (1991) cites evidence of the link between West and the author Charles Dickens which predates the opening of the Hospital in Great Ormond Street by 5 years. Dickens gave his patronage to West and became a principal supporter of the hospital in its early years. Dickens is actually cited in the minutes of the Committee of the Management of The Hospital for Sick Children dated April 8, 1852 and given thanks for his public support of the hospital (Kosky and Lunnon, 1991). Indeed Great Ormond Street Hospital featured in Dickens' last novel, Our Mutual Friend, as,

A place where there are none but children; a place set up on purpose for sick children; where the good doctors and nurses pass their lives with children, talk to none but children, comfort and cure none but children

(Dickens, 1865)

West's ambition finally became a reality when on Valentine's Day; February, 14 1852, the doors of The Hospital for Sick Children, Great Ormond Street, London, opened its doors to patients for the first time and during that first year Queen Victoria herself became the hospital's patron. West, although he may not have known this at the time, entered the halls of medical legend by becoming the father of paediatrics.

Charles West's Influence on the Development of Children's Nursing

One of the most famous of the Great Ormond Street Hospital children's nurses was Catherine J. Wood, who wrote, 'There is no more touching sight than to see Dr West making his rounds: the little patients welcomed him as their friend, and the fractious or frightened child could not long resist the magic of his smile or the winning gentleness of his manner'.

Wood had joined the hospital in 1863 at the age of 22, as a superintendent of one of the wards. After a number of associated roles, she became lady superintendent to the hospital in 1878 and remained in post for 10 years, creating the foundation of modern paediatric nursing (Kosky and Lunnon, 1991). This illustration of the first children's ward, above, dates from 1858, some 6 years after the opening of the children's hospital in Great Ormond Street and gives perhaps the very first insight into the notion of family centred care. In the foreground can be seen parents and nurses interacting together in partnership, whilst Charles West can be seen examining the leg of a child. This scene is interesting as it predates the era of Florence Nightingale and later photographs of the hospital wards at Great Ormond Street Hospital taken in the latter part of the 19th century are devoid of parental or family presence. Fear of parental borne infection and fomites gradually squeezed out lay care as Florence Nightingale's influence on hospital design and operating codes began to be applied universally. Furthermore it was Nightingale's quest to see nursing established as a profession for women, based on education and training, which left little room for amateurs! It was the Nightingale model of nursing which rose to prominence, one in which lay care quickly became subordinate to the health care professional. In the context of children's nursing, an inspection of the minutes of the first hospital committee meeting reveals that Charles West had aspirations for the Hospital in Great Ormond Street which are still applied to the contemporary hospital in the 21st century, namely the provision of health care to sick children, the application of research in the quest to better implement care and treatment to children and the education of doctors and children's and young people's nurses. The minutes of this committee meeting show that one of the founding aims of the hospital was to 'To disseminate among all classes of the community but chiefly among the poor a better acquaintance with the management of infants and children during illness by employing it (The Hospital) as a school for the education of women in the special duties of children's nursing'.

Hence in many respects children's nursing education predates that of adult nursing, because the Nightingale Training School did not open at St Thomas' Hospital until 1860. Despite this, the struggle by children's nurses in Britain for statutory training and a recordable, professional qualification was protracted and hard (Glasper and Charles-Edwards, 2002). It is important to stress that Charles West's children's hospital which he almost single-handedly developed at Great Ormond Street in 1852 was neither the first, the largest, nor possibly the best children's hospital in Europe. However, what West achieved was not solely the opening of a children's hospital, but the beginnings of a new medical science: modern paediatrics built on research and scholarly output. West's own considerable intellect was harnessed to push forward the frontiers of medical science in the quest for answers to the management of disease in childhood. Famous paediatricians such as Thomas Barlow (recognition of infantile scurvy), Dennis Browne (founder of the British Association of Paediatric Surgeons),

Mildred Creek (child psychiatry), Rodger Hardisty (child leukaemia research), and Roland Levinsky (bone marrow transplantation) all benefited from the legacy of Charles West and who relentlessly sought to increase the world's stock of knowledge related to childhood illness whilst working at Great Ormond Street throughout its long and distinguished history.

West's own emphasis on attracting staff that were among the intellectually elite of their generation also impacted nurses. Besser (1977), in describing the outstanding men of Great Ormond Street in his tribute to the 125 years of service of the hospital, reminds the reader of Charles West's publication

How to Nurse Sick Children, (1854) which appeared in 1854, some 5 years earlier than Nightingale's (1859) famous 'Notes on Nursing'. Of interest is that the first edition of his nursing book was published anonymously and he did not append his name to the book until 1860.

Although Besser fails to mention the development of children's nursing, the publication of a book to illuminate the art and science of nursing sick children at a point in history when the future configuration of the profession was still unclear is remarkable as is West's early commitment to the education of children's nurses. The emphasis by West on a scholarly approach to learning also resulted in children's nursing attracting high calibre students or probationers as they were referred to in the 19th century. Undoubtedly these probationer nurses would have benefited from the zealousness of the medical staff as they endeavoured to more fully understand the pathology that lay behind much of children's morbidity and mortality. The manifest failure of traditional medicine to fully address childhood illness for the first half of the 19th century would have left a knowledge vacuum that West and his colleagues strove to fill. These early children's nursing students would have learned the art and science of their profession within this climate of scientific inquiry. Even today within contemporary children's and young people's nursing education in the UK, there are eight applicants for every available university undergraduate place. Many children's hospitals were developed in the decades following the opening of The Hospital for Sick Children in Great Ormond Street, which Twistington-Higgins (1952) describes, quoting Charles West himself, 'as the mother of children's hospitals'.

Given West's own quest for patronage it is easy to understand why children's nursing became popular not only at Great Ormond Street but also in the many children's hospitals which were opened subsequently across the whole country and then later in Europe, North America and beyond. For example, the Royal Manchester Children's Hospital (1855), the Royal Hospital for Sick Children, Edinburgh (1860), the Birmingham Children's Hospital (1862), the Meyer Pediatric Hospital, Florence (1884), the Gaslini Children's Hospital, Genoa (1931), the Children's Hospital of Philadelphia, Pennsylvania (1885) and the Hospital for Sick Children in Toronto, Canada (1875) to name but a few (Stang and Joshi, 2006). Certainly royal patronage made the Great Ormond Street School of nursing very popular and a good coup for children's nursing occurred when The Princess Royal became a probationer at the Hospital for Sick Children in 1918. Although Princess Mary never registered as a children's nurse, she was a good role model. Princess Tsahai, the daughter of Emperor Haile Selassie of Ethiopia, came to England in 1936. The Princess trained as a children's nurse at Great Ormond Street. She returned home with the ambition of using the knowledge she had acquired to develop child health services there, but died of meningitis in 1942, aged 24. A memorial hospital bearing her name was later established in Addis Ababa. West was keen to keep children's nursing in the forefront of nurse education and he recognised the growing influence of Florence Nightingale on the development of the fledgling nursing profession. Although she had no recorded experience in the care of sick children the archives at Great Ormond Street show that West corresponded with her by letter seeking her advice on optimum ways of delivering nursing care to children. Despite this, Nightingale was an opponent of his initiative, believing that children should not be in hospital wards. Undoubtedly, Nightingale's preoccupation was with adult-focused general nurse education, although in her 'Notes on Nursing' she does mention sick children, stating, 'Children: they are affected by the same things (as adults) but much more quickly and seriously' (Nightingale, 1859, p. 72).

State registration for nurses in Britain was not supported by Nightingale and its introduction was effectively stifled until after her death in 1910 (Glasper and Charles-Edwards, 2002). The campaign for nurse registration was led by Mrs Ethel Bedford Fenwick, the former matron of St Bartholomew's Hospital. Despite commencing her nursing career as a paying probationer (student nurse) at The Children's Hospital in Nottingham in 1878, Mrs Fenwick did not support the inclusion of children's nurses in a proposed nursing register. Fortunately Catherine Jane Wood in her final year as lady superintendent at the Hospital for Sick Children wrote in an article in the Nursing Record that, 'Sick children require special nursing and sick children's nurses require special training' (Wood, 1888), thus leaving a legacy for children's nurses to use in the fight for recognition as a discrete nursing entity. Conflict between the 'branches of nursing' had been precipitated, when the British Nurses Association, led by Mrs Fenwick and the rival College of Nursing (later to become The Royal College of Nursing) decided on a joint strategy which was not to include those nurses who had trained only in a children's hospital on the proposed register of nurses, or on the supplementary register, which was to include male nurses, mental nurses and fever nurses. However after a number of acrimonious exchanges between senior children's nurses and those nurses seeking to exclude children's nursing from the proposed supplementary register, the Bill and Act for the State Registration of Nurses in which children's nursing became part of a supplementary register was passed in December 1919.

Charles West held a post as a senior paediatrician at Great Ormond Street until he resigned in 1877 after a series of disagreements with colleagues and members of the management committee. West's own notes held in the archive of Great Ormond Street show his bitter disappointment with the direction of travel of the children's hospital and how his views on hospital management led to his increasing unpopularity. West's interpersonal relationships with medical colleagues had been difficult and strained, perhaps Charles West attributed to his strong religious views as a Roman Catholic, although in West's own words, 'Neither by deed, word nor thought has my conduct ever been influenced by my religious opinions'.

This brief overview of the changing concept of childhood provides some insight into the nature of children's lives in earlier centuries.

THE ORIGINS OF FOUNDLING HOSPITALS AND DISPENSARIES

In Britain in the mid-18th century, many parents – faced with extreme poverty – abandoned their infants and children. They did so in the hope that they would be taken by adults who were in a better position to love, nurture and care for them (Schwartzman, 1978). Interestingly, the mortality rate among children who remained with their natural families was higher than among those who were abandoned and subsequently taken in by other adults. This was because the original home conditions for many children were squalid, with poor sanitation, overcrowding and high levels of poverty (Kosky and Lunnon, 1991). It is estimated that during the 1850s, 50,000 deaths occurred each year, of which over 21,000 were children less than 10 years of age.

👤 ACTIVITY

Consider the aims set out by Charles West in 1852 for the Sick Children's Hospital, Great Ormond Street (Miles, 1986a,b), and reflect on how they compare with the aims of the Alder Hey Children's Hospital, Liverpool, at the beginning of the 21st century.

The Sick Children's Hospital, Great Ormond Street
- To provide for the reception and maintenance and medical treatment of children of the poor during sickness and to furnish them with advice, that is, the mothers of those who cannot be admitted into the hospital.
- To promote the advancement of medical science generally with reference to the diseases of children and, in particular, to provide for the more efficient instruction of students in this department of medical knowledge.
- To disseminate among all classes of the community, but chiefly among the poor, a better acquaintance with the management of infants and children during illness by employing and training of women in the special duties of children's nursing.

Alder Hey Children's Hospital (2003)
Aim:
- To provide a comprehensive, high-quality child health service that promotes the integration of hospital and community care in a family-centred, friendly and safe environment.
Guiding principles:
- A range of services will be provided to meet all child health needs with the least possible delay.
- Parents will be involved with professionals in the planning and provision of care.
- Parents shall be encouraged to stay with their children in hospital at all times.
- Recreation, play activities and education will be provided according to individual needs.
- Opportunities for development and training will be provided to ensure highly motivated, well-trained and educated staff.
- Equal care and consideration will be given to all our patients so that their privacy, dignity and beliefs are respected at all times.
- Children and parents will be told the name and status of any person caring for them.
- http://www.alderhey.com/RLCH/home.asp

Thomas Coram (1668–1751) was born in Dorset and spent much of his life at sea. After working in the ship-building business he moved to London, where by 1732 he was a successful merchant. The sight of abandoned infants and children appalled Thomas Coram and in response to what he saw he applied for and was granted a Royal Charter by George II to open the Foundling Hospital, in Hatton Gardens in London in 1741 (Franklin, 1964). By taking abandoned infants and children into the Foundling Hospital, Coram wanted to prevent the murder of infants at birth and to stop the practice of parents abandoning their infants and children to die on the streets of London. The primary aim of the Foundling Hospital, which was not a hospital as we know it today, was the provision of care and education. The visionary work of Thomas Coram was widely recognised and many famous artists became patrons and governors of the hospital. Some of their artwork was displayed in the Foundling Hospitals during the 18th century. Today examples of the work of Hogarth, Reynolds and Gainsborough are now on view in the Foundling Museum, established in London in 1998.

There were many such hospitals and, as the name suggests, they were places to which children who were the illegitimate offspring of the poor or who had been abandoned by their parents were taken. Members of the public viewed the foundling hospitals with a high degree of suspicion, considering them to be places of death because of their high mortality rates. In 1756 the governors appealed to the House of Commons for financial assistance. Although granted, the assistance was conditional and required that the governors accepted all children offered to them. The number of sick and seriously debilitated infants and children arriving at the hospital increased dramatically. According to Franklin (1964), the indiscriminate admission of 14,934 babies over a 46-month period in the 1760s resulted in 10,389 deaths. The majority of the infants who died were under 6 months of age. Increasingly it was recognised that children who survived until their second birthday had a significantly improved chance of surviving childhood.

In the UK, the response to the growing problem of sick children involved the setting up of charitable dispensaries. Dr George Armstrong (1719–1789), a Scottish surgeon, is credited with the establishment of the first dispensary or 'ambulatorium' in Red Lion Square, London, in 1769. His work is an early example of ambulatory care and some today consider him to be the 'father of ambulatory care'. The main aim of dispensaries was to lower the toll of mortality among infants and children by providing advice and administering medicines to children of the poor, from birth to 10–12 years of age. This provision was designed to meet the needs of infants and children who, at that time, were often refused admission by most hospitals. Children were acknowledged to be susceptible to infection often as a result of poor nutrition.

As well as keeping children out of hospital, the work of Dr George Armstrong was based on the belief that to separate children from their families was to 'break their heart' (Miles, 1985). Accounts about the dispensaries suggest that cost of hospital care was a factor for many parents. Armstrong shared the concern that the economic pressure of looking after a child in hospital would place an intolerable financial burden on many parents. However, the overriding view of Armstrong was that children should 'remain at home, however humble, surrounded and affectionately nursed by their dearest relations, and by those who feel a natural and earnest interest in their welfare' (Miles, 1986a,b).

John Bunnell Davis founded the Universal Dispensary for Children in 1816. In 1823, it became the Royal Universal Dispensary, located in Waterloo Road in London (Franklin, 1964). It was intended to provide a centre-point of medical attention for the investigation of diseases in children and young people. Although initially teaching and home visits appeared central to the work of the dispensary, these elements gradually ceased. Other cities throughout the UK opened dispensaries based on similar principles, for example in Manchester in 1829 and Liverpool in 1851. The figures from the Universal Dispensary for Children during the first 3.5 years after its introduction demonstrate a significant improvement on the statistics from the foundling hospitals. It is reported that during this time 7820 sick infants were treated and 7030 cured, 300 vaccinated, 130 died and the remainder continued to receive ongoing care (Franklin, 1964). Charles West, the founder of the Hospital for Sick Children, Great Ormond Street, worked for almost 10 years as the physician from 1842. John Bunnell Davis died at the young age of 44 but is credited with being one of the most important influences on British paediatrics, having established an early version of a school of medicine linked to the Universal Dispensary for Children that he founded (Franklin, 1964).

Although dispensaries met with some success in reducing the mortality rate amongst infants and children, physicians were forming the opinion that specialist inpatient care was becoming increasingly necessary. In their first argument for such a provision they cited examples of the European cities where children's hospitals were already established. The number of children's hospitals in Europe had increased steadily throughout the 17th, 18th and 19th centuries, starting with the La Maison de l'enfant Jesus (which was an orphanage, although reported by some writers to be a foundling hospital; Guthrie, 1960), which opened in 1679. This institution was subsequently converted to L'Hôpital des Enfants Malades in 1802 at the Rue de Sevres in Paris. Other European cities that opened hospitals include St Petersburg in 1834, Vienna in 1837, Budapest in 1839 and Moscow in 1842. However, the mortality in such places was a cause for concern. The high mortality rate reported in L'Hôpital des Enfants Malades was attributed to infectious diseases and the scarcity of nurses with the necessary knowledge and skills (Lomax, 1996). Around this time, Louis Pasteur's work on microorganisms was gaining momentum and the knowledge and understanding of microorganisms and cross-infection steadily increased (Craig, 1977). Pasteur (1822–1895) provided the impetus for microbiology and contributed to the development of the first vaccines.

THE ESTABLISHMENT OF CHILDREN'S HOSPITALS

In London in 1850 it was estimated that children under the age of 10 years occupied approximately 3% of available hospital beds but that the deaths in the same age group accounted for 50% of all deaths in London (Franklin, 1964). In 1851, a public meeting approved the idea of establishing a children's hospital and the Hospital for Sick Children, in Great Ormond Street, opened in 1852 with 10 beds (Arton, 1982). In 1858 the purchase of a second house adjacent to the original provided much needed additional accommodation and the number of children who could be admitted rose to 75. The novelist Charles Dickens, a close friend of Charles West – the founder of the Hospital for Sick Children, Great Ormond Street – was himself a strong advocate of the idea of a children's hospital and his depiction of the nurse Sairey Gamp in his novel 'Martin Chuzzelwit' (Dickens, 1984) has been credited with providing ammunition that undermined the early working-class domiciliary nursing movement in favour of a medically dominated, nurse subservient workforce (Rafferty, 1995). Queen Victoria, who subscribed to the project, subsequently became its patron (Arton, 1982) and Lord Shaftesbury (1801–1885), the factory reformer and philanthropist, was another supporter of the venture to build a children's hospital. The slogan used at the time of fundraising in the late 19th century was 'children's health, the nation's wealth'. Today, as the Hospital for Sick Children, Great Ormond Street plans new and exciting developments, the centrality of the child continues to be reflected in its mission statement 'the child first and always'.

During his time at the Universal Dispensary for Children, West had had the opportunity to visit the homes of sick children and was aware of the acute problems, such as overcrowding and lack of ventilation, that made the home environment unsuitable for many of the children. Before establishing the Hospital for Sick Children, Great Ormond Street, he also visited the National Children's Hospital in Dublin, the first hospital in Britain entirely dedicated to the care of sick children.

The aims outlined by West in 1852 formed the basis for other similar institutions throughout the UK. They reflected a change in emphasis from reducing mortality to a stronger focus on teaching. This shift in emphasis acknowledged that specially trained children's nurses would be vital in the overall efficiency of care of sick children. By 1888 it was estimated that there were 38 hospitals for sick children in the UK (Franklin, 1964). Many general hospitals dedicated wards to the care of sick children. The newly founded children's hospitals, in common with adult hospitals, were voluntary hospitals that relied entirely on public money for support.

THE GROWTH OF CHILDREN'S HOSPITALS

Many hospitals were established during the 19th and early 20th centuries. One such was the Royal Manchester Children's Hospital, which was founded in 1829 as a dispensary and became a six-bedded hospital in 1855. Like many other early children's hospital, the demands on the hospital were great and in 1873 it moved to its present site to the north of the city centre. Booth Hall Infirmary, now known as Booth Hall Children's Hospital, opened in 1909 but its designation as a children's hospital came 6 years later in 1915 and Royal Patronage was granted in 1923.

Nottingham Children's Hospital, originally referred to as the Free Hospital for Sick Children, was founded in 1869. The aims of the hospital included the reception, maintenance and provision of medical treatment to children less than 10 years of age. The hospital moved to a new site shortly after its opening and, in 1978, moved again to its present site as part of the University Hospital, Queens Medical Centre (Crothall, 1978). Like many children's hospitals across the UK, it has an informative website detailing information about its history and current initiatives and future plans.

Similarly in Oxford, the new children's hospital was built as part of the John Radcliffe Hospital and in Portsmouth as part of Queen Alexandra Hospital.

Dr William Jackson Cleaver established the Sheffield Free Hospital for Sick Children in a rented property, Brightmore

House, in 1867. The opening of the hospital met with some degree of opposition, and the hospital accommodation was soon inadequate for the demands placed on it (Harvey, 1976). Like so many other children's hospitals it moved to a new site a few years later.

The Southampton Children's Hospital, the only dedicated children's hospital in the Hampshire region, was established in 1884, initially as The Shirley Children's Hospital and Dispensary for Women. In reality, the hospital was little more than a small house in Church Street, Shirley – then an outlying village of Southampton. Although the hospital moved to larger premises in Winchester Road, Southampton, in 1912, it was not until 1920, when a new wing was built, that the name was changed to the Southampton Children's Hospital and Dispensary for Women. Although the General Nursing Council established the Register for Nurses in 1919, the Southampton Children's Hospital did not found its own school to train Registered Sick Children's Nurses (RSCN) until 1936. The nurses undertook a 3-year course leading to part 8 of the professional register. Probationers following the Registered Sick Children's Nursing course at the hospital had to work, attending lectures and studying in their own free time. The classroom was very small and the nurses were educated in the art and science of children's nursing by the resident Sister Tutor.

The RSCN course was suspended during the early years of the Second World War and recommenced in 1944, the same year that the hospital became the Southampton Children's Hospital. Although the hospital flourished after the inauguration of the National Health Service in 1948, the training of Registered Sick Children's Nurses was discontinued in 1960, after the General Nursing Council decreed that the hospital was too small to adequately train RSCNs. For a short time the Children's Hospital continued to offer training for Enrolled Nurses. The hospital was closed in 1974, transferring its children to the newly built east wing of Southampton General Hospital. Since then, children's services at Southampton have grown and, as in Oxford and as in Portsmouth, a new separate children's hospital was developed as part of the Southampton General hospital.

In Ireland, the Adelaide, Meath and National Children's Hospitals were all voluntary hospitals. The Meath was founded early – in 1753. In 1821 a group of doctors from Dublin founded the first hospital in Ireland (also the first in Britain) entirely devoted to the care of children. It was this hospital that Charles West visited before setting up the Hospital for Sick Children, Great Ormond Street. The Adelaide was founded in 1839 and opened a school of nursing in 1859, the year in which 'Notes on Nursing' was published. The three institutions amalgamated in 1998.

In Wales, the opening of a new children's hospital early in 2005 replaced a multisite service with services for children and their families at a central location. With a strong emphasis on creating a suitable environment for children and appropriate facilities for parents, the new hospital offers a wide range of specialist services to the children of Cardiff, south of Wales and beyond.

From 1860 to 1883, three children's hospitals opened in Scotland. The Hospital for Sick Children in Edinburgh opened in early 1860 and credit for the founding of this hospital is given to two members of the medical profession – Charles Wilson and John Smith (Guthrie, 1960). John Smith visited the Paris Children's Hospital and is reported to have stated:

> There is no question whatever that it seemed inconceivable and altogether unaccountable that while almost every municipality on the continent of Europe possesses at least one, if not two, hospitals devoted to children's diseases, no such institution was to be found in the famous medical centre of Edinburgh

> **(Birrell, 1995)**

The development of the Hospital for Sick Children was similar to the development of the Great Ormond Street hospital: it started with limited facilities and gradually acquired larger premises. Guthrie (1960), writing about the early days of the hospital, notes that when it was first opened children were, to some extent, still regarded as miniature adults, with little or no consideration given to the unique diseases from which they suffered.

 POWERPOINT

Access the companion PowerPoint presentation and look up the history of the Royal Hospital for Sick Children in Edinburgh and then view the silent film on childcare in the 1930s, in particular section 2:
- http://www.lhsa.lib.ed.ac.uk/images/hc/healthycity.html

The Aberdeen Children's Hospital opened in 1877 to provide services for children in the city of Aberdeen, the surrounding counties of Aberdeen, Kincardine, Banff, Moray and the islands of Orkney and Shetland. It moved to a site at Foresterhill in Aberdeen in 1929. A new children's hospital, built within the Foresterhill complex, was opened early in 2004.

The Glasgow Hospital for Sick Children, which later became the Royal Hospital for Sick Children, opened in 1883. It moved to its Yorkhill site in 1914 and is the largest children's hospital in Scotland.

POWERPOINT

Access the companion PowerPoint presentation and view the archive material from the Royal Hospital for Sick Children in Glasgow, which provides an interesting account of nurses' training, working and living conditions 1883–1920.

Children's hospitals also opened in other parts of the world in the later part of the 19th century. Examples include the Children's Hospital of Philadelphia, which is the oldest hospital in the USA solely dedicated to the care of children. It was founded in 1895 during the Industrial Revolution. Francis

West Lewis visited the Hospital for Sick Children, Great Ormond Street, and on his return to the USA decided to open a similar institution devoted to the care of sick children and to finding cures and treating illnesses and injuries specific to children. The innovative research programmes have led to developments such as fetal surgery techniques and the hospital is recognised to be a leader in its field.

Allan Campbell founded the Adelaide Children's Hospital in 1876. The hospital is now merged with the Queen Victoria Hospital and is the first fully integrated Women's and Children's Hospital in Australia.

In 1904, the Children's Memorial Hospital opened in Montreal, Canada. It was the first hospital in Montreal whose sole mandate was the provision of care for sick children. Five years after it opened a new hospital was built and in 1920 the hospital became part of a teaching hospital affiliated to McGill University; it is now part of the McGill University Health Centre. It is a multicultural, bilingual institution that serves an increasingly diverse community.

THE ORIGINS OF EDUCATION AND REGISTRATION OF CHILDREN'S NURSES

Undoubtedly, Charles West, the Founder of Great Ormond Street Children's Hospital, was a formidable individual. Before founding Great Ormond Street Children's Hospital, he worked in The Universal Dispensary for Children in London. He resigned when he failed to persuade the management of the need to expand the facilities to include inpatient beds. It was during his time in the dispensary that he came to the conclusion that dispensaries did not have all the necessary facilities to cope with the problems of children. In his opinion, the dispensaries served only to accentuate the need for specialist hospitals (Miles, 1986a,b). Franklin, in his account of children's hospitals in the UK, pays this tribute to West, describing the way he dealt with children: 'the fractious or frightened child could not long resist the magic of his smile or the winning gentleness of his manner' (Franklin, 1964). Charles West's book 'How to nurse sick children' contains much of interest and he is very direct in his observation about what he considers to be the qualities of a sick children's nurse (West, 1854). This book was published 5 years before 'Notes on Nursing' by Florence Nightingale. West's book formed the basis of the theoretical teaching at Great Ormond Street. Although only 52 pages in length, it was considered very comprehensive and for many years remained the mainstay of teaching within the hospital, continuing in print until 1907 (Arton, 1982). It was recently reprinted by Great Ormond Street Children's Hospital.

In 1856, 2 years after the publication of his book, Charles West appointed a superintendent to oversee the training of pupil nurses. Catherine Jane Wood wrote the book entitled 'A Handbook for Nursing', which was considered an important adjunct to the original text written by West. Wood had many innovative ideas about how nursing should be organised and proposed patient allocation and an early version of the nursing process (Arton, 1982).

 SEMINAR DISCUSSION TOPIC

Read this extract from West's book and discuss what qualities children's nurses need in order to be able to provide effective care for children and families in the 21st century.

Indeed, if any of you have entered on your office without a feeling of very earnest love to little children – a feeling which makes you long to be with them, to help them – you have made a great mistake in undertaking such duties as you are now engaged in: and the sooner you seek some other mode of gaining an honest livelihood, the better. I do not mean this unkindly, for you may be very good, very respectable women, and yet be very bad nurses. You may be feeble in health, and then you will be unable to bear the confinement and fatigue upon attending upon the sick; or you may be fretful in temper, and may find your greatest trial to consist in the difficulty of subduing it, and in being as thankful to God for all his daily mercies, and as friendly with those who you live amongst as you ought to be; or you may naturally have low spirits and a child's prattle, instead of refreshing, may weary you. Now if any of these things are really the case with you, I would advise you not to be a children's nurse, and especially not to be a nurse in the Hospital for Sick Children.

(West, C., 1854. How to Nurse Sick Children. Brown, Green and Longman, London.).

 ACTIVITY

Consider the following extract from West's book 'How to Nurse Sick Children'. How valid are the comments in the light of current knowledge about the care of sick children?

At the Children's Hospital you know it is customary, unless otherwise ordered by the doctor, to place a child on its admission in a warm bath. For this now there are several reasons in addition to the very evident one of ensuring the child's perfect cleanliness. The warmth of the water is grateful and soothing to its feverishness, and that is one advantage; but another is than when stripped for the bath the nurse has the opportunity of carefully examining the whole of the child's body and thus of seeing whether there is any rash, or eruption as it is called, upon it, while the bath moreover helps to throw out any rash if it were about to appear.

Although part of the initial strategy, it was almost 26 years after the opening of Hospital for Sick Children, Great Ormond Street, before the first purpose-built training school for sick children's nurses opened under the tutelage of Catherine Jane Wood. She stated that 'sick children require special nurses and sick children's nurses need special training' (Wood, 1888) and demonstrated great determination in her efforts to ensure that children received appropriate care. Often forgotten in the general discussion about the origins of nurse training is the fact that children's nurse training started almost 10 years before the training of adult nurses (Miles, 1986a,b).

Florence Nightingale, on her return from the Crimea, was suffering from what many now believe to be post-traumatic stress syndrome. However, she and colleagues such as Mary Seacole were determined to professionalise nursing. Although Nightingale remained preoccupied with general nursing, she does make mention of the needs of children in her book 'Notes on Nursing', in which she states 'children; they are affected by the same things (as adults) but much more quickly and seriously' (Nightingale, 1859). However, she saw no need for a children's hospital, although it is known that she corresponded with Charles West, possibly because she was considered the 'official voice of nursing' at that time. There is evidence from the archives of Hospital for Sick Children, Great Ormond Street, that West and Nightingale corresponded on matters such as the optimum way to nurse children. This is surprising in view of the fact that Nightingale's knowledge of children, sick or well, was considered to be scant. This pattern of prominent individuals seeking advice about children from nurses who do not hold the requisite qualification or knowledge continues to the current day.

Nightingale used money given to her by the State, in recognition of her contribution during the Crimean war, to develop a school of nursing. The Nightingale School at St Thomas' Hospital in London contributed to the ascendancy of the generalist nurse with the subsequent denigration of other types of nursing, including children's nursing. The seeds of generic nurse preparation were sown and, like Hydra's teeth of Greek mythology, have returned to haunt the profession in the years since.

The battle for training and a professional recordable qualification continued for many years. Florence Nightingale opposed registration and its introduction occurred only after her death in 1910 (Baly, 1973). Baly describes how the Midwives Act, passed in 1902 and which mandated all midwives to undergo a period of formal training and to subsequently register with the Central Midwives Board, made the registration of general nurses an inevitability. The First World War slowed the progression towards registration but did not stop it. Mrs Bedford Fenwick, who was responsible for founding the British Nurses' Association, worked for more than two decades to develop a register and continued despite many obstacles, such as the introduction of Private Members bills during the war years. She, together with other colleagues, did not support the inclusion of children's nurses in the Registration Act (1919).

Conflict among the 'branches' of nursing was precipitated when the College of Nursing was founded in 1916. This organisation became the Royal College of Nursing; it was considered to be a rival group to the British Nurses' Association and had the backing of the medical royal colleges. The College of Nursing and the British Nurses' Association decided that nurses who had undergone training only in a children's hospital should not have their names included in the proposed register of nurses. There was also no attempt to include the names of children's nurses in the proposed supplementary register that was set up to include the names of male nurses, mental and fever nurses.

With little support from the nurses' organisations, staff in the sick children's hospitals took action. The matrons of the London children's hospitals produced a petition opposing the idea by the British Nurses' Association for a supplementary register without the names of children's nurses. The petition from the children's hospitals had the support of an eminent paediatrician from Great Ormond Street, Arthur Frances Voelcker. According to Twistington-Higgins (1952), Voelcker wrote in the petition that 'serious injury will be caused not only to children's nurses but to children's hospitals and the Empire'. He considered that to exclude the names of children's nurses from the supplementary register would be disadvantageous in terms of status, prestige and financial remuneration.

In 1919, the unified Nurses Registration Bill was presented to the House of Lords. In addition to the general part of the register, there were a number of supplementary parts, including one containing the names of nurses trained in the nursing of sick children. The supplementary part of the Register for sick children's nurses now remains part of the Register of Nurses in the UK (Barlow and Swanick, 1994). The supplementary register was set up to recognise the specialist nursing required by children, although the records of the debate that preceded its establishment suggest that at least one Member of Parliament was keen to ensure that sick children's nurses should not masquerade as registered nurses! The Registration Bill, passed in December 1919, enabled the setting up of the General Nursing Council (GNC) for each of the countries in the UK. Initially, a caretaker GNC was formed until elections were arranged from amongst the registered nurses.

One of the remits of the GNC was to create the register of nurses. Those whose names appeared on the register were required to have completed a course of study of a designated length, to an agreed standard and in different areas of nursing. Arton (1988) reports on the opposition to the supplementary register by Bedford Fenwick, who believed that the supplementary register for children's nurses would be short lived. However, after 85 years of existence the future of the children's nurse appears to be assured.

Closer examination of the progress of registration for children's nurses, however, reveals it to be fraught with difficulties. Although the original idea was to ensure that nurses, practising in different disciplines, would be of equal qualification, the struggle to establish equity between the different parts of the register continues to the present day.

The Register opened on 27 July 1921 but the process of compiling it was slow because Mrs Bedford Fenwick insisted on scrutinising each individual application. The first sick children's nurse (RSCN no. 1) to be listed on the Supplementary Register was Evelyn Margaret Hughes, who registered on 28 October 1921 following a 3-year course at Birmingham Children's Hospital. Agnes Coulton (RSCN no. 96) was a member of the caretaker GNC, having trained at the Infirmary for Children in Liverpool. She became the Lady Superintendent of the East London Hospital for Children and was a member of the Registration Committee.

TABLE 1.1 General Nursing Council Register in 1923

Type of nurse	Number
General nurses	10,887
Male nurses	24
Mental nurses	639
Sick children's nurses	191
Fever nurses	356
Total	12,097

From Arton, M., 1987. The caretaker General Nursing Council and Sick Children's Nursing 1920–1923. RCN History of Nursing Bulletin 2 (1), 1–7.

According to United Kingdom Central Council (UKCC) archives, of the 119 women who registered as a Sick Children's Nurse on the first published register, no fewer than 27 trained at the Hospital for Sick Children, Great Ormond Street. On 10 January 1923 the electorate for the forthcoming election for the GNC comprised all the registered nurses, as shown in Table 1.1. At that time a small victory for children's nurses occurred when Dr Addison, Minister for Health, was persuaded to include onto the GNC two nurses who had experience of caring for sick children.

Another remit of the GNC was to compile a syllabus of topics for examination. One of the criticisms of the English GNC was its generic focus, which from the perspective of sick children's nurses could be demonstrated in the content of the examination set in 1925.

 ACTIVITY

The GNC examination (Arton, 1992)
Read and consider the following questions:
1. Describe a case of acute nephritis. How would you nurse such a case? (Mention diet and nursing that might be ordered.)
2. Describe the nursing of a case of peritonitis.

 ACTIVITY

The 1931 hospital for sick children examination paper
Read the following questions in the examination paper and compare and contrast them with examination questions in your current programme of study.
1. A child of five has developed an acute attack of asthma. Give the symptoms and nursing care of the immediate attack. What general steps would you take to prevent occurrences?
2. Give in detail the treatment of a child of four years suffering from:
   • scabies.
   • threadworms.

In addition to completing the GNC examination, students were required to undertake a hospital examination before completing their training. A sample examination paper from the Hospital for Sick Children, Great Ormond Street, in 1931 has a clear child focus that is in stark contrast to the GNC questions above.

Many of the issues that emerged at the time of the introduction of registration persisted in the years that followed. The ratification of the Supplementary Register created difficulties for RSCNs striving to maintain equal status with their colleagues on the General Register. Despite the recognition that sick children require specialist nurses, many hospitals insisted that, to be promoted to a Ward Sister post, the individual required a general nurse qualification in addition to the RSCN. The establishment of the Association of Sick Children's Hospital Nurses was an attempt by a group of matrons from Sick Children's Hospitals to further the interests of sick children's hospital nurses by enabling discussion on matters pertaining to the nursing of sick children. The over-riding principle of the Association of Sick Children's Hospital Nurses was that 'children's trained nurses should nurse sick children' (Duncombe, 1979). The renaming of the Association of Sick Children's Hospital Nurses in 1953 to the Association of British Paediatric Nurses (ABPN) occurred in recognition that the initial title was too restrictive, focusing only on hospital-based nurses when in fact an increasing number of children were being cared for in the community.

Between the mid-19th century and the inception of the NHS in 1948, considerable advances were made in the provision of community nursing. Community children's nursing services were first introduced during the latter part of the 19th century (Whiting, 2000). The minutes of a meeting at the Nottingham Children's Hospital in the mid-1800s provides some of the earliest accounts of paediatric home care provision (RCN, 1984/85). According to Hunt and Whiting (1999), a similar system operated from Great Ormond Street in the 1880s following an application to the Management Committee of the hospital. Similar accounts are found in the records from Liverpool Children's Hospital in 1910 (RCN, 1984/85). According to Lomax (1996), there is limited information on the number of hospitals that employed nurses to visit children. Many hospitals found the expense of such schemes prohibitive and discontinued the service on these grounds. Great Ormond Street continued to provide a paediatric nursing service until the introduction of the NHS in 1948.

Following the introduction of the NHS, Rotherham is credited with the first appointment of a nurse involved exclusively in the care for sick children in the community in 1949 (Gillet, 1954). Much of the work involved the care of children with acute infections such as pneumonia and bronchitis. Building on the success of Rotherham, other home care schemes emerged (While, 1991). As early as the time of the Court Report (Department of Health and Social Security [DHSS] 1976) it was recognised that sick children required community care by nurses with the appropriate knowledge and skills. With the changing pattern of hospital care, including shorter admission stays and day surgery, growing numbers are currently being supported in the community. In addition, increasing numbers of children with complex and long-term needs are now being cared for at home (ACT/RCPCH, 1997).

In 1998 the government made the decision to introduce community children's nursing teams to commemorate the memory of Diana, Princess of Wales. A qualified children's nurse with a community qualification leads each team. Known as Diana, Princess of Wales Community Child Nursing Teams, there are approximately 110 within the UK. The key aims of the initiative are to:

- support children with life-limiting illnesses and their families
- provide high-quality, seamless care
- involve other agencies
- bring different services together to meet a multitude of needs.

 ACTIVITY

Consider the above aims and explore the potential benefits of the service to children and their families.

EDUCATION OF CHILDREN'S NURSES

Inevitably, the educational programmes for children's nurses have evolved over the years in response to changing perceptions about children and childhood and the increased knowledge and understanding about children's needs in health and illness. The work of John Bowlby (1952, 1953a,b, 1960, 1971, 1988) and James Robertson (1955, 1968, 1970, 1989), among others, added considerably to the knowledge base about the needs of infants and children, and subsequently to the impact of hospitalisation on these groups. Bowlby (1907–1990) and Roberston (1911–1988) have had a profound influence on how infants and children are cared for in hospital and other settings. In his work, Bowlby provided a theoretical framework to explain the process of attachment (Bowlby, 1953a) and separation (Bowlby, 1953b). Although some criticised the theories of attachment and separation, the original work provoked further studies that have shown the accuracy of Bowlby's original work on the effects of separation (Alsop-Shields et al., 2001). Robertson, influenced by Bowlby's work, became very interested in the effects of hospitalisation on the behaviour of young children. He firmly believed in the need to change practices within children's hospitals and, to this end, produced a series of compelling films as evidence for his claims. His series of films included 'A 2-year-old goes to hospital' (Robertson, 1953) and later – in 1969 – 'John, 17 months, 9 days in a residential nursery'. Although professionals initially refused to accept these films, they stimulated a significant amount of discussion and debate.

As concern mounted about the welfare of children in hospital, the government response was to commission a report on the welfare of children in hospital, universally known as the Platt Report (Ministry of Health, 1959). This report increased public awareness of the impact of separation on young children and led to the foundation, in 1961, of the organisation that became the National Association for the Welfare of Children in Hospital (NAWCH). This association became the Action For Sick Children (ASC) in 1990 when its role changed from being a pressure group to being an advisory one.

 ACTIVITY

Obtain a copy of the following article:
- Alsop-Shields, L., Mohay, H., 2001. John Bowlby and James Robertson: theorists, scientists and crusaders for improvements in the care of children in hospital. Journal of Advanced Nursing 35 (1), 50–58.

To what degree do you consider the work of Bowlby and Robertson influences today's care of children in hospital?

 POWERPOINT

Access the companion PowerPoint presentation and read the web pages describing the origins of Action For Sick Children and its ongoing contribution to the work with sick children and their families:
- http://www.actionforsickchildren.org

 SEMINAR DISCUSSION TOPIC

Does Action for Sick Children still have a role in contemporary child health?

Throughout the years since its inception, children's nursing has faced many threats to its continuation, with many attempts from within the nursing profession to introduce a generic preparation for nurses in the UK. The publication of the RCN-commissioned report chaired by Lord Horder in 1943 (RCN, 1946), just 5 years before the introduction of the NHS, made clear recommendations that sick children's nursing should become a post-registration qualification. Although never implemented, few doubt that this did a significant amount of damage to the continuation of the direct entry RSCN programme. Sir Alan Moncrieff, a paediatrician from the Hospital for Sick Children, Great Ormond Street, did much to mitigate the pernicious effects of the Horder Report when he addressed a meeting of the Association of Sick Children's Hospital Nurses in 1944 with a paper entitled 'The future of the nursing of sick children'. Central to his message was the belief that 'paediatric nursing is not a specialty but general nursing at a special age period'. Price (1993) draws attention to the similarities between past discussions about children's nurses and the ongoing debate about the current child health qualification.

In England, the damaging effects of the recommendations of the Horder Report were profound and sustained. As a result, the direct-entry RSCN programme was phased out during the mid-1960s. Many RSCNs holding single qualifications found it difficult to further their careers without obtaining a second qualification, usually in adult nursing. The impact of nurses leaving to gain a second qualification proved detrimental to the recruitment and retention of staff in children's hospitals. To alleviate the situation, some of the larger teaching hospitals introduced a 4-year combined course leading to the qualification of SRN on completion of the first 3 years and RSCN on successful completion of the fourth year.

However, an unexpected number of nurses leaving on successful completion of 3 years further exacerbated the issue of recruitment to children's nursing. To counter this difficulty, in 1968 several teaching hospitals introduced a new programme lasting 3 years and 8 months. This required students to complete the entire programme with one final examination from which, if successful, they received the award of SRN/RSCN and inclusion on Parts 1 and 8.

The 3-year programme in Ireland was discontinued in 1978 (Love, 1998). In Wales, the first recognised courses for RSCN commenced in 1976 with limited post-registration courses. Accelerated courses were introduced in 1990 but were replaced by flexible pathways leading to registration and inclusion on Part 15 of the Register (Davies et al., 2001). The Welsh Assembly acknowledged the need to employ additional children's nurses with the scheduled opening of the first Children's Hospital in Wales in 2005.

Only in Scotland did the 3-year direct entry continue. Combined courses leading to the award of RGN/RSCN were run in Scotland between 1950 and 1958. The programmes were 4 years and 3 months in length. The courses were subsequently discontinued in Scotland because of the high attrition rate. Just as the integrated schemes of training were discontinued in Scotland, in England they were gaining in popularity. In 1972 new comprehensive programmes were introduced in which all students gained experience in adult nursing, psychiatric nursing, obstetrics and community nursing.

The introduction of the United Kingdom Central Council and the four National Boards under the auspices of the Nurses, Midwives and Health Visitors Act (1974) led to significant changes in the education and registration of nurses. The culmination of the reforms resulted in the publication of Project 2000, an examination of how nurse education should be changed to meet the predicted demands of society in the forthcoming century. Eve Bendall, a well-known and respected children's nurse and previous head of the School of Nursing at the Hospital for Sick Children, Great Ormond Street, became the Chief Executive of the UKCC and Sheila Barlow, Director of Nurse Education at the Hospital for Sick Children, Great Ormond Street, became Vice President of the Project 2000 working group. Her efforts resulted in the shaping of the new registration in which children's nursing (Part 15) was introduced as a discrete entity. The English National Board (ENB) approved the first 14 Project 2000 sites in England in the year between April 1989 and April 1990; 10 of these sites offered the new child branch programme leading to inclusion on Part 15 of the Register. The programmes embraced the new educational curriculum in which all nurses followed an 18-month common foundation programme irrespective of their chosen branch.

It was anticipated that the new programmes would give all nurses equal status irrespective of their chosen branch and children's nurses were initially euphoric to see their direct entry register returned to them. But the initial euphoria was short lived, as once again overt discrimination against children's nurses became apparent. In the new programmes, the adult nurse continues to be perceived as a 'general' nurse and

TABLE 1.2	Geographical Breakdown of the Register	
Breakdown of the Register Country	**Number on Register**	**Percentage of Register**
England	470,536	72.89
Northern Ireland	20,968	3.25
Scotland	54,527	8.45
Wales	29,665	4.60
Overseas	28,974	4.48
Postcode not known	40,838	6.33

Nursing and Midwifery Council (NMC), 2004. Statistical Analysis of the Register (1 April 2002 to 31 March 2003). NMC, London.

children's nurses continue to experience difficulty undertaking shortened programmes such as the one leading to registration as a midwife. Employment overseas remains somewhat problematic for children's nurses. The changes in educational provision increase the opportunities for children's nurses who wish to work in Europe, but with the proviso that it must be a country where there is a reciprocal qualification (Smallman, 1998). The lack of equity between branches, to the disadvantage of all but adult nurses, continues to be demonstrated by the adult bias of many common foundation programmes (UKCC, 1999).

The publication of the UKCC (2001) document 'Fitness for Practice and Purpose' reopened the debate about the education of children's nurses. Central to the debate is the question of genericism versus specialism (Glasper, 1995). In the generic approach to nurse education, students would be required to undertake a general programme followed by a period of specialist preparation following initial registration (Barr and Sines 1996). Those in favour of genericism argue that children's nursing is a specialism and that education should therefore take place at the post-registration level. However, to suggest that children's nursing is a specialism is to fail to recognise the generic nature of the children's nursing curriculum (Glasper, 1995). Those opposed to genericism share the view expressed by Moncrieff (1944) that children's nursing is not a specialty but general nursing at a special age period.

For many years there has been inequity between the branches and, with relatively few registered nurses on Parts 8 and 15 of the Register, they have become a vulnerable group (Glasper, 1995). According to the Nursing and Midwifery Council (NMC) statistical analysis, of the 645,508 individuals on the Register (Table 1.2) only 36,314 are children's nurses (NMC, 2004). It should be noted that a percentage of these might hold dual qualification.

Gibson et al. (2003) acknowledged that there is evidence in literature to support the continuation of a children's nursing qualification and considered the need to make a distinction between generalist and specialist nursing to distinguish children's nursing from all other branches of nursing. To do so, competencies required by generalist children's nurses are first identified and then additional competencies are identified. The competencies cover areas such as knowledge, abilities, values and qualities. Gibson et al. contend that the development of these standards provides clear statements of what is required for a children's nurse to practice effectively. They suggest that this information can form the basis for identifying whether children's nursing is indeed a distinct and separate entity (Gibson et al. 2003). The debates relating to the future of children's nursing will undoubtedly continue but it is important to stress that each year the evidence base for children's nursing interventions increases.

Despite support for the continuation of a specific child field of practice qualification, The Nursing and Midwifery Council (NMC) for the UK commenced a consultation of the future configuration of pre-registration nursing in November 2007. The Association of Chief Children's Nurses (ACCN) of the UK, in preparation for a joint symposium with higher education institute children's nursing academics, undertook a SWOT analysis of the suggested changes to the existing register, with particular reference to one of the NMC's review criteria: 'marks relating to fields of practice (nature and number of branches versus no branches at all)'. Ellis et al. (2008) reported on the views of these senior children's and young people's nurses on the future configuration of the register concluded that the existing configuration of the NMC register should remain. This analysis of the NMC consultation was later extended to some of the other criteria of the review and involved members of the children's nursing academic community across the UK. The UK academic children's nursing departments were invited to participate in this review and Richardson et al. (2007) after an analysis of the data confirmed that academics favoured the retention of a direct entry children's nursing field of practice. The response to the NMC consultation by the children's and young peoples nursing community was extremely robust. In late 2008 the results of the consultation were published and, to the delight of children's and young people's nurses, the NMC made a decision to retain the field of practice.

Within the context of a four-field approach to nursing, children's pre-registration nursing curricula within the UK currently adheres to the 2010 NMC *Standards for pre-registration nurse education* which adopts a field specific focus and a broad appreciation of all fields. The fundamental skills and values required of children's nurses were outlined in the NMC standards, and field specific competencies. The 2010 standards supersede the 2004 *Standards of proficiency for pre-registration nursing education (CFP and branch nursing)*. The current UK programmes currently adopt a competency-based approach with 50% theory and 50% practice experience. The NMC's move to an all graduate status in 2010 in line with most of the Western world (World Health Organisation [WHO], 2009) also positions children's nursing firmly as a profession which continues to evolve. The UK does continue to adopt a four-field approach, i.e. adult, children's, mental health and learning disability, rather than an internationally accepted pre-registration 'generic' programme (WHO, 2009).

CONTEMPORARY CHILDREN'S NURSING IN THE UK

Due to a shortage of children's nurses and for those not registered as children's nurses but provide health care to children, an option to complete an 'Additional Registration' programme of study remains available in Northern Ireland and in varying formats across the UK. For example, a registered nurse who does not hold a children's nursing qualification can complete a process which releases them from their current NHS Trust and seconded by the DoH to complete a NMC (2010) approved undergraduate degree programme in children's nursing.

Today's children's nurse continues to care for the child and family within the acute setting and community. The Children's Community Nurse (CCN) is the principal registered children's nurse who directs and provides care to the child and family primarily within the child's home. Every child and young person has the right to expect care to be provided at home unless they need to be admitted to a hospital environment (RCN, 2014). Appropriate help and support from the CCN team should be available for parents and families to enable them to care for a child at home (RCN, 2009). A child's referral to a CCN team prior to or post hospital admission may influence the child's experience of hospital by reducing length of stay in hospital or need for hospitalisation.

Children's nursing, although allied to mental health and learning disability nursing because of the child-specific stage of human development, does remain different to adult nursing. It is both diverse and inspiring and remains a much-sought field of nursing which rightly continues to fight for equality. Disparity is evident within the NMC register of 2008 which holds 497,020 RN's, with only 19,164 children's nurses and 396,776 adult nurses. In 2015, change within children's nursing appeared imminent within UK nurse education due to a review by Lord Willis, who proposed it time for the nursing profession to find its voice (Raising the Bar, Shape of Caring: A Review of the Future Education and Training of Registered Nurses and Care Assistants, 2015). The review proposed nursing would be rights based when considering how the child and young person (CYP) could participate in the proposed four branch/field model of registered nursing. Children were regrettably only mentioned three times in the review. This was followed by a wide NMC consultation across the UK with nurses from all four fields, nurse educators and service users. May 2018 then provides UK nurse education providers with the NMC's *Future Nurse: Standards of proficiency for registered nurses*. The future of nursing is a four field 'people' approach, inclusive of direct entry undergraduate children's nursing (not CYP nursing). The 2018 NMC document is now in position to guide UK nurse educators on curricula which will produce the children's nurse of the future.

👤 ACTIVITY

Review the Nursing and Midwifery Council (2018) Future Nurse: Standards of Proficiency for Registered Nurses. NMC, London, NMC and other related documents.
   Access the suggested website:
• https://www.nmc.org.uk/standards/standards-for-nurses/

SUMMARY

The role of historical investigation gives health care researchers not only a window to the past but also a vehicle to make judgements about the future. The work of the RCN in promoting the History of Nursing Society is commendable and provides all nurses with the opportunity of learning from the past. Not to do so, to cite Plato, is folly, as those who do not are doomed to repeat the lessons of history.

REFERENCES

ACT, R.C.P.C.H., 1997. A Guide to Developments of Children's Palliative Care Services. Report of a Joint Working Party. Royal College of Paediatrics and Child Health, London.

Alsop-Shields, L., Mohay, H., Bowlby., J., 2001. James Robertson: theorists, scientists and crusaders for improvements in care of children in hospital. J. Adv. Nurs. 35 (1), 50–58.

Aries, P., 1962. Centuries of Childhood. Jonathan Cape, London.

Arton, M., 1982. Children first and always. Nursing Times 78 (40), 1687–1688.

Arton, M., 1987. The caretaker general nursing council and sick children's nursing 1920–1923. RCN History of Nursing Bulletin 2 (1), 1–7.

Arton, M., 1988. The supplementary register for sick children's nurses. Accident or Design 2 (4), 24–28.

Arton, M., 1992. Development of Sick Children's Nursing 1919–1939. University of Bath, MPhil thesis.

Avery, G., Briggs, J., 1989. Children and Their Books. Clarendon Press, Oxford.

Baly, M.E., 1973. Nursing and Social Change, third ed. Routledge, London.

Barlow, S., Swanick, M., 1994. Supplementary benefits. Paediatr. Nurs. 6 (3), 16–17.

Barr, D., Sines, D., 1996. The development of the generalist nurse with the pre-registration education in the UK: some points for consideration. Nurse Educ. Today 16, 74–77.

Birrell, J., 1995. A Most Perfect Hospital. Edinburgh Sick Children's NHS Trust, Edinburgh.

Bowlby, J., 1952. Maternal Child Care and Mental Health. World Health Organization, Geneva.

Bowlby, J., 1953a. Child Care and the Growth of Love. Penguin, Harmondsworth.

Bowlby, J., 1953b. Attachment. Penguin, Harmondsworth.

Bowlby, J., 1960. Separation anxiety. Int. J. Psychoanal. 41, 89–113.

Bowlby, J., 1971. Attachment, vol. 1. Penguin, Harmondsworth.

Bowlby, J., 1988. A Secure Base: Parent–Child Attachment and Health Human Development. Basic Books Inc., New York.

Children Act, 1989. HMSO, London.

Children (Scotland) Act, 1995. HMSO, London.

Craig, J., 1977. A Short History of the Royal Aberdeen Children's Hospital. University Press, Aberdeen.

Crothall, L., 1978. Let's Begin with the Children. Nottingham Children's Hospital, Nottingham.

Davies, A., Earles, C., Eaton, N., et al., 2001. Educating children's nurses in Wales. Paediatr. Nurs. 13 (6), 21–24.

Department of Health and Social Security (DHSS), 1976. Fit for the Future (The Court Report). The Report of the Committee on Child Health Services. HMSO, London.

Dickens, C., 1984. Martin Chuzzlewitt. Oxford University Press, London.

Duncombe, M.A., 1979. A Brief History of the Association of British Paediatric Nurses 1938–1975. Association of British Paediatric Nurses, London.

Ellis, J., Glasper, E.A., Horsley, A., McEwing, G., Richardson, J., 2008. The future of preregistration children's and young peoples nursing; a SWOT analysis. J. Children's Young People's Nurs. 2 (2, 06), 56–60.

Franklin, A.W., 1964. Children's hospitals. In: Poynter, F.N.L. (Ed.), The Evolution of Hospitals in Britain. Pitman Medical, London.

Gibson, F., Fletcher, M., Casey, A., 2003. Classifying general and specialist children's nursing competencies. J. Adv. Nurs. 44 (6), 591–602.

Gillet, J.A., 1954. Children's nursing unit. Br. Med. J. 4863, 684–685.

Glasper, E.A., 1995. The value of children's nursing in the third millennium. Br. J. Nurs. 4 (1), 27–30.

Glasper, E.A., Charles-Edwards, I., 2002. The child first and always: the registered children's nurse over 150 years. Part one. Paediatric Nursing 14 (4), 38–42.

Glasper, E.A., Lowson, S., 1998. Ambulatory care – the scope of practice. In: Glasper, E.A., Lowson, S. (Eds.), Innovations in paediatric ambulatory care: a nursing perspective. Macmillan, London.

Guthrie, D., 1960. The Royal Edinburgh Hospital for Sick Children. Churchill Livingstone, Edinburgh.

Harvey, P., 1976. Up the Hill to Western Bank, History of the Children's Hospital Sheffield, 1876–1976. The Centenary Committee. Sheffield Children's Hospital, Sheffield.

Hoffman, H., 1845. Der Struwwelpeter. Kindlers Literaturlexikon. [English Version 1994 the Struwwelpeter. Munich in Association with Ragged Bears Ltd, Singapore].

Human Rights Act, 1998. HMSO, London.

Hunt, M., Whiting, M., 1999. A re-examination of the history of children's community nursing. Paediatr. Nurs. 11 (4), 33–36.

Kosky, J., Lunnon, R.J., 1991. Great Ormond Street Hospital and the story of medicine. The Hospitals For Sick Children in association with Granta Editions, London.

Lomax, E., 1996. The control of contagious disease in nineteenth-century British paediatric hospitals. Soc. Hist. Med. 7 (3), 383–400.

Love, H., 1998. The Royal Belfast Hospital for Sick Children: A History 1948–1998. Blackstaff Press, Belfast.

Lowden, J., 2002. Children's rights: a decade of dispute. J. Adv. Nurs. 37 (1), 100–106.

de Mause, L., 1982. Foundations of Psychohistory. Creative Roots, New York.

de Mause, L., 1995. The History of Childhood: Untold Story of Child Abuse. Jason Aronson, Northvale, NJ.

Miles, I., 1985. A suitable case for treatment. Nursing Times May 48–50.

Miles, I., 1986a. The emergence of sick children's nursing. Part 1: sick children's nursing before the turn of the century. Nurse Educ. Today 6, 82–87.

Miles, I., 1986b. The emergence of sick children's nursing. Part 2: the emergence of sick children's nursing. Nurse Educ. Today 6, 133–138.

Ministry of Health, 1959. Committee of the Central Health Services Council. Report of the Committee on the Welfare of Children in Hospital (The Plest Report). Ministry of Health, London.

Moncrieff, A., 1944. The Future of the Nursing of Sick Children. The Association of Sick Children's Hospital Nurses. Great Ormond Street Archives, London.

Nightingale, F., 1859. Notes on Nursing: What It Is and What It Is Not. Duckworth, London (reprinted 1970).

Nursing and Midwifery Council, 2018. Future Nurse: Standards of Proficiency for Registered Nurses. NMC, London.

Nursing and Midwifery Council (NMC), 2004. Statistical Analysis of the Register (1 April 2002 to 31 March 2003). NMC, London.

Nursing Midwifery Council, 2010. Standards for Pre-Registration Nursing Education. NMC, London.

Power, K., 2002. Implications of the human rights Act. Paediatr. Nurs. 14 (4), 14–19.

Price, S., 1993. Children's nursing, lessons from the past. Nurs. Stand. 7 (50), 31–35.

Rafferty, A.M., 1995. The anomaly of autonomy: space and status in early nursing reform. Int. Hist. Nurs. J. 1 (1), 43–45.

Raising the bar, 'Shape of Caring': A review of the future Education and training of registered Nurses and Care assistants. 2015. Lord Willis, Independent Chair–Shape of Caring review Health Education England. Available at: http://hee.nhs.uk/wp-content/blogs.dir/321/files/2015/03/2348-Shape-of-caring-review-FINAL.pdf. (Accessed on 31/3/15).

Richardson, J., Glasper, E.A., McEwing, G., Ellis, J., Horsely, A., 2007. All change in children's and young people's nurse education: the views of senior practitioners. Journal of Children's and Young People's Nursing 1 (8), 377–383. http://eprints.soton.ac.uk/52546/.

Robertson, J., 1953. A Two-Year-Old Goes to Hospital. A Scientific Film Record. Concord Film Council. Suffolk, Ipswich.

Robertson, J., 1955. Young children in long-term hospitals. Nursing Times September 23, 63–65.

Robertson, J., 1968. The long-stay children in hospital. Maternal and Child Care 4, 161–166.

Robertson, J., 1969. John 17 Months, 9 Days in a Residential nursery (Film). Tavistock Institute for Human Relations, London.

Robertson, J., 1970. Young Children in Hospital, second ed. Tavistock, London.

Robertson, J., 1989. Separation and the Very Young. Free Association Books, London.

Royal College of Nursing, 2009. Breaking Down Barriers, Driving up Standards: The Role of the Ward Sister and Charge Nurse. RCN, London.

Royal College of Nursing, 2014. Health Care Service Standards in Caring for Neonates, Children and Young People. RCN, London.

Royal College of Nursing (RCN), 1946. Report of the Nursing Reconstruction Committee (Horder Report). RCN, London.

Royal College of Nursing (RCN), 1984/85. Changing Provision for Sick Children and Diseases in Childhood in Liverpool since 1850. RCN Bulletin 6. RCN, London.

Schwartzman, H.B., 1978. Transformations. Plenum Press, New York.

Scraton, P. (Ed.), 1997. Childhood in Crisis. UCL Press, London.

Seidler, E., 1990. An historical survey of children's hospitals. In: Granshaw, L., Porter, R. (Eds.), The Hospital in History. Routledge, London.

Singer, J.L., 1973. The Child's World of Make-Believe. Academic Press, New York.

Smallman, S., 1998. Children's nursing in Europe. Paediatr. Nurs. 11 (11), 6.

Soderback, M., Coyne, I., Harder, M., 2011. The importance of including both a child perspective and the child's perspective within health care settings to provide truly child-centred care. J. Child Health Care 15 (2), 99–106.

Stone, L., 1977. The Family, Sex and Marriage in England 1500–1800. Harper and Row, New York.

Twistington-Higgins, T., 1952. Great Ormond Street 1852–1952. Odhams Press, Watford.

United Kingdom Central Council (UKCC), 1999. Fitness for Practice. UKCC, London.

United Kingdom Central Council (UKCC), 2000. 1986 Project. A New Preparation for Practice. UKCC, London.

United Kingdom Central Council (UKCC), 2001. Fitness for Practice and Purpose. UKCC, London.

United Nations General Assembly, 1989. Convention on the Rights of the Child. UNICEF, Geneva.

Watt, S., Mitchell, R., 1995. Historical perspectives. In: Carter, B., Dearnum, A. (Eds.), Child Health Care Nursing. Concepts, Theory and Practice. Blackwell Science, Oxford.

West, C., 1854. How to Nurse Sick Children. Brown, Green and Longman, London.

While, A., 1991. An evaluation of a paediatric home care service. J. Adv. Nurs. 90 (12), 1413–1421.

Whiting, M., 2000. 1888–1988 100 years of community children's nursing. In: Muir, J., Sidey, A. (Eds.), Textbook of Community Children's Nursing. Baillière Tindall/Royal College of Nursing, London.

Wood, C.J., 1888. The training of nurses for sick children. The Nursing Record December 6, 507–510.

World Health Organisation (WHO), 2009. Nursing & Midwifery Human Resources for Health. Global Standards for the Initial Education of Professional Nurses and Midwives. WHO, Geneva.

2

Nursing, Children and Their Childhoods

Duncan C. Randall

LEARNING OUTCOMES

- Describe how theory influences the practices of children's nurses.
- Outline and debate the concepts of Family Centred Care in relation to the assumptions, concepts and practices of children's nursing.

- Consider how theories developed in adult and mental health nursing may have influenced children's nursing practices.
- Identify the main concepts in Pragmatic Children's Nursing and relate them to the practices of children's nurses in facilitating childhoods for children living with illness.

GLOSSARY

Atheoretical A hypothetical position in which theory is absent (i.e. that no theory is being used by nurses).

Child Person aged 0–18 years old. The various division of childhood such as neonate, infant, preschool child are only referred to where specifically indicated; otherwise it should be assumed that child refers to children of all ages.

Child's carers Person or persons deemed by a community or society to be responsible for a child's care. May be parents, mothers, fathers, but may also be grandparents or uncles and aunts.

Expressive collaborative morality Feminist morality put forward by Margaret Urban Walker in which people collaborate to accept or reject aspects of care, and where this agreement is expressed, discussed and public, as opposed to theoretical judicial morality in which learned judges (men) make pronouncements based on principles, laws and precedent.

Family Centred Care Philosophy of care proposed by Anne Cassey and expanded by Smith, Coleman and Bradshaw in which the family is taken as the unit of therapeutic care. The goal of children's nursing by implication is the care of the child within a family unit.

Nursing theory Organisation of thinking about children's nursing for the purpose of describing it, explaining relationships between aspects, predicting consequences, and/or prescribing nursing care for children.

Pragmatics North American philosophy founded by William James and Charles Peirce in the Metaphysical Club at Harvard in 1871 developed over the 20th and 21st centuries by writers such as John Dewy, WVO Quine and Richard Rorty. Pragmatics takes an Aristotelian view, which embraces pluralism and relativism.

INTRODUCTION

As a student of children's nursing you may be told by a more experienced colleague 'oh you don't need that theory stuff we just get on with it'. The suggestion here is that there is an 'atheoretical' position stating that children's nursing can be undertaken without theory and such theories are not required. Let us consider this 'atheoretical' position a bit more closely. The statement above of 'just getting on with it' reflects a naturalism stance where looking after children and therefore children's nursing is something that generally women are naturally good at. There is no need for education or theory as women are naturally just good at this sort of proxy mothering. This stance has some logical implications. Firstly, that children's nursing would be a female occupation, and secondly, that

nurses would not need to be educated, merely screened to make sure they were naturally nurturing.

There are some logical problems with this stance. We don't have any reliable and valid ways of knowing if someone is 'naturally nurturing' as the concept is vague and culturally constructed. Determining what a good mother is considered to be is dependent on a community social and political view of mothers (Blackford, 2004; Williams, 2007). The technological advances in nursing mean that children demand nurses who are not only kind, but are also competent and able to deliver complex technical care with compassion (Randall and Hill, 2012). To expect someone to just know, and get on with, giving intravenous drugs, for example, without education and specific training, is obviously a highly risky strategy.

Moreover, the real problem with this gendered 'atheoretical' stance is that it perpetuates a prejudicial patriarchal view of women, mothers and childcare. It casts women as servants, handmaidens, unthinking minions to medical colleagues, children and parents. It excludes men and their masculinities. It feeds an outdated patriarchal view of women undertaking 'domestic' private work away from the public gaze, work which is unseen by wider society and therefore undervalued, underfunded and vulnerable to being lost (Davies, 1995; Liaschenko, 1997).

Fundamentally this 'natural nurturing' stance is not an 'atheoretical' position as it relies on a set of concepts as described earlier, that can be organised into a coherent view: it's a theory of naturalism. So what is a nursing theory?

THEORY AND NURSING THEORY: FROM SILENT KNOWING TO CRITICAL THINKING

A theory is not a very fancy or highbrow thing; it is simply a way of organising ideas or:

> *A basic structure developed to organise a number of concepts that are focused on a particular set of questions.*
> *O'Toole (2003, p 705)*

A good way to get nurses to think about theory is to ask what happens when they admit a child. The questions on the admission sheet are normally organised under headings such as breathing, circulation, temperature control, washing (and dressing), elimination, communication and play (or work), all of which are *activities of daily living*, which were devised for the theory put forward by Roper, Logan and Tierney in 1980 (Roper et al., 2000). Nurses use this admission assessment to draw up plans of care, again often organised into plans to address certain activities of daily living. They are using theory, even if they perhaps at first do not recognise that they are. At first they may be what Carper (1978) called *silent knowers*. This is where nurses use a set of ideas or a theory without realising or critically thinking about the underpinning concepts and about the potential implication (Meleis, 2012).

The definition of theory given above (O'Toole, 2003) is a general definition; what then does theory mean in nursing to children's nurses? Afaf Ibrahim Meleis (2012) has defined nursing theory as:

> *… a conceptualisation of some aspect of nursing reality communicated for the purpose of describing phenomena, explaining relationships between phenomena, predicting consequences, or prescribing nursing care.*
> *(Meleis, 2012, p 29)*

Further, Jacqueline Fawcett set out that nursing theory should contain four elements which articulate the understanding of health, environment, person and nursing (Fawcett, 1995). This is where children's nursing starts to have some particular challenges. Randall (2016a) has argued nursing theories, which were designed and developed for adults (or to address a whole lifespan approach), do not account for how children and their childhoods are understood in relation to these four elements of a nursing theory. In particular, the conception of person is difficult when adapting theories designed for adults, or designed to address mental health issues to children. Does the person mean the child, or their family? Some authors deal with this problem by placing family in the environment; others argue that family is integral to the child as a person. Perhaps more important are the missing elements, which adult designed theories do not address, such as the process of growing up, of moving through childhood, in peer groups and the associated social expectations.

To address this gap, children's nurses devised and developed the philosophy of Family Centred Care.

FAMILY CENTRED CARE

The main proponents of Family Centred Care state that it is a philosophy of care (Cassey, 1988; Smith and Coleman, 2010). This philosophy of care places the family as a unit at the centre of care. Arguably this approach to care has been very successful in extending participation to children's parents. Children's nurses have used Family Centred Care to advocate for child appropriate environments, extended visiting hours and involvement in care by parents, and in securing child field of practice education for children's nurses. Unfortunately, children's nurses have been less successful in proving that they enact family centred care, nor in demonstrating its benefits. Linda Shields and her colleagues have produced two extensive systematic reviews using the Cochrane review process and have reviewed the qualitative evidence, but have not been able to demonstrate that Family Centred Care is anything more than a professional concept, one which nurses espouse, but which is not recognised either in their actions, nor by children or their carers (Shields et al., 2006, 2007, 2012).

Central to the Family Centred Care approach is a partnership continuum between nurses and parents (Fig. 2.1). Although later versions of the text on Family Centred Care have addressed the participation of children (Smith and Coleman, 2010), this has not addressed in detail the negotiation of care with children. Indeed Kelly et al. (2012) have suggested nurses are not good at upholding the rights of children despite more than two decades of Family Centred Care.

CHALLENGES TO FAMILY CENTRED CARE

The fact that we have not been able to evidence how nurses deliver Family Centred Care does not mean that it is not being delivered, nor that it is not a 'good' idea. It may be that it is alive and well and is being practiced, but that we have not been able to measure it or demonstrate that it is being practiced; the error may be in the measurement. However, there are other concerns we should consider.

No involvement	Involvement	Participation	Partnership	Parent/child led
Nurse led	Nurse led	Nurse led	Equal status	Parent/child led

Fig. 2.1 Family Centred Care: nurse/parent practice continuum. (Adapted from Smith, L., Coleman, V., [Eds.], 2010. Child and Family-Centred Healthcare: Concept, Theory and Practice, second ed. Macmillan, Basingstoke, Palgrave.)

Firstly, that Family Centred Care according to its main proponents is a philosophy rather than a theory. It does not claim to 'explaining relationships between phenomena, predicting consequences, or prescribing nursing care' but rather to offer an approach to partnership working with primarily parents.

Such a working partnership is of course desirable; however it may not always be possible, or in the child's best interests. Further there are some challenges which modern societies pose. The Institute for Patient and Family Centred Care (2010) defines a 'family' as:

...two or more persons who are related in any way— biologically, legally, or emotionally. Patients and families define their families.

Institute for Patient and Family Centred Care (2010)

The problem we face now is that often 'families' are fractured. A child may feel 'emotionally' that they want their father to participate in their care, but the father (or mother) may not live with the family, may well have formed a new family and live in another town or city far away.

Secondly, Family Centred Care assumes the family is the unit of nursing intervention and that we would plan for a family unit to support the family as a whole. This assumption can be challenged on a number of levels. There may not be a unified view of the 'family' about a child's condition (Burley Moore and Beckwitt, 2004). Other family members may not see the child's health problem as one which should or could affect them (other than obviously feeling empathy and hopefully a desire to support a family member, which may or may not be forthcoming as not all families like each other or have the capacity to support each other). A child's broken leg may with justification be regarded as a problem of a breach in a bone, caused by accident and not an indication of a systemic family problem giving rise to a nursing need. Indeed, it may seem highly prejudicial to imply that a child's physical health problem is somehow associated with a family problem. The obvious exception being family therapy in mental health conditions where, rightly, the family unit may well be the level of intervention (Alexander et al., 2013). Finally, the concepts of person, family and child centred care have not been well defined (Coyne et al., 2018), which makes putting them into practice difficult; for example, using them to devise an admission sheet, as discussed above, is not possible. The more adult orientated concept of person centred care assumes the singular 'person' in question is autonomous and a cognitively competent person with mental capacity. Family Centred Care as discussed previously assumes a unified 'family', despite the obvious tensions experienced in most families where individual members have different views, capacities and desires. Child centred care is an emerging concept, which has yet to be fully defined (see Carter et al., 2014), and which may also be underpinned by the assumption that a child can be seen as the object of care irrespective of other factors such as the carers capacities for caring. The emerging concepts of 'person' centred care may be welcomed as an attempt to empower people in their own care. However, without clear definitions and critical debate about some of the assumptions, it seems likely that these 'person' centred concepts will fall into the same dilemmas that have affected Family Centred Care. The lack of clarity and engagement of people has resulted in the concepts not being realised in practice (Shields et al., 2007, 2012), and the danger that these become professional concepts, much debated by professionals, but of little practical impact and unrecognised by people receiving care.

Despite these many challenges to Family Centred Care, it remains a central concept in children's nursing. What cannot be denied is the importance that family relationships have in children's childhoods. We will return to the family and its central role in children's lives below.

NURSING THEORY: SOMETHING BORROWED?

Nurses have often borrowed theories, and still continue to borrow theories from other disciplines (Meleis, 2012), such as safety theory from the airline industry (Yoder et al., 2015), change management theory from business (Herman et al., 2015) and social world theory from sociology (Neilson et al., 2013). As children's nurses we use child psychology theories on child development (Piaget, 1953) and public health theories (Keleher and Murphy, 2004). There are existing theories of nursing so why not just use one of these?

Nursing theories have been designed and developed to meet the needs of adults and adults with mental health problems. The nurses who constructed theories mainly have an adult acute nursing background (Benner, Orem) or mental health nursing background (King, Roy), few have a community nursing focus (Neuman), but even when nurse theorists have experience of children's nursing, such as Dorothy Johnston (who was professor of paediatrics at the University of California), their theories contain little that applies to children.

Children's nurses have attempted to adapt these borrowed nursing theories to fit the care of children, for example Dorothea Orem's self-care model (Burley Moore and Beckwitt, 2004), theories of human becoming and caring (Karnick, 2005; Lundqvist and Nilstun, 2009) and activities of daily living (Roper et al., 2000; MacDonald, 1988). However, the fact that none of these attempts has been widely adopted or built upon is perhaps indicative of how adapting a theory designed for adults and/or people with mental health nursing needs is unlikely to serve the needs of children (Randall, 2016b). At best, such attempts are a fudge or a fix which is created to try to address some of children's needs such as when we change 'Working' in Roper et al. theory to 'Playing', despite the obvious differences between work as an economic occupation and social construct for adults and the concepts of play as not only an occupation for children (without direct economic value or capital), but as an essential developmental process and social self-efficacy and self-worth activity (James et al., 1998 [Chapter 6]; Burghardt, 2010). This switching of concepts in the theory also ignores the relationship between aspects of the theory. Roper et al. (2000) theory is not just a list of daily activities but sets out the relationships between health and social care and personal relationships, which are very different for children, and the relationship between their play is different to that of adults to their work. As Meleis (2012) has argued, while borrowing theories from other disciplines may have been useful in the early evolution of nursing, nurses and nursing must design, develop and test its own theories in order to support the delivery of nursing care. Nursing adults with physical and mental health issues is different from nursing children. There are risks involved in using concepts and ideas developed in one field and applying them to another.

PRAGMATIC CHILDREN'S NURSING

To address these concerns and to design a nursing theory for children, Pragmatic Children's Nursing was developed (Randall, 2016a). The aim or focus of the theory is simple:

Children's nursing is about facilitating children who live with illness to live a childhood which as far as possible is similar to that of their peers in their communities.

Randall (2016a, p 40)

The theory is termed Pragmatic because it is based on the philosophy of Pragmatics. Thinkers such as Charles Peirce and William James, who founded the Metaphysical Club at Harvard in 1871, used the ideas of Alexander Bain to develop a North American philosophy tradition, which has been built upon in the 20th century by writers such as Richard Rorty, John Dewy and W.V. Quine (Murphy, 1990). There are a number of ways in which Pragmatics and children's nursing share common aspects and thus fit together very well. Firstly, Pragmatics is based on Aristotle's conceptions of reality being based on the relationships and the context of the phenomena. Unlike Plato who proposed a schema that there exists a

perfect understanding of a phenomena, we might not have reached that understanding, but it is out there somewhere. What this gives rise to in practical terms is two very different views; followers of the Plato tradition (most European philosophies) would suggest there is an ideal way to practice children's nursing, whereas North American pragmatists following Aristotle would suggest there are many ways to practice relating to the context. The pragmatic contextual and relativist position is very similar to sociological views on childhoods, which argue that children and their childhoods are socially and culturally constructed (Mayall, 2002; Corsaro, 2012). James and colleagues have argued that despite attempts to construct psychological stages of childhood unrelated to social circumstance, childhoods in different social, cultural, political and geographical spaces are very different (James et al., 1998). Many children's nurses would agree that one size does not fit all and that often practice is shaped and adapted to fit the circumstance of children and their carers.

Secondly, within Pragmatics it is recognised that practice changes over time and that it is bound by time or is temporal. James famously stated that we have to be ready to hold false what we believe today. The relativist approach in Pragmatics recognises the context of time, for what was good at one time may not be for us in this time (Rorty, 1994). We can understand that childhood, however it is viewed, is also limited to a certain time frame. Although the age of maturity is different in different countries and communities there is still an age of maturity, the expectation is that a child will be born, grow and reach adulthood, and that childhood is a period of time in life that will end. In addition, we know that childhoods change over time. The childhood I experienced in the 1970s has all but disappeared. New aspects of childhood have been created such as screen time, stranger danger, and fluid gender identities. In generations to come other aspects will emerge. Richard Rorty links this ever-evolving landscape to the American pioneers, who went West to uncover what for them were new vistas. Children's nursing is on a constant journey uncovering new and changing aspects of childhoods, as well as adapting care to children themselves as they progress through their childhood with their peers.

Lastly, Pragmatics is based on a process in which beliefs are linked to action and what works in definable and discernible ways, over both the short and long term (Murphy, 1990). Richard Rorty (1994) explores the understanding of 'what is good and for whom' in more depth. He points out as noted above that for us in this time and space we are unable to judge what may be good, or not for others in a different time and space. Not only can we not judge others from times past, such as fever nurses who isolated children from their parents (Lindsay, 2001), but also we cannot judge what might work for children and their carers in other countries and cultures (see Chapter 25), or what may work in a family or community for that child, family or people. However, Rorty recognises that this may leave us feeling frustrated in a relativist's quagmire of interests and counter interests, which can seem unprincipled and conflicted. He guides us from the swamp by suggesting that there are two questions here: one is practical, what is good for certain parties in a situation, and the other is political. In the political frame we might ask is this good for the sort of society or community we want to live in. For children's nurses a practice may suit a parent, be good for them, but not for the child. Not funding children's services might save a government money to the 'good' of tax payers, but would leave children uncared for and at risk of harm. Thus the practices of parents and of governments may be 'good' for them, but may not respect the rights of children to access health care. Children's nurses may have to challenge practices and policies to advocate for children.

In guiding our consideration of the politics and moral aspects of children's nursing Randall (2016a) has proposed that collaborative expressive morality as described by Margaret Urban Walker (2007) could assist nurses. Walker proposes that the cultures of communications used by women are more helpful in understanding moral conflicts. These tend to be collaborative, people discuss the issues together and either accept responsibility or reject it. In discussing the issues people express their views and unpack how the situation makes them feel. Walker criticises the more male-orientated theoretical judicial approach as being unresponsive and unable to deal with complexity, which changes with time. A good example of this in action is the difficulties nurses have when a case goes to the high court. A judgement based on principles of law is decreed (usually albeit not always by male judges), some discussion may occur, but the decision of the court is influenced by principle as well as discussion. It is thankfully rare that cases are referred to court (in comparison to the number of moral dilemmas presented in practice). Normally what actually happens is the medical and nursing teams discuss with the child (if possible) and their carers (parents) how to proceed. Within these conversations people will agree to accept responsibility. This might be overt, for example the child accepting that they have to eat fewer sweets to avoid a repeat of diabetic ketone acidosis, or less overt, for example the nurse takes the responsibility to contact a school nurse and work with them to advise the school to remove sugary snacks from the vending machines. As the child grows, changes school and takes more responsibility for their health the issues would be discussed again. These discussions are not based (generally) on principles per say, but on working out who will do what. They are however expressed and often the decision is written down. Walker is a feminist writer and using her work to influence children's nursing is in itself a political act recognising that women play a role in the nurturing of children, who are future citizens.

THE PROCESS OF LEARNING/GROWING IN PRAGMATIC CHILDREN'S NURSING

John Dewy (1944) a pragmatist writer has stated that to be alive an organism must change, that education is a process of change thus to be alive is to learn and to be changing over time. In childhood this process of change is perhaps obvious and more dramatic than at any other stage of the life span (Boyd et al., 2017). In *Pragmatic Children's Nursing* Randall (2016a) suggests that the theory relates to a process of learning, growth and healing in which children change over the course of their childhoods. This process can be linked to eight outcome measures (Fig. 2.4) set out by Randall (2016a).

Although Pragmatic Children's Nursing is not a staged theory (like Piaget's of cognitive development 1953) there are priorities and arguably phases. A child cannot play, be with their peers, attend class (i.e. access their childhood) if their cardiac output is so poor that they collapse. Thus to access a childhood, to learn and grow one has to have a stable internal environment. It is difficult, if not impossible, to learn very much if your physiological state is altered and you have an altered health status. Thus the work of children's nurses is to promote, restore and stabilise the child's health status/internal environment, such that they can join in the activities and maximise their cognitive abilities in being a child. It is not very helpful to stabilise a child's health status such as our example to give a blood infusion and stabilise cardiac output, if the child is about to have their arm amputated. The internal environment inside the confines of the child's body and the environment outside their body are obviously linked and influence each other to some extent. The first two phases are then linked. Once the nurse has attempted to restore and stabilise the child's health status, then it may be possible to negotiate care. It is difficult to negotiate care if the child is not stable. We might imagine a child who has a traumatic injury. We prioritise stabilising the child, to remove them from danger of further trauma and to stabilise their injury, before attempting rehabilitation, and returning to school. Although in Fig. 2.2 the flow chart suggests movement towards the right to recovery, this may of course not be the case, and a child may deteriorate such that the internal and external environment may again need to be assessed and issues addressed.

Children may also not recover if the disease process or trauma they have suffered are too great, and the internal environment deteriorates to a point where life is no longer sustainable. The process of dying and death of a child can be addressed in the theory by nurses attempting to stabilise the internal environment to manage symptoms, such as managing pain and in negotiating goals, which might be going to the cinema with friends. Pragmatic Children's Nursing allows for both the being and the becoming of childhoods. By this I mean it allows for children being children in the moment of their childhood, and the aspects of childhood, which are preparations for adulthood. As certainty of prognosis is poor in children's health care (Brook and Hain, 2008) it seems wise to both allow children to be children (to manage symptoms to allow interaction, learning, play) and

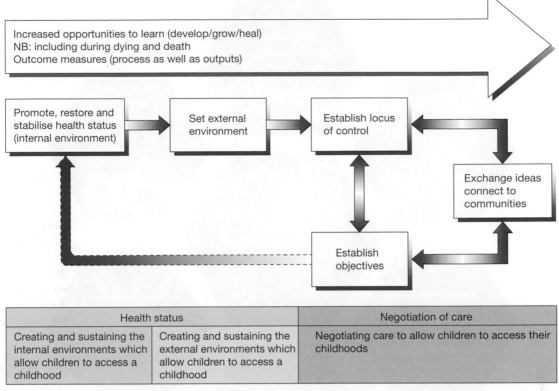

Fig. 2.2 Pragmatic approach to children's nursing.

Within the figure:

Increased opportunities to learn (develop/grow/heal)
NB: including during dying and death
Outcome measures (process as well as outputs)

Promote, restore and stabilise health status (internal environment) → Set external environment → Establish locus of control

Exchange ideas connect to communities

Establish objectives

Health status		Negotiation of care
Creating and sustaining the internal environments which allow children to access a childhood	Creating and sustaining the external environments which allow children to access a childhood	Negotiating care to allow children to access their childhoods

to prepare children for adulthoods (facilitate peer interactions and education). This being and becoming is central to childhoods (Randall, 2017) particularly where children live with life threatening or limiting conditions, in that a child may not live into adulthood (Shaw et al., 2015), but living their childhood, albeit a short one, is equally as important as producing adult citizens who are economically active and healthy.

NEGOTIATING CARE: A TRIPARTITE DISCUSSION

It can be argued that the work of children's nurses is to empower parents, perhaps mothers, to care for their child, to in effect make themselves redundant. Such that excellence in children's nursing might achieved when parents (carers) deliver all of the child's care. Equally some might argue that instead of being reliant on nurses or parents children living with illness should be empowered to care for themselves. Randall (2016a) has argued that this is a challenge to children's nursing for the nurse may disrupt the relationships between parents and child. When a child experiences illness, the reaction of their carer, their parents, is a part of the experience of childhood. Nurses taking a role of *loco parentis*, allowing parents to avoid, defer or delay their response to the child, might disrupt the child/parent relationship. In such an argument it is suggested that how one's parents (mother) responded is part of one's experience of childhood. The fact that your mother

(or grandmother, or father) was there for you taking care of you when you felt unwell affects your relationship with your carer (parents). You might have a memory of chicken soup, which you (re)tell yourself and adapt, but is part of your attachment to your mother is the fact that she made chicken soup for you, or did not this will affect your relationship? If professional nurses take on this role your relationship with your parents might be different.

While this argument is perhaps valid for minor childhood illness, it is difficult to see how any parent might be expected to care for their child in a highly technical acute care setting. If one's child were to develop cancer, as a society we don't think it reasonable that a parent learns how to administer chemotherapy. Such learning is highly technical, and requires a period of study. People would not undertake such study on the off chance they one day need it if their child fell ill. Equally caring for oneself has advantages in self-efficacy and esteem (Salinas, 2007), but a reasonable person would recognise that there are limits to this strategy. One can be so unwell (one's internal environment so disrupted) that making reasonable judgements with the ability to enact them might be impossible.

Thus we may agree that in children's nursing care there is a tripartite, consisting of children, carers (parents) and nurses. Randall (2016a) has stated that there are seven possible interactions (Fig. 2.3) between the three parties.

In Pragmatic Children's Nursing, the locus of control might move between these seven types of interactions (see Fig. 2.4): between child, carer and nurses, and the various

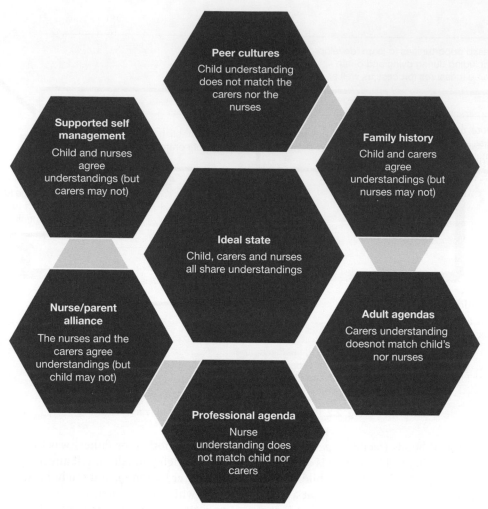

Fig. 2.3 Child, carer and nurse interactions. (Adapted from Randall (2016a).

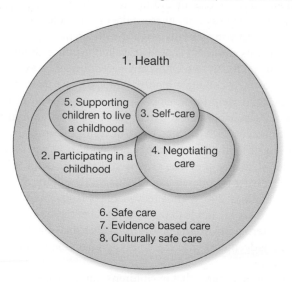

Fig. 2.4 Pragmatic Children's Nursing proposed outcomes.

combinations of the three parties. Sometimes a child might develop their own ways of dealing with illness often by discussing coping strategies with peers. In other situations a child might rely on a nurse's advice, which their carer might not be aware of, or a child and a parent might have their own way of dealing with a problem. We might want to propose an ideal state in which child, nurse and carers have a shared understanding and agree on an action. However, using Pragmatics we can allow that the different interactions might work in different ways for different people, at different times.

The political, moral and ethical questions which arise from accepting these positions or interaction types would be separate from the practices of children, nurses and carers in clinical contexts. This is why the exchange of ideas connecting communities is there. The negotiation of care does not happen in a social vacuum, rather how children are viewed in communities, what parents are expected to do, or not do, and the role of nurses, are all socially constructed. What this means is that communities decide what a child might be expected to be able to do when living with illness. In some cultures, children take responsibility for their own care at a young age, whereas in Western culture maturity is deemed to develop later, perhaps in adolescence. In some cultures, family members are expected to provide food and comfort for their child in hospital (Shields and Nixon, 2004) and nurses perform a more technical role; in Western Northern cultures (UK, USA, Canada and Europe) nurses are also expected to provide comfort and meet nutritional needs.

These socially constructed ideas about children, parents and nurses might work well in certain cultures at certain times. However, this does not mean nurses accept these practices uncritically. A peer culture in a community of young people with eating disorders might support and encourage each other to hide their behaviours from the nurses (and carers/parents). Parents might decide to not complete their child's course of antibiotics as the child seems improved, reserving some medication for the next time the child is poorly so they can give another 'short' course. Nurses force children to have bloods taken, forcibly holding them during the procedure in the belief that there is no other option (Bray et al., 2015). Remember as stated earlier the 'good' that we look for in Pragmatics must be discernible and must apply over the medium and longer term. We can discern that not completing a course of antibiotics may lead to bacteria resistance and thus while it may seem a good action for parents in the short term to not use antibiotics as prescribed, it can be argued that in the medium and longer terms this is not good for children and thereby their parents. We could make similar arguments for each of the examples set out above.

Moreover, there can be political arguments about the participation of children in their care and the respecting of their human rights, which might lead us to advocate for the ideal state where understanding is shared between nurses, children and carers. We should remember of course that the negotiation of care is also influenced by the internal and external environment aspects (health status of the child), which might mean at times a nurse needs to adopt a professional agenda interaction (perhaps typically in acute care settings). In addition, children are developing human beings so at times an adult agenda and/or a nurse/parent alliance might be appropriate (perhaps in neonatal nursing).

The locus of control may shift then between the parties of the tripartite. The locus of control should not be uncritically accepted and at time nurses may be called upon to challenge where the locus sits. What Pragmatic children's nursing calls for is that who has control is discussed and stated; it is a collaborative expressive process as set out by Urban Walker (see earlier). In some practice this is already clear such as in transition where the locus clearly shifts from carers to the child/young person (Royal College of Nursing CYP mental health forum, 2008). In other situations, it may be less clear, perhaps as children recover from an anaesthetic.

NEGOTIATION OF CARE: ESTABLISHING OBJECTIVES

At the same time as discussing and stating the locus of control in the collaborative and expressive way suggested above, nurses should be negotiating the objectives of care. In the pluralistic, relativist context driven Pragmatic Children's Nursing, children, carers and nurses may have different objectives. As for locus of control, what these are is not determined in a social vacuum, but rather in a context of how societies view children living with illness and/or disability. Randall (2016a) suggests that the nursing objectives being set are developed over time and build in a sequence in line with Vygotsky's (1962) conceptions of proximal development. This approach would suggest nurses discuss (or express their collaboration as Walker might put it) with children, where the child is situated both in terms of their childhood, peer and family relationships and in their illness trajectories. The objectives for care are then person centred (child centred) and focused on the nursing interventions. There are two assumptions, which sit behind Randall's assertions on setting care objectives. Firstly, that self-care by the child is preferred and secondly that parental care, delivered by the child's main carers, is preferred to 'professional' nursing care. Both of these have some obvious limits as some children will not have the cognitive abilities to manage their own health care. Some parents (carers) will not have the resources, capacities, skills, or motivation to take on proxy nursing roles. What Randall (2016a) is proposing is that where possible nurses should facilitate a child's self-care, because this promotes self-efficacy and self-esteem, as well as being useful learning for life (Salinas, 2007). Again where possible, nurses should facilitate parental participation and delivery of care as such practices are vital to children's experience of their childhood (Mayal, 2002).

OUTCOME MEASURES: HOW DO WE KNOW IF CHILDREN'S NURSING CARE IS OF GOOD QUALITY?

The outcome measures described by Randall (2016a) were designed to measure the quality of children's nursing services. The eight outcome measures should be applied at a service level, rather than necessarily at an individual child level. Although aspects might well apply to individual cases, because they are receiving care from the children's nursing service (see Fig. 2.4).

The first outcome measure relates to the health status of children and would measure the extent to which nurses are able to promote, restore and stabilise children's health status such that children can participate in their childhoods. Arguably this outcome measure is an overarching outcome to which the other outcomes would be instrumental in achieving the health outcome. Participating in a childhood measure relates to the duration of time children are away from the environments that their peers access relating to their experience of a childhood within their communities. This might include days missed from school, or social clubs. This outcome reflects the importance for children to be with their peers, and/or families doing social activities, skills and interactions, which are integral to a child's experience of childhood. There are obvious linkages with the outcome of supporting children to live a childhood. This outcome relates to plans of care, which demonstrate the nurses understanding of the child's position in their childhood, the child's carers abilities to meet the child's needs, and the effects that illness and/or disability have on children and their childhoods. Randall (2016a) also notes here that the outcome involves promoting parental or carer lead care, as to be cared for by one's parents (carers) is a part of childhood experience (see above). As previously discussed in negotiating care, the child's self-care should be promoted; the self-care outcomes would be demonstrated by nurses providing evidence of assessing and reassessing the child's capacity to self-care and encouraging and developing children's capacity to participate in their care. Similarly, the outcome for negotiating care would be demonstrated by a plan of care where the child, carers and nurses have defined responsibilities, and that such plans are regularly reviewed. All of the outcomes mentioned so far might be undermined if care were not safe, culturally safe and evidence based. In considering safe care outcomes Randall (2016a) suggests that nurses may, in some circumstances, have to advocate for the child and assume the responsibilities for the child. In delivering safe care, nurses would work with carers (parents) to help them acquire skills, attitudes and understandings to enable them to care for their child. However, if this facilitation fails, or nurses believe children are at risk of significant harm, then there should be clear referral pathways to social care and child protection services. To demonstrate, safe care procedures would need to be clearly stated and supported by programmes of education and audits. Linked to these safe care outcome measures would be measures to ensure that care is culturally safe (Ramsden, 2002), where children and their carers feel respected as individuals from a particular cultural background. Randall also notes that these outcome measures should include how nurses are able to challenge cultural practices, which might be harmful to children or undermine other aspects of their health care and/or nursing care. The outcome measures relating to evidence-based care would relate to the other outcomes, and include nurses demonstrating that their care is based on contemporary understanding about children, childhoods, parenting and health, education and social care of children.

These proposed outcome measures have not been tested and the relationships between the outcomes are speculative. Nor has there been work to ask children and their carers if these are acceptable measures of quality. So there is much to do to either validate these outcome measures or to refute them. To return to paraphrasing William James, we have to work with the quality measures we have today and stand ready to call them false tomorrow as we develop new ones.

CONCLUSIONS

One might argue that children's nursing has not been the subject of theory in the ways that adult and mental health nursing have. Perhaps the naturalism view of women as proxy mothers led to an assumption that women 'naturally' care for children, and as in most areas of the world nursing is a predominately female occupation, and that no theorising was required. This position of no theory or an atheoretical position is not sustainable, as the assumptions of a naturalism stance give rise to certain ideas, which are organised to describe, predict and prescribe nursing care for children. Thus the natural caring women approach is a theory. There is a history and continuing tradition of borrowing theories from other disciplines in nursing, and some children's nurses have borrowed theories from adult nursing and attempted to modify them or adapt them to fit children. However, these are at best adaptations of theories designed for adult or mental health nursing, not for children. None of these adaptations account for the process of childhood being both important in and of itself as it happens, and being a very important aspect of how people become adults. Recently Family Centred Care has been explored in more detail and while it was a very successful idea, helping many children have their needs as children considered in much more meaningful ways, the evidence that children want a family approach or that nurses deliver one has not been forthcoming.

Pragmatic children's nursing is the first attempt to design a children's nursing theory. Pragmatics is a North American philosophy, one which responded to the opening up of the West in North America, where pioneers discovered new vistas (new to the white Europeans). Mistakes were made and challenges faced, and although Pragmatic Children's Nursing theory is perhaps not fully formed and settled yet, it may have aspects which we need to work upon. New vistas will open up on the horizons as childhoods change with time. To follow the analogy just a little further, Pragmatic Children's Nursing will change over time and look different in different places, but it will be our theory of nursing, and it will give us the freedom to ensure that the children we look after live their childhoods.

REFERENCES

Alexander, J.F., Waldron, H.B., Robbins, M.S., Need, A.A., 2013. Functional Family Therapy for Adolescent Behaviour Problems. American Psychological Association, Washington. https://doi.org/10.1037/14139-000.

Blackford, H., 2004. Playground panopticism; ring-around-the children, a pocket full of women. Childhood 11 (2), 227–249.

Boyd, D.R., Bee, H.L., Johnson, P.A., 2017. Lifespan Development, sixth Canadian ed. Pearson Education. ISBN 0134431316, 9780134431314.

Bray, L., Snodin, J., Carter, B., 2015. Holding and restraining children for clinical procedures within an acute care setting: an ethical consideration of the evidence. Nursing Inquiry 22 (2), 157–167.

Brook, L., Hain, R., 2008. Predicting death in children. Archives of Disease in Childhood 93, 1067–1070.

Burghardt, G., 2010. Defining and recognizing play. In: Nathan, P., Pellegrini, A. (Eds.), The Oxford Handbook of the Development of Play. Oxford University Press, Oxford.

Burley Moore, J., Beckwitt, A.E., 2004. Children with cancer and their parents: self-care and dependent-care practices. Issues in Comprehensive Pediatric Nursing 27, 1–17.

Carper, B.A., 1978. Fundamental patterns of knowing in nursing. Advances in Nursing Science 1 (1), 13–23.

Carter, B., Bray, L., Dickinson, A., Edwards, M., Ford, K., 2014. Child-Centred Nursing: Promoting Critical Thinking. Sage, London.

Cassey, A., 1988. A partnership with child and family. Senior Nurse 8 (4), 8–9.

Corsaro, W.A., 2012. The Sociology of Childhood, third ed. Pine Forge Press, Sage, Thousand Oaks, California.

Coyne, I., Holmstrom, I., Soderback, M., 2018. Centeredness in healthcare: a concept synthesis of family-centered care, person-centered care and child-centered care. Journal of Pediatric Nursing 42, 45–56.

Davies, C., 1995. Gender and the Professional Predicament in Nursing. Open University Press, Buckingham.

Dewy, J., 1944. Democracy and Education: An Introduction to the Philosophy of Education. The Free Press Simon & Schuster Inc., New York.

Fawcett, J., 1995. Analysis and Evaluation of Conceptual Models of Nursing, third ed. F.A. Davis, Philadelphia.

Herman, S., Gish, M., Rosenblum, R., 2015. Effects of nursing position on transformational leadership practices. Journal of Nursing Administration 45 (2), 113–119.

Institute for Patient and Family Centred Care, 2010. What is meant by the word "family". Institute for Patient and Family Centred Care.

James, A., Jenk, C., Prout, A., 1998. Theorizing Childhood. Polity Press, Cambridge.

Karnick, P.M., 2005. Human becoming theory with children. Nursing Science Quarterly 18 (3), 221–226.

Keleher, H., Murphy, B., 2004. Understanding Health a Determinants Approach. Oxford University Press, Oxford.

Kelly, M., Jones, S., Wilson, V., Lewis, P., 2012. How children's rights are constructed in family-centred care: a review of the literature. Journal of Child Health Care 16 (2), 190–205.

Liaschenko, J., 1997. Ethics and the geography of the nurse-patient relationship: spatial vulnerabilities and gendered space. Scholarly Inquiry for Nursing Practice 11 (1), 45–59.

Lindsay, B., 2001. Visitors and children's hospitals, 1852–1948: a re-appraisal. Paediatric Nursing 13 (4), 20–24.

Lundqvist, A., Nilstun, T., 2009. Noddings caring ethics theory applied in a paediatric setting. Nursing Philosophy 10 (2), 113–123.

MacDonald, A., 1988. A model for children's nursing. Nursing Times 84 (34), 52–55.

Mayall, B., 2002. Towards a Sociology for Childhood: Thinking from Children's Lives. Open University Press, Birmingham.

Meleis, A.I., 2012. Theoretical Nursing: Development and Progress, fifth ed. Lippincott Williams & Wilkins, Philadelphia.

Murphy, P.J., 1990. Pragmatism from Peirce to Davidson. West View Press, Colorado.

Neilson, S., Kai, J., MacArthur, C., Greenfield, S.M., 2013. Using social world's theory to explore influences on community nurses' experiences of providing out of hours paediatric palliative care. Journal of Research in Nursing 18 (5), 443–456.

O'Toole, M.T., 2003. Millar-Keane Encyclopedia, Dictionary of Medicine, Nursing and Allied Health, seventh ed. Saunders, Philadelphia.

Piaget, J., 1953. The Origin of Intelligence in the Child. Routledge and Kegan Paul, London.

Ramsden, I., 2002. Cultural safety and nursing education in Aotearoa and Te Waipounamu. http://kawahakaruruhau.massey.ac.nz/RAMSDEN%20THESIS.pdf.

Randall, D., Hill, A., 2012. Consulting children and young people on what makes a good nurse. Nursing Children and Young People 24 (3), 14–19.

Randall, D., 2016a. Pragmatic Children's Nursing: A Theory for Children and their Childhoods. Routledge, Abingdon.

Randall, D., 2016b. Taking a new path: Time to move from family-centred care and adopt a pragmatic approach to children's nursing. Nursing Children and Young People 28 (8), 17.

Randall, D., 2017. Being and becoming: pragmatics and children living with illness. German Journal of Paediatric Nursing 6, 234–238.

Roper, N., Logan, W.W., Tierney, A.J., 2000. The Roper-Logan-Tierney Model of Nursing: Based on Activities of Living. Elsevier Health Sciences, Edinburgh.

Rorty, R., 1994. Truth Without Correspondence to Reality. Philosophy and Social Hope (1999). Penguin Books, London.

Royal College of Nursing Children and Young People's Mental Health Forum, 2008. Lost in Transition: Moving Young People Between Child and Adult Health Services. Royal College of Nursing, London.

Salinas, E., 2007. Evaluation Study of the Staying Positive Pilot Workshops: A Self-Management Programme for Young People with Chronic Conditions. University of Oxford, Expert Patient Programme.

Shaw, K.L., Brook, L., Mpundu-Kaambwa, C., Harris, N., Lapwood, S., Randall, D., 2015. The spectrum of children's palliative care needs: a classification framework for children with life-limiting or life-threatening conditions. BMJ Support and Palliative Care 5 (3), 249–258.

Shields, L., Nixon, J., 2004. Hospital care of children in four countries. Journal Advanced Nursing 45, 475–486.

Shields, L., Pratt, J., Hunter, J., 2006. Family centred care: a review of qualitative studies. Journal of Clinical Nursing 15 (6), 1317–1323.

Shields, L., Pratt, J., Davis, L., Hunter, J., 2007. Family-centred care for children in hospital. Cochrane Database Systematic Reviews CD004811. https://doi.org/10.1002/14651858.CD004811.pub2.

Shields, L., Zhou, H., Pratt, J., Taylor, M., Hunter, J., Pascoe, E., 2012. Family-centred care for hospitalised children aged 0–12 years. Cochrane Database of Systematic Reviews 10, CD004811. https://doi.org/10.1002/14651858.CD004811.pub3.

Smith, L., Coleman, V. (Eds.), 2010. Child and Family-Centred Healthcare: Concept, Theory and Practice, second ed. Palgrave Macmillan, Basingstoke.

Vygotskii, L.S., 1962. In: Hanfmann, E., Vakar, G. (Eds.), Thought and Language. MIT Press, Cambridge.

Walker, M.U., 2007. Moral Understandings: A Feminist Study in Ethics. Oxford University Press, New York.

Williams, A.N., 2007. Four candles. Original perspectives and insights into 18th century hospital child health care. Archives of Disease in Childhood 92, 75–79.

Yoder, M., Schadewald, D., Dietrich, K., 2015. The effect of a safe zone on nurse interruptions, distractions, and medication administration errors. Journal of Infusion Nursing 38 (2), 140–151.

3

Contemporary Child Health Policy: The Implications for Children's Nurses

E. Alan Glasper, Lesley Bloomfield, Kath Evans

LEARNING OUTCOMES

- Recognise the impact of child health policy on changes in care delivery for children and their families.
- Appreciate the role of children's nurses in the translation of policy into practice.
- Recognise the barriers to policy recommendations in contemporary health care settings.
- Understand that policies can be a powerful weapon for family advocacy.

- Appreciate the role of the complaint process in the clinical governance agenda.
- Recognise the learning opportunities that arise from complaints and accolades.
- Understand the role of the nurse in complaint investigations.

INTRODUCTION

The publication of the now famous government white paper 'Welfare of children in hospital' (Committee of the Central Health Services Council, 1959) was a wake-up call for those health care workers involved in the care of sick children in hospital. The knowledge and confirmation that children could be harmed by early psychological traumas provided the necessary stimulus for a growing interest in the adverse events of childhood. The work of John Bowlby and James Robertson (Bowlby, 1951; Robertson, 1962) had been highly influential in bringing to the public domain the negative effects on development that could occur following a child's stay in hospital. Many of the subsequent policy recommendations reiterated the central tenet of the 1959 welfare document now universally known as the Platt report after its chairman Sir Harry Platt. It would be naïve to suggest that all policy documents published since then have taken a proactive stance, as many have been reactive to events or practices that actually harmed children and their families during the process of care. Current practice is therefore the prime beneficiary of the cumulative successes or otherwise of the implementation of the various policies and reports published since 1959. To suggest that health care for sick children is at an optimum level would be imprudent, and this is exemplified through the necessity for periodic public enquiries when and where poor practice flourishes. Child health policy reviews will therefore continue to play an important part in the evolution of optimum child health care. Reviews and policies pertinent to child safeguarding are covered in another chapter.

THE ROLE OF HEALTH POLICY

The role of health policy is primarily concerned with maintaining or improving the health of individuals or groups within society. Increasingly, such policies are generated at local, national and international forums for the benefit of all. Despite this, it must be acknowledged that there are gross inequalities in health status among childhood populations both within and outside the UK.

SCENARIO

Louise is a second-year child field of practice student, who at a meeting of her weekly learning group reveals that a number of children have been admitted to her ward suffering from chest infections. These sick children are predominately from lower socioeconomic groups.

HEALTH INEQUALITIES

A report published in 1955 by a joint committee of The Institute of Child Health, The Society of Medical Officers of Health and The Population Investigation Committee (University of London, 1955) acknowledged that children from disadvantaged, lower socioeconomic, manual labouring families had a higher admission rate to hospital with infections. Overcrowding was cited as a causative agent and was additionally linked to the high level of readmissions in the same group of children. Of historical interest is the reporting of 10% of all admissions being cared for in adult wards, and 33% being admitted to wards that allowed no visitors. The final summary point in this report states: 'It is too soon to attempt an assessment of the effects of hospitalisation' (University of London, 1955, p 3).

Nearly half a century later, Utting (1997) revealed that approximately 15,300 children spent periods of more than a month per year as hospital inpatients. He particularly highlighted the vulnerability of certain categories of children, such as those with disabilities and emotional or behavioural difficulties. Carter (2002), in stating that children's nurses cannot be complacent about the negative effects of health care inequality on children, perhaps reinforces the reality that children's nurses can never be mere bystanders in the determination of health and social policy. To this end, children's nurses are helping in the process of setting and implementing policy, and are not simply following it. Utting's report was commissioned after continuing revelations of widespread abuse of children living away from home, but especially those living in children's homes. The thrust of Utting's report for the NHS was to establish methods of monitoring and safeguarding the welfare of children in hospitals and other NHS settings.

HOW DO GOVERNMENTS RESPOND TO POLICY REVIEWS?

The way in which, for example, the NHS responds to such reports is illuminating and the Utting report (Utting, 1997) can serve here as a case in point of how the process works in practice. The report, under the chairmanship of Sir William Utting, made over 150 recommendations. In response to the report, the government created a ministerial taskforce to advise it on how to respond appropriately to these recommendations. The ministerial taskforce duly reported to the government, which in turn translated some of the key findings into an action plan. This in turn was developed into a Health Service Circular, which was sent for action to, among others, all the chief executives of the NHS Trusts in England. (It is important to stress here that Scotland and Wales commission their own policy documents, whereas the Northern Ireland Assembly has thus far primarily followed the English precedent. As a general rule of thumb, UK child health policies are transferable across the four countries of the UK.) The changes, which primarily related to who might or might not work with children, had to be implemented by 1 April 1999. As with other similar reports, the wording used by the NHS Executive was 'Ministers expect' and in this example Regional Offices of the NHS required written confirmation by 31 March 1999 that action had been taken to comply with this circular.

Sadly, other reports and polices do not carry the weight of a Health Service Circular and it is for this reason that the reports and polices outlined in this chapter have had mixed success in changing mandatory policies towards children requiring health care. For example, the now famous Black Report – commissioned by Labour Secretary of State, David Ennals – was predicated on the inability of the NHS to alleviate ill health among the poorest and disadvantaged sectors of society; the reality is that the greatest improvements in health since the foundation of the NHS have been among the upper socioeconomic groups. The working party, under the chairmanship of Sir Douglas Black, an eminent and respected physician, uncovered significant weaknesses in the way that

health services were delivered. Black's account recommended sweeping changes, particularly in the child health domain. Among other measures, he advocated increases in child benefit, infant care allowances and free school meals. However, the incoming Conservative government, led by Margaret Thatcher, was not persuaded by the findings and it was to be a further 20 years before the report was taken seriously (Ham, 1999).

Black remained a strong supporter of the NHS until his death in 2002 (Tucker, 2002), and eventually the gauntlet he threw down was picked up by Sir Donald Acheson, the former Chief Medical Officer, whose report – published in 1998 (Department of Health [DoH], 1998) – confirmed that health inequalities still existed. For example, in the case of breast feeding, widely acknowledged to be the healthiest option for infants, Acheson revealed a striking difference between those mothers in the upper socioeconomic groups and those in the lower.

UK POLICY VARIATIONS

The individual countries within the UK can commission a report after specific problems arise within the child health arena.

SEMINAR DISCUSSION TOPIC

Analyse a local, national or international child health policy. In your learning group, discuss if the recommendations are met in your workplace. Are there variations in the way policy recommendations have been implemented?

THE WELFARE OF CHILDREN IN HOSPITAL (1959)

The Welfare of Children in Hospital, published in 1959 (Committee of the Central Health Services Council, 1959), was the first of many reports specifically aimed at alleviating the psychological traumas perpetrated on children during a hospital stay. The main background to the commissioning of the report, chaired by Sir Harry Platt (a famous orthopaedic surgeon), was the growing public concern over the way children were cared for in hospital. The numbers of academic papers suggesting that a stay in hospital could be detrimental to a child's psychological development forced the pace of change and formed a platform upon which the subsequent report would be based. The report was commissioned on 12 June 1956 and the final report was sent to Lord Cohen of Birkenhead, Chair of the Central Health Services Council, on 28 October 1958. The reason given for the delay in reporting was the sheer enormity of the task facing Platt's committee, which included one children's nurse, Miss MW Janes SRN, SCM, RSCN. The primary term of reference given to the committee by the Central Health Services Council was:

To make a special study of the arrangements made in hospitals for the welfare of ill children – as distinct from their medical and nursing treatment – and to make suggestions which could be passed on to hospital authorities.

Over the two and a half years of the study, the Committee met 20 times to collate the written and verbal evidence. The antecedents of the report have already been covered but suffice to say that the work of Bowlby and Robertson was crucial. Of considerable interest is the revelation within the report that the Central Health Services Council had issued no fewer than three memoranda to hospital authorities to allow daily visiting for children. The failure of some hospitals to implement this recommendation is as pertinent today as it was then and reflects the status and perceived importance of 'topdown' government reports.

The Platt report had profound and lasting effects on the welfare of children in hospital not only in the UK but also

 ACTIVITY

Access the full transcript of the Platt report from the book website and in your learning group discuss the similarities between this and more contemporary polices.

much further afield in countries such as Australia, New Zealand, Canada and the USA. The report made 55 recommendations, the majority of which can be summed up by one (recommendation 52):

> *Nurses (and all members of the child health care team) need training not only in the special aspects of disease in children but in the factors that influence the development of the normal child. Part of this training should take the form of practical experience in the care of well children both in nursery schools, etc. and in their homes. The emotional needs of children in hospital should be stressed in refresher courses for ward sisters.*

The last point was perhaps an acknowledgement that ward sisters were the gatekeepers who could facilitate or inhibit change. It is therefore ironic that in recommendation 10 Platt sows the seed of the demise of the RSCN direct-entry qualification when he states 'The Sister in charge of the ward should be RSCN as well as SRN'. Platt was not to know that the direct-entry single RSCN qualification was to disappear from England by the early 1960s, leading to shortages in the number of nurses holding a sick children's nursing qualification. If one could travel back in time to have a one-to-one with Sir Harry Platt, one could point out to him that the care a sick child receives is only as good as the nurse who delivers it.

 ACTIVITY

Conduct a SWOT analysis of the Platt report and debate the strengths, weaknesses, opportunities and threats that it posed to health care practitioners in the 1960s.

 SCENARIO

Louise is gaining experience in a children's medical unit where some of the nurses do not possess a children's nursing qualification.

PROFESSIONAL CONVERSATION 1

Harriet is a registered children's nurse on the Nursing and Midwifery Council's Professional Register.

Issues affecting skill mix on the children's medical unit:

I have been qualified for 4 years and I am really pleased that I decided to undertake a direct-entry children's nursing course at my local university. Some of my older colleagues who trained prior to the late 1980s have told me that this option was never open to them and that they had to undertake general nursing first. A few of these colleagues were actually seconded from the children's medical unit to undertake a post-registration children's nursing course. They said that more post-registration child branch places were made available in response to policy documents that stated that children should be cared for by people with specific training in the care of sick children. During one of my recent coffee breaks one of the adult field of practice nurses who works on my unit confided to me that she felt uncomfortable working with some of the sicker children because she did not feel that she had the right skills to do so.

• What do child health policy document recommendations have to say about skill mix?

OTHER HISTORIC POLICES AND REPORTS

The second edition policy chapter contained full discussions of a range of historic polices and reports and the second edition chapter can still be accessed through the student website, which accompanies this book. This is worth reading as many historical polices from the 1970s, 1980s, 1990s and early years of the millennium are still pertinent in contemporary practice.

Contemporary Health Care Polices for Children
Our Children Deserve Better: Prevention Pays (Report of the Chief Medical Officer)

On 24 October 2013, the Department of Health and Social Care published the report into children's health care by the then chief medical officer Professor Dame Sally C Davies. This imposing 352-page document was the most comprehensive policy document since the publication of the National Service Framework (NSF) for children, young people and maternity services in 2004. The report contained 24 primary recommendations. The full report with detailed discussions on each recommendation can be accessed via the website: https://assets.publishing. service.gov.uk/government/uploads/system/uploads/ attachment_data/file/255237/2901304_CMO_complete_ low_res_accessible.pdf.

ACTIVITY

In your learning group access the National Children's Day website and debate if it actually promotes a healthy childhood.

Recommendation five was linked to the importance of improving physical activity among schoolchildren.

ACTIVITY

In your learning group discuss school based physical activity programs and their relative success in tackling rising levels of obesity.

One of the first recommendations was that the Cabinet Office should consider initiating an annual National Children's Week to highlight the importance of child health. Although a full week was not achieved, a National Children's Day was implemented in 2014.

Standards for Children With Long-Term Conditions and Disabilities

Children with complex health needs have traditionally been poorly served by society. The National Service Framework (NSF) standard 8 and its exemplars, and other similar policies, set standards for disabled children and young people, and those with complex health needs. One of the exemplars cited within this NSF standard relates to the care of long-term ventilated children in the community. This is due to many factors, but the increased survival of pre-term babies is an important contributor.

ACTIVITY

In your learning group commence a debate to answer the following three questions:
- Why are these children important?
- Do they get a good deal?
- Does society value these children?

ACTIVITY

In your learning group discuss the changing relationship between Ebenezer Scrooge, Bob Cratchit and Tiny Tim from Charles Dickens' novel *A Christmas Carol* (1848), and determine if contemporary attitudes have changed in light of subsequent health care policy.

The National Service Framework for Children, Young People and Maternity Services

Standard 8, entitled *Disabled Children and Young People and Those With Complex Health Needs*, stipulated a range of standards the most important of which stated that

Children and young people who are disabled or who have complex health needs receive co-ordinated, high quality child and family-centred services which are based on assessed needs, which promote social inclusion and, where possible, which enable them and their families to live ordinary lives.

The vision of Standard 8 for disabled children and young people with complex health needs is among others:
- Children and young people who are disabled or who have complex health needs should be supported to participate in family and community activities and facilities.
- Children and young people and their families should be actively involved in all decisions affecting them and in shaping local services.
- Children and young people who are disabled or who have complex health needs must receive co-ordinated, high-quality child and family centred services which are based on assessed needs, which promote social inclusion and where possible, which enable them and their families to live ordinary lives.

What Do the Children and Young Peoples With Complex Health Needs Want for Themselves?
- To be listened to especially when decisions are made about them
- Have friends of the same age to share experiences
- Do all the 'stuff' other children do
- Be involved in out of school activities
- Be safe, especially from bullying
- Have control of spending money
- Live in a world without prejudice

Aiming High for Disabled Children: Better Support for Families HM Treasury; Department for Education and Skills

This 2007 policy is designed to help disabled children, young people and their families get the support they need to live ordinary lives. This report focuses on three priority areas to improve outcomes for disabled children:
- access and empowerment
- responsive services and timely support
- improving quality and capacity

There are, however, many polices and publications to support children and young people with complex health needs such as:
- Department of Health, 2001. Valuing People: A New Strategy for Learning Disability for the 21st Century. Department of Health, England.
- Department for Education and Skills and Department of Health, 2003. Together from the Start-Practical Guidance for Professionals Working with Disabled Children (Birth to Third Birthday) and Their Families. Department of Health, London.
- Department of Health, 2004. Disabled Child Standard, National Service Framework for Children, Young People and Maternity Services: Disabled Children and Young People and those with Complex Health Needs. Department of Health, England.

- Department of Health, 2007. Services for People With Learning Disabilities and Challenging Behaviour or Mental Health Needs. Department of Health, England.
- Department of Health, 2008. Better Care: Better Lives. Department of Health, London.
- Department of Health, 2009. Valuing People Now: A New Three-Year Strategy for People With Learning Disabilities. Department of Health, England.
- Department for Children, School and Families and Department of Health, 2009. Aiming High for Disabled Children: Best Practice to Common Practice. Crown Copyright.
- Emerson, E., Baines, S., 2010. Health Inequalities & People With Learning Disabilities in the UK: 2010. Improving Health and Lives: Learning Disabilities Observatory. DoH, UK.
- HM Treasury and Department for Education and Skills, 2007. Aiming High for Disabled Children: Better Support for Families. HM Treasury.
- Jonathan, M., 2008. Health care for all: the report of the independent inquiry into access to healthcare for people with learning disabilities. Tizard Learning Disability Review 13 (4), 28–34.

Child health policy for children with long term conditions is only as good as the children's nurse who delivers it! Use it for the benefit of these children you care for!

POLICES FOR TRANSITION OF YOUNG PEOPLE FROM CHILDREN'S TO ADULT SERVICES

There have been a number of policies and standards to enhance the experience of young people undergoing transition from child to adult health services. Transition polices have been necessary because continuing new developments in health have resulted in greater numbers of children, who in the past would not have lived beyond their early years, surviving into adulthood. There are more than 40,000 people aged under 18 in England who have complex health needs, caused by physical disabilities, special education needs, or life-limiting or life-threatening conditions.

 WWW

https://www.cqc.org.uk/publications/themes-care/transition-arrangements-young-people-complex-health-needs-children%E2%80%99s-adult

It is because the young adult thinks and functions so differently from the mature adult that there is a case for developing young adult health services that meet the developmental needs of young people, to ensure that they optimally provide them with the health care they need to help them reach full adulthood without mishaps.

For certain groups of young adults the transition from children's services to adults' services can be problematic and for many scary. Some children with long-term conditions may have been cared for by individual paediatricians and children's nurses since birth. Suddenly they have to leave the familiarity of this partnership when they reach 16 or thereabouts, and enter an adult medical world, where in some

cases they are expected to behave beyond their actual developmental age. In the case of young people with learning disabilities, for example, transition is often very challenging and at a period of their lives when they are also undergoing other profound physiological and psychological changes.

 WWW

https://www.mencap.org.uk/advice-and-support/children-and-young-people/education-support/transition-adult-services

Similarly, young people with mental health disorders such as those with attention deficit hyperactivity disorder (ADHD) are particularly vulnerable during the transition period, and disruption of care during transition can adversely affect the health, well-being and potential of this vulnerable group (Young et al., 2016).

Such is the concern about the optimum management of these young adults as they transition into adult health services that various organisations have published policies over recent years, which articulate strategies to ensure that their health does not adversely deteriorate in the wake of transfer.

The principal ones are:

Youth matters: Evidence-based best practice for the care of young people in hospital (1998). *Youth Matters* (Viner and Keane, 1998), coordinated through the consortium CCHS, aimed to raise awareness of the plight of young people in hospital. The report revealed that only 8% of health authorities contained adolescent provider units in their hospitals. Glasper and Cooper (1999) contrast the prominent position of young people in society with their invisibility in a hospital setting, where they have such a low profile, despite the fact that in morbidity terms they continue to be one of the most vulnerable groups in society. This report asked all health authorities to conduct a detailed survey to determine what provision should be made for young people in hospital. Despite a lack of progress following the publication of *Youth Matters*, Viner participated in a subsequent policy initiative on behalf of the Royal College of Paediatrics and Child Health, the Royal College of Psychiatrists and others in producing.

Bridging the gaps: health care for adolescents (2003).

 ACTIVITY

Find out if this survey was undertaken in your health area?
   Conduct your own survey in your own hospital or unit. Are you satisfied with the level of adolescent provision?

ACTIVITY

Access 'Bridging the gaps: health care for adolescents' (2003) using the link below and discuss progress made since its publication in your learning group.
   http://rcpch.adlibhosting.com/files/Bridging%20the%20Gaps%20-%20Health%20Care%20for%20Adolescents%202003-06.pdf

You're Welcome – Quality Criteria for Young People Friendly Health Services was first published in 2005 with the objective of helping commissioners and providers of health services to improve NHS and non-NHS health services for young people. A new and enhanced version of this was published on 15 April 2011. The Department of Health (DoH) hoped that these criteria would if implemented and greatly improve the care experiences of young people in the health service, leading to better health outcomes. *You're' Welcome* criteria was designed as an audit tool to allow hospitals to determine how young person friendly they were. The audit tool covered 10 themes, and theme eight was specifically entitled health issues and transition for young people. This theme had seven components, ranging from the identification of the health needs of young people as they emerged from transition into adult services, through to the promotion of healthy lifestyles and the care and support of young people with complex health needs. The prime message of *You're Welcome* was that all young people should be entitled to receive appropriate health care wherever and whenever they accessed it and the Department of Health expected health providers such as hospitals to use these standards and benchmarks for reviewing and measuring their own compliance. However, although some clinical commissioning groups insisted that their provider hospitals carry out a 'You're Welcome audit' many did not and like many polices it lay on the shelves of senior health care professional's offices gathering dust. Coles et al. (2013) also showed that teaching related to transition in the undergraduate nursing curriculum was poor. Despite this wealth of guidance, young people making the transition from children's to adults' services are in many cases still inadequately or inconsistently supported. Some believed that this can lead to disrupted care, and if young people subsequently disengage from services, can be financially costly both for the young person and for care providers. The *You're Welcome* criteria were updated and refreshed in 2017.

 ACTIVITY

Find out if your own local children's and young people's unit has undertaken a *You're Welcome* audit. Access the link to see the 2017 version of the audit tool:

http://www.youngpeopleshealth.org.uk/yourewelcome/

The Royal College of Nursing (RCN) *Lost in Transition*, published in 2013, called for action to ensure that all staff working with young people and young adults received specific training to facilitate the transition between services and that each health care area has an agreed transition policy in place, which clearly outlines transitional care arrangements.

🌐 **WWW**

https://www.swswchd.co.uk/image/Clinical%20information/Transition Lost%20in%20Transition%202013.pdf.

 ACTIVITY

Enquire from your lecturer how much of the undergraduate curriculum is devoted to transition.

The NICE Quality Statement on Transition (2016)

In 2016 The National Institute for Health and Care Excellence (NICE) published a standard on Transition from children's to adults' services, which can be accessed here: https://www.nice.org.uk/guidance/qs140/chapter/Quality-statements.

The quality standard has been designed to apply to young people in need of health or social care and applies to the period before, during and after a young person moves from children's to adults' services in all settings. Importantly, the standard also applies to young people with mental health problems, disabilities and long-term, life-limiting or complex needs, and those in secure settings or under the care of local authorities.

The Five NICE Quality Statements

1. Young people who will move from children's to adults' services should start planning their transition with health and social care practitioners by school year 9 (aged 13–14 years), or immediately if they enter children's services after school year 9.
2. Young people who will move from children's to adults' services have an annual meeting to review transition planning.
3. Young people who are moving from children's to adults' services have a named worker to coordinate care and support before, during and after transfer.
4. Young people who will move from children's to adults' services meet a practitioner from each adults' service they will move to, before they transfer.
5. Young people who have moved from children's to adults' services, but do not attend their first meeting or appointment are contacted by adults' services and given further opportunities to engage.

In the wake of such polices and standards some hospitals such as the University Hospital Southampton has developed and implemented transition programmes. Ready Steady Go, which is a structured and adaptable transition programme developed at Southampton, is designed to empower young people to take control of their lives and equips them with the necessary skills and knowledge to manage their own health care as they prepare to leave children's services and enter adult services (Nagra et al., 2015).

The Care Quality Commission (CQC) From the Pond Into the Sea (2014)

The CQC is taking an increased interest in transition arrangements for young people when they inspect children's and young people's services in NHS trusts. The CQC report on young person health care transition entitled *From the Pond Into the Sea* (https://www.cqc.org.uk/sites/default/files/CQC_Transition%20Report.pdf) indicates that greater emphasis will be given to transition arrangements, and providers will be encouraged to improve their services and importantly castigated when inadequate care is revealed, which fails to meet the needs of this vulnerable group. During forthcoming inspections CQC inspectors and their specialist advisers will seek evidence that children's and young people's services have:

1. good planning for transition
2. a good transition plan in place
3. health passports for young people
4. a lead professional to support young people and their families through transition
5. health care settings and services that are responsive to the needs of young people and their families when transferring to adult services
6. systems in place where the needs of parents as carers are assessed and addressed
7. processes in place which agrees responsibility for funding at an early stage in the process of transition

> ### 👤 ACTIVITY
>
> Select at random, from the Care Quality Commission website two inspection reports from hospitals that have been inspected and discuss in your learning group how well these children's and young people's units fared in meeting transition standards.

Facing the Future: Standards for Children With Ongoing Health Needs

This was published by the Royal College of Paediatrics and Child Health (RCPCH) in 2018. These standards attempt to improve transition of children with long-term conditions to adult health services. This was in response to the growing incidence of chronic illness and disability among the childhood population. The RCPCH standards are configured as 11 standards in total, with standards one to three focusing on the need to ensure that children and young people are given a timely and correct diagnosis, where all sectors of health and social care work effectively together in partnership with families in providing support and treatment as near to home as is possible. Standards four to eight have been designed to improve the long-term care and management of children and young people in the health service and with specific attention given to access to, and between specialist children's health services, optimum transition planning and the provision of high-quality mental health services. Standards nine to eleven have been developed to ensure that the whole system that is child health is well coordinated, and where the voice of the child and family is heard clearly by the board of every health organisation. This is to ensure that the health care journey of the child throughout their early and middle years and through adolescence to adulthood is fully integrated and functioning effectively and efficiently. Standard 6 states that

> *Service planners ensure there is a designated person within the child health service who is responsible for ensuring that developmentally appropriate transitional care is provided and coordinated by both child and adult services.*

Significant emphasis has been given to safe and effective transition from child to adult health services. The RCPCH has revealed that young people have concerns about their transition and that this is justified by evidence, which shows that young people do experience sub-optimum health care when transition arrangements are poorly implemented. The RCPCH standard therefore insists that services are jointly planned for all young people making a transition from children's to adult services, and that appropriate facilities are in place coordinated by a designated person from the children's health care team (often a senior children's nurse), who is responsible for transitional care. However, full implementation of the report findings was meagre, despite highlighting that in contrast to all other age groups mortality among young people in the UK did not fall significantly in the second half of the 20th century and the early years of the 21st century (https://www.rcpch.ac.uk/facing-future-service-standards).

All young people have to contend with the challenges of adolescence as they prepare for adult life. For young people with long-term health conditions, both physical and mental, these challenges can be exacerbated. There are now a number of polices and standards to help health care professionals to work with young people and their families to ensure that the process of transition to adult health services proceeds without undue complications.

POLICES TO PROMOTE GOOD PUBLIC HEALTH FOR CHILDREN AND YOUNG PEOPLE

Successive governments seek to enhance the health of the adult population by ensuring the health of children, who will become adults tomorrow, and to reinforce the commitment to a healthy start for all children in the country. Two polices will be considered here, one which aspires to improve care for all children and the other specifically to address obesity in childhood.

1. Healthy Lives, Healthy People

This early coalition-government policy revealed plans for the Healthy Child Programme, health visitors and the Family Nurse Partnership, and illuminated the pivotal contribution that these have made to the wider public-health priority of encouraging good health and well-being throughout life. Despite the meaningful aspirations of this policy, the Government reinforced its child health strategy in 2014 to help families have the best start in life.

In recognising that child health problems can start before birth, the Government envisages that all women should have a positive experience of maternity care and receive optimal services for themselves and their babies. It was committed to:

- Giving women a single, named midwife who will oversee their care during pregnancy and after they have had their baby.
- Making sure that every woman has one-to-one midwife care during labour and birth.
- Giving people expecting a baby a choice about where and how they give birth.
- Making sure that women who have postnatal depression, and women who have suffered a miscarriage, stillbirth or the death of a baby get more support from the NHS.

The Government also intended measuring how well the NHS looked after parents who had miscarried or suffered a stillbirth or cot death. From 1 October 2015, local authorities took over responsibility from NHS England for planning and paying for public health services for babies and children up to 5 years old. These services included health visiting and the Family Nurse Partnership programme. Local authorities more fully understand the needs of their local communities, so they are well placed to be able to bring together a range of different services for children and families and have more opportunities to reduce the health inequalities in their geographical areas.

Helping Parents to Keep Their Children Healthy

The health service wants to improve all children's chances in life by giving families the help they need to keep their children healthy and safe. The current Healthy Child Programme aims to:

- Help parents develop a strong bond with children
- Encourage care that keeps children healthy and safe
- Protect children from serious diseases, through screening and immunisation
- Reduce childhood obesity by promoting healthy eating and physical activity
- Encourage mothers to breastfeed
- Identify problems in children's health and development (such as learning difficulties) and safety (such as parental neglect), so that they can get help as early as possible
- Make sure children are prepared for school
- Identify and help children with problems that might affect their chances later in life

The Government also aspires to help mothers and young children in low-income families stay healthy through the Healthy Start programme. This gives pregnant women and mothers' vouchers every week to spend on milk, fruit and vegetables and formula milk. They can also get free vitamins.

Encouraging Healthy Living From an Early Age

The Government has also harnessed new technologies to give parents and people expecting a baby information and advice through regular emails, text messages and short videos on the NHS Information Service for Parents (https://www.nhs.uk/start4life/signups/new).

Improving the Health Visiting Service

The Government has expanded and strengthened the health visiting service to help every child get the healthiest possible start in life. This was achieved through the recruiting and training of an extra 4200 health visitors to increase the support and information available to families. However, there are still shortages of these vital public health nurses.

Protecting Through Immunisation

Immunisation is the most significant medical intervention that has been introduced in society to protect babies and children from infectious disease. Andre et al. (2008) have indicated that vaccines prevent almost 6 million deaths worldwide annually. They believe that a comprehensive vaccination programme is the epitome of a society's programme of public health interventions, a strategy that also reduces health inequities and poverty. They also suggest that it is misguided safety concerns in some countries that are responsible for a decline in herd immunity, because of a fall in vaccination uptake by parents, which has led to the re-emergence of diseases such as pertussis (whooping cough) and measles.

Much of this arose because of a scientific paper published in *The Lancet* by Wakefield et al. (1998), which implied a link between the measles, mumps and rubella (MMR) vaccine and a 'new syndrome' of autism and bowel disease. Although this paper was shown to be totally flawed by Godlee et al. (2011), the damage caused to the reputation of the MMR vaccine was incalculable. However, a Cochrane review published in 2005 (Demichelli et al., 2005) showed that there was no credible link between the MMR vaccine and any long-term disability, including Crohn disease and autism. Public disquiet about vaccines and especially the MMR vaccine was responsible for the 2012 outbreak of whooping cough, the largest for a decade, which prompted the DoH to launch a temporary immunisation programme to ensure that babies were protected against the disease. NHS England is now responsible for planning immunisation in England.

Supporting Mothers and Children With Mental Health Problems

It is recognised as important that mothers and children with mental health problems are enabled to access support as early as possible, to reduce the impact of poor mental health on a child and to prevent problems extending into a child's later years. To achieve this, the Government is committed to:

- Spending money on giving more people, including children and young people, better access to talking therapies such as cognitive behavioural therapy
- Ensuring that health visitors have special training to more easily identify the signs of postnatal depression in patients and to get them the help and support they need as soon as possible

Improving Chances for Children With Vulnerable Mothers

By supporting vulnerable mothers, the Government intends to:

- Increase a child's chances of developing healthily
- Make it less likely that a child will experience abuse and neglect

The Government has been working with the National Institute for Health and Care Excellence (NICE). In 2012 they produced new guidance on the social and emotional well-being of vulnerable children under 5 years old, in which they suggest that all health and early years professionals should develop trusting relationships with vulnerable families and adopt a non-judgemental approach (NICE, 2012). To help with the achievement of the NICE guidelines, the Government doubled the number of places on the Family Nurse Partnership. This is a voluntary, preventative programme for vulnerable, young first-time mothers and aims to improve:

- Pregnancy outcomes
- Child health and development
- Parents' economic self-sufficiency

It also offers intensive and structured home visiting, delivered by specially trained nurses, from early pregnancy until age two (DoH, 2012).

Providing Free School Meals

From September 2014 the Government pledged to provide free school meals for children in reception, year 1 and year 2 of infant school to help all children have a nutritionally healthy start to life. Advice was given to schools who need it most, as well as extra funding to increase capacity in school kitchens. Wood and Harper (2008) have examined the links between child nutrition and health, and cite studies that suggest that young children eating a healthy meal together at lunchtime can improve their development and social skills.

Public health polices for children and young people are designed to reinforce the commitment to giving all children a healthy start in life, and to ensure that the assets of the nation are invested in the health of all its children and young people.

2. Childhood Obesity: a Plan for Action, a Policy to Tackle the Childhood Obesity Epidemic

In recent years the Government has published strategies, which aspire to tackle rising levels of obesity in children.

In 2016 the Government published the first of its strategies to address childhood obesity and in June 2018 it published a further initiative to further strengthen the national childhood obesity plan.

WWW

https://assets.publishing.service.gov.uk/government/uploads/system/uploads/attachment_data/file/718903/childhood-obesity-a-plan-for-action-chapter-2.pdf

This plan contains a range of proposals to bring together various agencies in society to improve the nutritional content of the food and drink children in contemporary culture consume, often on a daily basis. Additionally, the government seeks to reinforce the information pertinent to these foods and drinks, which is available to parents, and to modify the way in which unhealthy food and sugary drinks are promoted across society. The Government hopes that this will impact on and improve strategies to tackle the emerging long-term illnesses, which attributed to obesity in childhood and then later in adulthood.

The third millennium has been increasingly characterised by excessive sugar and fat consumption, and what threatens the health of the nation most is the rising burden of childhood obesity. This is because obese children are susceptible to developing type 2 diabetes and liver problems, among other diseases, during their childhood. Fat children are more likely to experience bullying at school, suffer low self-esteem and a poorer quality of life, and most importantly are likely to become fat adults, who in turn have a higher risk of developing cancer, heart and liver disease. National childhood obesity rates reveal that the UK is now ranked among the worst in Western Europe. The incidence of childhood obesity is currently highest in families from deprived areas. Children growing up in such low-income households are more than twice as likely to be obese than those in higher income households. Although a significant percentage of obese children live in low-income households, children from disadvantaged Black and minority ethnic families are also likely to become obese. Government statistics show that in both the 4- to 5-year-old and the 10- to 11-year-old age groups, Black African children were the most likely to be overweight in 2015/16. Furthermore in 2015/16, Black African children aged 4–5 years of age were more than twice as likely to be overweight compared with Indian children, of whom 14.5% were overweight (https://www.ethnicity-facts-figures.service.gov.uk/health/preventing-illness/overweight-children/latest).

New figures cited in this report show that one-third of children are obese or overweight when they leave primary school. School letters sent to parents warning them that their children are overweight have been criticized by the parents, who have found the so-called fat letters offensive. However, the Guardian Newspaper has reported that although some parents object to these letters, the government is to retain them, partly because obesity is currently costing the NHS over 5 billion pounds per year in treatment costs (https://www.theguardian.com/society/2016/nov/03/chief-medical-officer-obesity-school-warning-letters-parents).

The government plan to tackle childhood obesity remains ambitious and seeks to configure polices which aspire to empower parents to make healthier choices for their children when shopping and when eating out in food venues. In particular, the government wants to eradicate some of the supermarket strategies, which shoppers find difficult to resist, such as promoting unhealthy food at the checkouts where so-called pester power prevails. This happens when children see chocolate bars or other sweets in open view whilst waiting at the checkout and pester their stressed parents into buying for them. Similarly, the government wants to change fundamentally the 'buy one get one free' deals to make them a health choice. Because of this, the government intends to ban price promotions, such as buy one get one free, and multi-buy offers, or unlimited refills of unhealthy foods and drinks in the retail sector, through legislation.

Most importantly the government intends to shield children from subliminal advertising, which encourages an appetite for unhealthy food. Hence, it plans to introduce a 9 pm watershed on TV advertising of high fat, high sugar and high salt products and similar protection for children viewing adverts online, with the aim of limiting children's exposure to this type of food. The government intends to put pressure on the food and advertising industries to harness their talents to help all parents find the healthier and easier choice for their children. The measures to be taken include:

Promoting Health Exercise

Exercise is central to maintaining a healthy weight and this new policy seeks to encourage every primary school to adopt the active mile initiatives such as the 'Fantastic Daily Mile'. Such initiatives have been shown to improve the physical, social, and mental well-being of children in school (WAVES

Collaboration and Barrett, 2014). It is envisaged that these types of physical interventions will encourage young people away from their device screens and into exercise because the 'Daily Mile' gets children out of the classroom for 15 minutes every day to run or jog, at their own pace, with their classmates, thus promoting fitness and enhanced concentration in the classroom (https://thedailymile.co.uk/).

The 2018 world cup series has probably raised the profile of football as an exercise in children, and Faude et al. (2010) believe that football training can be successful in improving the physical capacity, health-related fitness parameters and self-esteem in obese children as a standard exercise program. In this context playing football by overweight children can have significant health effects. However, successive governments have allowed many schools to sell their school playing fields for building land. For example, an article in the Times Educational Supplement cites data which shows that 65 local authorities in 2016 sought permission to sell or transfer 160 acres of school playing fields, which as a consequence has left many children deprived of space for sport and play (https://www.tes.com/news/exclusive-councils-sell-hundreds-acres-school-playing-field-land).

Reducing Sugar in Food and Drink

James et al. (2004) are adamant that energy imbalance is the reason for excessive weight gain and one of the contributory factors is linked to the drinking of carbonated drinks sweetened with sugar. Consequentially children who consume one regular carbonated drink a day have an average 10% more total energy intake than those that do not. In the United Kingdom more than 70% of adolescents consume carbonated drinks on a regular basis. Pivotal to the government's aspirations to reduce the amount of sugar in children's food and drink, the Soft Drinks Industry Levy (SDIL) was introduced in 2016 to put pressure on manufacturers to reduce the sugar content of soft drinks. The levy has encouraged the producers of added sugar soft drinks to reformulate their products to reduce the sugar content and to reduce portion sizes for added sugar drinks. The levy on sugary drinks came into force in April 2018 (https://www.gov.uk/government/publications/soft-drinks-industry-levy/soft-drinks-industry-levy).

As part of the overall plan to address childhood obesity the Government challenged industry to take 20% of sugar out of the food most commonly eaten by children by 2020, with a 5% reduction target for the first year. This has already led many parts of the food and drink industry to remove sugar from their most popular products such as breakfast cereals. The Government has noted that the effects are already being seen with an increasing consumer demand for healthier food and drink. However, despite some sections of industry meeting the 5% 1-year progress target, overall the 5% goal has not been achieved across the country. Because of this, the Government intends to continue to call for further progress on reducing the sugar content of foods and drink with particular reference to sugary milk drinks, which had not been included in the 2016 levy. Furthermore, it is the intention of the Government to evaluate the progress made towards a 20% sugar reduction in the foods most commonly eaten by children. If by 2020 the progress has been insufficient

the Government will impose more stringent actions on the industry, including mandatory and fiscal penalties.

However, obesity and weight gain in childhood is not just attributable to eating too much sugar, but reflects the whole complexity of the child's diet. The government report shows that on average overweight and obese children are eating up to an additional 500 calories per day. Work has already been initiated to implement a calorie reduction programme, which challenges all food and drink companies to reduce the calories by 20% in a range of everyday foods consumed by children by 2024. The Government also intends to monitor progress against the calorie target closely and will consider further additional steps if progress is not sufficiently achieved.

Energy Drinks

Crucially the Government is seeking to impose legislation on the sale of caffeine-loaded energy drinks to children. There are many concerns about the impact that high-caffeine energy drinks are having on the levels of caffeine and sugar that children in society drink. Seifert et al. (2011) show that these energy drinks have no therapeutic benefit, and many of the ingredients are poorly understudied and not regulated. The known and unknown pharmacology of agents included in such drinks, combined with reports of toxicity, raises concern for potentially serious adverse effects in association with energy-drink use among children. Currently all manufacturers have to label all energy drinks containing over 150 mg of caffeine as 'unsuitable' for children and this is because the regular consumption of caffeinated energy drinks has been linked with adverse health outcomes for children, such as headaches, sleeping problems, irritation and tiredness. These energy drinks are also laden with sugar in addition to caffeine, and may contain more sugar than full-sugar soft drinks, making them a prime suspect in adding to childhood obesity. Nevertheless, despite these concerns this new government publication shows that nearly 70% of UK adolescents (aged 10–17 years old) consume energy drinks on a regular basis, drinking them at a rate of over 50% of the European average. One of the reasons cited by the Government as the cause of this epidemic in the use of energy drinks is that that they are often cheaper than other soft drinks and, in some shops, can be bought for as little as 25 pence a can.

https://www.kingsfund.org.uk/blog/2018/06/second-government-childhood-obesity-plan?gclid=EAIaIQobChMI3vH-H1ZnN6wIVDrh3Ch1Bjg8rEAAYASAAEgIiW_D_BwE

The Government, in the face of what is becoming a childhood obesity pandemic, has set in motion a national ambition to halve childhood obesity and significantly reduce the gap in obesity between children from the most and least deprived areas by 2030. If the plan is successful it will have huge physical health benefits and in particular will reverse the emergence of type 2 diabetes in children. The Government knows that the task is daunting and will require all agencies and professionals including nurses, health visitors and schools to collaborate and work as one to tackle this new disease, which is damaging the nation's children. Such drastic action is necessary to eradicate the profound health effects of childhood obesity on both the individual child and society as a whole.

POLICIES TO IMPROVE THE WAY IN WHICH CHILDREN'S AND YOUNG PEOPLE'S SERVICES IN HOSPITALS ARE INSPECTED BY THE HEALTH CARE REGULATOR

The Care Quality Commission (CQC) is the Government appointed independent regulator of health and social care in England. Its primary function is to ensure that health and social care services provide people with safe, effective, compassionate, high-quality care. Through regular inspections, the CQC drives improvement in care services. There are similar arrangements in the other countries of the United Kingdom.

 WWW

https://www.cqc.org.uk/about-us/our-purpose-role/who-we-are.

Other countries outside the UK have similar bodies to maintain standards of health care. In the USA for example, various organisations perform accreditation and establish standards for health care delivery.

 WWW

https://www.jointcommission.org/about_us/about_the_joint_commission_main.aspx.

The CQC inspects health and social care institutions in five discreet domains namely:
- Safety (of service users)
- Effectiveness (of organisations)
- Caring
- Responsiveness (of organisations to service users)
- Leadership (of organisations and its effect on service delivery)

Using key lines of inquiry CQC inspectors and their specialist advisors assess each organisation's ability to deliver care to service users under the five domains of inspection. To achieve this agenda the CQC triangulates data, which it receives from the organisation in advance of the inspection with real-life data (from interviews with staff members and service users, and observations) collected during the inspection itself. The CQC inspection teams examine the results of the Friends and Family Tests, which most organisations participate in. The Friends and Family Test was first used in 2013 to allow service users an opportunity to anonymously give feedback to organisations about their experiences of care delivery. The CQC uses data from its inspections to produce reports, which are akin to holding a mirror to the organisation to show how they perform against each of the five inspection domains.

As part of the inspection process, the CQC assesses how individual providers comply with various children's and young people's health policies. Although most of these policies are not mandatory and at best can be seen as good practice, only some carry more weight than others, and the CQC does assess how polices for child health are implemented in organisations they inspect.

Each domain is given a rating ranging from:
- outstanding
- good
- requires improvement
- inadequate

Inadequate ratings for any domain require the provider to take steps to make improvements and many inadequate ratings reflect noncompliance to important polices, for example, policies related to nurse or medical staffing.

Although it is not the role of the CQC to drive policy formulation, it can as an organisation produce reports, which summarise policy direction, for example, *From the Pond to the Sea* discussed earlier, which reflects contemporary strategies to enhance children's transition to adult health services (https://www.cqc.org.uk/sites/default/files/CQC_Transition%20Report.pdf).

Children and young people make up about 20% of the population of England and Wales, but use medical services proportionally higher than other groups, for example as seen in a study by Lattimer et al., 1998.

In 2014 Dr Sheila Shribman, the former National Clinical Director for Children, Young People and Maternity Services, was commissioned by the CQC to investigate health care for children and young people. She produced a report entitled *Getting It Right For Children and Young People (Including Those Transitioning Into Adult Services): A Report On CQC New Approach To Inspection.* She believed that the needs of sick children had often been ignored in the adult-centric focused orientation of many general hospitals. She cited the Report of the Children's and Young People's Health Outcomes (Lewis and Lenehan, 2012), which had shown that there are variations in childhood ill health in differing parts of the country. Inequalities in child health, especially infant mortality, obesity, accidents and teenage pregnancy, are more common in those from disadvantaged backgrounds. Children, young people and their families find it challenging to make their voices heard and to be involved in decisions about their health. Worryingly, multidisciplinary team members are not adequately prepared to cope with the complexities of caring for sick children and some staff have limited experience of working with them, especially in areas such as disability and mental health (Glasper, 2012).

 WWW

https://www.cqc.org.uk/sites/default/files/20140730%20CQC%20response%20to%20Dr%20Shribman%20recommendations%20for%20publication.pdf

The CQC's new approach to inspection is now used to enhance the standards of care delivered to sick children and their families in hospital and reduce unacceptable variations in care delivery. One of Dr Shribman's initial comments in her report was aimed at destroying the myth that children and young people are simply little adults who eat less food and require smaller beds. She also highlighted the importance of care staff acknowledging the vulnerability of the sick child and in recognising the signs of the deteriorating child. This is exemplified by, and perhaps reflective of, Florence Nightingale's famous quotation that children 'are affected by the same things as adults but much more quickly and seriously' (Nightingale, 1859, p72) It is beyond the scope of this chapter to consider all 73 of Dr Shribman's recommendations, but a summary of the main aspects can be accessed from the website (https://www.cqc.org.uk/sites/default/files/20140730%20 CQC%20response%20to%20Dr%20Shribman%20recommendations%20for%20publication.pdf).

 ACTIVITY

In your learning group access the report from the CQC web-pages and discuss if Dr Shribman's assertions are still true.

POLICES THAT ARE CONCERNED WITH STAFFING AND WORKFORCE IN CHILD HEALTH AREAS

There are three primary policies concerned with workforce and staffing, which the CQC use in their inspections of children's and young people's services (2013).

1. Defining staffing levels for children and young people's services. RCN standards for clinical professionals and service managers.
2. British association of perinatal medicine service standards for hospitals providing neonatal care (third edition, 2010).
3. Facing the future – standards for acute general paediatric services (RCPCH, 2013).

Defining Staffing Levels for Children and Young People's Services. RCN Standards for Clinical Professionals and Service Managers (2013)

The Royal College of Nursing (RCN) has produced very sophisticated nurse staffing models for different departments within children's services (RCN, 2013). The Care Quality Commission also expects that infants, children and young people have the right to be cared for by sufficient numbers of staff with the right qualifications, skills and experience, and that all staff must receive appropriate training and supervision to meet the professional standards that allow them to practice. The RCN believes that these staffing standards are the minimal essential requirements for all providers of services to babies, children and young people. The RCN has developed 16 core-staffing standards, including that there will be a minimum of 70:30 per cent registered to unregistered staff and at least one nurse per shift in each clinical area will possess an advanced life support qualification. The RCN believes that there should be a minimum of two registered children's nurses at all times in all inpatient and day care areas.

https://www.rcn.org.uk/get-help/rcn-advice/staffing-levels

 ACTIVITY

In your learning groups access the RCN staffing policy and debate some of the impediments that some wards and departments might have in maintaining the standards.

British Association of Perinatal Medicine (BAPM) Service Standards for Hospitals Providing Neonatal Care (third edition, 2010)

BAPM have developed policies and standards for nurse staffing within neonatal units. These are summarised in the following sections.

Intensive Care

The ratio of neonatal nurses who are qualified in speciality (QIS) (which is the term used to describe a nurse who has undergone speciality training in the care of neonates) to baby should be one nurse:one baby. This nurse should have no other managerial responsibilities during the time of clinical care, but may be involved in the support of a less experienced nurse working alongside her in caring for the same baby.

High Dependency Care

The ratio of QIS neonatal nurses responsible for the care of babies requiring high dependency care should be one nurse:two babies. The more stable and less dependent babies may be cared for by registered nurses who are not QIS, but who are under the direct supervision and responsibility of a neonatal nurse who is QIS.

Special Care

The ratio of nurses looking after special care babies should be at least one nurse:four babies. It is essential that staffing in special care is sufficient to ensure that discharge is properly planned and organised including the adequate support for parents. Registered nurses and non-registered clinical staff may care for these babies under the direct supervision and responsibility of a neonatal nurse QIS.

https://www.rcn.org.uk/get-help/rcn-advice/staffing-levels

FACING THE FUTURE – STANDARDS FOR ACUTE GENERAL PAEDIATRIC SERVICES (RCPCH 2013)

The Royal College of Paediatrics and Child Health has produced a range of policies pertinent to the care of sick children and young people. In the context of this chapter, only the staffing standards for acute paediatric services will be considered. The primary goal of the RCPCH is to promote their policy, which stresses that it is essential that paediatrics is a 24 hours a day, 7 days a week specialty, with the most experienced doctors present at the busiest times. Their report gives ten standards for high quality, safe and sustainable acute general paediatric services:

1. A consultant paediatrician is present and readily available in the hospital during times of peak activity, 7 days a week.
2. Every child who is admitted to a paediatric department with an acute medical problem is seen by a health care professional with the appropriate competencies to work on the tier two (middle grade) paediatric rota within 4 hours of admission.

3. Every child who is admitted to a paediatric department with an acute medical problem is seen by a consultant paediatrician within 14 hours of admission, with more immediate review as required according to illness severity or if a member staff is concerned.

4. At least two medical handovers every 24 hours are led by a consultant paediatrician.

5. Every child with an acute medical problem who is referred for a paediatric opinion is seen by, or has their case discussed with, a clinician with the necessary skills and competencies before they are discharged. This could be: a paediatrician on the consultant rota, a paediatrician on the tier two (middle grade) rota, or a registered children's nurse who has completed a recognised advanced children's nurse practitioner programme and is an advanced children's nurse practitioner.

6. Throughout all the hours they are open, paediatric assessment units have access to the opinion of a consultant paediatrician.

7. All general paediatric inpatient units adopt an attending consultant system, most often in the form of the 'consultant of the week' system.

8. All general paediatric training rotas are made up of at least ten whole time equivalent posts, all of which are compliant with the UK Working Time Regulations and European Working Time Directive.

9. Specialist paediatricians are available for immediate telephone advice for acute problems for all specialties, and for all paediatricians.

10. All children, children's social care, police and health teams have access to a paediatrician with child protection experience and skills (of at least level 3 safeguarding competencies), who is available to provide immediate advice and subsequent assessment, if necessary, for children under 18 years of age where there are child protection concerns. The requirement is for advice, clinical assessment and the timely provision of an appropriate medical opinion, supported by a written report.

ACTIVITY

Access the RCPCH facing the future staffing standards and see if your own clinical area meets these standards.

POLICES THAT PROMOTE CHILD AND FAMILY INVOLVEMENT IN CARE

There have been a range of policies and standards produced by various bodies to promote the involvement of children, young people and their families in care delivery. The principal one is 'The 15 Steps Challenge', which was one of the final legacies of the Institute for Innovation and Improvement. It provided a useful tool to guide work with staff, children and young people and other stakeholders, and a framework to help view a clinical setting through the eyes of families who use NHS services.

The 15 Steps Challenge

The Fifteen Steps Challenge: Quality From a Patient's Perspective, was a series of toolkits that formed some of the resources available for the productive care work stream for NHS England. It was a quote from the parent of a child in hospital that initiated the 15 Steps Challenge philosophy 'I can tell what kind of care my daughter is going to get within 15 steps of walking on to a Ward'.

The Productive Series supports NHS teams to redesign and streamline the way they manage and work. This is intended to help achieve significant and lasting improvements in the quality of care delivered and to reduce costs, but also, for example, to provide extra time that nurses can devote to patients. Efficiency techniques previously used in car manufacturing, and safety techniques learned in the aviation industry have been adapted for the NHS. The Productive Ward Initiative, the first in the series to be published, focused on improving ward processes and environments to help nurses and therapists spend more time on patient care, thereby improving safety and efficiency. The 15 Steps Challenge was the final part of the series and was co-produced with patients, service users, carers, relatives, volunteers, staff, governors and senior leaders. The policy was designed to help examine care in a variety of settings through the eyes of patients and service users to help capture what good quality care looks, sounds and feels like. Initially launched in October 2012, an addendum to the toolkit suite facilitating the involvement of children, young people and their families was added in March 2013.

What is the 15 Steps Challenge?

Five toolkits make up the challenge:

- The 15 Steps Challenge for acute services
- The 15 Steps Challenge for mental health inpatient care
- The 15 Steps Challenge for children and young people's inpatient services (intended to be used alongside the adult toolkits but designed specifically for use in the care of children and young people)
- The 15 Steps Challenge for community services
- The 15 Steps Challenge for clinic and outpatient settings

Each toolkit provides a model for a service evaluation that consists of a series of questions and prompts to guide patients, service users, carers and NHS staff through their first impressions of a care setting. As with the other toolkits, the 15 Steps Challenge for children and young people's inpatient services is designed to help nurses and others gain an insight into how children, young people and their families feel about the care provided and what gives them confidence. This 'walking in the shoes of your patient' approach can help health professionals understand and identify the key components of high-quality care that are important to children and their families from their first contact with a care setting.

 ### ACTIVITY

In your learning group, explore how this child-focused toolkit can be used to conduct a service evaluation.

The purpose of the challenge is:

- To help staff, children and their families and others to work together to identify improvements that could enhance the child's experience of hospital.
- To provide a way of understanding their first impressions more clearly.
- To provide a method for creating positive improvements and dialogue about the quality of care delivered.

Bates and Roberts (2006) highlight the fact that the designing or redesigning of health care facilities and procedures based on the perceptions of service users has been key to the improvement of contemporary health care. The 15 Steps Challenge for children and young people's inpatient services, launched almost simultaneously with the Francis inquiry report into the events that occurred at Mid Staffordshire NHS Trust (Francis, 2013), was designed to accelerate the quest for the greater involvement of children and young people in service design and change.

This was reinforced by the publication of the Report of the Children's Outcomes Forum (DoH, 2012), which clearly articulates that all health organisations must demonstrate how they have listened to the voices of children and young people. As active citizens, children and young people take action and make contributions in everyday life that influence their personal circumstances and society. Hence the prime purpose of the 15 Steps Challenge toolkit is to help those using it gain an insight into how children, young people and their families feel about the care provided and what gives them confidence in managing illness. The toolkit is also designed to help hospital services more fully understand and identify the key components of high-quality care that are important to children and their families when they are receiving care in hospital from their first contact with the care setting. The toolkit was developed with the involvement of young people and is designed to support and involve young people in the 15 Steps Challenge process. It includes a useful poster, templates, observation guides, feedback sheets and certificates that can help with service evaluation. The toolkit helps provide a window into the NHS for children and families, facilitating the sharing of powerful insights into the things that matter most to them. The poster and guides concentrate on four themes for investigation that have previously been identified by families as important:

- Is the area being evaluated welcoming?
- Is it a safe place?
- Will it care for me?
- Is it well organised and calm?

The 15 Steps Challenge harnesses these key themes and aims to provide a tool for NHS organisations to guide work with staff, children, families and other stakeholders to give them a lens through which to view a clinical setting through the eyes of the child and family as they take the steps of the admission to hospital journey. The toolkit is designed to facilitate a service evaluation that documents clearly all the things that children and families might say matter to them during the admission process.

When conducting a service evaluation using the 15 step challenge it is felt that the involvement of children and young people in the process will help to enhance services. The toolkit includes a range of helpful tips on how to solicit and engage young people in the challenge. These include:

- Showing how children and young people may be contacted via local youth groups, schools and young people's councils.
- Using existing young patient or service user councils or forums such as the Young People's Executive (YiPpEe). The YiPpEe is a group of children and young people who advise hospital staff on what children and young people in hospital want and need (Oxford University Hospitals NHS Trust, 2018).

🌐 WWW

https://www.ouh.nhs.uk/get-involved/yippee.aspx

- Using, as appropriate, young people who are patients or service users and might like to get involved with the 15 Steps Challenge.
- Involving the patient experience team through Patient Advice and Liaison Services (PALS).
- Inviting, as appropriate, family members who have been complimentary or made a complaint about their experience in hospital.
- Preparing a clear explanation about the 15 Steps Challenge and why it is important to hear young peoples' views.
- Writing to young people formalising the date, time and details of the 15 Steps Challenge service evaluation.
- Discussing the nature of the clinical environment that will be visited to prepare children and young people to conduct the evaluation.
- Discussing and exploring behaviours that should be exercised within a clinical area, for example, the importance of hand hygiene and respect for the confidentiality of other child patients.
- Providing a briefing on the day of the visit to review the purpose of the evaluation and to remind all non-medical participants of hand hygiene and confidentiality.
- Creating an equal partnership in the process between adults, children and young people.
- Recognising and valuing ideas and suggestions from children and young people and ensuring that sufficient time is available for these to be expressed.
- Valuing the diversity children and young people offer.
- Making the process a rewarding and fun experience for children and young people.
- Providing a debrief on the day of the visit, thanking family members for their contribution and rewarding children with the certificate from the resource pack.
- Formally following this up with a letter of thanks including an example of a change that has been made as a result of their participation in the service evaluation.

Once the team has been assembled under the leadership of an appointed coordinator and a date agreed, an important stage in the challenge is to walk around the hospital areas being evaluated. Optimally the team should include a child and a parent, a staff member and a hospital board member. The purpose of the walk is to recognise and identify what the child/parent sees and to make notes on their first impressions.

The team uses a feedback sheet from the resource pack to make notes that are subsequently used to provide feedback to senior personnel in the hospital with a focus on good practice and areas for improvement.

It is recommended that the service evaluation is repeated at regular intervals to monitor whether improvements are being made and importantly sustained. It is now the responsibility of health professionals such as nurses to create the mechanisms to facilitate the effective engagement of children and young people, who are the current and future users of health care. If children's inpatient services are to deliver high-quality holistic care, the contributions of children and young people must be actively sought to ensure that there is true participation within this arm of the NHS. The engagement of children and young people through the 15 Steps Challenge will provide rich data that can be used to improve health outcomes and enhance services.

The materials are available from the national archive at:

WWW

http://webarchive.nationalarchives.gov.uk/20150401170344/http://www.institute.nhs.uk/index2.php?option=com_content&task=view&id=4644&pop=1&page=0&Itemid=6700.

ACTIVITY

The toolkit is free to download from NHS England via the archive. Download the kit and in your learning group use the poster to identify the positive and less positive aspects of the clinical areas where you are currently on placement.

POLICIES FOR ENHANCING THE MENTAL HEALTH OF CHILDREN AND YOUNG PEOPLE

With news of royal patronage for people with mental health problems by the Duke and Duchess of Cambridge and their bother Prince Harry it is timely to review perceptions of mental health in society. The quest by the Royals is to destigmatise mental illness and to bring it into line with physical health problems and therefore public acceptability.

WWW

https://www.theguardian.com/society/2017/mar/29/royals-launch-mental-health-campaign-videos-get-britons-talking

\The Duke and his brother Harry have endeavoured to raise the public profile of mental health for some time and have themselves publicly discussed the impact of their mother Princess Diana's death in August 1997.

The Care Quality Commission (CQC) Thematic Review on Children and Young People's Mental Health

In October 2017, the Care Quality Commission published phase one of a thematic review on children and young people's mental health (CQC, 2017).

This initial report represents a response to the call for a review of mental health services for children and young people

in England by the Prime Minister earlier in 2017. In compiling this initial report, the CQC has collated evidence from existing mental health reports, research and other forms of evidence, in addition to scrutinising the findings of its own inspections of children and young people's mental health services in England. The CQC also held meetings with young service users to identify the strengths and weaknesses of the current systems of care. The report reaffirms many of the issues raised in the *Five Year Forward View for Mental Health*, published in 2016, but especially the difficulties children and young people have in seeking appropriate support for their mental health concerns from Child and Adolescent Mental Health Services (CAMHS), which have struggled to meet demand in recent years (Mental Health Taskforce, 2016). The CQC report does not make recommendations as its primary goal is to identify the issues that children and young people face when engaging with mental health concerns and makes specific recommendations in its phase two report, which was published in 2019 (https://www.cqc.org.uk/publications/themed-work/are-we-listening-review-children-young-peoples-mental-health-services). The CQC aspires to raise awareness of some of the deficiencies in current service provision. There is variation in the quality of care, and some parts of the service do not function optimally, allowing some children to fall through the gaps in services. Despite this, the CQC highlight several examples of good care delivery.

It is widely acknowledged that emotional problems in childhood are increasingly a cause for concern, with up to 10% of children suffering from a diagnosable mental health disorder, and with half of all mental health conditions beginning before the age of 14. Children and young people today face emotional demands that did not exist in previous generations. The growth in social media and access to the internet, for example, has led to unexpected consequences, with Hawton et al. (2012) highlighting the effects of social media on self-harm and suicide rates among young people. A report from the Education Policy Institute has shown that more than a third (37.3%) of UK 15-year-olds are classed as extreme internet users, who use the internet for more than 6 hours outside of school on a typical weekday, and nearly a third (27.6%) were 6 years old or younger when they first used the internet (Frith, 2017). There is now a greater awareness of mental health problems in society and a growing expectation that mental health issues be viewed more positively. This has been helped by a high-profile royal campaign (Booth, 2017). However, accessing appropriate care for this group of children and young people is challenging, not least of which is because of the recruitment and retention crisis in the mental health workforce across the country. To tackle this crisis, the Government has committed to creating 2000 additional nurse, consultant and therapist posts in CAMHS (Glasper, 2017a; Health Education England, 2017). Expanding CAMHS is crucial if meeting the mental health needs of children and young people is to be achieved. However, CAMHS alone cannot meet all of the demand and it is for this reason that new initiatives – for example, giving teachers access to mental health first aid training – have been undertaken. This is because many children and young people with mental health disorders are not known to CAMHS and there is a growing recognition that schools are a fundamental route of referral to mental health services (DoH et al., 2017; Glasper, 2017b).

The CQC report is configured into four sections:

- What can we learn from young people's experiences of care?
- Where do services need to improve?
- What are the barriers to high-quality care?
- What good and outstanding practices can we learn from?

Learning From Young People's Experiences

Children who were interviewed by the CQC indicated that their experience of care was best when staff with the optimum toolkit of skills were available. Although the majority of CQC inspections of CAMHS across England have rated services as 'good' or 'outstanding', and many children and young people who use CAMHS services have a positive experience of mental health care, there remain too many variations. The CQC found that too many children and young people continue to face obstacles in accessing timely interventions, with Childline reporting a 34% increase in calls from children and young people about poor mental health services (Childline, 2017:8). Some of the children and young people told the CQC that there was a high turnover of staff, causing a lack of continuity in their relationships with members of the mental health team. Concerns were also expressed about how long they have to wait to access mental health support. In many cases this resulted in a deterioration in their mental health, with some reaching crisis point. Some children told the CQC that the care they received was not always age appropriate and that they wanted much more autonomy in decision making about their care, especially as they got older. They also said that some of the systems of care were inflexible and that informal methods of support, such as counselling groups or telephone provision, were not always available. Although the young people interviewed believed that stigma around mental ill health had improved, there were some for whom stigma was still linked to both having a diagnostic label of mental ill health and in accessing mental health services. Families and carers expressed anxiety and frustration about the fragmented nature of services. They told the CQC that they wanted more involvement with managing their children's mental health, particularly when self-harm was involved. Parents generally felt that communication between themselves and mental health professionals was inadequate and that information about their children's care was sub-optimal.

Where services need to improve. Of the 101 units inspected by the CQC, only one CAMHS specialist service, an inpatient unit, was rated as outstanding for safety. In some of the services inspected, the physical care environment was judged to be unsafe. Some inpatient units were deemed unclean, putting staff and patients at risk of infection. The CQC found that there were ongoing issues with waiting times for CAMHS services. Perhaps most worrying is the lack of specialist inpatient beds, resulting in some children and young people being inappropriately admitted to adult wards. In some geographical locations specialised care for children with severe and enduring mental health

problems is not available and this resulted in children being admitted to units some considerable distance from their own home or having to wait inordinate periods of time to access the specialist care and support they need. This is made worse through inadequate staffing levels and the CQC is adamant that safe, effective and compassionate care can be delivered only when there are sufficient numbers of staff with the right skill set to provide high-quality care. Young people were especially concerned that staff in emergency departments did not always have the right skills to manage them when they were experiencing a mental health crisis.

Barriers to high-quality care. The CQC found that a major barrier to the delivery of high-quality care is a lack of accurate data relating to the complexities of child mental health across the country. For example, services currently do not routinely gather data on children with mental health problems who are homeless or in relation to their sexual orientation. Such gaps in data collection make it difficult to completely capture the landscape of children's mental health to determine, for example, if there is sufficient provision of community mental health support. Furthermore, if clinical decisions pertinent to a young person's treatment are not fully communicated across the range of agencies that provide care, there is a danger that delays or mistakes in treatment can occur. There has been an increase in the demand for out-of-hours and emergency mental health care for children and young people and there is no doubt that CAMHS is under strain as it tries to meet demand, often with diminishing resources (Glasper, 2017a).

Learning from good and outstanding practice. Perhaps one of the most fundamental aspects of providing good care for children and young people with mental health problems is to involve them in the design of mental health services. The DoH's *Quality Criteria for Young People Friendly Health Services,* published in 2011, was designed to help commissioners and providers of health services to improve NHS and non-NHS health services. Services that have implemented this audit tool, which involves service users, have found it useful as a way of improving the patient experience and health outcomes for young people (Coles et al., 2013). The CQC has also revealed that strong links between schools and mental health services are an important feature of some services. The report states that several services have introduced 'crisis cards' or 'crisis plans' to ensure that children and young people can access support quickly when their mental health deteriorates.

This CQC report indicated that there is variation in the quality of mental health care delivered to children and young people and that there are barriers to accessing high-quality care.

 ACTIVITY

In your learning group discuss progress made since the CQC report and debate the success of any improvements, which have occurred.

GETTING IT RIGHT – DEALING WITH ACCOLADES AND COMPLAINTS

There are a range of policies and procedures for dealing with complaints and accolades from the families of sick children in health care environments.

Seeking Family Feedback on Their Experience of Health Care

What Is the Friends and Family Test?

Initially launched in 2013 by the coalition government, the Friends and Family Test (FFT) is an important feedback tool that supports the fundamental principle that people who use NHS services should have the opportunity to provide feedback about their experience. Listening to the views of patients and staff helps identify what is working well, what can be improved and how.

The FFT asks people if they would recommend the services they have used and offers a range of responses. When combined with supplementary follow-up questions, the FFT provides a mechanism to highlight both good and poor patient experience. This kind of feedback is vital in transforming NHS services and supporting patient choice.

So far, the FFT has produced more than 48 million pieces of feedback so far – and the total rises by around 1.2 million more every month – making it the biggest source of patient opinion in the world. Scores so far have told us that at least nine out of ten patients would recommend the NHS services they used to their loved ones. Patient comments also identify areas where improvements can be made so that providers can make care and treatment better for everyone.

How Does FFT Work?

NHS England core requirements for FFT are that every eligible patient be given the opportunity to answer the question at the point of discharge. This can be via SMS, IVM or paper survey. It is essential that the FFT is conducted in such a way that patient anonymity is respected and given high priority. Providers must submit monthly data to NHS England that include at least the number of responses in each category, the number of responses collected by each method and where specified in the area of care guidance – an eligible population.

The Friends and Family Test allows service users an opportunity to anonymously give feedback to organisations about their experiences of care delivery. The principal aim of the initiative was to make this feedback publicly available to enable service users to use that information in making their own decisions and choices about their care.

 WWW

https://www.england.nhs.uk/wp-content/uploads/2014/07/fft-rev1.pdf

Although standardised Friend and Family Test questionnaires have been made available through NHS England, other designs, which are aimed at improving inclusiveness, for example, for use with children and young people, are also obtainable from their website.

 WWW

https://www.england.nhs.uk/fft/fft-inclusive/

However, Sizmur et al. (2015) have raised some concerns about the current FFT, which shows that the actual test instrument is prone to bias from demographic factors and from the mode of administration. They believe, therefore, that the data from the FFT should be used with caution when using it to make comparisons between differing organisations.

Using Tops and Pants to Get Feedback From Children and Their Families

Manchester Children's hospital was one of the first to start using pants and tops daily on a washing line, using pants and tops shaped like a pair of shorts and a t-shirt that children in hospital could embellish with their own words to describe what was good (tops) and want was less desirable (pants) about their experiences during their stay in hospital.

 WWW

https://www.preparingforadulthood.org.uk/SiteAssets/Downloads/y1ko25ft636379738653108324.pdf

The so-called Pants and Tops proforma is a useful tool to encourage feedback from children and young people, who can write or draw their thoughts on the blank pants and tops. Many children's units use either this concept of something similar to solicit direct feedback from their child patients. The pants and tops daily washing line can be created using string with clothes pegs or paper clips for example in a range of wards and departments and it is a useful adjunct to the FFT.

⊕ **WWW**

http://www.mefirst.org.uk/resource/pants-and-tops-feedback-tool/

DEALING WITH COMPLAINTS

From one of our most recently constructed hospitals complaints have been made that there were not sufficient nursing conveniences, that nothing was at hand, that everything had to be sought. Where this is the case the hospital administration must be both inefficient and costly.

Florence Nightingale (1863)

Complaints are a fact of life. No organisation or profession can avoid them and it is not desirable to ignore or belittle them. Most complaints, if well handled, can have a very positive outcome. Complaints in the health service often indicate ways in which practice or processes can be improved or highlight matters that really concern children, families or carers.

If a family makes a complaint about any aspect of their child's care, nurses and the multidisciplinary team not only need to be involved in the investigation of that complaint, but also must also reflect back on the accuracy of their record-keeping, particularly records of any communication that they have had with the child or carers and multidisciplinary colleagues. Many hospitals use Datix, the incident reporting software to record complaints. The Nursing and Midwifery Council (2008) states 'You must keep clear and contemporaneous records of the discussions you have, the assessments you make, the treatment and medicines you give and how effective these have been'. If an aspect of care is not documented, how can there be any evidence that that care has taken place? Often a complaint is made after an issue has occurred and it would be difficult for any nurse to recall details of a particular case. Consequently, the investigator is reliant on what is documented.

Effective clinical governance processes ensure that all complaints are seen and dealt with as part of everyday business and that complaints are used to indicate improvements to services across the whole organisation. Where possible complaints should be dealt with at ward level to resolve this issue as quickly as possible for the child and family and then this will reduce the need for a formal process. If procedures and processes have been changed, complainants appreciate being informed of the changes. Consideration needs to be given by Trusts as to the most effective way to encourage staff to manage complaints as efficiently and effectively as possible. Complaints training can help staff understand the importance of this.

Criteria for Investigating Complaints

For an investigation under the NHS complaints procedure, a complaint must be about NHS services. Anyone making a complaint under the procedure is entitled to:

- A full and complete explanation of what happened and why, given in a language the complainant can understand.
- An apology if there was an error or omission on behalf of the staff.
- Information about the action that the organisation has taken or is proposing to take, if an error or omission has occurred, to try and prevent it happening again.

Complaints should be dealt with quickly and efficiently. Ideally complaints should be made as soon as possible after the incident has occurred, but normally within 6 months of the event or within 6 months from the time that it came to the complainant's notice. Occasionally, as a result of bereavement or prolonged illness, a Trust may decide to investigate a complaint if it is outside of these time limits.

Since April 2009 the new NHS Complaints Process has consisted of only two stages: Local Resolution and the Parliamentary and Health Service Ombudsman.

Local resolution is an essential stage of the complaint process. This is the stage at which nurses and other multidisciplinary colleagues can become involved, and take note of when families are becoming anxious or distressed or clearly need to sit down and talk through concerns. Even this informal process requires clear and accurate documentation. How local resolution is handled is for the individual organisation to decide. Staff need to be empowered and trained to act on concerns the moment they receive them. The sooner a complaint is responded to the more likely it will be resolved. Families often just want to be heard and to express their anxieties and

it is at this stage that the Patient Advice and Liaison Service (PALS) can be of great benefit.

Family advocates (PALS) are available to help families. The service is free to all patients, families, carers and friends and they can speak in confidence to trained staff; information will not be disclosed unless permission is given. If it is thought necessary to protect a child from serious harm or injury, then a decision needs to be made as to the way forward. PALS can:

- provide a listening ear
- help sort out any problems by liaising with staff
- support families in making their concerns heard
- guide families through the hospital complaints process if they wish to make a formal complaint
- link families to information and support services

Written complaints must receive a written response, unless otherwise agreed by the complainant. A range of individuals can provide this response; often it is the health care professionals themselves who will prepare a response for the Complaints Manager, and this will then be collated into a full response for the Chief Executive to sign. This is an important stage for nurses and multidisciplinary team (MDT) to be involved; they have often been working closely with the families and are able to provide their version of events. It is important to understand the full picture from beginning to end and to hear that story from all the individuals involved. People's perceptions can be very different and it is important to receive a balanced view.

The final letter at the end of local resolution must advise the complainant of his or her rights to refer their complaint to the Parliamentary and Health Service Ombudsman if they are unhappy with the outcome of the Trust's handling of their complaint. Finally, if something has gone wrong, the Parliamentary and Health Service Ombudsman must decide whether a Trust has been clear about the steps that have been taken to reduce the chances of a repetition of the event. At this stage it is essential for the investigations teams to take independent clinical advice if the complaint involves clinical issues. The type of advice obtained will depend upon the clinical issues in question, therefore independent advice may be sought from a range of health care professionals, for example, nurses, doctors, midwives, dieticians or pharmacists. There are then two options:

- To refer the complaint back to local resolution for further investigation and explanations from the Trust.
- To fast-track the complaint to the Ombudsman.

Complainants have a right to approach the Parliamentary and Health Service Ombudsman if they remain dissatisfied at the end of the current second stage of the NHS Complaints process. The Ombudsman considers the request and decides whether to investigate. As a result, the Ombudsman has become the last resort for a complainant, who remains dissatisfied after exhausting the initial two stages of the NHS complaints procedure. The Health Service Ombudsman's powers and duties are set out in the *Health Service Commissioner's Act 1993*. Jurisdiction was initially confined to the classic Ombudsman territory of maladministration (in the NHS), but was extended in 1996 to include clinical complaints and complaints about family health service practitioners.

Complaints in the NHS often stem from stressful events at a time when people feel vulnerable and scared. They may at times be unreasonable but must still be assessed objectively. Complaints can also be stressful for NHS staff, who might well feel that they did their best in difficult circumstances and that the only outcome is for them to be criticised. It is essential that Trusts are able to provide support for both the complainant and staff.

CONCLUSION

This chapter has endeavoured to portray the landscape of child health policy, but it should be stressed that successive governments will continue to address deficiencies in children's health care through new policy publications and it is therefore imperative that readers remain vigilant and check for new policies periodically.

REFERENCES

Andre, F.E., Booy, R., Bock, H.L., et al., 2008. Vaccination greatly reduces disease, disability, death and inequity worldwide. Bull. World. Health. Organ. 86, 140–146. https://doi.org/10.2471/BLT.07.040089.

Bates, P., Robert, G., 2006. Experience-based design: from redesigning the system around the patient to codesigning services with the patient. Qual. Saf. Health Care 15 (5), 307–310.

Booth, R., 2017. Royals launch campaign to get Britons talking about mental health. Guardian. https://tinyurl.com/kvefnnh (accessed 20 December 2017).

Bowlby, J., 1951. Maternal Care and Mental Health, World Health Organisation Monograph. Series No 2, Geneva.

Care Quality Commission (CQC), 2017. Review of children and young people's mental health services: phase one report. https://tinyurl.com/ya77azjx (accessed 20 December 2017).

Carter, B., 2002. Health inequalities; a blight on children's lives and futures. J. Child. Health. Care 6 (1), 4–6.

Childline, 2017. It turned out someone did care: Childline annual review 2015/16. https://tinyurl.com/y75flc3x (accessed 20 December 2017).

Coles, L., Glasper, A., Nicols, P., 2013. Are young people welcome in the English National Health Service? Issues Compr. Pediatr. Nurs. 36 (1–2), 144–167. https://doi.org/10.3109/01460862.2013.790738.

Committee of the Central Health Services Council, 1959. The Welfare of Children in Hospital. HMSO, London.

Demicheli, V., Jefferson, T., Rivetti, A., Price, D., 2005. Vaccines for measles, mumps and rubella in children. Cochrane. Database. Syst. Rev. 4. https://doi.org/10.1002/14651858.CD004407.pub2. Article No: CD004407.pub2.

Department of Health (DoH), Department for Education, Hunt J., 2017. Secondary school staff get mental health 'first aid' training. https://tinyurl.com/y9mmrjo4 (accessed 20 December 2017).

Department of Health (DoH), 2011. You're welcome: quality criteria for young people friendly health services. https://tinyurl.com/hejrhj6 (accessed 20 December 2017).

Department of Health (DoH), 2012. Report of the Children and Young People's Outcomes Forum. https://www.gov.uk/government/groups/children-and-young-peoples-health-outcomes-forum.

Faude, O., Kerper, O., Multhaupt, M., Winter, C., Beziel, K., Junge, A., Meyer, T., 2010. Football to tackle overweight in children. Scand. J. Med. Sci. Sports 20, 103–110. https://doi.org/10.1111/j.1600-0838.2009.01087.x.

Francis, R., 2013. Final Report of the Independent Inquiry Into Care Provided By Mid Staffordshire NHS Foundation Trust. Published http://tinyurl.com/6j47g6z.

Frith, E., 2017. For the Independent Commission on Children and Young People's Mental Health, Education Policy Institute. Social media and children's mental health: a review of the evidence. https://tinyurl.com/yccrb4mf (accessed 20 December 2017).

Glasper, A., 2012. A strategy to improve the health of children and young people. British Journal of Nursing 21 (17), 1040–1041.

Glasper, A., 2017a. Recruit and retain: planning to expand the mental healthcare workforce. Br. J. Nurs. 26 (19), 1080–1081. https://doi.org/10.12968/bjon.2017.26.19.1080.

Glasper, A., 2017b. Promoting mental health first aid literacy in secondary schools. Br. J. Nurs. 26 (16), 944–945. https://doi.org/10.12968/bjon.2017.26.16.944.

Glasper, E.A., Cooper, M., 1999. Hospitals need specialist inpatient adolescent units. Br. J. Nurs. 8 (9), 549.

Godlee, F., Smith, J., Marcovitch, H., 2011. Wakefield's article linking MMR vaccine and autism was fraudulent. BMJ 342, c7452.

Ham, C., 1999. Health Policy in Britain, fourth ed. Macmillan, Basingstoke. ch. 4.

Hawton, K., Saunders, K.E.A., O'Connor, R.C., 2012. Self-harm and suicide in adolescents. Lancet 379 (9834), 2373–2382. https://doi.org/10.1016/s0140-6736(12)60322-5.

Health Education England, 2017. Stepping forward to 2020/21: mental health workforce plan for England. http://tinyurl.com/yaakxgbs (accessed 20 December 2017).

James, J., Thomas, P., Cavan, D., Kerr, D., 2004. Preventing childhood obesity by reducing consumption of carbonated drinks: cluster randomised controlled trial [published correction appears in BMJ. 2004 May 22;328(7450):1236]. BMJ 328 (7450), 1237. https://doi.org/10.1136/bmj.38077.458438.EE.

Lattimer, V., George, S., Thompson, F., et al., 1998. General practice. Safety and effectiveness of nurse telephone consultation in out of hour's primary care: randomised controlled trial. Br. Med. J. 317 (7165), 1054–1059.

Lewis, I., Lenehan, C., 2012. Report of the Children's and Young People's Health Outcomes Forum. http://tinyurl.com/o4vj3pq (accessed 30 September 2014).

Mental Health Taskforce to the NHS in England, 2016. Five year forward view for mental health. https://tinyurl.com/gvc4or3 (accessed 20 December 2017).

Nagra, A., et al., 2015. Arch. Dis. Child. Educ. Pract. Ed 100, 313–320. https://doi.org/10.1136/archdischild-2014-307423.

NHS Education for Scotland (NES), 2013. Nursing and Midwifery Workload and Workforce Planning. Learning Toolkit, second ed. NES, Edinburgh.

Nursing and Midwifery Council, 2019. https://www.nmc.org.uk/standards/code/record-keeping/.

Nightingale, F., 1859. Notes on nursing: what it is, and what it is not. Edn. 1970. Duckworth and company, London Northampton General Hospital (2010) Fabio helps young NGH patients to have their say.

Robertson, J., 1962. Hospitals and Children, a Parents Eye View. Victor Gollanez, London.

Royal College of Nursing, 2013. Defining Staffing Levels for Children and Young People's Services. RCN, London. http://tinyurl.com/bwlfutg (accessed 30 September 2014).

Seifert, S.M., Schaechter, J.L., Hershorin, E.R., Lipshultz, S.E., 2016. Health effects of energy drinks on children, adolescents, and young adults [published correction appears in Pediatrics. May;137(5):null]. Pediatrics 127 (3), 511–528. https://doi.org/10.1542/peds.2009-3592. 2011.

Shribman, S., 2014. Getting it right for children & young people (including those transitioning into adult services): a report on CQC's new approach to inspection. http://tinyurl.com/k53ofsr (accessed 30 September 2017).

Sizmur, S., Graham, C., Walsh, J., 2015. Influence of patients' age and sex and the mode of administration on results from the NHS Friends and Family Test of patient experience. J. Health Serv. Res. Policy 20 (1), 5–10.

Tucker, A., 2002. Sir Douglas Black. The Guardian (Public health), Saturday September 14th.

University of London, 1955. An Account of Hospital Admissions in the Pre-school Period. Joint Committee of The Institute of Child health, Society of Medical Officers of Health and Population Investigation Committee.

Utting, W., 1997. People like Us: The Report of the Review of Safeguards for Children Living Away from home. The Stationary Office, London.

Viner, R., Keane, M., 1998. Youth Matters: Evidence-Based Best Practice for the Care of Young People in Hospital. Action for Sick Children. London.

Wakefield, A.J., Murch, S.H., Anthony, A., et al., 1998. Ileal–lymphoid–nodular hyperplasia, non-specific colitis, and pervasive developmental disorder in children. Lancet 351, 637–641.

Wood, Harper, 2008. http://citeseerx.ist.psu.edu/viewdoc/download?doi=10.1.1.455.6535&rep=rep1&type=pdf.

Young, R., et al., 2016. Leaving school: a comparison of the worries held by adolescents with and without intellectual disabilities. J. Intellect. Dis. Res 60 (1), 9–21.

4

Contemporary Childhoods and Health

Duncan C. Randall

LEARNING OUTCOMES

- Describe the main social and psychological theories that are associated with children and childhoods.
- Discuss the ways in which these theories impact on children's nursing.

- Describe how children acquire language and the understanding of personality formation in childhood.
- Discuss children's concept of health, illness and their internal bodies, and be able to use this information to offer explanations to children and families.

GLOSSARY

Accommodation Accommodation occurs when new information or stimuli cannot be assimilated in existing conceptions and cognitive abilities, forcing a reorganisation of conceptions and development of new cognitive abilities.

Assimilation Assimilation occurs when new information is incorporated into the child's existing schema. The new information can be used by the child by using their existing conceptions and cognitive abilities.

Continuous/discontinuous Processes of children's development, which are either *continuous*, that is, the child's abilities gradually become more complex and sophisticated over time without interruptions; or *discontinuous*, that is, the child obtains abilities at certain ages, during certain periods of childhood and the process can be broken into stages.

Developmental milestone Agreed points in time during childhood when cognitive and or physical abilities are obtained and can be demonstrated by children.

Developmental process The process during a socially proscribed period of childhood in which children's physical and cognitive abilities change. There is a social expectation that such processes result in the attainment of the physical and cognitive abilities assigned to adults (see maturation, later).

Language acquisition How children obtain the abilities to comprehend language and to express themselves through articulation of language.

Maturation Maturation of an ability can be deemed to have occurred when a child's abilities are equal to those expected of adults within a community. Although for some, maturation is the end of child development processes, others would argue that developmental processes continue to influence the life course of people and as such 'maturation' is a misnomer.

Nature Processes of children's development which are claimed to be 'natural', to occur irrespective of interventions by others (normally assumed to be adults).

Nurture Processes of children's development, which are claimed to be constructed by others (adults), such as child-rearing practice or education.

Personality A difficult concept to define but here taken to mean, the interaction of a person's traits, which indicate their approach to life in general – including interests, motivations, self-concepts and emotional patterns. Theories relevant to children were put forward by Freud and Erikson.

Pre-sociological theories of childhoods Theories and conceptions of children and childhoods, which are claimed to apply to all children irrespective of social/cultural or political context.

Sociological theories of childhoods Theories and conceptions of children and childhoods, which take into account the social/cultural and political context of children's lives as lived in communities. By implication such theories do not suggest a 'one size' fits all approach, but that there are many different views of children and their childhoods, both in communities and between different communities.

Stability Children's abilities are deemed stable (or not) if demonstrated in different social or environmental contexts (situations). The ability to hold a pen and draw a circle would be seen as stable if a child could demonstrate this in a pre-school setting and in their own home. If abilities are not stable this may indicate other mental or physical health problems. Children with hearing loss can attend in the quiet of a home setting, but are distracted in a school setting where there is a lot of background noise.

Zone of proximal development Conception advanced by Vygotsky to explain the learning of new skills and the development of cognition in which learning or development proceeds by incremental stages, each based upon cognition and skills already obtained. This means skills and cognition are built over time and that sudden development of skills or cognition not utilizing existing abilities is not possible. For example, children need to learn to balance on two feet before they walk; they do not (normally) go from crawling to walking without learning to balance first.

INTRODUCTION

The essential nature of children and their childhoods is a highly contested concept (James et al., 1998). Perhaps we should not be surprised by this; children and their nurturing to adulthood is an investment for any society in its future. Thus various arguments have raged across the centuries: nature versus nurture, continuous versus discontinuous development, the 'clinic' experimental method versus 'natural' observations. Often practitioners from various disciplines hold to certain positions with much fervor, but the empirical evidence is sometimes less than robust. We don't intend to detail all of these arguments, and certainly don't intend to offer any definitive resolutions to the debates. Instead we want to set out briefly some of the arguments and their underpinning philosophy, point briefly to where there are major areas of contention and move swiftly to the implication for children's nursing and children's nurses.

In part what we discuss here should help you as a children's nurse to place children in their childhood. As eluded to in Chapter 2, it is important not only to understand the position of children in the process of their childhood, but also in how others (mostly adults) consider children. It may be helpful to read this chapter alongside Chapter 5, which details physical development. Perhaps the division of the physical and the psychosocial is unfortunate, but it aids clarity to divide the two. However, we should remember that the physical aspects of development, how children's bodies and brains change over childhood, is occurring in a social/political context, which influences children's thinking and how we think about children.

THEORIES OF CHILDHOOD

James et al. (1998) have set out the ways in which we theorise childhoods. They point out that there have been a number of ways in which children have been seen by adults throughout human history and that these conceptions of children and their childhoods persist into our thinking and behaviours today. These conceptions of childhood can be placed in two categories, according to James and her colleagues, pre-sociological and sociological. These are explored below.

Pre-Sociological

The pre-sociological views are as James et al. (1998) argue, ideas about children and their childhoods in which the concept of a society and of social/cultural and political ideas about generations and children are not taken into account. These are conceptions about children, which are proposed to be applicable to all children, at all times, in all places. While some of these ideas were established in the late 18th century, they are often used by people today, and we can see aspects of these views of children in modern film, literary and media representations of children.

'The evil child'. The idea that children are 'evil' can be seen in films such as 'The Exorcist' (1973) and book such as William Golding's (1962) classic *Lord of the Flies*. Arguably this idea comes from religious perspectives that we are all 'evil' and that we are in need of saving. According to this view, children are born sinners and 'evil' and through religion are saved, but always have the potential to revert to sin.

'The innocent child'. Directly opposite to this view is Rousseau's conception 'Man is born free and everywhere he is in chains' (*Social contract*, 1762a). In *Emile* (1762b) Rousseau expanded upon this idea. In his vision, children are born innocent and are corrupted by the world (i.e. adults) around them. Further in Rousseau's utopia, children would be left to find their own way and in doing so would create a much improved world, free from 'adult' meddling. This is the ethos of Summerhill School, founded by A.S. Neill in 1921 and which continues to educate children in a democratic school where children choose to participate, or not.

⊕ **WWW**
- http://www.summerhillschool.co.uk/

'The Immanent child'. Also based on thoughts about education, John Locke in 1693 set out a less idealised view of children. Although not being the salvation of mankind, Locke moved away from the religious conception of children as evil. Instead he describes children as a blank page upon which adults, through education, write. The child is 'Immanent' and though education they are brought to reason, guided to be responsible citizens and thinking adults.

'The naturally developing child'. This is the view adopted by most psychologists, and expanded upon later. Psychologists propose that there is a 'natural' process, which children are a part of, and which occurs through childhood and inevitably results in adulthood. That children are both 'natural' and their progression through childhood is predictable. More recently this view has been contested both for the idea that there is a staged standardised progression in childhood and that there is a universal 'adult' state to be obtained. There are also concerns that this standard view of 'normal' means children are measured, and held as not succeeding, if they do not obtain in a timely fashion, arbitrary criteria of childhood development (Blackford, 2004). However, as discussed below, Piaget and his theories

remain a central part of child developmental assessment led by psychologists and influence many other aspects of children's health services.

'The unconscious child'. The writings of Freud also continue to influence our thinking about children and their childhoods. Now often controversial and contested, Freud's ideas on Ego and Id are still used to explain pathologies and problems in childhood. However, perhaps the main influence of Freud was in casting childhood as the period of time which influences adult life. The importance for Freud of childhood was how it led to pathologies in adulthood. This has led to retrospective examinations of childhood in Freudian psychoanalysis, but to little considerations of how to live less damaging childhoods.

Although these pre-sociological views are purported to be applicable irrespective of a child's culture or community, what we find is that to varying degrees, aspects of these views are held by people from different communities. The challenge for children's nurses is to understand these various views, which may differ from their own. In some communities the 'evil' child is a commonly held view of children and parents may adopt overly severe punishments in the belief that the child deserves such punishment, for what might be reasonable normal developmental behaviour (Azar et al., 2008, 2013).

 ACTIVITY

Find a copy of Peter Brooks 1963 film of *Lord of the Flies*, watch with a colleague, and debate the various images and views of childhood depicted in the film.
- How do these compare to your own experience of childhood?

Sociological Childhoods

James et al. (1998) offer sociological views of children and their childhoods as a more recent alternative view of children. Sociologists have in the past twenty years or so become more interested in childhood as a sociological issue. This understanding of children is based on how societies interact with younger generations. These views are related to sociological ideas and constructions. In opposition to pre-sociological views these sociological ways of understanding are contextual and relational. In other words, the view of children is based in a cultural/political and often geographical space. There is not a one size fits all approach but rather that different communities will have different views of children and their childhoods. The plural is used here on purpose to signify that within communities there are sub-populations of children, who may experience different childhoods, rather than the idea of one 'naturally' occurring process of childhood.

'The socially constructed child'. Writers such as Aries (1960) have argued that childhood as a distinct period in the life span is a relatively modern invention and that in other periods of history children were more integrated into adult societies. Thus childhood and children are constructed by societies. In *Teenage*, Jon Savage (2008) traces the modern development of the concept of youth and reveals the economic and social factors dating back to the early 20th century, which make fashion, music and film so important to young people. Sue Palmer (2006) in her book on *Toxic Childhood* puts forward a very different view of children's experiences growing up in the early 21st century. What this shows is that we as members of communities form a view of children and their childhoods, which informs our actions as children's nurses delivering care to our communities (see Chapter 2).

'The tribal child'. Some sociologists have attempted to highlight how children can be seen as a separate group in societies. They are often underrepresented and whose rights are vulnerable to being ignored (Kelly et al., 2012). They suggest children are a separate 'tribe', or are a minority group in need of adult protection and advocacy. This view leads to initiatives to empower children such as enlisting young people as researchers, or as public patient ambassadors (Coyne, 2008; Coad and Evans, 2008). The work of William Corsaro (2012) is helpful in understanding the limitations of such an approach. Corsaro's work with children in schools in Italy shows how children's peer cultures is a production and reproduction of cultures. The children produce their own cultures, for example, a playground game involving a forbidden crate. They also reproduce elements of adult society, the forbidden crate is turned into a bank and carried around, money is dispensed. The children are producing and reproducing culture they see around them. The extent to which we can say children are a separate tribe or minority group is then perhaps limited as they are clearly interacting and reacting to the cultures in which they live.

'The social structural child'. In Berry Mayall's work (2002, 2008), she describes a view of children in which children are seen as social agents, active in their communities and involved in the formation that society has of children. This is a development of the socially constructed child view where societies (we presume adults in these societies) determine how children are viewed. What Mayall and others argue (James et al., 1998) is that children, as well as adults in a society, determine the construction of childhoods. Rather than passive recipients of a social view of what it is to be a child, children also form and influence the view taken of them and their childhoods. Recent work in children's nursing has adopted Mayall's approach to argue children are active partners in their care, with useful contributions to be made to designing, monitoring and evaluating care (Moules, 2009; Carter et al., 2014; Randall, 2016). Further, Mayall sets out childhoods as relational, temporal and generational. How children experience childhoods is dependent on their relationships (in the main with one main adult carer), that childhoods are bound by time, they are temporal, they start at a point in time and finish around 18–19 years, perhaps 24 (The World Health Organization [WHO], 2014), but also that childhoods change over time. So children's nurses qualifying today will have experienced different childhoods to those of the parents they may encounter and to

the children in their care. This also implies that as we go forward in our careers as children's nurses we will have to keep up to date with how childhoods continue to change. Lastly, that childhood is experienced as a generation and in relation to other generations. That is to say children move through a childhood with their peers, but also compete with and are influenced by other generations for resources, influence and (re)producing cultures.

 ACTIVITY

Find a local children and young people participation group for a children's service in your area. These might be through the hospital Patient Advocacy and Liaison groups (PALs) or an advisory group to a children's hospice or CAMHS service.

If unable to find a local service perhaps look at the Royal College of Paediatric and Child Health participation programme (see https://www.rcpch.ac.uk/work-we-do/rcpch-us-children-young-people-families).

Review the material and projects undertaken with children and young people.

What view of children and childhoods emerges from this participation work?

PSYCHOLOGICAL THEORIES OF CHILDHOOD

Our understanding about children and childhood is developing. However, as discussed above an awareness of various understandings that people hold about children is useful in children's nursing. While some elements of child psychology continue to be contested, it remains a major influence on how children are assessed and treated for developmental and psychological problems. As a field of study, it is also highly influential in informing service design and nurses' interactions with children. The debates and discussion detailed below are not definitive nor do we suggest that they are uncontested or without controversy. Simply that as children's nurses attempting to understand contemporary childhoods you need to understand these approaches, including Freud; colleagues in nursing and from other disciplines will refer to them, use them as justification and may seek to impose these views as 'correct' or definitive. Understanding the debates helps nurses to engage in the conversation and advocate for children and young people.

The Nature–Nurture Debate

For any student considering developmental psychology, the nature–nurture debate is a key concept that underpins the work of almost all the major contributors. Thus an understanding of the nature–nurture concept is a useful starting point. Boyd and Bee (2012) describe this debate as about the relative contributions of biological and experiential developmental factors. Therefore, the nature perspective would argue that a personality characteristic, for example, moral behaviour, will develop naturally over time irrespective of external influences. By contrast, the nurture perspective would take the position that morality is a phenomenon that is learned. In reality, of course, there are few who would argue that any aspect of child psychological development is

entirely attributable to one or the other perspective, and it is increasingly acknowledged that the acquisition of any human characteristic is inevitably a synthesis of both inherited and environmental influences.

Cognitive Development

Although developmental psychology considers a variety of important domains, there is little doubt that the topic with the greatest influence for the child health care practitioner is that of cognitive development. From the outset it is important to acknowledge the perceived dominance within this field of Jean Piaget (1896–1980). However, although Piaget's invaluable contribution to developmental psychology is both acknowledged and valued, it is important to question the appropriateness of the domination of some of his assertions within the theory and practice of children's nursing.

Piagetian Perspectives

Piaget was a prolific author, whose worked spanned most of his very long and active life as a psychological theorist. Most students with some insight into Piaget's work will be familiar with his four stages of cognitive development, a summary of which is offered below (Figure 4.1, derived from Boyd and Bee, 2012; Daly et al., 2006; Meadows, 2006; Piaget, 1929, 1930; Piaget and Inhelder, 1969). Underpinning these four stages are concepts central to Piaget's view. Firstly that children think differently to adults, secondly that the maturation process advances at its own pace and cannot be altered. Piaget's view is dependent on the child developing schema, conceptual cognitive structures in which the child organises their understanding of the world. These schemas can be altered by assimilation, where new information is incorporated into an existing schema or by accommodation, where new information forces a change, revision or complete (re)creation of the schema.

Sensory Motor Stage: From Birth to Around 2 Years

Piaget identifies this first stage as characterised by the links formed between the infant and the environment as the infant comes to understand the relationship between actions, sensation and movement. Piaget divided the stage into six subsections (for more detail see Piaget and Inhelder, 1969, pp 4–12). These stages characterise the infant's development from being primarily reflexive/reactive (stage 1), through processes of trial and error, experiment and reinforcement (stages 2–5), to finally being able to actively understand and manipulate aspects of his or her world (stage 6). In other words, the infant has a gradually increasing awareness of the relationship between action and effect.

 WWW

• https://www.youtube.com/watch?v=ue8y-JVhjS0

Piaget saw a key concept within this stage as something he called 'object permanence'. This means that for the younger infant 'out of sight' is also 'out of mind'. In contrast, older infants (Piaget argued from around 8 months) realise that an object exists even when it cannot be seen. Also, throughout this first stage the child is described as egocentric, that is 'the child's initial universe is entirely centred on his [sic] own body' (Piaget and Inhelder, 1969, p 13).

Preoperational Stage: From Around 2 Years to Around 7 Years

Piaget viewed the next two stages as a vital period of transition. At the beginning of this second stage, Piaget argued that the child's behaviour is characterised by actions; by its end the child will have internalised these actions to allow the child to do mentally what was previously done physically. Piaget regarded achieving this as of pivotal importance and saw the preoperational period as dominated by organisation and preparation towards becoming 'operational' (Piaget and Inhelder, 1969, p 96). Consequently, the stage tends to be characterised negatively, by what children are not yet able to do, rather than what they can do now. Examples include their perceived inability to classify objects into groups, to think logically and to engage in moral reasoning. A key skill not yet achieved is that of conservation, that is the ability to realise that something might 'stay the same' despite a change in appearance. For example, a preoperational child would think the amount of juice in a short, fat glass becomes 'more' when poured into a tall, thin glass (Santrock, 2009).

⊕ WWW

- https://www.youtube.com/watch?v=gnArvcWaH6I

Also within this stage is a continued focus on the child's egocentricity, characterised particularly by the inability to be able to see the world from another's point of view or to distinguish another's point of view from their own (both visually and intellectually). Closely linked to this is Piaget's belief that these children could not conceptualise a world beyond their direct experience, that is what they had actually seen or experienced. Practically applied, it can be seen how such beliefs may limit perceptions of the preoperational child's abilities in a whole variety of conceptual domains. Piaget also noted that these children display animism, the attribution of 'life' to non-live objects.

Concrete Operational Stage: From Around 7 Years to Around 11 Years

Piaget saw this stage as characterised by children becoming 'operational', and thus being able to do many of the activities that they were working towards in the preoperational stage. He argued that operational children are capable of logical, systematic thought, and able to 'conserve' concepts such as number, mass, length, weight and volume. They are also able to classify and serialise objects/items, and to understand logical relationships between them. However, Piaget felt at this 'concrete' stage that children could only understand problems related to direct experience; they are not seen as capable of abstract or hypothetical thought, or the manipulation of variables.

Formal Operational Stage: From Around 12 Years Onwards

Piaget used the term 'propositional operations' to describe this final stage. He regarded these skills as congruent with preparation for adolescence, with the child able to think in abstract terms and capable of 'the handling of hypotheses and reasoning with regard to propositions removed from concrete and present operation' (Piaget and Inhelder, 1969, p 131). Thus young people are able systematically to explore the solutions to an abstract or hypothetical problem, including everything from algebra to decisions concerning their future'. An important extension of this is described as 'reflective abstraction' – self-awareness in relation to one's own strategies and thoughts.

👤 ACTIVITY

Before reading further, think about the following situation. Suppose you are admitting Jack, a 5-year-old child, to hospital for a course of intravenous antibiotics due to pneumonia:

- Consider Piaget's views on cognitive development. In what ways might your care of Jack be influenced if you assumed all of Piaget's assertions to be true?
- Think particularly about what explanations you might give to Jack regarding the treatment and care he will receive.
- Do you feel entirely comfortable with the approach you would take, or is there some conflict with your current experience and understanding of hospitalised children?

Critiquing Piaget

The 1970s and 1980s were characterised by a series of challenges to Piaget's perspective on child development, with a whole range of authors suggesting that Piagetian theory unreasonably limited our beliefs in children's abilities and that in reality, children were capable of far more than Piaget gave them credit for.

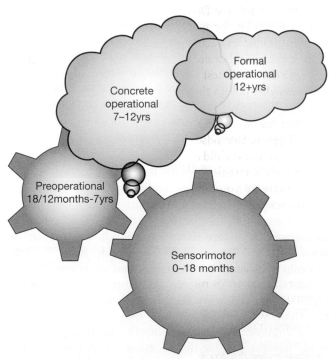

Fig. 4.1 Piaget stages of development. (adapted from Piaget and Inhelder 1969)

In respect of the preoperational child, various studies have demonstrated the ability of young infants to visually recognise their parents and distinguish them from strangers (see Taylor et al., 1999, pp 25–26). Boyd and Bee (2012) point out that with increasing sophisticated computer technologies, researchers can track the eye movements of infants; these 'looking' studies suggest very young infants can demonstrate object permanence. Studies particularly of imitation of tongue protrusion (sticking your tongue out) have demonstrated an infant's ability to recognise and imitate behaviour over time, with 6 week babies imitating the movement a few minutes later and 9 month olds delaying their imitation for up to 24 hours (see Boyd and Bee, 2012, p 112).

Similar critiques of Piagetian theory are found in respect of the preoperational child. For example, in his study of egocentricity, Piaget devised a test known as the 'three mountains experiment' (Piaget and Inhelder, 1956). The child was shown a three-dimensional model of three differently coloured mountains, positioned so that clearly different views of the mountains were visible from each of the four sides of the model (see Piaget and Inhelder, 1969 or https://www.youtube.com/watch?v=OinqFgsIbh0 for more detail). The child was given a series of four two-dimensional drawings representing the view from each side of the model, and asked to 'work out' which drawing represented the view of a doll positioned on the opposite side of the model to the child. The fact that most children aged under 7 years were unable to do this was central to Piaget's persistent belief in their egocentricity; their inability to see the world from another's point of view.

Yet in contrast, Donaldson (1978), one of Piaget's foremost critics, constructed another experiment where children were far more successful, using an intersection of two walls in a 'cross shape' (see Donaldson, 1978, pp 21–22 or Taylor et al., 1999, p 58, for more detail). Two policeman models were positioned in such a way that they could see behind most of the walls, but not all. In this study, children who got the three-mountain test wrong were frequently able to position a naughty doll so that the policemen were unable to see her; clearly they had to understand what the world looked like from the policemen's perspective to do this. Perhaps the key difference, Donaldson suggests, is that this experiment 'made sense' to the child and so was more readily understood. Clearly if children below 7 years are able to see another's point of view there are major implications for beliefs regarding their egocentricity.

👤 ACTIVITY

Gaining evidence of children's ability to see the world from another's perspective may be simpler even than Donaldson suggests:

- Take a favourite toy belonging to a child as young as 3 and position it facing the wall. Ask the child what the toy can see?
- Now move the toy to face in different directions in the room, and ask the same question.

Many 3- and 4-year-old children will happily tell you what the toy can or can't see. Yet these children are up to 4 years younger than those Piaget claimed were still egocentric.

In another of her critiques of Piaget's work, Donaldson also challenged some of his conservation experiments. For example, Piaget had conducted a study where children are asked to view two identical rows of sweets and say whether the rows are the same. The experimenter then repositions the sweets in one row so they are further apart, but leaves the same number. When re-questioned in Piaget's study, many children under 7 years insisted the row where the sweets have been moved now contained 'more'. Yet when Donaldson (1978) replicated the study using a 'naughty teddy' to move the sweets, significantly fewer children got the answer wrong than in a control group where, like in Piaget's original study, the researcher moved the sweets. Donaldson argued this was because the answer 'still being the same' now 'made sense', unlike the Piagetian version in which many children assumed the answer must now be different. Indeed, central to Donaldson's (1978) theories about Piaget was a recurrent theme that his experiments were designed in such a way that the children were often set up to fail, and that as a consequence children's abilities at a given age/stage were at significant risk of being underestimated.

For the concrete operational child numerous studies challenge Piaget's perspectives. One particular study with clear health care implications is by Alderson (1993). She interviewed 120 children, many of whom fell into Piaget's concrete operational age group, and demonstrated the ability of several of these children to make carefully considered and informed choices about non-essential surgery.

Arguably these critiques of Piaget's work cast sufficient doubt on his theories to make us question the use of these theories to influence and direct children's nursing. However, this can be challenging as Piaget's views continue to be influential in nursing and in other disciplines, and a coherent and comprehensive alternative view has yet to gain widespread interdisciplinary acceptance.

Carey: 'Novice to Expert Shift' Theory

One of the key theorists who offers a very different view to that of Piaget is Carey (1985). In her 'novice to expert shift' theory, Carey – writing from an empirical perspective – argued that there is nothing fundamentally different about the way in which children and adults think and come to an understanding of the world. She argued that it is knowledge, not maturation, that is the key. Where only a little knowledge of a topic exists, thinking is 'novice', and thus it is likely that a concept will be misinterpreted or only partially understood. In contrast, the expert thinker has a great deal of knowledge of a topic, and thus sophisticated understanding exists. Crucially though, Carey argued that both children and adults are capable of 'novice' and 'expert' levels of understanding simultaneously, depending on how much they know about a particular topic.

For example, Carey cites 3-year-old dinosaur 'experts' who can tell you not only the names of all the dinosaurs but their eating habits, habitat, chronology and relative size.

She similarly recognises young computer experts and chess players. Equally possible is novice thinking by adults when learning about a new topic for the first time, as evidenced, for example, by game-show contestants attempting to draw their internal anatomy. Thus, Carey argues that while children are far more likely to be 'novice' thinkers on a range of topics because their overall knowledge level is inevitably less, there is nothing about childhood thinking per se that limits children's understanding. Consequently, a child as young as 3 years may well be able to develop a sophisticated understanding of a topic provided the knowledge is imparted at an accessible level and pace.

What emerges when comparing Piaget's nativist perspective and Carey's empirical perspective is a polarity between their two views, which regard either maturation or learning as very much the dominant forces in child development. It is the interactionist perspective, however, that offers the possibility of bridging this nature–nurture gap. Thus the theories of Lev Vygotsky (1896–1934) perhaps offer the most useful tool for health care practitioners in seeking developmental theory to underpin their practice (Daly et al., 2006; Rushforth, 1999; Shayer, 2003).

Vygotsky and the 'Zone of Proximal Development'

Vygotsky (1978) was working in Russia at a similar time to Piaget, but his early death (aged just 38) and delayed translation of his work hindered his wider recognition for many years. Importantly, unlike Carey, his views were not in opposition to those of Piaget, and more recent authors have argued that there are rather more similarities than differences in their work (Shayer, 2003). Like Piaget, Vygotsky believed in the importance of maturation and biological processes, but he saw the interplay between these processes and the child's social world as being of prime importance. He saw thought processes as uniquely human and derived from children's early exposure to language, and from social and cultural influences conveyed to the child by both family and teachers. Indeed, the nature of the role of 'the teacher' is perhaps one of the key differences between Piagetian and Vygotskian perspectives.

Central to Vygotsky's work was his notion of the 'zone of proximal development', which he defined as:

> *The distance between the actual developmental level as determined by independent problem solving and the level of potential development as determined through problem solving under adult guidance or in collaboration with more capable peers.*

> *Vygotsky (1978, p 86)*

In other words, he saw the actual developmental level as the point of maturation that the child has already reached, but also recognised that at any given point in time the child had the potential for additional knowledge and understanding to be gained in that particular area of development. Thus the zone of proximal development looks at development 'prospectively', taking what the child knows as a starting point and using this to discern what the child is capable of achieving

in the immediate future. Vygotsky argued that you cannot determine any child's cognitive level without observing both what they already know and how they respond to instruction, hence the role of the nurses as teacher being so crucial (for more detail see Rushforth, 1999; Shayer, 2003; Taylor and Woods, 2005; Daly, 2006; Santrock, 2009).

If a Vygotskian perspective rather than a Piagetian perspective influences children's nursing, the key difference is that a child's developmental potential is not persistently viewed in negative terms but rather in positive ones. Piagetian 'tools to guide practice' are framed in terms of what children are unable to understand (e.g. Taylor et al., 1999, p 64). By contrast, a Vygotskian perspective encourages the nurse to find out what the child already knows and then to use this as a basis for working with the child and family to help the child to reach an enhanced level of understanding (Gaffney, 2000; Rushforth, 1999).

Vygotsky's work was further developed by Bruner (1972), who used the analogous term 'scaffolding' to describe the role of teachers (both professionals and parents) within the 'zone of proximal development'. Bruner saw this human scaffolding as a 'supportive mechanism', which was gradually withdrawn as the child strengthens in his or her own knowledge and understanding. Bruner believed that any topic could be meaningfully conveyed at some level to any child, provided it was appropriately individualised and congruent with what the child already knew and understood.

 ACTIVITY

Consider again Jack, the 5-year-old child admitted to hospital described earlier. Now reconsider his care from a Vygotskian perspective:
- What differences emerge when compared with the earlier Piagetian perspective?
- Which approach to Jack's care are you more comfortable with and why?

LANGUAGE DEVELOPMENT

It is difficult, if not impossible, to imagine education and learning, central to Vygotsky's proximal development, without language. Understanding then how children acquire the understanding of language and the skills to express themselves through language is key to developmental assessment and children's nursing practice. It is important then to understand the psychological processes underpinning language development, and the extent to which these can be influenced by a period of illness or hospitalisation.

The Empiricist Perspective

Skinner (1957) took a view of language development that is congruent with the empiricist perspective. He believed that children's earliest language development was shaped from their meaningless infant 'babbling', through a process of reinforcement. This involves parents praising, reiterating and thereby reinforcing sounds that most closely approximate to actual words (e.g. 'ma ma ma', 'da da da'). This is seen alongside the process of 'imitation', suggesting that children's verbatim copying of words, phrases and sentences uttered by adults enables them to construct sentences themselves.

This view of language development, sometimes referred to as the behaviourist perspective, sees children very much as a 'blank slate', on whom language is imposed. However, as Berk (2008) points out, the 3- or 4-year-old child typically has a vocabulary of around 14,000 words, which they can use correctly to construct sophisticated and grammatically correct, or near correct, sentences. If the behaviourist perspective alone was responsible for language development, it would rely on parents and others engaging in the equivalent of extremely intensive language tuition processes. Many contemporary psychologists agree that the empiricist perspective alone is insufficient to explain young children's sophisticated language development.

The Nativist Perspective

Interestingly, published in the same year as Skinner's work, was another seminal text. Chomsky (1957) proposed an opposing view of language development. Chomsky viewed children as far more active participants in the process of language acquisition. Although exposure to adult language was clearly important, he argued that they were effectively 'pre-programmed' to learn language via what he referred to as the language acquisition device (LAD). He saw this as a mental 'apparatus', which innately enables children to actively construct their vocabulary into grammatically sound sentence constructions (see also Daly et al., 2006).

Chomsky drew on the evidence of when children get things wrong to support his theory. For example, children who say they 'ridded' their bike, 'didded up' their shoes or 'maked a picture for Mummy' are using words they are unlikely to have been taught or even heard in that context. Rather, it appears that children have actively constructed the words by mistakenly interpreting or overgeneralising their grammatical understanding. For Chomsky, this was supportive of his view that a maturational process was primarily responsible for what he viewed as the unique human ability to construct language.

Perhaps one of the most persuasive arguments in support of Chomsky's perspective is the ease with which younger children can assimilate a new language or learn two languages simultaneously. However, critics of Chomsky's perspective have questioned whether it is realistic to suggest that children have an innate grammatical structure (Berk, 2008), and argue that it would be unsafe to underplay the role of both parents and teachers in the development of meaningful language and purposeful communication.

The Interactionist Perspective

These views have led to a third, interactionist perspective on language development. This viewpoint recognises both the inherent linguistic abilities of young children and the importance of education and social experience in informing and shaping these inherent processes. The perspective is supported by the work of Bruner (1983), who believes that a rich social environment is central to language acquisition, while at the same time acknowledging the importance of innate determinants of both linguistic and social behaviour. As an extension of this perspective, Vygotsky (1962) also argued that play is intrinsically linked to the language development process.

Vygotsky also acknowledged the fundamentally important contribution of both innate and social processes to language development. He further believed language was central to development of children's thought processes, with social exposure and language learning being gradually internalised by the child to become the human thought processes central to cognitive development. Thus, for Vygotsky, the acceleration of language learning was linked implicitly to accelerating cognitive developmental processes and children's abilities in a whole variety of other domains (Holaday et al., 1994).

It is important that beliefs regarding links between linguistic and cognitive ability are not applied universally. There are significant numbers of children with little or no verbal language but highly sophisticated cognitive development (e.g. some children with cerebral palsy). This can be at least partly explained by the observation that children's development of language comprehension occurs more rapidly than their ability to produce language (Berk, 2008); the latter requiring additional cognitive and neuromuscular skills. However, there are also clear indications that children with delayed language development can struggle with a whole range of cognitive processes. For these children there appears to be a link between language and reasoning, and thus enhancing a child's language development through the provision of speech and language therapy can be the key that 'unlocks' other aspects of their cognitive development (Wood, 1988). Furthermore, acceleration of language development, both comprehension and articulation, can enable many children to 'keep up' with their peers in mainstream education, when they would otherwise have lagged impossibly far behind.

Practical Applications

In considering these perspectives on language development, a number of important considerations emerge for practitioners caring for younger children, particularly in hospital settings. These include the following two key perspectives:

- The importance of providing a *stimulating environment*, which maintains the child's exposure to social language.
- The importance of knowing *normal developmental milestones* well enough to recognise a child whose language development may require additional support and intervention. More detail on this can be found in a range of texts on physical development and/or child assessment (e.g. Barnes, 2003).

👤 ACTIVITY

Sian, aged 3 years and 6 months, is admitted to your ward for routine surgery. She is the youngest of four children. During the admission process you observe that Sian is speaking only in single words, and also that these words are quite difficult for you to understand. You explore this concern with Sian's mother during the admission process, but Sian's mother seeks to reassure you, saying:

'Oh, I'm not worried, I think it's just that her older brothers do all the talking and translating for her – she'll get there in the end.'

When you ask whether Sian's health visitor is concerned, her mother says:

'Oh, I haven't seen her since Sian was about 12 months. If I don't know what I'm doing after four of them, then I never will!'

- Based on your experience and on your knowledge of speech and language development, are the mother's assumptions about Sian's language development correct?
- What actions should you take to ensure that your concerns are followed up?

PERSONALITY DEVELOPMENT

As with other aspects of psychological development, the development of personality has been linked very strongly to the nature–nurture debate, focusing on the extent to which personality is innately inherited and predestined, and the extent to which it is shaped by society and environmental influences. Ultimately, here also one is left to conclude that both factors play a part. Innate determinants are clearly influential, as attested by studies of twins reared apart who display markedly similar personality traits (see Santrock, 2009, for examples). However, experience undoubtedly also shapes personality, and two important theorists have contributed to these dimensions of our understanding of personality development, Erikson (1902–1994) and Freud (1856–1939). Although in many ways

their work currently receives less recognition than that of the cognitive developmental theorists, they offer perspectives that greatly influence our understanding of many phenomena, such as infant attachment, child-rearing practices, moral development and sex role identification. There are consequently clear implications for child health care delivery.

Erik Erikson

Erikson, like Piaget, offered a stage theory of development (Erikson, 1950). Importantly, when compared with Piaget, Erikson's theories offer a far more holistic view of the individual. Furthermore, his stages were not restricted to childhood, but rather reflected ongoing development throughout the lifespan, a psychological perspective that particularly gained popularity throughout the 1990s and remains popular today (e.g. Boyd and Bee, 2012; Santrock, 2009). Such a perspective is very important for nurses who care for adults as well as children, and can help children's nurses understand carers of children such as parents and grandparents.

The core of Erikson's work is his 'eight stages of man' (Erikson, 1965) in which he sets out a series of conflicts through which the developing individual needs to pass (Table 4.1). At any point in the process, a developmental conflict can have a negative effect on personality and future development. Importantly though, Erikson's stages cannot be seen as sequential. Although the age groups indicated are likely to represent the earliest point at which that stage becomes significant, the importance of each of the earlier stages is maintained to some extent throughout the lifespan, and is thus vulnerable at any point to deviation into the alternative path.

Basic trust versus mistrust. Trust is seen as the essential norm of babies' early experience, in the presence of food, sleep and other essential bodily functions. The infant's first real act of trust is 'to let the mother out of sight without undue anxiety or rage' (Erikson, 1965, p 239), arguably based on a certainty that she will always be there to meet his or her needs. This may explain why the younger infant seems to derive positive comfort from parental presence, but not to protest strongly in its absence, in opposition to Piaget's notion of 'object permanence' – 'out of sight' and therefore

TABLE 4.1	Erikson's Stages of Development in Childhood (1965)					
Oral Sensory	Basic Trust vs. Mistrust					
Muscular–Anal		Autonomy vs. Shame/Doubt				
Locomotor – Genital			Initiative vs. Guilt			
Latency				Industry vs. Inferiority		
Puberty					Identity vs. Role Confusion	
Young Adulthood						Intimacy vs. Isolation

Adapted from Erikson (1965)

'out of mind'. Thus trust is seen to depend on the quality of the maternal relationship (later theorists would include the father and significant others). Although it is part of normal development to recognise the possibility that these support figures may not always be present (hence the protest on separation made by the older infant), prolonged parental separation can be seen to be intrinsically linked to development of 'mistrust', which Erikson would argue can even perpetuate into adulthood. It can thus be seen how closely Erikson's perspective links with Bowlby's (1969) notion of 'attachment' and the need for the infant to have a close and continuous relationship with a 'mother figure' and significant others. It also links with the extensive work surrounding the harmful effects of hospitalisation by Robertson (1952) and others (see Taylor et al., 1999, for a summary, also see https://www.youtube.com/watch?v=s14Q-_Bxc_U). The widespread belief in the importance of parental presence with children in hospital is testament to the value placed on these theories, and beliefs in the harmful effects of separation.

Autonomy versus shame and doubt. The development of control within aspects of the younger child's world is seen as central to the development of autonomy. 'Shame and doubt' are seen as negative outcomes of this process. To use Erikson's own words:

> *For if denied the gradual and well-guided experience of the autonomy of free choice (or if, indeed, weakened by an initial loss of trust) the child will turn against himself …*
>
> ***Erikson (1965, p 244)***

From a nursing perspective the negative consequences of lack of autonomy for the child will be inappropriate endeavours to gain control in any way possible. Examples could include such phenomena as inappropriate toileting behaviour (e.g. soiling or constipation), or in an older child, more proactive processes of rebellion and even self-harm. Appropriate levels of autonomy are therefore vital for a child's healthy development, and these principles should be readily reflected in the care of sick or hospitalised children. Although many processes are essential to the child's well-being, choices such as 'which arm is used for a blood test', 'which parent accompanies them for a procedure' or 'whether something happens before or after breakfast', can all help to restore a sense of control for the child in what is often a very threatening and 'controlling' environment. The potential value of such choices to the child's well-being cannot be overestimated.

🔒 ACTIVITY

Consider Sanjay, a 4-year-old boy admitted to hospital following a fractured femur. He must stay on bed rest, on traction, for 5 weeks:

- What are some of the threats to Sanjay's autonomy that exist as a result of this experience?
- What are the realistic choices Sanjay can be given within his treatment and care delivery that can help to minimise the threats to his autonomy?

Initiative versus guilt. 'Initiative' links in many ways to the notion of autonomy, and characterises development of understanding and the child's active construction of the world, concepts congruent with Vygotskian theory. Erikson sees initiative as fundamental to all learning processes. The child is seen as deriving pleasure from actively setting out to achieve certain goals, and indeed doing so. Here, important links with Freudian theory (which Erikson readily identified as influencing his work) can be seen; these will be discussed more fully in the next section.

'Guilt' is closely linked with initiative, in that the child will frequently overstep boundaries. He or she will encounter a range of negative emotions as a result of external, and increasingly internal, regulation of his or her inappropriate behaviour. This stage can thus also be very closely linked to the child's moral development (Santrock, 2009). Erikson (1965, p 248) sees the consequence of these processes as the child becoming 'divided in himself' with internalised 'infantile' and 'parental' sets of guidelines emerging in parallel and influencing future aspects of behaviour. In the most extreme cases, children who encounter problems at this stage can require support from experts in child mental health. In contrast, however, most children show a more balanced adherence to 'both selves', requiring regular guidance, but gradually achieving a sense of individual responsibility and 'self-regulation' as they progress through childhood.

Industry versus inferiority. This stage is seen as concurrent with the school age child and reflects a central focus on learning and social development. These theories also have implications within the health care arena.

For many children, educational processes are continued in hospital settings and individualised programmes of learning are essential to ensure a child's self-esteem is not harmed by this different educational encounter.

Identity versus role confusion. This fifth, and final childhood stage is characteristic of the adolescent and with the development of self-identity. Adolescence can represents a particularly turbulent time for a child. Although the reality is that most adolescents 'make it', the potential negative outcome is 'role confusion', which can arise from any number of factors, for example, uncertainty regarding sexual identity or orientation, uncertainty about future career paths, or coping with delayed physical development. In extreme cases such situations can have a profoundly negative effect on the individual's personality development. However, most adolescents normally experience some elements of 'role confusion', responding by what Erikson (1965, p 253) describes as 'overidentification, to the point of apparent complete loss of identity'. Such overidentification and associated peer pressure might be important influential factors in experimentation with drugs, smoking, alcohol and sexual activity. Thus the need for carefully targeted and insightful health promotion is paramount.

For adolescents who are sick, this can be a particularly difficult time to cope with illness. For many chronically ill children, social and physical development can lag behind that of their well peers, leading to teasing and feelings of alienation.

Altered body image (e.g. hair loss in cancer) can also be particularly difficult for this age group to cope with. Even a brief hospital stay can be extremely traumatic, threatening privacy and dignity, new-found autonomy and the fragile sense of self-identity. Adolescent units are widely regarded as the ideal environment for this age group.

ACTIVITY

Consider Ania, an adolescent girl aged 13, recently diagnosed with leukaemia. She will require repeated hospital admissions and an extensive programme of chemotherapy:
- What might be some of the psychological challenges and risks Ania faces during her period of illness?
- How can both hospital- and community-based practitioners help Ania to minimise these risks and to emerge from her illness experience with a sense of 'identity' as opposed to 'role confusion'?

Sigmund Freud's Theory of Personality Development

Freud (1856–1939) belonged to a school of thought that is often referred to as psychoanalytic, in that it sought to explain individual differences in personality. Erikson represented the same school and his theories are more usually reported in texts after the earlier theories of Freud. Furthermore, Erikson regularly referred to Freudian theory in support of his own hypotheses about human development. However, whereas Erikson's holistic perspective remains widely respected, Freudian theory has been substantially critiqued and for many discredited, primarily because of his work being based on a few highly selective cases. However, Freudian ideas are still used by some and continue to influence children's health care services. Freud proposed that a child's personality has three facets the id, the ego and the superego (Freud, 1938/1973, 1923/1974). The id is the inherited component, biologically influenced and desiring immediate gratification of need. The ego is an emergent component, influenced by the environment. It regulates the id's desire for immediate gratification into socially acceptable channels. The superego is the final component, governing 'conscience'. It is therefore potentially in conflict with the desires of the id. Parallels can thus already be seen with Erikson's notion of conflict within the different stages of development, which expand Freud's fundamental notions of the relationship between id, ego and superego in mediating individual desires.

Freudian Stages of Personality Development

Freud (1938/1973) further argued that there were five key stages of personality development (see also Berk, 2008; Erikson, 1965; Santrock, 2009; Taylor et al., 1999):

1. The oral stage (birth to 1 year)

This stage is dominated by the id, with the gratification of hunger being the primary drive that is satisfied by sucking to take in nutrition. For Freud, lack of gratification of oral urges led to nail biting and thumb-sucking, which he regarded as deviant behaviours. Lack of oral gratification has also been used to explain cigarette smoking and excessive eating by older children and adults.

However, 'non-nutritive sucking' of either a dummy/pacifier or fingers is seen as normal within infant development. Indeed, for an infant unable to feed orally, a pacifier is regarded as essential to maintain the sucking reflex. Furthermore, infants clearly derive a great comfort from sucking, which often extends well into childhood.

2. The anal stage (1–3 years)

In this stage Freud argued that pleasure was primarily gained from the processes of passing urine or having a bowel action. He argued that the role of the ego was to learn that the pleasure had to be appropriately channelled in time or place via the process of 'toilet training'. Thus for Freud a child 'potty trained' too soon may later develop obsession with order and cleanliness (hence the expression 'anally retentive'), whereas a child not properly trained at all is likely to demonstrate untidiness and an acceptance of mess and squalor.

Criticisms of Freudian theory include a rejection of his singular acceptance of the domination of anal pleasure at this point in life. Certainly, it would appear not only that oral pleasures continue, but also that many other factors influence the child's experience of pleasure and his or her future personality development. However, in terms of Erikson's notion of autonomy, it can be seen that bladder and bowel function offers children powerful modes of exerting control over their parents or carers. At a conscious or subconscious level constipation is seen as having significant psychological components for many children, and is frequently linked to other behavioural problems (Smith and Ward, 2003).

ACTIVITY

Imagine you are caring for Matthew, a 4-year-old child who has been admitted with a history of severe constipation and soiling, which requires intervention under anaesthesia, as well as laxative drug therapy. No physiological cause for the problem has been identified. His older brother, Jacob, has severe Down syndrome and his parents are currently considering separating:
- How might you consider Matthew's problems in Freudian and Eriksonian terms?
- What advice and support might his parents be given to help overcome the problem?

---

3. The phallic stage (3–6 years)

This stage is perhaps the one that caused the greatest controversy when Freud's theories were first published. He argued that pleasure is now derived from genitally focused desires. He suggested that boys feel sexual desire for their mother, but fear their father's disapproval. Consequently, they end up identifying with the father and adopting the father's personality characteristics, behaviours and beliefs. For girls the reverse situation exists, that is paternal desire and maternal identification. Freud refers to these phases respectively as the oedipal phase and the Electra complex, and saw the resolution of this conflict as effectively the development of the superego and the individual's personality.

These theories have been widely and controversially used to describe a whole range of phenomena, including promiscuity, frigidity and deviant sexual behaviour. Evidence to support such beliefs remains minimal but many psychologists nevertheless retain some respect for aspects of Freudian theory. Links can be seen between the Eriksonian notion of 'guilt' and Freudian beliefs that morality and the conscience were products of the child's resolution of his or her desires for the opposite sex parent.

4. The latency period (6 years to puberty)

For Freud, this stage was one in which sexual desire and instinct were repressed, hence the preference for friends of the same sex. Curiously, as the title 'latency' suggests, Freud believed little of importance would happen in the absence of sexual development. For Erikson, by contrast, this latency was put to good use in the notion of 'industry' as the child focuses on the processes of academic learning and ongoing social development.

5. The genital stage (puberty onwards)

This stage is characterised by the emergence of adult sexual desire, and all the repressed sexual desires of childhood can now be appropriately channelled into sexual relationships with partners. This forms an important part of Erikson's views of the adolescent's search for identity, although for Erikson it was balanced by recognition of other important factors in adolescent development. Nevertheless, sexual identity is recognised as a vital part of adolescent development and the perceived appropriateness or inappropriateness of various sexual activities would appear to be an ongoing and cyclic process within different cultures and generations (Wilton, 2000).

MORAL DEVELOPMENT

In common with other models of development Kolberg (1969) developed a staged model of development with regard to children's moral understanding. Kolberg posed a moral dilemma to children in which Heinz's wife is dying. There is a drug which can help her, but Heinz can't afford the drug, so he decides to steal it.

Kolberg asked children if Heinz should do this; if not, why not? The resultant staged approach is outlined in Table 4.2. It is generally accepted that very few individuals reach stage 6. However, it is useful to bear in mind that as children move through their childhood they acquire more understanding and social skills that allow them to perhaps move through these stages so that older children may achieve levels 4 and 5. Understanding the moral development that children may have acquired can be helpful in motivating them to adhere to treatment regimens and adopt healthy lifestyles when coping with illness.

CHILDREN'S CONCEPTUALISATION OF HEALTH, ILLNESS AND THEIR INTERNAL BODIES

One example of applying cognitive developmental theory to practice is consideration of the ways in which children conceptualise health and illness concepts. Since the middle part of the 20th century, numerous authors have researched children's ability to understand the concepts of health and illness. The seminal work within the field was arguably that of Bibace and Walsh (1980, 1981), who offered a stage theory of children's conceptualisation of illness that was very closely aligned to Piaget's earlier described stage theory of cognitive development. Thus preoperational children (aged 2–7 years) were seen as having an illogical or magical understanding of illness, and concrete operational children (aged 7–11 years) were seen as having a limited and largely external understanding with little awareness of internal biological processes. It was only the formal operational child (aged 11+ years), who was viewed as likely to have any detailed understanding of illness physiology (see Vacik et al., 2001 for a fuller summary).

However, it is now recognised that such studies, although offering useful tools in terms of understanding the way in which children conceptualise health and illness, were also misrepresenting younger children's potential to gain enhanced understanding of these health and illness concepts. Kister and Patterson (1980) noticed that children who better understood 'contagion' were less likely to display 'imminent justice explanations' (the belief that illness was a punishment). This and more recent studies questioned

TABLE 4.2 **Kolberg's Stages of Moral Development (1969)**		
Stages	**Description**	**Example Behaviour**
Pre-conventional Morality		
1	Punishment orientation	Obeys rules to avoid punishment
2	Reward orientation	Conforms to social norms to receive rewards/praise
Conventional Morality		
3	Good child orientation	Conforms to social norms to avoid disapproval
4	Authority orientation	Upholds social norms from sense of duty and to avoid censure
Post-conventional Morality		
5	Social contract	Uphold socially agreed principles sense of public 'good'
6	Ethical principle orientation	Self-determined ethical principles upheld irrespective of social norms

Adapted from Kolberg (1969)

the Piaget approach of maturation in which children were seen as not cognitively able to understand some of the complex ideas involved in health and illness. More recent research recognises children's potential to understand far more than earlier researchers gave them credit for. There are now a range of papers, which offer insights with useful application to child health nursing practice on a variety of subjects, including McDonald and Rushforth (2006), Myant and Williams (2005, 2008), Piko and Bak (2006), Fox et al. (2008), and Franck et al. (2008).

Yet various studies (e.g. Burbach and Peterson, 1986; Crisp et al., 1996; Veldtman et al., 2000) have repeatedly failed to demonstrate a clear link between illness experience and understanding of health and illness concepts. The potential for misunderstanding and misconception remains clear, leading Ireland (1997) to advocate the 'gather, give, gather' model of explanation giving, drawing on Vygotsky's (1962) proximal development ideas. In other words, find out what the child already knows, give the explanation and then (because we know how readily misunderstandings can occur despite good explanation) recheck the child's understanding to ensure that the explanation has been safely received. It has been suggested that health care practitioners often have an inadequate understanding of how children conceptualise health and illness (Rushforth, 1996; Vacik et al., 2001). Thus developing the understanding and skills to tailor health information to individual children's conceptions of health and illness should be a part of all children's nurses learning.

👤 ACTIVITY

Suppose Chloe, a 4-year-old girl, tells you after her appendectomy that the reason her tummy hurts is 'because I have been naughty':

- What might be the reasons for her beliefs?
- How can you help her to realise this is not the case, and understand the real reasons for what has happened and why?
- What theories are influencing giving your explanation?

SUMMARY

Advances in the fields of sociology, childhood studies and psychology have led to a deepening of our understanding of the progression of children through their childhoods and to what might be termed maturity. The work of child psychology theorists of the early-to-mid 20th century continue to influence children's nursing. People nurses work with in multi-disciplinary teams may well also be heavily influenced by such theories. This is despite wide-ranging and significant concerns about the veracity of such theories in application to the social/cultural and political worlds of children.

As we point out above childhoods are temporal and will continue to change with the cultures of societies over time. This ever-changing landscape of childhood demands of children's nurses that they continually scan the horizon as new understanding emerges. In particular, new ideas about growing up and the development of the structures of children's bodies may emerge from the increased understanding and focus on the interaction of genetics, epigenetics and proteomics, and the sociology of childhood, with the political focus on childhoods and the implications for populations and economies.

Arguably we should be mindful that despite the importance of childhood as a period of the lifespan there has been a woeful lack of attention to the scientific study of how children's bodies, minds and social worlds develop, whereas the beginnings of life (embryology) and the transitions into adulthood, have received some more attention. The processes and underpinning mechanisms of how children develop their thinking in their communities remains poorly understood. This means that children's nurses have to amass evidence to support their practices as best they can from a number of disparate fields (child psychology, education, social care, developmental anatomy and physiology).

It is clear however, that attempting to understand the process of child development over the period of childhood remains a central underpinning aspect of children's nursing. We may only have bits of the whole puzzle, but we still have to relate these developmental and social changes to the nursing care of children.

ACKNOWLEDGEMENT

This chapter was prepared using material written by Helen E. Rushforth from 'The dynamic child: children's psychological development and its application to the delivery of care', Chapter 11 in Glasper and Richardson (eds.), 2010. We are very grateful to Helen for allowing us to use this material.

REFERENCES

Alderson, P., 1993. Children's Consent to Surgery. Open University Press, Buckingham.

Aries, P., 1960. Centuries of Childhood translation of Enfant Et La Vie Familiale Sous L'ancien Régime (1973). Penguin, Harmonsworth.

Azar, S.T., Okado, Y., Stevenson, M.T., Robinson, L.R., 2013. A preliminary test of a social information processing model of parenting risk in adolescent males at risk for later physical child abuse in adulthood. Child Abuse Rev. 22, 268–286.

Azar, S.T., Reitz, E.B., Goslin, M.C., 2008. Mothering: thinking is part of the job description: application of cognitive views to understanding maladaptive parenting and doing intervention and prevention work. J. Appl. Dev. Psychol. 29, 295–304.

Barnes, K., 2003. Paediatrics: A Clinical Guide for Nurse Practitioners. Butterworth-Heinemann, Edinburgh.

Boyd, D., Bee, H., 2012. Lifespan Development, sixth ed. Pearson Education, New Jersey.

Berk, L., 2008. Child Development, eighth ed. Pearson Education, New Jersey.

Bibace, R., Walsh, M., 1980. Development of children's concepts of illness. Pediatrics 66 (6), 912–917.

Bibace, R., Walsh, M., 1981. Children's Concepts of Health, Illness and Bodily Function. Jossey-Bass, San Franscisco.

Blackford, H., 2004. Playground panopticism; ring-around-the-children, a pocket full of women. Childhood 11 (2), 227–249.

Bowlby, J., 1969. Attachment and Loss, vol. 1. Hogarth Press, London.

Bruner, J.S., 1972. The Relevance of Education. Allen and Unwin, London.

Bruner, J.S., 1983. Child's Talk: Learning to Use Language. WW Norton, New York.

Burbach, D., Peterson, L., 1986. Children's concepts of physical illness: a review and critique of the cognitive developmental literature. Health Psychol. 5, 307–325.

Carey, S., 1985. Conceptual Change in Childhood. MIT Press, Cambridge, MA.

Carter, B., Bray, L., Dickinson, A., et al., 2014. Approaches to nursing children, young people and their families. In: Carter, B., Bray, L., Dickinson, A., Edwards, M., Ford, K. (Eds.), Child-centred Nursing: Promoting Critical Thinking. Sage, London.

Chomsky, N., 1957. Systematic Structures. Mouton, The Hague.

Coad, J., Evans, R., 2008. Reflections on practical approaches to involving children and young people in the data analysis process. Children and Society 22, 41–52.

Corsaro, W.A., 2012. The Sociology of Childhood, third ed. Pine Forge Press, Sage, Thousand Oaks, CA.

Coyne, I., 2008. Children's participation in consultations and decision making at health service level: a review of the literature. Int. J. Nurs. Stud. 45, 1682–1689.

Crisp, J., Ungerer, J., Goodnow, J., 1996. The impact of experience on children's understanding of illness. J. Pediatr. Psychol. 21 (1), 57–72.

Daly, M., Byers, E., Taylor, W., 2006. Understanding Early Year's Theory in Practice: An Accessible Overview of Early Year's Theory. Heinemann, Oxford.

Donaldson, M., 1978. Children's Minds. Fontana Press, Glasgow.

Erikson, E., 1950. Childhood and Society. WW Norton, New York.

Erikson, E., 1965. Childhood and Society, revised edn. Penguin, London.

Fox, C., Buchanan-Barrow, E., Barrett, M., 2008. Children's understanding of mental illness: an exploratory study. Child. Care Health Dev. 34 (1), 10–18.

Franck, L., Sheikh, A., Oulton, K., 2008. What helps when it hurts: children's views on pain relief. Child Care Health Dev. 34 (4), 430–438.

Freud, S., 1973. An Outline of Psychoanalysis (Original Work Published 1938). Hogarth Press, London.

Freud, S., 1974. The Ego and the Id (Original Work Published 1923). Hogarth Press, London.

Gaffney, A., 2000. Pain and Piaget: qualitative change with age in the content area about children's ideas of pain. Irish J. Psychol. 21 (3–4), 194–202.

Golding, W., 1962. Lord of the Flies. Faber and Faber, London.

Holaday, B., LaMontagne, L., Marciel, J., 1994. Vygotsky's zone of proximal development: implications for nurse assistance of children's learning. Issues Compr. Pediatr. Nurs. 17, 15–27.

Ireland, L.M., 1997. Children's perceptions of asthma: establishing normality. Br. J. Nurs. 6 (18), 1059–1064.

James, A., Jenk, C., Prout, A., 1998. Theorizing Childhood. Polity Press, Cambridge.

Kelly, M., Jones, S., Wilson, V., Lewis, P., 2012. How children's rights are constructed in family-centred care: a review of the literature. J. Child Health Care 16, 190–205.

Kister, M., Patterson, C., 1980. Children's conceptions of the causes of illness: understanding contagion and use of imminent justice. Child Dev. 51, 839–846.

Kolberg, L., 1969. Stage and sequence: the cognitive developmental approach to socialisation. In: Goslin, D.A. (Ed.), Handbook of Socialisation Theory and Research, ninth ed. Rand McNally, Chicago.

Locke, J., 1693. Some Thoughts Concerning Education. Bureau of Publications, Teachers College, Columbia University, New York. 1964.

Mayall, B., 2002. Towards a Sociology for Childhood: Thinking from Children's Lives. Open University Press, Birmingham.

Mayall, B., 2008. Conversations with children: working with generational issues. In: Christensen, P., James, A. (Eds.), Research with Children: Perspectives and Practices, second ed. Routledge, Abingdon, pp. 109–125.

McDonald, H., Rushforth, H., 2006. Children's views of nursing and medical roles: implications for advanced nursing practice. Paediatr. Nurs. 18 (5), 32–36.

Meadows, S., 2006. The Child as Thinker, second ed. Routledge, London.

Moules, T., 2009. 'They wouldn't know how it feels' – characteristics of quality care from young people's perspectives: a participatory research report. J. Child Health Care 13 (4), 322–333.

Myant, K., Williams, J., 2005. Children's concepts of health and illness: understanding of contagious illness, non-contagious illness and injuries. J. Health Psychol. 10 (6), 805–819.

Myant, K., Williams, J., 2008. What do children learn about biology from factual information? A comparison of interventions to improve understanding of contagious illnesses. Br. J. Educ. Psychol. 78 (2), 223–244.

Palmer, S., 2006. Toxic Childhood: How the Modern World Is Damaging Our Children and What We Can Do About It. Orion, London.

Piaget, J., 1929. The Child's Conception of the World. Routledge and Kegan Paul, London.

Piaget, J., 1930. The Child's Conception on Physical Causality. Kegan Paul, Trench, Trubner and Co, New York.

Piaget, J., Inhelder, B., 1956. The Child's Conception of Space. Routledge and Kegan Paul, London.

Piaget, J., Inhelder, B., 1969. The Psychology of the Child. Routledge and Kegan Paul, London.

Piko, B., Bak, J., 2006. Children's perceptions of health and illness: images and lay concepts in pre-adolescence. Health Educ. Res. 21 (5), 643–653.

Randall, D., 2016. Pragmatic Children's Nursing: A Theory for Children and Their Childhoods. Routledge, Abingdon.

Robertson, J., 1952. A two-year-old goes to hospital (film). In: Taylor, J., et al. (Eds.), (1999) Nursing Children: Psychology, Research and Practice, third ed. Stanley Thornes, Cheltenham.

Rousseau, J.J. 1762a. The Social Contract. Wordsworth edition (1998) introduction by Matravers D. Wordsworth Edition Limited, Herfordshire.

Rousseau, J.J., 1762b. Emile: or On Education, Introduction, Translation and Notes. Bloom, A. (1997) USA Basic books.

Rushforth, H., 1996. Nurses' knowledge of how children view health and illness. Paediatr. Nurs. 8 (9), 23–27.

Rushforth, H., 1999. Practitioner review: communicating with hospitalised children. JCPP (J. Child Psychol. Psychiatry) 40 (5), 683–691.

Santrock, J., 2009. Life-Span Development, twelfth ed. McGraw Hill College, Boston.

Savage, J., 2008. Teenage: The Creation of Youth 1875–1945. Pimlico, London.

Shayer, M., 2003. Not just Piaget, not just Vygotsky, and certainly not Vygotsky as an alternative to Piaget. Learn. InStruct. 13 (5), 465–485.

Skinner, B.F., 1957. Verbal Behaviour. Appleton Century Crofts, New York.

Smith, L., Ward, C., 2003. Childhood constipation and encopresis. In: Barnes, K. (Ed.), Paediatrics: A Clinical Guide for Nurse Practitioners. Butterworth-Heinemann, Edinburgh.

Taylor, J., Muller, D., Wattley, L., Harris, P., 1999. Nursing Children: Psychology, Research and Practice, third ed. Stanley Thornes, Cheltenham.

Taylor, J., Woods, M., 2005. Early Childhood Studies, second ed. Hodder Arnold, London.

Vacik, H.W., Nagy, C.M., Jessee, P.O., 2001. Children's understanding of illness: students' assessments. J. Pediatr. Nurs. 16 (6), 429–437.

Veldtman, G., Matley, S., Kendall, L., et al., 2000. Illness understanding in children and adolescents with heart disease. Heart 84 (4), 395–397.

Vygotsky, L.S., 1962. Thought and Language. MIT Press, Cambridge, MA.

Vygotsky, L.S., 1978. Mind in Society. Harvard University Press, Cambridge, MA.

Wilton, T., 2000. Sexualities in Health and Social Care: A Textbook. Open University Press, Buckingham.

World Health Organization, 2014. Heath for the World's Adolescents: A Second Chance in a Second Decade. Geneva World Health Organization. Available from http://apps.who.int/adolescent/second-decade/files/1612_MNCAH_HWA_Executive_Summary.pdf.

Wood, D., 1988. How Children Think and Learn. Blackwell, Oxford.

5

Physical Growth and Development in Children

Janet Kelsey

LEARNING OUTCOMES

- Define growth and development and understand how they can be assessed.
- Demonstrate an understanding of the anatomy and physiology of the newborn baby.

- Gain an overview of the development of the child from birth to adolescence.
- Be aware of the importance of assessing child development and the detection of deviations from normal.

INTRODUCTION

The physical development of the child is only one aspect of its whole development, which includes cognitive, social and emotional elements. Inherited attributes and environmental factors will affect physical development. These factors interact to cause effects on the child's development from conception to adulthood.

Babies and children vary considerably in exactly when and in what way they progress in all areas of development. It is not always appropriate to assign exact ages in months and years to stages of development, although an approximate age range is possible.

ACTIVITY

- Write down what you think is meant by the terms 'growth' and 'development'.
- Why might it be important to you as a nurse to have some understanding of the growth and development of children?

FACTORS AFFECTING GROWTH AND DEVELOPMENT

- Genetic/chromosomal factors: inherited rate of growth and individual differences
- Endocrine system
- Environmental factors
  - Illness: children grow more slowly during periods of illness, but there might be increased growth to catch up after recovery
  - Nutrition: poorly nourished children grow more slowly and do not reach their full potential size; malnutrition can have a permanent effect on some parts of the brain and nervous system

- Socioeconomic status
- Environment: exposure to environmental pollutants, the ability to practise skills, for example crawling, walking

Other factors also govern growth and physical changes. Hormones are the most important of these (Table 5.1).

PHYSICAL GROWTH AND DEVELOPMENT

The development of children is 'multidimensional and multidirectional' (Chamley, 2005). Physical growth and maturation are dynamic processes governed by complex interactions between genetics and environmental factors. Maturation, however, is sequential, appears in all children and describes those aspects of development genetically pre-determined.

Growth is defined as an increase in the size of and number of cells that results in an increase in size and weight of the whole, or any of its parts. In clinical practice, growth of the infant is generally measured by estimating the weight, length, head circumference, and in certain circumstances, skin-fold thickness.

Pattern of Growth

Growth begins prenatally with the release of the ovum and fertilisation resulting in the zygote, which implants into the uterine wall to develop as an embryo; from the 9th week of development the embryo is known as the fetus and continues to develop for 40 weeks until birth. Growth continues through childhood into adulthood and finally old age. As the child develops they get larger and more complex. Growth proceeds in a continuous pattern but is not smooth; the most rapid growth takes place in utero, the first 2 years of life and during adolescence. However, acceleration and deceleration occur in response to illness and changes in nutrition or environment.

TABLE 5.1	**The Hormones Involved in Growth and Physical Development**	
Gland	**Hormone**	**Aspects of Growth**
Thyroid	Thyroxine	Normal brain development and overall rate of growth
Adrenal	Adrenal androgen	Involved in some changes at puberty, particularly the development of secondary sex characteristics in girls
Testes	Testosterone	Formation of male genitals before birth. Also triggers the sequence of changes in primary and secondary sex characteristics at puberty in the male
Ovaries	Oestradiol	Development of the menstrual cycle and breasts in girls. Less important than testosterone for secondary sex characteristics in boys
Pituitary	Growth hormone activating hormone	Rate of physical maturation. Signals other glands to secrete hormones

Infants grow very quickly in the first year of life, adding 25–30 cm to their height and gain weight at an equally rapid rate, doubling birth weight by the age of 5–6 months and tripling it by the end of the first year. The birth size of a normal infant is determined by the mother. Inherited factors, however, are one of the greatest influences affecting the final stature of the child. Although children tend to attain a stature between those of their parents, some children take after one parent, a grandparent or even a more remote member of the family.

Measuring Growth
Length/Height

An infant's recumbent length is measured supine on a measuring board, placing the head firmly at the top of the board and the heels of the feet at the foot-board (Figs 5.1 and 5.2).

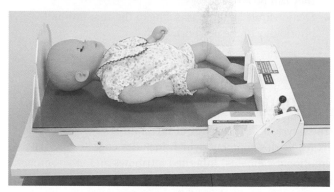

Fig. 5.1 Infant length.

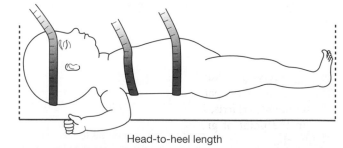

Head circumference   Chest circumference   Abdominal circumference

Head-to-heel length

Fig. 5.2 Measurement of the head, chest, abdominal circumference and the recumbent length.

CLASSIC CLUES: HEIGHT

The height of an infant increases by around 12 cm during the first 6 months of life at a rate of approximately 2.5 cm/month. By the age of 1 year, the height has increased by almost 50% and by the age of an infant at 2 years is about half as tall as he or she will be as an adult (Chamley, 2005). There is a rapid increase in size during the first 2 years, which then settles down to a slower and steadier rate: 5–7.5 cm in height per year and 3 kg in weight per year. Adolescence then brings a 'growth spurt', following which height and weight are slowly gained until adult size is achieved.

Height is the measurement taken when children are measured upright. Shoes should be removed and the child should stand as tall and straight as possible with the head in mid-line and the line of vision parallel to the floor. The most accurate measurement of height is gained by using a wall-mounted stadiometer (Fig. 5.3). It might be useful to remember that the height will be less when measured in the afternoon than in the morning. This effect can be reduced by applying modest upward pressure under the jaw or mastoid process.

CLASSIC CLUES: WEIGHT

Infants lose weight after birth typically 10% of their body weight in the first 3–4 days, which should be regained by the 10th postnatal day. On average, an infant gains 600–800 g in weight per month. An infant's weight at 6 months will therefore be almost double the birth weight. By the first year of life, weight has tripled and by the second year birthweight has quadrupled slowing to a gain of approximately 2.25–2.75 kg/year through to toddlerhood to 1.8–2.7 kg/year. Adolescence is a time of rapid change with increases in weight reflecting increases in lean body mass and fat.

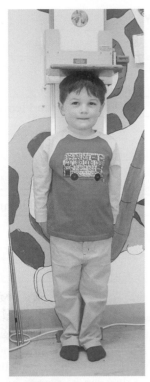

Fig. 5.3 Child height.

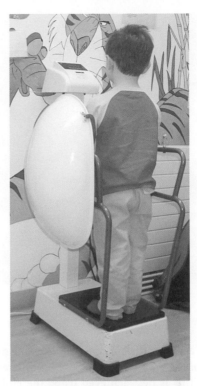

Fig. 5.4 Child weight.

Weight

Infants should be weighed naked and preferably at the same time of the day. Older children can be weighed in light clothing without their shoes (Fig. 5.4).

Head Circumference

This measurement is important because the size of the skull is closely related to the size of the brain. It is usually recorded in children who are under 3 years of age or in cases where the growth of the brain/skull is under observation. It is advisable to use a non-elastic, paper, disposable tape measure for this measurements (Harris, 2015). The head should be measured around the point of greatest circumference, this is usually slightly above the eyebrows and pinna of the ears and around the occipital prominence at the back of the skull. The Royal College of Paediatrics and Child Health provide growth charts based on the World Health Organization (WHO) Child Growth Standards, and describe the optimal growth for healthy, breastfed children.

 WWW

• https://www.rcpch.ac.uk/resources/growth-charts

CLASSIC CLUES: HEAD CIRCUMFERENCE

The head growth of an infant is rapid. In the first 6 months the circumference increases by between 8 and 9 cm. By the first year there is an increase of 33% in the overall size of the head.

Surface Area

The child's surface area can be calculated once the height and weight of the child is known using the body surface area nomogram. This measurement is important for the prescription of some drugs.

 ACTIVITY

Find a copy of the body surface area nomogram and calculate the body surface area for:
• A newborn weighing 3 kg and 50 cm in length
• A 6-year-old child weighing 20 kg and with a height of 115 cm

Skinfold Thickness

Skinfold thickness is a quick and easy method of measuring subcutaneous fat that allows for the estimation of an individual's body fat. The most common site for measuring skinfold thickness is the triceps; others include the subscapularis, suprailiac, abdomen and upper thigh. The measurement is made by pinching the skin between two fingers and measuring the skinfold thickness using specially designed callipers (Fig. 5.5).

ACTIVITY

Two groups of factors that strongly influence normal growth and development are heredity and environment. From your observations of children, give two examples from each group.
  Go to:
• https://www.rcpch.ac.uk/resources/growth-charts
  Look at the range of charts available for different children.

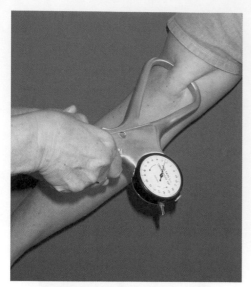

Fig. 5.5 Skinfold thickness.

Bone Age

Bone age is a method of measuring skeletal maturity; the appearance of the epiphyseal centres is compared with standard charts. This is best achieved using the child's left wrist and hand, where the 20 bones can be judged against that recognised as the normal pattern of development.

Assessment of Growth

Centile charts have been developed using statistics of children's growth patterns. They give estimations of expected height, weight and head circumference for boys and girls at different ages. An infant usually has a similar centile at birth for head circumference and weight. Children of large parents tend to be towards the 90th centile and those of small parents tend towards the 10th; most will remain on these centiles for the rest of their lives.

 ACTIVITY

Centile charts provide a useful measure of normal growth. Different charts are available for boys and girls, for different age groups and for different cultures. Children may need to be assessed if they are above the 97th or below the 3rd centile. Some show height and weight measurements only, whereas others also show head circumference. To ensure that you understand the format of a percentile chart, look at a chart in your practice area and answer the following questions:

- What sex, age and measurements does it cover?
- Which percentiles does it show?
- Where on the chart would you find a child of abnormal growth?
- If Helen is 3.5 years and 98 cm tall, which centile is she on?
- How many children fall below the 50th centile and how many above?
- John is on the 90th centile. Is he above or below the average for his age?

ACTIVITY

Plot the following weight, height/length and head circumferences on to growth charts from your practice area.

John (Male)			
Age	Weight (kg)	Head (cm)	Length (cm)
Birth (40 weeks)	3.5	34	51
6 weeks	5	38	56
20 weeks	7.25	42	66
36 weeks	9.75	46	72

Rebecca (Female)			
Age	Weight (kg)	Head (cm)	Length (cm)
Birth (37 weeks)	2.6	34	50
4 weeks	4	36	52
12 weeks	6.25	41	61
40 weeks	9.25	44.25	68

Some children resemble one parent more than the other in final size. If only their weights are recorded, they may appear to have faltering growth if father is small, or gaining weight excessively if father is tall. If weight is plotted against head circumference then they can be seen to be running in parallel, i.e. the whole of the child's size is approaching that of a particular parent.

Growth charts give an early warning of some problems, such as obesity, which will be indicated by the child's weight starting to deviate upwards even though the head circumference remains on the same centile.

Changes in Shape and Proportion

After 2 years, the rate of growth slows down and the child gains approximately 2.7 kg in weight each year until adolescence. Changes in proportion and shape take place at the same time. An adult's head is an eighth of his total height but in a 2-year-old the head is a quarter of the total body length. In addition to this, a 2-year-old has a large body and shorter legs in proportion to that of an adult (Bee, 2013).

If a child is growing and their shape is altering, then there must be changes occurring in the child's bones, muscles and fat. Bones increase in number, become longer and grow harder. Although bones are not all formed at birth, the newborn baby has virtually all the muscle fibres that will ever be needed. As a child grows, the muscle fibres get longer, thicker and less watery.

Development

Development refers to the changes that occur throughout the lifespan. The increasing complexity of the individual involves changes in structure and function and the emergence of an individual's capacities through learning, growth and maturation. Maturation can be defined as an increase in competence and adaptability, a change in the complexity of a structure that makes it possible for that structure to work. Many of the debates about child development have centred on the nature versus nurture controversy. The former believe that human behaviour is guided by inborn factors and argues that differences are a result of heredity. Those who err towards nurture stress the importance of acknowledging the influence of a child's physical and social environment. According to them, individual differences are a result of the child's life experiences. The reality is probably somewhere in between. What is certain is that development is a complex process in which many variables play a part.

Measuring Development

Development is measured using developmental scales. It is divided into four major areas:

1. Physical: growth, vision, hearing, locomotion, coordination.
2. Cognitive: language and understanding.
3. Psychosocial: adapting to the society and culture to which the child belongs.
4. Emotional: control of feelings and emotions.

The most widely used tool for screening development for a long time was the Denver Developmental Screening Test (Denver scale), which suggests milestones according to the age. Charts by Sheridan (1997) and Frankenburg and Dodds (1967) (the Denver Developmental Screening Test) were developed to show what can be expected at key stages of development. However, these are now dated and the practice of child health surveillance and screening has changed in the UK since the introduction of the Healthy Child Programme (HCP). The emphasis is on a review at 2.5 years with early detection and action as the basis. The programme encourages opportunistic questions by health care professionals with onward referral on basis of need.

⊕ WWW

- https://www.e-lfh.org.uk/programmes/healthy-child-pro-gramme/
  Enrol on the on the e-LfH Hub to deepen your knowledge.

Differences in Rate

There may be individual differences in the rate and timing of developmental progress, for example, three perfectly normal infants may sit unaided at 5, 6 or 9 months. However, the sequence of developmental progress is always the same. A child may be consistently early, average or slow in development, for example. a child whose bone development is slower probably walks later and eventually reaches puberty later.

The development of walking can be used to illustrate the factors that influence growth and development (Bee, 2013):

- Newborn infants held with the sole of the foot on a table move their legs in a reflex walking action.
- By 8 weeks: infants briefly hold their head up if held in a standing posture.
- At 36 weeks: infants pull themselves up and remain standing by grasping furniture.

- At 48 weeks: infants walk forwards if both hands are held, or sideways if holding furniture.
- By 52 weeks: infants walk forwards if held by one hand.
- At 13 months: infants walk without help.

Factors Required for the Development of Walking

A complex set of changes occurs in the muscles, bones, and nervous system:

- Nutrition: for growth
- Environment: in which to practise walking
- Genetics: were the parents early walkers?
  The child's ability to walk (or not) will also affect other areas of development such as social, emotional and intellectual.

👤 ACTIVITY

From your experience of your own childhood, can you think of areas where the rate and timing of the development for certain skills was different between yourself and others? Make some notes about your ideas.

Developmental Assessment

In the main, developmental assessments are performed by the child's health visitor and GP, although there might be occasions when a paediatrician will also perform them. However, all health care professionals should be competent to carry out an opportunistic developmental assessment. These assessments include the evaluation of:

- locomotion or gross motor development referring to large muscle skills
- fine motor or manipulation skills: referring to small muscle skills
- hearing and speech
- vision
- social development, for example feeding, dressing and social behaviour

To assess deviations from normal, it is first necessary to know about normal development. The development of a child between the ages of 0–18 months is very complex. These are the major milestones and their approximate age of appearance:

- smile: 1–2 months
- laugh: 6 months
- sits (with support): 6 months
- sits (without support): 8–9 months
- crawls: 8–9 months
- stands/walks: 12 months
- pincer grip: 12 months
- delicate pincer: 18 months
- walks backwards: 18 months

👤 ACTIVITY

Watch a video showing different aspects of child development; find one at your university library or your local health promotion centre.

TABLE 5.2   Interlinked Aspects of Development

Skill	Information	Activity	Next Stage
Drawing	Holding pencil	Drawing	Writing
Running	Spatial awareness	Running	Football, dancing

All aspects of development are interlinked. Skills are acquired sequentially; an example of this is the sequence of development of motor skills, which is often described as cephalocaudal, that is head (cephalo) to toe via the spine (caudal). So, initially, head control is developed before the baby is able to sit independently; this is followed by crawling and finally by control of the lower limbs for standing and walking. Each new skill usually appears at the most appropriate time to make use of information coming in to carry out activities to prepare for the next stage (Table 5.2).

It is important to know about child development to:

- teach and advise parents
- have reasonable expectations of the child
- be able to plan suitable activities and play
- be able to identify limits and capabilities
- be able to recognise deviations from the norm and be alert to regression (behaviour from an earlier stage of development), disability and abnormality

TRANSITION FROM INTRAUTERINE TO EXTRAUTERINE LIFE

This demands considerable effective physiological changes by the baby to ensure survival. Simultaneously, they have to make major adjustments in their respiratory and circulatory systems, as well as gaining control of their body temperature. The baby emerges to encounter light, noise, cool air, gravity and tactile stimuli. Adaptation to extrauterine life involves the onset of respiration, circulatory changes and thermal adaptation.

Onset of Respiration

Regular respirations begin 60–90 seconds after complete expulsion from the mother as a result of both chemical and thermal stimulation. Thermal stimulation is caused by the sudden cooling of the infant leaving the warm environment of the uterus (37.7°C) and entering the cold atmosphere of the outside environment (approximately 21°C). This cooling excites sensory impulses in the skin that are transmitted to the respiratory centre. In addition, low levels of oxygen, high levels of carbon dioxide and low pH initiate impulses that excite the respiratory centre. At term, approximately 100 mL lung fluid is present within the respiratory tract. Some fluid is expelled through the mouth, assisted by the pressure on the thorax during vaginal delivery; the remainder is absorbed via the pulmonary lymphatics during the first 24 hours of life. The first breath requires a large pressure to open the terminal airways and overcome the initial stiffness of the lungs.

Circulatory Changes

Separated from the placenta, the infant must make major adjustments within the circulatory system to divert deoxygenated blood to the lungs for reoxygenation. The transition from fetal to postnatal circulation involves the closure of the foramen ovale, the ductus arteriosus and the ductus venosus.

Fetal blood pressure (BP) is low as a result of low vascular resistance in the placental circuit. A systolic BP of around 76 mmHg is found at birth; this level rises to 96 mmHg by 4 weeks. Coughing, crying and straining raise the BP.

THE NEWBORN BABY

Measurements

The average measurements at the 50th centile are shown in Table 5.3. The weight of the infant at birth also correlates with the incidence of perinatal morbidity and mortality. At birth, head circumference head is usually 2–3 cm greater than the circumference of the chest.

Appearance

- Head: one-quarter the body size (Fig. 5.6)
- Plump
- Prominent abdomen
- Lies in an attitude of flexion
- Lusty cry used to evoke a response from attendants with a view to controlling environment

The Skin

The skin has a film of vernix caseosa – a white sticky substance that is absorbed within a few hours and thought to have a protective function. The skin is thin and delicate; it is prone to blistering, infection and excoriation. Lanugo (downy hair) covers the skin and is plentiful over the shoulders, upper arms and thighs. Colour depends on ethnic origin.

Sebaceous glands are active late in fetal life and early infancy because of the high levels of maternal androgens. Plugging of the sebaceous glands causes milia. The epidermis and dermis are loosely bound to each other and very thin; friction such as removing sticky tape can separate the layers and cause blistering. The eccrine sweat glands (found mainly on the palms of the hands and the soles of the feet and forehead) are functional at birth and respond to heat and emotional stimulus. By the age of 43 weeks, palmar sweating can be used in pain assessment. The mature baby has many skin creases on its palms and soles; the nails are fully formed and adhere to the fingertips. Melanin levels are low at birth therefore the skin of the newborn is lighter than that it will be as a child, which means that young babies are more susceptible to the harmful effects of the sun. The hair is soft and silky; there may be lots or nearly none. The same is true for the eyebrows. The cartilage of the ears is

TABLE 5.3	**Newborn Measurements**	
	Girls	**Boys**
Weight on 50th centile	3.4 kg	3.5 kg
Length on 50th centile	50 cm	51 cm
Occipitofrontal circumference on 50th centile	34.5 cm	35 cm

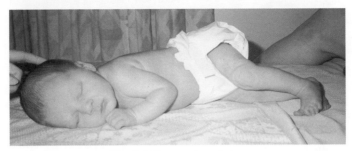

Fig. 5.6 The newborn baby.

well formed. The cord stump necroses and falls off within the first 10 days of life.

Genitalia and Breasts

In both sexes the breasts may be enlarged in the period immediately after birth. They may also discharge clear fluid. This is due to the stimulation caused by maternal hormones; these effects subside in the first few weeks of extrauterine life (MacGregor, 2000). There are nodules of breast tissue around the nipple. The testes are descended and the scrotum has plenty of rugae; the prepuce is adherent to the glans penis. The labia majora cover the labia minora.

Thermoregulation

Heat regulation is critical to the newborn baby's survival. The baby's capacity for heat production is adequate, but several factors predispose to excessive heat loss. The newborn's large surface area increases the possibility of heat loss to the environment, although this is normally partially compensated for by their flexion position, which effectively decreases the amount of surface area exposed to the environment. The subcutaneous fat layer is thin, giving poor insulation. This also allows transfer of core heat to the environment and cooling of blood. The hypothalamus in the brain has the capacity to promote heat production in response to stimuli received to thermoreceptors. Babies cannot shiver, nor are they able to voluntarily increase muscle activity to generate heat. Infants do produce heat by non-shivering thermogenesis and that generated by the heart, liver, brain and skeletal muscles.

Noradrenaline (norepinephrine) is secreted by the sympathetic nerve endings in response to chilling and stimulates fat metabolism in brown adipose tissue (BAT); this is unique to the newborn baby. BAT has a greater capacity for heat production through intensified metabolic activity than ordinary adipose tissue. BAT is situated between the scapulae, around the neck, in the axilla, behind the sternum, and around the kidneys, trachea, oesophagus, adrenal glands and some

arteries. However, this process does require energy, so the infant's oxygen requirement will increase. The regeneration of this tissue also requires good nutrition; a poor calorie intake will mean that the brown fat is not replaced and the infant will be less able to maintain body heat in a cool environment. Healthy, clothed infants will maintain their temperature provided the environmental temperature is maintained between 18°C and 20°C, nutrition is adequate and movements are not restricted. The temperature of the newborn is 37.5°C and by the age of 13 years it has reduced to 36.6°C; this is because infants produce more heat per kilogram body weight than older children. The temperature regulatory system is immature in the newborn infant, rendering infants and small children susceptible to temperature fluctuations. Factors such as environmental temperature, increased activity, crying or infection can cause a rapid increase in body temperature in the infant.

Eyes

At birth, the eyeball is too short for its lens; therefore babies focus best at approximately 20 cm (Fig. 5.7). As the eyeball continues to grow, distance vision is achieved. The ciliary muscles are immature, limiting the ability of the eyes to accommodate and fixate for any length of time. Babies have been shown to demonstrate visual preferences for some colours rather than others. No tears are present and eyes are easily infected. Corneal, papillary and blink reflexes are present.

Hearing

Once the amniotic fluid is drained from the external ear canal the acuity is similar to that of an adult. Babies can detect pitch, loudness and timbre of sound in addition to location and changes in complex sounds. The internal and middle ear is larger in proportion at birth and the external canal small. The mastoid process and the bony part of the external canal have not yet developed. The tympanic membrane and facial nerve are close to the surface and easily damaged.

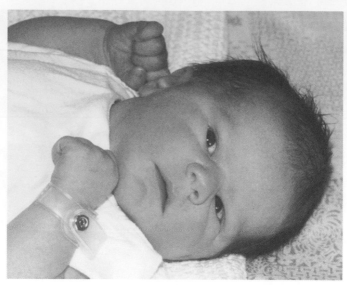

Fig. 5.7 The eyes.

Respiratory System

The respiratory system is developmentally incomplete. The lungs mature after birth and new alveoli continue to grow for many years. The number of alveoli at birth is estimated between 20 and 150 million, increasing to 300 million by approximately 3–4 years of age. After this the alveoli increase in size and number up until about 8 years of age; then from 8 years, size only until as in adults a 3000 mL volume and surface area of 75 m² in adolescence is reached (Meadow and Newell, 2002; Neill & Knowles, 2004; Crawford, 2011). This means that infants and young children have a relatively small alveolar surface area for gaseous exchange. Airway resistance in children is high due to the small diameter of the respiratory tree. The lumen of the peripheral airways is narrow, which predisposes the infant to airway obstruction. The infant's breathing is mainly abdominal: the abdomen distends, the diaphragm contracts and the thorax expands. The chest wall is very compliant and therefore easily distorted, which can increase the work of respiration.

Babies under 6 months of age are obligatory nose breathers and do not convert automatically to mouth breathing when nasal obstruction occurs. Respiratory rate is 30–60 per minute. Respirations are shallow and the pattern alters during sleeping and waking. Many term babies have periods of rapid breathing alternating with periods of breathing at a slower rate, or they may not breathe for periods of up to 15 seconds – this is normal as long as the colour and heart rate do not change significantly and the infant then begins to breathe again spontaneously (MacGregor, 2000). Periods of apnoea, when breathing ceases for more than 20 seconds, are only common in babies under 32 weeks' gestation unless there is an underlying condition.

Cardiovascular System

The heart rate is roughly 120–160 beats per minute (bpm) and fluctuates with respiratory function, activity and sleep. It reaches a maximum at 1 month, after which there is a gradual slowing until adult levels at 12–16 years of age. Peripheral circulation is sluggish and there may be mild cyanosis of hands and feet with mottling of skin when exposed.

Normal blood pressure ranges between 50/25 and 70/40 mmHg. The amount of total circulating blood is 80 mL/kg or approximately 300 mL at birth. Haemoglobin (Hb) = 15–20 g/dL; 70% is fetal Hb, which is replaced by adult Hb in the first 2 years of life. Mean cell volume (MCV)/100 L = 135 femtolitres = 10–12 g.

Breakdown of excess red blood cells in the liver and spleen predisposes to jaundice in the first few weeks. Prothrombin levels are low due to a lack of vitamin K. Colonisation of the intestine promotes synthesis of vitamin K. The white cell count is initially 18×109/L and reduces rapidly. Cardiac output is related to the heart rate and the stroke volume; as children have smaller hearts the stroke volume is reduced. The heart then needs to beat faster in order to oxygenate their body tissues.

Renal System

The newborn baby's kidneys weigh 23 g; this will have doubled by 6 months and trebled by the end of the first year (Sinclair, 1991, cited in MacGregor, 2000). The renal system is functional before birth but the workload is minimal. The infant is not able to concentrate or dilute urine very well in response to variations in fluid intake, and cannot compensate well for high or low solutes in blood. The ability to excrete drugs is also limited. However, the newborn can excrete amino acids and conserve sodium and glucose. The glomeruli are immature; they are resistant to aldosterone, which results in limited ability to concentrate the urine. This lack of ability to conserve or excrete water makes the baby vulnerable to dehydration. The glomerular filtration rate is 30 mL/min/m² at birth and doubles during the first 2 weeks of life, continues to rise to 100 mL/min/m² at 9 months, and reaches adult values at 1 year (Kanneh, 2004; Davenport, 1996, cited in MacGregor, 2000). Dehydration, hypotension and hypoxaemia all produce a fall in glomerular filtration rate, so renal function becomes compromised very quickly in a crisis. Urine is voided by reflex emptying of the bladder. The first urine is passed either at birth or during the first 24 hours and then increases in frequency as the fluid intake increases. Healthy neonates pass 1–3 mL/kg/h of urine rising within a month to 5 mL/kg/h. Neonatal urine is diluted at birth but the ability to concentrate develops in the first month with the lengthening of the loop of Henle and an increased response to antidiuretic hormone. After birth, the kidneys increase in size in proportion to body length, the weight doubling in the first 10 months as a result of tubular growth.

Endocrine System

The endocrine system produces limited quantities of antidiuretic hormone from the posterior pituitary gland, thus making the infant more susceptible to dehydration. The effect of maternal hormones may cause the labia to be hypertrophied and the breasts engorged.

Gastrointestinal System

This system is structurally complete but functionally immature. The teeth are usually still buried in the gums. Sucking pads in the cheeks give them a full appearance. Sucking and swallowing reflexes are coordinated. At birth the system is sterile and the development of stable flora is dependent on diet and takes time. Breast milk exposes the infant to microorganisms in the milk and from the skin of the breast and nipple. As diet changes and weaning commences the flora change.

The stomach's capacity at birth is approximately 10–30 mL, although this increases rapidly in the first few weeks of life up to 150 mL by 1 month. The cardiac sphincter is weak, making the baby prone to regurgitation or possiting and gastric emptying time is 2.5–3 hours. Hydrochloric acid is present in the stomach at birth but, due to swallowing of amniotic fluid, the pH is nearly neutral. Acid secretion commences within 8 hours of birth and digestion in the stomach is then reliant on the action of hydrochloric acid and rennin to cause the formation of curds by coagulating the casein in milk. Human milk contains e-fructose, a bacterium that raises the acidity of the gut inhibiting the growth of *Escherichia coli* bacteria. Adult levels of acid secretion are reached by the age of 10 years.

Intestine

At birth the intestines are thin walled and the villi continue to develop up until puberty by which time the length of the intestine has doubled. The breakdown of most food occurs in the intestine. In the young infant the colon has a small volume and therefore results in frequent bowel movements. Food reaches the caecum in about 4 hours. The breakdown of protein into large polypeptides is brought about by pepsin and hydrochloric acid. Subsequent breakdown into amino acids occurs by the action of the pancreatic enzymes, trypsin, chymotrypsin and polypeptides, and by enzymes derived from the small intestinal mucosa, such as enterokinase. Hence enzymes are available to catalyse proteins and simple carbohydrates but deficient production of pancreatic amylase impairs utilisation of complex carbohydrates. A deficiency of pancreatic lipase until 4–5 months of age reduces the infant's capacity to convert fat into fatty acids and glycerol. The gastrocolic reflex opens the ileocaecal valve so that feeding is often accompanied by emptying of the bowel and meconium, which is present in the large colon from 16 weeks gestation, is normally passed within 24 hours and totally excreted within 48–72 hours. Meconium is blackish in colour, tenacious and contains bile, fatty acids, mucous and epithelial cells. Following passage of the meconium, the stools change to brownish yellow, their frequency and consistency depending on the method of feeding. Breastfed babies' stools are loose, bright yellow and inoffensive. Bottle-fed babies' stools are paler, semi-formed and have a sharper odour; there is an increased tendency to constipation.

The liver occupies 40% of the peritoneal cavity at birth (MacGregor, 2000). There is decreased activity of the enzyme glucuronyl transferase, which is needed to conjugate bilirubin resulting in physiological jaundice of the newborn. The liver also stores less glycogen, leaving the infant susceptible to hypoglycaemia.

Absorption of Minerals and Vitamins

Vitamin B is absorbed from the terminal ileum. Iron, calcium, magnesium, sodium, potassium, ascorbic acid, folic acid and water-soluble vitamins are absorbed from the proximal small intestine.

 ACTIVITY

Find out what advice is given to the parents of newborns regarding feeding. How does this relate to the absorption capabilities of the infant's stomach and intestines?

Reflect on Your Practice
- Explain to a junior nurse or parent why newborn babies are at risk of jaundice.

Immunological Adaptations

There are three main immunoglobulins: G (IgG), A (IgA) and M (IgM). Infants are unable to produce their own immunoglobulins until 5 weeks old. IgG can cross the placenta so that at birth the baby's level is as high as the mother's. Breast milk, and especially colostrum, provide the infant with additional IgG. This gives passive immunity for the first few months of life, which gives the infant protection against most of the major childhood illnesses such as diphtheria, measles, poliomyelitis and rubella for about 12 weeks, provided the mother has antibodies to these diseases. The fetus can manufacture IgM and IgA but it takes 2 years to achieve adult levels. IgA protects against infections of the respiratory and gastrointestinal tract and eyes. The thymus gland, where lymphocytes are produced, is relatively large at birth and continues to grow until 8 years of age.

Reproductive System

Spermatogenesis does not occur until puberty. The total complement of primordial follicles containing primitive ova is present in the ovaries at birth.

Skeletomuscular System

All muscles are present at birth, although the muscle tissue is 35% water. The long bones are incompletely ossified allowing for growth at the epiphyses. The bones of the skull are incompletely ossified, essential for growth of the brain and moulding during labour. Moulding is resolved within a few days of birth. The posterior fontanelle closes within 6 weeks and the anterior fontanelle remains open for up to 18 months. This allows assessment of intracranial pressure by palpation.

In ventral suspension the head droops below the plane of the body (Fig. 5.8) and when the infant is pulled to sit there is marked head lag (Figs 5.9 and 5.10).

Neurological System

Compared with other systems this is very immature both anatomically and physiologically at birth. The most fully developed parts of the brain are the medulla (or hindbrain) and the midbrain. The least developed part is the cortex. This is no surprise when you consider the function of these areas of the brain and the abilities of the newborn/older child:

- The medulla is in the lower part of the skull and regulates sucking, breathing, heart rate, body temperature and muscle tone.

- The midbrain governs attention, sleeping, eating and eliminating. This part of the brain is similar to the brain of lower animals, that is the primitive reflexes are in control.

- The cortex governs perception, body movements, complex thinking and language. It follows that development of certain areas of the cortex sets limits on the development of the child's motor and perceptional skills.

The nerve cells or neurons of the brain are present at birth but the neurons of the cortex are not well connected. Over the first 2 years of life, the number and density of the dendrites, and speed of the synapses, increase rapidly, along with the size of individual neurons and the total weight of the brain; by 4 years of age the brain has tripled its weight. At birth the spinal cord is not fully myelinated. Myelination continues rapidly in the first 6 weeks postnatally and by 3 months the cerebellum is almost completely myelinated. Myelination and growth of connective tissue continues until adolescence. After birth, brain growth is rapid, requiring constant and adequate supplies of oxygen and glucose. The immaturity of the brain renders it particularly vulnerable to hypoxia, biochemical imbalance, infection and haemorrhage. Temperature instability and uncoordinated muscle movement reflect the incomplete state of brain development and incomplete myelination of the nerves.

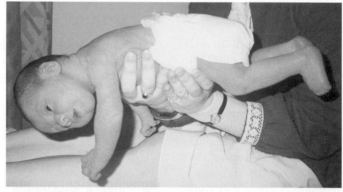

Fig. 5.8 In ventral suspension, the head droops below the plane of the body.

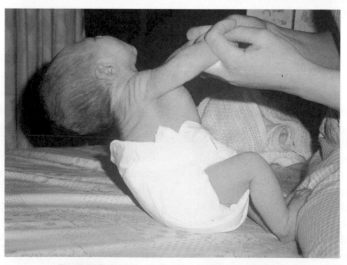

Fig. 5.9 Pulled to sit, there is a marked head lag.

A neonate is equipped with many reflexes, the presence of which indicates normality and integrity of the neurological and skeletomuscular system. Reflexes are automatic physical responses triggered involuntarily by a specific stimulus. Many of these reflexes are still present in adults (e.g. the knee jerk, automatic eye blink when a puff of air hits the eye, and the involuntary narrowing of the pupil when exposed to a bright light).

The newborn infant also has a set of 'primitive' reflexes. These are controlled by the more primitive parts of the brain: the medulla and the midbrain. By about 6 months, when the portion of the brain governing more complex activities such as perception, body movement, thinking and language has developed more fully, these primitive reflexes begin to disappear, as if superseded by the higher level brain functions.

Some primitive reflexes are essential for survival, such as the breathing reflex and the reflexes involved in eating. Infants who are touched on the cheek will automatically turn towards the touch and search for something to suck on; this is the rooting reflex (Fig. 5.11). The suck reflex is demonstrated when infants locate a suitable object that fits in the mouth and automatically begin to suck and swallow.

There are other primitive reflexes that do not have an obvious use. Infants who are confronted with a loud noise or some kind of physical shock will throw their arms outward and arch

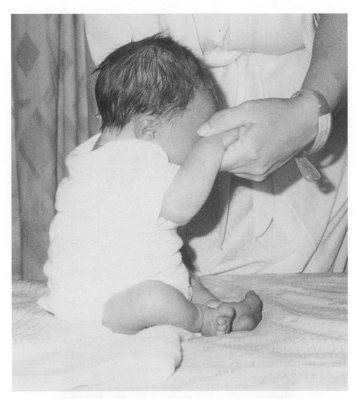

Fig. 5.10 Pulled to sit, there is a marked head lag.

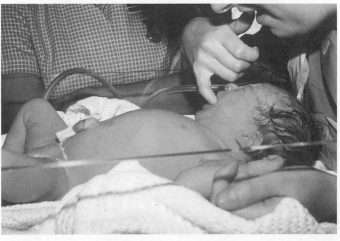

Fig. 5.11 The rooting reflex.

their back; this is the startle reflex. The Moro reflex occurs when the baby suffers a change in equilibrium or sudden jarring, which causes tension and abduction of the extremities and fanning of the fingers, followed by flexion and adduction of the extremities and the infant may cry (Fig. 5.12). The step reflex can be demonstrated by holding the baby so the sole of the foot touches a hard surface; this causes a reciprocal flexion and extension of the leg simulating walking (Fig. 5.13). If you touch an infant on the bottom of the foot, the Babinski reflex will be demonstrated when the toes are first splayed out and then curled in. If you touch an infant on the palm of the hand, his or her fingers will curl around your hand and hold on tightly; this is called the grasp reflex.

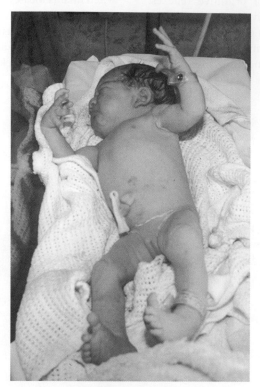

Fig. 5.12 Moro reflex.

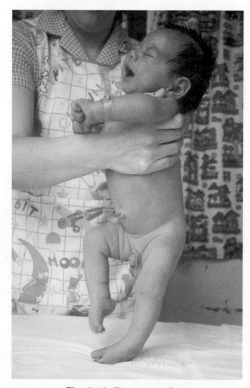

Fig. 5.13 The step reflex.

These reflex patterns are interesting not only because they may be remnants from our evolutionary past but because their presence past the age of roughly 6 months may signal the existence of some kind of neurological problem. The Babinski reflex is used as a diagnostic tool by neurologists who suspect the existence of some dysfunction.

1 MONTH TO 2 YEARS

Aged 1 Month

After birth, the rate of weight gain and growth in length accelerates to reach a maximum velocity between 4 and 6 weeks. The velocity of growth then declines rapidly until 4–5 years. Weight has a similar growth curve to height. Other organs show variations in their growth curve.

Posture and Large Movement

When the baby is pulled to sit, the head lags until the body is vertical (Fig 5.14), when the head is held momentarily erect before falling forward.

When held sitting, the back is one complete curve (Fig. 5.15).

In ventral suspension, the head is in line with the body and the hips are semi-extended (Fig. 5.16).

Vision and Fine Movement

- Pupils react to light.
- Turns head and eyes to light source.
- Follows pen torch briefly with eyes at 25 cm.
- Shuts eyes tightly when light is shone in them.
- Fixes and follows.
- Watches mother's nearby face when she feeds or talks to him with increasingly alert facial expression.

Hearing and Speech

- Startled by sudden noise.
- Stops whimpering and (usually) turns towards sound of nearby soothing voice, but not when screaming or feeding.

- Cries lustily when hungry or uncomfortable.
- Guttural noises when content.
- Coos responsively to mother's talk from 5 to 6 weeks.

Social Behaviour and Play

- Sucks well.
- Sleeps most of the time when not being fed or handled.
- Expression still vague: more alert later, progressing to social smile and responsive vocalisations at 5–6 weeks. Hands are normally closed but fingers are grasped when palm is touched.
- Stops crying when picked up and spoken to. Turns to regard nearby speaker's face. Needs head support when being carried, dressed or bathed. Passive acceptance of bath and dressing routines gradually changes to an increasing awareness and response.

Infant Assessment

There is a requirement for local authorities to commission five universal health visiting checks for families. The first

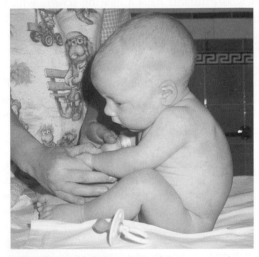

Fig. 5.15 When held sitting, the back is one complete curve.

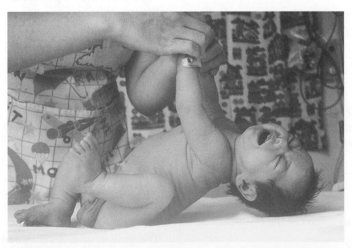

Fig. 5.14 When pulled to sit, the head lags until the body is vertical.

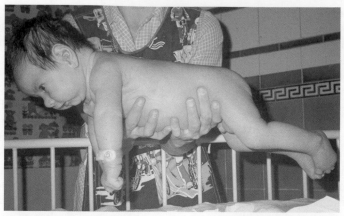

Fig. 5.16 In ventral suspension the head is in line with the body and the hips are semi-extended.

check happens at 28 weeks of pregnancy, and the rest continue up until the age of 2.5 years, forming part of the Healthy Child Programme. At 6–8 weeks a physical examination and a general assessment of alertness, vision and motor function should take place.

All newborn infants have a hearing screen, which is followed up as a targeted service according to the UK National Screening Committee (UK NSC), which recommends that all eligible newborn babies in England are offered screening to identify those with bilateral (both ears) moderate or worse permanent childhood hearing impairment (PCHI). Hearing is usually assessed soon after birth or within 4 weeks if a hospital-based programme or 5 weeks if community-based. (Public Health England, 2018a,b).

 ACTIVITY

Look at the requirements of the health child programme. Consider the comments made, do you think these universal checks are being carried out in your local area? https://publichealthmatters.blog.gov.uk/2017/03/01/continuing-the-mandation-of-the-universal-five-health-visiting-checks/

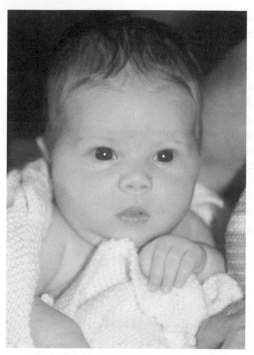

Fig. 5.17 Aged 6 weeks.

Vision

The infant turns to regard the speaker's face (Fig. 5.17). The infant holds gaze and follows to 90 degrees – failure to do so is not normal, but may be due to distraction. Infants who do not follow should be rechecked.

Motor Function

When placed prone, infant will lift their head for a few seconds. Infants who normally sleep prone are more advanced at this than others. Infants who fail this test should be retested 2 weeks later.

Other Assessments

Testes (boys)
- Assessed for developmental dysplasia of the lips
- The heart rate and sound
- Any matters of concern raised by parents or professionals

Age 6 Weeks Upwards
Sleep

At 3–7 months infants sleep through the night with two or three short naps during the day. Rapid eye movement (REM) sleep is less frequent by 6 months and levels off at 25%–30% total sleep time. There are four stages to sleep:
1. Drowsiness
2. Sleeping: easily wakened
3. Sleep becomes increasingly deeper: heart rate stable, muscles relaxed, brain waves slow
4. Deepest: difficult to rouse from sleep

A single night-time sleep contains all four stages arranged in cycles. The length of the sleep cycle gradually increases with age.

Skeletal System

The growth and development of bone consists of two processes, which occur at the same time: the creation of new cells and tissue and the consolidation of these tissues into a permanent form. The number of bones increases in the hand, wrist, ankle and foot. New centres of ossification in bones of hand and wrist are present at 5–6 months. These are useful for determining skeletal age. The length of the bones, particularly the long bones of the arms and legs, also increases to attain increase in height. Infant bones contain much more water than those of the adult, which makes them softer and more malleable (this ability to bend enabled the fetus to curl up inside the uterus). The bones of the skull are joined together as the fontanelles fill with bone; this process is usually complete by the age of 2 years. The ossification process takes place throughout infancy to adulthood. Girls mature faster than boys. At birth, girls are 5–6 weeks ahead in level of skeletal maturity.

3 Months
Posture and Large Movement

- Supine: prefers to lie with head in midline, limb movements smooth (Fig. 5.18).
- Pulled to sit: little or no head lag (Fig. 5.19).
- Held sitting: the back is straight except for lumbar region (Fig. 5.20).
- In ventral suspension: head held well above line of body (Fig. 5.21).
- Prone: lifts head and upper chest, uses forearms for support, buttocks flat (Fig. 5.22).

Vision and Fine Movement

- Visually alert, responds to nearby human face.
- Turns head deliberately to look around.
- Follows hanging ball at 30 cm through 180 degrees.
- Watches movements of own hands and demonstrates finger play.
- Recognises feeding bottle and makes eager movements as it approaches.
- Defensive blink present.
- Holds rattle for a few seconds but doesn't look at it at the same time.

Hearing and Speech

- Sudden loud noises still cause distress, eyes close tightly and the infant cries.
- Definite quietening or smiling in response to mother's voice.
- Vocalises happily when spoken to, can also vocalise when playing alone.
- Cries when uncomfortable or angry.
- Sometimes sucks or licks lips when food is being prepared.
- Demonstrates excitement when hears people approaching.

Social Behaviour and Play

- Intense gaze at mother's face when being fed.
- Reacts to familiar situations by showing excitement.
- Enjoys bathing.
- Responds with obvious pleasure when played with.

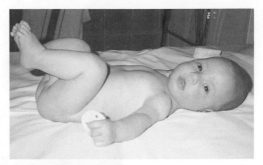

Fig. 5.18 When supine, prefers to lie with head in midline, limb movements smoother.

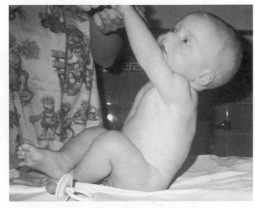

Fig. 5.19 Pulled to sit, there is little or no head lag.

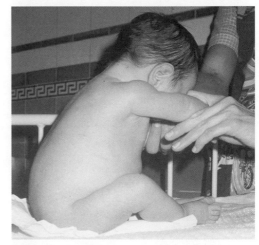

Fig. 5.20 Held sitting, the back is straight except for the lumbar region.

6 Months
Posture and Large Movement

- Supine: raises head to look at feet, lifts legs into vertical and grasps feet (Fig. 5.23).
- When hands are held: braces shoulders and pulls self to sit (Fig. 5.24).
- Held sitting: head firmly erect, back straight. Can sit momentarily alone (Fig. 5.25).

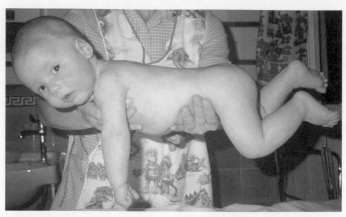

Fig. 5.21 In ventral suspension, the head is held well above the line of the body.

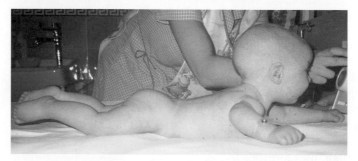

Fig. 5.22 When prone, lifts head and upper chest and uses forearms for support; the buttocks are flat.

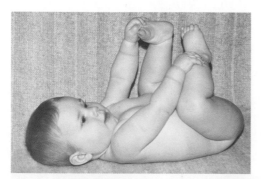

Fig. 5.23 When supine, raises the head to look at the feet, lifts legs into the vertical and grasps the feet.

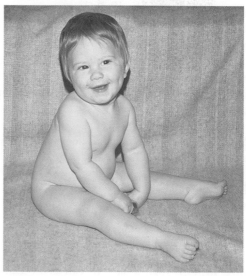

Fig. 5.25 Held sitting, the head is firmly erect and the back is straight. Can sit momentarily alone.

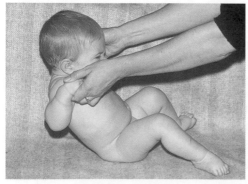

Fig. 5.24 When the hands are held, braces shoulders and pulls self to sit.

- Held standing: bears weight on feet and bounces up and down.
- Can stand momentarily when holding on to furniture (Fig. 5.26).
- When placed prone: lifts head and chest well up, supporting him- or herself on extended arms (Fig. 5.27).

Vision and Fine Movement

- Visually insatiable, moves head and eyes eagerly when attention attracted.
- Shows interest and watches adult movements at a distance.
- Eyes move in unison.
- Immediate fixation on interesting small objects at 30 cm.
- Uses whole hand to palmar grasp and passes object from one hand to the other.
- When toys fall outside visual field: does not follow them.

Hearing and Speech

- Turns immediately to mother's voice.
- Vocalises tunefully to self and others.
- Using single or double syllables: 'adah', 'goo', 'aroo'.
- Laughs and chuckles.
- Screams with annoyance.
- Demonstrates different responses to mother's tone of voice.

Social Behaviour and Play

- Reaches out and grasps small toys.
- Takes everything to mouth.
- Plays with feet and hands.
- Puts hands around bottle and pats it.
- Shakes rattle deliberately to make sound.
- Manipulates objects attentively passing from hand to hand.
- Friendly with strangers but does show some anxiety if approached too quickly.

8 Months (Fig. 5.28)

Vision

Near vision should demonstrate that the infant can see a small pellet about 20 cm away and he or she usually reaches out for it.

Motor Function

- From the prone position: infants should get up on their wrists.
- When pulled from supine: they should be able to sit spontaneously for a minute or two.
- Children can normally sit without help at 8 months (Fig. 5.29); they should be able to take their weight on their legs when they are held standing.
- If a cube is placed in front of them, infants should grab it with their whole hand (Fig. 5.30). Infants should transfer objects from one hand to the other.

Hearing

The distraction method is the hearing test used at this age. The distracter holds the infant's attention while the tester produces

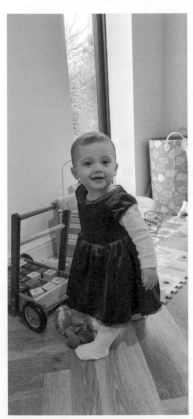

Fig. 5.26 When held standing, bears weight on feet and bounces up and down. Can stand momentarily holding on to furniture.

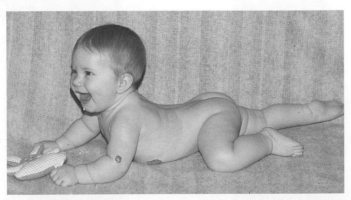

Fig. 5.27 When placed prone, lifts head and chest well up, supporting self on extended arms.

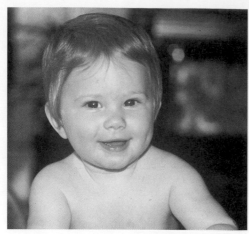

Fig. 5.28 Aged 8 months.

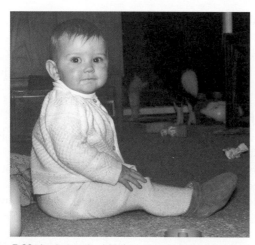

Fig. 5.29 An 8-month-old infant can sit without being held.

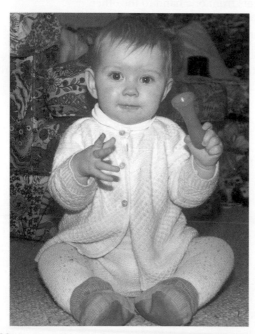

Fig. 5.30 An 8-month-old infant picks up and explores objects presented to them.

a sound. Careful attention to detail is essential to produce reliable results. The most common reasons for failure to respond to sound are tiredness, lack of interest, distraction, ear wax, otitis media and lack of familiarity with the test sounds. Infants who fail this test should be retested 2 months later. At 8 months, infants normally respond to their own name.

1 Year (Fig. 5.31)
Posture and Large Movement
- Crawls on hands and knees, shuffles on buttocks or bear walks.
- Usually able to stand alone, may walk.

Vision and Fine Movement
- Looks in correct place for toys dropped out of sight.
- Recognises familiar people at 7 m distance.

Hearing and Speech
- Turns immediately to own name.
- Comprehends simple instructions associated with gesture, for example 'come to mummy'.

Social Behaviour and Play
- Drinks from a cup.
- Waves 'bye-bye', plays 'pat-a-cake'.
- Helps with dressing, for example holding out arm for sleeve.

18 Months
Posture and Large Movement
- Walks competently, starts and stops safely.
- Walks upstairs with hand held.

Vision and Fine Movement
- Picks up small sweets, beads, etc., with delicate pincer grasp (Fig. 5.32).

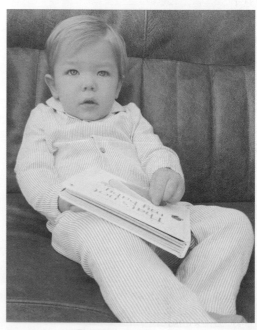

Fig. 5.31 Aged 1 year.

- Beginning to show a preference for using one hand.
- Enjoys simple picture books, recognises objects.
- Builds tower of three cubes (Fig. 5.33), knocks it down.

Hearing and Speech
- Uses 6–20 words and understands more.
- Attempts to sing.

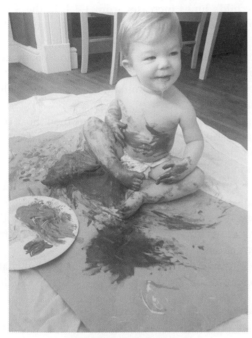

Fig. 5.32 Aged 18 months.

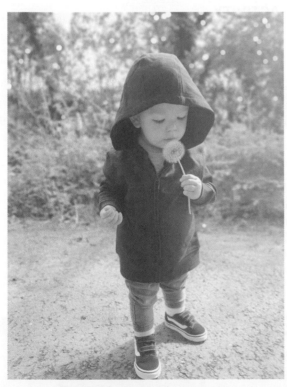

Fig. 5.33 Vision and fine movement.

Social Behaviour and Play
- Holds spoon, gets food safely to mouth (Fig. 5.34).
- Takes off clothes, but unable to dress self.

The Physiological Changes of a Toddler
The physical appearance is squat with a pot-belly and slightly bowed legs (Fig. 5.35); by preschool children become more slender and graceful.

The rate of increase of head circumference slows with head and chest having roughly the same circumference by 1–2 years of age. In the second year the increase in head circumference

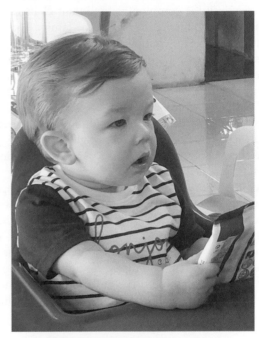

Fig. 5.34 Social behaviour and play.

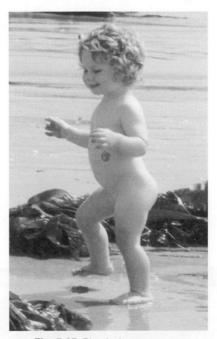

Fig. 5.35 Physical appearance.

is 2.5 cm. By 5 years the rate of increase has reduced to 1.25 cm a year. Between 12 and 18 months the anterior fontanelle closes (Chamley, 2005). Between the ages of 2 and 6 years epiphyses emerge in the skeleton.

Myelinisation of the spinal cord is almost complete by 2 years of age and brain growth is 75% complete. As specific areas of the brain develop, the child progresses developmentally; for example, as the cortex develops then better control of the arms, legs and feet is gained.

During infancy, the capacity of the stomach increases to allow digestion of three meals a day and milk in the evening. Bowel movements have reduced to one or two a day, although bowel irregularity is common as the infant changes from a bland simple weaning diet to that of the family. Young children cannot control their bowel until they develop central nervous system control, although the tendency to defaecate after breakfast is often taken advantage of. Children have daytime control of their bowel movements from about 24 to 30 months old (MacGregor, 2000).

The skin matures during early childhood, with the epidermis and the dermis becoming more tightly bound together, thus the effectiveness of the skin as a barrier to infection and against fluid loss is improved.

The child's ability to maintain body temperature improves, with the capillaries constricting and dilating in response to cold and heat and shivering as an effective means of thermogenesis.

The volume of the respiratory tract increases but the internal structures of the ear and throat continue to be short and straight with the lymphoid tissue of the tonsils and adenoids large, which predisposes the young child to otitis media, tonsillitis and upper respiratory tract infections.

Metabolism

This is affected by an assortment of intrinsic and extrinsic factors. The basal metabolic rate (BMR) is highest in newborns. BMR closely relates to the proportion of surface area (SA) to the body mass, which decreases with maturity. The rate of metabolism determines caloric and protein requirements (Table 5.4) – during illness, needs can be high.

There is an increased metabolic rate (about twice that of an adult) and an increased respiratory demand for oxygen consumption and carbon dioxide elimination. The proportion of energy intake used to build and maintain tissue changes as the child grows:

- Birth: 40%
- 3 months: 40%
- 1–2 years: 20%
- 9–11 years: 4%–10%

Respiratory System

Overall lung growth has been measured in children using annual radiographs. Lung width and length follows a similar growth curve to overall height, with an adolescent growth spurt. Boys are on an average larger than girls in all lung dimensions.

The number of alveoli increases after birth reaching 90% at age 4 years. By the age of about 10 the increase in alveoli ceases and is followed by an increase in size. The total capacity of a child's lungs increases from 1.4 L in the 5-year-old child to 4.5 L at the time of puberty (MacGregor, 2000). The ribs lie more horizontally in infants and contribute less to chest expansion. This results in infants and young children breathing diaphragmatically and respiration rate therefore is observed by watching abdominal movement rather than the movement of the chest.

The muscles are more likely to fatigue than those of adults and young children are more prone to respiratory failure. Anything that impedes diaphragm contraction or movement, for example, abdominal distension, can contribute to the development of respiratory failure. The sternum and ribs are cartilaginous, the chest wall is soft and the intercostal muscles are poorly developed. In the event of illness, the infant's chest wall may move inwards instead of outwards during inspiration (retractions).

Smooth muscle is present throughout the lungs at birth and bronchospasm can occur even in the very young infant.

Lymphatics: B and T Cell Systems

The total amount of lymphoid tissue in the body (thymus, lymph nodes and lymphoid tissue of gut) increases throughout childhood.

 ACTIVITY

What childhood illness is a particular indicator of this growth and what common surgery is carried out?

 ACTIVITY

Think of the implications of malnutrition and understimulation on a young infant.

Dental Eruption

Deciduous teeth begin to appear at the following ages (Fig. 5.36):

- Incisors: 6–9 months
- Canines: 16–19 months
- 1st molars: 10–15 months
- 2nd molars: 16–27 months

TABLE 5.4	Recommended Daily Requirements of Calories and Protein	
	Energy Allowance (kcal/kg)	Protein (g)
0–6 months	108	13
6 months to year	98	14

Salivary Glands

These start to function at 2–3 months; hence this is when babies start drooling.

Normal Observations
Respiration

- 1–11 months: 30/min.

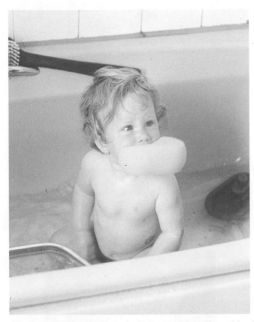

Fig. 5.36 The pain and irritation of teething is relieved by biting.

Heart Rate: 3 Months to 2 Years

- Resting awake: 80–150 bpm.
- Sleeping: 70–120 bpm.
- Exercise or fever: up to 220 bpm.

Temperature

- 37.5°C.

Blood Pressure

Table 5.5 shows blood pressure by age.

GENERAL TRENDS IN HEIGHT AND WEIGHT GAIN DURING CHILDHOOD

Weight Gain

Table 5.6 shows weight gain by age.

Height

Table 5.7 shows height gain by age.

The Preschool Child

During this period the child grows 6–8 cm and gains 2 kg each year. The child has 20 deciduous teeth at 2.5 years.

The 2-Year-Old

- Walks, runs, stops and starts to avoid collisions.
- Squats to play and rise again (Fig. 5.37).

TABLE 5.5	Blood Pressure (mmHg) by Age	
Age	Girls	Boys
3 months	89/51	91/50
6 months	91/53	90/53
12 months	91/54	90/56

TABLE 5.6	Weight Gain by Age
Age	Weight Gain
Birth to 6 months	Weekly 140–200 g
	Doubles by end of 4–7 months
6–12 months	Weekly 85–140 g
	Triples by end of first year
Toddlers	Yearly 2–3 kg
	Quadruples age 2.5 years
Preschoolers	Yearly 2–3 kg

TABLE 5.7	Height Gain by Age
Age	Height Gain
Birth to 6 months	Monthly 2.5 cm
6–12 months	Monthly 1–5 cm
Toddlers	By age 2 years 50% adult
Preschoolers	Yearly gain 7.5 cm
	Birth length is doubled by 4 years

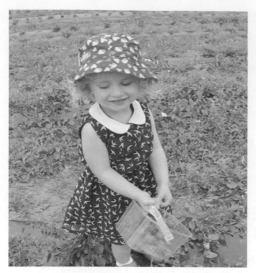

Fig. 5.37 The 2-year-old.

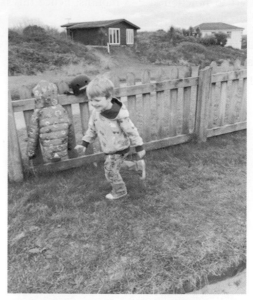

Fig. 5.39 A 3-year-old enjoys riding on toys.

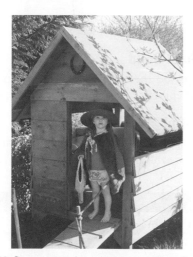

Fig. 5.38 Spontaneously engages in make-believe play.

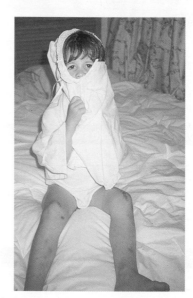

Fig. 5.40 At 3 years, children start trying to dress themselves.

- Climbs on furniture to look out window or open door.
- Attempts to throw and kick a ball.
- Operates a sit-and-ride toy.
- Has difficulty with spatial awareness.
- Has strong sense of identity. Will resist things being done to them.
- Temper tantrums common.
- Holds a pencil like a rod and copies straight lines.
- Usually dry by day.
- Spontaneously engages in make-believe play (Fig. 5.38).

The 3-Year-Old

- Speech is well developed (girls better than boys).
- Understands sharing, turn taking.
- Is nimble and can judge distances.
- Jumps, stands briefly on one leg.
- Rides a tricycle and other toys (Fig. 5.39).
- Motor skills well established, can climb stairs with alternate feet (coming down puts both feet on the same step).
- Is clean and dry and can self-feed.
- Can build a tower of eight or nine cubes.

- Holds a pencil using almost a mature grasp, copies circles, cuts with scissors.
- Can attempt to dress self, can pull on clothes overhead, pull up pants but needs help with buttons (Fig. 5.40).
- Joins in active make-believe play (Figs 5.41–5.43).

The 4-Year-Old

- Self-care skills are developing, is willing to attempt to brush own hair (Fig. 5.44) and brush own teeth (Fig. 5.45).
- Holds a pencil in a mature grasp (Fig. 5.46) and copies circles and crosses as well as drawing an accurate body shape.
- Matches and names four primary colours.
- Gives full name, home address and sometimes age.
- Enjoys jokes, knows several nursery rhymes.

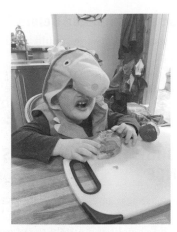

Fig. 5.41 Joins in make-believe play.

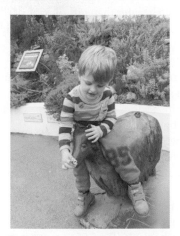

Fig. 5.42 Joins in make-believe play.

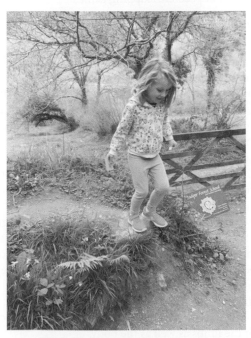

Fig. 5.43 Joins in make-believe play.

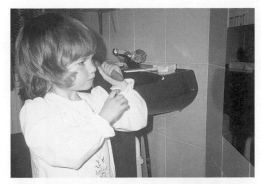

Fig. 5.44 A 4-year-old learning to brush her hair.

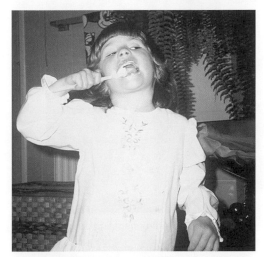

Fig. 5.45 Learning to clean her teeth.

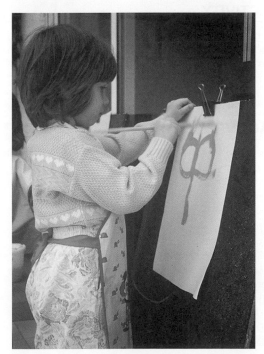

Fig. 5.46 Demonstrating a mature grip.

- Walks and runs skilfully and negotiates objects at speed without running into them.
- Can balance (Fig. 5.47), hop and climb up and down stairs.

- Enjoys the company of and is aware of the feelings of other children.
- Looks forward to treats and has some concept of time.
- 'Lordosis' (pot belly) disappears.

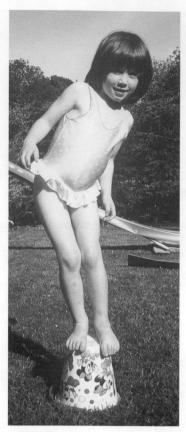

Fig. 5.47 Demonstrating balance.

ACTIVITY

The child's need for sleep varies at different ages:
- Find out how much sleep you would expect a 1-year-old and a 4-year-old to require.

ACTIVITY

Between the ages of 1 and 5 years growth slows considerably compared with the first year of life:
- What would be considered an average weight gain per year?
- What would be considered an average height gain?
- Birth weight is quadrupled by what age?
- Adult height is twice the child's height at what age?
- Brain growth is what percentage complete by 2 years?
- At what age should myelination of the spinal cord be complete?
- What age should the anterior fontanelle close?
- At what age would you expect a child to be:
  - Dry by day?
  - Dry by night?
- What energy (k/cal/g) and protein (g) requirements are needed for a 1–3-year-old daily?
- What would you expect the normal pulse, respirations and BP to be of a 4-year-old?
- At what ages would you expect to see a growth spurt in children?

Child Assessment Completed Before 5 Years

Assessments of hearing and vision should be completed either before or soon after starting school.

A pre-school hearing screen should be performed with follow-up by the audiology services if there are any concerns. All children should also be screened for visual impairment between 4 and 5 years of age by an orthoptist-led service.

PHYSICAL GROWTH FROM 5 YEARS TO ADOLESCENCE

Physical changes are less obvious than 0–5 years. Children grow taller, change shape and acquire new skills. By the age of 5 years the child's height and weight are increasing steadily at the rate of 5 cm and 2–3 kg/year. Boys are on average 2.5 cm taller and 1 kg heavier than girls during early school years; however by 12 years of age girls are both taller and heavier than boys in their peer group.

- The 5-year-old is able to:
  - Draw a recognisable person or house, and write his or her own name
  - Hop, skip, swing, jump, balance, climb, dance and throw a ball (Figs 5.48–5.50)
  - Ride a two-wheel bicycle
  - Choose friends
  - Undress and dress, except for laces and ties (Fig. 5.51)
  - Perform domestic and dramatic play alone or with friends (Figs 5.52 and 5.53)
- Age 6: swings by arms and skips with rope (Fig. 5.54)
- Age 7: 'walks the plank' (Fig. 5.55), uses a bat and ball (Fig. 5.56)
- Age 8–10: hopscotch, skipping games

Skeletal Growth

The growth of the trunk and extremities exceeds that of the head.

The centre of gravity lowers and body proportions become slimmer. Growth hormone stimulates longitudinal growth in a dose-dependent manner; however other influences on growth are socioeconomic, emotional and genetic factors. Problems are caused by ill-fitting shoes, chairs of the wrong height and carrying heavy loads, such as school bags.

Muscle growth occurs in tandem with bone growth increasing in size due to their diameter increasing along with an increase in length and width. The muscles are, however, immature and susceptible to damage.

Growth is reflected in limb length. Girls stop growing sooner than boys because of epiphyseal unity, which is under the control of oestrogen secretion. Boys' longer growth is reflected in their greater height and longer arms and legs. The extremities grow first, followed by neck, hip, chest, shoulder, trunk and depth of chest, hence the long-legged, gangly appearance of teenage boys with trousers and jumpers that never fit the limbs as well as the body.

ACTIVITY

Assessment of growth: go to the web site of the Royal College of Paediatrics and Child Health and search for growth charts for the latest information.

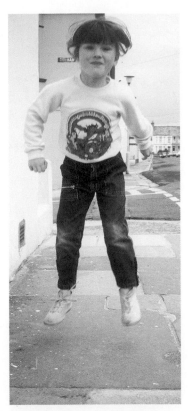

Fig. 5.48 A 5-year-old learning sophisticated motor skills.

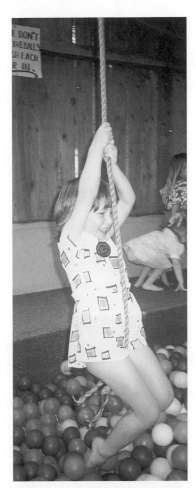

Fig. 5.50 A 5-year-old learning sophisticated motor skills.

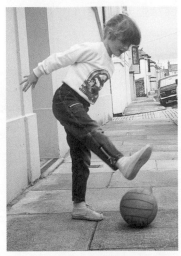

Fig. 5.49 A 5-year-old learning sophisticated motor skills.

Teeth

Children start to lose their deciduous teeth and permanent teeth appear at about the rate of four per year between the ages of 7 and 14 years.

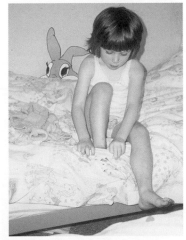

Fig. 5.51 Dress and undress except for laces and ties.

ACTIVITY

Find out the sequence of teeth eruption for permanent dentition from a recommended textbook.

Head

- 6 months (Fig. 5.57).
- 5 years (Fig. 5.58).
- 10 years (Fig. 5.59).
- 13 years (Fig. 5.60).
- 16 years (Fig. 5.61).

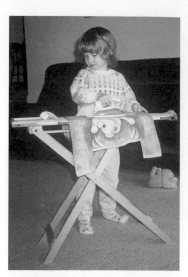

Fig. 5.52 Performs domestic and dramatic play alone or with friends.

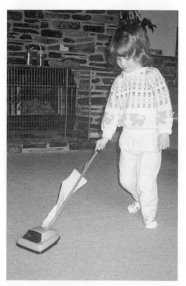

Fig. 5.53 Performs domestic and dramatic play alone or with friends.

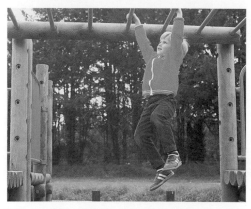

Fig. 5.54 Aged 6, swings by the arms and skips with a rope.

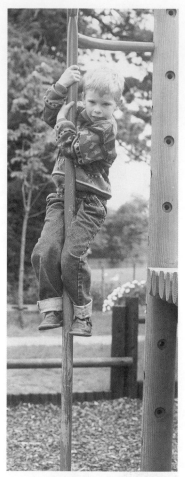

Fig. 5.55 Aged 7, greater strength and body control.

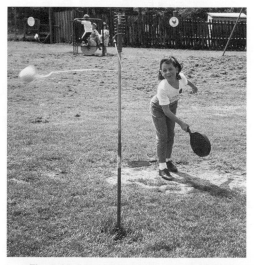

Fig. 5.56 Aged 8–10, uses a bat and ball.

The shape of the child's face changes from infancy to adult-hood. Facial proportions change and the face grows faster in relation to the cranium. The frontal sinuses become visible on x-ray. When the permanent teeth erupt, they force the shape of the jaw to change to accommodate them. In adolescence, both the jaw and the forehead alter, the jaw grows forward and the forehead becomes more prominent. This changes the overall shape of the face from a rounded appearance to one that is longer and more angular. The head and eyes are extra-large in children; by the age of 8 years the child's head is 90% of its adult size. As facial remodelling continues and the

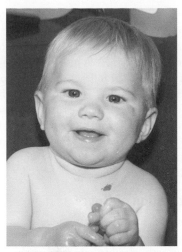

Fig. 5.57 Aged 6 months.

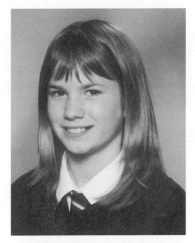

Fig. 5.60 Aged 13 years.

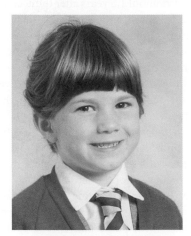

Fig. 5.58 Aged 5 years.

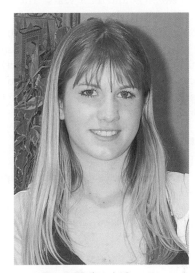

Fig. 5.61 Aged 16 years.

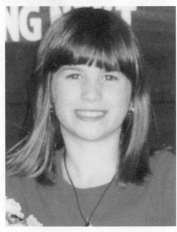

Fig. 5.59 Aged 10 years.

Cardiovascular System

This participates in the muscular growth spurt – its weight nearly doubles (this is more pronounced in boys). The systolic BP rises at an accelerated rate during puberty, and pulse rate decreases. Blood volume, Hb, and red blood cell count rise more in boys than girls; by adulthood, women have one million fewer red cells per mL than men.

Respiratory System

The size and capacity increase; the respiratory rate decreases. Boys take in more air at one breath than girls, due to the increased chest and shoulder size.

Peak flow rate measures the maximum flow achieved in expiration after a maximum inspiration. Normal ranges of peak flow rates are:
- 5 years: 150 L/min
- 10 years: 240 L/min
- 15 years: 400 L/min

jaw reaches adult size, there is hypertrophy of the laryngeal mucosa and enlargement of the larynx and vocal cords.

Body Mass

Muscle growth follows that of bone and is therefore greater in boys.

Skin

Oestrogen causes the skin of the female to develop a soft smooth, thicker texture. The sebaceous glands are particularly active and the eccrine and apocrine sweat glands become fully functional. Body hair takes on the characteristic distribution patterns and the texture changes.

ADOLESCENCE

Puberty is triggered by a chain of hormonal effects that bring on visible physical changes. The biology of puberty is triggered by hormonal influences and is controlled by the anterior pituitary in response to a stimulus from the hypothalamus (Fig. 5.62).

Sexual Maturation of Girls

The average age for appearance of breast buds is 10–11 years, with a range between 9 and 11.5 years. The appearance of pubic hair usually follows breast development by about 2–6 months, although in about one-third of girls the appearance of pubic hair may occur first. There is often an increase in normal vaginal discharge associated with uterine development. Menarche usually occurs 2 years after the appearance of breast buds with a critical weight of 45 kg or 17% body fat required before menarche begins.

Development of the Breasts (Fig. 5.63)

- *Stage one.* Elevation of papilla.
- *Stage two.* Small area of elevation around papilla, enlargement of areolar diameter.
- Stage three: Further development of breast and areola with no separation of their contours.

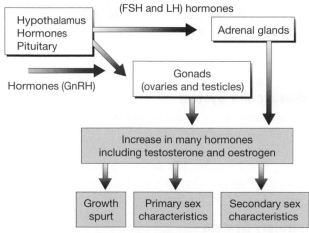

Fig. 5.62 The hormones produced in adolescence.

- *Stage four.* Projection of areola and papilla to form a secondary mound (may not appear in all girls).
- *Stage five.* Mature configuration, projection of papilla only caused by recession of areola into general contour.

Growth of pubic hair follows the same pattern as for boys, with stage one having no pubic hair, through stages two and three when the hair goes from sparse and downy to more coarse and curly, and stages four and five when the hair becomes denser, curled and finally adult in quality, with spread of hair to the thighs. Fig. 5.64 shows the pubertal changes for girls.

Sexual Maturation of Boys

Maturation begins in boys with an increase in the rate of growth of the testes and scrotum at about age 12 years of age. There is slow growth of pubic hair at about the same time and, approximately 1 year later, accelerated growth of the penis. Ejaculation occurs about 1.5 years after the accelerated growth of the penis begins. Body and facial hair usually appear about 2 years after the beginning of pubic hair growth. The lowering of the voice occurs quite late in puberty. Some changes also occur to the male breast, which includes an enlargement of the areola; but this usually disappears within a year or so.

Marshall and Tanner (1969) describe the developmental stages of genital development in boys as:

- *Stage one: Prepubertal.* No pubic hair – essentially the same as in childhood.
- *Stage two: Pubertal.* Initial enlargement of the scrotum and testes with reddening of the scrotal skin.
- *Stage three.* Penile lengthening, thinning of the scrotal skin, testicular enlargement, which begins between 10.5 and 14.5 years with pubic hair spread sparsely over the entire pubis.
- *Stage four.* Glans enlargement, penile broadening, testicular enlargement, scrotal increase in size and deepening of pigmentation with more abundant pubic hair but restricted to the pubic area.
- *Stage five.* Adult size and shape with spread of hair to inner thighs.

Spermatogenesis is active from the time of penile growth; and ejaculate can be produced from 1 year after its onset. Fig. 5.65 shows the pubertal changes for boys.

👤 **ACTIVITY**

Look up www.cua.edu and search for pubertal processes.

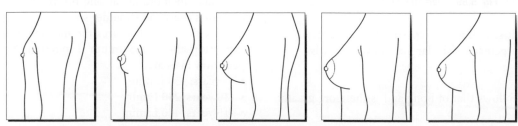

Fig. 5.63 Development of the breasts.

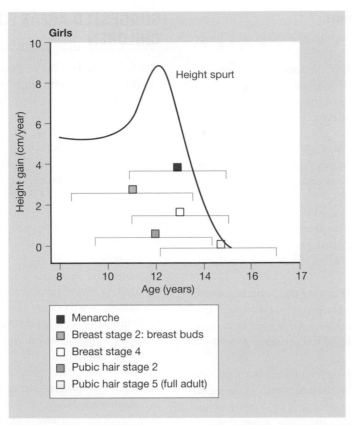

Fig. 5.64 The pubertal changes for girls (Chimlea, 1982 [cited in Bee, 2013]; Garn, 1980; Tanner, 1962).

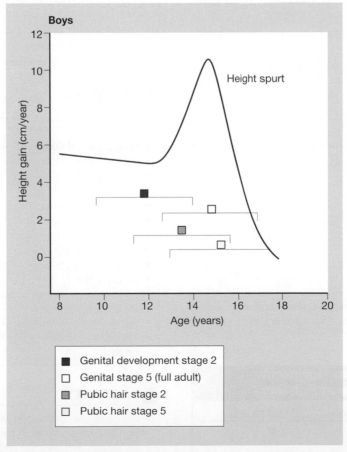

Fig. 5.65 The pubertal changes for boys (Chimlea, 1982 [cited in Bee, 2013]; Garn, 1980; Tanner, 1962).

The Adolescent Growth Spurt

The internal organs grow, including the lungs and heart, which increases physical endurance.

The lymphoid system, including the tonsils and adenoids, decreases in size, improving asthma, in some teenagers.

The growth of the skeletal system is reflected in limb growth. Boys' longer growth is reflected in their greater height and longer arms and legs.

Muscle mass increases in boys and girls. For girls, this peaks at menarche then slows; for boys it continues, resulting in a higher lean body mass in boys and peaking at approximately 25 years.

Adolescence is a time of continued brain growth. There is no actual increase in number of neurons, but growth of the myelin sheath continues until at least puberty, thus enabling faster neural processing, which corresponds with the development of cognitive abilities.

The rate of growth may double during the pubertal growth spurt. The final 20%–25% of linear growth is achieved; this can be as much as 5.5 cm in a peak year. Girls gain an average of 5–20 cm in height and 7–25 kg in weight; boys gain 10–30 cm in height and 7–30 kg in weight.

Both the growth spurt and onset of menstruation are occurring earlier now than they used to. Since 1850, the age at which menarche occurs has been declining in Western countries, probably the result of better nutrition, fewer diseases and good medical care. For example, in the United States, girls first menstruated at 13–15 years; this is now 11–13 years. This means that girls are reaching the 'critical weight' of 45 kg, which must be attained before menstruation can begin, earlier than in former times.

A more recent example can be seen at La Scala opera house, which was built between 1776 and 1778 with seats that were 33 cm wide; this means of course that this must have been the average size of the bottom. In 1975 aircraft seats were 60 cm wide. (Do you know how wide they are today? Watch the TV commercials to find out.) What does this say about the size of our bottoms?

ACTIVITY

What size do you think the knights of yesteryear were?

ACTIVITY

Look up the hormonal changes and sequence of sexual maturation at puberty in a recommended textbook and in Table 5.8.

TABLE 5.8 Timings for Hormonal Changes/Developments at Puberty

	Boy (Years)	Girl (Years)
Begins as early as	10.5	7.5
Begins as late as	16	11.5
Average onset	12	10
Peaks	14	12

SUGGESTED AREAS FOR OBSERVATION OF CHILDREN

The following is a list of placement areas where the theory of child development can be observed in practice. The list is not exclusive and you may visit other areas where you can observe children:

- Child health clinics
- Developmental screening
- Home visits with health visitor
- School health checks
- Practice nurses
- Family centres
- Mother and toddler groups
- Play groups
- Nurseries
- Schools
- Youth centres/organisations, for example Cub Scouts, Girl Guides, youth centres
- Voluntary-sector child-oriented organisations, for example riding for the disabled, youth enquiry service, play centres, toy libraries

When observing and interacting with children, consider their developmental progress using a developmental screening chart as a framework. Please use it simply as a guide to your observation; do not feel you have to test the child or check every item. Do not attempt any of the specific screening tests, such as hearing, physical examinations of the hips and testicles and checking of reflexes. Do not record any information that might compromise the confidentiality of the child, for example, name, address.

The following three activities can help to focus your findings when observing children.

ACTIVITY

Complete the following worksheet as a record of your findings.

Developmental Observation Exercise
- Practice area
- Age of child
- Gender
- Context of observation
- Background of child (if applicable)
- Social behaviour and play
- Hearing and speech
- Fine motor and vision
- Gross motor
- Feeding and nutrition (if applicable)
- Physical appearance
- Personality and demeanour
- Additional comments (e.g. reasons for any developmental issues)

ACTIVITY

If you have the opportunity, when out with the health visitor, weigh and measure three babies or young children and plot their heights and weights on the percentile chart. Be sure to ask the permission of the child's parents before you undertake this exercise.

ACTIVITY

The ways in which family life affects development are many. Through daily incidents and decisions parents affect their child's development in both positive and negative ways. Think of some examples in which parents can affect their child's development:

- Sean is 5 months old and cannot sit unaided
- Sue is 2 years old and screams when her mother dresses her, but she cannot cope on her own
- John is 6 years old and is slow in beginning to read
- Gill has just begun her periods and her body is changing
- Gary is 16 years old with no qualifications, out every night and surly

REFERENCES

Bee, H., 2013. The Developing Child, thirteenth ed. Pearson Education, Essex.

Chamley C, Carson P, Randall D, Sandwell W (2005) Developmental Anatomy and Physiology of Children: A Practical Approach. Churchill Livingstone. Edinburgh.

Crawford, D., 2011. Understanding childhood asthma and the development of the respiratory tract. Nurs. Child. Young People. 23 (7), 25–34.

Frankenburg, W.K., Dodds, J.B., 1967. The Denver developmental screening test. J. Pediatr. 71, 181–191.

Garn, S.M., 1980. Continuities and Change in Maturational Timing. Constancy and Change in Human Development. Harvard University Press, Cambridge, Mass.

Harris, S.R., 2015. Measuring head circumference: update on infant microcephaly. Can. Fam. Physician 61 (8), 680–684.

Kanneh, A., 2004. Control of body fluids in childhood in the biology of child health. A reader in development and assessment. In: Neill, S., Knowles, H. (Eds.). Palgrave, New York.

MacGregor, J., 2000. Introduction to the Anatomy and Physiology of Children. Routledge, London.

Marshall, W.A., Tanner, J.H., 1969. Variations in pattern of pubertal changes in girls. Arch. Dis. Child. 44, 291.

Meadow, R., Newell, S., 2002. Lecture Notes in Paediatrics, seventh ed. Blackwell Science, Oxford.

Neill S, Knowles H, (2004)The Biology of Child Health. A Reader in Development and Assessment. Red Globe Press.

Public Health England, 2018a. Guidance Our Approach to Newborn Hearing Screening Standards. https://www.gov.uk/government/publications/newborn-hearing-screening-programme-quality-standards/newborn-hearing-screening-programme-standards-format-and-scope. (Accessed 09/07/18.)

Public Health England, 2018b. Guidance Healthy Child Programme 0 to 19: Health Visitor and School Nurse Commissioning. https://www.gov.uk/government/publications/healthy-child-programme-0-to-19-health-visitor-and-school-nurse-commissioning. (Accessed 09/07/18.)

Royal College of Paediatrics and Child Health. https://www.rcpch.ac.uk/resources/growth-charts. (Accessed 09/07/18.)

Sheridan, M., 1997. From Birth to Five Years, Children's Developmental Progress. Revised and Updated by Marion Frost and Dr Ajay Sharma. Routledge, Cornwall.

Tanner, J.M., 1962. Growth at Adolescence. Blackwell Scientific Publications, Oxford.

6

Death and Dying in Childhood

Rachel Cooke, Duncan C. Randall

LEARNING OUTCOMES

- Describe the concepts of death and dying relating to death in childhood and social and cultural reactions to death in childhood.
- Outline children's understanding of death and dying as it develops through childhood.

- Discuss the how parents and siblings of children who are dying, or who die, may understand and react to childhood death.
- Summarise social attitudes to death and dying in childhood.

GLOSSARY

Anticipatory grief Advice to people in preparation of bereavement, preparing for dying and death in a child or parent/carer.

Bereavement The objective reality of something lost, that is what happens to you?

Brain stem death The irreversible cessation of brain-stem integrative function whether induced by intra-cranial events or the result of extra-cranial phenomena, such as hypoxia which allows a medical practitioner to diagnose death (Academy of Medical Royal Colleges, 2008).

Circulatory death Simultaneous and irreversible onset of apnoea and an absence of a central pulse and of heart sounds on auscultation (Academy of Medical Royal Colleges, 2008).

Death A lack of life, a state in which growth and change no longer occurs (Dewy, 1944) and a living human being

ceases to exist (Academy of Medical Royal Colleges, 2008).

Grief Complex set of psychological and physical reactions to loss, that is how you feel?

Life limiting or threatening condition A condition which can potentially limit a child's life to less than current life expectancy for individuals in their community or which is associated with the potential for the child's health status to deteriorate, for treatment to be ineffective and which may result in the child's death (see Shaw et al., 2015).

Loss To be deprived of, to fail to get, to die or be destroyed.

Mourning The observable expression of grief according to culturally specific rituals: what you do (Wilson, 1993).

Short life A life of less duration than the normal life expectancy, often associated with a life where death occurs in childhood, that is under 18 (see Shaw et al., 2015).

INTRODUCTION

Death at any age can be difficult to determine; this may seem a contrary statement, but with advancing technologies death has become less certain (see activity, later). Death in childhood is as with most matters of childhood further complicated by the social standing of children and their childhoods and their developing physical and psychological systems.

If we take the technological aspects to begin with, technological advances in the mid-20th century mean that we can now ventilate people, feed them artificially and keep their bodies 'alive'. When previously if you didn't breathe you were considered dead. Still in English law a fetus does

not become a person until they have taken a spontaneous breath. To determine death people looked to see if a person was breathing, but with the invention of artificial ventilation not breathing is no longer a certain sign of death. With the development of pacemakers, bypass surgery and ECMO (Maslach-Hubbard and Bratton, 2013) we can no longer say that not having a heart beat is a sign of death; similarly we can replicate the functions of the kidney with dialysis. While there are no artificial mechanical solutions to replicate the function of the liver we can offer transplantation (to some children, in some countries at least [Kelly, 2015]) so a poorly functioning liver no longer places a child on a certain path to death. It is possible that brain function may be replicated in computer systems in the near future (given Moore's law on the exponential increases in computing power, and the development of 3D computer chips and nano technologies). Thus the certainties of death in the past have been superseded by technological advances and new nursing practices (such as care of children who have a transplanted organ or tissue [Mendes-Castilo et al., 2017]).

Predicting death in people is also a very challenging, if not impossible task, yet determining prognosis and likely duration of illness and deterioration towards death are perhaps the most pressing concerns for children and their carers/families (Grinyer, 2012; Brook and Hain, 2008). Predicting death in children and during childhood is again more complex (Brook and Hain, 2008). Whereas in adulthood the process of certain illness has been studied, often conditions of childhood, which can be fatal, have attracted less attention. Lists of conditions thought to be life limiting and/or life threatening have been complied (Hain and Devins, 2014). These categorise the medical conditions using International Disease Classification (IDC10). However, the authors of this directory warn that this is not an exhaustive list, nor is it predictive of death, just of increased likelihood of a short life or of the threat of death. Given the poor predictability Grinyer (2012) has warned against clinicians attempting to make definitive prognostic predictions.

Although the predictability of prognosis is challenging, the scale of palliative care needs has been estimated and appears to be increasing (Fraser et al., 2011). In the decade 2000/01 to 2009/10 the prevalence of children living with life-limiting or life-threatening conditions increased in England from 25 per 10,000 of child population to 32 per 10,000. Fraser et al.'s (2011) work showed variation over the age range and between genders with a greater increase prevalence in boys. This work also showed a significant difference in rates in different ethnic groups in England: South Asian (48 per 10,000), Black (42 per 10,000) and Chinese, mixed and 'other' (31 per 10,000) populations compared to the White population (27 per 10,000).

The death of a child is not part of a family's scripted life story. We don't expect a child to die before their parents, as it feels as if a child's death is against the natural order of things, nor do we expect children to face grief. Professionals and people in the wider communality may also struggle to accept child death.

We will all experience grief at some time and it is important to remember that it isn't an illness but part of life.

As children's nurse we understand the needs of children and young people have social, cognitive, emotional, physical and spiritual needs and therefore understand the different approaches required to support a bereaved child and families. Not all approaches in supporting children need to be intense therapy (Fig. 6.1).

The death of every child deserves to be treated with respect and professionals have a duty to support and engage with families at all stages.

Providing bereavement support is an essential component of bereavement care delivery; however, there is currently little evidence-based guidance for health professionals and others

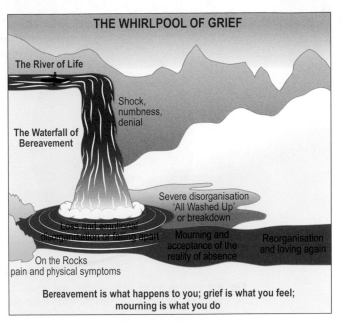

Fig. 6.1 The whirlpool of grief. (Wilson, R., 1993. Good Grief: Exploring Feelings, Loss and Death With Over Elevens and Adults. Jessica Kingsley, London.)

providing this support. Without bereavement support, parents, siblings and significant others 'are left to navigate the grief process without the support' (Thrane and Jones, 2012; Grinyer, 2012).

> **ACTIVITY**
>
> Listen to the podcast from the infinite monkey-cage debate with a friend is a strawberry alive?
> https://www.bbc.co.uk/sounds/play/b02ykcwh
> Write a short piece of reflection on the question:
> • Is severe disability in childhood a living death?

CHILDREN'S CONCEPTS OF DEATH

It has been calculated that by the time children reach 16 years old 4%–7% will have experienced the death of a relative (Talwar et al., 2011). It is generally thought that the concept of death for children contains four dimensions which are universality, irreversibility, non-functionality/cessation of life and the causality of death (Nguyen and Gelman, 2002; Yang, 2013; Vázquez-Sánchez et al., 2018). The acquisition of these concepts/dimensions is influenced by developmental process but also cultural aspects such as children's literature, schooling, family rituals and geographical location (Cox et al., 2005; Vázquez-Sánchez et al., 2018).

The analysis of drawing by Vázquez-Sánchez et al. (2018) of children in Spain aged 9–11 years showed children's understanding of causation of death. Media exposure to violent content in films and games may explain why violent and accidental death was often represented,

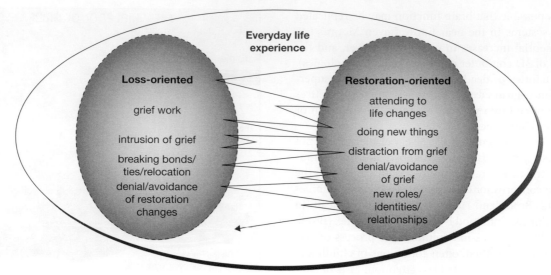

Fig. 6.2 Dual process model. (Stroebe, M.S., Schut, H., 1999. The dual process model of coping with bereavement: rationale and description. Death Studies 23 (3), 197–224.)

but children also demonstrated their understanding of illness as a cause of death in childhood. The concept of a good death was seen in these drawings in line with work by Yang (2013). Anxiety about death and understanding of metaphysical aspects were also present in these drawings by healthy children. Children's understanding of death as a concept emerges then during childhood; it is thought that around the age of 5 children begin to recognise the finality and irreversibility of death, that between 5 and around 9–10 years children's understanding of death may be influenced by experience, media exposure and cultural practice, but by 10 years most children have a more adult conception of death as irreversible, permanent and inevitable (Cox et al., 2005).

> 👤 **ACTIVITY**
>
> Read *Badgers Parting Gifts* by Susan Varley (or watch video https://www.youtube.com/watch?time_continue=56&v=tR-TRABhJTbo)
>   Discuss with students in your group:
> - What ideas about death are portrayed in the book or video?
> - What emotions/ mood is conveyed in this work in particular about Badger's death?
> - How could you use this book or video with children and their carers?

THEORIES OF GRIEF IN CHILD LOSS

When considering the context and factors that impact upon grief reactions, it is important to consider holistic perspectives. Child death, loss of a child and bereavement is understood differently in different communities (Hedayat, 2006). Recent developments in grief theory recognise that human diversity accounts for both risk factors and coping styles. However,

it is also essential that the differences between the loss of a child and other types of bereavement are acknowledged, as child loss carries an increased risk for the development of complicated grief and will impact on the coping strategies of parents (Rossetto, 2015). Early theorist on grief and bereavement suggested that grief is a staged process through which people move to an eventual resolution (Kubler-Ross, 1970; Parkes, 1975) as might be seen in Fig. 6.1. Moving though the whirlpool might involve certain tasks as suggested by Worden (2008). Firstly to accept the reality of the loss, second to work through the pain of grief. Then to adjust to life without the deceased person and finally to develop and maintain a connection to the deceased person while moving on with life.

As an alternative to the linear stage-based model, Stroebe and Schut (1999, 2010) developed a dual process model of bereavement (Fig. 6.2). They identified two tasks associated with bereavement which are loss and restoration. Bereaved people attempt to perform their 'everyday' lives while dealing with loss-orientated and restoration-orientated activities.

There has been a movement away from the idea that successful grieving requires 'letting go', with writers such as Klass et al. (1996) offering an alternate approach, where they argue that after a death bonds with the deceased do not necessarily have to be severed, and that there is a potentially healthy role for maintaining continuing bonds with the deceased.

Patterns of grief are variable for some resilient individuals, significant grief may be limited to a few weeks (Bonanno and Kaltman, 2001); for most people the acute experience of grief subsides over time. For a sub-group of people, around 10%–15%, the symptoms of distress following the death of a family member or friend are more intense and persistent (Prigerson et al., 2009). Failure to find meaning in, or make sense of the death over a lengthy period of time is associated with more complicated grief. Intense search for meaning is more likely when the death is unexpected or untimely, for example the sudden death of a child (Neimeyer and Burke, 2012).

With all the different approaches to grief theory it is important to reassure the bereaved that what they are experiencing is 'normal'. Lindemann (1944) explored the difference between pathological (complicated) and normal (uncomplicated) grief reactions. The 'normal' reactions as classed as follows:

Feelings: numbness, sadness, anger, guilt, anxiety, despair, loneliness, powerlessness, relief

Physical sensations: shock, fatigue, hollow stomach, aching limbs, dry mouth, breathlessness

Thoughts: disbelief, confusion, disorientation, obsessional preoccupation, visual/auditory hallucinations

Behaviours: sleep disturbance, lack of appetite, absent-mindedness, crying, sighing, over activity, searching, visiting the grave

What Is Unique About a Death of a Child? Parental Grief

Acceptance of grief can be a difficult concept for parents; some consciously (or unconsciously) hold on to the intensity of early grief as a mark of loyalty to their child. That is why it is important to reassure them of the continuing bonds with their child. As previously mentioned Lindemann (1944) that describing patterns of grief reactions can be reassuring, particularly for those who are grieving for the first time. In terms of most grief theories the loss of a child would be defined as complicated grief or prolonged grief disorder. This condition can be associated with severe mental and physical health problems such as insomnia, substance misuse, depression, depressed immune function, hypertension, cardiac problems, cancer, suicide, and work and social impairment. Bereaved people in this cohort report higher use of medical services and more frequent hospitalisation than people with similar losses whose grief is less intense and of shorter duration. These effects have been observed for between 4 and 9 years after the death (Neimeyer and Burke, 2012). Stroebe et al. (2007) identify the range as varying from 9% to 20% in an adult population to over 50% in those who had lost a child. Lannen et al. (2008) indicate that 'unresolved grief' in parents who have lost a child to cancer report significantly worsening psychological and physical health including sleep disturbance and greater use of medical care and sick leave.

Most bereaved parents will turn to family, friends and their local communities for support and will not necessarily need the input of health professionals. Where parents seek added support however, this may be in the form of emotional support (consoling demonstrating empathy), information support (advice or guidance say on registering a death) and practical support (arranging a visit from an undertaker or religious leader to discuss funeral arrangements). Support may be provided formally or informally through counselling, support groups, or the provision of literature. Professionals who have known the family and the child who has died can assist them to; accept the reality of the loss and work through the pain of grief so that they can start to adjust to the environment in which the deceased is missing, renegotiate the relationship with the deceased child such that it continues albeit in a different way. 'Letting go' of the relationship with the deceased is not a requirement. Bereaved individuals are able to maintain bonds with the dead person by remembering them, talking about them and sometimes talking to them.

Children's nurses can provide support to bereaved parents by:

* maintaining a presence if that is the family's wish
* providing comfort
* acknowledging what has happened
* acknowledging the emotions the parents are experiencing
* normalising these emotions
* listening to parent's stories sympathetically and non-judgementally

It is important to state that families will differ in their preferred means of support. Some will just want to be left alone. Others might want to share their feelings quite openly. In some cases, no one individual or health discipline can meet all the family's needs in terms of providing bereavement support.

Health professionals need to recognise the significance they may have in a family's life. Many children are treated over long periods of time and the hospital may become something of a second home. Health professionals also care for families during the intense highs and lows of serious illness and may even be present at the time the child dies. The significance of this cannot be overstated. These relationships cannot be abruptly ended and many (but not all) families will want ongoing contact with people they feel truly understand what they have experienced. A follow-up appointment with the child's paediatrician should always be offered to discuss the child's illness and treatment, the results of any outstanding investigations including postmortem examinations and how the family is coping. This is an opportunity to address ongoing concerns, normalise feelings associated with grief, provide advice on how to support siblings and offer information on potential sources of support for the family should they require it. Parents almost universally find these meetings helpful although it may be difficult for them to return to the hospital. They may therefore need a number of opportunities to respond to invitations to attend. Clinicians who write to families and then follow up with a telephone call appear to have greater success in achieving a meeting with families. Some paediatricians may feel they are intruding on a family by telephoning, but most parents will appreciate this gesture of ongoing support. A social worker may be very helpful in facilitating this process.

The ideal timing of such a follow-up visit is unknown. However, many bereaved parents state that it is after the time of the funeral (6 weeks to 3 months after the death) when the loss is felt more severely. Many of the practical tasks required up to that point will have been completed and family and friends have returned to their own lives, leaving the bereaved parent to feel abandoned (Grinyer, 2012).

The issue of whether or not to acknowledge the anniversary of the child's death may cause staff concern. In general, families appreciate some sort of contact at this time. As described earlier, doctors, nurses and social workers have cared for the family at a time of great significance and families will generally appreciate knowing they are in the thoughts of those staff members.

For all bereaved individuals, grief is experienced in the context of their 'whole being', including their physical, emotional, cognitive, behavioural and spiritual manifestations. When grief is complicated and prolonged, evidence suggests that intervention is both indicated and effective (Currier et al., 2008). However, the available evidence suggests that only a minority of people will require specialist bereavement interventions and that for the remainder, intervention is not effective. With the loss of a child, bereaved parents more commonly fall into the first group. Therefore, targeting scarce resources for people who will benefit most from them is important.

Parents should be informed of expected follow-up contacts such as regular scheduled phone calls and letters. In-person meetings should be offered, especially if there is a postmortem examination.

Strategies to facilitate follow-up bereavement support by staff include having condolence notes in the Emergency Department (ED) so that caregivers may complete the notes close to the time of death or at a later time and can then be mailed out as scheduled. Completing condolence letters not only helps the family feel connection with the personnel who cared for their child, but also helps the staff feel a sense of closure (Thrane and Jones, 2012). A bereavement checklist can facilitate coordination of bereavement efforts (O'Malley et al., 2014).

Corden, et al. (2002) have also undertaken some work on the financial consequences of a child's death. The resultant financial impact was that families would lose child benefit, and if paid, disability living allowance and invalid care allowance. Reduction of income of 14% occurred in highest earning families and a reduction of 25% of net monthly income for two-parent middle income households. This was increased to a reduction of 72% for single mothers (single parent households are usually mothers). In addition, they had to pay for funerals, although they could use Social Fund assistance for this. There was also, specifically after a period of caring for the dying child, difficulty in reengaging with work and subsequent gaps in National Insurance and other contributions. The work also highlights the psychological impacts of the immediate loss of finance and how support might be offered to address financial issues with the possibility of continuation of payments for a period of time. Randall's analysis of the financial implications of living with the dual possibility of continued care for a child with a life limiting/threatening condition, often with severe disability, and a future where a child dies, showed the complexity of living with the two futures (Randall, 2017). Families in this study spoke of losing their livelihoods, transport and homes, as well as the impact on siblings when a child dies:

> *There isn't an end date on anybody's life but equally we have to prepare for two futures. We lose the house, we lose the car very quickly and that's the reason we've got our own dog and not a working dog from someone else because if the dog was under eight we'd have to give it back and I don't think the other two would cope very well with losing the house, the car, the dog and their sister at the same time*
>
> **Female Participant 16 (Randall, 2017)**

 ACTIVITY

> Write a short reflection on a child that you have looked after and their carers who live with a life-limiting condition. What might be the effects on parents of living with this child?
>   Share and discuss your reflection with colleagues.
> • What social and practical assistance is there for bereaved parents in your area?

Siblings, Grief

Bereaved siblings have been identified as the 'forgotten mourners' as they adjust to the loss of the sibling relationship and the broader changes in parenting and family dynamics as a result of the loss. Some important questions to consider when working with bereaved children and their families are seen in Fig. 6.3. Not all families are open in their communication. We might consider the ACT 2011 approaches as described by Grinyer (2012) which includes four possible approaches:

Closed awareness. Where children are not included and others who know about the illness/death conceal it.

Suspected awareness. The child is aware something is wrong but not certain what is happening, not included by others who are aware.

Mutual pretence. The child and others are all aware, but no one talks about the illness/death or acknowledges it.

Open awareness. Everyone knows and talks openly/acknowledges the illness and or death.

These approaches can also be seen in parents and other carers in communication with health professionals and children when a child lives with a life-limiting/threatening condition. Nurses need to be mindful that they have a public duty to be honest and truthful, but that how communication is facilitated can be crucial to establishing and maintain relationships. It is possible to not only be open, honest and truthful with children, but also respectful of people's cultural, religious and personal preferences, as well as mindful of how people process information. All of the 'truth' all at once may be too much for people to understand, and cause more distress than inform. However, children's nurses do have a duty to help parents and children to deal with death. It may be useful to discuss how children can sense emotional atmospheres and understand changes in families' lives from very young ages. For some children sensing these things in their family and not receiving an explanation can lead them to feel they have done something wrong, are to be punished' or they may invent other explanations. Open and honest communication about death can be positive, and help children to cope with life changes and death. This is not to deny the challenging emotional work required by parents and other carers (including nurses) when talking to children about the sadness people feel at losing a person. Children need to know why others in the family are sad. Children must be told that it is the death that has made their family members sad. Without an explanation, children may think the sadness is caused by something that they did or said. Start by saying '... A very, very sad thing has happened ...' or 'Mummy and Daddy are sad because ...'.

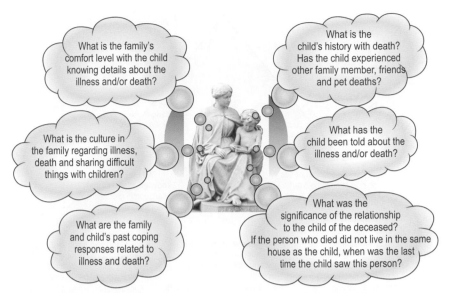

Fig. 6.3 Questions to consider when working with bereaved children.

Modelling of sad feelings and behaviours lets children know that it's okay to be sad. Children also need to be taught that people express sadness in different ways (i.e. some may cry, some may want alone time, some may share more than others) and these happen at different times for different people and all of this is OK.

Children's Understanding of Death

As discussed earlier, children's conceptions of death changes during the course of childhood. The Alder centre has drawn up some helpful guidance on the needs of children at various ages, used here with kind permission. It should be remembered that age in childhood is a useful, but approximate measure and individual difference should also be considered.

All bereaved children and young people have the need for information, explanation and reassurance (Level 1, Irish childhood bereavement pyramid [Fig. 6.4]). Depending on their personalities, the circumstances of the death, family functioning and a child's stage of development, there may be additional needs. These include a need for help with normalising the experience (Level 2); a need for extra help with feelings or behaviours that are disrupting day to day life (Level 3) or for a very small number, needs which include addressing suicidal thoughts/behaviour and other clinical issues (Level 4). Another key factor to keep in mind is the resilience of the bereaved child. Resilience refers to the child's approach to control in their lives and their sense of hope about the future. Those with a strong sense of resilience believe that they can control their fates by their own actions. Research has shown that bereaved children may have a stronger belief that their lives are controlled by external factors and therefore developing the skills and coping strategies they need to deal with their bereavement may be more of a challenge. It can be helpful if bereavement support promotes that sense of resilience or mastery in the child.

Some children may develop bereavement responses that cannot be met by Level 1 support and will require additional support.

This will be influenced by key factors which can include:
- Reaction and coping style of parent/parents and other family members – a family that is coping well will be a better support for a child.
- The beliefs exhibited by parents or others about grieving, for example silence – 'we don't talk about our loss' or exclusion – 'children don't need to be included in rituals etc.'
- Child's developmental age – which may differ from chronological age.
- Child's relationship to the deceased – loss of someone close and familiar impacts on all parts of life and routine and may hurt more.
- Circumstances of the death – sudden, traumatic deaths can be more difficult to process, but this is not always the case and can be influenced by the developmental stage of the child and the reaction of the adults around them.
- Effect on the family unit – need to move house, change school, lose friends and for people with less resources such changes can be very difficult.
- Level of self-esteem/self-worth – some children have greater resilience than others. Bereavement responses should be contextualised in relation to the factors leading up to the death, the family circumstance and other day-to-day aspects of the child's life.
- Childs culture/belief systems – this can be different for every child and may differ from the cultural practice and beliefs of the family and or community.

These factors at Level 2 or 3 it may be considered for a child where they are exhibiting some of the reactions identified earlier (Table 6.1A–D). While symptoms such as

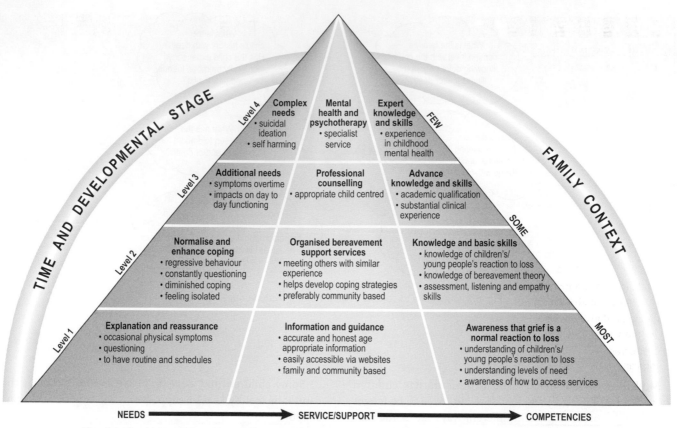

Fig. 6.4 The Irish childhood bereavement care pyramid. (Irish Childhood Bereavement Network, 2018. The Irish Childhood Bereavement Care Pyramid. Available from: https://www.childhoodbereavement.ie/wp-content/uploads/2018/05/ICBN-PYRAMID-OL.jpg.)

separation distress, depression, anxiety, behavioural issues and social withdrawal are, to some degree, aspects of the usual response to bereavement in childhood, these do not necessarily lead to psychological or pathological problems. Bereavement itself does not significantly increase the risk for psychiatric disorder in children. However, research has found that there are particular circumstances where the usual resources of child/family can be overwhelmed. In these situations, the child or family struggle to deal adequately with the demands created by the death and its aftermath. This is particularly relevant in cases of suicide and traumatic death.

In the following scenarios some bereaved children may require extra support (Levels 3–4):
- Parental death following divorce/separation or parental mental illness
- Death from inherited and transmitted conditions
- Difference (e.g. living in a different cultural context)
- Pre-existing mental health issues (in the child)

Children obviously need help and support around the time of bereavement, but children may need to revisit their bereavement and 're-negotiate' their loss in the context of their changing cognitive abilities.

In the main, children adjust to the bereavements that they experience in life within the context of their family and community, but a good understanding of their needs and reactions is essential to their support. Those who care for them need to understand and respond to 'normal' grief in order to identify the possibility of situations where children may develop maladaptive behaviours.

 ACTIVITY

You have cared for Darren over a number of years on the children's medical ward of a local hospital. He lived with Duchene muscular dystrophy diagnosed when he was 7 years old. Darren has died at age 13, after a short respiratory illness. He was a lively and active boy with a huge social media following. His parents and teachers would like you to talk to his classmates in his local secondary school about how they might be feeling and normal grief reactions as they cope with losing Darren.

Plan a session to deliver to the class:
- Consider what you might do if you become aware of delayed or complex bereavement issues as you talk to the young people.
- What preparation might be needed by the teachers, children and school community?

TABLE 6.1A   Ages and Grief Reactions: 3–6 Years

Child Development	Grief Reactions	Therefore Children Need
Literal, concrete thinking	Confused by ambiguous statements/ euphemisms	To be told, repeatedly, the dead person is not coming back
Memory not developed	Psychosomatic symptoms, e.g. tummy ache, headache	To be told simple, brief, clear, honest facts repeatedly
Believe what they are told, fact and fantasy confused	Talk about events to imaginary friends – using imagination to fill in missing facts	Questions answered in a brief, straightforward, concrete way. No euphemisms – e. g. gone to sleep
Thinking moves from specific to general	Make unrelated connections, e.g. Dad died from head injury: I have a headache = I will die	As time goes on, to be given more information appropriate to their age/understanding
Difficulty taking viewpoint of others	Eating/sleep problems, nightmares – fear of monsters/dark	To be reassured they are not to blame for what happened
Communication based on direct experience – unable to make sense of experience	Regressive behaviour – baby talk, tantrums, clinginess, bed wetting	To be given lots of love, cuddles, sympathy, reassurance and support
Imitate others; learning to trust, forming basic attachments	Fear of separation and abandonment	To be reassured they'll still be looked after, cared for and loved
Egocentric thinking – view world from own perspective	Act out their thoughts and feelings in play	Their routine maintained and consistent boundaries given
Hard to verbalise thoughts, feelings and experiences	Difficulty putting their thoughts and feelings about events into words	To be provided with safe ways to express their thoughts/feelings
Not emotionally/cognitively able to understand/cope with events or make sense of experience	React casually to loss because of games/ cartoons where person is not really dead	Opportunities to: say goodbye; remember the person who has died; make the death 'real'

TABLE 6.1B   Ages and Grief Reactions: 6–9 Years

Child Development	Grief Reactions	Therefore Children Need
Think logically	Confusion if given ambiguous statements/ euphemisms	To be told simple, brief, honest facts about the death
Criticism or failure hard to manage	Psychosomatic symptoms, e.g. tummy ache, headache	Questions answered in a brief, straightforward, concrete way
Begin to use words to express thoughts and feelings	Concerned about separation from, or safety of/death of remaining family members/self	As time goes on, to be given more information appropriate to their age and understanding
Important being part of a group	Eating/sleep problems – nightmares, sleepwalking	To be asked if they wish to be involved in decisions
Magical thinking	Think their words/actions caused the death to happen	To be reassured they are not to blame for what happened
Increasingly independent	Regressive behaviour – tantrums, clinginess, bedwetting	To be given lots of love, cuddles and sympathy
Developing ability to reason	Morbid curiosity about causes/physical process of death	To be given permission to play, relax and have fun
Problem solve, question and observe	Frustration if can't find words to express themselves – leads to temper/aggression/ withdrawal	Their grief heard – and held – it is normal to feel shocked, angry, upset and guilty
Developing a conscience, a moral sense	Suicidal thoughts – join dead person/survivor guilt	To be provided with safe ways to express their thoughts and feelings
Begin to understand the other person's perspective	Good behaviour to make amends, bring loved one back or to please adults	Opportunities to: say goodbye; remember the person who has died; make the death 'real'

TABLE 6.1C   Ages and Grief Reactions: 9–12 Years

Child Development	Grief Reactions	Therefore Children Need
More advanced verbal and cognitive skills – work things out for themselves	Conflict with carers if feel not given all the information	To be given concrete facts about the death – questions answered in a brief, straightforward way
Want to be responsible for own actions/decisions	Psychosomatic symptoms, e.g., tummy ache, headache	To be asked if they wish to be involved in decisions but not burdened with responsibilities
View things as black/white, right/wrong, wonderful/terrible	Concerned about separation from, or safety of/death of remaining family members/self	Opportunities to talk at an appropriate time to a trusted family member/close friend
Easily influenced by peers	Eating/sleep problems, nightmares	To talk but not in front of friends – don't like to be different
Begin to reflect on own experience	Think their words/actions caused the death to happen	To be reassured they are not to blame for what happened
Independent	Regressive behaviour – childish talk, clinginess	To be given lots of love, cuddles, sympathy balanced with space
Begin to be self-aware and self-conscious	Lack of concentration; spends time on own, daydreams	To be given permission to play, relax and have fun
Begin to react against authority	Withdrawn and/or aggressive – refuses to cooperate	Their grief heard/held – normal to feel shocked/angry/upset/guilty
Early puberty often brings on 'teenage' problems	Suicidal thoughts – join dead person/survivor guilt	To be provided with safe ways to express thoughts and feelings
Want to be given responsibilities	Good behaviour to make amends, bring loved one back or to please adults	Opportunities to: say goodbye; remember the person who has died; make the death 'real'

TABLE 6.1D   Ages and Grief Reactions: Teenagers

Child Development	Grief Reactions	Therefore Children Need
Thinking changes from concrete to abstract, able to reflect on situations	Seek dangerous experiences in order to gain control over death/court death themselves	To be given facts about the death and questions answered in an appropriate way
Emotionally drained as they develop separate sense of identity	Psychosomatic symptoms, eating disorders, depression, sleep problems	To be involved in decisions, to cooperate with adults but not burdened with responsibilities
Become concerned about the future/unknown	Concerned about separation from, or safety of/death of remaining family members/self	Opportunities to talk at an appropriate time to a trusted family member/close friend
Want to be responsible for their own actions/decisions	Put grief on hold because of academic pressure – exams	To be allowed to talk/grieve in their own time, in their own way
Peer pressure and group identity predominate	Sense of omnipotence undermined, become vulnerable	To be reassured they are not to blame for what happened
Time of biological, emotional, psychological, social change	Regressive behaviour – needy, clinging – but also adolescents	To be given lots of love, cuddles, sympathy balanced with space
Ask 'big' questions about life and death	Protect parents/adult carers (parenting the parents)	To be given permission to go out, relax and have fun
Difficulties re: communicating with parents/carers	Mood swings – even more than normal!	Their grief heard/held – normal to feel shocked/angry/upset/guilty
React against authority	Lack of concentration – spends time on own, daydreams	To be provided with safe ways to express thoughts and feelings
Develop self-concept, self-esteem; become self-conscious	Good behaviour to make amends, bring loved one back or to please adults	Opportunities to: say goodbye; remember the person who has died; make the death 'real'

Alder Centre, see: https://aldercentre.org.uk/bereavement-care-services. Used by kind permission.

SUMMARY

In many cultures death remains a taboo subject and death in childhood especially so. Technological advances in the late 20th century mean that we have the technical ability to sustain life. The lack of discussion in communities about death and death in childhood and the perception that modern medicine can and should be able to prevent children dying has led to high media profile cases in which families and communities and health care professionals have been in conflict over how to deal with dying and death in children. Many people argue that the duration of a life is less important than the quality of that life. Some children and some parents will have to cope as best they can with loss of a loved one. How people react to such a loss is highly dependent on their circumstances, existing mental and physical conditions and the cultural and religious beliefs. Most people will learn with time to accept their loss and develop a relationship with those who have died. Some people will need extra help and support to deal with complex or delayed grief and this may affect children as well as adults.

Although death in childhood remains a contested, challenging and emotional issue what we can be certain of is that when children are with us they are children with the same needs of love, play and learning. Those that leave us are never truly gone for they live in our memories.

REFERENCES

Academy of Medical Royal Colleges (2008) A code of practice for the diagnosis and confirmation of death available from file:///F:/2T%20Storage/documents/RCM%202008%20Code_Practice_Confirmation_Diagnosis_Death_1008-4.pdf.

Bonanno, G.A., Kaltman, S., 2001. The varieties of grief experience. Clinical Psychology Review 20, 1–30.

Brook, L., Hain, R., 2008. Predicting death in children. Archives of Disease in Childhood 93, 1067–1070.

Corden, A., Sainsbury, R., Sloper, P., 2002. When a child dies: money matters. Illness, Crisis and Loss 10 (2), 125–137.

Cox, M., Garrett, E., Graham, J.A., 2005. Death in Disney films: implications for children's understanding of death. Journal of Death and Dying 50 (4), 267–280.

Currier, J.M., Neimeyer, R.A., Berman, J.S., 2008. The effectiveness of psychotherapeutic interventions for bereaved persons: a comprehensive quantitative review. Psychological Bulletin 134, 648–661.

Dewy, J., 1944. Democracy and Education: An Introduction to the Philosophy of Education. The Free Press. Simon & Schuster Inc., New York.

Fraser, L.K., Miller, M., Aldridge, J., 2012. Life-limiting and life-threatening conditions in children and young people in the United Kingdom; national and regional prevalence in relation to socioeconomic status and ethnicity. Final Report for Children's Hospice UK October 2011. University of Leeds, Leeds. Available from: https://www.togetherforshortlives.org.uk/wp-content/uploads/2018/01/ExRes-Childrens-Hospices-Ethnicity-Report-Leeds-Uni.pdf.

Grinyer, A., 2012. Palliative and End of Life Care for Children and Young People: Home, Hospice and Hospital. Wiley-Blackwell, Chichester.

Hain, R., Devins, M., 2014. Directory of Life-Limiting Conditions, vol. 1.3. Available from: https://www.togetherforshortlives.org.uk/wp-content/uploads/2018/01/ExRes-Directory-of-Life-Limiting-Conditions.pdf.

Hedayat, K., 2006. When the spirit leaves: Childhood death, grieving and bereavement in Islam. Journal of Palliative Medicine 9 (6), 1282–1291.

Kelly, D.A., 2015. Liver and biliary disease in childhood. Medicine 43 (11), 631–635.

Klass, D., Silverman, P.R., Nickman, S.L. (Eds.), 1996. Continuing Bonds: New Understanding of Grief. Taylor and Francis, Washington.

Kubler-Ross, E., 1970. On Death and Dying. Macmillan, New York.

Irish Childhood Bereavement Network, 2018. The Irish Childhood Bereavement Care Pyramid. Available from: https://www.childhoodbereavement.ie/wp-content/uploads/2018/05/ICBN-PYRAMID-OL.jpg.

Lannen, P.K., Wolfe, J., Prigerson, H.G., et al., 2008. Unresolved grief in a national sample of bereaved parents: Impaired mental and physical health 4 to 9 years later. Journal of Clinical Oncology 26 (36), 5870–5876.

Lindemann, E., 1944. Symptomatology and management of acute grief. American Journal of Psychiatry 101 (3), 141–149.

O'Malley, P., Barata, I., Snow, S., American Academy of Pediatrics Committee on Pediatric Emergency Medicine, Emergency Nurses Association Pediatric Committee, and The College of Emergency Physicians Pediatric Emergency Medicine Committee, 2014. Death of a child in the emergency department. Pediatrics 134, e313–e330.

Maslach-Hubbard, A., Bratton, S.L., 2013. Extracorporeal membrane oxygenation for pediatric respiratory failure: history, development and current status. World Journal of Critical Care Medicine 2 (4), 29–39.

Mendes-Castio, A.M.C., Bousso, R.S., Sloand, E., 2017. The family management styles framework as a toll of tailoring interventions for pediatric transplant recipients and their families: a case study. Comprehensive Child and Adolescent Nursing 40 (1), 39–52.

Neimeyer, R.A., Burke, L.A., 2012. Complicated grief and the end-of-life: risk factors and treatment considerations. In: Werth, J.L. (Ed.), Clients Near the End-of-Life: A Practical Guide for Mental Health Professionals. Springer, New York (2103).

Nguyen, S.P., Gelman, S.A., 2002. Four and 6 year olds biological concept of death: the case of plants. British Journal of Developmental Psychology 20, 495–513.

Parkes, C.M., 1975. Determinants of outcome following bereavement. Omega 61, 303–323.

Prigerson, H.G., Horowitz, M.J., Jacobs, S.C., et al., 2009. Prolonged grief disorder: psychometric validation of criteria proposed for *DSM-V* and *ICD-11*. PLOS Med 6 (8), e1000121. https://doi.org/10.1371/journal.pmed.1000121.

Randall, D., 2017. Two futures: financial and practical realities for parents of living with a child who has a life-limiting or threatening condition. Comprehensive Child and Adolescent Nursing 40 (4), 257–267. https://doi.org/10.1080/24694193.2017.1376360.

Rossetto, K.R., 2015. Bereaved parents' strategies and reactions when supporting their surviving children. Western Journal of Communication 79 (5), 533–554.

Shaw, K.L., Brook, L., Mpundu-Kaambwa, C., Harris, N., Lapwood, S., Randall, D., 2015. The spectrum of children's palliative care needs: A classification framework for children with life-limiting or life-threatening conditions. BMJ Support and Palliative Care 5 (3), 249–258.

Stroebe, M., Schut, H., 1999. The dual process model of coping with bereavement: rationale and description. Death Studies 23 (3), 197–224.

Stroebe M and Schut H (2010) The dual process model of coping with bereavement: A decade on Journal of Death and Dying 61(4) 273–289.

Stroebe, M., Schut, H., Stroebe, W., 2007. Health outcomes of bereavement. Lancet 370, 1960–1973.

Thrane, S., Jones, B., 2012. Communication with families after the death of a child. Journal of Hospice and Palliative Nursing: JHPN: The Official Journal of the Hospice and Palliative Nurses Association 14 (1), 6–10.

Talwar, V., Harris, P.L., Scheleifer, M., 2011. Children's Understanding of Death: From Biological to Religious Conceptions. Cambridge University Press, New York.

Vázquez-Sánchez, J.M., Fernández-Alcántara, M., García-Caro, M.P., 2018. The concept of death in children aged from 9 to 11 years: Evidences through inductive and deductive analysis of drawings. Death Studies 43 (8), 467–477.

Wilson, R., 1993. Good Grief: Exploring Feelings, Loss and Death With Over Elevens and Adults. Jessica Kingsley, London.

Worden, J.W., 2008. Grief Counseling and Grief Therapy: A Handbook for the Mental Health Practitioner, fourth ed. Springer, New York.

Yang, S.C., 2013. Assessment and quantification of Taiwanese children's views of a good death. Omega: Journal of Death and Dying 66 (1), 17.

USEFUL RESOURCES

Department of Health, 2005. When a Patient Dies: Advice on Developing Bereavement Services in the NHS. DH, London.

Murray, J.A., 2001. Loss as a universal concept: A review of the literature to identify common aspects of loss in diverse situations. Journal of Loss and Trauma 6, 219–241.

Neuberger, J., 2004. Dying Well: A Guide to Enabling a Good Death. Radcliffe Press, Oxford.

American Academy of Pediatrics Committee on Pediatric Emergency Medicine, 2014. American College of Emergency Physicians Pediatric Emergency Medicine Committee, Emergency Nurses Association Pediatric Committee. Death of a child in the emergency department. Pediatrics 134 (1), 198–201.

Cochran, D., Saleem, S., Khowaja-Punjwani, S., Lantos, J.D., 2017. Cross-cultural differences in communication about a dying child. Pediatrics 140 (5), e20170690 pii.

Falkenburg, J.L., Tibboel, D., Ganzevoort, R.R., et al., 2016. Parental physical proximity in end-of-life care in the PICU. Pediatr. Crit. Care Med. 17 (5), e212–217.

7

Ethical and Legal Aspects of Child Health Care

Louise M. Terry, Jim Richardson

LEARNING OUTCOMES

- Achieve an overview of the major ethical and legal principles in child health care.
- Recognise how these principles can be applied in everyday children's and young people's nursing and how they impact on the well-being of children and their families.

- Appreciate dimensions surrounding some current ethico-legal debates in relation to clinical practice and research involving children.
- To understand consent issues.
- To appreciate what a 'duty of care' entails and to reflect on the impact and consequences of negligence.

INTRODUCTION

This chapter will explore aspects of legal and ethical issues in relation to the nursing care of children and young people. The law of the land must be obeyed and anyone who does not will have to answer for this, ultimately in a court. The law in relation to children is complex and seeks always to protect the best interests of the child within a family context. In order to facilitate an understanding of how the law governs the delivery of health care to children and young people, key principles will be identified and examined. As the law is constantly evolving to meet changes in society, it will be important for professionals to continue to be familiar with current requirements. Ethical issues are subsidiary to the law, but new interpretations arising from ethical debates may also feed into law making. Ethics is concerned with examining what is right and wrong or appropriate in the circumstances. Consideration of the United Nations Convention on the Rights of the Child (1989) will be used as a framework to help develop an understanding of subtle and sometimes challenging situations, which can arise in practice. This element is made even more interesting by the rich range of beliefs and values found within a modern multicultural society. Overall, this chapter will explore principles of law and ethics in relation to real-life clinical nursing practice and examples for practice will be used to illustrate these.

THE UN CONVENTION ON THE RIGHTS OF THE CHILD AND *THE HUMAN RIGHTS ACT (1998)*

The General Assembly of the United Nations adopted the convention on the Rights of the Child in November 1989; this came into force in the UK in January 1992. The vast majority of the world's nations have ratified this Convention and the document is intended to be applicable to a range of very different countries and contexts. This sometimes makes some of the articles seem a little less relevant to the UK context. However, closer examination will show that this is not, in fact, the case. For example, the article which prohibits the kidnap of children is actually relevant to those children who are removed from the UK against their will by a parent who is a second country national or those children who are removed from the UK for the purposes of forced marriage. The document is based on a number of articles which lay down the rights of any person under the age of 18. These rights protect the child and young person and require that others, individuals, organisations and states observe their duty to protect children and promote their rights. Each of these rights can be classified into three categories:

(i) Protection – these articles are concerned with protecting children and young people from harm. It must be clear that harm is not just a physical issue but might also be psychological, social or cultural damage. For example, to deprive a child of education negatively affects their life chances and their ability to reach their maximal potential.

(ii) Participation – in these articles the objective is to ensure that the child and young people's voice is heard in relation to matters which affect them. One of the Children's Commissioners made it a priority to lobby for better toilet conditions in schools. This was mocked in the media as trivial, but arose directly from what school children wanted. This demonstrated that the children were actually listened to, and their concerns about their experience of school taken into account.

(iii) Promotion – this aspect of the Convention seeks to enhance the role and image of children and childhood in society. This will help to engage young people in the active role of being a citizen. There can be a tendency to stereotype young people as illustrated by the recent debate about the 'snowflake generation'. Positive developments in this area include the current discussion about reducing the voting age in the UK from age 18 to age 16 years.

WWW

You can access the UN Convention at:
- https://www.unhcr.org/uk/protection/children/50f941fe9/united-nations-convention-rights-child-crc.html

ACTIVITY

Read through the summary of the Convention on the Rights of the Child. Make notes against each article on its relevance to:
(1) clinical children's and young people's nursing practice, and
(2) clinical research involving children.

When you have done this, consider to what extent the requirements of these two fields of practice differ from each other in their ethical requirements.

UN Committee on the Rights of the Child State's Report (2016) and Activity

The Human Rights Act of 1998, which came into effect on 2 October 2000, highlighted the potential of some areas of health and social care practice to affect the rights and freedoms promised under the Act. Power (2002) discusses Article 3, among others of the Act, which relates to torture and degrading treatment or punishment and highlights the implications for child health nurses, especially when restraining children for health care interventions.

WWW

You can find the text of the *Human Rights Act* at:
- https://www.legislation.gov.uk/ukpga/1998/42/contents

The implementation of these policies is beginning to make an impact on the way in which children are cared for in hospital and the Child Friendly Hospital Initiative spearheaded by UNICEF has been embraced by a number of children's hospitals in the UK, such as The Royal Hospital For Sick Children Glasgow.

WWW

You can find details of the Child Friendly Hospital initiative at:
- http://www.childfriendlyhealthcare.org

THE FOUR PRINCIPLES OF HEALTH CARE ETHICS

Although the Nursing and Midwifery Council (NMC) Code of Professional Conduct (NMC, 2015) provides explicit guidance on consent for all nurses, Section 3.9 discusses children in particular. Additionally, the Royal College of Nursing (RCN) has issued guidelines for nurses involved with research (RCN, 2018). These and other guidelines implicitly or explicitly use the four principles of health care ethics first proposed by Beauchamp and Childress in 1979. The British Medical Association (BMA, 2010) published a Toolkit to support consent, rights and choices with children and young people.

1. Autonomy

The primary interpretation of this word is self-determination. The complexity of this concept is increased by its link with liberty. Personal liberty, although a common value of Western life, may have different value in other countries and other social groups, where decisions may be made by a group, such as a family, rather than espousing individual rights. Autonomy and childhood have in the past been perceived as mutually exclusive, but there is now a growing awareness that children are able to make their own decisions if given information in an age-appropriate manner (BMA, 2010).

When the term 'autonomy' is applied to contemporary health care practice and research the focus is on the right to informed consent (Behi, 1995). Although every individual has this right, it must be appreciated that some, but especially children, may not be able to articulate this or may be prevented from doing so. When this conveniently matches the decision of the health care professional or guardian, this inclusion in decision making is seen as an example of good practice. When it does not, the rights of the child may be diluted on the basis that adults know best. Although this paternalistic approach within both treatment and research is in decline, competent children remain a group whose rights to consent or refuse consent are easy to overlook.

In the case of younger, pre-autonomous children, respect for autonomy is shown by ensuring that parents agree to give proxy consent to treatment and research. The cases detailed below demonstrate the loving commitment of parents to the well-being of their child and their deep sense of betrayal if their child is harmed by health professionals.

Another element of autonomy which needs to be considered is that of where parents are exercising autonomy on behalf of their children who do not have the competence themselves to exercise autonomy. This does not pose a problem when parents and professionals are working together to promote the best interests of their child. However, recently, there have been a number of cases where a child has had a severe and complex health problem that is likely to be life-limiting, yet the parents want to continue all curative measures which the health professionals judge to be futile; therefore a palliative approach would be better, in the health professional's opinion. In these challenging situations, it is important that the nurse can navigate between the natural wishes of the parents to preserve the life of their child who is often technology dependent but which is not in accord with the judgment of health care and legal professionals who focus on the child and have identified that there is no possibility of improvement or recovery and the child is suffering distress and pain. In these charged situations proposals to withdraw life-sustaining equipment to allow the child to die naturally are highly contested and then a legal decision is sought and enacted. In this context, these families will need highly skilled nursing care, as whatever the decision made there is no question of care being withdrawn. This will continue until the child's death and beyond.

2. Beneficence

Beneficence means the duty to do good to others, to act in their best interests. However, if this principle was universal and we were required always to do good to everyone, the duty would be too onerous. Beneficence is a constituent part of a special duty of care such as that which exists between a nurse and patient or between a parent and child (Charles-Edwards, 1995).

One of the ambiguities at the heart of health care is the duty to act in the patient's best interests, while avoiding the danger of following only the principle of beneficence and ignoring that of autonomy – 'the doctor knows best' phenomenon. The contemporary insistence that patient (and parent) must be given an informed choice attests to this and to the anachronism of paternalistic attitudes: 'Partnership between patient and healthcare professional is the way forward' (Kennedy, 2001, p 13).

3. Non-Maleficence

Florence Nightingale is reported to have said 'first do the patient no harm' and non-maleficence simply means to do no harm. However, this has to be tempered with the reality that inadvertent harm may befall a child during a caring intervention, which may not have been foreseen. It is the duty of every nurse to avoid harming others, and this is reflected in the use of policies, procedures and protocols that are designed to minimise this. Some hospitals include this philosophy in their mission statements, for example, The Great Ormond Street Hospital for Children has as its motto 'The child first and always'.

4. Justice

When applied to health care, justice is used in the context of an equitable use of health care resources. There is consequently a dichotomy between wanting to give the best for each patient (beneficence) and the recognition of competition for scarce resources among the whole of the client group. At times, parents may believe that decisions to withdraw treatment from a terminally ill child are driven by resource considerations rather than the best interests of the child. If the parent is in denial over the terminal nature of their child's condition, the parents may reframe the clinical decision as a 'justice' issue as in the case of Alfie Evans. In 2018, an 'Alfie's Army' staged protests and called for 'Justice for Alfie'.

Advocacy

For the sake of completeness, it will be useful to consider the role advocacy might have in such ethically demanding situations. Advocacy is an idea that is widely discussed in nursing circles (Wheeler, 2000). The concept is based on the fact that there will always be some who will need someone else to speak out on their behalf to protect their best interests. Although all of us are likely to require such assistance at some point in our lives, there are certain groups in society who have been identified as potentially in need of such help. Children who have not yet achieved the developmental skills for autonomous decision making are an obvious example of this and need nurses to advocate for them (RCN, 2017a,b).

Although advocacy is usually assumed to be benign in character and well-intentioned (Willard, 1996), it must be recognised that the basis of advocacy is that the advocate has the power to speak with effect, whereas the person advocated for does not. This power gradient must be recognised and acknowledged for what it is if advocacy is to be constructive. Checks and balances must be in place to ensure that paternalism, at best, and abuse, at worst, is avoided. With a realistic view of its potential advantages and disadvantages, advocacy can be a strong contributor to child well-being. Parents have long been advocates!

Scenarios: Apply the ethical principles noted above to the following scenarios:

- 14-year-old Sam has been suffering from lethargy, unusual tiredness and a tendency to bruise easily. Bloods drawn by his GP have yielded a very pathological result. Sam needs further investigation for a potentially serious illness. He absolutely refuses to tell his parents about this situation or to allow his parents to be told by a member of the care team.
- 6-year-old Grace has been brought to Children's Emergency Department by a paramedic crew following the school making a call to emergency services. She has painfully swollen eyes and blurred vision. It seems that a religious leader within Grace's community ordered her parents to apply a substance to Grace's eyes, which caused stinging and swelling in order to 'drive the devil out'. This is a safeguarding issue under the category of faith-based practices.
- Baby X is the 4-month-old first-born baby of refugee parents. He has a bilateral deformity of his feet, which requires management involving manipulation under anaesthetic and serial splinting with plaster casts. His parents speak little English and have very poor home conditions. They seem bewildered and upset. Through an interpreter, it becomes clear that Xavier's parents have little faith in the effectiveness of the treatment he is receiving. In their culture it would be expected that X's condition would be addressed through prayer and the support of a traditional healer.

👤 ACTIVITY

Consider the rights and responsibilities of each of the individuals/agencies involved in the above situation. Think about the ethical implications and consequences of the available courses of action. Which ethical principles might be involved in this scenario? Look at The Code (Nursing and Midwifery Council, 2015). How would you advocate for the child in these cases?

Conducting Research and Protecting the Rights of Children and Their Families

The BMA (2018) states:

Children and babies should be eligible for inclusion in research and innovative therapy, with appropriate safeguards. To fail to do research would lead to stagnation of current practice and the continuation of medical management by using untried or unproven remedies on the basis of belief rather than best evidence.

The need for pharmaceutical products specifically designed for use by children has long been recognised. These need to be developed with the involvement of children and young people once initial studies involving adults have proved the safety and efficacy of the product.

Available from: https://www.bma.org.uk/advice/employment/ ethics/children-and-young-people/children-and-young- peoples-ethics-tool-kit/14-research-and-innovative-treat- ment

Likewise, the Royal College of Paediatrics and Child Health (RCPCH) notes the importance of child health research. It has published a charter on conducting research with children. The child should be involved in the decision and feel that their voice has been heard (UNICEF, 2011).

 ACTIVITY

Obtain and read in detail the Royal College of Paediatrics and Child Health's Infants', Children's and Young People's Child Health Research Charter. Available from: https://www. rcpch.ac.uk/resources/infants-childrens-young-peoples-child- health-research-charter

A number of questions related to research with children and young people have been raised and discussed by Alderson (1995):

- Are children likely to suffer any harm as a result of the research, in the form of emotional distress or intrusion?
- Do the benefits of the research clearly outweigh these possible risks?
- Who will benefit from the research – children or just the researchers?
- Are children given the proper information about the research?
- Are children offered the opportunity to refuse to participate or answer particular questions?

THE LEGAL SYSTEM AND KEY LEGAL PRINCIPLES

The legal system of England and Wales differs from that of Scotland and Northern Ireland. All share a common law tradition in which both judge-made law (case law) and parliament-made law (statutes) play a part. Judges interpret statutes (Acts of Parliament) and use previous case law

(precedents) to guide their decisions. If no statute exists, judges rely on legal principles and precedent to reach a decision. The Civil courts are separate from the Criminal courts.

The Family Division of the High Court hears cases involving child medical treatment decisions. Appeals against the decision can go to the Court of Appeal (Civil Division) and then to the Supreme Court. In cases involving disputes over the treatment of children, the child will be represented by a guardian *ad litem*, usually from the Child and Family Court Advisory and Support Service (CAFCASS); the Official Solicitor may act as guardian *ad litem*. The guardian *ad litem* will try to ascertain the views of the child, if he or she is able to express them. Once a child is over 16 years, but lacks capacity in relation to the decision that has to be made, their case may be transferred from the High Court to the Court of Protection (COP), if the COP powers are more appropriate to resolve the dispute than the Children Act. Claims for compensation for negligently caused harm are heard in the civil courts unless the negligence was criminally culpable. The Magistrates courts, which have a 'bench' of three lay Justices of the Peace, hear many criminal cases and some family cases, for example, contact disputes.

 ACTIVITY

Attend a session at your local Magistrates court to see justice in action.

Cases involving breaches of the 1950 European Convention for the Protection of Human Rights and Fundamental Freedoms can be heard in all British courts since the *Human Rights Act 1998* (HRA) came into force in 2000. Appeals from the Supreme Court can go to the European Court of Human Rights (ECHR), but the future relationship between the UK and the ECHR is uncertain due to 'Brexit' (the UK leaving the European Union). Also, the HRA may be repealed or rewritten post-Brexit. Although the UK ratified the 1989 United Nations Convention on the Rights of the Child, this is not yet part of domestic law although government suggests it is 'compliant'.

ACTIVITY

Visit the Houses of Parliament or listen to/watch a House of Lords debate on radio or television.

WWW

Look at the European Court of Human Rights website on:
- http://www.echr.coe.int

Who Is a Child?

The *Family Law Reform Act 1969* confirms that a child or 'minor' is any person who has been born but is under the age of 18.

SEMINAR DISCUSSION TOPIC

Should unborn children have rights? If so, what rights would you give them? Does the journey down the vaginal tract into the outside world change their moral status?

Who Has Parental Responsibility?

1. The gestational mother (who may or may not be the biological mother).
2. The biological father if he:
   - was married to the gestational mother (or, where the legislation permits, in a civil partnership with) when the child was born (divorce does not remove parental responsibility);
   - has since married the gestational mother;
   - is with the child's mother, jointly registered or re-registered the child's birth if the child was born after 1 December 2003, when relevant parts of the Adoption and Children Act 2002 came into force;
   - has a court arrangements order (pre-2014 this was a residence order);
   - has a court order that gives him parental responsibility;
   - has a formal 'parental responsibility agreement' with the mother.
3. The husband of the gestational mother is presumed to be the legal father of the child, but this can be rebutted by evidence, for example, DNA samples. If the child was conceived using in vitro fertilisation treatment in a licensed clinic and the husband of the gestational mother consented to the use of another man's sperm, he will be the legal father.
4. The same sex partner of the gestational mother will have parental responsibility if she:
   - has a formal 'parental responsibility agreement' with the mother;
   - is married to or in a civil partnership with the gestational mother or later marries or enters a civil partnership or later enters into such a formal relationship.
5. A guardian of the child.
6. Someone who holds a child arrangements order/residence order in respect of the child.
7. A local authority that has a care order in respect of the child.
8. Someone who has an emergency protection order in respect of the child.
9. Any person who has adopted the child.
10. The criminal justice system in the case of an imprisoned child.

There is a presumption by the courts that it is in the child's best interests to know his/her biological parentage: *Re H and A (Paternity: blood tests)* CA 21 [2002] 1 FLR 1145.

SEMINAR DISCUSSION TOPIC

In the case of *Re G (Children)* [2014] EWCA Civ 336, after their relationship broke down, the biological mother of twins, who had been born to her lesbian partner, sought a shared residence order which would give her legal parental responsibility for the twins. The biological mother had previously had a child conceived using the same sperm donor so all three children were full biological siblings. They disagreed over who had been the primary carer for the first year of the twins' lives before the relationship broke down. The gestational mother accepted that the biological mother should have a part to play in their lives, but wanted to be the only legal parent. What are your views as to whether there should be 'a non-biological parent with parental responsibility and a biological parent without it' as the judge asked?

Decision-Making Regarding Children

The *Children Act 1989* reflects the following legal principles:
1. The welfare of the child is paramount.
2. The child's views, in the light of his or her age and understanding, are to be taken into account.
3. There should be partnership with parents and other family members and support for the child within the family whenever possible.

Achieving consensus between parents and the medical team over the welfare of the child can be problematic. Since the case of *Re A (Conjoined twins: medical treatment)* [2001] 1 FLR 1 when the parents of conjoined twins opposed the separation of the conjoined twins, which would result in the inevitable death of the weaker twin, more parents have challenged medical decisions in court. In the case of Alfie Evans, his parents repeatedly went to court asking for permission to take him abroad for experimental treatment or prolonged care. His father asked the Pope for help and the Italian government made Alfie an Italian citizen. However, since Alfie was both resident and domiciled (i.e. had his permanent home) in the UK, the UK courts retained jurisdiction over the case and the welfare of Alfie remained their paramount concern.

Determining the welfare of the child requires establishing what harm the child has experienced or might experience in the future. Sometimes, different courts interpret the harm threshold differently. Some women of African origin attending charismatic churches in the UK have been led to believe that they were pregnant, and back in Africa they have had 'labour' and been presented with a baby. On returning to the UK, these babies have been found to have no biological connection to the 'mother'. In *Re E (a child) (fact-finding hearing: assessment of biological parents)* [2011] EWHC 3453 (Fam), the baby was removed due to the risk of future harm from believing he was a 'miracle' and not knowing his true medical history. In *Re A (a Child) (Fact finding hearing: biological parents)* [2014] EWHC 75 (Fam) the judge ruled that the child could stay with the 'parents' despite having no biological links.

Consent to Treatment

Respect for autonomy is one of the principles underpinning the need to obtain consent before performing any health care intervention. Another is the right to bodily integrity. Lord Donaldson in *Re W (a minor) (medical treatment)* [1993] Fam 64 explains that consent has a clinical purpose of ensuring patient cooperation with treatment, and a legal purpose of providing a 'flak jacket' against criminal charges of assault or battery (e.g. *Offences Against the Person Act 1869 s47* – liability for causing actual bodily harm), or civil claims for damages for trespass to the person. Failure to adequately inform or advise may give rise to negligence claims. In *Schloendorff v Society of New York Hospital* (1914), Cardozo said 'Every human being of adult years and sound mind has a right to determine what shall be done with his own body.' Increasingly, children's rights to determine what is done to them are being recognised in both law and ethics (Terry and Campbell, 2001).

 ACTIVITY

Does your ward have information leaflets telling children what to expect from their stay? If not, why not design one? If you have got information leaflets, are they available in the languages your patients speak?

There are three forms of consent:
1. Orally, for example the patient says 'I need my dressing changed'.
2. Implied, for example the patient holds out his or her arm for a cannula to be inserted.
3. In writing, for example a signed consent form.

Each form is equally valid unless statute law expressly says otherwise, as in the *Human Fertilisation and Embryology Act 1990*, which requires written consent. The law also prohibits certain procedures regardless of patient or family wishes. For example, the *Female Genital Mutilation Act 2003* and the *Serious Crime Act 2015* criminalises acts relating to the excision, infibulation or mutilation of the whole or any part of the labia majora, labia minora or clitoris in the UK or overseas.

Obtaining Valid Consent

Consent to medical or surgical treatment is usually obtained by a clinician, but this duty can be delegated to a nurse who is suitably knowledgeable and competent to do this task. For consent to be valid, it must be:
- given by a competent person
- freely given
- informed

 ACTIVITY

Observe how different practitioners inform patients and help children make decisions.

The Giving of Consent by a Competent Person

The competent person may be the child or someone with parental responsibility. The law treats the giving of consent to treatment differently depending on the age of the child. For instance, consent for very young children is very different from that for mature adolescents. Each situation will be considered in turn.

The infant or very young child.

The obvious decisional incapacity of the child means that decisions will be made on its behalf usually by one or both parents. Usually, the consent of only one person with parental responsibility is required. Parental decisions should be made in the child's best interests and the welfare of the child is paramount. The ethical principles of beneficence (doing good) and non-maleficence (avoiding harm) underpin the decision (Beauchamp and Childress, 2013). Doctors have dual obligations: to act in accordance with a responsible body of medical opinion when identifying treatment options and to act in the best interests of the incompetent patient (*Re S [Sterilisation: Patient's Best Interests]* [2000] 2 FLR 389).

When there is doubt or conflict over what constitutes a child's best interests, the court may be asked to decide. Education and communication are preferable to litigation, which can polarise views because of the adversarial nature of legal decision making in this country. The child might even be lost to medical scrutiny as in the case of Asha King. His parents took him overseas for proton beam treatment that his UK doctors did not consider appropriate for his condition.

 SEMINAR DISCUSSION TOPIC

Find a recent news report on Asha and how the proton beam treatment helped him. Should this treatment have been considered as 'experimental' or 'research'? Also read about Alfie Evans. Discuss whose opinion should count most when deciding what experimental treatment a child should have. Discuss the impact of the 'Alfie's Army' protests upon the patients, relatives and staff at Alder Hey Children's Hospital.

 REFLECT ON YOUR PRACTICE

How can you show respect for a person's personal, religious or cultural beliefs while ensuring that you practise within legal and professional boundaries?

 ACTIVITY

Next time the media discloses a contentious medical treatment case, read reports in different newspapers. Does your opinion change as you read the different versions?

The school-age child.

Normal childhood development leads to increasing ability to act autonomously (BMA, 2010). Alderson and Montgomery (1996) suggest that children as young as 5 years should be deemed as autonomous unless the evidence or the complexity of the decision suggests otherwise. Thus a young child might be able to consent to a grazed knee being cleaned, but not consent to x-rays and surgical resetting of a broken limb.

Nurses can help educate even very young children about medical treatment in a variety of ways. The child's views can be obtained, even though decisions will ultimately be taken in the child's best interests.

SCENARIO

Jake, a 6-year-old boy, is admitted for a tonsillectomy. His parents insist he is not told any details of his surgery, so he is not able to be fully informed and prepared by the health professionals.
- Identify the difficulties this could cause and evaluate possible interventions by health care professionals.
  Note: In June 2018, the UK government indicated that it was planning to save money by stopping procedures like tonsillectomies.

The mature minor under 16 years old.

Maturity and insight into medical treatment has to be measured on an individual basis. A 10-year-old child who has undergone years of treatment for leukaemia might be sufficiently competent to make his or her own decisions regarding further chemotherapy. In *Gillick v West Norfolk and Wisbech AHA* [1986] AC112 at p 114, the House of Lords held that a child under the age of 16 can consent to medical treatment if she had 'sufficient understanding and intelligence to enable her to understand fully what was proposed'. It is for the doctors to decide whether the child has a 'full understanding and appreciation of the consequences both of the treatment in terms of intended and possible side effects and equally important, the anticipated consequences of a failure to treat' (*Re R [A minor] [Wardship: consent to treatment]* [1992] Fam 11 at p 26 per Lord Donaldson MR). In this case, the girl who suffered from psychosis was deemed incompetent due to her fluctuating understanding.

'Gillick competent' children can consent to medical treatment even if their parents are opposed to it: 'parental right yields to the child's right to make his own decision' (per Lord Scarman), although their rights to refuse treatment are more limited. Their confidentiality should be upheld so their parents have no right to know that they have sought treatment. Nurses should encourage children to involve their parents, particularly when surgery is proposed but they also need to encourage children to develop their autonomy. In the case of *Westminster City Council v M and F and H* [2017] EWHC 518 (Fam), involving 40 volumes of evidence, the judge held that the 15½-year-old child's parents 'be distanced from any involvement in his medical care, physiotherapy or therapeutic support in order that H may be afforded the opportunity to assert his most basic of rights, his own personal autonomy'. Both parents had misrepresented, exaggerated and fabricated his medical symptoms. In *PD v SD, JD and X County Council* [2015] EWHC 4103 (Fam), a 16-year-old's parents could not understand or accept his gender dysphoria and the court agreed that his Article 8 rights meant they had no right to be informed about his medical treatment.

The 16–17-year-old child.

The *Family Law Reform Act 1969* s8 (1) states that:
> *The consent of a minor who has attained the age of 16 years to any surgical, medical or dental treatment which, in the absence of consent, would constitute a trespass to his person, shall be as effective as it would be if he were of full age; and where a person has by virtue of this section given an effective consent to any treatment, it shall not be necessary to obtain any consent from his parent or guardian.*

'Treatment' includes diagnosis, anaesthesia and ancillary procedures.

ACTIVITY

Compare and contrast examples of completed consent forms. Can you identify weaknesses?

The parent of questionable competency.

Competency can be affected by learning disabilities, mental illness or other conditions. Where the parent is obviously incompetent, consent must be obtained from another person with parental responsibility, or the court. In the case of adults and children over 16 years, competency requires being able to comprehend and retain the information given and weigh it in the balance to reach a decision: *Re C (Adult: refusal of treatment)* [1994] 1 FLR 31 approved in *Re MB (Medical treatment: consent)* [1997] 2 FLR 1097. Although Anglo-Welsh law does not fully recognise the concept of the emancipated minor, marriage or fighting for one's country have been deemed to free minors from parental control. Regardless of her age, the girl who becomes a mother has parental responsibility for her child. Her parents will not automatically have parental responsibility for the grandchild. In cases where the child-parent's ability to consent for her own child is doubtful, it may be necessary to apply to the court. In London Borough of Brent v C [2016] EWHC 1335 (Fam) a 13-year-old conceived (the boy was similar age) and at 14 years gave birth. She made it very clear she did not want any responsibility for the child, who was fostered. At 6 months old, the child was diagnosed as having a progressive, inherited neurological fatal condition. The local authority (LA) failed to apply for a care order until the child was nearly 5 years old, so the LA kept approaching the mother for consent for medical procedures as she remained the only person with legal parental responsibility. The mother was a child herself so the LA failed in their duty to protect her and they had breached the dying infant's Article 8 rights under the European Convention on Human Rights.

Freely given consent.

Duress can invalidate consent, even if it has been applied in the best interests of the patient. Persuasion is acceptable, coercion is not and is likely to cause a breakdown in the relationship between the various parties. Even adults can be placed under duress to accept or reject treatment as in the case of *Re T (Adult: refusal of treatment)* [1993] Fam 95, whose Jehovah's Witness mother persuaded her to reject blood transfusions. A court later allowed transfusion on the grounds that *T* was incompetent due to pain and pethidine at the time of her decision and was placed under duress. Children may be less able than adults to withstand emotional pressure. Regarding *Re E (A minor)(Wardship: medical treatment)* [1993] 1 FLR 386, a 15-year-old Jehovah's Witness boy with leukaemia who refused blood transfusions, Brazier and Bridge (1996) question whether his refusal was 'free choice'.

Duress of circumstances is inadequately recognised within medicine. A 14-year-old may appear 'Gillick competent' but her fear of 'what my parents will say if they find out' might mean she does not fully consider the risks of abortion.

 SCENARIO

A 15-year-old girl underwent a termination of pregnancy without her parents' knowledge. Complications arose and she underwent an emergency hysterectomy. On arrival in intensive care, a decision had to be made about notifying her parents, but a senior manager was strongly opposed to this on confidentiality grounds. Discuss and justify your reasoning.

🌐 **WWW**

Look at the recommendations regarding the principles underpinning the use of patient information given to Caldicott guardians on:
- https://www.ukcgc.uk/manual/contents

Informed consent.

The World Medical Association's Declaration of Helsinki 1964 states:

If it is at all possible, consistent with patient psychology, the doctor should obtain the patient's freely given consent after the patient has been given a full explanation.

Difficulties arise over provision of information. A balancing act is often performed, which can leave the patient or parent under informed. The House of Lords decision in *Sidaway v Board of Governors of the Bethlem Royal Hospital and the Maudsley Hospital* [1985] AC 871 meant that for years the standard was how much information would the 'reasonable' doctor disclose. In 2015, this changed when the Supreme Court decision ruled on *Montgomery v Lancashire Health Board and GMC* (2015) UKSC 11 SC 11 March 2015 saying:

The doctor is therefore under a duty to take reasonable care to ensure that the patient is aware of any material risks involved in any recommended treatment, and of any reasonable alternative or variant treatments. The test of materiality is whether, in the circumstances of the particular case, a reasonable person in the patient's position would be likely to attach significance to the risk, or the doctor is or should reasonably be aware that the particular patient would be likely to attach significance to it. (paragraph 87)

The law now says:
- Patients must be told about all material risks involved in any recommended treatment and of any alternative or variant treatments, procedures or diagnostic tests.
- Patients have a right to refuse to be informed of risks.

- Doctors can withhold information if they reasonably believe its disclosure will be seriously detrimental to the patient's health (the therapeutic exception).

The health care professional is under a duty to:
- Consider patient-specific characteristics as well as known facts relating to the risk of the proposed treatment.
- Provide information in a way that is comprehensible to the specific patient.
- Not to abuse the therapeutic exception.

 ACTIVITY

Read the Terry and Deegan article: Terry, L., Deegan, M., 2015. Informing clients of risk: Immediate implications of a landmark supreme court decision. British Journal of Midwifery 23 (7), 516–521.

Substitute words like 'child', 'parents', 'nurse' for words like 'woman', 'midwife' and discuss what the implications will be for informing children and parents about medical treatment options.

REFUSAL OF TREATMENT

Refusal by Parents

Decisions should be made in the best interests of the child. Cases may arise in which it is obvious that the parents' decision is coloured by personal preferences or beliefs and seems clearly contrary to the child's best interests. In the case of a life-threatening emergency, treatment can be given in the child's best interests to save 'life and limb' under the common law doctrine of necessity. In other cases, if doctors believe treatment is appropriate and persuasion has failed, they can refer the decision to the courts. A Specific Issue Order can be given under the *Children Act 1989* or the court can exercise its inherent jurisdiction and make a declaration as to lawfulness of treatment.

 ACTIVITY

When a child's treatment is the subject of dispute, a guardian *ad litem* will want to meet the child:
- What arrangements exist in your hospital regarding such meetings?
- How can you ensure that your professional responsibilities under The Code (NMC, 2015) are fulfilled?

In *Re B (A minor) (Wardship: medical treatment)* [1981] 1 WLR 1421, where the child had Down syndrome and needed life-saving emergency surgery but the parents refused consent, the Court of Appeal concluded 'it is not for this court to say that life of that description ought to be extinguished'. *Re J (A minor) (Wardship: medical treatment)* [1991] Fam 33 at p 55, which involved a severely brain-damaged baby, held that 'the correct approach is for the court to judge the quality of life the child would have to endure if given the treatment'. *Re A (Conjoined twins)* shows how difficult it is to determine 'best interests'. Sanctity of life, quality of life, the parents' views and the lawfulness of the operation were all considered. Lord Justices Ward and Brooke held the separation was not in Mary's best interests, although it was allowable. Lord Justice Walker was, according to Foster (2000), '… scarily clear [that] a short, terribly disabled and possibly painful life was a life not worth living' consequently, separation (and death) was in Mary's best interests. In *An NHS Trust v Child B, Mr & Mrs B* [2014] EWHC 3486 (Fam), the court authorised blood transfusions for a young child who required skin grafts following accidental burns, against his Jehovah's Witness parents' religious objections. The judge said, 'even a small risk of death is a risk which points powerfully towards the provision of available treatment subject to any counterbalancing risks consequent on such treatment'.

> ### ⚙ SEMINAR DISCUSSION TOPIC
>
> In the case of *Re C (A child) (HIV testing)* [1999] 2 FLR 1004, the baby's mother was HIV positive and breast-feeding her infant against medical advice. She refused to allow the baby to be HIV tested or to be given prophylactic medication. The doctors obtained a court order for the child to be tested, in his best interests, but the mother went abroad with the baby before this could be done.
> - Discuss the baby's rights versus the mother's.

In other cases, it is much less certain which viewpoint is the correct one. As Ham and Pickard, 1998 (p 22) point out, differences of opinion:

> … *reflect the individualistic values to which medicine has always subscribed, particularly in the case of clinicians who have reached the top of the hierarchy and feel they possess sufficient expertise to act on the basis of their own judgement.*

In *Re MM (Medical treatment)* [2000] 1 FLR 224 the child, *MM*, was a temporary resident in the UK while his Russian parents studied here. There was no definite diagnosis of his immunological condition and the parents seemed as knowledgeable as the doctors. The parents wanted to continue his existing treatment, because if started on immunoglobulins as English doctors wished, he would have to continue with them, but they would be difficult to obtain in Russia. Using telephone conferencing, the judge was able to help the parents and doctors reach a compromise position.

In other cases, compromise may seem unachievable. In The Matter of AB (A Child) [2018] EWHC 3, the child's parents were reported as 'uncooperative, rude and aggressive and intimidating of medical and nursing staff' to the extent the local authority started care proceedings. However, eventually the parental behaviour adjusted and they discontinued activities such as withholding pain medication and excessive suctioning that caused harm to the child. Finally, the child was able to be discharged home for the rest of his short life with a full local authority-funded support package. The nurses' evidence that 'that when with [his parents] AB can be more settled, particularly in his mother's arms or on his mother's lap, that he may find some sounds more soothing than a noisy hospital environment' helped the court decide.

Refusal by Children

Young children lacking understanding may struggle and fight against those delivering necessary care. In such circumstances, when explanations or reassurances have failed to help, minimal restraint in the child's best interests is allowable. Guidance is available from the Department of Health (1993) and the Royal College of Nursing (2017a,b).

> ### 🧑 ACTIVITY
> #### *Reflect on Your Practice*
>
> How would you give a 2-year-old child an intramuscular injection when she is fighting, crying and her mother can't stand injections either?

The *Children Act 1989* (s38, 43, 44) gives the court powers to order medical or psychiatric examination and treatment, but if the child is of sufficient understanding to make an informed decision, the child has the right to refuse medical/psychiatric examination. If a competent child refuses examination, the doctor will be unable to make a diagnosis and recommend treatment. A competent child is unlikely to refuse examination because he or she will recognise the need for diagnosis. Consequently, a refusal of examination could be evidence of incompetence. The child's welfare is the paramount consideration, although the court should take into account the factors in s1 (3) of the *Children Act 1989*. The child's wishes are only one factor to be considered.

The courts have held that a child's refusal of treatment can be overridden by anyone with parental responsibility or by the court. In *Re W (A minor) (Medical treatment)* [1993] Fam 64, a 16-year-old girl with anorexia refused force feeding. As the *Family Law Reform Act 1969* s8 does not use the word 'refuse' her powers to refuse treatment were not absolute – others could give permission. In An NHS Foundation Hospital v P (A child) [2014] EWHC 1650 (Fam) the 17½-year-old girl refused treatment for a paracetamol overdose. The psychiatrist held that she had capacity under the *Mental Capacity Act 2005*. As the time threshold for commencing treatment was passing, an application was made to the out-of-hours judge who held that 'the wishes and feelings … of a young person who is almost an adult' are not 'decisive' and there was a 'very strong presumption' to take steps to save her life.

In *Re M (Child: refusal of medical treatment)* [1999] 2 FLR 1097, a 15½-year-old girl refused consent to a heart transplant. Although her mother had consented, doctors wanted judicial backing and obtained it when the judge held *M* to be incompetent. Mason et al. (2011, p 74) suggest this represents 'the outermost reaches of acceptable paternalistic practices'. In *Re M* (at p 1099) the court was told 'no other medical option was available', although life-saving alternatives such as mechanical hearts, which may have been medically better as well as more acceptable to the patient, did exist, at the time

(Rogers, 2000a). When treatment is refused, particularly if it involves physical maim, alternatives should be sought and considered before resorting to enforcement of the doctor's preference against the wishes of the mature minor.

A risk in *Re M* was non-compliance with antirejection medication once she reached adulthood. The boy in *Re E* exercised his right to refuse further blood transfusions once he reached 18 and died. Bailey-Harris (2000, p 137) believes 'teenagers with deeply held convictions' should be regarded as mature and 'entitled to their full autonomy rights'. In 2008, a 13-year-old, Hannah Jones, refused a heart transplant against medical advice. In her case though, doctors respected her autonomy, but kept the door open for her to change her mind if she so wished. A year later, she accepted the transplant. In 2017, she graduated with a university degree, and in 2018, was reunited with her surgeon during a television programme.

The Mentally Ill Child

If the child has mental illness, statutory powers under the *Mental Health Act 1983* allow enforced treatment, although there is marked reluctance to use them because of the stigmatising nature of mental illness and being sectioned. Reluctance to use these powers left one child barricaded in her room, manipulating her family and not receiving the psychiatric help she needed before the court was eventually asked to exercise its jurisdiction (*South Glamorgan CC v W and B* [1993] 1 FLR 574). In *Re C (A minor) (Detention for medical treatment)* [1997] 2 FLR 180, an order was made under s100 of the *Children Act 1989* so that a 16-year-old with anorexia could be returned to a clinic for treatment. She had a history of absconding and was at risk of significant harm.

END-OF-LIFE ISSUES

Lord Justice Hoffman, in *Airedale NHS Trust v Bland* [1993] AC 789 (at p 834), felt that whether 'it would be lawful to provide or withhold the treatment or care is a matter for the law' not doctors. This reflects public opinion that doctors are accountable and patients have protectable rights. Imminent, unavoidable death constitutes well-established grounds for ending treatment (*Re C (A baby)* [1996] 2 FLR 43, concerning a baby left brain-damaged following meningitis). Establishing brainstem death is difficult in very young children, but in *Re A* [1992] 3 Med LR 303, it was accepted that the 2-year-old was brainstem dead and that it was appropriate to disconnect the ventilator. In *Re C (A minor) (Wardship: medical treatment)* [1989] 3 WLR 240, it was appropriate to withhold treatment enabling a baby with severe hydrocephalus to 'die peacefully with the greatest dignity and the least of pain, suffering and distress'. *Re J (A minor) (Wardship: medical treatment)* [1991] Fam 33 (at p 53) held that 'it is settled law that the court's prime and paramount consideration must be the best interests of the child'. There is a 'strong presumption' in favour of preserving life except in 'exceptional circumstances', with Lord Justice Taylor stating 'it cannot be too strongly emphasised that the court never sanctions steps to terminate life' (p 53). In *Re C (Medical treatment)* [1998] 1 FLR 384, concerning a

terminally ill child with spinal muscular atrophy type 1, the court held that 'whilst the sanctity of life is vitally important, it is not the paramount consideration. The paramount consideration here is the best interests of little C' (at p 393). The Orthodox Jewish parents wanted reventilation to remain an option because of their vitalist approach to sanctity of life.

Among other factors, the court will consider 'whether the life of this child is demonstrably going to be so awful that in effect the child must be condemned to die' (*Re B (A minor) (Wardship: medical treatment)* 1981 1 WLR 1421 [at p 1424]). However, pain alone is no defence for ending life unlawfully, as Dr Cox found after he gave his patient potassium chloride to end her intolerable pain (*R v Cox* [1992] 12 BMLR 38).

In *A National Health Service Trust v D & Ors* [2000] FLR 677, the resuscitation status of a severely disabled child was considered. The court listed the four principles to be applied:

1. The paramount consideration is the best interests of the child.
2. The court has a clear duty to respect the sanctity of life, which imposes a strong presumption in favour of taking all steps to preserve it.
3. Actions to accelerate death or terminate life cannot be approved by the court.
4. The court cannot order a doctor to give treatment that the doctor is unwilling to give and which is contrary to the doctor's clinical judgement.

Lady Hale, in the Court of Appeal case of *Re A (A child)* [2016] EWCA Civ 759 said

decision-makers must look at [the child's] welfare in the widest sense, not just medical, but social and psychological; they must consider the nature of the medical treatment in question, what it involves and its prospects of success; they must consider what the outcome of that treatment for the patient is likely to be; they must try and put themselves in the place of the individual patient and ask what his attitude towards the treatment is or would be likely to be; and they must consult others who are looking after him or are interested in his welfare, in particular for their view of what his attitude would be.

> ### 👤 ACTIVITY
>
> In *Re A (Conjoined twins)*, Lord Justice Ward held that 'Mary may have a right to life, but she has little right to be alive' (p 54); in effect, Mary's twin, Jodie, had a stronger right to life than Mary. Discuss the rights of the two children.

Conflict Between Parents and Doctors

In *R v Cambridge District HA, ex parte B* [1995] 1 FLR 1055, the father of 'Child B' obtained a judicial review of the Health Authority's decision not to fund further treatment for his daughter, a 10-year-old suffering from leukaemia. His refusal to accept the doctor's non-treatment decision represented a 'direct challenge' to the doctors involved in her care (Ham and Pickard, 1998). The court held that further treatment would not be in her best interests. If the court decides the doctor's stance is contrary to the patient's best interests, it can order the transfer of the patient to another doctor. This option was considered in *Re T* (the child needing a liver transplant). Doctors at Great Ormond Street Hospital requested the transfer of the conjoined twins in *Re A* on the grounds that they had the necessary expertise to do the separation, although they also said they might accede to the parental wishes not to operate (Rogers, 2000b).

Parents may be concerned that their child is being used as a teaching tool and not receiving appropriate care, as in the case of a baby with Goldenhar syndrome. When the parents sought to remove the child from the hospital, a child protection order banning this was obtained (Mahendra, 2002).

Parents and doctors may conflict over when the child's condition should be considered terminal. In *Royal Wolverhampton Hospitals NHS Trust v B* [2000] 1 FLR 953, Bodley, J. concluded that the breakdown in trust between the parties required that the doctors were given permission to not treat the child dying from chronic lung disease due to prematurity if they thought fit, not just because this was in the patient's best interests but as 'a kindness to the parents' (p 957). The cases of babies Charlotte Wyatt ([2005] EWHC 693) and Luke Winston Jones ([2004] EWHC 2713) involved parents challenging medical decisions not to provide life-prolonging treatment and resuscitation.

Good Care and Communication Seem Vital to Prevent Conflicts

In the David Glass case, doctors gave David, a severely disabled boy with respiratory failure, the respiratory depressant diamorphine against his mother's clearly expressed objections (*R v Portsmouth NHS Trust ex parte Glass* [1999] 2 FLR 905). The family was outraged and, en masse, invaded the ward and resuscitated David amid scenes of violent disorder during which two doctors and the mother of another child were injured. Three of them were later jailed for assault (*R v (1) Davies (2) Wild (3) Hodgson* (2000) CA 28 July 2000 unreported). In March 2004, the European Court of Human Rights ruled that 'the decision to impose treatment on the first applicant (David) in defiance of the second applicant's (his mother's) objections gave rise to an interference with the first applicant's right to respect for his private life, and in particular his right to physical integrity' (*Glass v The United Kingdom* Application No 61827/00 ECHR 9 March 2004 paragraph 70). The Court concluded that the situation was not one of such urgency that treatment could proceed without the mother's consent, because it was clear that the hospital had had sufficient time to secure a police presence on the ward and 'the doctors and officials used the limited time available to them in order to try to impose their views on [the mother]' (paragraph 81). In regard to the fact that the doctors' notes indicated the mother had consented at one point to the therapeutic use of diamorphine, even though a solicitor's letter the next day made her opposition clear, the Court held 'it cannot be stated with certainty that any consent given was free, express and informed' (paragraph 82).

The UK government was ordered to pay compensation to David and his mother jointly, because the Court recognised 'the stress and anxiety' she suffered in her own right, as well as

'feelings of powerlessness and frustration in trying to defend her own perception of what was in the best interests of her child' (paragraph 87). David was discharged into the care of his GP a few hours after the violent incident and was still alive at the time of writing. The final word perhaps belongs to Judge Casadevall: 'In the particular circumstances of [this case] maternal instinct has had more weight than medical opinion.'

 WWW

Find the Glass v United Kingdom judgement on the European Court of Human Rights website:
• http://hudoc.echr.coe.int/eng?i=001-61663

Conflict Between Parents

An exception to the rule that only one person with parental responsibility need consent arose in *Re J (Child's religious upbringing and circumcision)* [2000] 1 FLR 571, when the non-practising Muslim father of a child wanted him to be circumcised against the non-practising Christian mother's wishes. The court ordered that circumcision required the consent of both parents, or when old enough to decide for himself, the child's consent.

In *F v F* [2013] EWHC 2683 (Fam) the father of two girls aged 15 and 11, asked the court to order that they should receive the MMR vaccine. Previously, in light of suggestions of a link between the vaccine and autism, the parents had agreed they should not receive the triple vaccine. The father had changed his mind as Andrew Wakefield's research was thoroughly discredited. The court held that immunisation was in the children's best interests.

CONSENT TO NON-THERAPEUTIC, CONTROVERSIAL OR EXPERIMENTAL TREATMENT

Although the incompetent patient has a right not to be subjected to non-consensual touching, which is waived only if inhumane not to, children have been allowed to donate bone marrow to siblings or other relatives, with minimal, or no interference by the courts. Child B's sister was the donor for the failed bone marrow transplant (*R v Cambridge District HA, ex parte B* [1995] 1 FLR 1055). In most such cases, providing the parents, doctors and child (if old enough to be involved) agree, the courts are not involved. In the Australian case of *Re GWW and CMW* (1997) 21 Fam LR 612, a 12-year-old boy was allowed to donate bone marrow to his aunt. It was clear that this was his own, voluntary decision. Although Month (1996) argues that preventing children from donating bone marrow may not be in their best interests, it is important for nurses to be alert for signs of duress or distress. In the American case of *Hart v Brown* (Super, 1972) 29 Conn Supp 368, permission was given by the courts for a kidney donation from a healthy 7-year-old to his seriously ill, identical twin brother.

An example of controversial treatment is the use of plastic surgery to alter the facial features of Down syndrome children. One retired consultant paediatrician has called for such surgery to be outlawed, like female circumcision (Jones, 2000).

Where conventional medicine holds no hope, and death is certain, experimental treatment might be allowed. In *DS v (1) JS (2) An NHS Trust and PA v JA (2) An NHS Trust and Secretary of State for Health* [2002] EWHC 2734 (Fam) the court allowed two sufferers of variant Creutzfeld–Jakob disease (JS, an 18-year-old and JA, a 16-year-old, neither of whom had capacity any more to make their own decisions) to be given an untested treatment – pentosan polysulphate – directly into their brains, even though the procedure itself might kill them.

For activities; core response.

In your response to the ethical questions relating to the scenarios in this chapter you might consider:

- The United Nations Convention on the Rights of the Child requirements, for example right to be protected from harm. However, while we are required to demonstrate respect for the religious beliefs and practices, the best interests of the child are paramount and practices, which cause harm to the child, must be prevented. All this can be done in a manner which also demonstrates a respectful attitude to the family and their community.
- Doing good (beneficence). There are other cultural practices, which are defined as illegal in the UK. Eradication of these practices has been most successfully achieved by educating communities and mobilizing them to stop these practices themselves. This also conveys respect by avoiding patronizing actions.
- Avoiding harm includes action taken to reduce the risk of harm to the child or young person, for example working with communities to reduce the incidence of female genital mutilation or forced marriage.
- Advocacy – everything the children's nurse does is orientated towards speaking on behalf of Grace and promote her well-being.
- Justice requires that all people are treated equally, are treated with respect, and given true and accurate information. A central idea within this context is fairness.
- Autonomy requires that the person who is competent to do so is able to make decisions on behalf of themselves. The child who is not competent to undertake this is protected by a parent doing so on their behalf. As the child develops towards become a young adult, they become progressively more able to exercise competence. However, young people are unique and variable in the rate and stage at which they fully acquire this ability.

It is important to realise that an ethical analysis rarely provides a single, clear response to clinical questions especially as these situations are often complex and dynamic. However, an ethical analysis can help to identify the best possible response and to secure consensus on this, that is, majority or unanimous agreement on a course of action.

Explore podcasts as an activity, for example, child specific Moral Maze/Inside the Ethics Committee episodes.

NEGLIGENCE

Health care interventions are not always successful. Where consent to risks has been sought and given, if those risks come about, the 'flak jacket' protects against being sued. When harm is caused through negligence, either by an omission to act appropriately or by errors in the actions performed, the injured child, or his or her family, might make a claim for compensation in the Civil Courts under the Tort of Negligence. To win compensation, the claimant must prove the following:

- The patient was owed a duty of care by the defendant.
- The defendant (doctor, nurse, hospital) breached the duty of care by failing to reach the standard required of them by law.
- The breach caused harm of a type that was foreseeable.

A request for patient records may indicate that a negligence action is being considered.

 WWW

Read the NHS guidance on accessing patient information on:
- https://www.nhs.uk/NHSEngland/thenhs/records/healthrecords/Pages/what_to_do.aspx

Duty of Care

A duty of care is owed once the hospital, doctor, surgeon, nurse or other person undertakes to perform certain tasks for the child. It is owed once the patient presents for treatment (*Barnett v Chelsea and Kensington HMC* [1968] 1 All ER 1068) and may continue after the patient has been transferred from one professional to another, has left the GP's surgery or hospital, or the nurse has left the patient's house.

Breach of the Standard of Care

Many nurses act in an extended role. The court will decide whether the health care professionals, or other carers, have met the standard that the law expects them to meet. The standard of care is found in *Bolam v Friern Hospital Management Committee* [1957] 1 WLR 582 (the 'Bolam test'):

> *The test is the standard of the ordinary skilled man exercising and professing to have that special skill. A man need not possess the highest expert skill. It is a well-established law that it is sufficient if he exercises the ordinary skill of an ordinary competent man exercising that particular art.*

The key words are 'exercising' and 'professing':
- Professing is what you say you are, for example children's nurse, doctor.
- Exercising is what you do: what task were you actually doing?

REFLECT ON YOUR PRACTICE

Read the article: Terry, L., Carr, G., Halpin, Y., 2017. Understanding and meeting your legal responsibilities as a nurse. Nursing Standard 32 (12), 52–62.

Are you checking why you are doing what you are doing in clinical practice? Could you justify your actions or inactions in a court of law?

The court will hear expert witness evidence to determine what standard was acceptable. In *Bolitho v City and Hackney HA* [1998] AC 232, a child was left brain-damaged following a respiratory arrest. The ward sister had asked the doctor to attend with a view to preventively intubating him, but the doctor failed to arrive. The House of Lords held that not only should a responsible body of opinion uphold the act or omission, but there must be a logical basis to the opinion given. This reflects the trend for evidence-based health care.

Learners and their instructor must together meet the standard of the qualified person; inexperience is no excuse – the standard goes with the post. In *Wilsher v Essex AHA* [1986] 3 All ER 801, a junior doctor misplaced a catheter and miscalculated the oxygen for a premature baby, who then suffered retrolental fibroplasia.

Written standards, guidelines, protocols, and Do Not Attempt Resuscitation (DNAR) policies are useful for providing consistent care. They need updating regularly and can be used as evidence in a court of law – failure to comply with standard guidance may be seen as proof of a failure to meet the relevant standard of care.

 ACTIVITY

Attend a hearing of the NMC Professional Conduct Committee. Places are limited so book in advance.

Causation of Foreseeable Harm

Experts for the claimant will provide evidence to persuade the court 'on the balance of probabilities' that the breach of the standard of care caused the harm complained of. The defence will produce its own experts. The question the court asks is 'But for the negligent act or omission, would the harm complained of have occurred?' In *Barnett v Chelsea and Kensington* HMC [1968] 1 All ER 1068, a doctor who failed to examine three men who fell ill after night duty was found to have breached his duty of care. However, this breach did not cause the death of one of the men, which was held to be inevitable due to arsenic poisoning.

Where there are multiple possible causes of the harm, as in *Wilsher v Essex AHA* [1986] 3 All ER 801, unless the claimant can prove on the 'balance of probabilities' that one was the cause, the claim will fail. In *Wilsher*, the blindness could have been caused by several factors, not just the excess oxygen, so the child's claim failed. Likewise, in *Temple v South Manchester Health Authority* [2002] EWCA Civ 1406, negligent treatment of a 9-year-old's diabetic ketoacidosis had not, on the balance of probability, caused his irreversible brain damage. Where there are two equal acts of negligence, either of which could have resulted in the harm complained of, but science cannot provide the necessary proof, *Fairchild* [2002] 3 WLR 79 now holds that the court can decide that both were 'material causes'.

Compensation may sometimes be recovered for psychiatric damage. In *North Glamorgan NHS Trust v Walters* [2002] EWCA Civ 1792, a mother was compensated for suffering psychiatric injury caused by the shock of seeing the distressing final 36 hours of her son's life following a negligent failure to diagnose his acute hepatitis.

The doctrine of *Res Ipsa Loquitur* (the thing speaks for itself) simplifies the proof of negligence and causation. If forceps are left inside a patient after an operation, there was obvious negligence and the subsequent peritonitis will be attributed to this.

Unforeseeable harms cannot be protected or insured against, so claimants will not be able to recover compensation for harms no one knew existed. If the professional should have known, liability can be established; continuing professional development is important.

 WWW

Read the NHS Litigation Authority advice on how to reduce negligence in the NHS:
- https://resolution.nhs.uk/

Accurate record keeping is vital. This is your defence when asked to justify your actions or inactions months or years later. In *Juliff v (1) Dr Hillard (2) Dr Trigg (3) Dr Lukaszewicz* (2001) QBD 24 June unreported, the medical notes were 'conscientiously, properly and accurately recorded' and demonstrated that the defendants had 'discharged their duties with conspicuous care and conscientiousness'. They were not to blame for the child's stroke, which followed a difficult-to-diagnose case of meningitis.

 REFLECT ON YOUR PRACTICE

Look at a nursing record you made a week ago. How clearly can you recall the patient's care? How well could you do this if asked in 8 years' time when a solicitor's letter arrives?

 ACTIVITY

How can record keeping in your practice area be improved?

Vicarious Liability

Under the doctrine of vicarious liability, the employer will be held liable for the employee's negligence providing the employee was working within the course and scope of his employment. In *Townsend v Worcester and District HA* [1995] 23 BMLR 31, the defendants were vicariously liable for brain damage caused by the excessive force applied to the baby's head during a forceps delivery.

Limitations for Legal Actions

In the case of negligent harm occurring during pregnancy, delivery, or any time in childhood, the child retains a right to sue for 3 years after becoming an adult or becoming aware of the negligent act, if no legal action has commenced before then.

Duty of Candour

From November 2014, a statutory duty of candour came into effect. It is a legal duty requiring hospital, community and mental health trusts to inform and apologise to patients if there have been mistakes in their care that have led or may lead to harm.

WWW

https://resolution.nhs.uk/wp-content/uploads/2018/09/NHS-Resolution-Saying-Sorry.pdf

CRIMINAL LIABILITY

Gross Negligence Manslaughter

Where negligence causes death, criminal charges of gross negligence manslaughter might follow, as in *R v Adomako* [1993] 3 WLR 927 in which an anaesthetist's negligence led to his patient's death.

ACTIVITY

Visit your local Coroner's court, particularly if there is a paediatric case being heard.

Murder

Intentional neglect resulting in death may constitute murder or attempted murder. In *R v Arthur* [1981] 12 BMLR 1, Dr Arthur prescribed sedation and nursing care only for a Down syndrome baby rejected by his parents. Initial charges of murder were reduced to attempted murder when a post-mortem revealed the baby would have died anyhow because of his medical condition.

Deliberate Harm by Parents, Carers or Others

Child protection issues are covered in a separate chapter of this book.

Applying your new understanding, read the following description of a situation that occurred in 2018. Have a go at applying everything that has been covered in this chapter (children's rights, ethical, legal and research principles). Think about:

- The child's best interests.
- The rights of the child (including the right to privacy).
- The role of the health care professionals, in particular, children's nurses.
- The role of the parent as a spokesperson not just for her child but for others.
- The use of the media (including social media) in medical treatment campaigning.
- The role of the criminal law in protecting its citizens from harmful activities/products.
- Research into the effectiveness of unproven/experimental therapies and the particular concerns where children are involved.
- The duties of all those involved including health care professionals, researchers, media, government agencies, and the legislature.
- How should this situation have been handled?
- What are the lessons for the future?

Billy Caldwell (12-year-old at the time of events in June 2018) has severe epilepsy. In 2016, Billy received treatment with cannabis oil in the United States of America. His mother, Charlotte, reported that prior to this treatment, which is not recognized in the UK, Billy was having 100 seizures a day. This is a life-limiting and life-threatening condition. Following this, Billy was prescribed cannabis oil by a GP in County Tyrone, Northern Ireland. In 2018, the Home Office ordered the GP to stop. Billy's family started lobbying the Home Office to have this decision reversed. There are a small number of families with children with severe epilepsy who also wish their child to receive the same treatment. As Billy's supply was dwindling, Charlotte went to Toronto, Canada. On her return to the UK at Heathrow Airport on Monday, 11 June 2018, she declared that she was carrying cannabis oil. The oil was immediately confiscated by customs officials. The situation received intense media publicity. The following Friday, Billy was admitted to hospital with recurrent seizures and it was reported that he was likely to die. Eventually the Home Office agreed that one of the bottles of cannabis oil could be released by Customs and Billy received treatment. Later, the Home Office agreed that Billy will be granted a lifetime license to have cannabis oil therapy.

SUMMARY

The world of health care practice and research remains a moral minefield. Additionally, it is important for all health care professionals to remember that the law is not static. Changes to legislation and new cases testing out the boundaries of care occur regularly. It is your duty to keep yourself up-to-date to ensure that you continue to practise safely, ethically and within the law. Child health nurses, working within their philosophy of family care, are often at the forefront of activity and therefore open to criticism. It is incumbent upon all nurses to make themselves aware of the ethical and legal dimensions of any research or clinical care they might be involved with no matter how peripherally. It will not be possible to protect the rights of the child unless they do so. If we do not learn the lessons of the past then we are destined to repeat them.

REFERENCES

Adoption and Children Act 2002. The Stationery Office, London.
Alderson, P., Montgomery, J., 1996. Health Care Choices: Making Decisions with Children. Institute of Public Policy Research, London.
Alderson, P., 1995. Listening to Children. Children, Ethics and Social Research. Barnardos, Ilford.

Bailey-Harris, R., 2000. Patient autonomy – a turn in the tide? In: Freeman, M., Lewis, A. (Eds.), Law and Medicine: Current Legal Issues, vol. 3. Oxford University Press, Oxford, pp. 127–140.

Beauchamp, T.L., Childress, J.F., 2013. Principles of Biomedical Ethics, seventh ed. Oxford University Press, Oxford.

Behi, R., 1995. The individual's right to informed consent. Nurse Researcher 3 (1), 14–23.

Brazier, M., Bridge, C., 1996. Coercion or caring: analysing adolescent autonomy. Leg. Stud. 16, 84–109.

British Medical Association (BMA), 2010. Children and Young People Toolkit. BMA, London.

Charles-Edwards, I., 1995. Moral, ethical, and legal perspectives. In: Carter, B., Dearmun, A.K. (Eds.), Child Health Care Nursing. Blackwell Scientific, London, pp. 61–74.

Children Act 1989. HMSO, London.

Department of Health (DoH), 1993. Guidance on permissible forms of control in children's residential care. HMSO, London.

Family Law Reform Act 1969. HMSO, London.

Foster, C., 2000. Rocks and hard places. Solicitors' J. 922–923.

Gillick v West Norfolk and Wisbech AHA [1986] AC 112, 1985 3WLR 830, 3 All ER 402 HL.

Ham, C., Pickard, S., 1998. Tragic Choices in Health Care. The case of Child B. King's Fund, London.

Human Rights Act 1998. The Stationery Office, London.

Jones, R.B., 2000. Parental consent to cosmetic facial surgery in Down's syndrome. J. Med. Ethics 26, 101–102.

Kennedy, I., Chair, 2001. Learning from Bristol: The Report of the Public Inquiry into Children's Heart Surgery at Bristol Royal Infirmary Inquiry 1984–1995. Final Report. Cmd 5207. The Stationery Office, London. Available from: http://www.bristol-inquiry.org.uk.

Mahendra, B., 2002. Facing up to a child's dilemma. New Law J. 152 (7024), 426.

Mason, J.K., McCall Smith, R.A., Laurie, G.T., 2011. Law and Medical Ethics, sixth ed. Butterworths, London.

Mental Health Act 1983. HMSO, London.

Month, S., 1996. Preventing children from donating may not be in their best interests. Br. Med. J. 312, 241–242.

Nursing and Midwifery Council (NMC), 2015. The Code. NMC, London.

Power, K., 2002. Implications of the human rights act 1998. Paediatr. Nurs. 14 (4), 14–19.

Rogers, L., 2000a. Mini heart pump to end transplants. Times 9 April 2000.

Rogers, L., 2000b. Doctors may not operate on twins. Sun. Times 2000.

Royal College of Nursing (RCN), 2017a. Getting it Right for Children and Young People. RCN, London.

Royal College of Nursing (RCN), 2017b. Three Steps to Positive Practice: A Rights Based Approach when Considering and Reviewing the Use of Restrictive Interventions. RCN, London.

Royal College of Nursing (RCN), 2018. Using and Doing Research. RCN, London. Available from: https://www.rcn.org.uk/library/subject-guides/using-and-doing-research-a-novices-guide.

Royal College of Paediatrics and Child Health (RCPCH). Health's Infants', Childrens' and Young People's Child Health Research Charter. Available from: https://www.rcpch.ac.uk/resources/infants-childrens-young-peoples-child-health-research-charter.

Terry, L.M., Campbell, A., 2001. Are we listening to children's views about their treatment? Br. J. Nurs. 10 (6), 384–390.

UNICEF, 2011. Every Child's Right to Be Heard. UNICEF, London.

Wheeler, P., 2000. Is advocacy at the heart of professional practice? Nurs. Stand. 14 (36), 39–41.

Willard, C., 1996. The nurse's role as patient advocate: obligation or imposition. J. Adv. Nurs. 24 (1), 60–66.

Promote, Restore and Stabilise Health Status in Children: A Systems Approach to Childhood Conditions, Disease and Disability

8

Inherited Conditions and the Family

Maggie Kirk, Emma Tonkin

LEARNING OUTCOMES

- Appreciate the impact that a genetic illness may have on family life.
- Apply core principles of inheritance and genetic variation to understand how genetic conditions can be passed on in families.

- Evaluate the role of the children's nurse in helping families to access genetic information and services, and supporting their decision making based on this.
- Appreciate some of the ethical issues surrounding the application of genetic technologies of relevance to children and their families.

GLOSSARY

Allele The different versions of a gene that may exist, because of small differences in the DNA sequence. An individual inherits two alleles for each gene, one from each parent.

Autosome A 'numbered' or non-sex chromosome, named according to size from 1 (largest) to 22 (smallest).

Carrier An individual who has a genetic alteration within a gene that predisposes to disease, but who may not display any symptoms of the disease. Such individuals are usually heterozygous for a recessive condition.

Chromosome A single long strand of DNA. Humans usually have 46 chromosomes comprising one pair of sex chromosomes and 22 pairs of autosomes (non-sex chromosomes).

DNA (deoxyribonucleic acid) The molecule in the cell nucleus that carries the genetic information for the development and function of an individual and from one generation to the next. DNA consists of two strands folded in a double helix. Each strand comprises a sugar and phosphate backbone and a sequence of four different types of chemical bases. The particular sequence of the four bases is known as the genetic code.

Dominant A characteristic that is evident in an individual even when there is only one altered copy of a particular gene present.

Expressivity The severity or extent to which the signs and symptoms of a condition differ between individuals with the same condition.

Gene The basic functional unit of inheritance, composed of a sequence of DNA at a specific location on a chromosome. Individuals have two copies of each gene.

Most genes code for assembling a specific protein or part of a protein.

Genetics The study of heredity and the structure and composition of single genes.

Genome All of the genetic information contained on an individual's chromosomes as well as mitochondrial DNA. This equates to around three billion bases of DNA, which contains 20,000 or so genes and other intervening and regulatory (non-coding) sequences.

Genomics The study of the complete set of genetic material including all the genes and non-coding DNA in the human genome, including their interactions with each other, the environment, and other psychosocial and cultural factors [1].

Genomic health care This involves the use of genomic information and technologies at any stage of the health care continuum, to determine disease risk and predisposition, diagnosis and prognosis, and to inform the selection and prioritisation of therapeutic options. Genomic health care also takes into account the potential ethical, psychological and social implications of genomic information and the application of genomic technologies' [2].

Genotype The entire genetic make-up of a person, or the genetic make-up in relation to a specific gene or genes.

Hemizygous Having just a single copy of a gene or DNA sequence, rather than the usual two. Males are normally hemizygous for most genes on the sex chromosomes.

Heterozygote An individual who has two different versions of an allele for a particular gene or DNA sequence.

Homozygote An individual who has the same version of an allele for a particular gene or DNA sequence on both chromosomes.

Karyotype An individual's collection of chromosomes.

Mitochondrial DNA The small amount of genetic material in mitochondria (cell organelles) found in the cytoplasm of cells. Harmful alterations to mitochondrial DNA can result in absence or impairment of enzymes crucial to energy manufacture within the cell.

Multifactorial Traits or conditions that are the result of interactions between different genes, and between genes and the environment.

Mutation An acquired or inherited change in the usual DNA sequence in a gene. The alteration may be beneficial, neutral or harmful.

Penetrance The proportion of people with a particular genetic alteration who will show signs and symptoms of a clinical condition. A condition that is not always manifest even though the individual has the associated genotype, is said to have reduced penetrance.

Pharmacogenetics The study of how different people respond to drugs due to their genetic make-up, in order to identify new, more specific and more effective drug targets with fewer side effects.

Phenotype The observed characteristics of an individual.

Precision medicine An approach that takes into account individual variability in genes, environment, and lifestyle to better understand disease prediction and risk, onset and progression, informing better selection of targeted therapies and associated diagnostics.

Recessive A characteristic that is apparent in an individual only when the associated genetic alteration is present in both copies of a particular gene.

RNA (ribonucleic acid) A single stranded molecule made by the cell that is essential for cellular function. RNA is produced when a DNA sequence is copied. It contains the same information as DNA and is an intermediate step in the production of protein.

Sex chromosomes The X and Y chromosomes in humans. Females have two X chromosomes, males have one X and one Y chromosome.

INTRODUCTION: THE REVOLUTION IN GENETICS AND GENOMICS

The interest that we have in how characteristics are passed down through the generations is demonstrated at a typical family gathering following the birth of a new baby. We like to identify who the baby most resembles, what features he or she may have inherited from a particular 'side' of the family. As the child grows and develops, the attribution of characteristics may be broadened from the mainly physical (he has his mother's eyes) to include aspects of temperament (she has her father's quick temper). With the advances in knowledge and understanding of the role that inheritance plays in our health and development, we can be increasingly more specific about the contribution of each parent to the features observed in their children. The range of features for which an underlying genetic component has been identified is also increasing, such as longevity or sports performance. Of course parents (and grandparents) take pride in the positive attributes, but how do they feel when a child has inherited a less desirable characteristic, such as a degenerative or life-limiting condition? In order to help you understand the complexities associated with such a diagnosis, in this chapter we shall explore how genetics can impact on family life, the science underpinning this, and the implications for children's nurses.

With the advances in genomic research and technologies we are beginning to appreciate far more the extent of the role that genes play in health and illness – and it is far more extensive than most people imagined, and more complex. Genes and environment interact along a continuum, with relatively rare disorders at the one end where genes alone will dictate the existence of disease, and at the other end, a few diseases in which environmental factors only play a part (Fig. 8.1). Most diseases, though, represent the outcome of the interactions between different genes, and between genes and the environment. Alongside our growing understanding of the nature and function of these genes and their interactions, we are also gaining knowledge of the role of some genes in protecting against disease, and of others in influencing our responses to medicines.

What is driving the rapid increase in knowledge and understanding are the numerous large-scale national and international genome research programmes, often backed by substantial government investment, that have followed the iconic Human Genome Project. That ambitious international project, completed in 2003, deciphered the sequence of the chemicals that make up the DNA within the human blueprint (genome). This has been followed by an exponential rise in the pace of gene discovery along with improvements in genomic data collection technologies, allowing for more

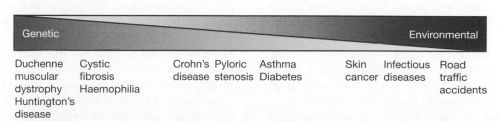

Fig. 8.1 The contribution of genetic and environmental factors to health and disease.

rapid and more economical identification of variations within the whole genome. Analyses of these variations offer insights into the molecular underpinnings of health and disease, with the potential for more cost-effective and improved diagnostic, treatment and management approaches, better targeted to an individual's genetic make-up. The clinical implications of such approaches and their impact on health care are profound. England's Chief Nursing Officer offers her perspective on the implications of this for nurses:

> *As nurses and midwives we play a key role throughout the patient journey. That journey is set to be revolutionised through advances in our understanding of DNA. We need to be ready to make the best use of this huge step forward in personalised medicine.*
>
> *Imagine being able to give an individual a drug or advice to mitigate problems, or to effectively target diseased cells without affecting healthy cells. These are the possibilities of DNA-based care (or genomics). Understanding how a person's DNA can affect their health will change how your patient is diagnosed, and how you manage and treat their condition.*
>
> **Bayliss-Pratt (2017; http://bit.ly/2vlkD1S)**

However, achieving the benefits of 'genomic health care' depend on an informed health care workforce, including nurses and midwives, confident in integrating genetics and genomics into daily practice. Recognising the importance of establishing this, the Nursing and Midwifery Council makes two statements with reference to genomics in its 2019 Standards of Proficiency for Registered Nurses. In relation to promoting health and preventing ill-health, it identifies that at the point of registration, the registered nurse should be able to demonstrate a knowledge of genomics and apply this to an understanding of global patterns of health and well-being outcomes (Nursing and Midwifery Council [NMC], 2018). The ability to demonstrate and apply a knowledge of genomics when undertaking full and accurate person centred nursing assessments and planning care has also been identified. Both statements about genomics are brief, but if we pause to reflect on the wider knowledge and skill set needed to adopt these standards in context of child- and family-centred care, the NMC statements represent 'the tip of the iceberg'. Some awareness of the advances in genomics, its possibilities and potential pitfalls in application to health care can help nurses in differentiating fact from fantasy for their families. The potential for misuse of new knowledge and technologies has also to be considered. What is vitally important is that children's nurses have a sound understanding of the impact of inherited disease on family life. This needs to be underpinned by a grasp of core genetic principles and an appreciation of the nurse's professional role in supporting families at times of crisis and in everyday life. With earlier genetic testing and more prompt, targeted and improved treatments, children with life-limiting conditions, who were seen more by nurses in paediatric intensive care, are now being seen in ambulatory paediatric and adolescent care settings, as well as transitioning to adult services. Cystic fibrosis (CF) provides an early example of this. In 1962 the predicted median survival age was 10 years, but 50 years later, by 2012 the predicted mean survival age for cystic fibrosis was 43.5 years. In 2019 it is 47 years (Cystic Fibrosis Trust, 2018). De Montalembert et al. (2014) note a similar pattern in people with sickle cell disease, where improved clinical outcomes have transformed a fatal disease of childhood to a long-term condition, but which also brings challenges in the transition from paediatric to adult services.

GENETICS AND GENOMICS: THE PARADIGM SHIFT

With the ever-improving capacity to analyse whole genomes, there has come a broadening of interest to study genetic variation and its associations with common diseases such as cancer, diabetes and asthma as well as responses to medication, rather than focusing on the rarer hereditary diseases from single gene and chromosomal conditions. The insights gained are driving a shift from health care approaches aimed at acute intervention to preventive care and individualising clinical care, with interventions more precisely tailored to an individual's genotype. It is also bringing a greater emphasis on the relevance of genomics to 'mainstream' health care rather than considering it the province of regional genetics centres and specialist health professionals. The development of 'precision medicine' strategies in the United States (US) and devolved United Kingdom (UK) governments is testimony to the perceived potential and benefits of this paradigm shift in health care provision.

In the UK there has been unprecedented government investment in genomics research and education, starting with the publication of the Genetics White Paper in 2003 (Department of Health, 2003). The 100,000 Genomes Project, launched in 2012, is an example of its investment. This flagship initiative to collect 100,000 whole genomes from 75,000 people met its target in late 2018 (Genomics England, 2018). The overall aim of the project is to accelerate the uptake of genomics medicine in the NHS. Its focus has been on patients with cancer and on patients with a rare disease and their families.

The inclusion of rare diseases in the 100,000 Genomes Project is an important one given the level of interest in exploring the genomics of common conditions. A rare disease is one that affects less than one in 2000 of the general population. However, there are between 6000 and 8000 known rare diseases, so collectively they are more common than people might think – and new rare conditions continue to be described in the literature on a regular basis. It is estimated that one in 17 people, or 7% of the population, will be affected by a rare disease at some point in their lives. This represents about 3 million people in the UK. At least 80% of rare diseases are genomic in origin, with half of new cases being found in children (Department of Health, 2013). These include the inherited single gene and chromosomal conditions and this is the focus of this chapter. How do such conditions affect family life?

THE IMPACT OF GENETIC DISEASE ON FAMILY LIFE

Family functioning is affected when a child becomes ill because of the usual stresses and practical problems associated with this. If the illness becomes prolonged, or if the child has a chronic condition, in particular one that is degenerative, these stresses are exacerbated. What part might the fact that a disease is 'genetic' play in this? Does it make any difference to the family?

The question of whether genetic conditions bring added stresses is an important one. Application of new genomic technologies is leading to new gene discoveries and an increase in the number of children for whom a genetic diagnosis becomes possible, whether newly affected by a condition or with an existing, previously undiagnosed condition. At the time of writing, the Deciphering Developmental Disorders (DDD) project has identified over 30 new genes not previously associated with developmental disorders and has been able to provide diagnoses for 454 of the 1133 families who have participated in the research (https://www.ddduk.org/). Depending on the current policies surrounding the testing of children, there could also be an increase in the number of children for whom predictive testing would reveal a high risk of developing a condition in the future, such as cardiomyopathy. There are clear advantages to using these new technologies; Dame Sally Davies, Chief Medical Officer for England notes that for patients with rare diseases, it can shorten their 'diagnostic odyssey' helping to identify therapeutic options faster and improve outcomes (Davies, 2017). However, the immediate impact for families might be less positive, at least initially.

A mother's account of her experiences following the diagnosis of two of her sons with adrenoleucodystrophy offers a powerful insight into how genetic diseases can impact on family life (McGowan, 1999). Adrenoleucodystrophy is a degenerative metabolic disorder inherited as an X-linked condition; the variable range of symptoms is associated with a build up of fatty acids. McGowan says: 'The diagnosis of an inherited condition can drop a bombshell into family relationships' (p 197). She states earlier that: 'We now take nothing for granted, such as the simple hopes that our sons will become teenagers or adult men' (p 195). In their research surveying parents of children with confirmed, probable or possible mitochondrial disease, Senger et al., (2016) found that parents experience more guilt, worry, sorrow, anger and long-term uncertainty and have fewer emotional resources than parents of children with other chronic conditions.

Two mothers tell their stories of the impact of a genetic disease on family life on the website *Telling Stories, Understanding Real Life Genetics* (www.tellingstories.nhs.uk). Sarah talks movingly of how she felt on being told her son's diagnosis of Niemann–Pick disease, a lipid storage condition:

It's such an overwhelming thing to be told that your son's got a genetic disorder because your children's lives are mapped out and you have hopes and dreams for them and to be told that things are going to be different for one of your children – it's very hard.

Rachel has two children with cystic fibrosis. She writes:

How has it changed our life? In every way imaginable. Not expecting grandchildren. Spend a lot of time at the hospital. Daily routine is EXTREMELY different from that of parents of healthy children, we spend 2–2½ hours a day doing physio, three hours a day giving intravenous medicine at the moment, and have to give my son a total of 26 doses of oral medications per day, and my daughter a total of 11 doses of oral medications per day.

My marriage has been put under intense strain from all the emotional stress involved in caring for our children. Our children can't live a normal life, and we can't be normal parents. We don't think the thoughts that normal parents would. We don't take their health or life expectancy for granted. We try to make every moment count for them, because we don't know how many they have. We take tons of photos, to remember as much as we can of them growing up.

In her seminal paper, Whyte (1992) studied four families caring for children with cystic fibrosis. In addition to describing the stresses associated with the 'chronic burden of care', she analyses the part that the genetic nature of the illness plays and has concluded that it has a profound effect. The assault on self-image and self-esteem of parents who feel they are unable to produce healthy children can be devastating, and the implications of this for future childbearing are keenly felt. Related to this are the tough decisions that parents may have to face about their reproductive options. This is especially challenging when parents may be considering an option to terminate a pregnancy following prenatal diagnosis. If they have an existing child with the condition, there may be worries that this could devalue that child, and explanations to the child could be difficult.

👤 ACTIVITY

What circumstances can you think of where genetics will have an impact on family life? Make a list of the instances and compare these with those shown in the companion PowerPoint presentation. Read Rachel's story in full at: http://www.tellingstories.nhs.uk/index.php/joys-story?id=213.

So how do families with children affected by, or at risk of, genetic conditions adapt to the situation? Canam (1993) describes the tasks that parents have to face in adapting to chronic childhood illness:

- Accept the child's condition.
- Manage the condition on a day-to-day basis.
- Meet the normal developmental needs of the child.
- Meet the developmental needs of other family members.
- Cope with continuous stress and periodic crises.
- Assist family members to manage their feelings.
- Educate others about the child's condition.
- Establish a support system.

We will consider each of the stages in relation to genetic diseases.

Accepting the Condition

Canam (1993) identifies acceptance as the first phase in the process. Seeking answers and a reduction of uncertainty are integral to this, but a definitive diagnosis is not always available, particularly if the condition is rare. If the condition is one that is already 'in the family' the difficulties can vary. Many families may be accepting, with an established support system, but other parents have to cope with accusations of 'irresponsibility'.

One factor that can have an impact on accepting a condition is its visibility. The shock of a major physical abnormality can be profound and the reactions of others on first meeting the child serve as a reminder of this. Lack of visibility can also make it more difficult for the family and others to accept. When the condition is associated with behavioural problems (such as autism or Tourette syndrome), its physical invisibility frequently presents problems with tolerance and understanding from others, both within and outside the family.

Fanos (1999) reported how acceptance by siblings may be influenced by the visibility of a condition in an affected brother or sister. She noted that the visibility of ataxia-telangiectasia (a recessive condition characterised by unsteady gait and involuntary movements) caused less resentment of the time given to the child, less guilt or tendency to idealise the affected sibling, than children with cystic fibrosis. However, it was associated with more embarrassment and shame.

Manage the Condition on a Day-to-Day Basis

The problems of coping with the practical matters of everyday living when a child (or any family member) has a chronic illness have been widely reviewed (see Chapter 44). A crucial factor in dealing with the problems are resources, including time, energy, money, and social support systems, and the availability of all of these over an extended time. The extent of the resources needed will vary according to the specific condition. With a condition such as cystic fibrosis, for example, the child will need daily physiotherapy, regular visits to clinics, careful supervision of diet and may require frequent periods of hospitalisation. Medication will need to be given and regular supplies maintained. The extra workload may make full- or even part-time employment impractical for one parent. In managing the condition on a day-to-day basis, the parent may then have to adjust to reduced career prospects, loss of role and problems with self-esteem. The latter may be a factor in feelings of guilt at having passed on a condition to the child.

Meet the Normal Developmental Needs of the Child

The nature of the condition and how debilitating it is will clearly be a significant factor in how well the developmental needs of the child can be met. The instinctive desire to protect

the child can be further fuelled by feelings of guilt, predisposing to 'spoiling' and children may take advantage of this. Labelling of the child by the family or by others can further compromise the situation.

> ### PROFESSIONAL CONVERSATION
>
> *I was enjoying my placement with the community paediatric team. I enjoyed meeting the families and seeing their care from another perspective, it is so different to the hospital setting. This particular visit was to see Lucy and her son Gareth. I knew them from previous admissions to the ward. Gareth is 7 years old and he has multiple problems – developmental delay, some autistic features and feeding problems. The reason for today's visit was to discuss the genetic test results that Lucy was to have been given at the genetic clinic earlier that week.*
>
> The nurse spent the first few minutes catching up with Gareth's progress, his feeding and his toilet training. Then she asked about the test results:
>
> *Lucy started to cry as she explained that all the tests had come back negative. I did not understand why she was crying – surely this was good news to hear Gareth does not have a genetic condition. I listened while she talked about the guilt that she is responsible for Gareth's problems, her description of her pregnancy, wondering if she had done something during this time that caused it all. I tried to reassure her reminding her that the geneticist had told her that it was not her fault. She turned to me and said 'How can they say that if they do not know what did cause his problems?', I did not know what to say.*
>
> *Reflecting on this visit later I realised that my response to Lucy had been very naive. I had not thought about her position and that a positive result showing that her son had a serious genetic condition could be preferable to a negative one, which left her with so many unanswered questions and a guilt that seemed could only be erased if she could replace it with certainty.*

Meet the Developmental Needs of Other Family Members

Fanos (1997) reminds us that the accessibility of a parent for the psychosocial support of a child is a crucial factor in his or her well-being. If the condition is an autosomal dominant one, a parent may already be trying to cope with their own illness, or that of the partner. With one (or more) child affected by a condition, the accessibility of the parents will be compromised – more so when they are grieving the death of an affected child. With frequent hospital stays, the availability of a parent on a day-to-day basis will also be severely limited. In a later study of the impact on siblings of boys with severe combined immunodeficiency disorder, most expressed distress over the prolonged absence of the mother during hospitalisation of the ill brother (Fanos and Puck, 2001). They concluded that parents need help in balancing the needs of well siblings with those of an affected one.

PROFESSIONAL CONVERSATION

The Bradley family was well known to me – various members had been back and forth to the cystic fibrosis clinic over the years. Teresa was just 15 when she came and asked me about carrier testing for cystic fibrosis. Because newborn CF screening wasn't introduced in the UK until 2007, she'd missed out on testing when she was a baby of course. Her cousin has the condition and her mum, older sister and another cousin are carriers, as well as her aunt and uncle of course. The family has always talked openly about cystic fibrosis and Teresa said she felt it was now her turn to be tested. I was a bit concerned because of her age, although she is quite mature and sensible, but also because I wondered how she might feel if she turned out not to have the gene. With so many of her family being carriers (in fact, all of the older females and the uncle) a negative result might exclude her from 'the gang'. I don't think the family had registered this and I know they would not knowingly exclude her but the potential for her to feel left out needed to be raised.

Cope With Continuous Stress and Periodic Crises

Sickle-cell disease and cystic fibrosis (both autosomal recessive conditions) are typical examples of how the pattern of the illness is one of continuous stress, managing the condition on a daily basis with a regime of medication and other therapy, interspersed with crises, both familial and medical. A child with sickle-cell having an acute episode (where the abnormally shaped red blood cells can cause severe pain, infarction and necrosis) and a chest infection in a child with cystic fibrosis require prompt hospitalisation and aggressive clinical intervention. The gradual deterioration of a child with a degenerative condition such as Duchenne muscular dystrophy (X-linked) as he becomes increasingly dependent on his family also provokes continuous stress.

The day-to-day fluctuations in condition and the uncertainty this brings make a major contribution to stress (Locker, 1991; Nereo et al., 2003). To this symptomatic uncertainty is added the trajectory uncertainty of being able to predict the course and outcome of the disease. This is not only because of individual variation in gene expression, but also because of advances in management in a fast-moving research field, underpinning hopes for more effective treatments or even cure (through gene or stem cell therapy) in the future.

 ACTIVITY

Watch Pamela's story on the *Genetic Disorders* UK website: https://www.geneticdisordersuk.org/beginners-guide-to-genetics/films-about-genetic-disorders/pamelas-story/.

She is a young girl with sickle cell anaemia. Pamela describes what it is like to live with the uncertainty of her condition.

Then read Tony's story on the *Telling Stories* website: http://www.tellingstories.nhs.uk/index.php/all-stories/120-tonys-story.

What are the common issues for Pamela and Tony?

The National Institute for Health and Care Excellence has published a quality standard for managing the care of people in hospital with acute painful episodes of sickle cell disease (SCD). You can view it at: https://www.nice.org.uk/guidance/qs58.

ACTIVITY—cont'd

Sickle Cell Disease in Childhood: Standards and Recommendations for Clinical Care produced in 2019 by clinicians, parents and carers, the Sickle Cell Society and UK Forum on Haemoglobin Disorders, the NHS Sickle Cell and Thalassaemia Screening Programme, and Public Health England: https://www.sicklecellsociety.org/paediatricstandards/.

Managing the Family's Feelings

It is important to acknowledge the positive contribution that the child makes to the family, irrespective of the nature of the condition. Kearney and Griffin (2001) conceptualise the experiences of parents of children with developmental disability as being a dynamic between joy and sorrow. Although there are undoubtedly negative experiences, these can be balanced by positive feelings such as hope and humour. As McGowan expresses it: 'My sons are special people, beyond their genetic flaw …' (McGowan, 1999, p 199).

Nonetheless, the sorrows can be profound and long-lasting, and other feelings such as guilt, blame, anger, fear, anxiety and depression can also be difficult to cope with. One factor that may be more apparent in families with a child affected by a genetic condition is the feeling of guilt. This can take the form of 'survivor guilt' in unaffected family members, including children. In one study examining the long-term psychological effects of genetic testing for a hereditary colorectal cancer, some children with a negative result and a positive-testing sibling demonstrated an increase in symptoms of anxiety at follow-up (Codori et al., 2003).

The guilt that parents can feel can be overwhelming. In his book about his daughter Alex, Frank Deford recounts eloquently the impact of genetic disease on family life (Deford, 1983). Alex had cystic fibrosis and she lived until she was 8 years old. The story of Alex's life, of the family's struggle with her disease, and of her death is indescribably moving and essential reading for any children's nurse. Deford captures some of the feelings that many parents may experience in this situation:

Ultimately, whether in my dealings with Carol [his wife], with Alex herself, with anyone involved with the disease – or with myself, for that matter – the major emotion pressing upon me was the feeling of inadequacy … And I could not explain how I felt, because of the shame, nor could I ever escape, because of the guilt.

Deford (1983, p 96)

He goes on to say:

When our child was dying – when she was dying because of the genes we passed on to her – no matter how irrational it may have been to flagellate ourselves, there were times, in the mustiest corners of self-awareness, when we had to. Had to. I could not forgive Carol any more than I could forgive myself. After all, we quickly enough assume credit for the genes that make our children attractive and bright – she takes after me. It's only human nature, then, that we also accept the responsibility when we pass on genes of destruction.

Deford (1983, p 94)

Of course, such feelings are not the prerogative of parents in this situation. Many parents will blame themselves for contributing in some way to their child's condition. However, with genetic disease, particularly the single gene disorders and chromosomal conditions, the cause may be clearly attributable to one or both parents. Furthermore, as the condition may be passed on to future generations, this may be accompanied by ongoing guilt and fear that subsequent children will also inherit it.

Educate Others

There are thousands of single gene disorders and chromosome abnormalities and most are rare. However, even the more common ones are unfamiliar to most health professionals outside the specialist genetics service. The families tend to become the experts, demonstrating knowledge and understanding of the condition and using this to educate others involved in the care of the child. Many contribute to the work of support groups such as Contact a Family (www.caf.org.uk), Genetic Alliance UK (https://www.geneticalliance.org.uk/), and their websites can provide a valuable education resource for other families. The *Telling Stories* website (www.tellingstories.nhs.uk) is developed with patients and carers, using family stories primarily as an education resource for health professionals. One of the common themes of storytellers on this website is the importance they place on health care professionals being informed and they are happy to play a part in this. Yvonne's granddaughter has a syndrome without a name (SWAN, www.undiagnosed.org.uk). Yvonne echoed many when she told us:

> *Please don't be afraid to ask the parents and to talk about the child's needs ... We deal with the child each day and we are aware of the changes which you don't see. Please listen to us. Don't be afraid to say that you don't know.*

> *http://www.tellingstories.nhs.uk/index.php/all-stories/130-yvonne-story*

Establish a Support System

With any enduring illness, the health care system becomes a major part of the family's environment and they need to become socialised into it. The success of this depends in part on the quality of information available and on accessible and effective multi-agency communication. Support groups can thus be life savers. However, family centred care is core to good quality support and Christian (2011) emphasises the importance of children's nurses creating partnerships with parents and families, providing quality care to improve lives and reduce the impact of the care-giving burden.

Marianne's son James was born with Edwards syndrome and he died aged 3.5 years. She describes how the specialist nurses and the respite care team became part of the family 'and they loved him and he could see that they loved him and that was really important because we were leaving the most precious gift with them whenever we left the house'.

Marianne goes on to talk about the support that most helped her family:

> *I think what's helped me the most has been my friends that have had children with Edwards; my husband and I are really supportive of each other; we've had an amazing network of nurses caring for him. Respite is a major thing, a major thing for families – I mean we were exceptionally lucky in the respite that we got – and to give families that break.*

> *http://www.tellingstories.nhs.uk/index.php/all-stories/191-mariannes-story*

◼ SEMINAR DISCUSSION TOPIC

The Human Fertilisation and Embryology Act 2008 amends the law related to assisted reproductive treatment and embryo research. Section 14 (4)(9) of the Act (p10) states that:

Persons or embryos that are known to have a gene, chromosome or mitochondrion abnormality involving a significant risk that a person with the abnormality will have or develop— (a) a serious physical or mental disability, (b) a serious illness, or (c) any other serious medical condition, must not be preferred to those that are not known to have such an abnormality.

https://www.legislation.gov.uk/ukpga/2008/22/pdfs/ukpga_20080022_en.pdf

The explanatory notes (p 19) reiterate that it is:

... a condition of a treatment licence that embryos that are known to have an abnormality (including a gender-related abnormality) are not to be preferred to embryos not known to have such an abnormality. The same restriction is also applied to the selection of persons as gamete or embryo donors. This would prevent assisted reproduction technology being used to select an embryo with a view to increasing the chance of giving birth to a child that had or would develop a serious medical condition, or to select a donor to increase the chance of a child having a serious medical condition.

https://www.legislation.gov.uk/ukpga/2008/22/pdfs/ukpgaen_20080022_en.pdf

There is no further explanation to qualify the terms 'serious medical or mental disability,' 'serious illness,' or 'other serious medical condition'.

How would you define these terms? Would your friends, family or colleagues define the terms differently?

What are the implications of the Act for those who might be identified as meeting the terms of this subsection of the Act?

The phases of adaptation we have described can be 'worked through' by families, with time and support. However, it is important to note that individuals within a family will progress at different rates, and the progress itself may not be linear as individuals move back and forth across the stages. Whyte (1992) identifies that a crucial aspect of the process is the synchrony with which partners move through these phases.

Many of the challenges facing families that we have outlined so far apply to other diseases, and not just genetic disease, but the distinction between these is becoming blurred as advances in genetics research increasingly are revealing the genetic component of common diseases. The next section explains how genes can be passed on through the generations and how 'faulty' genes may lead to disease and ill health.

IT RUNS IN THE FAMILY: THE ROLE OF GENETIC FACTORS IN DISEASE

There are over 4000 simply inherited serious genetic conditions, such as cystic fibrosis, sickle cell disease and Duchenne muscular dystrophy. Together with the chromosomal alterations such as Trisomy 21 (Down syndrome), they account for about 10 to 20 people with a genetic condition per 1000 population. However, by the age of 60, about 60% of the population is likely to have been affected by a disease that is partially genetically determined. Our genes, at least in part, determine nearly all of our characteristics, including how we respond to infection, and so they play a fundamental role in our health. But what are genes and how can they lead to ill health that can be passed on through the generations?

Genes

Almost every cell of the body contains a complete set of genes, each one representing a chemical instruction to make one or more proteins, protein sub-units or RNA molecules for different cell functions, guiding development from embryo to adult. It is estimated that we have about 20,000 genes, which direct the development, growth and function of every cell in the body, its tissues and organ systems. There are genes that control other genes, switching them on or off according to the cell type and the functions it performs. For example, in the pancreas, the gene providing the instructions for the manufacture of insulin might be turned on, whereas genes for making keratin, a structural protein found in hair and nails, would be switched off. There are also genes that control cell growth and division; faults in these genes can lead to different types of cancers.

Genes are made up of DNA.

The genes themselves are located on the chromosomes, each chromosome being made up of two enormously long strands of DNA, joined together and tightly coiled into a double helix. The genes are spaced along the DNA molecule and are an integral part of it.

DNA molecules consists of four different chemical bases (nucleotides), A, C, G and T. A gene has hundreds or thousands of these bases; some, like the dystrophin gene (associated with Duchenne muscular dystrophy), have millions. Each chromosome is made up 100–1000s of genes. If the DNA molecule that comprises one chromosome was likened to a tower of Lego, then the tower could be built using only four colours of Lego blocks – but the tower could be about 100 million blocks high.

It is the order or sequence of the four nucleotides within a gene along the length of a DNA molecule that contains the instructions to make specific proteins or protein sub-units, in the form of a chemical code. A block of three nucleotides (a triplet) represents the code for one amino acid, the building blocks of proteins. Essentially, each gene is made up of a series of three-letter words (using a four-letter alphabet), which when deciphered, gives us a sequence of amino acids.

Alterations to the Genetic Make-Up

The sequence of the chemical bases that make up the DNA in each of the 23 pairs of chromosomes is the same in every person for about 99% of the human genome. However, there are variations in the remaining genetic material and it is these variations that make us unique.

Some of the variations occur by chance in the body (somatic) cells or in the sex cells (eggs or sperm). Alterations that occur in the latter can be passed on to future generations. Although many alterations are repaired, some are not. Of these, many will have no effect, some may confer an advantage to the genome, but others may be harmful, particularly if the number of alterations (or mutations) increases with increasing age and exposure to environmental hazards. These mutations are effectively gene errors. Diseases or conditions that are caused by harmful alterations within a single gene are referred to as single gene disorders. If clinical signs or symptoms of a single gene condition are present when just one allele of the gene pair is altered, the condition is said to be dominant. If the disease occurs only when both alleles have been altered, the condition is described as recessive.

The nature of the gene error can also vary. Some arise when a single nucleotide from an entire gene sequence is accidentally replaced by a different nucleotide. The mutation associated with the most common type of sickle cell disease is a classic example of this type of 'point' alteration. Sickle cell disease has a global incidence of between 300,000 and 400,000 newborns each year, the majority in sub-Saharan Africa. The genetic alteration can be advantageous for some carriers, providing resistance to malaria for a short time. In the UK, it is most common in families of African or African-Caribbean origin, but rare in those of North European origin. It is one of the most common inherited conditions affecting around one in every 2000 babies born in the UK and there are between 12,500 and 15,000 people with SCD.

Haemoglobin is formed from four chains of amino acids, two α chains, and two β chains, each of which is associated with a haem group that binds with oxygen. In the most common type of SCD both genes on the chromosome pair (chromosome 11) that provide the code for the β chains have the same alteration. A single base (A) within the gene is replaced by a different base (T). This alters the code so that the amino acid valine is assembled instead of glutamine, and this single alteration is sufficient to change the normal β-globin structure of haemoglobin (Fig. 8.2). The result is that the red blood cells become abnormally shaped in particular conditions such as during an infectious illness, dehydration or in reduced oxygen levels. The sickle-shaped cells can block capillaries, causing painful

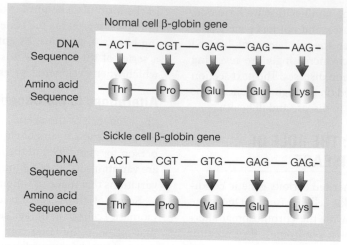

Fig. 8.2 The sickle cell mutation. *DNA*, Deoxyribonucleic acid.

TABLE 8.1 **Examples of Single Gene Conditions Seen in Childhood**		
Autosomal Dominant	**Autosomal Recessive**	**X-Linked Recessive**
Achondroplasia	Cystic fibrosis	Haemophilia A and B
Marfan syndrome	Sickle cell disease	Alport syndrome
Osteogenesis imperfecta	Thalassaemia	Fragile X
Tuberous sclerosis	Phenylketonuria	Red–green colour blindness
Neurofibromatosis type 1	Spinal muscular atrophy (Werdnig–Hoffman disease)	Duchenne muscular dystrophy
Gilles de la Tourette syndrome (Tourette's)	Congenital deafness	Glucose-6-phosphate dehydrogenase deficiency

infarctions during sickling episodes, and the disturbances to blood flow can also cause leg ulcers. Internal organs are compromised, and splenomegaly may be apparent. Premature destruction of the abnormally shaped cells also leads to anaemia, and a loss of immune function predisposes the child to infection. Early diagnosis is crucial to improve survival and testing for SCD is offered as part of the newborn screening programme. Sickle cell disease has a recessive phenotype, although people with one altered gene 'carriers' may show some signs of the disease, but it is very much milder.

How Genes Are Passed on Through Families

Single gene disorders show characteristic patterns of inheritance sometimes referred to as Mendelian patterns, as they are passed on through generations, depending on whether the associated phenotypes are dominant or recessive, and located on an autosome or the sex chromosomes (Table 8.1).

Because an autosomal dominant trait is invariably manifest in the affected person, the family tree will typically show someone affected with the condition in each generation, and with both sexes affected in similar numbers (Fig. 8.3). Each child of an affected parent has a one in two or 50% chance of inheriting the altered gene, but unaffected parents do not transmit it.

 ACTIVITY

Visit the Genomics Education Programme's Family History channel: (https://vimeo.com/channels/familyhistory) and watch both videos on sudden death (*The Conversation* and *The Pedigree*). Helen Evans is concerned about the risk to her daughter following the sudden death of her son and the strong family history. Listen to The Pedigree video again and try drawing Helen's family tree yourself.

What type of inheritance pattern do you think is most likely in this family?

In contrast, an autosomal recessive trait can be carried through generations 'hidden' from view, because carriers usually show no symptoms. Often, the first indication of the condition being 'in the family' is when an affected baby is born of parents who are both carriers. When both parents are carriers, with each conception there is a one in four or 25% chance that the baby will be affected by the condition, and a one in two or 50% chance that the baby will be a carrier. However, the chance of both parents being carriers is usually quite rare, but higher when parents are more closely related by blood – such as first cousins. Such consanguineous marriages are more common in some populations, such as among North Africa, the Middle East, western Asia and South India communities. Some conditions are associated with a higher

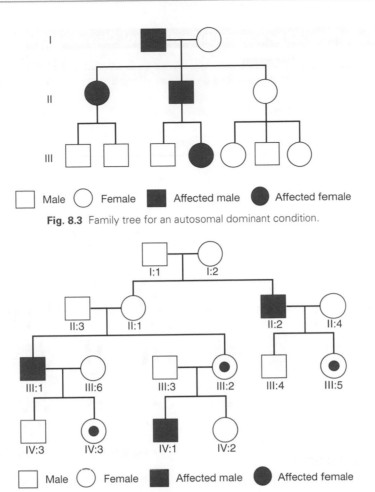

Male Female Affected male Affected female

Fig. 8.3 Family tree for an autosomal dominant condition.

Male Female Affected male Affected female

⊙ Female who is an obligate carrier of the gene alteration

Fig. 8.4 X-linked inheritance.

carrier frequency in particular populations, such as cystic fibrosis in white northern Europeans (in the UK, this frequency is approximately one in 25).

When the gene under question is located on the X chromosome, the pattern (known as X-linked inheritance) is somewhat different. X-linked inheritance can be either recessive or dominant, although the latter is much rarer. X-linked recessive conditions result from gene alteration on the X chromosome, but as females have two X chromosomes, they usually have a second unaltered copy of the gene on the other chromosome of the pair to compensate. Males have only one X chromosome and are said to be hemizygous for X-linked genes. If they have a gene alteration on this chromosome, they will develop the condition. Males pass on their Y chromosome to their sons so male-to-male transmission is not seen in X-linked conditions such as haemophilia, but all daughters of affected males will inherit the altered gene (Fig. 8.4). Women who are carriers have a 50% chance of passing on the altered gene to their sons (who will then be affected) and their daughters will have a 50% chance of being carriers themselves. The characteristic features of the three types of inheritance can be summarised as shown in Table 8.2.

There are occasions when a family history does not seem to follow the typical pattern. Alterations to mitochondrial DNA show that a mother-to-child inheritance as mitochondria are passed on in the woman's egg cell at the time of conception. Each egg cell may contain a mix of fully functioning and malfunctioning mitochondria and the balance between the two is important in determining whether and to what extent an individual may show signs of disease. Males pass very few mitochondria on to their children.

New mutations in the sex cells of a parent can account for the appearance of a dominant trait in a family even though neither parent is affected. Some dominant traits can also be affected by penetrance and expressivity. Traits associated with a reduced penetrance may not be expressed in an individual, and when they are expressed, the severity of expression may also vary. Neurofibromatosis is a dominant condition with variable expression such that it may have gone undetected in an individual at first and thus appear to 'skip' a generation in affected families. However, closer examination might reveal, for example, some of the characteristic pigmented patches (café-au-lait spots) on the skin. Finally, non-paternity can also account for an otherwise puzzling family tree, and this situation has to be dealt with sensitively.

TABLE 8.2   The Family Tree: Characteristic Features of Classically Inherited Diseases

Dominant Inheritance	Recessive	X-Linked
Usually more than one successive generation affected	Usually only one generation affected	More than one generation affected
People of both sexes affected	People of both sexes affected	Males affected more severely generally than females
Male to male transmission evident	Offspring of two healthy parents affected	No male to male transmission

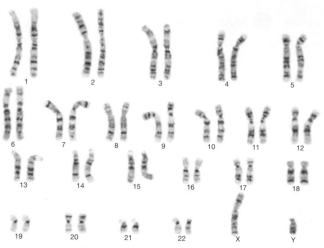

Fig. 8.5 A typical male karyotype.

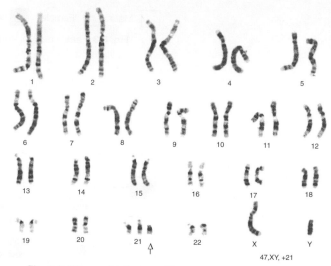

47,XY, +21

Fig. 8.6 Trisomy 21 *(arrowed)* karyotype (Down syndrome).

DNA Is Packaged Into Chromosomes

Chromosomes are the more visible elements of inheritance, seen under the microscope as tightly packed coils of DNA. Cells have 23 pairs of chromosomes, one member of each pair being inherited from the mother and one from the father. We inherit one set of 23 chromosomes, and thus one set of genes, from each parent, passed on through the egg and sperm cells. The total chromosome number of 46 is restored with the fusion of the egg and sperm to form the embryo.

When the chromosomes are examined in the genetics laboratory, they are set out in a systematic way, according to their matched pairs, arranged in order of size, and aligned with the shorter arm of the chromosome (designated p) above the longer one (q). This arrangement is the karyotype (Fig. 8.5).

Members of a pair of chromosomes will have the same genes in the same order along the chromosome and are referred to as being homologous. However, the form of a particular gene may be a little different on each chromosome – these different forms are known as alleles. The alleles we inherit govern our traits such as blood group, haemoglobin structure, skin colour, whether we can smell or taste certain substances and so on. For example, the ABO gene encodes for the production of specific antigens on the surface of red blood cells. It is located on chromosome 9q, at the same location (or locus) on each chromosome of the pair and the three different types of allele (A, B, O) that can occur here form the basis for the ABO blood type classification. If both chromosomes have identical alleles (e.g. A) the person is said to be homozygous at that locus and will be blood group A. If the alleles

are different (e.g. one is A and the other B) the person will be blood group AB and is heterozygous at that locus.

As well as errors that occur in the DNA sequence, at 'gene level', we can also have errors at the level of the chromosome, involving part or whole chromosomes. Such errors account for more than 50% of all spontaneous first trimester losses, 20% of second trimester losses, and occur in about one in 160 live births. The errors involve alterations either to the number or structure of chromosomes.

Alterations to chromosome number are the most common. Polyploidy is the term given to cells that contain a multiple of 23 chromosomes. In humans, triploid (69 chromosomes) and tetraploid (92 chromosomes) conceptions can occur, but are incompatible with survival. An embryo that is aneuploid has missing or additional chromosomes, most commonly one additional chromosome (trisomy). The general rule is that we can tolerate additional genetic material more readily than a loss, so monosomy (loss of one chromosome) is not compatible with life. The exception to this is Turner syndrome, a condition seen only in girls where there is a loss of one X chromosome.

The most common form of aneuploidy is trisomy and while most trisomic fetuses are spontaneously aborted, some survive to term and beyond. Down syndrome, and its association with increased maternal age, is the most well-known (Fig. 8.6). Trisomies of the sex chromosomes (XXX female, XYY male or XXY male with Klinefelter syndrome) have much less severe consequences, and many people with this condition may be undiagnosed until after puberty, or at fertility clinics.

TABLE 8.3　Some Examples of Chromosome Rearrangements

	Example	Karyotype
Numerical		
Gain of a whole chromosome	Down syndrome (Trisomy 21)	47,XX (or XY) +21
		Gain of an autosome (Chr 21)
	Klinefelter syndrome	47,XXY
		Gain of a sex chromosome
Loss of a whole chromosome	Turner syndrome	45,X
		Loss of a sex chromosome
Structural		
Translocation	Balanced Robertsonian translocation	45,XY t(14;21)
		Chr 14 and 21 have fused to form one chromosome
Deletion	Cri du chat	46,XX (or XY)5p–Partial deletion on short arm of Chr 5
Microdeletion	22q	46,XX (or XY)22q–Microdeletion on long arm of Chr 22

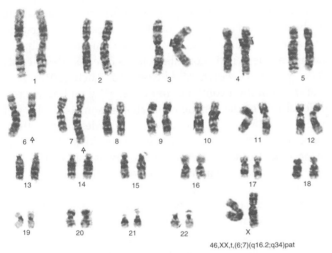

46,XX,t,(6;7)(q16.2;q34)pat

Fig. 8.7 Karyotype of a reciprocal translocation. Genetic material has been exchanged between one of each pair of chromosomes 6 and 7 *(arrowed)*.

Structural alterations occur when chromosome material becomes rearranged following breakage and abnormal reconstitution. Parts of a chromosome may become detached and lost, duplicated, or rearranged (Table 8.3). Breaks can be caused spontaneously, or by certain viruses, drugs or radiation. The effects of these depend on the nature of the rearrangement and whether there is an overall loss or gain of genetic material. For example, a gene that spans a break site will be broken and can no longer provide the entire instructions required for the protein that it encodes.

A translocation occurs when there is an exchange of material between two different (non-homologous) chromosomes (Fig. 8.7). These are the most clinically significant of the structural chromosome rearrangements. Occasionally, genes located at the breaks of the two different chromosomes become joined together and a novel protein is produced as a result. In most cases, there is no net loss or gain of chromosomal material during the exchange process, and the translocation is thus said to be 'balanced'. It is estimated that 1 in 500 individuals has a balanced translocation, usually with no health consequences for the individual. However, problems arise during the formation of the egg or sperm cells, and some may carry unbalanced chromosomes, often causing early pregnancy loss or multiple abnormalities in the infant.

Genetic Testing

The US National Institutes of Health describes genetic testing as 'a type of medical test that identifies changes in chromosomes, genes, or proteins. The results of a genetic test can confirm or rule out a suspected genetic condition or help determine a person's chance of developing or passing on a genetic disorder' (https://ghr.nlm.nih.gov). More than 1000 genetic tests are currently in use, and more are being developed. Different reasons for genetic testing include:

1. Diagnostic: carried out on individuals who either have, or are suspected of having, a particular condition because of clinical signs or symptoms.
2. Predictive/presymptomatic tests, carried out on healthy people to detect if they have a gene alteration associated with a particular condition for which there is a family history. The result can indicate whether they will or might develop the condition in the future. They are usually only offered to adults.
3. Carrier: identifies healthy individuals with a single copy of an altered gene, or a balanced translocation, who might pass on the genetic alteration to their children.
4. Prenatal diagnostic tests: carried out in pregnancy where there is an increased chance of the baby being affected by a serious genetic condition. The procedures are usually invasive, via amniocentesis or chorionic villus testing, but non-invasive genetic diagnosis using fetal DNA in maternal blood can be used in specific circumstances.
5. Newborn blood spot screening test: offered to all newborn infants in the UK to detect a range of conditions, including cystic fibrosis, sickle cell disease and inherited metabolic diseases. Blood is collected via a heel prick. The aim is early diagnosis of serious conditions which can be ameliorated with early intervention.
6. Direct-to-consumer testing: tests sold directly to the public, usually from a website.

In the UK, genetic testing is usually conducted through accredited NHS laboratories, is free and the process is voluntary. The term 'genetic laboratory' test could be applied where the test involves the direct analysis of genetic material (nucleic acid or chromosomes, e.g. see Figs 8.5–8.7) or the analysis of biochemical parameters, such as the concentration of metabolites or the activity of enzymes, to diagnose a genetic condition or make predictions about the genetic make-up of a person. Genetics information can also be obtained from clinical examination, imaging and family history. For instance, a sigmoidoscopy in a young person at risk of inherited bowel cancer through familial adenomatous polyposis (FAP) could be defined as a genetic test in that it gives 'genetic information'. There are benefits and limitations to testing and it is important that individuals and parents have full, balanced information and are supported professionally in making a decision about whether or not to undergo genetic testing.

Cystic fibrosis provides a useful example to illustrate how 'finding' the gene can help in understanding the underlying disease mechanism and in providing a direct genetic test. Children with cystic fibrosis generally fail to thrive and are prone to recurrent respiratory infections, amongst other problems. When the gene associated with CF was identified in 1989, it was found to be one that codes for a transmembrane regulator protein (known as CFTR). The normal protein helps to control the flow of chloride ions across cell membranes and so produces good-quality mucus secretions. If this flow is compromised, sodium and water balance will be affected leading to abnormal secretions and a build-up of thick mucus. Although other mutations can occur, most mutations in Europe (70%) show a deletion of three bases at a specific position of the *CFTR* gene. This results in the loss of the amino acid phenylalanine from the protein product and this deletion may be detected using direct analysis of DNA.

Understanding how genes that contribute to ill health can be inherited, how they can then be detected to inform a diagnosis and then communicating this and other information to parents and children is part of the role of professionals within the genetics service. However, with the integration of genetics into mainstream services and increasing demand for genetic information, there is a growing need for all health professionals to develop competence in this area. The next section looks at the role of the children's nurse in relation to this.

GENETICS REFERRAL AND THE FAMILY JOURNEY: THE ROLE OF THE CHILDREN'S NURSE

There are a variety of reasons why a referral is made to the specialist genetics service and health professionals should be alert to any 'red flags' for referral (Box 8.1). Typical reasons include: that a child has developmental delay, learning difficulties or other health concerns, which might be due to a genetic condition and specialist advice is sought for assessment and diagnosis; that there is a known genetic condition in the family and advice is sought about how it might affect any children; that a woman is pregnant and there is some chance that the baby has a genetic condition because of family history or as a result of prenatal screening tests; following a positive newborn screening test result. Nurses have a crucial role in alerting colleagues to a possible need for referral through their awareness of family history, or potential familial link. Referrals are usually made by a general practitioner (GP) or paediatrician to the regional genetics centre. The very first clinical genetics service began at Great Ormond Street Hospital in 1946. There are currently 21 regional centres across the UK, comprising clinical and laboratory services (for a map with contact details, visit https://www.bsgm.org.uk/healthcare-professionals/list-of-genetic-clinics/). The centres are staffed by multidisciplinary teams and patients are usually seen by a clinical geneticist and/or a genetic counsellor at outpatient clinics, although home visits are sometimes made.

Clinical geneticists are medical doctors who have undergone substantial further specialist training. Genetic counsellors are registered health professionals (some are nurses) who have also undergone training in genetics. Genetic counselling has been defined as 'the process of helping people understand and adapt to the medical, psychological and familial implications of the genetic contributions to disease' (Resta et al., 2006, p 79). However, Middleton and Patch (2018) note that the definition continues to evolve. They outline the traditional role of the genetic counsellor as someone who will assess an individual's risk of a genetic disorder, prepare them for genetic testing, communicate the results and assist the management of the patients' genetic disease, as well as prepare and support the individual to contact their relatives also at risk of the same disease.

Families can expect the following at a typical appointment:
- Reasons for the referral will be discussed.
- A family tree will be drawn, for which the patient may be asked medical details of other family members.
- A medical examination may be carried out.
- The findings will be explained and options discussed.
- Tests may be offered.
- A plan will be discussed and agreed with the patient/carer.
- They may be invited to participate in a research programme.
- A follow-up letter will be sent confirming the key points of the discussions.

🌐 WWW

Read the patient information leaflet about the clinical genetics appointment, prepared by Unique, a rare chromosome disorder charity support group. It outlines why referrals are made, who patients might see and what to expect before, during and after the appointment:
- https://www.rarechromo.org/media/familyguides/English/A%20Clinical%20Genetics%20appointment%20FTNW.pdf

Think about how you would summarise the key points to tell your patients about what 'having a referral' means.

Barr and Millar (2003) argue that genetic counselling should be seen as an integral part of the adaptation process that parents and other family members journey through. The

BOX 8.1 Red Flags for Referral to Genetics Specialists

General Red Flags for Clinical Practice

One or more of these red flags that may indicate a high genetic risk in your patient:

- The patient is unusually young to have the condition.
- The condition does not commonly occur in patients of this sex.
- There is an absence of typical environmental factors that are usually associated with the condition.
- There is a strong family history of the condition.
- The presentation is more severe than usual.
- The patient is affected bilaterally in paired organs.

Red Flags for Suspicion of a Genetic Condition in a Baby or Child

- The infant/child has signs of developmental delay – in motor skills, speech and/or cognition.
- The infant/child has multiple congenital abnormalities.
- The child has similar problems to other family members.
- The infant/child has unusual physical (dysmorphic) features (or features very different from either parent).
- The child/infant has failure to thrive or overgrowth.
- The child/infant has a small or large head.
- There is a history of recurrent spontaneous miscarriage in the family.
- The infant/child has a combination of unusual problems.

From Gen-Equip: Genetics Education for Primary Care. Available from: https://www.primarycaregenetics.org/?page_id=2157&lang=en.

role of the children's nurse is then to journey with the family, helping family members 'prepare for, engage in and move on' irrespective of the information provided at the genetic clinic. To do so effectively, the nurse has to be equipped with sufficient knowledge and understanding of genetics to be able to support the family, placing genetics information into context as a part of that journey. Appropriate nurse education and preparation in genetics and genomics is fundamental to this.

NURSE EDUCATION AND STANDARDS IN GENETICS/ GENOMIC

The international literature on nursing competence in genetics and genomics widely acknowledges low levels of genomics literacy among nurses (Calzone et al., 2018). However, there are efforts being made globally to address deficits in knowledge and skills and the UK, along with the US, has been leading developments in this. In 2011 the Nursing and Midwifery Professional Advisory Board convened a Task and Finish Group to consider genetics and genomics and the future for nursing and midwifery. It set out a vision which included that 'every nurse and midwife recognises and acts on the importance of genetics/genomics in the care they provide to people and families':

- recognising the issues of particular relevance to their area of practice;
- recognising the limits of their own competence;
- knowing where and how to seek the most appropriate help and advice;

and that 'every nurse and midwife is competent to a minimum standard in genetics/genomics through education provision' (Task and Finish Group, 2011, p 9). Education provision is coming to the forefront of policy in the UK. The Precision Medicine strategies for England and Wales both acknowledge the importance of education and development of the NHS workforce. Health Education England's Genomics Education Programme (https://www.genomicseducation.hee.nhs.uk/) offers practical support to all health professionals, including nurses, with education resources and free courses (online and university based).

Earlier in this chapter, we likened the NMC's standards that include genomics to the tip of the iceberg. Further detail is necessary on what nurses should include in their practice in order to make a nursing assessment and plan care that incorporates genetics/genomics. The extent of the knowledge and skills required in genetics by all nurses in the UK has been set into a competency framework (Kirk et al., 2014). Building on an earlier framework created in 2003, the authors worked with stakeholders (including professional and client groups) to identify the knowledge, skills and attitudes in genetics that nurses should demonstrate.

⊕ WWW

Read the paper online (open access):
- https://onlinelibrary.wiley.com/doi/pdf/10.1111/jan.12207. Discuss in your learning group if you think the competencies are relevant for children's nurses.

Eight competency statements were constructed, representing the minimum standard that should be achieved by nurses at the point of registration (Box 8.2). Identifying people who might benefit from genetic services and information was acknowledged as the key competency, and requires all nurses to have some skills in family history assessment. The role of the nurse in providing ongoing care and support to the family is also emphasised. The framework suggests learning outcomes and practice indicators for each competency statement to aid curriculum development.

▶ REFLECT ON YOUR PRACTICE

- How confident are you that you could demonstrate these competencies in your practice?
- How can you address any deficit you identify in your skills?

Although the competencies apply to all nursing professionals, the situations in which children's nurses in particular need to use genetic knowledge and skills was earlier outlined by the Association of Genetic Nurses and Counsellors (2002). These include where the children's nurse would need to:

- provide supportive, informed communication at the time of diagnosis or receipt of definitive results;

BOX 8.2   The Eight Core Genomics Competency Standard Statements for Nurses

1. Identify individuals who might benefit from genetic services and/or information through a comprehensive nursing assessment:
   - that recognises the importance of family history in assessing predisposition to disease;
   - recognising the key indicators of a potential genetic condition;
   - taking appropriate and timely action to seek assistance from and refer individuals to genetics specialists, other specialists and peer support resources;
   - based on an understanding of the care pathways that incorporate genetics services and information.

2. Demonstrate the importance of sensitivity in tailoring genetic/genomic information and services to the individual's culture, knowledge, language ability and developmental stage:
   - recognising that ethnicity, culture, religion, ethical perspectives and developmental stage may influence the individual's ability to utilise information and services;
   - demonstrating the use of appropriate communication skills in relation to the individual's level of understanding of genetic/genomic issues.

3. Advocate for the rights of all individuals to informed decision making and voluntary action:
   - based on an awareness of the potential for misuse of human genetic/genomic information;
   - understanding the importance of delivering genetic/genomic education and counselling fairly, accurately and without coercion or personal bias;
   - recognising that personal values and beliefs of self and individuals may influence the care and support provided during decision making and that choices and actions may differ over time.

4. Demonstrate a knowledge and understanding of the role of genetic/genomic and other factors in maintaining health and in the manifestation, modification and prevention of disease expression, to underpin effective practice:
   - which includes core genetic/genomic concepts that form a sufficient knowledge base for understanding the implications of specific conditions that may be encountered.

5. Apply knowledge and understanding of the utility and limitations of genetic/genomic information and testing to underpin care and support for individuals and families prior to, during and following decision making, that:
   - incorporates awareness of the ethical, legal and social issues related to testing, recording, sharing and storage of genetic/genomic information;
   - incorporates awareness of the potential physical, emotional, psychological and social consequences of genetic/genomic information for individuals, family members and communities.

6. Examine one's own competency of practice on a regular basis:
   - recognising areas where professional development related to genetics/genomics would be beneficial;
   - maintaining awareness of clinical developments in genetics/genomics that are likely to be of most relevance to the client group, seeking further information on a case-by-case basis;
   - based on an understanding of the boundaries of one's professional role in the referral, provision or follow-up to genetics services.

7. Obtain and communicate credible, current information about genetics/genomics, for self, patients, families and colleagues:
   - using information technologies and other information sources effectively to do so, and
   - applying critical appraisal skills to assess the quality of information accessed.

8. Provide ongoing nursing care and support to patients, carers and families with genetic/genomic healthcare needs:
   - being responsive to changing needs through the life-stages and during periods of uncertainty;
   - demonstrating awareness about how an inherited condition and its implications for family members might impact on family dynamics;
   - working in partnership with family members and other agencies in the management of conditions;
   - recognising the potential expertise of individuals, family members and carers with genetic/genomic health care needs that develops over time and with experience.

Kirk, M., Tonkin, E., Skirton, H., 2014. An iterative consensus-building approach to revising a genetics/genomics competency framework for nurse education in the UK. J. Adv. Nurs. 70 (2), 405–420.

- act as a trusted and informed carer for children growing up with genetic conditions (such as muscular dystrophy or cystic fibrosis), as they may be probing increasingly for information about the condition, its prognosis and effect on life plans;
- help parents deal with feelings of anger, guilt or blame as they acknowledge their own genetic contribution to the child's illness or consider prenatal diagnosis in a future pregnancy;
- enhance awareness of conditions, which may mimic non-accidental injury or abuse, such as osteogenesis imperfecta or conditions that result in failure to thrive;
- facilitate referral to local genetic services when appropriate.

The need for clear and accurate information, delivered sensitively and at a pace and level appropriate to the understanding and needs of family members is fundamental, but this is not always achieved (Chapple et al., 1997; Fallowfield and Jenkins, 2004; McGowan, 1999). The family nurse can help in 'going over' information with the family, working with them at their own pace – and is in the ideal position to recognise that individuals within the family may be at different stages of adaptation. Preparing families for genetic counselling, helping them to have realistic expectations, is an important aspect of placing genetic information into context.

Skirton (2001) stresses the importance of certainty in the family's quest for a diagnosis, but there will be many times when a diagnosis is not available. However, as noted earlier, as more genetic tests become available, there will be circumstances where families who had not previously been given a diagnosis will be recalled, or invited to join research programmes and a definitive diagnosis may become possible, such as in the DDD project. These families may well experience a re-adaptation, particularly where a genetic cause can now be attributed to one or both parents.

Part of giving reliable information includes the need to avoid false reassurance, but at the same time provide a balanced perspective, helping the family to maintain hope. Support groups can be particularly helpful, but information about these needs to be delivered at an appropriate time, and the nurse needs to be aware of the type and quality of information available.

At the heart of effective communication is the relationship that the nurse has with the family. Trust is central to this, developed through open, honest communication and practice within an ethical framework as indicated by the competence standard statements. Some of the ethical issues surrounding the application of genetic technologies are of particular relevance to children's nurses.

ETHICAL ISSUES FOR CHILDREN'S NURSES

Although the benefits that new genetic technologies may bring to help people with or at risk of a genetic disease are to be welcomed, there are also concerns about potential harms. An increase in genetic testing may challenge personal privacy, undermining the 'right not to know'. Some authors voice concern that it has the potential to promote discrimination, and devalues the existence of people with a disability (see, e.g. Ward, 2002). Newell (2000) claims that the prediction that an embryo is at risk of an increasing number of 'defects' is regarded as a standard basis for a decision to terminate the pregnancy on 'therapeutic' grounds.

The application of new genetic technology in reproductive decision making provokes fierce debate on occasion. One aspect of this is the selection of embryos during in vitro fertilisation, on the basis of its genotype for the purposes of helping an existing child. This could potentially help families such as McGowan's, where a bone-marrow transplant from a sibling with appropriate genotype could help her sons. She states that:

> At this stage, my husband and I have rejected such options as we feel it is not right for us to have a child for such reasons … I really believe that people should be valued for more than just their genes.
>
> *McGowan (1999, p 197)*

👤 ACTIVITY

Yasmin and Michael have a happy, stable relationship. They are about to decide whether to start a family. Draw a decision tree (like a flow diagram) for the couple, starting with the question 'shall we have children?' and assuming that their initial decision is that they will. Work through all the subsequent decisions they have to make, up until the final decision of 'shall we have another child?'

Try and include all possible options, incorporating your knowledge of current reproductive technologies. What decisions might they have to make in the pre-conceptual and antenatal periods? What decisions might they face in the immediate postnatal period? Which do you think might be the most difficult?

Once you have done this, you might like to draw another decision tree, but this time think of a couple facing this decision back in the 1950s. How has the nature of reproductive decision making changed? Does increased choice bring greater freedom?

Certainly, a common concern is about whether and where a line should be drawn between using genetic information to prevent harm (negative eugenics) and to promote desirable characteristics (positive eugenics). Iredale (2000) reviews these issues and concludes that nurses need to play an active role in promoting good genetic health, underpinned by an appreciation of the history of genetics and the eugenics movement. Professional practice also has to incorporate the ethical principles of privacy, confidentiality, informed consent and non-discrimination.

👥 SEMINAR DISCUSSION TOPIC

People with cystic fibrosis (CF) are susceptible to infections and can pose a higher risk of cross-infection to each other, so should not mix. When there is more than one person with CF in a school (child or staff) who are not siblings, the school will conduct a risk assessment and put a plan in place to minimise the infection risk between the individuals concerned. This will be developed in liaison with health professionals, parents and individuals with CF.

In 2012, Colman Chadam, an 11-year-old boy in California, was not allowed to attend his school because of his genetic make-up. He is a carrier for cystic fibrosis but does not have the condition. His parents had disclosed his CF status at the start of the school year on his confidential medical record; it had not been an issue at previous schools. There were two children at school with CF and the school divulged Colman's CF status to their parents. The school then barred Colman on the basis of cross-infection risk. Over several years, his parents fought the decision through the US legal system, on the grounds of discrimination. A settlement was agreed in August 2018. The case had a high media profile in the US.
- What are the ethical issues in this case and for whom?
- What approach should the school have taken if Colman had actually had CF?
- What do you think might have been the impact of this case for other parents and children in the school?

One of the key ethical issues for children's nurses is the genetic testing of children, in particular predictive testing for conditions of early and later adult onset, and carrier testing. Early identification of at-risk children might facilitate earlier surveillance and treatment, and would remove uncertainty but there are potential disadvantages. Clarke (1997) raised concern about the child's loss of autonomy as an adult to make their own decisions, which might differ from that of the parents. He also noted the potential psychosocial consequences for the child, which might include labelling, fatalism, damage to self-esteem and alteration to family dynamics.

This issue was more recently considered by the British Society for Human Genetics (BSHG, 2010). Its report includes parental decision making, children's choice and disclosure of carrier status. The focus is on caution, taking time to assess the balance of harms and benefits, with health care professionals and parents being enabled to spend time discussing the optimal timing of a predictive genetic test and discussing within the family where appropriate. Parents are encouraged to talk to children about their family history from a young age, so that they grow up knowing about it. The key recommendation was that unless testing has current medical benefit, it should be deferred until a child is old enough to make their own decision, with a stress on the importance of evidence for the benefit of testing being sufficiently strong and clear to outweigh the need for caution.

The BSHG report and recommendations are somewhat at odds with the views of the British public reported by (Shkedi-Rafid et al., 2015). They conducted an email survey of 2998 participants to explore attitudes towards testing of children for genetic conditions of adult onset for which no treatment or preventive measures were available during childhood and testing for carrier status to inform future reproductive risks. Just under half (47%) agreed that children should be tested for adult onset conditions and 60% agreed they should be tested for carrier status. They were also asked about their level of agreement in favour of four arguments for deferring testing for adult onset conditions:

1. It removes the child's ability to decide in the future if they want to be tested.

2. The child may feel stigmatised or discriminated against as they grow up.
3. The child may be misinformed about the genetic condition if they are not involved in the decision about testing.
4. There is no benefit to testing now; the test should be done only where there is a benefit.

The researchers found that option 1 received the least support (37% agreeing) and option 4 had the most support (46% agreeing). This study finding is important as it reminds us that parents may not share the same views as health care professionals, as this may not be based solely on incomplete understanding of the benefits and potential harms of testing.

Following this study, (Fenwick et al., (2017) conducted in-depth interviews with health care professionals (n=34) with experience in dealing with parents who had asked for testing for their children when there was no medical benefit, to explore how they managed such requests. Three themes emerged from their analysis: future autonomy, balancing no medical benefit and best interests, and reframing the request as when, not whether to test. They felt that this latter approach was useful in engaging parents in complex discussions and they recommended that health care professionals (HCPs) should adopt the strategy of finding the right time for testing rather than focusing on whether or not to test.

The issue of genetic testing of children (with or without any immediate medical benefit) is likely to persist as whole genome testing becomes more affordable and more reliable, and newborn screening expands. Although birth profiling was considered and shelved in the UK (Human Genetics Commission, 2005), the benefits of whole genome screening of the newborn continue to be debated (Ulm et al., 2015). However, as part of its long-term plan, from 2019 the NHS is offering whole genome sequencing to seriously ill children with rare genetic conditions and certain cancers. The role of the children's nurse, acting as an advocate, is central to upholding the rights of children in relation to genetic testing.

PROFESSIONAL CONVERSATION

I was asked to go and see Rebecca at home because the neonatal screening test on her baby George had revealed her son to have Duchenne muscular dystrophy. Of course, this meant there were quite a few implications for the family. Rebecca could be a carrier of the condition, and her siblings could also, so it would be important to make sure that Rebecca understood this, and understood how she might want to take this into account for further reproductive decisions. I would also need to make sure that Rebecca understood what being a carrier would mean for herself in terms of her own health. Lots to tell her – lots to ensure she understands. The headache for me is that Rebecca is only 13-years-old herself.

SUMMARY

The advance in genetics knowledge and related technology is transforming health care, moving a hitherto specialist subject, with its focus on rare conditions, into mainstream services. Understanding how genetics can affect families is increasingly important for children's nurses as they support families in their care. Being able to interpret and communicate information about genetics accurately, honestly and sensitively is a central feature of the role. A wider appreciation of the ethical issues that may arise, not only for children and their families, but also for wider society, is also important. Education is core to this and it is important that this is relevant and of practical value to nurses. Practical tips are always helpful and members of the Association of Genetic Nurses and Counsellors offer the following advice for nurses on how to integrate genetics/genomics into practice (Kirk and Tonkin, 2009):

- Familiarise yourself with how genetics fits into your area of practice and concentrate on this.
- Learn key warning signs to look for in the patient group you are most in contact with.
- Do not assume that all patients consider having a genetic condition in the family to be a problem.
- Be aware of ethical issues and family dynamics and do not assume everyone wants to be tested.

- Be honest and do not say to a patient that you understand their result when you do not.
- Speak to genetic counsellors who are always happy to advise.
- Know who your contacts are in the regional genetics service and make use of them.
- Never be afraid to pick up the phone and ask for advice.

ACKNOWLEDGEMENTS

We wish to dedicate this chapter to the late Emer Parker, in memory of her commitment to her work supporting families as a specialist genetics nurse and in recognition of her contribution to the two previous editions of this chapter.

GLOSSARY

1. Consensus Panel on Genetic/Genomic Nursing Competencies, 2009. Essentials of Genetic and Genomic Nursing: Competencies, Curricula Guidelines, and Outcome Indicators, second ed. second ed. American Nurses Association, Silver Spring, MD.
2. Genetics in Nursing & Midwifery Task and Finish Group, 2011. Task and Finish Group Report to the Nursing and Midwifery Professional Advisory Board of the Department of Health Genetics/Genomics in Nursing and Midwifery.

REFERENCES

Association of Genetic Nurses and Counsellors (AGNC), 2002. Education Working Group. Education in genetics for health professionals not working in specialist genetic units. Report E, Reports for the Genetics Policy Unit Department of Health. AGNC, Birmingham.

Barr, O., Millar, R., 2003. Parents of children with intellectual disabilities: their expectations and experience of genetic counselling. Journal of Applied Research in Intellectual Disabilities 16, 189–204.

Bayliss-Pratt, L., 2017 Are we ready for the revolution in personalised medicine? Health Education England http://bit.ly/2vlkD1S.

British Society for Human Genetics, 2010. Report on the Genetic Testing of Children 2010. British Society for Human Genetics, Birmingham.

Calzone, K.A., Kirk, M., Tonkin, E., et al., 2018. The global landscape of nursing and genomics. Journal of Nursing Scholarship. https://doi.org/10.1111/jnu.12380.

Christian, B., 2011. Pediatric nursing research: creating partnerships with parents to improve the health of children and adolescents. Journal of Pediatric Nursing 26 (1), 95–96.

Canam, C., 1993. Common adaptive tasks facing parents of children with chronic conditions. Journal of Advanced Nursing 18, 46–53.

Chapple, A., Campion, P., May, C., 1997. Clinical terminology: anxiety and confusion amongst families undergoing genetic counselling. Patient Education and Counseling 32, 81–91.

Clarke, A.J., 1997. The genetic testing of children. In: Harper, P.S., Clarke, A.J. (Eds.), Genetics, Society and Clinical Practice. BIOS, Oxford, pp. 15–29.

Codori, A.M., Zawacki, K.L., Petersen, G., et al., 2003. Genetic testing for hereditary colorectal cancer in children: long-term psychological effects. American Journal of Medical Genetics 116A, 117–128.

Cystic Fibrosis Trust, 2018. Cystic Fibrosis Strength in Numbers. UK Cystic Fibrosis Registry Annual Data Report 2017. Cystic Fibrosis Trust. https://www.cysticfibrosis.org.uk/registryreports.

Davies, S.C., 2017. Annual Report of the Chief Medical Officer 2016, Generation Genome. Department of Health, London.

Deford, F., Alex, 1983. The Life of a Child. Viking Press, New York.

Department of Health (DoH), 2003. Our Inheritance, Our Future. Realising the Potential of Genetics in the NHS. The Stationery Office, London.

Department of Health (DoH), 2013. The UK Strategy for Rare Diseases. The Department of Health, London. Available from: https://www.raredisease.org.uk/uk-strategy-for-rare-diseases/.

Fallowfield, L., Jenkins, V., 2004. Communicating sad, bad and difficult news in medicine. Lancet 363, 312–319.

Fanos, J., 1997. Developmental tasks of childhood and adolescence: implications for genetic testing. American Journal of Medical Genetics 71, 22–28.

Fanos, J., 1999. 'My crooked vision': the well sib views ataxia telangiectasia. American Journal of Medical Genetics 87 (5), 420–425.

Fanos, J., Puck, J., 2001. Family pictures: growing up with a brother with X-linked severe combined immunodeficiency. American Journal of Medical Genetics 98 (1), 57–63.

Fenwick, A., Plantinga, M., Dheensa, S., Lucassen, A., 2017. Predictive genetic testing of children for adult-onset conditions: negotiating requests with parents. Journal of Genetic Counseling 26 (2), 244–250.

Genomics England, 2018. The UK has sequenced 100,000 whole genomes in the NHS. Press release 5 December 2018. Available from: https://www.genomicsengland.co.uk/the-uk-has-sequenced-100000-whole-genomes-in-the-nhs/.

Human Genetics Commission (2005) Profiling the newborn: a prospective gene technology? London: Human Genetics Commission.

Iredale, R., 2000. Eugenics and its relevance to contemporary health care. Nursing Ethics 7 (3), 205–214.

Kearney, P.M., Griffin, T., 2001. Between joy and sorrow: being a parent of a child with developmental disability. Journal of Advanced Nursing 34 (5), 582–592.

Kirk, M., Tonkin, E., Skirton, H., 2014. An iterative consensus-building approach to revising a genetics/genomics competency framework for nurse education in the UK. Journal of Advanced Nursing 70 (2), 405–420.

Kirk, M., Marshallsay, M., 2013. Providing nursing care and support to individuals and families with genetic/genomic healthcare needs. Nursing Standard 28 (16–18), 39–46.

Kirk, M., Tonkin, E., 2009. Understanding the role of genetics and genomics in health 2: implications for nursing practice. Nursing Times 105 (46), 19–23.

Locker, D., 1991. Living with chronic illness. In: Scambler, G. (Ed.), Sociology as Applied to Medicine. Baillière-Tindall, London, pp. 81–92.

McGowan, R., 1999. Beyond the disorder: one parent's reflection on genetic counselling. Journal of Medical Ethics 25, 195–199.

de Montalembert, M., de Guitton, C., 2014. Transition from paediatric to adult care for patients with sickle cell disease. British Journal of Haematology 164 (5), 630–635.

Middleton, A., Patch, C., 2018. Genetic counselling in the era of genomic medicine. British Medical Bulletin. https://doi.org/10.1093/bmb/ldy008.

Nereo, N., Fee, R., Hinton, V., 2003. Parental stress in mothers of boys with Duchenne muscular dystrophy. Journal of Pediatric Psychology 28 (7), 473–484.

Newell, C., 2000. Biomedicine, genetics and disability: reflections on nursing and a philosophy of holism. Nursing Ethics 7 (3), 227–236.

Nursing and Midwifery Council (NMC), 2018. Future nurse: standards of proficiency for registered nurses. Available from: https://www.nmc.org.uk/globalassets/sitedocuments/education-standards/future-nurse-proficiencies.pdf.

Rare Disease UK, 2018. Understanding Children and Young People's Experiences. London Rare Disease, UK.

Resta, R., Biesecker, B.B., Bennett, R.L., et al., 2006. A new definition of genetic counseling: National Society of Genetic Counselors' Task Force report. Journal of Genetic Counseling 15, 77–83.

Senger, B.A., Ward, L.D., Barbosa-Leiker, C., Bindler, R.C., 2016. The parent experience of caring for a child with mitochondrial disease. Journal of Pediatric Nursing 31 (1), 32–41.

Shkedi-Rafid, S., Fenwick, A., Dheensa, S., Lucassen, A.M., 2015. Genetic testing of children for adult-onset conditions: opinions of the British adult population and implications for clinical practice. European Journal of Human Genetics 23 (10), 1281–1285.

Skirton, H., 2001. The client's perspective of genetic counselling – a grounded theory study. Journal of Genetic Counselling 10 (4), 311–329.

Task and Finish Group, 2011. Genetics/Genomics in Nursing & Midwifery. Report to the Department of Health Nursing &

Midwifery Professional Advisory Board. Available from: http://www.dh.gov.uk/en/Publicationsandstatistics/Publications/PublicationsPolicyAndGuidance/DH_131946.

Ulm, E., Feero, W.G., Dineen, R., et al., 2015. Genetics professionals' opinions of whole-genome sequencing in the newborn period. Journal of Genetic Counseling 24 (3), 452–463. https://doi-org.ergo.southwales.ac.uk/10.1007/s10897-014-9779-3.

Ward, L., 2002. Whose right to choose? The new genetics, prenatal testing and people with learning difficulties. Critical Public Health 12 (2), 187–200.

Whyte, D., 1992. A family nursing approach to the care of a child with a chronic illness. Journal of Advanced Nursing 17, 317–327.

USEFUL WEBSITES

UK

The Genomics Education Programme is an excellent site for news and activities about genomics, learning resources and information on genomics courses (some are free to access): https://www.genomicseducation.hee.nhs.uk/.

Genomics England has up-to-date news on the 100,000 Genomes Project as well as stories from families involved in this, and other useful learning resources: https://www.genomicsengland.co.uk/.

This slide set from the CNO England outlines why genomics education matters to nurses and midwives in the 21st century: https://hee.nhs.uk/sites/default/files/documents/Genomic%20Education%20Matters%20to%20all%20nurses%20and%20midwives%20FINAL.pdf.

The Public Health Genetics Foundation, University of Cambridge provides a good quality resource with a regular 'round up' of current papers and events: http://www.phgfoundation.org.uk.

The Genesense website from the University of Plymouth provides a useful resource for health professionals that seeks to demystify genetics: http://www.genesense.org.uk.

Genetic Alliance UK (www.geneticalliance.org.uk/) is a large national charity that represents over 200 patient organisations. The website is comprehensive, with sections on living with a genetic condition, learn about genetics, services and testing, research and innovation.

Genetic Disorders UK is a national charity which aims to support those with a genetic disorder. Their website has some excellent learning resources, including children/family stories and a database of genetic conditions written in accessible terms: http://www.geneticdisordersuk.org/.

Unique is a small charity supporting families with some rare types of conditions. They have a range of useful factsheets: https://www.rarechromo.org/.

Other Countries

An excellent glossary from the US National Human Genome Research Institute: www.genome.gov/glossary/index.cfm. Visit their wider site (https://www.genome.gov), for extensive educations links and resources.

From the US National Cancer Institute, another helpful glossary: https://www.cancer.gov/publications/dictionaries/genetics-dictionary.

The Genetics Genomics Competency Center (http://genomicseducation.net/) is a US-led repository of education resources for nurses and other health professionals. An added strength is that all resources have been quality reviewed.

This Genetics Home Reference site provides clear information and a good glossary: http://ghr.nlm.nih.gov/.

The Genetics Education Program for Nurses developed at the Cincinnati Children's Hospital provides a number of free resources, including a free module, Genetics is Relevant Now: http://www.cincinnatichildrens.org/ed/clinical/gpnf/default.htm.

Australia's New South Wales Government Health Centre for Genetics Education website has some useful resources, including a wide range of Fact Sheets, free to download: http://www.genetics.edu.au/.

9

Contemporary Issues in Genomics and Other 'Omic' Technologies for Children's Nursing: An Introduction

Emma Tonkin, Maggie Kirk, Alex Murray

LEARNING OUTCOMES

- To appreciate the role of genomic and environmental factors in the predisposition to, and development of, a condition.
- To acknowledge the developments in new technologies and the associated implications for health care and children's nursing and take action to keep up to date.
- To be more confident in using genomics knowledge when talking to patients, families and colleagues.
- To appreciate the ethical considerations (for the individual, other family members and the health care team) associated with genomic information.

GLOSSARY

[As the current edition has the glossary associated with the chapter and some terms are already in the genetics chapter the following sentence has been included in the abstract: Glossary terms have not been duplicated so you may need to refer to the previous chapter for some definitions]

100K Genomes Project A UK initiative to sequence 100,000 whole genomes from NHS patients with a focus on rare diseases and cancer. The long-term vision was to use the knowledge generated to develop infrastructure across the NHS and create a new genomic medicine service to bring the predicted benefits of genomics to everyone.

DDD project 'deciphering developmental delay' A UK study to assess the effectiveness of using microarray and sequencing technology on DNA samples from children and adults with undiagnosed developmental disorders to make new diagnoses.

Epigenome The set of chemical tags found across the DNA molecule and associated histone proteins that regulate which genes are active or silenced in a cell. These modifications occur in response to the environment, do not involve alterations to the DNA sequence and can be heritable or reversible. Epigenetics is the study of phenotypic change in an individual as a result of these tags and epigenomics is the study of modifications and their outcomes across an individual's entire genome.

Exome The exon containing component of a genome. Exons make up around 1.5% of the human genome.

Exon The coding segments of genes that are usually copied ('transcribed') and then converted ('translated') into a functional protein. Between exons are non-coding regions of DNA (called introns), which are cut out during transcription. The exons are spliced together to form the transcript, which is a template from which a functional protein can be made.

Genome editing A range of technologies (including CRISPR-Cas9) used to alter the DNA of an organism.

Incidental finding Results that are outside the original purpose for which a test or procedure was conducted, for example, a previously undiagnosed medical condition that is discovered (unintentionally) during an evaluation for a different medical condition.

Mitochondria Organelles used by cells to produce energy. Primarily passed on through the maternal line (via the egg), mitochondria contain DNA (1% of the human genome) which contains 37 genes.

Mitochondrial transfer/replacement therapy: An *in vitro* fertilisation based technique that replaces faulty mitochondria in a mother's egg with healthy mitochondria from a donor egg to prevent or ameliorate disease.

Microarray A high-throughput laboratory method used to genotype multiple regions of a genome or to measure the expression levels of different genes in a particular population of cells. Each array can contain thousands or tens of thousands of microscopic dots of DNA attached to a solid surface.

Microbiome The set of microorganisms present, for example, on a body (or part of a body).

Next generation sequencing (NGS) Also known as high-throughput sequencing describes a number of modern technologies that can be used to read the chemical sequence of DNA and RNA much faster and more cheaply than original methods. Millions of DNA bases (letters of the genetic code) can be read ('sequenced') simultaneously.

Personalised medicine The use of new approaches (including genomic technology) to better manage patients' health and targets therapies to achieve the best outcomes in the management of a patient's disease or predisposition to disease.[1] (Personalised and Precision are often used interchangeably. Precision medicine tends to now be the preferred term as it does not imply that treatments are developed specifically for the individual, which may be inferred from 'personalised'.)

Pharmacogenomics The study of how different people respond to drugs due to their genetic make-up, in order to identify new, more specific and more effective drug targets with fewer side effects. Pharmacogenomics and pharmacogenetics are often used interchangeably.

Primary finding The result actively sought by the practitioner and patient and the purpose for undertaking the test. (Sometimes referred to as 'main' or 'pertinent finding'.)

Secondary finding An additional result actively sought by the practitioner and patient that was not the primary target of the test.

Variant of unknown (or uncertain) significance (VUS) A variation in a genetic sequence for which the association with disease risk is unclear based on the available evidence. (Sometimes referred to as an 'unclassified variant'.)

INTRODUCTION: GENOMICS – WHAT IS ALL THE FUSS ABOUT?

Genomics today contributes very modestly to the routine care of a pregnant patient. Yet by the time the child born of that pregnancy reaches adulthood, it is likely that knowledge of his or her genetic makeup will not just guide the treatment of most health problems but help prevent or at least postpone or lessen, the very manifestation of many of them.

Elias Zerhouni, M.D. (in Guttmacher et al.[2004])

In the preceding chapter *Inherited Conditions and the Family* we introduced genomics and how the study of traits, human variation and specific diseases have shifted from a focus on the individual genes involved (genetics) to the recognition that each needs to be studied and understood in the wider context of the entire genome and the environment. In many ways, the completion of the first full human genome sequence in 2003 was the initial step in a long and ongoing journey to improve health outcomes as illustrated in Fig. 9.1. Knowing the order (sequence) of DNA bases across all 23 pairs of chromosomes and the mitochondrial DNA is enabling scientists to understand how the human genome is usually organised. More than 20,000 protein-coding genes have been identified (Willyard, 2018) along with a catalogue of sequences that influence when, by how much and in what tissue a gene is turned on ('gene expression'). The position of each gene along the DNA sequence is known, although there still remains a great deal of work to be done in understanding the purpose of the majority of the genome that was often incorrectly referred to in the past as 'junk DNA'. Knowledge of how the human genome is organised ('structured') helps inform our understanding about its functionality ('biology'), for example how specific variations in the DNA sequence can change which genes are turned on and off, or alter how the product of a gene works. From this, we are building a picture of how the products of different genes interact; the mechanism by which they work; the biological pathways in which they are involved and the environmental factors that influence all of this. The 'normal' or usual process(es) can then be compared and contrasted to that of the disease process, and it is this knowledge that is helping to advance the science of medicine and the effectiveness of health care to move from a model of intervention to one that in the longer term is more focused on prediction and prevention.

Each human genome is unique to the individual. Although we all share the same set of genes (with the exception being that women won't have the genes carried by men on the Y chromosome), about one in every 1000 bases ('letters') of the 3 billion letters of DNA code that make up a genome will be different between any two individuals. These differences can cause normal variation like eye colour, influence how we respond to medicines and protect, predispose or directly cause a specific disease. Each whole genome or section of DNA that is sequenced provides information on those individual variations, and it is this information that provides the foundation for genomic based health care. Back in 1998, Bell outlined how such information would lead to:

- New disease classifications based on the molecular mechanisms that cause disease rather than the clinical manifestation.
- The possibility of earlier detection of disease with an increasing range of genetic tests.
- Greater opportunities for prevention by identifying individuals and sub-populations who might be more at risk, and identifying ways of modifying or preventing this risk.
- Better targeted and more effective treatments using genotype to identify subtypes of populations who are more likely to display an enhanced response or increased toxicity to a treatment.

[1]https://www.england.nhs.uk/healthcare-science/personalisedmedicine/.

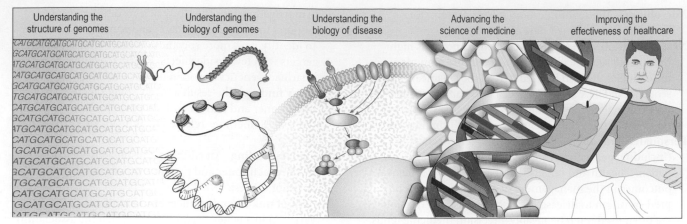

| Understanding the structure of genomes | Understanding the biology of genomes | Understanding the biology of disease | Advancing the science of medicine | Improving the effectiveness of healthcare |

Fig. 9.1 The pathway from genome to genomic health care. (From Green, Guyer, NHGRI, 2011.)

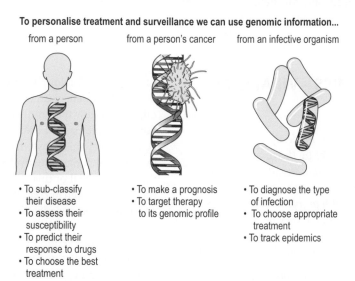

To personalise treatment and surveillance we can use genomic information...

from a person   from a person's cancer   from an infective organism

- To sub-classify their disease
- To assess their susceptibility
- To predict their response to drugs
- To choose the best treatment

- To make a prognosis
- To target therapy to its genomic profile

- To diagnose the type of infection
- To choose appropriate treatment
- To track epidemics

Fig. 9.2 Examples of how genomic information is being used within health care. (Genomics Education Programme, Health Education England, 2019.)

- New types of treatment with rational drug development based on an understanding of the pathogenesis.

Whilst we have yet to realise the full potential of genomics to transform health care (the authors of Fig. 9.1 [Green and Guyer (2011)] predicted that the majority of progress would be made after 2020), genomics is already changing clinical practice.

A key component of this chapter will be to look at the different ways genomic technology is currently applied to the identification and care of children with an alteration in a single gene or region of DNA. However, genomics offers health care many additional opportunities beyond diagnosis and this chapter will also delve deeper into the potential of genomics (as outlined by Bell [1998] and illustrated in Fig. 9.2) and other associated 'omic' areas of science that are of growing importance and of relevance to children's nursing. These include the fields of pharmacogenomics, epigenomics and microbial genomics. Pharmacogenomics is being used to personalise treatments through testing that can help determine the right drug and the right dose for a particular individual. Epigenomics is providing information about the way the environment can modify how genes work and is

beginning to provide the biological mechanism for some of the social factors that have been known for years to be pivotal in influencing health outcomes. And knowledge about the genomes of microbes is expanding opportunities for the diagnosis, prevention and treatment of infectious disease as well as for tracking infectious outbreaks.

Because genomic based health care is rapidly evolving it is important that all children's nurses have a fundamental understanding of the field which can be built on as progress is made and applied as needed to the care of individual children and their families.

ACTIVITY

Introducing Genomics in Health Care

Watch the video from Health Education England for a broad overview about the role that genomics is playing in NHS health care: https://www.youtube.com/watch?time_continue=463&v=KiQgrK3tge8L.

Implications for Health Care

Whilst current health care is predominantly focused on intervention after the onset of disease, the vision is to use genomics to provide more opportunities for prediction and intervention before the onset of symptoms, that is, prevention and in disease situations to deliver more precise treatments. So how far have we come since Bell's predictions in 1998 and the sequencing of the first human genome in 2003? Fig. 9.2 illustrates some of the current possibilities of genomic-based health care and a selection of examples are provided below and throughout this chapter.

New Disease Classifications

Being able to identify disease subtypes has clear implications for patient care. A rare form of diabetes known as 'maturity onset diabetes of the Young' (MODY) has four main causes, but can result from alterations in one of 14 genes (Naylor et al., 2018). Identification of this subtype of diabetes can allow children and young people to be switched from insulin to oral hypoglycaemic agents, or for some, no treatment at all. Similarly, there are now known to be multiple subtypes for the heart rhythm condition long QT syndrome that can cause sudden early death. Identification of a patient's subtype not only has implications for the selection of drug treatment, but also for management. Different triggers have been identified and should therefore be avoided by that specific group, but are not a concern for those with a different subtype. For example, strenuous exercise in Type 1, loud noises (alarms and phones ringing) in Type 2 and depression and sleeping in Type 3 (Strauss, 2010). Genomic technology is also being used to understand the molecular basis for cancer and as a result more precisely classify the disease beyond the primary organ location.

Improvement in disease classification is also important for research and development as it enables clinicians and researchers to focus therapy development to a particular biological pathway and clearly define the most appropriate patient group to include in clinical trials.

Earlier Detection

The large number of genetic conditions (around 7000); the potential for variation in presentation between individuals with the same condition; the frequent lack of clinical expertise and the size and complexity of the human genome, has meant that many individuals and families in the past have experienced a 'Diagnostic Odyssey'. A study by EURORDISCARE (2004) of eight rare diseases described a 5- to 30-year delay in diagnosis for 25% of patients. High-throughput technologies are now being used to speed up diagnosis and remove or reduce that delay and the associated uncertainty for patients and their families.

The ability of some methods to detect the presence of very small amounts of DNA means that prenatal screening and testing can be offered earlier in pregnancy. The technology provides future possibilities for the earlier diagnosis of a range of conditions, as well as the ability to track disease.

Opportunities for Prevention

As we learn more about sequences across the human genome that increase a person's susceptibility to common conditions (including those that may develop later on in life), we will begin screening individuals and populations where there are evidence-based interventions available to justify screening. Interventions could include lifestyle changes to reduce susceptibility or early access to therapies. Already it is possible to identify family members who have an inherited predisposition to certain cancers. Identification of their increased risk status provides individuals with the choice to enter targeted surveillance programmes or take prophylactic measures.

A rare hereditary cancer condition known as multiple endocrine neoplasia type 2 (MEN2) is associated with a very high risk of medullary thyroid cancer (MTC) and adrenal tumours called phaeochromocytomas. The onset of MTC can be as young as only a few months of age so prophylactic thyroidectomy is recommended for children known to be affected. The age of surgery depends on the subset of the condition, with those at highest risk (type 2B) of very early onset MTC being advised to have surgery in the first year of life.

Regular screening starts in childhood for conditions such as VHL (von Hippel-Lindau), FAP (familial adenomatous polyposis) and MEN1 (multiple endocrine neoplasia type 1) and it is likely that screening by whole body MRI will be recommended from birth for children with Li Fraumeni syndrome (LFS) in the near future.

Better Targeted and More Effective Treatments

In humans, identification of a particular genotype (genetic sequence) can predict an individual's response to a medication; in a tumour sample provide a target for a therapy, and in a microbe inform selection of a treatment for the specific infection. In addition to improving treatment efficacy, genomic testing can reduce the risk of an adverse drug response in an individual.

New Types of Treatment

Along with disease stratification informing the design and development of new treatments, new technologies for gene-based therapies, where cells are re-engineered to correct the disease-causing alteration, are being developed and trialled.

Currently, most testing for inherited (single gene and chromosomal) conditions and reporting of results occurs within regional specialist genetic/genomic centres. Specialist doctors and counsellors work with the health professionals in other clinical disciplines in the management of patients. One challenge to this approach is the finite capacity of the current specialist genomic services to manage the increasing number of conditions and markers that can be tested for, and the associated increase in patients and family members that are being tested. Burton (2011) discussed the need for clinical specialties to develop sub-specialties in inherited conditions so that pathways become more 'mainstream'. Similarly, the expansion of genomics to encompass other clinical applications like pharmacogenomic testing and tumour profiling is a further driver for the wider health service to develop knowledge and skills in genomics. Certainly within the United Kingdom, genomics is shaping the future of the National Health Service.

Following the successful completion of the 100,000 Genomes Project (www.genomicsengland.co.uk), an initiative to test the feasibility of embedding genomics throughout the NHS in England, there is now significant restructuring taking place to deliver a National Genomic Medicine Service, with the Devolved Nations also developing their own strategies for delivering genomic based health care.

ACTIVITY

The 100,000 Genomes Project: Jessica's Story

Although the 100,000 Genomes Project stopped recruiting in 2018, analysis of samples is continuing. Jessica was one of the first children to receive a definitive diagnosis through this programme. Watch Jessica's story online through a short video from Genomics England (https://www.youtube.com/watch?v=hxou7ayQSZQ) and listen to her parents talking about what having a diagnosis has meant to them.

MAINSTREAMING GENOMICS IN PAEDIATRIC CARE. WHAT ARE THE IMPLICATIONS FOR CHILDREN'S NURSING?

Providing care for children with a genetic diagnosis, or those awaiting a diagnosis will continue. However, as a result of mainstreaming genomic service, the on-going advancement in our understanding of what the human genome does and the developments in genomic technologies, the scope of practice for children's nurses will expand. Testing and return of results within the paediatric environment is likely to increase and become more visible. Genomic tests will move beyond the diagnosis of rare conditions to include monitoring and managing infections and 'point of care testing' at the bedside to inform treatment selection. Over the long term, tests may also come into use that will be able to identify those at increased susceptibility to common health problems. Children's nurses, particularly those working in community settings, will play an important role in discussing the implications of these tests and the potential to reduce risks through changes to lifestyle and behaviours. Where test results have implications for other family members, pathways and processes may need to be developed to ensure that everyone who needs to be told has the opportunity to receive that information. The delivery of care will also change as more is understood about the pathogenesis of conditions and as treatment options are developed. Genomics will be an explicit component of core activities (communication, collaboration, observation and 'doing' Fig. 9.3) that are already part of everyday nursing practice.

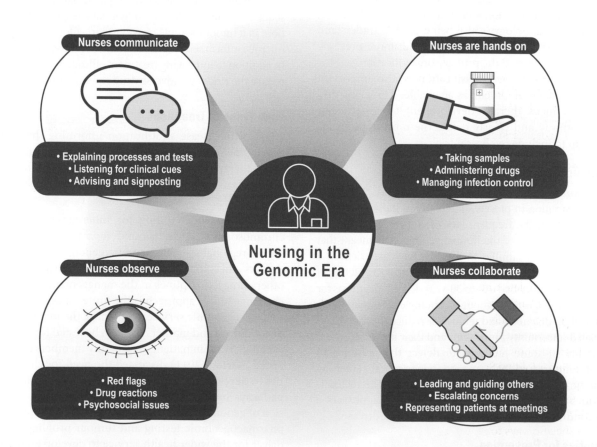

Fig. 9.3 Core nursing activities illustrated through a genomics lens. (Genomics Education Programme, Health Education England, 2019.)

ACTIVITY

What Does Genomics Have to do With Nursing?

Watch this introductory video (https://www.youtube.com/watch?v=LaHSMJGUco8) from the UK's Genomics Education Programme which looks at how nurses contribute to genomic health care, through collaboration, communication and observation. How do you see genomics fitting into your role?

As a result, the nurse will need to be familiar with both the technology and the implications for the child and their family. Children's nurses will need to provide support during periods of uncertainty and stress when families may feel overwhelmed by their child's illness, communicating and helping make sense of information that may be unfamiliar and hard to grasp, and directing them to additional sources of information and support.

PROFESSIONAL CONVERSATION

Support

As a children's nurse working on intensive care, I frequently worked with children and their families at very stressful times in their lives. Sometimes this was when a genetic diagnosis had just been made or when they were awaiting results of a genetic test. I can remember as a nurse, not quite knowing what to say and how to support and answer family's difficult questions in an open and honest way. There is often a lot of uncertainty and unanswered questions at the point of genetic testing or upon receipt of results in relation to prognosis and what the future will hold. Parents are not only worried about their child but also other family members who may be at risk. It is important that nurses are aware of the support available to these families and help facilitate the family in contacting their local genetic counselling service. As a genetic counsellor, I now understand how important it is to give as much information as possible in relation to the condition and use our knowledge to make accurate risk assessments. It is also important we acknowledge and use our skills to support families when we are unable to provide answers to questions. There are lots of support services available to families and it is important that they have access to these, if they wish.

Lisa McGrath RN (Child) BA (Hons) & GCRB Registered Genetic Counsellor.

Having an incomplete understanding of new technology or the implication of a test result creates uncertainty for both the patient and their family and those providing care. As a nurse it will be important throughout your career to regularly consider what you know and are able to do. If there are gaps (as illustrated in Unfolding Scenario – Simon's Story [Part 1]), it will be up to you to seek ways in which you can develop your competence to ensure you continue to provide safe and quality care. Opportunities may arise in the future to develop your role in specific ways to incorporate genomics. The eight core competency standards in genetics/genomics that should be achieved by all nurses (Kirk et al., 2014) are provided in the previous chapter (Box 8.2).

UNFOLDING SCENARIO

Simon's Story (Part 1) – My Role in Simon's Care and the Importance of Keeping Up-to-Date

I have been the nurse for Simon and his family since he was diagnosed with a bone cancer in his leg called osteosarcoma when he was 7 years old. He was initially treated with surgery to remove the tumour, but it came back and he had to have his leg amputated. He did well after that, but when Simon was 9 years old, he developed a cough and it was found that the disease had spread to his lungs. Since then he has been on different chemotherapy treatments but Simon's cancer has continued to progress. It has been decided that we are going to use genomic testing to look for changes in Simon's tumour that might help us select the next treatment option.

When I was attending Simon's case conference, I knew immediately that I did not have an adequate knowledge of the testing planned. I have always found that nurses need to have a great depth of knowledge so that they can not only understand a concept, but also explain it in lay language to the patient and their family. Even more important in this case is that Simon, although he is young and has been through a lot, he is still involved in treatment and needs to understand what this option involves in addition to his parents.

The oncologist I work with helped me learn about driver mutations that give tumours a growth advantage and how some therapies target specific variants. I also spoke with our genetic counsellor who helped me understand the testing techniques and the risk of finding inherited (germline) findings, which may have relevance not just to Simon but the family. Both were very generous with their time and pointed me to education resources both here and abroad that could help me learn this content quickly. By the time Simon and his parents came for his first visit to talk about tumour/normal sequencing and precision medicine, I was nervous but ready to provide more detailed information and answer their questions. Why wasn't the oncologist doing all the education? They covered the essence of what would be done, but with a clinic full of patients, they did not have the time to cover the nitty gritty details or spend the time needed to make sure Simon and his parents understood.

I could see why his parents were anxious; what if the test did not give Simon another treatment option. What then? I sat there realising what was at stake and how important this information would be.

Nurses support patients and families undergoing genomic testing and may be involved in communicating information about the test and/or test result to them. The need for nurses 'to be familiar with the basics of genome sequencing to appreciate both the power and the limitations of the data' was highlighted by Conley et al. (2013). For the same reasons, it is equally important that nurses are also familiar with other genomic technologies that are being used clinically.

MAKING IT POSSIBLE – GENOMIC TECHNOLOGIES

The term 'genomic technologies' encompasses a range of DNA-based methods that can be used to analyse and manipulate DNA. From a clinical perspective the main focus currently is on methods that enable alterations in the genome of an individual to be identified either as part of a population-based initiative like antenatal and newborn screening programmes, or specific testing as part of a diagnostic pathway.

Identifying Changes in the Human Genome

Changes to a patient's genome can take many forms. Genomic technology can be used to:

- identify a change in chromosome number
- identify a change in chromosome structure and determine the extent of the rearrangement ('imbalances')
- locate the precise points where a rearrangement occurs
- detect single-letter (base) or multi-letter changes in the DNA code

Previously microscopy-based techniques were used to look for changes in the number and structure of chromosomes, but these techniques could only identify visible (at high magnification) large scale alterations of at least 5–10 million bases (Mb) in size (Riegel, 2014). Because of developments in DNA based technology particularly array-based comparative genomic hybridisation, these changes are now being detected at much higher resolution providing a more precise location of the alteration. The ability to then identify which gene(s) are located in the region provides clinicians

---

OVERVIEW AND ILLUSTRATION OF ARRAY-BASED COMPARATIVE GENOMIC HYBRIDISATION (ARRAY-CGH) (FIG. 9.4)

Thousands of fragments from across the human genome are applied as dots to a glass slide in a precise and documented way. This is the 'microarray'.

Test DNA from a patient and a normal reference ('control') DNA are each labelled with a different fluorescent dye (Cy5 and Cy3 respectively in Fig. 9.4).

The two sets of DNA are then mixed and allowed to stick ('hybridise') simultaneously to the microarray. The fluorescent signals from the patient and reference DNAs are then measured and compared at each of the individual dots.

Where there is no difference between the patient and reference DNA both signals will be equal ('balanced'). Where there is a loss or gain of DNA in the patient sample, there will be less or more fluorescent signal (respectively) compared to the reference signal.

Because the precise location within the human genome of each fragment (dot) on the microarray is known. The location and extent of the patient's loss or gain can be determined.

How precisely the rearrangement can be located within the genome will depend on how many fragments are used in the microarray and the distance between adjacent fragments (e.g. every 0.06–100 thousand bases (Kb).

Microarray

As a trainee genetic counsellor one of the things I noted was that often the first test done in children who have developmental delay, physical abnormalities or behavioural concerns is a microarray test (see Overview and Illustration of Array-Based Comparative Genomic Hybridisation [Array-CGH] box for more information). In some situations, I found that the findings of this test can be difficult to interpret alongside the child's presentation. When a deletion or duplication is found in a child it could have occurred for the first time in the child or been inherited from either parent. Parents that I have spent time with are often keen to know whether the deletion or duplication came from one of them, particularly as they are concerned about the consequences for any subsequent or future children. Parents might find this time of waiting for genetic results particularly anxiety provoking. In my experience many of the deletions or duplications found can be very variable, a parent might have the same finding as the child and not have any concerns, whereas the child might have various symptoms. For children's nurses it is important to be aware that this can be difficult for parents to understand, as there is often a great deal of uncertainty associated with these test results. Having an understanding of what a microarray test is and what it can and can't do is useful for children's nurses as this can help them provide better support for parents. Children's nurses should be aware of the various implications of microarray testing such as the impact of having a deletion or duplication might not become clear until the child is older, which causes uncertainty. The findings of these tests can also affect other family members. Nurses can support parents in helping them to think through informing other members of the family about the results.

The following website provides details about various deletions and duplications found via microarray testing: https://www.rarechromo.org.

Dr Verity Leach, PhD, Master's in Genomic Counselling, BSc.

---

and families with further information that can inform diagnosis and management.

Similarly, the original method used to read the sequence of bases along a section of DNA was inefficient. High costs and an inability to generate and analyse large amounts of DNA sequence data resulted in a testing process that was diagnosis led. The patient's phenotype was used to guide the selection of candidate gene(s) for testing and in conditions where more than one gene was known to be involved, for example, the heart rhythm condition long QT syndrome, testing was often sequential. One candidate gene was tested and excluded before the next and subsequent genes were looked at. When looking for a specific sequence alteration in a gene, the approach is to either use other methods to identify the presence of an alteration and then use sequencing to identify the exact change, or to use DNA sequencing as the first choice to directly identify the alteration. Over time and with development of new technologies including Next Generation Sequencing methods, it has become much more cost effective and feasible to test multiple genes simultaneously or even sequence a patient's entire

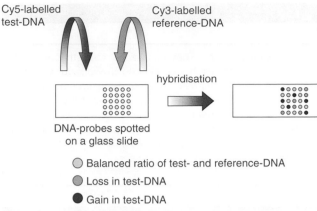

Cy5-labelled test-DNA

Cy3-labelled reference-DNA

hybridisation

DNA-probes spotted on a glass slide

● Balanced ratio of test- and reference-DNA

● Loss in test-DNA

● Gain in test-DNA

Fig. 9.4 Illustration of array-based comparative genomic hybridisation. (From Muller et al., 2012.)

genome. This is particularly useful in situations where it is not possibly to prioritise one gene over a number of candidates, or where there is a clinical need to identify the cause of a condition as soon as possible in order to inform care and management of a patient. Mestek-Boukhibar et al. (2018) and French et al. (2019) both describe studies to develop whole genome sequencing (WGS) services for critically ill children that would work within the UK's National Health Service infrastructure. In their study of children (195 families) in neonatal and paediatric intensive care units, French et al. (2019) found that WGS provided a diagnosis in 21% of cases and informed management including decisions around palliative care, in 65% of cases. Importantly, in 90% of cases the child's phenotype was a poor predictor of the gene identified suggesting the potential for unnecessary tests and interventions if a molecular diagnosis is not made. WGS has been shown to be an appropriate first line tool for some acute and long-term clinical situations, and both England (Department of Health and Social Care, 2019) and Wales are implementing WGS for seriously ill children with a suspected genetic condition during 2019/2020. Clearly, it is important for the children's nurse to be aware of WGS

NEXT GENERATION SEQUENCING (NGS): 'BIGGER, BETTER, FASTER'

NGS is also known as 'second generation', 'high-throughput' or 'massively-parallel' sequencing.

Cost: in 2019 sequencing a whole human genome costs approx. £1000 (NHGRI, 2019).[a]

Sequencing time: approximately 1 day.

NGS can be carried out on as little as a single copy of a person's DNA.

Methods vary but essentially the DNA is cut into hundreds of millions of pieces and from this the sequencing process generates multiple copies of short sequence reads that overlap. (The number of reads of a given DNA base is referred to as the 'depth of coverage'. The greater this is, the more accurate the sequence read should be.)

Software is used to align the overlapping sequence data against a reference sequence and identify differences. The time this takes will vary from case to case.

The ability to accurately identify differences is affected by the quality of the sequence and coverage across the genome.

Further analysis is undertaken to identify differences that may be disease causing. The time this takes will depend on the methods used.

The 100K Genomes Project undertaken by Genomics England, sequenced whole genomes at a read depth of 15x or greater, covering 97.3% of the genome (Davies, 2017).

---

services and the implications of testing in this way, to better support families in this situation.

How a test is selected will be dependent on clinical pathways, local decision making and the testing infrastructure available. A comparison of the broad approaches from single gene to whole genome is provided in Table 9.1. As NGS becomes more readily available the major challenge comes not from generating the sequence but from analysing and interpreting the findings. Starting with a candidate gene or group of genes selected on the basis of the presenting features of the patient remains a very valid approach to analysing whole or clinical exome sequence (WES/CES) or WGS data, and can be a quicker route to diagnosis. If no disease-causing alteration is found, then the remaining sequences can be interrogated. Alternatively, the whole data set can be analysed in a disease 'agnostic' approach. Determining which change in the DNA sequence is disease causing is of course fundamental. Sequence data from parents and/or other unaffected family members are used to exclude non-disease-causing variants. However, Mestek-Boukhibar et al. (2018) provides an indication of the scale of this challenge as their WGS of 24 child-parent trios generated an average of 5.8 million genomic variants per trio. Further laboratory testing and/or comparing sequence variants with known changes submitted to clinical databases is undertaken to aid interpretation.

Even though sequencing a human genome is quite straightforward, there is still a great deal to learn. Genes are still being identified; the molecular basis of many genetic conditions is yet to be identified and the roles played by the majority of the non-coding genome is unknown. It is for these reasons that some individuals and families do not get a result, and others are left with uncertainty about whether an identified change is pathogenic or not when the report returned refers to a VUS – variant of unknown significance. As more information is added to databases and better algorithms for sequence interpretation are developed, periodic reanalysis of the patient data should be undertaken in an attempt to clarify the variant's significance. This leaves the family with more uncertainty, within an uncertain time frame.

Other Clinical Applications of DNA Technologies
Tumour Profiling

Cancers arise when normal cellular processes are overridden and a cell divides and proliferates in an uncontrolled manner. This happens as a result of changes in the DNA that can be inherited or have accumulated in the cell and which then produce proteins that don't function or behave differently. Tumour profiling can use NGS alongside other tests to provide

PROFESSIONAL CONVERSATION

Inconclusive Result

The technology is changing very fast in genomic testing and patients are getting more and more information, but sometimes they get no information or uncertain information. I took a telephone call from somebody who had been part of a large genome sequencing project that was looking for an answer to why they had a child with a possible genetic disorder. They wanted to know what was going to happen to their child, whether they had a chance of having another child with the same problem or if their brothers and sisters could have a child with the same problem. They had had a result that was uncertain and more research was needed to work out whether the genetic variation that had been found caused the condition in their child. They were understandably disappointed but also wanted to be certain that doctors, laboratory scientists and researchers were going to carry on analysing the data and looking for an answer for them. They had consented for this to happen and hoped they would get an answer soon.

Dr Chris, Patch – Clinical Lead for Genetic Counselling, Genomics England, UK; and Reader in Genomic Healthcare, King's College, London.

TABLE 9.1   Comparison of Approaches to Detect Disease-Causing Alterations

Focus of Test What Is Looked At?	How Is the Test Selected/ Approached?	Advantages	Limitations and Implications for Families
Single gene analysis	Analysis based on a suspected diagnosis for which a specific gene or group of genes are known to be associated	Focused approach Low data analysis burden	Can be slow if multiple genes are analysed sequentially before the disease-causing alternation is identified Long wait for test results
Multi-gene panel	Analysis based on a suspected diagnosis, for which a number of genes are known to be associated	Multiple genes are analysed simultaneously in a single test	Panel may not contain all of the causal genes associated with a diagnosis Diagnosis may be missed
Whole exome sequencing (WES) or clinical exome sequencing (CES) Only the segments of genes that provide the template to make a functional protein 'exons' and the immediately adjacent splice sites are sequenced (~1.5% of the entire genome) In CES only the exons from known disease-causing genes are included	Analysis can be targeted based on a suspected diagnosis or Analysis can be disease 'agnostic' (hypothesis free)	Faster than WGS to complete the test and analyse the data Cheaper than WGS If targeted analysis fails to identify a causative change the data is available to reanalyse and look at remaining exons Secondary findings that would be clinically relevant to the patient (and potentially other family members) can be looked for and reported back to the patient	Requires additional steps to 'isolate' the exons Results can be complicated to interpret High data analysis burden High data storage requirement Exons analysed may vary between laboratory New genes identified after testing will be missing from the data set produced Families need to understand that: • a negative result does not mean there is no risk of disease • other conditions might be identified-importance of informed consent
Whole genome sequencing (WGS) The complete DNA (genome) of the individual is read. This can be: • germline (the inherited genome) • somatic (the genome from a specific tissue, e.g. tumour)	Analysis can be targeted based on a suspected diagnosis or Can be disease 'agnostic' 'hypothesis free'	Can detect disease-causing alterations that are located away from exons and splice junctions If targeted analysis fails to identify a causative change the data is available to reanalyse the remainder of the genome Secondary findings that would be clinically relevant to the patient (and potentially other family members) can be looked for and reported back Reanalysis in the future may provide additional health information	Results can be complicated to interpret High data analysis burden High data storage requirement (one genome is ~200 GB of data) Families need to understand that: • a negative result does not mean there is no risk of disease • other conditions might be identified–importance of informed consent

information on the unique characteristics of a child's cancer. This information can then be used to guide the selection of treatment(s) that the cancer is likely to respond to, identify drug resistance, as well as aid the prediction of whether a cancer may return or spread to other areas of the body.

When NGS is used, the somatic sequence derived from tumour cells is compared with the patient's 'normal' germline genome to look for the cancer specific changes.

◎ UNFOLDING SCENARIO

Simon's Story (Part 2) – Tumour Profiling Informing Treatment

Simon's parents had been reading a lot online about cancer treatment and had learned about targeted cancer treatment, so they were happy when our team had told them that testing to identify potential treatment(s) was an option for Simon. Today's visit was to learn the findings from the genetic testing that was done on Simon's tumour (somatic genetic testing) to see if there is a genetic variant in his tumour that could be treated with a therapy that targets that gene. I reminded Simon and his family about the purpose of today's visit, what kind of genetic testing was done, and what the possible test outcomes were. I had never realised until Simon that genetic testing could be done on a tumour to help guide treatment. I also had not understood that there are different kinds of tumour (somatic) testing and the most informative tumour test is when the tumour testing is performed with a companion normal sample from blood or saliva that can identify inherited genetic changes.

👤 ACTIVITY

Somatic and Germline Testing

Review this resource on tumour (somatic) testing https://www.jax.org/education-and-learning/clinical-and-continuing-education/tumor-testing/sdm and answer the following questions. What is the difference between somatic and germline genetic testing? What are the risks, benefits, and limitations of this kind of genetic testing?

Testing of Cell Free DNA (cfDNA) Circulating in a Person's Blood

As a cell dies, fragments of DNA from the cell enter the blood stream. These fragments are collectively known as cell free DNA (cfDNA). The sensitivity of some genomic technologies means that there are now a growing number of clinical applications that take advantage of the presence of cfDNA (Ranucci, 2019). Cell free tumour DNA (cftDNA) can be found in varying amounts circulating freely in a patient's blood and can be used to detect the presence of tumour post-surgery or post-treatment, and as a tool for earlier detection of recurrence over the long term. cftDNA can also be tested to look for changes in the genome of the cancer cells that may indicate or confirm resistance to a particular therapy. cfDNA is also being used to monitor the status of transplants by looking for higher than normal levels of donor-derived cfDNA in a recipient's blood.

Non-invasive prenatal testing (NIPT). Cell free fetal DNA (cffDNA) can be detected in the maternal circulation from early pregnancy and is cleared within hours of delivery, making a blood sample taken from the pregnant women, pregnancy specific. Currently in the UK, NIPT using cffDNA is recommended as part of the antenatal screening pathway for Down (trisomy 21), Edwards (trisomy 18) and Patau (trisomy 13) syndromes (UK National Screening Committee, 2016). Early identification of an increased risk for an affected pregnancy provides the woman (and her family) with choices around additional testing, termination and planning for the birth of that child. Although NIPT is a screening test and requires confirmation of a positive test through invasive sampling of the amniotic fluid or chorionic villus (which carries a risk of miscarriage), the greater accuracy of this approach compared with other screening tests means that NIPT is predicted to reduce the numbers of invasive tests offered. Microarray technology (see Overview and Illustration of Array-Based Comparative Genomic Hybridisation [Array-CGH] box and Fig. 9.4) can be used to look for a change (increase) in signal of one of the chromosomes that would indicate the presence of an extra copy ('trisomy'). Similarly, NIPT can also be used to determine the sex of a fetus if there is a known risk of a sex-linked condition. Some centres are using the presence of cffDNA to develop tailored non-invasive diagnostic tests for pregnancies in families with a known genetic condition and so the use of this technique and range of applications is expected to grow.

Identifying Variants Associated With Common Conditions, Response to Medication and Other Human Traits

The most common type of variants within the human genome are single base-pair differences known as single nucleotide polymorphisms (SNPs), which occur, on average, once every 1000 nucleotides of DNA. Although not usually involved in disease, SNPs are often located in close proximity to genes and are inherited together. As a result, some SNPs have been found to be markers of disease or predictors of other traits.

DNA technologies including array-based assays can be used to detect SNPs and are used in genome-wide association studies (GWAS) to identify regions of the genome associated with a trait of interest. GWAS often involve hundreds or thousands of unrelated individuals with a particular trait, plus control samples being tested for millions of different SNPs. For example, Grove et al. (2019) combined and reanalysed data from multiple studies involving 18,381 individuals with autistic spectrum disorder (ASD) and 27,969 controls to identify five variants associated with ASD. As of May 2018, more than 69,000 associations between SNPs and traits have been identified (European Molecular Biology Laboratory [EMBL], 2019). The range of traits associated with locations right across the genome is strikingly illustrated in Fig. 9.5. Examples of traits studied that would be of interest to the children's nurse include early spontaneous pre-term birth, childhood onset asthma, juvenile idiopathic arthritis, attention-deficit hyperactivity disorder and metabolic side effects of antipsychotic drugs (EMBL, 2019).

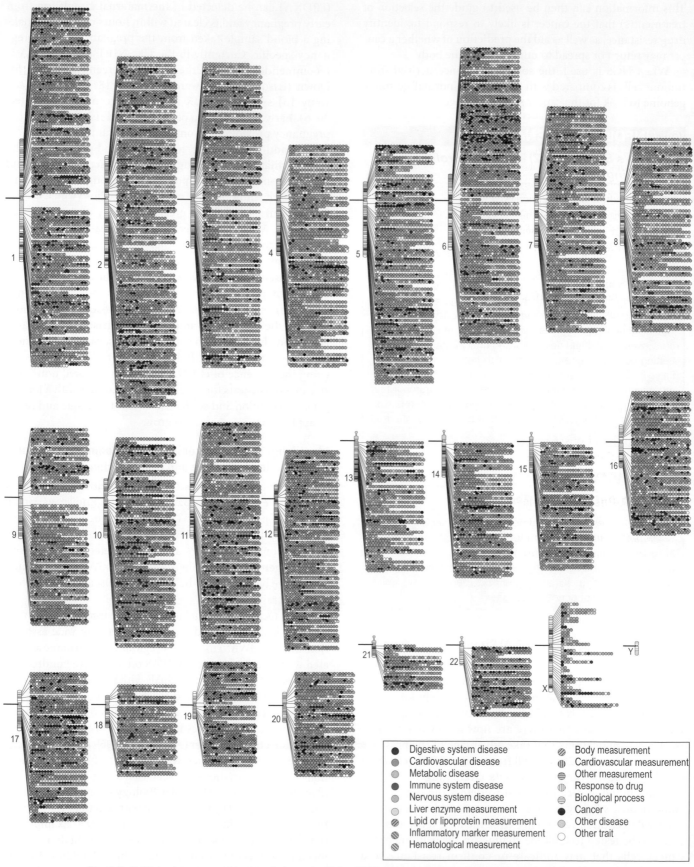

Fig. 9.5 Published genome-wide associations as of May 2018. Chromosomes 1–22 and the X-chromosomes are annotated for each association based on 17 different trait categories. (NHGRI-EBI GWAS Catalogue.)

While the individual effects of most of the SNPs that have been identified as being associated with common diseases or traits, for example, breast cancer, coronary heart disease, height and weight are small, their cumulative effects may be much more significant. A polygenic risk score (PRS) is a quantitative measure of this cumulative effect and while these are not routinely used in clinical practice at present, they may have some clinical utility in the future.

The area where polygenic risk scores have come closest to clinical practice is in the field of breast cancer, where researchers have used panels of SNPs to test women with a family history of breast cancer, with the aim of stratifying their risk more accurately. Those in the higher risk categories may benefit from earlier screening whereas those at lower risks may not. The utility of the PRS seems to be even greater when used in combination with traditional risk assessment tools and other information, for example, mammographic density.

With the advent of the new genomic technologies and initiatives such as the 100,000 Genomes Project, vast amounts of genomic variation data with associated phenotypic information is evermore available to researchers and it seems certain that the discovery of new disease-associated SNPs will continue for the foreseeable future. It is easy to imagine numerous potential roles for PRS in all areas of health care. These could include targeting dietary/exercise interventions to those at highest risk of obesity or diabetes, behavioural intervention to those at increased risk of childhood onset mental health problems or intensive anti-smoking advice/support to parent of those most susceptible to asthma.

Using DNA-Based Technology to Reduce and Remove Disease

Pre-implantation genetic diagnosis and nuclear transfer. Although prenatal genetic testing of at-risk pregnancies in families with a known genetic condition is an option, the risk of miscarriage of an unaffected pregnancy (as a result of the testing procedure) or the termination of an affected pregnancy may be unacceptable. Pre-implantation genetic diagnosis (PGD) is one alternative. Genetic testing is used alongside IVF (in vitro fertilisation) treatment to identify and implant only embryos that are unaffected. Regulated by the Human Fertilisation and Embryology Association, more than 600 conditions have been licensed to date to be tested by this method. All of these conditions are associated with autosomal and X-linked conditions. Within cells, mitochondria are involved in energy production and contain a small amount of DNA (mtDNA) encoding 37 genes. Mitochondria are typically passed on to offspring through the egg (although very recent data from Luo et al. [2018] suggests rare occurrences of paternal mitochondrial transmission), and as a consequence, genetic conditions that result from an alteration in mtDNA show a maternal pattern of inheritance. Disease severity and age of onset within families can vary depending on the proportion of altered mitochondria present in each person. Some mitochondrial disease can be life-limiting in the first few days of life.

Two in vitro methods have now been developed that use donor mitochondria (Fig. 9.6). In maternal spindle transfer, the mother's DNA is removed from one of her eggs and inserted into a donor egg with healthy mitochondria (that has had its DNA 'spindle' removed). This is then fertilised with sperm from the father, before implantation. In pronuclear transfer the mother's egg is fertilised using the father's sperm. The pronuclei containing the DNA is then transferred to a fertilised donor egg that has had its pronuclei removed and then implanted.

SEMINAR DISCUSSION TOPIC

'Three-Person' Children

In 2015, the UK became the first country to approve laws allowing the creation of babies from three people, in order to prevent inheritance of multi-systemic, progressive, life-limiting genetic disease known to be carried in the mother's mitochondria. The technique (mitochondrial replacement therapy) uses a modified version of in vitro fertilisation (IVF) to combine the healthy mitochondria from a donor woman with the DNA from the egg and sperm cells of the couple. Thus, as well as inheriting the DNA from both parents, the baby also inherits the mitochondrial DNA from the donor woman in a permanent change to the germ-line. The first baby created through this technique was born in Mexico in 2016.

In April 2019, the BBC News reported the birth of a 'Three-person baby boy' in Greece. (https://www.bbc.co.uk/news/health-47889387?intlink_from_url=https://www.bbc.co.uk/news/science_and_environment&link_location=live-reporting-story). A similar approach was used to that for mitochondrial replacement therapy whereby the nucleus of the woman's egg cell, containing her genetic material, is transferred to an enucleated donor egg. However, in this case, the technique was used in an attempt to overcome fertility issues in the woman rather for prevention of rare mitochondrial disease.

Do you think the two applications of this technique (fertility and disease prevention) are morally similar? What do you see as the potential ethical issues arising from these uses of the technology?

In the UK, children are able to trace the identity of egg or sperm donors once they reach the age of 18. Should they also be able to trace mitochondrial donors?

Further reading to guide discussion: Dimond, R., 2015. Social and ethical issues in mitochondrial donation. Br. Med. Bull. 115, 173–182.

Gene editing CRISPR-Cas9. Alongside many studies and clinical trials to use gene-based therapies to overcome genetic disease, there is now significant focus on developing and testing a very specific group of methods that could be used to edit out known mutations to remove disease. One of a number of techniques for manipulating an organism's DNA, the CRISPR-Cas9 system is showing great promise. Often likened to a 'molecular scissor' CRISPR-Cas9 can be targeted to a specific location in the genome. Once the DNA has been cut, the DNA can be repaired in a way that replaces the unwanted sequence.

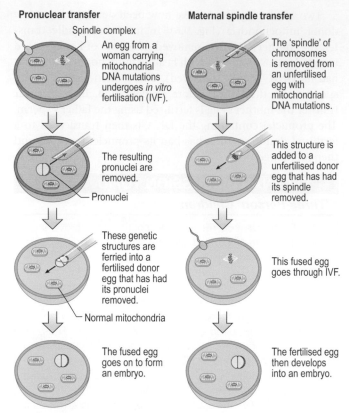

Pronuclear transfer

Spindle complex

An egg from a woman carrying mitochondrial DNA mutations undergoes *in vitro* fertilisation (IVF).

The resulting pronuclei are removed.

Pronuclei

These genetic structures are ferried into a fertilised donor egg that has had its pronuclei removed.

Normal mitochondria

The fused egg goes on to form an embryo.

Maternal spindle transfer

The 'spindle' of chromosomes is removed from an unfertilised egg with mitochondrial DNA mutations.

This structure is added to a unfertilised donor egg that has had its spindle removed.

This fused egg goes through IVF.

The fertilised egg then develops into an embryo.

Fig. 9.6 Using donor mitochondria to remove the chance of a mitochondrial disorder. (Callaway, Nature, 2014.)

Because blood stem cells are easily accessible, blood disorders (both inherited and cancer) are an early target for this method. Bone marrow stem cells can be taken from the patient, re-engineered in the laboratory and replaced back into the patient after ensuring none of the original stem cells remain. For inherited disorders of haemoglobin like sickle cell and beta thalassaemia, some studies are looking at using CRISPR technology to turn the fetal haemoglobin gene back on to compensate for alterations in the adult form of the gene. Trials are also underway in Leber congenital amaurosis type 10, the most common form of inherited childhood blindness. How this technology could be used in conditions affecting multiple organ systems, and/or where there is limited access to the tissue remains unclear.

SEMINAR DISCUSSION TOPIC

Gene Editing

In 2015 at Great Ormond Street Hospital, at the age of 11 months, Layla Richards became the first person in the world to be treated for drug-resistant acute lymphoblastic leukaemia using gene-edited immune cells. All conventional treatments had failed, but she responded well to this new experimental technique, which involved adding in genes to the immune cells that enabled them to recognise specific cell markers on the malignant cells, and destroy them. Layla's recovery was reported through international media and was heralded as an example of the therapeutic potential of gene-editing technology.

In late 2018, the birth of twin girls (referred to as Lulu and Nana) in China was announced by the leader of a research team that had used the CRISPR gene-editing tool in human embryos to target a specific gene *(CCR5)* with the aim of conferring resistance to infection by HIV. The *CCR5* gene has also been reported by other scientists to influence cognition, although Dr He stated that this had not been an aim of the research. The response to the announcement through the international media was one of deep concern and shock and Dr He's research was condemned by the Chinese authorities.

Why do you think the international reactions to the use of gene-editing techniques in these two cases were so different? What differentiates them? Think about both the scientific/clinical differences and the ethical ones.

Further reading to guide discussion:

Nuffield Council on Bioethics, 2018. Genome editing and human reproduction: social and ethical issues (Short guide). Nuffield Council on Bioethics, London. Available from: http://nuffieldbioethics.org/wp-content/uploads/Genome-editing-and-human-reproduction-short-guide-website.pdf.

Tanya Bridgen, 2018. Genome-edited babies: An unexpected reality (Blog), http://www.phgfoundation.org/blog/genome-edited-babies-an-unexpected-reality.

PHG infographic on gene editing. Available from: http://www.phgfoundation.org/infographic/what-is-genome-editing.

PHARMACOGENOMICS

Combining the fields of pharmacology and genomics, pharmacogenomics looks at how people respond differently to different drugs based on their genetic makeup. This information can be used to select the most appropriate medicine based on a prediction of how that person is likely to respond. Within a population for any one particular drug, there may be a range of responses (Fig. 9.7), each affecting different proportions of the population. In general it is difficult to predict who will respond to the drug in the expected way, who will have a limited or no response to the medicine and who will have an adverse drug reaction (ADR).

Drugs are broken down in the body ('metabolised') by proteins. Variations in the sequences of genes encoding some of these important proteins can result in an alteration in function of that protein, which in turn leads to a change in the metabolism process. As a consequence, a drug may be broken down too fast and lost from the body before the therapeutic benefit is received, or too slowly resulting in more side effects. On occasions the change in metabolism may lead to a toxic build up of the drug (or a downstream product) that can result in an ADR.

Once the sequence variant(s) of a particular protein have been identified and linked to an altered drug response, genomic technology can be used to identify the variants within a patient group prior to prescribing (Fig. 9.8). Test results may indicate when a dose needs to be adjusted (because of fast or slow metabolism) or whether a different drug should be selected because the risk of an ADR. This approach to prescribing is another example of precision (or personalised) medicine.

Some variations are more frequently associated with a specific ethnic heritage. Knowing this can be useful because dosage is often standardised across the population and is frequently based on clinical trial data with limited ethnic diversity.

Although the field of pharmacogenomics is still relatively new, and the applications within paediatric clinical practice are limited, there are some established tests. Children should be screened for hypersensitivity to the antiretroviral Abacavir prior to commencing treatment. Genotyping in children with acute lymphoblastic leukaemia to identify poor metabolisers of thiopurines, enables adjustment of their 6-mercaptopurune dose to avoid toxicity (Hawcutt et al., 2013). It is anticipated that with robust clinical trials to identify variants that can precisely predict outcomes, the numbers of available tests will grow and play important roles in dose individualisation and drug safety.

OTHER 'OMIC' TECHNOLOGIES

At the beginning of this chapter we discussed the importance of understanding the biology of the genome, as well as the 'normal' and disease states in order to move forward the science of medicine and improve the effectiveness of health care (see Fig. 9.1). This is being achieved not just through the study of DNA, but also through a broader group of 'Omic' technologies (that includes genomics), which are used to characterise and measure different biological molecules across different tissues, time points and disease states, in order to build a more comprehensive picture. These technologies include: *transcriptomics, proteomics* and *metabolomics*. Cataloguing the additional chemical modifications that occur across the genome in response to environmental cues is also a critical component of this work and is discussed further in the *epigenomics* section (see later). We will not discuss these technologies in detail but provide brief descriptions of each,

as they offer useful insight into the science that is providing the evidence to underpin future clinical applications to diagnose and treat complex diseases.

Transcriptomics

When a gene is read ('expressed'), the copy of the sequence that is created as messenger RNA (mRNA) is referred to as the transcript. All of the exons sequences (protein coding segments) in the gene are stitched ('spliced') together and the intervening sequences ('introns') are removed. The transcript provides the template for protein synthesis. The transcriptome is the total set of mRNA produced by a cell, population of cells or organism of interest, and transcriptomics is the study of the transcriptome. Different combinations of genes may be expressed in different cells and at different times.

Proteomics

Proteins (the products of genes), are manufactured using mRNA templates. Proteomics is the study of the proteome, which is the set of proteins produced by a cell, population of cells or organism of interest.

Scientists can predict, from a DNA sequence, the location of genes based on a number of features (including exons and introns). Transcriptomics can provide evidence that a predicted gene is functional (because it is expressed), as well as information on the different transcripts that may be produced from a single gene as a result of different combinations of exons being spliced together. Multiple forms of a protein can be produced from one gene because of the different transcripts that can be generated. The field of proteomics provides both the technology to identify the individual forms of a protein as well as techniques to investigate their function(s).

Metabolomics

Metabolism is the set of chemical reactions that take place in a cell, population of cells or organism. The study of both the substrates and products involved (that reflect the activity taking place in the cell[s] or organism), is referred to as metabolomics.

Microbial Genomics – the Human Microbiome and Diagnostic Pathogen Genomics

It is not just the study of the human genome that is important for health services. Microbes (including bacteria, viruses

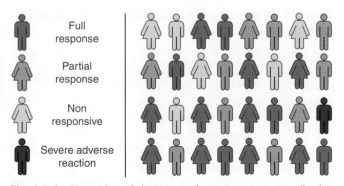

Fig. 9.7 An illustration of the range of responses to a medication within a population. (Pharmacogenomics (2007) PHG Foundation.)

Full response

Partial response

Non responsive

Severe adverse reaction

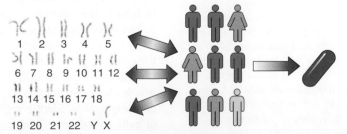

Fig. 9.8 Genomic information can be used to select the right drug tand/or right dose for individuals within a population. (Pharmacogenomics (2007) PHG Foundation.)

and yeasts) colonise our bodies and the combination and levels of microbes present can vary according to body site. Using DNA and other 'omic' technologies it is now possible to catalogue the human microbiome and there is a growing interest in understanding how the microbiome can influence different diseases and what role(s) the changing composition of the microbiome may play. Investigating how the paediatric gut and skin microbiomes develop and how these can differ, for example, between pre-term and term births, vaginal microbiome exposure compared to those born by caesarean section, or between breast and formula feed infants, may in the future offer opportunities for clinical applications to improve long-term health outcomes. Ihekweazu and Versalovic (2018) discuss the development of the gut microbiome through childhood and the impact of imbalances in the microbiome on brain development, inflammatory bowel disease/syndrome, asthma, allergy, obesity and autism.

Diagnostic pathogen genomics is a relatively new field, but one, which is growing quickly. As the name suggests, sequencing technologies are used to identify and characterise organisms for the purpose of diagnosis and treatment of infectious disease as well as tracking outbreaks. Some examples of its use includes identification of COVID-19 positive individuals; detect antimicrobial resistance in HIV and TB; characterisation of mycobacteria; strain analysis of circulating seasonal influenza; *Enterovirus* characterisation; *Clostridium difficile* sequencing and strain typing; and resistance and virulence determination of bacterial hospital associated infections.

Pathogen genomics in a paediatric setting is most relevant in relation to outbreaks and infection control. For example, an Influenza outbreak in a school or *C. difficile* infection on a ward, where the strain and sequence of the pathogens would help determine the variation in strains between infected individuals and the root of infection.

👤 ACTIVITY

Genomics and Infection Tracking

Towards the end of the video clip from the earlier activity (*Introducing Genomics in Healthcare*) the narrator mentions the application of genomics in tracking outbreaks of infectious disease. Whole genome sequencing of the microorganisms involved allows very precise classification of the pathogen. Watch Controlling MRSA by DNA Sequencing (https://www.youtube.com/watch?v=DvFbmCNvZQI) and listen to researchers at the Wellcome Sanger Institute in Cambridge, UK, talk about how they used bacterial whole genome sequencing to explore in more detail an outbreak of MRSA in a Special Care Baby Unit. They were able to track precisely the origins of the specific strain and the course of the outbreak. A staff member who was found to be a carrier of MRSA was identified and treated and the outbreak was thus contained. Further detail is available on the Sanger Institute's your genome website from Tracking superbugs: https://www.yourgenome.org/stories/tracking-superbugs.

EPIGENOMICS

All of the cells in the human body contain the same genetic material yet each cell type and tissue is unique because of the different combinations of genes that are turned on or off at any given point in time. Epigenetic modification is one mechanism for regulating gene activity that does not involve alteration of the DNA code. Histones are proteins used by the cell to package the very long molecules of DNA into the tightly wrapped structures we know as chromosomes. Both histones and the DNA molecule contain chemical tags collectively known as the epigenome and the presence or absence of these tags can result in genes being silenced or activated.

What is important in this biological process is that these tags are the body's response to external signals from the environment including diet, stress, lifestyle and chemical exposures. The DNA code for every individual essentially remains fixed, but the epigenome is flexible, adjusting as necessary to the ever changing environment throughout a person's life.

Epigenetic modifications can be both heritable and potentially reversible and therefore have consequences both for the individual and subsequent generations. Epigenetic modifications are required for normal growth and development, but are also associated with a number of disease processes including cancer and developmental delay (Fig. 9.9). Epigenomics is adding to our understanding of illness particularly around the modification of lifestyle to improve health outcomes; Fessele and Wright (2018) in their article on epigenetic control, acknowledge the benefit to nursing practice of having a 'foundational understanding' of core concepts in epigenomics.

How Do Epigenetic Modifications Work? Health and Ill-health

Genes are silent when the DNA is tightly packaged and are active when the DNA is unwound. The two main epigenetic mechanisms used for regulating gene expression are DNA methylation and histone modification (see Fig. 9.9). Specific sequences usually found at the start of genes ('promoter regions') are recognised by factors in the cell that trigger a gene being turned on ('expressed'). DNA methylation of these regions can prevent those factors accessing the gene as well as alter the way in which the DNA is packaged, making the gene inaccessible. Similarly, when histones are modified the presence of these tags result in that region of DNA becoming tightly wrapped and the genes in that area are unavailable to be read. In the absence of tags, the DNA relaxes and genes can be turned on. Epigenetic modifications are passed on through every (mitotic) cell division and are used to ensure that all of the cells in a particular line express the same set of genes.

Together these modifications provide a unique epigenetic profile that regulates the physical structure of the DNA and gene expression. Identifying and cataloguing the epigenome of cells and tissues is an important part of understanding genome biology as discussed at the beginning of this chapter (see Fig. 9.1).

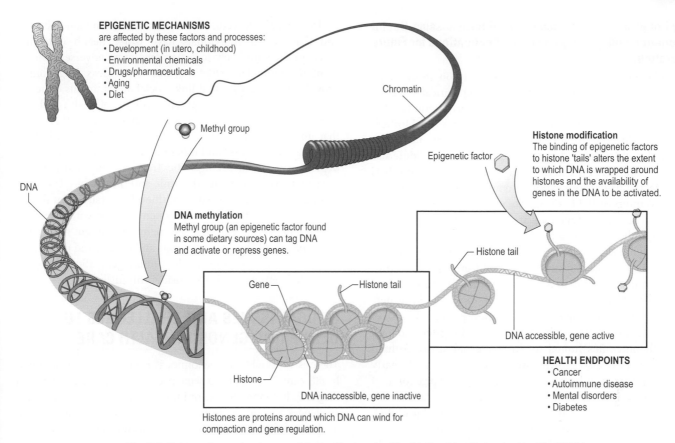

Fig. 9.9 Epigenetic mechanisms and their effect on health. (National Institutes for Health, 2018.)

Developmental Delay

There are a number of conditions associated with developmental delay where epigenetic modification is known to be the underlying disease mechanism (Egger et al., 2004) (see Table 9.1). For example, in Fragile X syndrome a DNA sequence in the promotor region of the *FMR1* gene gets longer (compared to individuals that do not have the conditions) and as a consequence becomes a target for methylation that results in the gene being silenced. As males have an X and Y combination of sex chromosomes they are always affected by this alteration. Only one set of genes from the X chromosome is required for human development. In females, methylation is the mechanism used to tightly and permanently silence all gene expression from one of the pair of X chromosomes present. The X chromosome inactivated in each cell is randomly selected and this helps explain why some females who carry an alteration for an X-linked recessive condition (like Fragile X syndrome) will display signs and symptoms even though they also have an unaltered/'normal' copy of the gene. This unaltered version will be permanently turned off in a proportion of cells. The number and type(s) of cells present that don't have a working copy will dictate the severity of the condition in that female.

Cancer

Exposure to different environmental triggers throughout the life course can result in the accumulation over time, of epigenetic tags. Another outcome of these modifications is cancer. Tumour suppressor genes are normally involved in slowing down cell division or triggering cell death. Modifications that lead to the suppression of these and other important genes, along with additional changes that activate genes when they shouldn't be on, can lead to the altered cell behaviour and abnormality in growth and division seen in cancer (Portela and Esteller, 2010). Tests are being developed that look for specific epigenetic signatures associated with different cancer types and prognoses. In addition, the cancer epigenome is seen as a potential target for therapeutic drug development, for example, by inhibiting the tagging process in order to reactivate the key genes that have been silenced. Whilst such drugs could provide an opportunity to hit multiple gene targets simultaneously the challenge will be in directing such therapies to only the cancerous cells. As the tags are present across the genome, any treatment that also alters the epigenome of normal cells could be very harmful.

👤 ACTIVITY

Epigenomics

Visit the Epigenetics module of the University of Utah's Genetic Science Learning Center website (https://learn.genetics.utah.edu/content/epigenetics/). Browse the nine sections and watch the short introductory video on epigenetics (The Epigenome at a Glance). Learn more about how the epigenome is re-programmed (Epigenetics and Inheritance). There are two interactive sections for you to explore, one on gene expression and how it can be modified (Gene Control), and one looking at mothering (Lick Your Rat).

Early Programming, Intergenerational Transmission, Social Epigenetics and Reprogramming – Implications for Future Generations

Some epigenetic traits are established early-on in development and can be affected by events during critical stages of development, including the prenatal and early periods, with the effects on health becoming apparent in later life. Mothers and their children share the developmental environment (Fig. 9.10) and studies have demonstrated the effect of different events on long-term outcomes. The classic example of this is data collected from those exposed to famine during the Dutch Hunger Winters of 1944–45. Sons of women, who experienced famine during early pregnancy and were born with a normal birthweight, had higher rates of obesity in later life, compared to others who were exposed mid and late gestation (Ravelli et al., 1976). In a more recent study, children exposed to prenatal maternal hardship and distress as a result of an extreme ice storm in Quebec, Canada, in 1998 appear to have persistent distinctive and altered methylation patterns (Cao-Lei et al., 2014) and are being followed over the long-term to look for health outcomes linked to this maternal stress. Animal experiments have also shown parental behaviours in the early postnatal period can be crucial in shaping the epigenome of offspring (see *Activity Epigenomics* for more information on the highly nurturing behaviour in rats producing calm adults).

Importantly, it is not only the intrauterine and early childhood environments that affects health outcomes in children. Epidemiological studies have provided evidence of both paternal contribution and inheritance across generations of these epigenetic traits. In a Swedish study, Kaati and colleagues (2002) found that low levels of nutrition during important stages in childhood growth of fathers, reduced cardiovascular disease deaths in their children, whereas diabetes increased in children whose paternal grandfather had excess food during this same critical period in childhood.

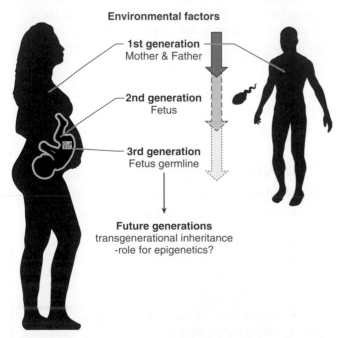

Environmental factors

1st generation
Mother & Father

2nd generation
Fetus

3rd generation
Fetus germline

Future generations
transgenerational inheritance
-role for epigenetics?

Fig. 9.10 How the environment affects three generations at a time. (Ling and Rönn, 2019)

That social and economic circumstances influence health, and that poorer individuals have worse health outcomes (because they are likely to experience more adverse environments throughout their lifetime) are not new ideas. Epigenomics provides a mechanism that links social determinants of health with the concept of developmental origins of health and disease (DOHaD). The study by McGuinness et al. (2012) is one that links global changes in the epigenome with markers of cardiovascular disease and inflammation, and socio-economic deprivation. Because epigenetic traits are not written into the genetic code, they are dynamic and modifiable. Trying to counteract the effects of early childhood adversity, poor diet or environmental exposures could potentially prevent, reverse, or slow the process of epigenetic silencing, and might reduce the development of chronic conditions and cancer, and potentially have implications for the health of future generations. (See the associated Seminar topic to consider this further.)

ETHICAL ISSUES AND CHALLENGES TO DELIVERING GENOMIC HEALTH CARE

There is no doubt that genomics is beginning to revolutionise health care. The ability to sequence a child's DNA to provide a diagnosis for a rare disease or inform treatment choices presents challenges beyond the technical issues around obtaining a high quality sample and reading the exome, or entire DNA of that child.

Interpretation and Use of Data

Variants of unknown (or uncertain) significance. The identification of alterations and prediction of whether or not they are likely to be disease causing is dependent on software algorithms, the availability of other clinical/sequencing data to support or refute a finding, and scientific expertise to interpret the prediction. Genes and mutations are still being identified and there is still a great deal that we do not know about the genetic code. Where a result is inconclusive (see Professional Conversation – Inconclusive Result box) the child and their family are left with uncertainty. Reanalysis of the DNA sequence data can be undertaken periodically (as algorithms and databases are updated) in an attempt to make a clear diagnosis. However, this then introduces the challenge of long-term data storage and the associated questions around privacy – who will have access to the data and will it be used for anything else (subject to consent by the participant or their parent/guardian if that person is a child)? Many large-scale sequencing projects have agreements in place with the wider scientific community (publically funded and commercial), to share anonymised data for the purposes of scientific discovery, diagnostic test and therapy development. For individuals who were children when the sequence was first generated, is the consent still valid once they are older and should they be re-consented for both research participation and clinical reanalysis as an adult?

Secondary and incidental findings (as illustrated in Simon's Story [Part 3]) can have a significant impact even when the possibility of such findings have been raised during pre-test discussion. At times of high stress, for example, when parents are faced with a critically ill child, consent for a test may be given without fully appreciating the extent of potential findings. The

SEMINAR DISCUSSION TOPIC

Epigenetics and the Role of the Children's Nurse in Promoting Health and Well-Being

In the previous chapter, *Inherited Conditions and the Family*, we described how harmful alterations to the genome, passed on by parents, can impact adversely on the health and development of the child. We acknowledged that nurses have a role in supporting parents who experience the feelings of guilt and blame that can ensue, helping them to understand the mechanisms underpinning inherited conditions and helping them to accept that they did not choose the genes they passed on to their offspring, any more than their own parents did.

Epigenetics potentially adds another dimension to this role as it runs contrary to our previous understanding of the independence of genome inheritance and the influence of environment, as captured in the phrase 'nature versus nurture'. The epigenome (the chemical framework around the DNA molecule itself) regulates gene activity through controlling gene expression (see Fig. 9.9). Modifications to the epigenome can result in variations in gene expression, without changing the DNA itself. Where the modifications have a harmful effect on gene regulation, the consequences can lead to problems with health and well-being across the lifespan. Furthermore, although they can be re-programmed, the alterations to the epigenome can be passed on through generations. These modifications can be caused by physical and psychosocial environmental factors including stress, trauma, social and physical adversity, diet and lifestyle behaviours, war, famine and natural disasters.

The epigenome thus acts as a mediator between the genome and the environment, underlining the importance of a nurturing environment and a healthy start in life that is linked not just to the inherited genome. It provides the link between 'nature' and 'nurture'.

Much of the research literature has focused on adverse pre- and post-natal conditions in relation to infant development and is helping to inform care in neonatal intensive care units and long-term infant well-being programmes. Understanding the potential contribution of the epigenome to child development, and the range of factors that might modify it, is important for children's nurses in relation to their health education and health promotion roles, and in developing effective intervention programmes.

However, is there a potential source of tension here? A core principle in genetic counselling in relation to inherited conditions is to be non-directive and non-judgemental in communications aimed at providing support for decision making, understanding results and adjusting to diagnoses. To what extent should this stance be applied, particularly where there is evidence that the modifying factor is a poor lifestyle choice? How can the nursing role as a health educator in promoting a 'healthy epigenome' here be compatible with the non-directive, non-judgemental approach adopted to diffuse feelings of guilt and blame around the inherited genome? Finally, how far should the children's nurse take the role of health promotion in championing the health of infants and children, when the influence of poverty, deprivation and other national and global factors on the epigenome can have far-reaching consequences for them and across future generations?

American College of Medical Genetics and Genomics have recommended that alongside the primary condition, analysis and reporting should be undertaken on 56 genes associated with clinically actionable conditions (Green et al., 2013). As part of the 100,000 Genomes Project participants could 'opt-in' to analysis of a much smaller subset of these genes including seven with childhood onset that would be looked for in child participants (bowel cancer: *APC*; other cancer predispositions: *VHL*, *MEN1* and *RET*; and familial hypocholesterolaemia: *LDLR*, *APOB* and *PCSK9*). Identification of pathogenic mutations can have implications for biologically linked family members, and support is often required to help families communicate and disclose this information to others.

Sequencing – Just Because We Can, Does It Mean We Should?

With the ability to sequence whole genomes, some advocate for the sequencing of babies at birth so that their unique health-related data is available to them from the beginning and right through their life course (Fig. 9.11). The potential benefits are that clinically actionable single-gene disorders could be identified; predictions could be made early on regarding susceptibility to common conditions in later life allowing interventions to be implemented; variations in drug response would be known ahead of any medication being prescribed and the sequence would provide a reference to compare against should cancer develop. Friedman et al. (2017) considered the sequencing of babies within the context of newborn screening and came to a

UNFOLDING SCENARIO

Simon's Story (Part 3) – Implications for Other Family Members

I was delighted when Simon and his family were scheduled to return for the results of the genetic testing as I had learned that there was a driver genetic variant identified in Simon's tumour that had a targeted agent we could treat him with. The challenge was that Simon was also found to have an inherited (germline) genetic variant that affects the function of a gene associated with Lynch syndrome. Pathogenic variants in this particular gene increase the risk for early onset colon, endometrial and ovarian cancer as well as many other cancers. In retrospect, this was not surprising given the family history. This was going to be a lot of information for the family, so we pre-planned a tag team approach first talking about Simon's cancer treatment, and then reviewing the results of the germline test. We had a genetic counsellor participate in that discussion. On the one hand Simon and his parents were happy to have a treatment plan customised to his own tumour, but his parents were stunned by the news of the germline finding, understood this would have been transmitted from one of them, and immediately expressed guilt that they had passed 'cancer' on their son. The genetic counsellor was terrific in explaining things and discussing that the parents needed to be tested to verify which side of the family this was coming from. Having had the discussion with our team ahead of time, she also appreciated that Simon's parents were going to be focused mostly on the treatment of their son. So we needed to respect that and schedule additional times to talk with them to continue to give them information and make recommendations for the at risk family members.

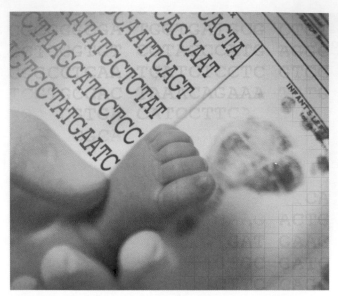

Fig. 9.11 Should babies have their genomes sequenced? (Courtesy: National Human Genome Research Institute, NIH.)

number of conclusions including that, at that time, the 'ability to interpret genomic variants does not justify the use of genome wide or large multi-gene sequencing panels in population-based newborn screening'. The BabySeq Project (https://www.genomes2people.org/research/baby-seq/) is a randomised clinical trial currently taking place in the US to determine how genomics can be used in clinical paediatrics and assess the impact on the child and their family of having this information available to them.

Genomics testing is not just available through the UK's National Health Service (and other health care providers). Commercial companies now offer direct to consumer genomic tests that can provide both ancestry and health-related results (based on single nucleotide polymorphisms). Test results can raise concerns or cause confusion if they are not understood and if there is no knowledgeable support available.

The complexity of sequence data and the potential applications for that information (many of what are still to be defined), mean that ideally, everyone should have some knowledge and understanding around genomics. This would allow people to engage with the issues and debates around the technology (e.g. sharing of clinical data with third parties or the ethical implications of gene editing), to ensure that policies are robust and acceptable to the public. More importantly, it will allow individuals and families to benefit from the technology, when there is a clinical reason for testing as they would have a better understanding of the implications and limitations of the findings and may be in a better position to act on results.

SO WHAT DOES ALL THIS MEAN FOR CHILDREN'S NURSES?

- The incidence of inherited/genetic conditions in children means that children's nurses should already be familiar with core genetic principles. Genomics is an extension of this field so build on these principles.

🧑 ACTIVITY
Direct to Consumer Genetic Testing

Personalised (direct to consumer, DTC) genetic testing kits have become increasingly popular in the UK and elsewhere. Kits can be ordered online through companies such as 23andme and AncestryDNA, where individuals then collect and return a saliva sample. For 23andme (https://www.23andme.com/en-gb/) for example, as well as receiving information about ancestry, consumers can also opt for information about health predispositions for conditions such as Type 2 diabetes and coeliac disease, 'wellness', carrier status and traits. There has been controversy over the availability of DTC testing and concerns have been expressed by specialist health professionals about individuals who take a test in this way. What do you think?

Watch the video from the Sanger Institute presenting the views and experiences of people who have considered, or undertaken Direct-to-Consumer genetic testing (https://www.yourgenome.org/video/direct-to-consumer-genetic-testing).

Do you feel you have the knowledge and skills to support individuals or families who have taken a DTC test and are stressed or confused about their results?

- A rapidly increasing raft of tests that use genomic technology including NIPT, newborn screening and genome/exome sequencing, has implications for diagnosis, including for previously undiagnosed conditions. The children's nurse should:
  - promote equity of access to these tests, including across all cultural groups
  - support informed consent
  - be able to explain nature of testing so parents/families/older children can understand what is being tested, why results may take a long time, what not finding anything actually means, why other conditions might be identified
  - be mindful of opportunities for families to participate in research
  - be aware that the field is very fast moving so families without a diagnosis should not give up hope of finding one
- There are ethical issues around ownership and privacy of genomic information (as for genetic), but also in relation to new technologies and alteration to germline.
- The growing use of genomic technologies in decisions around therapeutic options, to identify optimum treatment regimens and avoidance of harm because of adverse drug reactions, is an area for nurses to be aware of and be able to talk about.
- A greater understanding of the interactions between environment (including social) and the epigenome, and the subsequent influence on health and disease may in the longer term underpin management of children in NICU/PICU and provide the children's nurse with a significant role in public health to benefit early childhood development and long-term health of both current and future generations.

All of this may seem daunting to nurses with little previous education around genetics or genomics. Genomics is complex, the field is a fast-moving one and this chapter has really just touched on the 'basics'. You do not need to be an expert in genomic health care to deliver high quality care and support to children and their families. However, as the quote from Elias Zerhouni at the very beginning indicated, genomics isn't going to go away and you will need to know and understand sufficient information to be able to support families and explain 'the basics' to them. Most importantly, know where to go to get good quality, accurate and up to date information.

ACKNOWLEDGEMENTS

The authors would like to thank everyone who contributed 'Professional Conversations' for this chapter and to Dr Kathleen Calzone, Research Geneticist, National Institutes of Health, National Cancer Institute, USA for the unfolding scenario 'Simon's story' and Bree Gatica-Wilcox, Biomedical Scientist, Pathogen Genomics Unit, Wales for the information provided in relation to Diagnostic Pathogen Genomics.

REFERENCES

Bell, J., 1998. The new genetics in clinical practice. Br. Med. J. 316, 618–620.

Burton, H., 2011. Genetics and Mainstream Medicine. PHG Foundation. ISBN 978-1-907198-07-6.

Cao-Lei, L.L., Massart, R., Suderman, M.J., et al., 2014. DNA methylation signatures triggered by prenatal maternal stress exposure to a natural disaster: project ice storm. PLoS One 9 (9), e107653.

Callaway E (2014). Reproductive medicine: The power of three. Nature 509, 414–417.

Conley, Y.P., Biesecker, L.G., Gonsalves, S., et al., 2013. Current and emerging technology approaches in genomics. J. Nurs. Scholarsh. 45 (1), 5–14.

Davies, S.C., 2017. Annual Report of the Chief Medical Officer 2016, Generation Genome. Department of Health, London.

Department of Health and Social Care, 2019. The UK Strategy for Rare Diseases: 2019 Update to the Implementation Plan for England. Available from: https://assets.publishing.service.gov.uk/government/uploads/system/uploads/attachment_data/file/781472/2019-update-to-the-rare-diseases-implementation-plan-for-england.pdf. (accessed July 2019).

EURORDIS Rare Diseases Europe. Survey of the Delay in Diagnosis for 8 Rare Diseases in Europe ('EURORDISCARE 2'). Available from: www.eurordis.org/sites/default/files/publications/Fact_Sheet_Eurordiscare2.pdf.

Egger, G., Liang, G., Aparicio, A., Jones, P.A., 2004. Epigenetics in human disease and prospects for epigenetic therapy. Nature 429 (6990), 457–463.

European Molecular Biology Laboratory (EMBL), 2019. NHGRI-EBI GWAS Catalog. Available from: https://www.ebi.ac.uk/gwas/docs/diagram-downloads.

Fessele, K.L., Wright, F., 2018. Primer in genetics and genomics, article 6: basics of epigenetic control. Biol. Res. Nurs. 20 (1), 103–110.

French, C.E., Delon, I., Dolling, H., et al., 2019. Whole genome sequencing reveals that genetic conditions are frequent in intensively ill children. Intensive Care. Med. 45 (5), 627–636.

Friedman, J.M., Martina, C.C., Goldenberg, A.J., et al., 2017. Genomic newborn screening: public health policy considerations and recommendations. BMC Med. Genomics 10 (1), 9.

Green, R.C., Berg, J.S., Grody, W.W., et al., 2013. ACMG recommendations for reporting of incidental findings in clinical exome and genome sequencing. Genet. Med. 15 (7), 565–574.

Green, E.D., Guyer, M.S., National Human Genome Research Institute. 2011. Charting a course for genomic medicine from base pairs to bedside. Nature 470, 204–213.

Grove, J., Ripke, S., Als, T.D., et al., 2019. Identification of common genetic risk variants for autism spectrum disorder. Nat. Genet. 51 (3), 431–444.

Guttmacher, A.E., Collins, F.S., Drazen, J.M. (Eds.), 2004. Genomic Medicine: Articles from the New England Journal of Medicine. Johns Hopkins University Press, Baltimore.

Hawcutt, D.B., Thompson, B., Smyth, R.L., et al., 2013. Paediatric pharmacogenomics: an overview. Arch. Dis. Child. 98, 232–237.

Ihekweazu, F.D., Versalovic, J., 2018. Development of the pediatric gut microbiome: impact on health and disease. Am. J. Med. Sci. 356 (5), 413–423.

Kaati, G., Bygren, L.O., Edvinsson, S., 2002. Cardiovascular and diabetes mortality determined by nutrition during parents' and grandparents' slow growth period. Eur. J. Hum. Genet. 10, 682–688.

Kirk, M., Tonkin, E., Skirton, H., 2014. An iterative consensus-building approach to revising a genetics/genomics competency framework for nurse education in the UK. J. Adv. Nurs. 70 (2), 405–420.

Luo, S., Valencia, A., Zhang, J., et al., 2018. Biparental inheritance of mitochondrial DNA in humans. Proc. Natl. Acad. Sci. U.S.A. 115, 13039–13044.

McGuinness, D., McGlynn, L.M., Johnson, P.C.D., et al., 2012. Socio-economic status is associated with epigenetic differences in the pSoBid cohort. Int. J. Epidemiol. 41, 151–160.

Mestek-Boukhibar, L., Clement, E., Jones, W.D., 2018. Rapid Paediatric Sequencing (RaPS): comprehensive real-life workflow for rapid diagnosis of critically ill children. J. Med. Genet. 55, 721–728.

Müller, M.H., Reimann-Berg, N., Bullerdiek, J., Murua Escobar, H. 2012. Genetic characterization of dogs via chromosomal analysis and array-based comparative genomic hybridization (aCGH). Tierarztl Prax Ausg K Kleintiere Heimtiere. 2012; 40(1) 55–58.

Naylor, R., Knight Johnson, A., del Gaudio, D., 2018. Maturity-onset diabetes of the young overview. In: Adam, M.P., Ardinger, H.H., Pagon, R.A., et al. (Eds.), GeneReviews [Internet]. University of Washington, Seattle. Available from: https://www.ncbi.nlm.nih.gov/books/NBK500456/.

Portela, A., Esteller, M., 2010. Epigenetic modifications and human disease. Nat. Biotechnol. 28, 1057–1068.

Ranucci, R., 2019. Cell-free DNA: applications in different diseases. In: Casadio, V., Salvi, S. (Eds.), Cell-free DNA as Diagnostic Markers. Methods in Molecular Biology, vol. 1909. Humana Press, New York.

Ravelli, G.P., Stein, Z.A., Susser, M.W., 1976. Obesity in young men after famine exposure in utero and early infancy. N. Engl. J. Med. 295, 349–353.

Riegel, M., 2014. Human molecular cytogenetics: from cells to nucleotides. Genet. Mol. Biol. 37 (1 Suppl. l), 194–209.

Strauss, S., 2010. At the heart of genetic testing. Nat. Biotechnol. 28, 1003–1005.

UK National Screening Committee, 2016. UK NSC Non-Invasive Prenatal Testing (NIPT) Recommendation. Available from: https://legacyscreening.phe.org.uk/policydb_download.php?doc=570. (accessed July 2019).

Willyard, C., 2018. New human gene tally reignites debate. Nature News. Avaialbe from: https://www.nature.com/articles/d41586-018-05462-w (accessed July 2019) ISSN 1476-4687 (online).https://www.england.nhs.uk/healthcare-science/personalisedmedicine/

10

Homeostasis and the Deteriorating Child

Liz Gormley-Fleming, Anna Haviland

LEARNING OUTCOMES

- Understand how homeostasis is maintained in children and young people in relation to fluids and electrolytes.
- Detail the transportation of fluids and electrolytes in the body.
- Be able to explain the clinical manifestations of fluid loss on the child and young person and describe the principle of management and nursing care.
- Recognise the deteriorating sick child or young person and know the signs of sepsis.
- Be able to deploy a range of tools used for communication and assessment in the hospital setting.

INTRODUCTION

The aim of this chapter is to provide the reader with an understanding of the homeostatic mechanism within the bodies of infants, children and young people. This is essential knowledge for the children's and young person's nurse. Application of knowledge of physiology and the altered physiological state when caring for the sick child or young person will demonstrate safe and effective care. The second part of this chapter is concerned with recognising the deteriorating child and consideration of planning safe, effective evidence-based care.

Homeostasis is the ability of the human body to maintain internal stability through biochemical and physiological pathways. This tightly controlled system ensures optimal cell function and enzyme activity.

The homeostatic balance is maintained through a series of interrelated mechanisms that involve all the organs and body tissues. An example of some of the physiological variables, which are maintained within narrow parameters, are outlined in Table 10.1. Occasionally more than one mechanism may be involved. An example of this is the maintenance of blood pressure. A series of fine adjustments of hormone levels, the cardiovascular and the neuromuscular systems combine to maintain blood pressure within normal parameters.

Homeostasis is maintained within a narrow range of accepted norms through continual changes in the internal physiological processes. These changes occur automatically. This feedback system is triggered by variations outside the normal parameters. The impact of an imbalance to the homeostatic state can be profound. In fact, it should be considered that any episodes of ill health should be regarded as a result of its disturbance (Marieb and Hoehn, 2018). There will

be a risk to the well-being of the child and potential significant harm if not detected and treated appropriately.

This section will consider:

- Regulation of homeostasis.
- Homeostatic mechanisms (diffusion, active transport, hydrostatic osmotic colloid pressures, exocytosis, receptor mediated endocytosis and pinocytosis, osmoregulation).
- Production of energy – cell respiration: Krebs cycle, glycolysis, electron transport chain.
- Systematic approach – respiratory, GI, endocrine, renal and thermoregulation.

REGULATION OF HOMEOSTASIS

The maintenance of homeostasis is achieved by control systems. These detect a change in the internal environment and respond to that change. In order to respond to the change, the control system must have a detector/receptor, control centre and effector (Waugh and Grant, 2018). These control system functions are outlined in Fig. 10.1. The detector/receptor sensors cells as identified by Mulryan (2011) are:

- *thermoreceptors*, which monitor body temperature;
- *chemoreceptors*, which monitor the concentration of chemicals, for example carbon dioxide;
- *baroreceptors* that monitor pressure, e.g. blood pressure;
- *osmoreceptors* that monitor pressure and the amount of water within the body, for example concentration of urine.

Feedback Mechanism

Feedback systems are either positive or negative with the majority being the latter. The feedback mechanism enables the cell or organism to self-regulate and achieve a state of equilibrium.

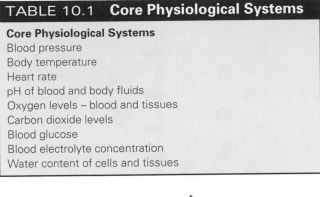

TABLE 10.1 Core Physiological Systems
Core Physiological Systems
Blood pressure
Body temperature
Heart rate
pH of blood and body fluids
Oxygen levels – blood and tissues
Carbon dioxide levels
Blood glucose
Blood electrolyte concentration
Water content of cells and tissues

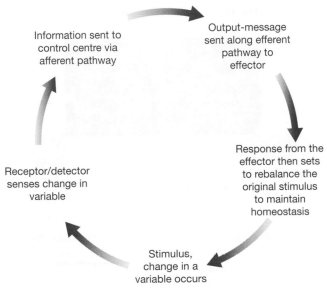

Fig. 10.1 Control system.

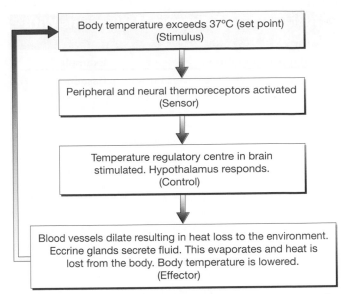

Fig. 10.2 Negative feedback mechanism of temperature control.

Negative Feedback Mechanisms

A negative feedback system requires a mechanism to alter its functionality. Any alteration away from the control systems' normal parameter set point is required to be reversed. This reversal will return the variable back to its normal parameter set point. If the variable increases, negative feedback will reduce the variable until it reaches the set point; if it decreases, the negative feedback system will increase until it achieves its set point. Body temperature is an example of a physiological function that is maintained by the negative feedback mechanism (Fig. 10.2). Blood glucose regulation is also maintained by negative feedback mechanism.

Positive Feedback Mechanism

There are fewer positive feedback mechanisms in the body and they are usually control events that are infrequent that do not require continuous adjustments. In a positive feedback mechanism, the output is amplified. An example of a positive feedback mechanism is childbirth. During the birth process, the baby's head pushes against the cervix. This then activates neurons that signal and enable a release of oxytocin from the pituitary gland. Oxytocin increases the contractions in the uterus, which responds by releasing more oxytocin. The resulting effect of this is stronger contractions and this positive feedback mechanism continues until the baby is born.

The ejection of breast milk is also as a result of the positive feedback mechanism. The baby sucks from the nipple, generating a sensory impulse, which is then transmitted to the hypothalamus leading to the release of oxytocin from the posterior pituitary (Waugh and Grant, 2018). When the oxytocin releases the breast, the milk ducts contract resulting in the myoepithelial cells, which surround the glandular cells, to eject milk.

The blood clotting mechanism is another example of the positive feedback mechanism.

Homeostatic Mechanisms

The movement of substances within and between cells occurs through various processes: diffusion, osmosis, exocytosis and osmoregulation. Fluid in the body is present in a dynamic state and is located in several compartments. Several mechanisms of transport enable cells to move material into and out of the cell.

These are: diffusion, osmosis, active transport, pinocytosis, phagocytosis, endocytosis and exocytosis. Energy is required for some of this in the form of adenosine triphosphate (ATP), but not for all. An overview is presented in Table 10.2.

Diffusion

Diffusion is the process of movement of small molecules from an area of high concentration to an area of lower concentration via a semipermeable membrane, for example, cell wall, capillary wall. An example of this is oxygen diffusing across the cell wall of the alveoli into the blood. The oxygen concentration in the alveoli is high, thus it moves to an area of low concentration – the blood (Fig. 10.3). These cells are small enough to diffuse across, whereas the cells in the blood are too large to diffuse.

Facilitated diffusion (facilitated transport or passive mediated transport) is concerned with the spontaneous passive movement of molecules or ions across the semipermeable membrane via specific transmembrane integral proteins. The protein molecules are known as carriers and are substance specific. The carrier binds itself to the substrate and then deposits the substrate in the other side of the cell wall (Clancy and McVicar, 2009; Ball

TABLE 10.2   Transport Mechanisms With the Cell

Mechanism	Definition	Example
Diffusion	Molecules move from an area of greater concentration to an area of lesser concentration	Gaseous exchange in the alveoli
Osmosis	Movement of water from an area of high concentration to an area of lower concentration through a semipermeable membrane	Absorption of water on the nephron
Active transport	Movement of molecules from an area of lesser concentration to an area of greater concentration. This requires energy in the form of ATP	Uptake of glucose by the cell
Filtration	Movement of water and a dissolved substance from an area of high concentration to an area of lower concentration	Formation of urine
Pinocytosis (drinking)	The process where a cell takes in molecules by engulfing them	Reabsorption of protein in the renal tubules. Drug absorption
Phagocytosis (eating)	Invagination of a molecule	While blood cells engulfing bacteria
Exocytosis	Vesicles within the cell join with the cell membrane and then expel their content within the cell	Secretion of hormones from the beta cells in the pancreas
Endocytosis	Takes in molecules from outside the cell	Neurotransmission

ATP, adenosine triphosphate.

and Bindler, 2006). The direction and rate of flow of the solute is dependent on the concentration gradient both inside and outside the cell. If the solute is of greater concentration, then it will bind to the carrier protein in the cytoplasm. It will then travel outside the cell and the opposite will occur if the concentration of the solute is greater outside of the cell. Saturation is an important concept when considering facilitated diffusion. The process is 'saturable'. This means that the concentration gradient will increase until it reaches a point where the carrier molecules are occupied and the substance will reach a saturation point. This will be achieved irrespective of the concentration gradient. An example of this is the transportation of chloride across the membrane of a red blood cell in one direction and bicarbonate ions in the opposite direction.

Active Transport

Active transport requires energy to move molecules from areas of low concentration to high concentration (Brady, 2015). For

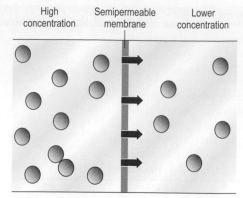

Fig. 10.3 Diffusion – simple diffusion.

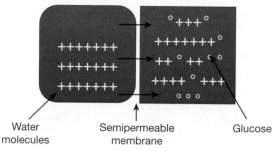

Fig. 10.4 Osmoregulation.

example, this might be potassium, calcium or sodium. Particles move across the concentration gradient. The energy used is harvested from adenosine triphosphate (ATP) via cellular metabolism. Disorders of metabolism may interfere with this process. The sodium-potassium pump is an example of active transport. Sodium and potassium ions are moved along the plasma membrane simultaneously: potassium moves in and sodium moves out. Active transport is said to move against a concentration gradient (Scanlon and Sanders, 2015).

Osmosis, Osmotic Pressure and Osmoregulation

Osmosis is the spontaneous movement of water or other solvents down its concentration gradient. The flow is from an area of high concentration to low concentration (Blows, 2012). The molecules will cross the semipermeable membrane until the concentration is equal on both sides (Fig. 10.4). The osmotic pressure pulls water from the low concentration into the area of high concentration until equilibrium is achieved. The fluid on either side of the semipermeable membrane will be of the same concentration but not necessarily of the same volume. This is called osmoregulation.

The osmolarity of plasma is maintained within very narrow parameters. If the water concentration of the plasma increases, water will move down the concentration gradient across its membranes and into the red blood cell. If this is allowed to continue the red cell may swell and then rupture. The plasma is hypotonic in this situation.

If the water concentration of the plasma is reduced and the plasma is more concentrated than the intracellular fluid within the red blood cell, the plasma is said to be hypertonic. This leads the blood cell to shrink as water is transported passively by osmosis from the blood cell into the plasma.

The serum sodium level reflects the osmolarity of the body fluids. The serum sodium concentration reflects the proportion of water and sodium in the extracellular compartments. Sodium levels are maintained at high extracellular and low intracellular levels by the sodium-potassium pump, which moves both these electrolytes across their expected concentration gradient (Ball and Bindler, 2006).

Understanding osmotic pressure is important when replacing fluids in a child who is dehydrated. All human cells have a concentration of sodium chloride 0.9%. Using this as a reference point, consideration of other sodium chloride concentrations within other solutions can be used to describe the terms below.

Isotonic fluids are normally used, for example, sodium chloride (NaCl) 0.9%. An isotonic solution is a solution that has a sodium chloride concentration equal to that within cells. The bloods plasma is equal to that (isotonic) of the red blood cell. This will provide rehydration without damaging the cells and there should be no shifting of fluids between the intra- and extra-cellular space.

Hypotonic solution is a solution with a sodium chloride concentration less than that within the cells. An example of this is distilled water which has 0% sodium chloride. This will enter the red blood cell causing it to swell and eventually rupture.

A hypertonic solution is a solution with a higher concentration of sodium chloride than that in the cells. For example, a 3% sodium chloride solution would be hypertonic to human cells and would cause water to leave the red blood cells, which would then shrivel up and die.

Exocytosis, Endocytosis and Pinocytosis

Exocytosis is an active form of cell transportation whereby the cell expels its contents by joining its vesicles within the cell to the cell membrane (Clancy and McVicar, 2009). As this requires energy it is a form of active transport. The pancreas releases glucagon by exocytosis when the blood glucose level drops. Endocytosis is the opposite, the cell wall in this case invaginates the protein from outside the cell by engulfing it.

There are three main types of endocytosis: receptor mediated endocytosis, phagocytosis and pinocytosis. If the material taken in by the cell is a particulate, then this process is called phagocytosis, for example, a bacterial cell. If the material is a liquid, it is called pinocytosis. Molecules that are transported across the cell membrane by receptor mediated endocytosis bind with specific receptors embedded within the plasma membrane. The cell then folds on itself to form an endosome (Brady, 2015) and is incorporated into the cell as a coated vesicle. The receptor then releases the molecules within the cell (Roiger, 2012).

Production of Energy

All body cells require energy to function. Energy is produced in the form of adenosine triphosphate (ATP). As the body is unable to store ATP, it is synthesised from carbohydrates.

👤 ACTIVITY

Revise the structure of the cell and describe the function of each component.

Cell Respiration

Cell respiration is the term given to the production of energy within the cell. It involves both respiratory gases, oxygen and carbon dioxide. The purpose of cell respiration is to produce ATP. Glucose is produced from the breakdown of food. This is transported into the cells by insulin, which has been produced from the beta cells in the pancreas. This glucose is potential energy and when this is broken down to CO_2 and H_2O in the presence of oxygen, the energy is released in the form of ATP and heat (Scanlon and Sanders, 2015). Each of these products have a function in the body. CO_2 is a waste product that is then carried in the blood to the lungs where it is exhaled. The water formed becomes part of the intracellular fluid. The heat that is produced has a role to play in maintaining normal body temperature and the ATP is required for cellular functions, for example, mitosis and muscle contraction. Cell respiration involves three stages:

1. Krebs cycle
2. Glycolysis
3. Cytochrome transport system

Krebs cycle. Krebs cycle occurs in the mitochondrial matrix and is concerned with glucose oxidation. It is fuelled mostly by pyruvic acid during glycolysis and by fatty acids from fat breakdown. Carbon dioxide and ATP are released via this second cycle of cell respiration, which is aerobic.

Pyruvic acid enters the mitochondria by active transport as it is a charge molecule with the assistance of protein molecules (Marieb and Hoehn, 2018). In a series of actions, these molecules are broken up and the carbons are converted into CO_2. The first CO_2 molecule is then removed by an enzyme, which contains the vitamin thiamine (Scanlon and Sanders, 2015). A two-carbon molecule called an acetyl group remains, which then combines with a molecule called a coenzyme A. This forms acetyl coenzyme A (Acetyl CoA).

Acetyl CoA is now ready to enter the Krebs cycle and is further broken down by the mitochondrial enzymes. Two more carbons are removed as CO_2 and this is then condensed with a four-carbon acid called oxaloacetic acid to produce a six-carbon citric acid. As citric acid is the first substrate of this cycle it is sometimes referred to as the citric acid cycle.

In the next steps of Krebs cycle, the atoms of citric acid are rearranged to produce intermediate molecules called keto acids. The acetic acid that enters the cycle is broken apart by carbon in a process called decarboxylation. This is then oxidised and simultaneously generates: nicotinamide adenine dinucleotide (NADH) + hydrogen (H+) and flavin adenine dinucleotide (FADH2) NADH +. Riboflavin is necessary to enable this process (Scanlon and Saunders, 2015). By the end of this cycle acetic acid is completely disposed of and oxaloacetic acid is regenerated.

The product of Krebs cycle is two CO_2 molecules and four molecules of the reduced coenzymes (three of NADH + H+ and one of FADH2). Some of the released hydrogen is attributed to the addition of water at certain parts of the cycle. There is enough energy released to synthesise one molecule of ATP (two per glucose) (Scanlon and Saunders, 2015). The four-carbon molecule oxaloacetic acid is regenerated after the formation of CO_2. This then reacts with the next acetyl

TABLE 10.3 **Cell Respiration Summary**

Location	Molecules Involved in Process	Outcome of Process	Required Minerals and Vitamins
Krebs cycle Mitochondria Aerobic process	Glucose/glycerol or excess amino acids form pyruvic acid Acetyl CoA from fatty acids or excess amino acids	ATP 3 NADH2 and 1 FADH2 molecules to carry hydrogen to cytochrome transport system CO_2	Thiamine Niacin Riboflavin
Glycolysis (cytoplasm)	Glucose – ATP	2 ATP 2NADH2 2 Pyruvic acid-aerobic Lactic acid-anaerobic	Niacin
Cytochrome transport system Mitochondria Aerobic	NADH2 and FADH2 from glycolysis and/or Krebs cycle	ATP Metabolic water	Iron Copper

Acetyl CoA, Acetyl coenzyme A; *ATP,* adenosine triphosphate; *FADH2,* flavin adenine dinucleotide; *NADH2,* .

coenzyme A to continue this self-perpetuating cycle. The waste products of Krebs cycle are excreted from the body as water and carbon dioxide.

Although this pathway is concerned with carbohydrate oxidation, breakdown products of carbohydrates, fats and protein may also feed into Krebs cycle and be oxidised for energy.

At times of illness, the demand for energy is increased. If the body is not able to provide sufficient energy, an imbalance will occur. To conserve energy the body will respond by reducing its function to core functions, hence why vasoconstriction occurs.

Glycolysis. Glycolysis is an anaerobic process occurring in the cytoplasm of the cell. A six-carbon glucose molecule is broken down into two three-carbon molecules of pyruvic acid. This requires two molecules of ATP to initiate this process. The energy required to commence this process is called the energy of activation (Scanlon and Sanders, 2015). This is enough to make the glucose molecule unstable, hence why it breaks down. As a result of this action four molecules of ATP are released. Two pairs of hydrogen are removed by nicotinamide adenine dinucleotide (NAD), which is a carrier molecule that contains the vitamin niacin. These two become 2NADH2 and are transported to the cytochrome system.

When exercising, if there is no oxygen present in the muscle cell, pyruvic acid is converted to lactic acid and this leads to muscle fatigue. If oxygen is present, the pyruvic acid continues into the next Krebs cycle.

Cytochrome transport system. This is also known as the electron transport chain. Unlike glycolysis and Krebs cycle who do not use oxygen directly, the cytochrome transport system performs the final catabolic reactions in the mitochondrial cristae (Marieb and Hoehn, 2018). Krebs cycle produces substrate from reduced coenzymes for the cytochrome transport system so these pathways are coupled and are considered to be aerobic.

Most of the components in the cytochrome transport system are proteins that are bound to metal atoms. Some are flavins, which are derived from riboflavin; others contain sulphur. The highly coloured cytochromes contain either iron or copper. The hydrogen pair are brought to the cytochromes by NAD and FAD (flavin adenine dinucleotide). It is then split into its proton and its electron. These are passed from one cytochrome to the next and eventually to oxygen. As the hydrogen ions accumulate, they create a concentration gradient. They flow to an area of less concentration through an enzyme called ATP synthase (Scanlon and Saunders, 2015). This releases enough energy to synthesise 25 molecules of ATP.

The final phase in this system is the formation of water. Each oxygen atom will have gained two electrons and they react with two of the H+ ions to form water. This metabolic water contributes to the intracellular water and prevents acidosis. If the H+ ions did not react with oxygen to form water they would accumulate and decrease the pH of the cell.

The relationship between eating and breathing is fundamental in understanding the concepts of cell respiration. They are co-dependent. Energy from food can only be released if we are breathing.

A summary of cell respiration is presented in Table 10.3.

Gastrointestinal System

The fluid in the body is in a dynamic state, it continually enters and leaves. It enters via food and fluids and leaves via the skin, urine, faeces and during respiration. In the absence of water, chemical reactions, metabolic processes and regulatory systems become severely compromised and eventually cease to function (Tortora and Derrickson, 2009). A healthy adult can survive for around 10 days without water; a healthy child will survive only 3–4 days without water.

Fluid is stored in several compartments. The major fluid compartments contain:

- the intracellular (ICF) fluid; fluid inside the cell;
- the extracellular fluid (ECF) fluid outside of the cells. Extracellular fluid consists of intravascular and interstitial fluids. Intravascular fluid is the fluid with the blood vessels. Interstitial fluid is the fluid between the cells, outside of the blood and the lymphatic system;
- transcellular fluid.

The percentage of body weight that is composed of fluid varies with age (Table 10.4). The ICF and ECF fluid percentages also fluctuate with age.

TABLE 10.4 Percentage of Body Water From Birth to Adulthood

Age	% Body Water	Extracellular Fluid	Intracellular Fluid
Newborn	80	45%	30%
Infant	75	25%	30%–40%
Child	60	10%–15%	40%
Young person	50		

Intracellular Fluid

Intracellular fluid comprises the body water that exists inside the tissue cells that make up the child's body, and accounts for 35%–40% of the total body water. The intracellular fluid is contained within the cell. It is largely controlled by the cell because there is selective uptake and the discharge mechanisms present in the cell membrane (Waugh and Grant, 2018). The composition of the ICF is different from the ECF. For example, sodium levels are 10 times higher in ECF than ICF. This occurs from the selective action of the sodium/potassium pump that maintains levels across the concentration gradient. As water can pass freely in and out of the cell membrane any change in the concentration of the ECF will have an immediate effect on the intracellular water level. The infant has a high daily fluid requirement and has little in reserve in their intracellular compartment (Lissauer and Clayden, 2012). This makes them vulnerable to dehydration.

Extracellular Fluid

Extracellular fluid (ECF) accounts for 20%–45% of the total body weight in children and is further subdivided:
- plasma-water in the blood vessels
- lymph-water in the lymphatic vessels
- specialised fluids – cerebrospinal fluid (CSF), synovial fluid, aqueous humor
- tissue fluids
  It may be further subdivided into:
- intravascular fluid compartment – inside blood vessels
- interstitial fluid – in-between tissue cells

Neonates and children have a higher proportion of ECF than adults as their brains and skin are both rich in interstitial fluid. Extracellular fluid is fundamental to the regulation and balance of body fluids and electrolytes because it is the changes in this compartment that act as a trigger for the activation of regulatory systems in the quest to maintain homeostasis. As every cell in the body is in contact with ECF and directly dependent on its composition for its own survival, very slight changes will have an impact and the potential for permanent damage (Waugh and Grant, 2018). For example, a decrease in plasma calcium level will affect the intercalated discs in the cardiac muscle thus impacting on the ability of the heart to pump effectively.

When fluid status is compromised extracellular fluid deficit-dehydration occurs. The situations that most often cause loss of fluid are:

TABLE 10.5 Signs of Dehydration in the Infant/Child

Clinical Sign	Moderate Dehydration	Severe Dehydration
Body weight	5%–10%	>10%
Appearance	Drowsy, complaining of thirst	Drowsy, limp, cold, clammy, cool peripheries
Respiratory rate	May be increased and deep	Increased and deep
Capillary refill time	Prolonged >2 seconds	Prolonged >2 seconds
Radial pulse	Rapid and weak	Rapid, thread, possibly not palpable
Mucous membranes	Dry	Very dry
Eyes	Sunken	Very sunken
Skin turgor	Slow to react	Very slow to react
Urine output	Reduced	Oliguric
Anterior fontanelle	Sunken	Very sunken

- gastroenteritis
- infections: septicaemia, meningitis, respiratory
- metabolic disorders
- food intolerance
- burns
- haemorrhage
- renal disease
- pyrexia
- radiant heat loss, e.g. phototherapy
- excessive drainage from drainage tubes

The disorders listed above will be covered in more detail in the relevant section of this textbook. An outline of the three major types of dehydration will be discussed and their management outlined in Table 10.5.

The three types of dehydration are:
- isotonic/isonatraemic dehydration
- hypotonic/hyponatraemic dehydration
- hypertonic/hypernatraemic dehydration

Isotonic/isonatraemic dehydration. This type of dehydration is commonly seen in young children with gastroenteritis. Fluid loss is greater than fluid intake hence the imbalance. Sodium loss is proportionate to water loss. Therefore the serum sodium is within normal limits even if the circulating blood volume is lower.

Management. In the majority of these cases, oral rehydration will be the preferred treatment as dehydration will be mild, <5% loss of body weight. Feeds can be substituted with glucose-electrolyte solution. The glucose in these solutions enhances sodium and water absorption. The solution should be administered until vomiting and diarrhoea has subsided. There is no need to reintroduce a normal diet gradually (Lissauer and Clayden, 2012).

Hypotonic/hyponatraemic dehydration. Hyponatraemic dehydration occurs when sodium losses are greater than the loss of water, and the plasma sodium decreases. Water shifts from the extra to the intracellular compartments. The increase in intracellular volume will lead to an increase in cerebral volume. With acute hyponatraemia, the cells most vulnerable to osmotic fluid shift into their intracellular compartment are brain cells. Ultimately, cytotoxic cerebral oedema, with its associated raised intracranial pressure (ICP), occurs. Cerebral function is altered, and this is reflected in an abnormal score on the Glasgow Coma Scale. Unrelieved, cerebral neuropathy resulting from the increased ICP can cause seizures, coma and death. Careful monitoring of serum sodium levels in children is essential (Au et al., 2008). Normal serum values are presented in Table 10.6. This type of dehydration can occur due to iatrogenic causes (treatment related), burns or renal disease.

Hypertonic/hypernatraemic dehydration. The loss of sodium is proportionally greater than water loss. This occurs from a high insensible water loss (pyrexia, environmental heat, profuse diarrhoea). The extracellular fluid becomes hypertonic with respect to the intracellular fluid and water shifts into the extracellular space from the intracellular space to compensate. The extracellular component remains normal initially, thus delaying the obvious signs of dehydration: sunken eyes, depressed fontanelle, tissue elasticity. The risk of this type of dehydration is the fact that water is drawn out of the brain. This can lead to cerebral shrinkage, microhaemorrhages and convulsions (Lissauer and Clayden, 2012). Hyperglycaemia may be present but is normally transient.

The signs of dehydration will be depended on the degree of dehydration. Table 10.6 provides an outline of the clinical signs of dehydration.

Management of dehydration. The management will depend on the percentage of dehydration, degree of shock present and the underlying cause. An overview is provided in Table 10.7. If maintenance fluids are required then these will be calculated according to the weight of the child (Table 10.8).

> **ACTIVITY**
>
> With reference to the descriptions of dehydration, explain why a dehydrated child might manifest abnormal physical features of the skin and mucous membranes.

> **ACTIVITY**
>
> Calculate the maintenance fluids required for a 26-kg child for a 24-hour period.

Amino Acid Metabolism

In addition to normal fluid balance for maintaining homeostasis, amino acid metabolism is a prerequisite for normal growth and development. Amino acids are subunits of protein and are made up of elements of carbon, hydrogen, oxygen and nitrogen (Scanlon and Sanders, 2015). There are approximately 20 amino acids that are necessary to make human protein. The majority of these are obtained from our diet. Children require eight essential amino acids and the neonate requires three additional amino acids (Table 10.9).

Amino acids are used for growth, repair, and are synthesised into plasma protein, enzymes, antibodies or hormones to produce energy via Krebs cycle and the cytochrome transport chain.

If our diet contains more amino acids than it requires, these will be converted into simple carbohydrates by glucogenesis and fat by lipogenesis and stored as a potential source of energy if required. Nitrogenous elements are excreted via the kidneys (Marieb and Hoehn, 2018).

Proteins are made from amino acids that join together and these protein chains vary in size from a few to many thousand. They may appear as single strands to complex

TABLE 10.6	Clinical Chemistry reference values for neonates, children and young people				
Electrolytes	**Range**	**Neonate**	**< 1 year**	**Child**	**Young person**
Sodium	133–146 mmol/L				
Potassium	3.5–505 mmol/L				
Chloride	95–106 mmol/L				
Bicarbonate	19–28 mmol/L				
Urea			0.8–5.5 mmol/L	2.5–6.5 mmol/L	
Creatinine		21–75 µmol/L	13–39 µmol/L (1 month to 4 years of age)	29–53 µmol/L	40–90 µmol/L
Calcium			< 4 weeks 2.0–2.7 mmol/L	>4 weeks upwards 2.2–2.7 mmol/L	
Magnesium	0.6–1.0 mmol/L				
Phosphate			1.3–2.6 mmol/L	0.9–1.8 mmol/L	
Glucose		2.5–5.5 mmol/L		3.0–6.0 mmol/L	
Glycated haemoglobin (HBA₁C)	20–42 mmol/L 4–6%				

Adapted from Royal College of Paediatrics and Child Health 2016 reference ranges.

TABLE 10.7 Types of Dehydration and Outline Management

Level of Dehydration	Clinical Indicators	Signs of Dehydration	Management
Mild dehydration	<5% body weight loss	Not overtly evident	Oral rehydration solution (NICE, 2009).
Moderate dehydration	<5%–10% body weight loss	Clinical signs of dehydration present	Oral/NG rehydration trial for 6 hours. If not successful, then intravenous rehydration is required. This will include fluids to replace the % dehydration and maintenance fluids. For maintenance fluids see Table 10.8. Monitor plasma sodium and potassium levels. Assess condition as per PEWS score. Weigh child.
Severe dehydration	>10% weight loss	Signs of hypovolaemic shock present	Immediate resuscitation. Intravenous administration of NaCl 0.9% initially. Replace fluid deficit with 0.45% NaCl and 2.5% dextrose (Lissauer and Clayden, 2012). Maintenance fluids. Replace electrolytes. Monitor plasma sodium and potassium levels. Strict fluid balance. Close observation as indicated by PEWS score/GCS. Weigh child.

TABLE 10.8 Maintenance Fluid Requirements for Intravenous Administrations

Body Weight	Fluid (mL/kg/24 h)	Sodium (mmol/kg/24 h)	Potassium (mmol/kg/24 h)
First 10 kg	100	2–4	1.5–2.5
Second 10 kg	50	1–2	0.5–1.5
Subsequent kg	20	0.5–1	0.2–0.7

TABLE 10.9 Essential Amino Acids for Newborns and Children

Essential Amino Acids in Childhood	Essential Amino Acids for Newborn Infants
Isoleucine	Cysteine
Leucine	Histidine
Lysine	Tyrosine
Methionine	Plus
Phenylalanine	
Threonine	
Tryptophan	
Valine	

multi-dimensional structures incorporating other molecules, for example, haemoglobin. Protein synthesis occurs in the ribosome of the majority of cells. This is controlled by deoxyribonucleic acid (DNA) and ribonucleic acid (RNA). Some proteins require trace elements to function normally, for example, iron and zinc. The impact of changes in pH can be very significant. The hydrogen ions disrupt the internal stabilising forces, and changes the shape of the protein leaving it unable to function (Waugh and Grant, 2018). Likewise, the impact of body temperature may be profound to enzyme activity. When body temperature is less than 37° C activity is reduced, and when above 37° C activity is initially increased, then reduces significantly, altering the shape of the protein (Brady, 2015).

Glucose is converted by the process of glycogenesis and is then stored in the liver and muscles. After eating, the serum glucose level rises and if this was to remain high it would be excreted in the urine via the kidneys. Glycogenesis requires insulin. The pancreatic beta cells secrete insulin and this stimulates the hepatocytes and the skeletal muscle cells to synthesise glycogen (Scanlon and Sanders, 2015). Glycogen is broken down into glucose when energy is required. This is oxidised during cellular respiration to produce ATP. Epinephrine (adrenal glands) and glucagon (alpha cells of the pancreas) control this process.

The skeletal muscle releases energy from glucose that has been catabolised via glycolysis and from Krebs cycle (Marieb and Hoehn, 2018).

Respiratory System and Acid Base Balance

Respiration in the child occurs via the respiratory system and gas is exchanged in the alveoli via the process of diffusion. There are important differences in the anatomy and physiology of the respiratory system of infants, children and young people. Table 10.10 provides an outline of the anatomical differences.

Respiration is controlled by the apneustic and the pneumotaxic centre in the medulla oblongata. The level of CO_2 is the stimulus to breathing. Chemoreceptors located in the carotid and aortic bodies, and in the medulla itself, detect changes in the blood gas and pH levels. Sensory impulses travel along the glossopharyngeal and vagus nerves to the medulla and an increase in respiratory rate is the initiated response (Gormley-Fleming and Peate, 2015;

TABLE 10.10	**Anatomical Differences Between Infant/Child/Young Person's Airway**
Airway	**Breathing**
Large head, short neck, inability to support head.	Infants rely mainly on diaphragmatic breathing, ribs lie more horizontal and contribute less to chest expansion.
Large tongue.	
Floor of mouth easily compressible.	Muscles are more likely to fatigue than adults type 2 muscle fibres.
Infants <6–8 months are obligatory nasal breathers.	
Smaller airway diameter.	Sternum and ribs are cartilaginous.
Epiglottitis is horseshoe shaped, projects posteriorly – 45-degree angle.	Chest wall is soft and the intercostal muscles are poorly developed.
Larynx is high and anterior.	Increased metabolic rate, increased respiratory demand for oxygen and carbon dioxide elimination.
Trachea is short and soft.	
Cricoid is the narrowest portion of the neck.	Lung compliance and high chest wall compliance in neonate.
Cricoid ring is lined by pseudostratified ciliated epithelium loosely bound to areolar tissue.	Small amount of elastic and collagen tissue in child's lung.

Scanlon and Sanders, 2015). The child will bring more air into the lungs and this will diffuse into the blood via the alveoli to correct the hypoxic state.

Oxygen is the major stimulus for respiration in the neonate, in certain cardiac conditions and chronic respiratory disease. Although this is not common in children and young people it must be a consideration when assessing respiratory status and administering oxygen therapy.

If there is decreased oxygen and carbon dioxide exchange in the lungs, the pH will decrease. This is caused by an accumulation of CO_2. This is corrected by the kidneys, but the blood oxygen level will continue to decrease. The oxygen level will eventually fall so low that it provides the stimulus to increase both the rate and depth of respirations.

The mechanical or nervous control of breathing is located in the medulla and pons in the brain stem. Inspiration and expiration control centres are located here. The inspiration centre generates impulses, which travel along nerves to the respiratory muscles. This is an automated response. The respiratory muscles contract and inhalation occurs. As the lungs inflate the baroreceptors in the lung tissue note this stretching and the sensory impulses are sent to the medulla and this results in the depression to the respiratory centre. This action prevents overinflation of the lungs. There is a decrease in the impulses sent to the respiratory muscles and this brings about exhalation, which is under the control of the pneumotaxic centre. This cycle continues. Infants have a higher metabolic rate and therefore greater demand for oxygen, which is the main reason for their increased respiratory rates. Thus oxygen levels are more significant in infants and children and they decompensate quickly if oxygen levels are not stabilised. As children age, the mechanisms of breathing change (Gormley-Fleming, 2010).

The interruption of any of these stages will lead to a reduction in circulating oxygen.

Peripheral chemoreceptors located in the carotid sinus and the aortic arch also detect the rising CO_2 level, hydrogen ions and decreased O_2 levels (Watson and Fawcett, 2003). This too increases respiratory rate in an attempt to remove excess CO_2.

Oxygen is dissolved in the blood plasma (Po_2 value). This is 1.5% (Scanlon and Sanders, 2015) of the total. The remaining amount, 98.5% is transported around the body attached to the haemoglobin in the red blood cell – Sao_2. This oxygen-haemoglobin bond is formed in the lungs as the Po_2 is high. As this bond is relatively weak, it breaks on entering the tissues and oxygen is released. The lower the oxygen concentration in the tissues the more oxygen the haemoglobin will release. Active tissues receive as much oxygen as possible to continue cell respiration. The amount of oxygen released from haemoglobin is also dependent on the body temperature and a high level of PCo_2.

If the SAo_2 is high this indicates that the Po_2 is high and conversely if the Po_2 decreases, then the SAo_2 also decreases (Brady, 2015). Normal oxygen saturation for a child is 95%–99% (Gormley-Fleming, 2010). Caution is required when determining the acceptable level for a neonate due to their sensitivity to hyperoxia leading to the potential development of retinopathy of prematurity (Rudolph et al., 2011).

Acid Base Balance

The relative concentration of hydrogen ions in the body is measured in concentration units called pH units. The acidity of blood is measured by pH. This is the H+ concentration in the blood. As this is a negative logarithm the higher the H+ concentration, the lower the pH and vice versa (Gormley-Fleming, 2013). The normal values are presented in Table 10.11.

The cells and fluids within the body all have a pH close to neutral.

As already identified, respiration affects the pH of the body fluids because it regulates the amount of CO_2 in these fluids. Excess carbon dioxide lowers the blood pH when it reacts with water to form carbonic acid. This ionises into H+ ions and HCO_3 ions.

The more H+ ions present in the blood the lower the pH and the fewer H+ ions the higher the pH (Scanlon and Sanders, 2015). Any change to the pH can have catastrophic implications. CO_2 is considered an acid gas because of its reaction with water to form carbonic acid (Blows, 2012). Carbonic acid can liberate H+. For this reason alone, any CO_2 retention will create respiratory acidosis. The main causes of respiratory acidosis in the infant and child occurs as a result of respiratory failure due to illness or any other cause, for example, asthma, inadequate mechanical ventilation, CNS depression.

TABLE 10.11	Blood Gas Values (Arterial) for Neonates/Children and Young People		
	Neonate	**Child**	**Young Person**
pH	7.31–7.47	7.35–7.42	7.35–7.45
Po$_2$	4.3–8.1 kPa	11–14 kPa	10.6–13.3 kPa; 79.5–99.8 mmHg
PCo$_2$	3.8–6.5 kPa	4.0–5.5 kPa	4.7–6.0 kPa; 35.3–45 mmHg
HCO$_3$	15–25 mmol/L	17–27 mmol/L	22–28 mmol/L

Adapted from Peate I., Gormley-Fleming, E., 2015. Fundamentals of Children's Anatomy and Physiology: A Textbook for Nursing and Healthcare Students. Wiley-Blackwell, Oxford.

Respiratory alkalosis occurs when the respiratory rate increases, and the CO$_2$ is exhaled very rapidly. This results in decreased H+ ion formation and increases the pH. Respiratory acidosis occurs as a result of hyperventilation; an infant with prolonged crying has the potential to become alkalotic.

 ACTIVITY

> Consider which of the respiratory gases is the more important as the regulator of respiration, and why.

Base Excess

A positive base excess is indicative of metabolic alkalosis and a negative base excess indicates metabolic acidosis. A negative base excess is usually only treated when it is less than 6 mmol/L and the pH is also low. In the presence of acute respiratory acidosis, the bicarbonate may initially be normal, but subsequently rise in an attempt to compensate and normalise the pH.

If pH and PaCo$_2$ are indeed moving in opposite directions, then the problem is primarily respiratory in nature.

If the pH and HCo$_3$ are moving in the same direction, then the problem is primarily metabolic in nature.

The arterial Pao$_2$ normal range is 11–14 kPa (8–10 kPa in neonates). A high reading will likely be an indicator of respiratory alkalosis and a low reading respiratory acidosis.

The following terms need to be understood in order to interpret blood gases:

- **pH (potential hydrogen)**: the pH determines the acidity or alkalinity of the blood
- **Po$_2$**: partial pressure of oxygen dissolved in plasma
- **PaCo$_2$**: this relates to the partial pressure of carbon dioxide (CO$_2$) dissolved in plasma. This is the respiratory component of the blood gas
- **HCO$_3$**: bicarbonate is also known as a 'base' and is present in blood within range of 22–28 mmol/L. This is the renal component of the blood gas

Thermoregulation

Thermoregulation is an important aspect of homeostasis. Controlled by the preoptic area in the anterior and posterior parts of the hypothalamus, thermoregulation is a negative feedback mechanism. The anterior hypothalamus response to an increase in temperature and conversely the posterior hypothalamus is stimulated when there is a decrease in temperature.

Excess heat is lost through the skin by convection, conduction, radiation and evaporation.

Humans maintain their core temperature within narrow parameters and the metabolic rate of the human body decreases with age. The temperature of the fetus is higher than that of its mother as it has a higher metabolic rate. The fetus passes the heat energy to its mother through the placental interface and the amniotic fluid (Power, 1989). As soon as the baby is born it is essential that it generate heat to deal with the hostile environment it has been born into, where the ambient temperature is lower that the in utero temperature. Heat generation is essential for survival as the newborn needs to compensate for this loss of energy. Cold stress is the term used to describe the infant's response to cold and this has serious physiological implications if left untreated.

Heat generation in the newborn infant occurs through shivering and non-shivering thermogenesis. The shivering response of the newborn is immature, as the musculature system is also immature, thus it is unable to achieve the desired response (Gormley-Fleming, 2015). Hence it is essential to dry the baby at birth and maintain a thermoneutral environment.

Non-shivering thermogenesis enables heat to be generated due to the presence of brown fat. Brown fat has a plentiful supply of mitochondria, glycogen stores, fat vacuoles, blood and a well-developed sympathetic nerve system (Asakura, 2004; Tucker & Blackburn, 2013). Brown fat starts to appear at 29 weeks gestation making the premature infant very vulnerable to heat loss.

In the presence of cold, there is an increase in noradrenaline, and this acts on brown fat causing lipolysis. As a result of this, the brown fat converts into free fatty acids. This produces heat and in turn increases the core temperature due to the rich blood supply of brown fat. Brown fat increases the basal metabolic rate and the heat that has been generated is rapidly transported around the body. This process of thermogenesis requires energy and is demanding on oxygen and glucose. This can lead to hypoglycaemia and metabolic acidosis.

A newborn has significantly more sweat glands than an adult. The newborn does not have the same ability to sweat so is unable to maintain its core temperature by this mechanism as the eccrine glands are immature. The ability to sweat does not occur until the baby is at least 3 weeks old. Therefore heat cannot be lost through this mechanism.

All newborns have the ability to lose water through the transcutaneous route. The more premature the infant the greater the insensible water loss is through their skin. This increases the potential for temperature loss as the evaporation of water requires energy. Infants are unable to constrict their surface blood vessels, unlike older children, so cannot conserve heat in this manner. In the older child, the receptors in the skin can detect the change in ambient temperature. Heat loss and heat production messages can be sent to and received by the hypothalamus via the automatic nervous system.

As the infant matures the neural network in the skin provides an accurate measure of the ambient temperature. This is done by the activation of the heat receptor in the dermis, which then passes a signal along the sensory nerve pathway to the hypothalamus (Gormley-Fleming, 2015). This will then either initiate the shivering reflex or deactivate the sweating mechanism.

Shivering requires energy as the muscles contract approximately 10–20 times per second (Cedar, 2012). Conversely, when the child exercises muscle activity generates heat and the metabolic rate is increased. This may lead to sweating as a means of heat loss via evaporation. An acclimatised adult will lose up to 10–12 litres of water per day. This is less for a child. Solute is also lost in sweat with sodium being the main electrolyte followed by potassium, magnesium and calcium.

In the presence of infection, the immune system releases endogenous pyrogens. The autonomic nervous system is activated via the hypothalamus and an increase in body temperature occurs. The increasing body temperature in the presence of infection will impede bacterial growth (Cedar, 2012).

The thermoregulatory function in children is immature until the age of 5 years approximately, as the autonomic nervous system is then mature (Neill and Knowles, 2004). Because children have a large body surface area, they are at an increased risk of hypothermia and this risk decreases with age. Thermoregulation is important in maintaining homeostasis and an understanding of this is essential for the children's and young person's nurse.

Endocrine System

There are a number of key areas in the endocrine system, which have a significant impact on homeostasis and it is not possible to cover all in detail within this text. The areas that will be covered are:

- control of glucose
- fluid control

Control of Glucose

This is maintained by the hormones glucagon and insulin. Both are produced by the pancreas. There is a very narrow parameter of glucose level in the maintenance of good health (4–6 mmol/L).

Glucagon. Produced by the alpha cells in the pancreas, glucagon stimulates the liver by acting on the enzyme phosphorylase to convert glycogen to glucose. This is known as glycogenesis. The use of fats and excess amino acids for energy is also triggered by this process. The overall effect of glucagon is to raise the blood glucose level making all food types available as sources of energy. In order to trigger the stimulation of glucagon, hypoglycaemia must occur. This can result from exercise, stress or delaying meals. The release of cortisol and epinephrine from the adrenal glands have a similar action to glucagon and can also trigger the release of glucose from glucagon (Clancy and McVicar, 2009).

Insulin. Insulin increases the transport of glucose from the blood into cells by increasing the permeability of the cell membrane to glucose (Scanlon and Sanders, 2015). Produced by the beta cells in the islets of Langerhans, insulin is secreted when blood glucose levels rise. Insulin is also required for the metabolism of other food types, the synthesis of lipids and protein. The serum level of lipids will rise and accumulate as excess fatty acid if insulin is not present. As a vital hormone, insulin is essential to sustain life.

In the event of the body failing to produce sufficient amounts of insulin, fats and proteins will be converted into glucose and this will result in the production of ketones leading to ketoacidosis. The serum glucose level increases and will spill into the urine (glycosuria) as the renal threshold is exceeded. Glycosuria leads to water loss via the urine from its hyperosmolar effect. The resulting impact of this will be an increased thirst. Weight loss occurs from the breakdown of protein and fats as energy sources. These are classic signs of type 1 diabetes mellitus.

Diabetic ketoacidosis (DKA) manifests as metabolic acidosis due to the presence of ketone acid, glycosuria and electrolyte imbalance (Lissauer and Clayden, 2012). Whether it results from infection or non-compliance with treatment, DKA may be life-threatening. Ketones are organic acids (acetone and acetoacetic acid), which can be used in cell respiration, but not by all cells. Hence, they accumulate in the blood and lower the pH of the blood. The kidneys excrete ketones, but also excrete more water leading to further dehydration and increasing acidosis. If insulin is not administered along with intravenous fluids and electrolytes, ketoacidosis may progress to coma and death. The care of a child with DKA is discussed in Chapter 20. Caring for a child with diabetes and endocrine disorders.

Fluid Control

Vomiting can lead to a loss of gastric acid and diarrhoea leads to a loss of mucous, which is also alkaline. Both can lead to alkalosis in the young child. Electrolytes and water is also lost. The osmoreceptors in the hypothalamus detect the rising osmolarity of the blood.

As part of the compensatory mechanism, urine output is depressed by the actions of anti-diuretic hormones (ADH) angiotensin and aldosterone.

The composition of the urine is altered here as sodium and water are reabsorbed. This will determine the volume of urine formed and its osmolality. The amount of water reabsorbed is influenced by ADH, whereas the amount of sodium reabsorbed is controlled by aldosterone. There is a resistance to aldosterone in the distal convoluted tubules and this continues until the nephron matures. The child will attempt to self-regulate as their thirst will be increased, but a young baby will not be able to do so.

A fundamental aspect of the role of the children's nurse is to correctly assess the state of hydration of their patients.

Renal System

Homeostasis of the body fluids and serum chemistry is the key role of the kidneys. In order to achieve this, accurate development and formation of the renal system is required.

The renal system matures during childhood and interruption at any stage of this process can lead to homeostatic imbalance impacting on the well-being of the child and young person.

This is achieved by:

- filtration of the blood
- tubular reabsorption
- secretion of waste

For the purposes of this chapter only the hormones concerned with regulation of homeostasis will be discussed. These are:

- atrial natriuretic peptide
- aldosterone
- angiotensin
- ADH

Atrial Natriuretic Peptide

Atrial natriuretic peptide (ANP) is a powerful vasodilator and a polypeptide protein. This hormone is secreted by the myocytes in the cardiac muscle in response to increasing blood volume, which has stretched the walls of the atria or by increasing blood pressure (Marieb and Hoehn, 2018; Scanlon and Sanders, 2015). The subsequent impact of this fluid increase is an increase in blood pressure. ANP has a diuretic effect and a natriuretic effect (salt excreting). It inhibits the ability of the collecting ducts to reabsorb sodium ions, therefore more sodium is excreted in the urine and this also leads to more water being excreted. The loss of water reduces the blood pressure and blood volume. ANP is an antagonist to the hormone aldosterone. ANP stimulates the smooth muscle of the blood vessels, which stimulates vasodilation furthering the reduction in blood pressure. This occurs from the direct and indirect action of ANP in this case as it inhibits renin induced generation of angiotensin II (Marieb and Hoehn, 2018).

If the circulating fluid volume is reduced due to haemorrhage or gastrointestinal losses, the amount of blood that is returned to the heart is reduced, so there is less pressure exerted on the walls of the atria and this is felt by the baroreceptors. Cardiac output is also reduced, blood pressure is reduced slightly and this subsequently reduces the blood volume returned to the heart. The heart rate will increase initially in an attempt to compensate and increase the circulation. Respiratory rate will also increase in an attempt to improve the amount of oxygen in the circulation (Waugh and Grant, 2018). There is a fluid shift from the interstitial space to the intravascular compartment and further vasoconstriction occurs. At this point the child will still be exhibiting normal vital signs as they can compensate up to 20%–25% loss of circulating volume before signs of shock become evident (Elliot et al., 2010). Urinary output will be reduced, and capillary refill time will be increased (Advanced Paediatric Life Support [APLS], 2016). The pulse pressure will also begin to reduce. Failure to recognise these often-subtle changes will lead to further decompensation and ultimately cell death.

Aldosterone

This hormone is the most influential in the renal regulation of the sodium ions. Produced in the adrenal cortex of the adrenal gland aldosterone is the main mineralocorticoid. The trigger to releasing aldosterone is the renin-angiotensin mechanism. Elevated levels of potassium in ECF will also stimulate the adrenal cortex to release aldosterone (Marieb and Hoehn, 2018). Through a negative feedback mechanism, aldosterone stimulates the reabsorption of Na+ by the renal tubules and the excretion of potassium in the urine. When aldosterone concentration is high, all the remaining filtered Na+ will be actively reabsorbed in the distal convoluted tubules and collecting ducts. Consistent with its central role in maintaining blood pressure and blood volume, water will always follow Na+. This water comes from the intracellular. Aldosterone increases the extracellular fluid volume. If aldosterone release is inhibited, the amount of Na+ that is reabsorbed is virtually nothing. If large amounts of Na+ are excreted in the urine it follows that the volume of water will also be large. The reverse is not true, as in order to maintain water balance, the urine excreted can leave a very low Na+ (Blows, 2010; Scanlon and Sanders, 2015).

Angiotensin

ACTIVITY

Consider a child with the diagnosis of Addison's disease. What advice would you give them and their family in relation to eating and drinking?

Angiotensin stimulates the adrenal cortex to release aldosterone. If the blood flow to the renal system is reduced or if the serum Na+ level decreases, the kidneys secrete renin. Renin converts the plasma protein angiotensinogen, which has been produced by the liver to angiotensin I. Angiotensin-converting enzyme (ACE), mainly from the lungs, converts angiotensin I to angiotensin II (Waugh and Grant, 2018). Angiotensin II results in vasoconstriction and the net result of this is an increase in blood pressure.

Antidiuretic Hormone

ADH is a hormone that is produced in the hypothalamus. Also known as vasopressin, it increases the reabsorption of water in the distal convoluted tubules, which decreases the amount of urine formed. The water is reabsorbed in the distal part of the convoluted tubule and collecting ducts of the nephron as the permeability of the cells is increased. As the water is reabsorbed into the blood, the urine output is reduced and the blood volume is increased thus maintaining blood pressure (Neill and Knowles, 2004). The stimulus for secreting ADH is a decreased water content in the body. The osmoreceptors in the hypothalamus detect the increase in sodium, sends impulses to the posterior pituitary to increase ADH production and decrease the amount of water that is excreted as urine (Scanlon and Sanders, 2015). In the case of fluid loss from the body or haemorrhage, ADH will be released in large amounts leading to vasoconstriction of the arterioles, which will lead to an increase in blood pressure.

ACTIVITY

After studying this section, you should be able to diagrammatically present the negative feedback system for the hormones that regulate the water content in the body.

To conclude this section, homeostasis is very complicated and involves all body systems. Nutrition and fluid intake are the foundation to maintaining a homeostatic balance. Each body system must work within its own boundary and yet sustain its interrelationship with other systems in order to maintain normal function. The next section will consider the deteriorating child.

RECOGNITION AND CARE OF THE DETERIORATING CHILD

Recognition of the deteriorating child is an essential skill for nurses (Large and Aldridge, 2018). Detecting deteriorating patients, ensuring patient safety, and initiating interventions are key aspects of quality care and it is vital that the multidisciplinary team understand and manage the needs of the deteriorating patient effectively, in addition to appreciating potential barriers to care delivery and the effects these barriers can have (Royal College of Nursing [RCN], 2017). The role of the children and young people's nurse regarding the assessment and recognition of the deteriorating child and the subsequent care required is well-known, and the relationship between effective assessment and timely interventions to improve outcomes has been harnessed historically in the formulation of early warning scores, the analysis and review of emergency situations, and the audit of patient outcomes to support and detect the deteriorating child (Chapman, 2013). Reviewing episodes of patient care and developing strategies from these episodes enables the multi-disciplinary team to avoid future detrimental situations, improve patient care and address any issues with escalation and intervention, as well as enhancing team communication (Gluyas, 2017).

Assessment of the Patient

Recognising deterioration begins with performing an effective assessment of the patient. It is known that a structured assessment process is effective in giving health care staff significant information on the patient's status and to highlight areas of concern in the patient's condition (RCN, 2017). When changes in the patient's condition indicate potential or apparent deterioration, holistic assessment of the patient, followed by effective communication and escalation to the multi-disciplinary team and also the instigation of clinical interventions will aid in the prevention of further deterioration (Gill et al., 2016; McKay et al., 2013).

The monitoring of vital signs (temperature, blood pressure, pulse rate, respirations, capillary refill time, oxygen saturations) is crucial for monitoring a patient's condition (McKay et al., 2013). Even subtle changes in a patient's vital signs can indicate deterioration and it is proven that changes in a patient's clinical status can be observed hours prior to clinical deterioration (Gill et al., 2016). Performing vital signs as part of the patient's assessment is an effective way of detecting signs of deterioration, and

also measuring the effectiveness of clinical interventions that are instigated when deterioration is detected (RCN, 2017). The frequency that vital signs will be measured is proportional to the clinical diagnosis and clinical status and it is essential that nurses are aware of their patient's clinical vulnerability and the risk each patient has of deterioration (RCN, 2017).

To aid nurses and the multi-disciplinary team in the assessment of the sick child or young person, early warning scores or trigger tools have been formulated to allow health care staff to detect deterioration and allow staff to escalate patients' clinical status more effectively (Smith and Bowden, 2017). Areas of risk relating to patient deterioration are considered to be: 'family concerns; high-risk therapies; elevated early warning scores; communication concerns and clinician concerns' (Brady et al., 2013). The role of early warning systems is to assist in the detection of patient deterioration as well as taking into account parental and clinician concerns (Roland, 2017). The tools use vital signs and other observations to highlight areas of concern and suggest possible actions to be followed with regards to assessment findings, such as the frequency that observations should be performed or who should be contacted.

However, although these tools have allowed the nurse to assess and recognise deterioration, these tools do not substitute clinical judgement and therefore nurses must appreciate that although vital signs are used to detect deterioration, nurses must also use other clinical methods of assessment, in addition, to complete a patient assessment (RCN, 2017; Gluyas, 2017).

To ensure an effective patient assessment is performed, an ABCDE approach should be used. As stated by the Advanced Life Support Group (2016), ABCDE assessment is based on the following structured assessment:

A – Airway
B – Breathing
C – Circulation
D – Disability
E – Exposure

This approach will allow nurses to detect deterioration as well as gaining other essential information about the patient's clinical situation (RCN, 2017; Smith and Bowden, 2017). The measurement of vital signs is incorporated into the ABCDE assessment approach in addition to other observations such as blood sugar measurement, neurological status, skin condition and colour, and signs of rashes or wounds. When performing an ABCDE assessment it is important to remember that if at any time during the assessment, it becomes clear that the patient is in need of urgent clinical interventions, the assessment should be halted and emergency care summoned (Barker et al., 2015). Documentation of findings of the ABCDE assessment is key to highlight trends in deterioration or the effectiveness of the any interventions (Smith and Bowden, 2017).

 ACTIVITY

Using the titles of the ABCD approach:
- List the corresponding observations or assessments that take place with each aspect of the ABCDE assessment.
- Describe the correct process to perform the observation or assessment in line with current evidence-based guidelines.

Situational Awareness

Even though a robust and structured assessment approach using the ABCDE method of assessment is recommended in order to detect patient deterioration, an awareness of the patient's condition, environment and other factors must be acknowledged. Having an appreciation of all potential or actual concerns regarding the patient allows the nurse or member of the multi-disciplinary team to incorporate concerns other than those assessed using the ABCDE approach into any interventions that may be deemed necessary to treat the patient (Advanced Life Support Group, 2016). Whereas the process of the ABCDE assessment is known as a technical skill in patient assessment, situational awareness is known as a non-technical skill (Cooper et al., 2013).

The concept of situational awareness requires an individual to be mindful and attentive to the surrounding situation, and communicate and implement the subsequent management of the situation based on this awareness (Gluyas, 2017). Therefore situational awareness is an on-going process and an important skill when observing the deteriorating patient as it allows the nurse to gain an insight into aspects of the patient that may be missed if they rely solely on the measurement of vital signs and the process of the ABCDE assessment.

Situational awareness includes 'perception, comprehension, and projection' (Fore and Sculli, 2013). It implies that nurses need to be familiar with all aspects of the patient's situation, and have the ability to envisage potential outcomes based on knowledge and observational findings. It is interesting to note that poor situation awareness is a precursor to an increase in patient risk and poor patient outcomes (Fore and Sculli, 2013).

Nurses have a key role in using situation awareness along with a structured assessment process to highlight patient deterioration, use developed cognitive processes from what is detected to communicate and advocate for the deteriorating patient, to promote effective interventions and favourable patient outcomes. It is also ideal to consider the family in the process of situational awareness and in the recognition and care of the deteriorating child (Gill et al., 2016; NHS Improvement, 2016). Using information from the family and their perceptions based on their situational awareness can assist the nurse and the clinical team in the management of the deteriorating child or young person.

ACTIVITY

- Think about the concept of situational awareness – how do you use situational awareness in your current practice?
- Reflect on a time that you have used situation awareness in practice.
- Focus on you what you perceived, what you understand from your perceptions, and your actions based on your awareness of the situation.

Human Factors

It is also imperative to consider the cognitive processes, subsequent actions and the resulting clinical decisions and behaviours health care workers make on the care of the deteriorating child or young person. The concept of human factors in the management of patient risk is another non-technical skill, which relates to the characteristics that affect the functioning of individuals in situations and the impact these have on patient care and the avoidance of risk (Advanced Life Support Group, 2016). Regardless of experience, knowledge, or skills, humans will make errors (Norris et al., 2012). Therefore it is imperative that when caring for patients, health care professionals are aware that mistakes can occur and that there is a need to be constantly aware of this risk. When faced with a deteriorating patient an understanding of the concept of human factors needs to be included as part of situational awareness and being aware of what can go wrong, and how human behaviour or decisions can contribute to this should also be appreciated (Advanced Life Support Group, 2016). If mistakes do occur it is vital that duty of candour is performed. Duty of candour relates to the requirement of clinical practitioners to be transparent regarding care that is delivered and that all errors must be discussed with relevant individuals such as patients and their families (Care Quality Commission [CQC], 2018). The details of the duty of candour conversation must include an apology, a factual account of what happened, an account of what further enquiries are needed, and the discussion must be fully documented (CQC, 2018). Staff involved in errors must also be supported appropriately and given the opportunity to reflect or debrief on the incident so that future errors can be avoided.

In order to avoid the risks associated with human error in health care, national and local organisations strive to create and establish tools and workplace processes to avoid human error. Tools such as early warning scoring or trigger tools, communication tools such as SBAR (Situation, Background, Assessment, Recommendation) (NHS Improvement, 2018), and practices such as such as post-incident debriefing sessions are now used across health care settings to promote effective human management and the avoidance of human error (Advanced Life Support Group, 2016). When creating these systems, Norris et al. (2012) states that the following should be considered:

- 'Physical abilities' – such as stress responses, workload, staffing levels
- 'Perceptual abilities' – the documentation used in the clinical area, the effectiveness of the documentation, physical responses to the environment, environmental effects (temperature, lighting levels, etc.)
- 'Cognitive abilities' – situational awareness, mental models (how things are supposed to work), recalling information, previous errors made, previous experiences
- 'Social/interpersonal traits' – team-working, communication

As with a structured patient assessment process, effective situation awareness and the systems in place to eradicate patient risk must not be used independently of each other when caring for the deteriorating patient (Gluyas, 2017). It is imperative that all systems are used in conjunction with each other to not only ensure an accurate assessment of the patient's clinical situation, but also an assessment of other relevant circumstances and the potential risk to the patient. Only then can all information be communicated to senior health care staff and interventions to assist the child or young person be decided.

Barriers to Detection and Recognition of the Deteriorating child

Although the processes to support and treat the deteriorating child and young person are well known, episodes of deterioration can still go undetected leading to increased patient risk and poor patient outcomes. The National Patient Safety Agency (NPSA) (2007) collected information regarding the main themes that contributed to undetected patient deterioration. These were found to be 'a lack of monitoring of clinical observations; a lack of recognition of the importance of the deterioration and/or no interventions initiated to treat the patient; and delays in the patient receiving medical assessment and intervention' (NPSA, 2007). Even with systems in place to encourage patient assessment, awareness of the potential issues that can occur, tools such as early warning scores to clarify assessment findings, and communication tools such as SBAR to ensure effective communication, there are still problems ensuring deteriorating children receive the best possible care.

Distraction appears to be a potential barrier when caring for the deteriorating patient. Findings from Endacott et al. (2014) indicate that when faced with a stressful situation such as patient deterioration, individuals tend to focus on an area or skill that they feel comfortable with. This then becomes the task that distracts them from being involved or increasing their awareness of what else may be happening around them. This trait is particularly noted in staff with less experience. A way of avoiding this is to ensure that there is effective leadership in place to support staff and encourage individuals to increase their situational awareness, as well as debriefing after stressful situations experiences in order to promote learning and development for future practice (Advanced Life Support Group, 2016).

Automation of knowledge and complacency can also contribute to not recognising the deteriorating child. Using early warning scoring or trigger tools has been shown to be effective at monitoring and detecting the deteriorating child (Ennis, 2014). These early warning tools have now become embedded in nursing practice and used as effective methods of recording vital signs, detecting clinical trends in observations and empowering staff to highlight any concerns. However, they have also contributed to a loss of skill when faced with deterioration, which is not detected by early warning tools (Fore and Sculli, 2013). It is important to be aware of the limitations of any tool used in patient assessment and to appreciate the nurse's role in using their clinical judgement alongside early warning tools (RCN, 2017).

Complacency when assessing and caring for a patient can also relate to previous clinical knowledge and experience and a subsequent lack of recognition of patient deterioration. According to Rassmussen (1983) and Gluyas (2017), nursing tasks are performed by either:

- 'Skill-based actions' – vital signs, assessment, situational awareness and being familiar with the tasks required and able to complete them routinely.
- 'Rule-based actions'– 'Pattern-match' the current situation to previous experience.
- 'Knowledge-based actions – actions undertaken in a new or unfamiliar situation based on a mental model (what is perceived to be needed) of the required action'.

It is easy for nurses and health care workers to maintain skill-based actions and rule-based actions as these have familiar connotations to the individual and are simple to perform. However, if nurses rely too much on skill or rule-based actions, vital signs or key observational findings can be missed and patient deterioration can go unrecognised. By matching the current situation to previous experiences (as in pattern-based matching) the findings of the current situation can be forcibly matched to previous experiences with the possibility that any mismatches will be cognitively discarded even though they may be of vital importance all because they do not match previous experiences (Rassmussen, 1983; Gluyas, 2017).

It is therefore vital to maintain an appreciation of our previous skills and experiences, but not to become complacent when assessing and caring for the deteriorating child by ensuring the assessment remains patient focused and all assessment findings are deemed important.

Communication is a vital skill needed in all aspects of health care but when caring for the deteriorating child it is imperative that all key information is transferred to the relevant members of the multi-disciplinary team. Poor communication results in poor patient care and can result in medical errors (Tschannen et al., 2013) and poor communication does not just relate to the inability of an individual to share information with another. Roberts et al. (2014) discovered clinical themes relating to poor communication methods in health care including lack of assertiveness when sharing information, a reluctance to share information due to doubting personal ability to detect deterioration, or a lack of empowerment to share communication with a senior staff member or colleague. To overcome communication barriers it is important to remember that in line with the NMC Code of Conduct (2018) nurses have a responsibility to advocate for their patients and this would include timely and effective communication with all members of the multi-disciplinary team to ensure that the deteriorating child receives relevant clinical interventions; it is also imperative to include parents and family members. Although family members will not be completing formal assessment of patients, close knowledge of their child allows them to have an advantage when identifying slight changes in a patient's condition. Asking parents and families of their concerns can be used to assist nurses and the multi-disciplinary team in detecting deterioration or just appreciating that there may be something wrong that requires further investigation (Gill et al., 2016)

Care of the Deteriorating Child

The process of caring for the deteriorating child must have a robust approach, which includes effective detection and the subsequent actions that follow in order to deliver effective interventions. Joffe et al. (2011) and McKay et al. (2013) discuss the stages that need to be followed in order to ensure there is effective recognition of deterioration and subsequent appropriate interventions. These stages are:

- deterioration is detected
- staff are empowered to seek assistance
- priority responses to the situation begins
- interventions are initiated

Throughout these stages, robust patient assessment and situational awareness must be used. These initial measurements and evaluation of the circumstances will influence the subsequent patient outcomes. Barriers to effective recognition also need to be appreciated to avoid inaccurate assessment or poor situational awareness and the risk of human error.

Following detection of patient deterioration staff must be empowered to call for assistance and effectively communicate their clinical findings. It is recognised that structured communication tools, such as SBAR and closed loop communication, aid in team communication and that these tools can be effectively utilised when caring for the deteriorating child (NHS Improvement, 2018). Reluctance of staff to share information is an on-going concern but for this to be avoided the causes of poor communication must be addressed. Whether it may be that the nurse doubts their own ability, does not equate their findings to patient deterioration, or that they just are reluctant to communicate information to a senior individual, all potential issues must be appreciated (Tschannen et al., 2013). These issues are being factored into assessment systems such as early warning tools to empower nurses to be able to follow a process. One such process used is that the nurse must update all aspects of deteriorating child or young person to the nurse in charge. This allows the senior nurse to support junior staff when there is clinical deterioration as well as facilitating the nurse to effectively communicate to more senior colleagues as appropriate (Rabøl et al., 2011). It is known that the proficiency and confidence of senior nurses is a major influence in effective multi-disciplinary team working (Clements et al., 2015). Therefore, including senior nurses in the assessment findings of the deteriorating child does not serve to deskill junior members of the nursing team, but instead encourages all essential information to be fully and effectively communicated, thus avoiding the barrier of poor communication.

Leadership, seen as another non-technical skill (Cooper et al., 2013), is a vital role for all nurses and clinicians. Leadership is an essential aspect of nursing as it serves as a way of encouraging ourselves and others to deliver effective care (Carragher and Gormley, 2017). When caring for a deteriorating patient, advocating for the child/young person and the family and leading on communicating all concerns effectively (whether it is at the initial stage of deterioration or when interventions are taking place) will allow priority clinical reviews – based on accurate assessment – as well as precise interventions. It should not be just up to senior nurses to be leaders – as discussed by the Kings Fund Leadership Review (2012). It is suggested that all aspects of leadership should come from all clinical staff as their role is delivering health care and they are aware of what works effectively and what needs improvement. When caring for the deteriorating patient leadership should not just end with detection of deterioration but should continue and all aspects of positive actions praised and any aspects of poor practice addressed. Interestingly, Roland (2017) suggests that the main state of intervention that needs constant adjustment and review is the stage when priority responses to the situation need to occur. When caring for the deteriorating child leadership needs to focus on effective assessment and situational awareness, effective team communication, on-going leadership and effective clinical interventions based on the patient's needs. It is the nurse's role to advocate for the patient during this process and also lead on any necessary areas for development, and encourage and develop colleagues during similar experiences.

CASE STUDY

You are caring for Evie who has been admitted to your ward with difficulty in breathing. Evie is a 5-year-old girl who has a 1-week history of coughing, wheezing, fever, poor appetite and lethargy. Following examination Evie is found to be suffering from pneumonia and has a right lower lobe consolidation. She has been admitted to the ward for intravenous antibiotics and has currently had 1 days' worth of treatment.

Evie's parents approach you because Evie has suddenly become sleepier, her oxygen saturation has decreased, and she has decreased urine output.

1. Using an ABCDE assessment, what initial assessment of Evie would you perform?
2. What assessment tools would you use and why? What are the limitations of the tools?
3. What information would you like from the parents?
4. Considering situational awareness and human factors, what other information do you need to be aware of when assessing Evie?
5. Who would you liaise with following the patient assessment and, using SBAR as your communication tool, what would you say?

The doctor comes to review Evie and states that they are concerned that she is suffering from sepsis.

1. What is sepsis and what is the Sepsis 6?
2. How do you now assess and treat Evie following this diagnosis?
3. What support do the parents require and how will you achieve this?
4. As the nurse who is looking after Evie, what is your leadership role when working with the multi-disciplinary team and the nurse in charge of the ward to ensure Evie and her family receive the best care?

REFERENCES

Advanced Life Support Group, 2016. Advanced Paediatric Life Support: A Practical Approach to Emergencies (APLS), sixth ed. Wiley-Blackwell.

Asakura, H., 2004. Fetal and neonatal thermoregulation. J. Nippon Med. Sch. 71, 360–370.

Au, A.K., Ray, P.E., McBryde, K.D., 2008. Incidence of postoperative hyponatraemia and complications in critically ill children treated with normotenic solution. J. Pediatr. 152, 33–38.

Ball, J.W., Bindler, R.C., 2006. Child Health Nursing. Partnering with Children & Family. Prentice Hall, New Jersey.

Barker, M., Rushton, M., Smith, J., 2015. How to assess deteriorating patients. Nurs. Stand. 30 (11), 34–36.

Blows, W.T., 2012. The Biological Basis of Clinical Observations, second ed. Routledge, London.

Brady, P.W., Muething, S., Kotagal, U., et al., 2013. Improving situation awareness to reduce unrecognized clinical deterioration and serious safety events. Pediatrics 131 (1), 298–308.

Brady, M., 2015. Homeostasis. Chapter 2. In: Peate, I., Gormley-Fleming, E. (Eds.), Fundamentals of Children's Anatomy and Physiology: A Textbook for Nursing and Healthcare Students. Wiley-Blackwell, Oxford.

Care Quality Commission (CQC), 2018. Regulation 20: Duty of Candour (accessed 2 July 2018). Available from: https://www.cqc.org.uk/guidance-providers/regulations-enforcement/regulation-20-duty-candour#full-regulation.

Carrager, J., Gormley, K., 2017. Leadership and emotional intelligence in nursing and midwifery education and practice: a discussion paper. J. Adv. Nurs. 73 (1), 85–96.

Cedar, S.H., 2012. Biology for Health: Applying the Activities of Daily Living. Palgrave Macmillan, Basingstoke, UK.

Chapman, S., 2013. Situation awareness is key to detecting deteriorating patients. Nurs. Child. Young People 25 (4), 11.

Clancy, J., McVicar, A., 2009. Physiology and Anatomy for Nurses and Health Care Practitioners: A Homeostatic Approach, third ed. Hodder Arnold, London.

Clements, A., Curtis, K., Horvat, L., Shaban, R.Z., 2015. The effect of a nurse team leader on communication and leadership in major trauma resuscitations. Int. Emerg. Nurs. 23, 3–7.

Cooper, S., Cant, R., Porter, J., Missen, K., Sparkes, L., McConnell-Henry, T., et al., 2013. Managing patient deterioration: assessing teamwork and individual performance. Emerg. Med. J. 30, 377–381.

Elliot, B., Callery, P., Mould, J., 2010. Caring for children with critical illness. In: Glasper, E.A., Richardson, J. (Eds.), A Textbook of Children's and Young People's Nursing, second ed. Churchill Livingstone Elsevier, Edinburgh.

Endacott, R., Bogossian, F.E., Cooper, S.J., et al., 2014. Leadership and teamwork in medical emergencies: performance of nursing students and registered nurses in simulated patient scenarios. J. Clin. Nurs. 24, 90–100.

Ennis, L., 2014. Paediatric early warning scores on a children's ward: a quality initiative. Nurs. Child. Young People 26 (7), 25–31.

Fore, A.M., Sculli, G.L., 2013. A concept analysis of situational awareness in nursing. J. Adv. Nurs. 69 (12), 2613–2621.

Gill, F.J., Leslie, G.D., Marshall, A.P., 2016. The impact of implementation of family initiated escalation of care for the deteriorating patient in hospital: a systematic review. Worldviews Evidence-Based Nurs. 13 (4), 303–313.

Gluyas, H., 2017. Errors in the nursing management of a deteriorating patient. Nurs. Stand. 32 (12), 41–50.

Gormley-Fleming, E., 2010. Assessing and vital signs-a comprehensive review. In: Glasper, E.A., Aylott, M., Batterick, C. (Eds.), Developing Practical Skills for Nursing Children and Young People. Hodder Arnold. London.

Gormley-Fleming, E., 2013. Pulse oximetry. In: Glasper, E.A., Coad, J., Richardson, J. (Eds.), Children and Young People's Nursing at a Glance. Wiley-Blackwell, Oxford.

Gormley-Fleming, E., Martin, D. (Eds.), 2018. Children's and Young People's Nursing Skills at a Glance. Wiley-Blackwell, USA Oxford.

Joffe, A.R., Anton, N.R., Burkholder, S.C., 2011. Reduction in hospital mortality over time in a hospital without a pediatric medical emergency team limitations of before-and-after study designs. Arch. Pediatr. Adolesc. Med. 165 (5), 419–423.

Large, C., Aldridge, M., 2018. Non-technical skills required to recognise and escalate patient deterioration in acute hospital settings. Nurs. Manag. 25 (2), 24–30.

Lissauer, T., Clayden, T., 2012. Illustrated Textbook of Paediatrics, fourth ed. Mosby Elsevier, Edinburgh.

Marieb, E.N., Hoehn, K., 2018 Eleventh edition. Human Anatomy & Physiology. Pearson International, San Francisco.

McKay, H., Mitchell, I.A., Sinn, K., et al., 2013. Effect of a multifaceted intervention on documentation of vital signs and staff communication regarding deteriorating paediatric patients. J. Paediatr. Child Health 49, 48–56.

Mulryan, C., 2011. Acute Illness Management. Sage Publication, London.

National Institute for Care and Excellence (NICE), 2009. Diarrhoea and Vomiting Caused by Gastroenteritis in Under 5s: Diagnosis and Management. Clinical guideline [CG84]. Published date: April 2009.

National Patient Safety Agency, 2007. Recognising and Responding Appropriately to Early Signs of Deterioration in Hospitalised Patients. NPSA, London.

Neill, S., Knowles, H., 2004. The Biology of Child Health. A Reader in Development and Assessment. Palgrave Macmillian, Basingstoke.

NHS Improvement, 2016. Patient Safety Alert NHS/PSA/RE/2016/005: Resources to Support Safer Care of the Deteriorating Patient (Adults and Children). Available from: https://improvement.nhs.uk/documents/177/Patient_Safety_Alert_Stage_2_-_Deterioration_resources_July_2016_v2.pdf.

NHS Improvement, 2018. SBAR Communication Tool- Situation, Background, Assessment, Recommendation. Available from: https://improvement.nhs.uk/resources/sbar-communication-tool/.

Norris, B., Currie, L., Lecko, C., 2012. The importance of applying human factors to nursing practice. Nurs. Stand. 26 (32), 36–40.

Nursing & Midwifery Council (NMC), 2018. The Code: Professional Standards of Practice and Behaviour for Nurses and Midwives. Available from: https://www.nmc.org.uk/standards/code/.

Peate, I., Gormley-Fleming, E., 2015. Fundamentals of Children's Anatomy and Physiology: A Textbook for Nursing and Healthcare Students. Wiley-Blackwell, Oxford.

Power, G.G., 1989. Biology of temperature: the mammalian fetus. J. Dev. Physiol. 12, 259–304.

Rassmussen, J., 1983. Skills, rules, and knowledge; signals, signs, and symbols, and other distinctions in human performance models. IEEE Trans. Syst. Man Cybern. 13 (3), 257–266.

Rabøl, L.I., Andersen, M.L., Østergaard, D., Bjørn, B., Lilja, L., Mogensen, T., 2011. Descriptions of verbal communication errors between staff. An analysis of 84 root cause analysis-reports from Danish hospitals. BMJ Qual. Saf. 20 (3), 268–274.

Roberts, K.E., Bonafide, C.P., Weirich Pains, C., et al., 2014. Barriers to calling for urgent assistance despite a comprehensive pediatric rapid response system. Am. J. Crit. Care 23 (3), 223–229.

Roiger, D., 2012. Anatomy and Physiology. Foundations for the Health Professions. McGraw Hill, Columbus OH.

Roland, D., 2017. Paediatric early warning systems: myths and muses. Paediatr. Child Health 27 (5), 242–246.

Royal College of Nursing (RCN), 2017. Standards for Assessing, Measuring and Monitoring Vital Signs in Infants, Children and Young People. The Royal College of Nursing, London.

Rudolf, M., Lee, T., Levene, M., 2011. Paediatrics and Child Health, third ed. Wiley-Blackwell, Oxford.

Scanlon, V.C., Sanders, T., 2015. Essentials of Anatomy and Physiology, seventh ed. F.A. Davis Company, Philadelphia.

Smith, D., Bowden, T., 2017. Using the ABCDE approach to assess the deteriorating patient. Nurs. Stand. 32 (14), 51–61.

The Kings Fund, 2012. Leadership and Engagement for Improvement in the NHS. The Kings Fund, London.

Tortora, G.J., Derrickson, B.H., 2009. Principles of Anatomy and Physiology, twelfth ed. Wiley, Hoboken, New Jersey.

Tschannen, D., Schoville, R., Schmidt, P., Buehler, K., Borst, S., Flaherty-Robb, M., 2013. Communication practices among nurses in the acute care setting. J. Commun. Healthc. 6 (3), 171–179.

Tucker Blackburn, A., 2013. Maternal, Fetal and Neonatal Physiology, fourth ed. Elsevier, St. Louis.

Watson, R., Fawcett, T.N., 2003. Pathophysiology, Homeostasis and Nursing. Routledge, London.

Waugh, A., Grant, A., 2018. Ross and Wilson. Anatomy and Physiology in Health and Illness. Elsevier, Edinburgh.

11

Respiratory Illness in Children

Janet Kelsey, Lee-Anne Rylatt

LEARNING OUTCOMES

- Demonstrate an understanding of the anatomy and physiology of the respiratory tract.
- Gain an overview of the nature of respiratory illness in children.

- Appreciate the role of the nurse in caring for children with respiratory illness.
- Identify the signs of respiratory distress.
- Use relevant literature and research to inform the nursing care of children with respiratory illness.

INTRODUCTION

The most common illnesses in infants and children in the UK are disorders of the respiratory system. Respiratory tract infections in children, although common, are not usually serious. Frequent infections occur in children because the immune system has not been exposed to common pathogens and therefore infections tend to develop with each new exposure. The risk of infection is also increased in children because the respiratory tract is relatively short. Most of these infections do not cause a serious problem to the child; however, children are particularly vulnerable to respiratory problems because of their small resting lung volumes, lower oxygen reserves, relatively high oxygen requirements and the immaturity of their respiratory system (Akers, 2015). Respiratory disease in early childhood can interfere with the development of the lungs and cause permanent lung damage. Acute respiratory failure can result from any airway, pulmonary or neuromuscular disease that impairs oxygen exchange or elimination of carbon dioxide.

Some respiratory problems are more common at specific ages. The same organism can cause different illnesses at different ages. For example, the respiratory syncytial virus (RSV) frequently causes bronchiolitis in infants, with approximately 1 in 3 infants developing bronchiolitis in the first year of life (National Institute for Clinical Excellence (NICE 2015)), but causes only a sore throat and cold symptoms in older children (NHS Health 2020).

The majority of infections (80%) are restricted to the upper respiratory tract and approximately 20% of these will become severe and require medical intervention. These include conditions such as bronchiolitis, laryngotracheobronchitis, pneumonia and acute asthma (Morton and Phillips, 1992; Thompson, 1990). Respiratory infections account for over a third of all paediatric consultations in primary care in the United Kingdom and the United States (hay et al., 2005, Fendrick et al., 2003). These are major causes of morbidity in children and a common reason for admission to hospital (Mighten, 2011).

Respiratory illness accounts for 30%–40% of acute medical admissions to hospital of children, with RSV estimated to account for 20% of hospital admissions in preschool children. Reeves et al (2019) estimated an annual average of 20,359 RSV-associated admissions in infants in England from mid-2010 to mid-2012 and the cost of treating respiratory symptoms to the NHS being estimated at £30 million per year (Mighten, 2011).

Anatomy and Physiology of the Respiratory Tract

The human body requires a constant supply of oxygen. Children have a higher metabolic rate than adults, and thus an increased need for oxygen, which demands that their respiratory system functions effectively. The respiratory system consists of the lungs, the airways, the chest wall and the pulmonary circulation. The lungs (Fig. 11.1) are situated in the thorax; the sides of the thorax are bounded by the rib cage, linking the ribs are the intercostal muscles. At the base of the thorax is a flexible sheet of muscle known as the diaphragm.

The primary function of the respiratory system is the exchange of gases between the environmental air and the blood. There are three steps in this process: the movement of air in and out of the lungs; the movement of gases between air spaces in the lungs and the blood; and the movement of blood from the capillaries surrounding the lungs to the body's organs and tissues. The first two processes are functions of the respiratory system, the third is performed by the cardiovascular system (West, 2012).

The respiratory system can be divided into the upper and lower airways. The upper airways consist of the nasopharynx and the oropharynx. These structures are lined with highly vascular, ciliated epithelium. This warms and moistens the inspired air and removes foreign particles from it as it passes into the lungs. During quiet respiration, air passes

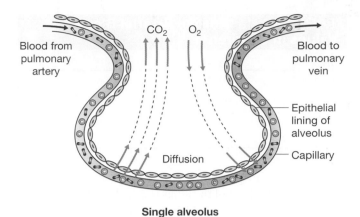

Single alveolus

Fig. 11.2 A single alveolus.

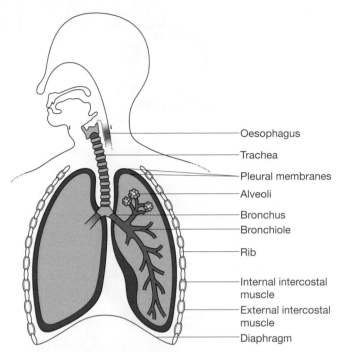

Fig. 11.1 Basic structure of the lungs.

through the nose, nasopharynx and oropharynx to the lower airways (Akers, 2015). During exercise or when the nose is obstructed, the mouth and oropharynx are used for ventilation; however by this route the air is not filtered or humidified as efficiently as via the nasopharynx. The larynx connects the upper and lower airways; it is a cartilaginous structure that prevents collapse of the airways during inspiration. Air then flows into the trachea, which is supported by U-shaped cartilage. The trachea divides into the two main bronchi, which in turn divide into bronchioles; there are 16 divisions in total, ending in the terminal bronchioles. This multiple subdivision causes a decrease in the velocity of the air flow into the lungs, which allows for maximum gaseous exchange to take place. The bronchioles have cartilage within their walls until the 10th division. The terminal bronchioles continue to divide into smaller respiratory bronchioles, and then into the alveolar ducts. These lead to the alveolar sacs, which are made up of numerous alveoli. The alveoli (Fig. 11.2) are the primary gas-exchange units of the lungs; it is here that oxygen enters the blood and carbon dioxide is removed (West, 2012).

 POWERPOINT

Access the companion PowerPoint presentation.

There are 20-million alveoli at birth; the number of alveoli continues to increase until the child is approximately 8 years old (Crawford, 2011), at which point the lungs contain around 500 million alveoli in the fully formed lungs of the adult (West, 2012). This means that infants and young children have a relatively small alveolar surface area for gaseous exchange. Each alveolus has a network of capillaries wrapped around it. The walls of the alveoli and the capillaries are only one cell thick. A thin layer of liquid covers their surface, which aids gaseous exchange between the inhaled air and the circulating blood.

Inhalation involves the diaphragm contracting and flattening and the external intercostal muscles contracting, pulling the ribcage upwards and outwards. This increases the volume inside the thorax, decreases the pressure inside the lungs, and air is sucked in. When the diaphragm relaxes it domes up into the thorax and, as the external intercostal muscles relax, the rib cage drops down and moves inwards. This increases the pressure inside the lungs and forces air out. The internal intercostal muscles contract during strenuous breathing to pull the rib cage down to produce a forced expiration. There are two main considerations in infants and children. First, in the newborn, the diaphragm is not able to contract as effectively as in an older infant or child because it is attached higher at the front and is therefore longer. Second, infants and children have a relatively round thoracic cavity due to the horizontal position of the ribs; this places increased dependence on the diaphragm and abdomen as the primary means of ventilation.

POWERPOINT

Access the companion PowerPoint presentation.

WWW

See respiratory movements online, Review the section on how your lungs work:
- https://www.blf.org.uk/support-for-you/how-your-lungs-work

Lung Volumes

The total capacity of a child's lungs increases from 1.4 L in the 5-year-old child to 4.5 L at the time of puberty:
- At the end of quiet respiration, the air that remains in the lungs is termed the **functional residual capacity.**
- Following forced expiration, between 0.5 and 1.5 L (depending on age) of air remains trapped in the alveoli; this minimal volume is called the **residual volume.**
- The additional volume of air forced out of the lungs during a forced expiration of between 0.5 and 1.5 L is known as the **expiratory reserve volume.**
- During quiet respiration, the amount of air in the lungs increases from 0.7 L at 5 years (or 2.25 L at puberty) at the end of expiration to 0.8 L at 5 years (or 2.55 L at puberty)

TABLE 11.1   Normal Arterial Blood Gas Values in Children

pH	7.35–7.45
pCO_2	4.7–6.0kPa
pO_2	10–13kPa
HCO_3	22–26 mmol/L
BE	+2––2

at the end of inspiration; this 0.1 L (0.3 L at puberty) of air moving in and out of the lungs is called the **tidal volume.**

- The **vital capacity** of the lungs is the amount of air moving when the patient is performing forced inspiration and forced expiration, which will be the sum of the inspiratory reserve volume, the expiratory reserve volume and the tidal volume. This volume is related to the size of the patient; at age 5 years it is approximately 1 L and this increases to 3 L at puberty. The vital capacity can be increased if the patient stands up because the volume of blood in the lungs is reduced.

- The **peak flow** is the maximum velocity of air flow produced in a forced respiration. When this value is low it suggests that expiratory respiratory muscle activity is weak or that there is an obstruction to expiratory air flow due to some form of bronchoconstriction such as asthma.

Nervous Control of Breathing

The respiratory centre is situated at the base of the brain and is made up of the medulla oblongata and the pons. The control of breathing has both automatic and voluntary components. Voluntary control allows for breathing to be integrated with voluntary actions such as blowing, singing and speaking. Automatic control involves input from two types of receptors: those that monitor the pH, carbon dioxide and oxygen levels in the blood; and those that monitor breathing patterns and lung function.

Chemoreceptors assess the level of carbon dioxide and oxygen in the blood, messages are transmitted to the respiratory centre and ventilation is adjusted to maintain arterial blood gases within a normal range (Akers, 2015) (Table 11.1). How much oxygen is in the blood depends on the:

- haemoglobin concentration in the blood (Hb g/dL);
- oxygen saturation of the haemoglobin (SaO_2);
- partial pressure of oxygen (PaO_2).

The central chemoreceptors located in the medulla oblongata monitor the carbon dioxide level in the blood by assessing the number of free hydrogen ions in the cerebrospinal fluid circulating around the medulla. This is important because the carbon dioxide level in the blood affects the pH level of the extracellular fluid of the brain. These receptors are extremely sensitive in the short-term but long-term elevation of carbon dioxide levels, such as can occur in chronic respiratory disease, causes desensitisation of these receptors.

The carotid and aortic bodies are chemoreceptors that are sensitive to oxygen levels in the carotid artery and aorta, respectively. They are less responsive than the central chemoreceptors and are activated only when the oxygen level falls below 60 mmHg. Therefore hypoxia is the main stimulus for ventilation in persons with chronic hypercarbia (Mighten, 2011).

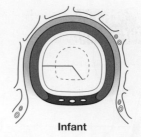

Infant

1 mm oedema = 16 fold resistance increase

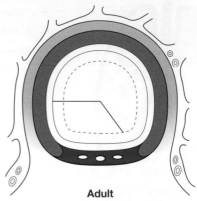

Adult

1 mm oedema = 2.4 fold resistance increase

Fig. 11.3 Anatomical differences between the airways of an infant and of an adult.

⏩ REFLECT ON YOUR PRACTICE

How would you explain to a junior nurse the importance of the correct level of oxygen administration when assisting a child with a chronic respiratory condition experiencing an acute respiratory illness?

⏩ POWERPOINT

Access the companion PowerPoint presentation.

The anatomy and physiology of the respiratory and cardiovascular systems of children differs from that of adults. This influences the care given to children and hence must be considered when assessing and managing children with respiratory problems.

It is important to remember that anatomical differences influence the degree to which children respond to respiratory illness because of the smaller diameter of the airways (Fig. 11.3 and Table 11.2). Poiseuille's law states that: resistance to airflow is inversely proportional to the fourth power of the radius. In other words, a small amount of mucous or oedema in the airways will significantly increase resistance to airflow and therefore increase the work of breathing.

RESPIRATORY ASSESSMENT AND EXAMINATION OF THE CHEST

A calm manner should always be adopted when assessing any child with respiratory problems. The 'hands-off approach'

TABLE 11.2 **The Differences in the Anatomy and Physiology of the Respiratory and Cardiovascular Systems of Children**

Factor	Nursing Considerations
Airway	
Large head, short neck, inability to support head.	Assistance required to maintain position of comfort.
Large tongue.	Airway is easily obstructed by tongue; proper positioning is often all that is necessary to open the airway.
The floor of the mouth is easily compressible.	Care is required when positioning the fingers when holding the jaw.
Infants less than 6 months old are obligate nose breathers.	Obstruction of the nasal passages by mucus can compromise the infant's airway.
Smaller diameter of all airways in a 1-year-old child. Tracheal diameter is less than the child's little finger.	Small amounts of mucous or swelling easily obstruct the airways; child normally has increased airway resistance.
The epiglottis is horseshoe shaped and projects posteriorly at 45%. The larynx is high and anterior.	Tracheal intubation can be more difficult. A straight blade laryngoscope is used; cricoid pressure may be necessary to facilitate intubation.
The trachea is short and soft. The cricoid cartilage is the narrowest portion of neck.	Airway of infant can be compressed if neck is flexed or hyperextended. Tube displacement is more likely. Provides a natural seal for the endotracheal tube.
The cricoid ring is lined by pseudostratified ciliated epithelium loosely bound to areolar tissue.	Particularly susceptible to oedema. Uncuffed tubes are preferred in pre-pubertal children.
Breathing	
Infants rely mainly on diaphragmatic breathing. The ribs lie more horizontally in infants and contribute less to chest expansion. Their muscles are more likely to fatigue compared with adults.	Children are more prone to respiratory failure. Anything that impedes diaphragm contraction or movement, e.g. abdominal distension, can contribute to the development of respiratory failure.
Sternum and ribs are cartilaginous; chest wall is soft; intercostal muscles are poorly developed.	Infant's chest wall may move inwards instead of outwards during inspiration (retractions) when lung compliance is decreased; greater intrathoracic pressure is generated during inspiration. The compliant chest wall may allow serious parenchymal injuries to occur without rib fracture.
Increased metabolic rate (about twice that of an adult); increased respiratory demand for oxygen consumption and carbon dioxide elimination.	Respiratory distress increases oxygen demand, as does any condition that increases metabolic rate, e.g. fever.
Lung compliance and high chest wall compliance in the neonate.	Respiratory function inefficient during episodes of respiratory distress.
Smaller amount of elastic and collagen tissue in the paediatric lung.	May contribute to the increased incidence of pulmonary oedema, pneumomediastinum and pneumothorax in infants.
Circulation	
Child's circulating blood volume is larger per unit of body weight (70–80 mL/kg), but absolute volume is relatively small; 70%–80% of newborn's body weight is water, compared with 50%–60% of an adult body weight; about half of this volume is extracellular.	Blood loss considered minor in an adult may lead to shock in a child; decreased fluid intake or increased fluid loss quickly leads to dehydration. Acute blood loss produces symptoms when 20%–25% of circulating volume has been lost. Dehydration will compromise peripheral perfusion when 7%–10% of the infant or child's body weight and 5%–7% of the adolescent or adult body weight is lost.
Stroke volume is small and relatively fixed in infants. Cardiac output is directly related to heart rate.	Stroke volume cannot increase to improve cardiac output. Response to volume therapy is therefore blunted.
By the age of 2 years the myocardial function and response to fluid is similar to that of an adult.	Tachycardia is the child's most efficient method of increasing cardiac output. However, ventricular rates of >180–220 beats/min compromise diastolic filling time and coronary artery perfusion.
Systemic vascular resistance rises after birth and continues to do so until adulthood.	Children's normal values for blood pressure increase with age.

Cosby, 1998; cited by Dolan & Holt, 2000.

can generate a lot of useful information gained through careful observation and this is particularly useful in very young children, who may resist physical examination. It is always important to leave the child with his or her carer in an upright position. Although observations focus on the respiratory status of the child, it is important to note the child's general appearance, level of engagement with the carer, colour, hydration status and temperature. In addition, the ability of infants to feed should be noted. If at any time you feel the child needs immediate intervention, for example, they are having difficulties breathing, then the assessment should be stopped and emergency care given to stabilise the child; evaluating whether the child is breathing spontaneously and able to maintain their airway is crucial (Akers, 2015).

Assessment follows the ABC criteria for assessment in conjunction with neurological observations and provides a framework for rapid and effective nursing assessment of the child with respiratory problems. The survey should therefore include assessment of the following:

A: Airway

Patency of the airway is assessed, observing for spontaneous ventilation, and look, listen and feel. Note any presence of inspiratory noises. If the child is able to speak or is crying this indicates that the airway is patent. If there is no evidence of air movement then chin-lift or jaw-thrust should be carried out and the basic life support algorithm commenced.

B: Breathing

To assess the adequacy of breathing the chest should be examined and the following assessed:
- The effort of breathing including respiratory rate, recession, grunting, use of accessory muscles and nasal flaring.
- The efficacy of breathing, including breath sounds and chest expansion/abdominal excursion.
- The effects of inadequate respiration, including heart rate, oxygen saturation, skin colour and mental status.

Assessment of breathing therefore involves examination of the chest for the following:
- Respiratory movements.
- Number rhythm, depth and quality of respirations.
- Character of breath sounds utilising the skills of palpation, auscultation and percussion.

Chest wall movement should be symmetric bilaterally and coordinated with breathing.

On inspiration, the chest rises and expands (Fig. 11.4A); on expiration, the chest descends and decreases in size (see Fig. 11.4B). In children less than 6–7 years of age, respiratory movement will be mainly abdominal or diaphragmatic; in older children respirations are mainly thoracic.

To observe for chest expansion, stand at the child's head or feet, and looking down the midline, note any asymmetry of movement. Decreased movement on one side may be the result of foreign body obstruction, pneumonia, pneumothorax or atelectasis.

Respiratory movements can be felt by placing each hand flat against the chest or back with thumbs in the midline along the lower costal margin (Fig. 11.5). The hands move with the chest wall during respiration. The amount of respiratory excursion is evaluated and asymmetry is noted.

> ## ⯮ POWERPOINT
>
> Access the companion PowerPoint presentation.

Palpation is carried out for voice conduction (vocal fremitus). Place the palmar surface of the hand on the child's chest and feel for vibrations as the child speaks. At the same time, move the hand symmetrically on either side of the sternum and vertebral column. Vocal fremitus is usually most prominent at the apex and least prominent at the base of the lungs. Absent or diminished vocal fremitus in the upper airway may

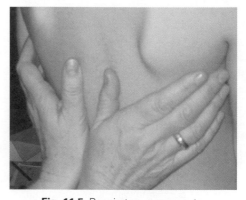

Fig. 11.5 Respiratory movements.

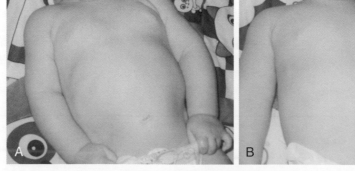

Fig. 11.4 Chest expansion. **(A)** On inspiration the chest rises and expands. **(B)** on expiration the chest descends and decreases in size

indicate asthma or foreign body obstruction. Increased vocal fremitus may indicate pneumonia or atelectasis.

During palpation other abnormal vibrations that indicate pathological conditions are noted. These include pleural rub, which is felt as a grating sensation and is synchronous with respiration and crepitation, which can be felt as a coarse crackly sensation and is the result of air escaping from the lungs to the subcutaneous tissue. This may be caused by injury or surgical intervention. Both crepitation and pleural rub can often be heard as well as felt.

The sinking-in of soft tissues relative to the cartilaginous and bony thorax may be noted in some respiratory disorders. This is recession and is described as intercostal, subcostal, substernal, clavicular and suprasternal/tracheal tug, and it demonstrates increased work of breathing:

- Intercostal, subcostal or sternal recession show increased work of breathing.
- Recession is more easily seen in younger children whose chest wall is more compliant.
- In children over 6 or 7 years, recession suggests severe respiratory problems.
- The degree of recession gives an indication of the severity of the breathing difficulty.

Nasal flaring is also an indication of increased work of breathing. The enlargement of the nostrils helps to reduce nasal resistance and maintain airway patency; it is usually described as either minimal or marked. Head bobbing in the infant is a sign of dyspnoea.

Respiratory rates should be measured over a full minute (Table 11.3). It should be remembered that young children breathe diaphragmatically and therefore are observed by watching abdominal movement rather than the movement of the chest. A decreasing rate or rhythm may indicate deterioration rather than improvement in the child's condition A resting rate of >60 breaths/min is a sign of respiratory distress in a child irrespective of age (National Institute of Clinical Excellence [NICE], 2015). Tachypnoea at rest indicates a need for increased ventilation.

Respiratory Rate

Further information about the severity of the child's illness may be gained by measurement of oxygen saturation (SaO_2) levels with a pulse oximeter (Fig. 11.6), however, oximeter probes must be selected according to age and size of child.

For further information see: https://www.england.nhs.uk/2018/12/risk-of-harm-from-inappropriate-placement-of-pulse-oximeter-probes/ and consider how you would choose the correct probe. A saturation of less than 92% while breathing air, or less than 95% when breathing oxygen, is low. Children whose normal oxygen saturations fall outside the normal limits should be recorded along with their normal expected range, for example, a child with a cyanotic heart lesion. Rajesh et al. (2000) evaluated respiratory rate as an indicator of hypoxia in infants <2 months of age and concluded that a respiratory rate of >60/min is a good predictor of hypoxia. The infants should be treated with oxygen should the facility to measure SaO_2 not be available. It should be remembered that pulse oximetry is less accurate when the SaO_2 is less than 70%, when shock is present, and in the presence of carboxyhaemoglobin. If there is evidence of respiratory or circulatory failure then arterial blood gases are needed.

> ### 🌐 WWW
>
> Learn about the oxyhaemoglobin dissociation curve at:
> - https://www.medicalexamprep.co.uk/understanding-oxygen-dissociation-curve/

The effectiveness of breathing is also assessed by observing breath sounds. Auscultation allows assessment of breath sounds for pitch, intensity, quality, location and duration. Breath sounds are best heard if the child inspires deeply. Normal breath sounds are vesicular, soft and low pitched on inspiration followed by a shorter sound on expiration; bronchial or tubular are similar to the sounds heard upon auscultation over the larynx during respiration; and bronchovesicular is a mixture of bronchial and vesicular sounds. Vesicular are heard over most of the chest, except over the larynx and trachea, and in infants, over the upper chest. Infants' breath sounds are bronchovesicular in the upper chest because of increased transmission (West, 2012). Fluid, air or solid masses in the pleural space all interfere with the conduction of breath sounds.

Consolidation or solidification of a portion of the lung caused by pneumonia, for example, will result in tubular or bronchial breathing being heard over the posterior chest due to increased transmission between the trachea and the periphery of the chest (British Thoracic Society [BTS], 2011).

TABLE 11.3 Normal Ranges of Respiratory Rate in Children	
Age (Years)	**Respiratory rate**
Neonate	25–50
<1 year	20–45
1-2 years	20–40
2-7 years	20–30
8-11 years	15–25
12 years>	12–24

Adapted from RCN (2017).

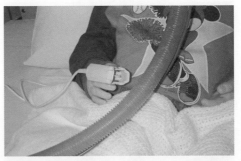

Fig. 11.6 Measurement of oxygen saturation levels. Ensure probe is appropriate size.

Alert, diminished or absent breath sounds are always abnormal. Percussion or tapping of the lungs (Fig. 11.7) is carried out to determine the presence and location of air, liquid and solid material in the lung and to evaluate the densities, position and landmarks of the underlying organs. Normally, the percussion note in a lung full of air is resonant. When there is fluid in the chest, for example, pleural effusion, the note becomes flat. With pneumonia where there is an increased amount of fluid, but not in the chest, the note becomes dull. With excess air, for example, asthma, the note is hyper-resonant. It is normal to find dullness over the liver and heart.

> ### 🔧 ACTIVITY
>
> To help discriminate between hollow and flat sounds:
> Try tapping various parts of an internal wall, see if you can distinguish between the hollow sound of the unsupported plaster board and the flat sound of the solid wood or concrete support.

Voice sounds are also part of auscultation of the lung. Normally, vocal resonance or voice sounds are heard, but the sounds are muffled and indistinct. Hearing clear distinct sounds is an abnormal finding and is caused by the same conditions causing abnormal vocal fremitus.

Various respiratory illnesses produce adventitious sounds that are not normally heard over the chest; these are not alterations in normal breath sounds but are additional abnormal sounds.

The effects of inadequate respiration can be seen by examining heart rate, skin colour and mental status. These are linked to the examination of circulation and disability.

C: Circulation

Adequacy of circulation is assessed by examining the cardiovascular status and looking for the effects of circulatory inadequacy on other organs.

Vital Signs

The child's vital signs should be appropriate for the child's age and clinical condition. A child normally has a faster heart rate (Table 11.4) and respiratory rate, and a lower arterial pressure than an adult. The child's heart rate and pulse volume should be assessed by palpating both central and peripheral pulses.

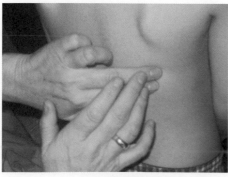

Fig. 11.7 Percussion.

It is important to note that normal vital signs are not always appropriate when a child is seriously ill; indeed a normal heart rate and respiratory rate may indicate cardiopulmonary arrest is imminent. Hypoxia produces tachycardia and is to be expected; bradycardia is a sign of respiratory failure and a preterminal sign. Absent peripheral and weak central pulses are signs of advanced shock and hypotension in children.

An accurate pulse should be measured for a full minute and be consistent with the apex beat. If measuring the heart rate of children less than 2 years of age, a stethoscope should be placed over the apex of the heart and the beats counted for a full minute. Sinus tachycardia is common in the unwell anxious child, and further assessment should be carried out to identify the cause.

Blood Pressure (*Table 11.5*)

The size of the child's limb must be taken into consideration when taking blood pressure. Make sure the width of the blood pressure (BP) cuff is about two-thirds the length of the child's upper arm (Fig. 11.8). The BP cuff should encircle 90–100% of the upper arm circumference (but not more than 100%) (British Hypertension Society, 2017). A cuff that is too large may produce a reading that is too low; a cuff that is too small may give a false high reading (Cook and Montgomery, 2010).

Children in early shock may have a normal blood pressure reading initially; hypotension is often a late sign and preterminal sign of circulatory failure. Small quantitative changes in the child's blood pressure may indicate significant qualitative changes in the child's clinical condition. It is therefore imperative that accurate and current observations are taken into account when assessing the child's circulatory status.

Skin Perfusion and Body Temperature

The skin colour and temperature should be consistent over the trunk and limbs. Clinical signs of poor perfusion include peripherally cool skin, pallor, mottling, peripheral cyanosis and capillary refill >2 seconds. By the time central cyanosis is visible in acute respiratory distress, respiratory arrest

TABLE 11.4	**Normal Heart Rates**
Age (Years)	**Beats/min**
<1	110–160
2–5	95–140
5–12	80–120
>12	60–100

TABLE 11.5	**Systolic Blood Pressure by Age**
Age (Years)	**Systolic Blood Pressure**
<1	70–90
2–5	80–100
5–12	90–110
>12	100–120

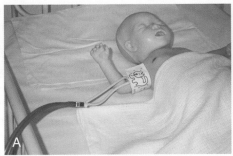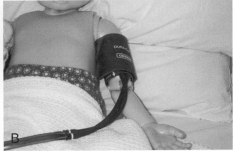

Fig. 11.8 Observation of a child's blood pressure. The Size of the BP cuff must be appropriate for the size of the child.

is very close. Capillary refill is a quick and easy method for determining the efficacy of respiratory function. A central capillary time is measured on the chest which is pressed for 5 seconds and the time taken for blood to return to the area is estimated in seconds. A capillary refill time of greater than 2 seconds in a child and 3 seconds in a neonate is a sign of poor oxygenation. Ambient temperature should always be considered in the interpretation of capillary refill.

The normal circadian range of an infant's temperatures over the 24-hour period has been described as ranging from 36°C at night to 37.8°C during active periods in the day (Table 11.6). In addition, there is now recognised that there is a variable fluctuation between individuals of 0.5°C (Mackowiak et al., 1992). Therefore we should accept individual variations in normal body temperature, recognising that time of day and age of child may affect expected normal values. Considering the variations in temperatures reported in the literature it may be more useful to consider temperature in terms of hypothermic, normothermic or fever (Table 11.7).

D: Disability

Parents are usually the first to recognise any changes in their child's level of consciousness and it is therefore important to listen to what they say. A hypoxic child may be irritable or agitated early on, but increasingly lethargic later. They might fail to recognise or interact, for example, maintain eye contact with the parents, or might not respond to stimuli, for example, unfamiliar nurses. A progressive drop in level of consciousness is a late sign of hypoxia and may be an indication of impending respiratory distress. Other factors that may lead to a decreasing level of consciousness are shock, sepsis, ingestion of depressants, metabolic abnormalities, hypothermia and head injuries. The level of consciousness should be assessed using the AVPU scale:

A – alert
V – responds to voice
P – responds to pain
U – unresponsive

Any problem with ABC must be addressed before assuming that a decrease in conscious level is due to a primary neurological problem.

The final but integral part of the child's assessment is their medical history. Factors to be taken into consideration include the following symptoms:

TABLE 11.6 Normal Variations in Temperature Related to Age

Age (years)	Temperature (°C)
<1	37.5–37.7
2–5	37.0–37.2
5–12	36.7–36.8
>12	36.6

TABLE 11.7 Temperature ranges

Classification	Neonates	Paediatrics*
Low temperature (or hypothermia)	<36.5°C	<36°C
Normothermia	36.5–37.5°C	36–37.5°C
Low grade fever (or normothermia)	37.6–37.9°C	37.6–37.9°C
Fever (or hyperthermia)	≥ 38°C	≥ 38°C

The Royal Childrens Hospital Melbourne (2019)

- Is the child breathless?
  - When? At rest, walking, talking, sleeping, feeding?
- Does the child have a cough?
  - What type?
  - How long has the child had this?
- When do the symptoms occur – daytime, night-time?
- Are the symptoms improving or worsening?
- Are there any aggravating or precipitating factors? Does anything relieve the symptoms?
- Are the symptoms associated with anything, for example, feeding? Is the child able to take feeds?
- How long has the child been unwell; has this happened suddenly; did it occur over time?
- Does the child have a sore throat?
- Is there any nasal discharge; has the child a cough; is the cough productive; what colour is the sputum; how long have these been present?
- Has the child's sleep been affected?
- Is the child's breathing noisy, in what way? Ask the parents to describe any noises they have heard.
- What has the child's activity level been like?
  Less specific symptoms to observe for include:
- pyrexia

TABLE 11.8   Terminology Used to Describe Different Patterns of Respiration

Term	Description
Tachypnoea	Increased rate
Bradypnoea	Decreased rate
Dyspnoea	Difficulty in breathing
Apnoea	Cessation or inability to breathe
Hypoventilation	Decreased and irregular depth of respirations
Hyperventilation	Increased rate and depth
Hypercapnia	Increased levels of carbon dioxide
Hypoxia	Low level of oxygenation
See-saw	Chest falls on inspiration and rises on expiration
Cheyne–Stokes	Altered rate and depth of respirations with periods of apnoea

- urinary output
- anorexia
- vomiting
- diarrhoea
- abdominal pain
- meningism

In addition, the family will be asked about the child's previous medical history, family and social history, environmental factors and developmental history including immunisation status. It is of interest to note that Elphick et al. (2001) found 'wheeze' to be a commonly chosen word used by parents to describe their child's noisy breathing. However, there was wide variation in what parents meant by this term, with many using the word inappropriately. The authors conclude that:

This highlights the need for accurate history taking, as parents' initial response may be to use words that they perceive as being a medical term. The responsibility lies with the doctor to ensure that interpretation of the language used by parents reflects accurately the noise they mean to describe (Elphick et al., 2001) (Table 11.8).

Summary

The diagnosis of acute respiratory disease in childhood is largely a clinical one. It rests on history and examination with the aid of chest radiograph when necessary. The clinical signs of respiratory failure include those demonstrating evidence of a significant increase in the work of breathing, for example, severe retractions or grunting, inadequate ventilation rate, apnoea or gasping, reduced or absent inspiratory breath sounds and alterations in level of consciousness and evidence of compromise in systemic perfusion, for example, significant tachycardia, bradycardia and extended capillary refill. Central cyanosis is a late sign of severe hypoxia and requires urgent treatment (NICE, 2015).

MANAGEMENT OF RESPIRATORY ILLNESS IN CHILDREN

The aims of the management of respiratory disease are applicable to all respiratory illnesses in addition to the disease-specific treatments. These aims of management are to:

- monitor the child's vital signs, effort and efficacy of breathing and effect of inadequate respiration, that is, oxygen saturations, colour and mental status;
- facilitate respiratory effort and maximise oxygen delivery to maintain O_2 saturations above 92%:
  - position the child for maximum comfort and to facilitate respiratory movements
  - decrease oxygen demand by reducing stress, minimal handling and fever
  - provide humidified and monitored supplemental oxygen by age-appropriate means, that is, head box for infants, mask for older children.
- minimise intrusive examinations and treatments;
- prevent complications such as hypoxia;
- promote hydration and prevent dehydration by utilising nasogastric or intravenous fluids to maintain adequate fluid intake;
- evaluate the effect of pyrexia on the child and administer antipyretics as appropriate;
- provide nutrition;
- instigate appropriate pharmacological interventions;
- communicate effectively with the child and family;
- provide psychological support for the child and family;
- provide opportunistic health education;
- prevent spread of infection;
- provide clear and explicit discharge advice.

RESPIRATORY INFECTION

Infections of the respiratory tract are described in a number of ways depending on the area of involvement (Fig. 11.9). However, the infections tend to spread from one area to another because of the continuous nature of the mucous membrane that lines the respiratory tract and the shorter distance between the anatomical structures in children. In addition, the short, open eustachian tube allows easy access to the middle ear. Infections of the respiratory tract may therefore involve more than one structure.

The largest percentage of infections accounting for acute illness in children is caused by viruses. Infants under 3 months of age have a lower infection rate, which then rises between the ages of 3 and 6 months and remains high through the toddler years. However, by the age of 5 years viral infections are less frequent, although the incidence of *Mycoplasma pneumoniae* and group B streptococcal infections rises.

Upper Respiratory Tract Infection

The average child has between four and twelve upper respiratory tract infections a year and 90% of these are viral, requiring symptomatic management only. Of the remaining 10%, group B haemolytic streptococcus is common and requires treatment with penicillin. However, we should always remain vigilant for the possibility that a child with a mild upper respiratory tract infection may have an accompanying illness such as meningitis.

Whooping Cough

Pertussis or whooping cough is a highly infectious, acute respiratory infection caused by *Bordetella pertussis*. It occurs mainly in non-immunised children. However, a previously infected

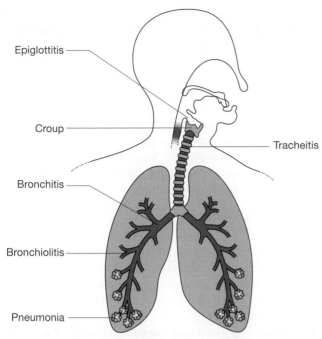

Fig. 11.9 Anatomic location of respiratory infections.

person can become re-infected with pertussis, but subsequent infections are usually less severe. Although vaccination does not always prevent infection, it usually attenuates the disease (Public Health England [PHE], 2016).

Characteristics of whooping cough (Waters and Halperin, 2010) are as follows in three key stages:

- Stage 1: Catarrhal Phase
  Lasting 1–2 weeks; conjunctivitis, malaise, sore throat and dry, unproductive cough.
- Stage 2: Paroxysmal Phase
  Commencing around 1 week after stage 1; lasting between 1 and 6 weeks; characterised by episodes of coughing, usually reasonably well between episodes and undisturbed sleep.
- Stage 3: Convalescent Phase
  Lasts up to 3 months and sees a gradual improvement in cough frequency and severity.

The name of the infection is derived from the characteristic 'whoop' that occurs, which is caused by sharp inhalation of breath during bouts of paroxysmal cough. In young infants, the 'whoop' may be absent and coughing spasms may be followed by periods of apnoea and/or cyanosis (NICE, 2017a).

Specific treatment. The management of whooping cough includes administration of antimicrobial therapy, if the onset of cough is within the previous 21 days. A macrolide antibiotic is the first-line recommended treatment, for example, clarithromycin (NICE, 2017a; PHE, 2016), as this may reduce the period of infectivity. However, it does not alter the course of the illness. Household and other close contacts should also be treated and individuals should be advised to rest, take adequate fluids and use paracetamol or ibuprofen for symptomatic relief (NICE, 2017a).

Croup Syndromes

Croup is a general term that applies to any condition producing inspiratory stridor. Stridor is a harsh vibratory sound

caused by partial obstruction of the upper airway. Croup syndromes include laryngotracheobronchitis (LTB), spasmodic croup, bacterial tracheitis and epiglottitis. LTB and croup are often used synonymously.

LTB is common cause of upper airway obstruction in children and is usually mild, but sometimes can be serious (British Medical Journal [BMJ], 2017a). It is an acute inflammation of the upper and lower respiratory tract. The symptoms are initially in the larynx causing stridor and then in the trachea and bronchi leading to a cough and wheeze that occurs in around 3% of children aged 6 months to 3 years, usually occurring in the winter months. The peak incidence is during the second year of life with boys more affected than girls (Johnson, 2014).

Characteristics of croup. Croup is usually preceded by an upper respiratory tract infection:
- Rhinorrhoea
- Coryza
- Low-grade fever
- Sudden onset – often at night
- Lethargy and fatigue
  It presents with:
- inspiratory stridor
- barking cough
- harsh cry/hoarseness
  If obstruction is severe there is:
- tachypnoea
- stridor
- intercostal, supraclavicular, substernal and suprasternal inspiratory retractions
  As the condition worsens there is:
- cyanosis
- increased respiratory effort
- restlessness
- reduced stridulous sound and asynchronous chest wall and abdominal movements (NICE, 2017b)

These symptoms are a result of oedema of the larynx and trachea. They are usually triggered by recent infection with the parainfluenza virus, although other pathogens can be involved (respiratory syncytial virus, adenovirus, enterovirus and rhinovirus).

Specific treatment.
- Maintain airway; less than 5% require intubation and this is usually due to gradual deterioration rather than acute obstruction.
- Nebulised and/or oral glucocorticoids – usually nebulised budesonide and oral dexamethasone.
- Inhaled steroids reduce upper airway oedema, which has a rapid and sustained effect.
- Nebulised adrenaline has been shown to provide temporary relief to patients with croup, but is not thought to have long-term benefits (BMJ, 2017a; NICE, 2017b).

⚓ ACTIVITY

Review Poiseuille's law and consider the effect of a distressed child with a more turbulent airflow.

EVIDENCE-BASED PRACTICE

Cold humidified air (mist therapy) is not effective in improving clinical symptoms in children with moderate croup. Discuss.

 WWW

Childhood immunisation: familiarise yourself with the guidance notes for professionals:
- https://assets.publishing.service.gov.uk/government/uploads/system/uploads/attachment_data/file/699392/Complete_immunisation_schedule_april2018.pdf

Epiglottitis

This is mainly seen in children aged 2–5 years, however it can manifest at any age (BMJ, 2017b). The infection is usually caused by *Haemophilus influenzae* B and the condition is becoming rare as a result of the introduction of the HIB immunisation of infants (NICE, 2017b; Guardiani et al (2010)).

Characteristics of epiglottitis (BMJ, 2017b):
- Sore throat
- Short history
- Fever
- Stridor
- Dyspnoea
- Systemically unwell: pale, toxic, lethargic
- May drool and be unable to swallow but have minimal cough
- Child often adopts the characteristic posture of sitting upright, mouth open and their chin thrust forward, known as tripod positioning
- Extreme anxiety

The infection causes inflammatory oedema of the supraglottic area, increasing airway resistance, and narrowing the supraglottic aperture. The glottis is not normally inflamed as the process affects the supraglottic structures. Further compromise can occur from secretions, potentially resulting in complete airway obstruction (BMJ, 2017b). If the condition is suspected, examination of the mouth must be avoided because acute or total airway obstruction could result. The child should be examined only with an experienced anaesthetist ready to intubate if required. Most children require intubation, whereas only 20% of adults require this procedure (BMJ, 2017b). Do not lie the child down, because this forces the epiglottis to fall backwards, leading to complete airway obstruction. Radiography of the neck is justified only if diagnosis is in doubt and should take place only if the child is stable; radiography in lateral position may also precipitate respiratory arrest due to complete airway obstruction. It is also not advisable to perform any procedure that may increase the child's anxiety (e.g. taking a blood specimen) as this could precipitate airway spasm and cause death (BMJ, 2017b).

Specific treatment. If epiglottitis is suspected, then emergency intubation should be performed to protect the airway, ideally in the operating theatre environment (BMJ, 2017b). Intravenous antibiotics are required immediately following intubation; empiric regimes include ampicillin and ceftriaxone combinations (BMJ, 2017b). Recovery is usually rapid once the airway is established and antibiotic therapy given.

Apnoea

Temporary cessation of breathing can be the result of central respiratory depression or from mechanical obstruction. It can occur in the first 2 days of infections, particularly respiratory syncytial virus and pertussis (NICE, 2017a). When apnoea is associated with cyanosis or unconsciousness then possible causes that need to be considered are seizures, congenital heart disease or airway obstruction.

Aspirated Foreign Body

Usually occurs in toddlers who are mobile and put small objects in their mouths. Small beads, coins and foodstuffs are the most common objects aspirated. Peanuts are the most dangerous because they swell in the airway, becoming firmly embedded and difficult to remove because they fragment. Initially, the child may suffer from acute choking, but the aspiration of a foreign body may not be recognised. Obstruction may be complete or incomplete. Incomplete obstruction usually allows the passage of air either in both directions or one only. Complete obstruction prevents either inspiration or expiration (BMJ, 2017c).

Characteristics of aspirated foreign body:
- Acute onset
- Respiratory distress
- Wheeze and unilateral decreased breathing sounds
- Persistent cough
- Asymmetry of chest
- Mediastinal shift
- Dull percussion if collapse has occurred (BMJ, 2017c)

Specific treatment. A bronchoscopy under general anaesthetic to remove the foreign body is required. It is important that this is performed as soon as possible to prevent coughing, moving the object back up into the trachea, which may lead to more severe obstruction of the airway (BMJ, 2017c).

 ACTIVITY

Look at your local health education literature to find the advice given to parents regarding suitable toys for toddlers, and first aid in the event of aspiration of a foreign body.

 WWW

Read the advice from the Child Accident Prevention Trust:
- http://www.capt.org.uk

Bronchiolitis

This condition is the most common cause of severe respiratory infection in infancy, usually occurring in the winter months. It is a viral infection with 75% of cases due to respiratory syncytial virus; other pathogens implicated include adenovirus, parainfluenza and rhinovirus. It occurs predominantly in children under 1 year, peaking between 3 and 6 months. One in three infants will develop bronchiolitis and 2%–3% of these require hospitalisation (NICE, 2015). By the age of 2 years 90% of children are immune to respiratory syncytial virus. In 2011/2012 in England there were 30,451 secondary care admissions for the management of bronchiolitis. Between 2015/16 to 2017/18 the emergency admission rate for children under 2 years per population was 3281.6 per 100,000 population in England (Public Health England, 2020). In 2009/2010 there were 72 recorded deaths of children from bronchiolitis, within 90 days of hospital admission (NICE, 2015). Variations in admissions for children with bronchiolitis may reflect epidemiological factors including:

- socio-economic deprivation
- being born prematurely
- maternal tobacco smoking during pregnancy
- household tobacco-smoking status

The infection causes inflammatory obstruction of the small airways and necrosis of the cells lining the lower airways. The ciliary damage impairs the clearance of secretions and this combined with increased mucosal secretion, submucosal oedema and desquamation of cells results in obstruction at the bronchiolar level with atelectasis and hyperinflation. The child is often able to inhale, but has difficulty exhaling. Air becomes trapped below the obstruction and interferes with gaseous exchange. Hypoxia and in severe cases hypercapnia may occur.

Characteristics of bronchiolitis (NICE, 2015). Diagnoses of bronchiolitis should occur if the child has coryzal prodrome lasting 1–3 days, followed by tachypnoea, recession or both, accompanied with either a wheeze or crackles on chest auscultation.

- Initial coryza
- Fever
- Tachycardia
- Tachypnoea
- Irregular breathing, recurrent apnoea
- Cough
- Subcostal and intercostal recession
- Irritability
- Poor feeding and oral intake
- Widespread wheeze and crepitations
- Hyperventilated chest
- Cyanosis/pallor

Apnoea may occur without other clinical signs and in cases of such presentation, consideration of a diagnosis of bronchiolitis must occur (NICE, 2015).

The typical appearance of a baby with acute bronchiolitis is therefore one of:

- marked breathlessness
- rapid respirations
- distressing cough
- retraction of lower ribs and sternum
- wheezing depending on degree of airway obstruction

Many infants with bronchiolitis can be managed at home; however, careful assessment is required in deciding which infants need hospitalisation. The National Institute for Clinical Excellence (2015) guidelines for the management of bronchiolitis recognise that a respiratory rate of >60/min,

and a fluid or breastfeeding intake of less than 75% of usual volume, or presentation of clinical dehydration requires hospitalisation (Table 11.9).

Emergency hospital admission is required if severe respiratory distress is present, a respiratory rate of >70/min, apnoea, central cyanosis and O_2 saturations that are persistently less than 92%. Oxygen supplementation is required in these children and fluid intake should be supplemented via nasogastric or oral gastric routes if fluid requirements cannot be achieved by mouth (NICE, 2015).

Specific treatment.
- Because of the risk of apnoea, small infants should be nursed using apnoea monitors or O_2 saturation monitors.
- Antibiotics, bronchodilators and steroids have no positive effect on this condition (NICE, 2015).
- Some infants (2%) suffer recurrent apnoea attacks, exhaustion or hypercapnia and hypoxia, and require mechanical ventilation.

REFLECT ON YOUR PRACTICE

What advice have you witnessed being given to children's families regarding the spread of RSV?

ACTIVITY

Review the effect of a raised temperature on an infant's metabolic rate and oxygen requirements.
- Why is this important in infants with bronchiolitis?

POWERPOINT

Emma's scenario is repeated on the companion PowerPoint presentation. Work through it here or on the PowerPoint. Answers are provided at the end of the chapter or on the presentation.

SCENARIO

Emma is 3 months old; she is admitted to the assessment ward accompanied by her anxious parents. The GP visited her at home and organised for an emergency admission.

Emma has had a runny nose for 2 days and is off her feeds. She has felt hot since yesterday evening and over the past few hours she has become quite pale. However, her mother reports that Emma is not as irritable as last night and has at last stopped crying:

- What framework would you utilise to assess Emma's physiological status?
- What observations do you need to carry out?
- What would you expect these observations to be?
- Would you categorise Emma's present condition as mild, moderate or severe?
- Is there any information in the history given that would cause concern?
- What care would you expect to be initiated?
- What ongoing care would Emma require?

TABLE 11.9   Assessment of Illness Severity

Clinical Parameter	SEVERITY	
	Mild	Moderate to Severe
Activity level	Alert	Reduced level of consciousness, exhausted or fatigued
Heart rate	<140/min	>140/min
Respiratory rate	<50/min	>50/min
Oxygen saturation	>92%	<92%
Temperature	<380	>380
Recession	Mild	Marked
Nasal flaring	None	Some
Feeding	Taking three-quarters or more than half of normal feeds	Taking less than one-half of normal feeds
Colour	Pink	Pallor, mottling, cyanosed or grey
Level of hydration	Normal	Evidence of dehydration
Apnoea	None	Temp in chart is 38 °C, history of apnoea
Capillary refill	<2 s	>2 seconds

Lower Respiratory Tract Infection

Pneumonia

Pneumonia is an infection of the lower respiratory tract most commonly due to bacterial or viral pathogens, such as RSV, parainfluenza and influenza. Pneumonia can be classified according to its anatomical distribution:

- Lobar pneumonia occurs when there is involvement of a large portion of or an entire lobe of a lung.
- In bronchopneumonia there is patchy consolidation involving several lobes of the lungs.
- Interstitial pneumonia involves the walls surrounding the alveoli and bronchioles; this type of pneumonia is usually caused by viral or mycoplasmal infections (Forster et al., 2004).

Pneumonia is also classified by the infective pathogen, for example, streptococcus or mycoplasma. The incidence of bacterial pneumonia is highest amongst children less than 2 years of age, with boys affected more than girls (2:1 ratio) (Clark et al., 2007). Viral infections with RSV are also common in this age group; this is the most common cause of viral pneumonia. Children who were born prematurely, are chronically sick or have congenital abnormalities are at greater risk (BTS, 2011). NICE (2013) guidelines on the management of fever advise practitioners to consider pneumonia in children who present with a fever, tachypnoea, crackles in chest, nasal flaring, recession, cyanosis and oxygen saturations of less than 95% in air.

Bronchopneumonia

This condition occurs in young children and older children with chronic conditions that affect their respiratory function

(Meadow and Newell, 2002). A large number of different organisms can be responsible. Bronchopneumonia usually follows another respiratory illness such as bronchiolitis, whooping cough or viral infection.

Characteristics of bronchopneumonia (Meadow and Newell, 2002):

- Tachypnoea
- Dry cough initially, then productive with purulent sputum
- Fever
- Fretfulness
- Intercostal/subcostal recession
- Grunting in infants
- Nasal flaring
- Generalised crepitations
- Cyanosis in severe cases

Lobar pneumonia

Lobar pneumonia accounts for 17.6% of cases (Clark et al., 2007) and around 90% of cases of lobar pneumonia are caused by *Streptococcus pneumoniae*.

Characteristics of lobar pneumonia (Meadow and Newell, 2002):

- Sudden illness
- High fever
- Flushed
- Tachypnoea
- Cyanosis in severe cases
- Respiratory distress
- Intercostal/subcostal recession
- Grunting in infants
- Nasal flaring
- Pleuritic pain – child leans forward towards affected side
- May have referred pain in abdomen or shoulder tip

Specific Treatment

All children with a clear diagnosis of pneumonia should receive antibiotics as bacterial and viral pneumonia cannot reliably be distinguished from one another (BTS, 2011). Supplementary oxygen should be administered if saturation levels are below 92%. Nasogastric tubes can compromise breathing; however if they cannot be avoided, the smallest tube should be passed down the smallest nostril. Careful monitoring of fluid intake must occur, and fluid therapy should occur if individuals cannot maintain the required intake due to breathlessness or vomiting. Physiotherapy is no longer considered beneficial in children with pneumonia.

SEMINAR DISCUSSION TOPIC

There is an increased risk of pneumonia in the first year of life if parents smoke.
- What other potential health risks are there to children in a smoking household?
- Should smoking be banned completely?

Tuberculosis

The Incidence of TB in children has been decreasing since 2007, both in UK born and non UK born children, although there was a slight rise in 2019. Rates in UK born children of Black African and South Asian ethnicities were 9-14 times higher than for children of white ethnicities.

In 2019, 169 children (<15 years) were notified with TB in England, a rate of 1.7 per 100,000 (95% CI 1.1-1.6). This rate was slightly higher than in 2018 and is the first increase following an annual decline since 2012 (Public Health England 2020).

TB is a curable infectious disease caused by bacteria, spread by droplets containing the bacteria, by someone who is infected with TB. Most children are infected by someone close to them but outbreaks also occur in other meeting places, such as schools.

Common presenting symptoms (World Health Organization [WHO], 2014):
- Cough and respiratory symptoms
- Mild dyspnoea
- Weight loss and anorexia failure to thrive
- Fever may occur
- Fatigue and reduced playfulness

These are gradual in onset and increase in severity as the disease progresses. Investigations include chest radiography, tuberculin test, and sputum testing. Careful history, exposure and contact with the source must be taken. Treatment is by antituberculosis drugs for between 6 months to 1 year, depending on the associated complications, under the care of a clinician with experience in tuberculosis care.

ASTHMA

The changes in prevalence of asthma in children are difficult to determine because of changes in diagnostic practice, but however defined, asthma and wheezing in children has increased dramatically over the past few decades and is the most common long-term medical condition in the UK (RCPCH, 2017). Asthma is thought to affect between 10% and 11% of children in the UK. The UK has one of the highest prevalences for emergency admission and death rates in childhood asthma in Europe (RCPCH, 2017). This increase is thought to be due to environmental factors (RCPCH, 2017). It is difficult to diagnose asthma in the very young because it is hard to distinguish between asthma and other causes of wheezing. Epidemiological studies suggest that up to 30% of all children under the age of 3 years have had an acute episode of wheezing (BTS, 2016). This makes asthma the most common medical condition of childhood. In 2016, 1410 people died from asthma (adults and children) in the UK due to asthma (Office for National Statistics, 2017); 80% of these are thought to be preventable.

Asthma is a chronic inflammatory condition of the airways, the cause of which is still not completely understood. Asthma is described as, 'airway obstruction that is reversible, airway inflammation and increased airway responsiveness to a variety of stimuli'.

The aetiology of asthma is multi-factorial (BTS, 2016). There is often a family history of atopy, asthma or allergies, and in addition to this, there are precipitating factors such as infection, allergic triggers, tobacco smoke or physical or emotional stress. Some of the possible reasons for an exacerbation of an asthma attack are:
- Predisposing factors (NICE, 2013)
  - a strong genetic factor
  - maternal smoking
  - not breast-fed for the first 4 months of life
  - family atopy
- Indoor triggers
  - allergy to house-dust mite
  - allergy to animal dander
  - tobacco smoke
  - moulds and fungal spores from *Aspergillus fumigatus*
- Outdoor triggers
  - allergy to pollen
  - cold weather
  - air pollutants
  - industrial chemicals
- Other possible triggers
  - viral infection
  - exercise
  - food allergies
  - stress, emotion and laughing.

Use of paracetamol in the first year of life and in later childhood is associated with risk of asthma, rhinoconjunctivitis, and eczema at age 6 to 7 years (Beasley et al., 2008).

Asthma is a hyper-responsiveness of the airways induced by a trigger (Akers, 2015). It commonly presents as a lower airway obstruction; the wheezing is generated by turbulent airflow causing oscillation of the bronchial wall. Three factors are involved in the asthmatic response:
1. Bronchospasm
   - narrowing of the bronchial walls due to contraction of the smooth muscle;
   - more severe in the smaller bronchi and bronchioles, where there is no cartilage in the walls.
2. Inflammation
   - causes the airways to become hyper-responsive and narrow easily in reaction to a wide range of stimuli;
   - further narrowing of the airways by the invasion of the mucosa, submucosa and muscle tissue by inflammatory cells.
3. Inflammatory cells
   - mainly eosinophils, but also contain neutrophils macrophages and mast cells;
   - contain chemical mediators, including histamine, prostaglandins and leukotrienes, which cause vasodilation and increased capillary permeability;
   - result in mucus production and oedema.

The lumen of the airways is therefore narrowed by contraction of the smooth muscle, mucosal oedema and the hypersecretion of mucus (Fig. 11.10) (Akers, 2015).

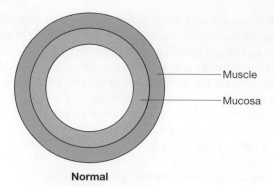

Normal

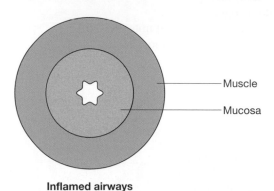

Inflamed airways

Fig. 11.10 The asthma response.

SCENARIO

It is 6 pm and Jason, a 12-year-old boy, is to be admitted to the children's ward. His mother is with him. Jason is a known asthmatic and he is prescribed regular medication. He was sent home from school earlier in the day with an acute exacerbation of his asthma. He is breathless and unable to carry out a conversation:

- What additional equipment would you get ready prior to Jason's arrival on the ward?
- When they arrive, what questions would you ask Jason and his mother?
- What observations would you carry out?
- What are the normal ranges for these observations for a child this age?
- What medications should have been administered during the day?
- What treatment should be given?
- What advice should be given to Jason and his mother before discharge from hospital?

Characteristics of Severe Asthma

- Too breathless to talk
- Chest recession/use of accessory muscles
- Respiratory rate >40 breaths/min (children aged between 1 and 5 years) or respiratory rate >30 breaths/min (children 5 years and over)
- Heart rate >140 beats/min (children aged between 1 and 5 years) or >125 beats/min (children 5 years and over)
- Peak flow reduced to between 33% and 50% of (best or predicted)

- Wheezing may or may not be a prominent feature
- Use of accessory muscles of respiration
- Spo_2 less than 92%
  British Thoracic Society (BTS) (2019).

Characteristics of Life-Threatening Asthma

- Conscious level depression
- Agitation or confusion
- Exhaustion
- Poor respiratory effort
- Cyanosis
- Oxygen saturation levels <92% in air
- Silent chest
- Peak expiratory flow rate (PEF) <33% (best or predicted)
- Hypotension
  British Thoracic Society (BTS) (2019).

There are two phases of the asthmatic response (Akers, 2015). The first phase occurs within minutes of the exposure to the stimuli, reaches a peak in about 30 minutes and subsides after approximately 2 hours. It includes oedema, mucus secretion and bronchospasm-induced wheezing. The second phase occurs about 4–12 hours after the exposure; it reaches a peak after about 4–8 hours, but can last for more than 24 hours. This inflammatory reaction can lead to damage of lung tissue. The airways are hypersensitive to allergic stimulation in this phase, which can result in further inflammation and bronchoconstriction.

🌐 WWW

Read the most recent audits on the prevalence of asthma in the UK:
- https://www.asthma.org.uk/about/media/facts-and-statistics

Principles of Asthma Management

The initial treatment of acute asthma Children with life-threatening asthma or Spo_2 levels includes (NICE, 2013):
- beta 2 agonists are recognised as the first line treatment.
- Pre-measured dose inhaler (PMDI) and spacer use are the preferred options in children with mild to moderate asthma.
- Individualised drug dosing should be administered according to severity of symptoms and patient response.
- If symptoms are refractory to beta 2 agonist medications, practitioners should add ipratropium bromide 250 micrograms mixed with the beta 2 agonist solution.
- Repeated doses of ipratropium should be given early to treat children who are poorly responsive to beta 2 agonists.
- Consider adding 150 mg magnesium sulphate to each nebulised salbutamol and ipratropium in the first hour in children with a short duration of acute severe asthma symptoms presenting with an SpO_2 <92%. (BTS, 2019).
- Discontinue long acting beta 2 agonists when short acting are required more than 4 hourly.

The early use of steroids is recommended; therefore oral soluble prednisolone should be given early in the attack, as it can prevent the relapse of symptoms and reduce the need for hospital admission; up to 3 days is normally sufficient. Magnesium sulphate may be considered (BTS, 2019).

Intravenous drugs may be necessary because inhaled drugs are not effective during severe asthmatic attacks because the airways are completely obstructed by inflammation and mucus (Akers, 2015). ECG monitoring should be used if frequent doses of nebulised salbutamol or intravenous salbutamol are given.

In cases of severe or life-threatening asthma, which is not responding to beta 2 agonists and steroids, then aminophylline can be given in a high dependency setting (BTS, 2016).

Children may require intravenous fluids to avoid dehydration if severe asthma is prolonged and they are not tolerating oral fluids.

Humidified oxygen may be required to maintain the child's oxygen saturation. The method of oxygen administration chosen depends on the child's age and condition. Transcutaneous measurement of oxygen saturation is used for continuous oxygen assessment if the child is hypoxic, so that oxygen therapy can be titrated against the oxygen saturation levels. Arterial blood gas monitoring may be necessary if the child shows signs of severe respiratory distress; this will help determine if the child is in respiratory failure and needs respiratory support. If necessary, assisted ventilation using endotracheal intubation may be used for a short period of time, usually 8–12 hours.

 POWERPOINT

Access the companion PowerPoint presentation.

The decision to admit the child to hospital or to discharge the child home is often difficult. Children can be discharged when stable on 3–4 hourly inhaled bronchodilators that can by continued at home. PEF should be >75% of best or predicted and Spo_2 >94%. Follow-up should be arranged by primary care services within two working days and follow up in a paediatric asthma clinic within 1–2 months. Clear guidelines are available from (BTS. 2019).

 WWW

Read the guide produced by NICE at:
- http://www.nice.org.uk
  Look up the resources for children with asthma to help gain their compliance:
- https://www.asthma.org.uk/advice/resources/#children

DISCUSSION OF THE SCENARIOS

Bronchiolitis Scenario: Emma

What framework would you utilise to assess Emma's physiological status?

Assessment follows the ABC criteria for assessment in conjunction with neurological observations and provides a framework for rapid and effective nursing assessment of the child with respiratory problems. The survey should therefore include assessment of:
- airway
- breathing
- circulation
- disability

What observations do you need to carry out?
- Vital signs: temperature, pulse and respiration. Remember that normal vital signs are not always appropriate when a child is seriously ill; indeed a normal heart rate and respiratory rate may indicate cardiopulmonary arrest is imminent.
- Respiratory rates: should be measured over a full minute.
- Assessment of breathing: involves examination of the chest including observation of respiratory movements, number, rhythm, depth and quality of respirations, and character of breath sounds utilising the skills of palpation, auscultation and percussion.
- Remember that the degree of recession gives an indication of the severity of the breathing difficulty and nasal flaring is a further sign of increased work of breathing. A resting rate of greater than 60 breaths/min is a sign of respiratory distress in a child irrespective of age and an oxygen saturation of less than 92% while breathing air is low.
- The child's heart rate and pulse volume should be assessed by palpating both central and peripheral pulses for 1 minute. The skin colour and temperature should be consistent over the trunk and limbs. Clinical signs of poor perfusion include peripherally cool skin, pallor, mottling, peripheral cyanosis and capillary refill >2 seconds. Remember that by the time central cyanosis is visible in acute respiratory distress, respiratory arrest is very close.

What would you expect these observations to be?
- Mum reports Emma as struggling to get her breath and you count her respirations as 52 breaths/min.
- Her peripheral temperature is 38°C.
- Her pulse is 155 beats/min on an apex recording.
- Her oxygen saturations are 90% in air.
- She has marked recession and nasal flaring.
- She is pale and her capillary refill time is 3 seconds.

Would you categorise Emma's present condition as mild, moderate or severe?

Most likely she would be classed as severe because her pulse rate is above 140/min, her oxygen saturations are below 92% in air, she has marked recession and nasal flaring. She has also become pale and stopped crying, which may be an indication of fatigue.

Is there any information in the history given that would cause concern?

Emma has not been eating for 2 days. You need to ask exactly how much feed she has taken. You also need to ask when she last had a wet nappy and assess if her anterior fontanelle is sunken. You are assessing her state of hydration. She has had a reduced fluid intake, a raised temperature and fewer wet nappies, therefore you would expect her to be dehydrated. If you cannot remember how to classify dehydration, please review this now.

Emma has stopped crying, which may indicate that she is becoming fatigued and that her decreased oxygen saturation is altering her mental status. You would need to assess her against the AVPU scale.

What care would you expect to be initiated?

- Regular observations of vital signs and capillary refill, continuous monitoring of oxygen saturations.
- Humidified and monitored oxygen therapy.
- Obtain a specimen of nasopharyngeal aspirate to determine cause of bronchiolitis.
- Nursing assessment of state of hydration to include amount of feed taken, urine output, temperature of peripheries, peripheral pulses, skin turgor, temperature gap, capillary refill time, state of mucous membranes and specific gravity of urine.
- Assessment of ability to feed orally and care planned accordingly to progress to either orogastric/nasogastric or intravenous fluids as condition determines.
- If oral feeding continues then reduce feed volume and increase frequency offered as condition determines returning to normal feeds and frequency as condition improves.
- If oral feeding discontinues then commence mouth care.
- If intravenous fluids are initiated then commence care of intravenous infusion and intravenous cannula site.
- Monitor urine output. Minimum required for an infant is 2 mL/kg/h. Weigh nappies before and after use; 1 g = 1 mL.
- Manage fever as appropriate. Remember that an increase in temperature raises basic metabolic rate and increases oxygen demand.
- Prevent spread of infection.

What ongoing care would Emma require?

Continuation of all above care and in addition:

- minimal handling
- care of family to include all aspects of family-centred care
- education of family regarding ongoing care needs at home
- discharge planning including outpatient appointment, health visitor liaison and referral to community team as appropriate, discharge summary, completion of health visitor red book, medication and provision of written information/advice

Asthma Scenario: Jason

What additional equipment would you get ready prior to Jason's arrival on the ward?

- Oxygen
- Nebuliser
- Oxygen saturation monitor
- Equipment for intravenous therapy
- Extra pillows

When they arrive, what questions would you ask Jason and his mother?

- What is his normal medication?
- What medication has he taken today, how frequently and when was it last given?
- What may have triggered this attack?
- Is his condition worsening or improving?
- How long has been breathless?
- Has he been in hospital recently for asthma?
- Response to treatment previously?
- How much has he had to drink today?

What observations would you carry out?

- Vital signs: temperature, pulse and respirations. Remember that normal vital signs are not always appropriate when a child is seriously ill; indeed a normal heart rate and respiratory rate may indicate cardiopulmonary arrest is imminent.
- Respiratory rates: should be measured over a full minute.
- Assessment of breathing involves examination of the chest including observation of respiratory movements, number, rhythm, depth and quality of respirations, and character of breath sounds. The child's inability to speak is a relevant factor when assessing their respiratory distress.
- Remember that the degree of recession gives an indication of the severity of the breathing difficulty and nasal flaring is a further sign of increased work of breathing. A resting rate of >60 breaths/min is a sign of respiratory distress in a child irrespective of age and an oxygen saturation of less than 92% while breathing air is low.
- The child's heart rate and pulse volume should be assessed by palpating both central and peripheral pulses for 1 minute. The skin colour and temperature should be consistent over the trunk and limbs. Clinical signs of poor perfusion include peripherally cool skin, pallor, mottling, peripheral cyanosis and capillary refill >2 seconds. Remember by the time central cyanosis is visible in acute respiratory distress, respiratory arrest is very close.
- The child's level of consciousness should be noted. Is the child agitated or becoming lethargic?

What are the normal ranges for these observations for a child this age?

- Normal respiratory rate 15–20 breaths/min
- Normal heart rate 80–120 beats/min
- Temperature 36.6°C–36.8°C
- Oxygen saturation level 95%–98%
- Capillary refill <2 seconds

What medications should have been administered during the day?

What treatment should be given?

- Continue oxygen via face-mask or nasal prongs.
- If required give intravenous hydrocortisone.

- Monitor Jason's vital signs.
- Position Jason for maximum comfort.
- Prepare for intravenous cannulation and infusion.
- Provide psychological support for Jason and his mother.

What advice should be given to Jason and his mother before discharge from hospital?

The following answers are based on British Thoracic Society Guidelines Network (British Thoracic Society (BTS), 2016):

- Continue with beta 2 agonist as prescribed.
- Continue with oral prednisolone for up to 3 days.
- Contact GP if asthma not controlled on prescribed treatment.
- Provided written asthma action plan.
- Check inhaler technique.
- Arrange GP follow-up.

REFERENCES

Advanced Life Support Group, 2016. Advanced Paediatric Life Support: A Practical Approach, sixth ed. Wiley and Blackwell, Oxford.

Akers, 2015. The respiratory system. In: Peate, I., Gormley-Fleming, E. (Eds.), Fundamentals of Children's Anatomy and Physiology. E Wiley Blackwell, Chichester, pp. 216–231.

Beasley, R., Clayton, T., Crane, J., et al., 2008. Association between paracetamol use in infancy and childhood, and risk of asthma, rhinoconjunctivitis, and eczema in children aged 6–7 years: analysis from Phase Three of the ISAAC programme. Lancet 372, 1039–1048.

British Hypertension Society, (2017). https://bihsoc.org/wp-content/uploads/2017/11/GOSH-BP-flowsheet-Children-E-Brennan-May-2017-1.pdf accessed 2/12/20.

British Medical Journal, 2017a. Best Practice Croup. Available from: https://bestpractice.bmj.com/topics/en-gb/681.

British Medical Journal, 2017b. Best Practice Epiglottitis. Available from: https://bestpractice.bmj.com/topics/en-gb/452.

British Medical Journal, 2017c. Best Practice Foreign Body Aspiration. Available from: https://bestpractice.bmj.com/topics/en-gb/653.

British Thoracic Society (BTS), 2011. British Thoracic Society guidelines for the management of community acquired pneumonia in childhood. Thorax 66 (Suppl. 2), 11–23.

British Thoracic Society (BTS), 2016. British Guideline on the management of asthma. A national clinical guideline. Available from: www.sign.ac.uk.

British Thoracic Society, 2019. SIGN 158 British Guideline on the Management of Asthma. https://www.brit-thoracic.org.uk/quality-improvement/guidelines/asthma/ accessed 3/12/20.

Child Health Committee, 1997. The Specific Health Needs of Children and Young People. 2nd report. Child Health Committee, London.

Clark, J.E., Hammal, D., Hampton, F., et al., 2007. Epidemiology of community-acquired pneumonia in children seen in hospital. Epidemiol. Infect. 135, 262e9.

Cook, K., Montgomery, H., 2010. Assessment. In: Trigg, E., Mohammed, T.A. (Eds.), Practices in Children's Nursing. Churchill Livingstone Elsevier, London, pp. 67–80.

Crawford, D., 2011. Understanding childhood asthma and the development of the respiratory tract. Nurs. Child. Young People 23 (7), 25–34.

Elphick, H.E., Sherlock, P., Foxall, G., et al., 2001. Survey of respiratory sounds in infants. Arch. Dis. Child. 84, 34–39.

Fendrick, A., Monto, A.S., Nightengale, B., Sarnes, M., 2003. The economic burden of non-influenza-related viral respiratory tract infection in the United States. Arch. Intern. Med. 163, 487–494.

Forster, J., Ihorst, G., Rieger, C.H., et al., 2004. Prospective population-based study of viral lower respiratory tract infections in children under 3 years of age (the PRIDE study). Eur. J. Pediatr. 163, 709e16.

Guardiani, E., Bliss, M., Harley, E., 2010. Supraglottitis in the era following widespread immunization against Haemophilus influenzae type B: evolving principles in diagnosis and management. Laryngoscope Nov120 (11), 2183–2188. https://doi.org/10.1002/lary.21083.

Hay, A.D., Heron, J., Ness, A., ALSPAC study team, 2005. The prevalence of symptoms and consultations in pre-school children in the Avon Longitudinal Study of Parents and Children (ALSPAC): a prospective cohort study. Fam. Pract. 22, 367–374.

Johnson, D., 2014. Croup. BMJ Clinical Evidence 09, pii 0321.

Mackowiak, P., Wasserman, S.S., Levine, M.M., 1992. A critical appraisal of 98.6°F the upper limit of the normal body temperature and other legacies of carl Carl Reinhold August Wunderlich. J. Am. Med. Assoc. 268, 1578–1580.

Meadow, R., Newell, S., 2002. Lecture Notes in Paediatrics, seventh ed. Blackwell Science, Oxford.

Mighten, J., 2011. Children's Respiratory Nursing. John Wiley and Sons Inc.

Morton, R.J., Phillips, B.M., 1992. Accidents and Emergencies in Children. Oxford University Press, Oxford.

National Institute for Clinical Excellence (NICE), 2013. Asthma Quality Standard. Available from: https://www.nice.org.uk/guidance/QS25.

National Institute for Clinical Excellence (NICE), 2015. Bronchiolitis in Children: Diagnosis and Management. Available from: https://www.nice.org.uk/guidance/ng9.

NHS Health, 2020. NHS Health A-Z Bronchiolitis. https://www.nhs.uk/conditions/bronchiolitis/causes/: accessed 2/12/20.

National Institute of Clinical Excellence (NICE), 2017a. CKS Whooping Cough. Available from: https://cks.nice.org.uk/whooping-cough#!topicsummary.

National Institute for Clinical Excellence (NICE), 2017b. CKS Croup. Available from: https://cks.nice.org.uk/croup#!topicsummary.

Office for National Statistics, 2017. Death Registrations in England and Wales, Summary Tables: 2016. Available from: https://www.ons.gov.uk/releases/deathregistrationsinenglandandwalessummarytables2016.

Public Health England, 2016. Guidelines for the Public Health Management of Pertussis in England.

Public Health England, 2017. Tuberculosis in England 2017 Report (Presenting Data to End of 2016) Vrown Copyright.

Public Health England, 2020. The 2nd Atlas of Variation in Risk Factors and Healthcare for Respiratory Disease in England. https://fingertips.phe.org.uk/documents/Bronchiolitis.pdf: accessed 3/12/20.

Public Health England, 2020. Tuberculosis in England 2020 Report. https://assets.publishing.service.gov.uk/government/uploads/system/uploads/attachment_data/file/934954/TB_Annual_Report_2020.pdf: accessed 3/12/20.

Rajesh, V.T., Singh, S., Kataria, S., 2000. Tachypnoea is a good predictor of hypoxia in acutely ill infants under 2 months. Arch. Dis. Child. 82, 46–49.

Reeves, R.M., Hardelid, P., Panagiotopoulos, N., Minaji, M., Warburton, F., Pebody, R., 2019 Jun. Burden of hospital admissions caused by respiratory syncytial virus (RSV) in infants in England: a data linkage modelling study. J. Infect. 78 (6), 468–475. https://doi.org/10.1016/j.jinf.2019.02.012. Epub 2019 Feb 26.

Royal College of Nursing, 2017. Standards for Assessing, Measuring and Monitoring Vital Signs in Infants, Children and Young People. RCN, London.

Royal College of Pediatric and Child Health, 2017. The State of Child Health Report 2017. Available from: https://www.rcpch.ac.uk/sites/default/files/2018-05/state_of_child_health_2017report_updated_29.05.18.pdf.

Thompson, S.W., 1990. Emergency Care of Children. Jones & Bartlett, Boston.

The Royal Childrens Hospital Melbourne, 2019. Clinical Guidelines Temperature management. Available from https://www.rch.org.au/rchcpg/hospital_clinical_guideline_index/Temperature_management/ accessed 3/12/20.

Waters, V., Halperin, S., 2010. Chapter 230: Bordetella species. Mandell, Douglas, and Bennett's Principles and Practice of Infectious Diseases – Online. Elsevier.

West, J.B., 2012. Respiratory Physiology: The Essentials. Lippincott Williams and Wilkins, Philadelphia.

World Health Organization (WHO), 2014. Guidance for National Tuberculosis Programmes on the Management of Tuberculosis in Children, second ed. Geneva.

Caring for Children and Young People With Cardiovascular Problems

Kerry Louise Gaskin, Amanda Daniels

LEARNING OUTCOMES

- Review the embryonic, fetal and developmental anatomy and physiology of the cardiovascular system in children and young people (CYP).
- Identify the causes of congenital, inherited and acquired heart disease in CYP.

- Consider the evidence-based assessment and management of CYP with congenital, inherited and acquired heart disease, adopting a family centred approach to care.

INTRODUCTION

The incidence of congenital heart disease (CHD) is eight per 1000 live births in the United Kingdom and relates to malformation or disease present at birth, including congenital arrhythmias, structural anomalies and some forms of cardiomyopathy (Health Quality Improvement Partnership, 2017) and accounts for about one-third of all major congenital anomalies (van der Linde et al., 2011). Inherited conditions, also known as genetic heart conditions, are familial; these are generally different from congenital heart conditions, although congenital conditions can occur as part of a genetic syndrome (British Heart Foundation, 2018). Acquired heart disease such as Kawasaki disease and most cardiomyopathies develop after birth.

The cause of CHD is not always known, although a range of teratogens are believed to contribute to an alteration of form or function of the cardiovascular system including recreational substances (tobacco, alcohol and marijuana) and prescribed drugs (some common drugs including certain antidepressants, antiepileptic and antibiotics); maternal disease or illness such as unstable pre-gestational diabetes, rubella, influenza and obesity (Lynch and Abel, 2015).

To understand the cause of these problems, it is important to have a good understanding of anatomy and physiology of the cardiovascular system. This chapter will begin by reviewing embryological, fetal and developmental anatomy and physiology.

THE ORIGINS AND DEVELOPMENT OF THE EMBRYONIC AND FETAL HEART

The heart and its corresponding blood vessels develop from the splanchnopleuric mesoderm (embryonic tissue adjacent to the endoderm) in the cardiogenic region. The underlying endoderm contributes to this development by signalling to the primitive angioblastic cords to converge and form a pair of lateral endocardial tubes, which are then gradually fused and reshaped as the embryo grows and folds. This gradual, but carefully orchestrated, fusion of these tubes shapes the single primitive heart tube, which is then remodelled by a sequential process of septation and folding that transforms the single lumen into the four chambers of the definitive heart. The initial chambers are primitive and require considerable development.

The primitive heart tube consists of endothelium, which is shaped by a series of definitive expansions, shallow ridges and crevices (sulci). By the 22nd day a thick mass of splanchnic mesoderm surrounds this heart tube, differentiating into the loosely organised myocardium and cardiac jelly, a layer of thick acellular matrix synthesised by the developing myocardium (Schoenwolf et al., 2014). The visceral pericardium lies externally to the myocardium. It evolves from mesothelial cells, which are derived independently from the splanchnopleuric mesoderm. These cells are believed to migrate onto the surface of the developing heart from the regions of the septum transversum or the sinus venosus.

Approximately from the 23rd day, the single heart tube begins to elongate, simultaneously loop and fold. This displaces the bulbus cordis to the right and adjusts the position of the primitive ventricle to the left, allowing the primitive atrium to move in an upward direction. The complex cardiac folding is believed to be completed by the 28th day of embryonic life. This highly organised looping of the primitive heart tube may be intrinsically motivated and possibly influenced by the state of hydration of the cardiac jelly, active migration and development of the primitive myocytes (cardiac muscle cells), and local haemodynamic forces initiated by the embryo's circulating blood. This early cardiac morphogenesis includes the formation of the coronary vascular plexus, which later forms the coronary vessels (Schoenwolf et al., 2014).

The mesoderm, mesodermal growth factors and other factors expressed in the developing myocardium influence tissue differentiation and regulate the course of atrial and ventricular development. The cardiac neural crest contributes to the formation of the primitive ventricular outflow tracts. The internal septation of the heart, and the formation of the heart valves, are attributed to the development of the mesenchymal tissue at the atrioventricular and proximal outflow regions of the heart. The structural developments in the heart and blood vessels may play a role in regulating the functions of the cardiovascular system. For instance, marginal increases in blood pressure may contribute to the development of the embryonic myocardium and the smooth muscle of the blood vessels.

The primitive heart begins to contract on approximately the 22nd day (Hill, 2018) and blood begins to circulate through the primitive vessels within the next 2 days. The first blood cells found in the embryo's circulation are formed in the yolk sac, although embryonic and later fetal haematopoiesis occurs in the liver, spleen, thymus and, of course, eventually the bone marrow.

The Developing Atria and Atrial Septation

The right atrium is remodelled during the fourth and fifth weeks of gestation. This initiates the gradual incorporation of the enlarged right sinus horn and the development of the venae cavae. A single pulmonary vein sprouts from the posterior wall of the left atrium and then divides to form the right and left pulmonary veins, which grow in the direction of the primitive lungs, where they join the smaller pulmonary veins, which develop around the primitive bronchial tissue. The right and left pulmonary veins are eventually reconstructed forming, in most instances, four pulmonary veins.

The anatomical divisions between the atria and the common atrioventricular canal separate the systemic from the pulmonary circulation. This separation also depends on the gradual fusion of the septum primum and the septum secundum. The septum primum establishes a firm interatrial muscle and the septum secundum contributes to the development of the foramen ovale, or oval window. If the septum secundum formation and covering of the perforations in the septum primum fails, a secundum atrial septal defect (ASD) occurs (Hill, 2018).

Division and shaping of the common atrioventricular canal by the septum intermedium (the middle segment of the intraventricular septum) into the right and left atrioventricular canals ensures that the right atrioventricular canal aligns the right atrium with the right ventricle and the left atrioventricular canal aligns the left atrium with the left ventricle. The division and reshaping of the common atrioventricular canal initiates the development of the primitive left ventricle, which establishes a firm contact with the proximal portion of the truncus arteriosus, a major vessel, which ultimately divides to form the future aorta and the main pulmonary artery. The four main cardiac valves begin to form in the fifth week of gestation, almost immediately following the division of the atrioventricular canal, and the septation of the truncus arteriosus, and is initially supported by growth and shaping of ventricular muscle from

below. However, proliferating cells, which surround these orifices eventually, form the distinctive mitral and tricuspid valves.

The Developing Ventricles and Ventricular Septation

The right ventricle is derived predominantly from the inferior aspects of the bulbus cordis and the right aspect of the conus cordis. The left ventricle develops mainly from the primitive ventricle and the left wall of the conus cordis. Corresponding outflow tracts, namely, the main pulmonary artery and the aorta, complete the morphogenesis of the heart and its major vessels. The intraventricular septum is formed by the developing right and left ventricular walls opposing one another. The growth of the muscular part of the septum halts just before its superior edge meets the inferior membranous surface of the septum intermedium in the middle segment of the intraventricular septum. This temporary arrest in growth is associated with a number of developmental benefits including ventricular enlargement and formation of the ventricular trabeculae (ridges in the myocardium), which shape the ventricular chambers and their respective outflow tracts so that the heart can function as a competent mechanical pump.

The truncus arteriosus, which serves as the main cardiac outflow pathway, is divided by a septum, which shapes the distal aspects of the right and left outflow tracts for the right and left ventricles, respectively. As the aorta separates from the main pulmonary artery, three distinctive swellings (tubercules) evolve, initiating the development of the semilunar valves, also known as the aortic and the pulmonary artery valves, which direct the intracardiac blood flow.

The final stage in the intracardiac development involves the growth of the membranous interventricular septum, which is originally derived from the inferior endocardial cushion. As the membranous septum fuses with the muscular interventricular septum at about 8 weeks of gestation blood flow between the right and the left ventricles ceases. The aorta and the pulmonary artery ensure that both ventricles can now function autonomously with respect to their own outflow tracts. In instances where fusion between the membranous and muscular parts of the septum fails a septal or intraventricular septal defect (VSD) will persist. This is the most common type of congenital cardiac anomaly that occurs in children.

The Development of the Valves

The atrioventricular valves begin their development in the fifth week of gestation with the formation of cusps within the atrioventricular canals. Generally, the left atrioventricular valve has only two cusps, which form the bicuspid valve, also known as the mitral valve. In contrast, the right atrioventricular valve usually, but not always, develops three cusps, which shape the tricuspid valve. The free edges of these cusps attach to the sinew-like chordae tendineae, which insert into the ventricular papillary muscles. The design of these valves ensures that during diastole the cusps fold back allowing the blood to flow uninhibited from the atria to the ventricles. Significantly, during systole, the tight closure of these cusps prevents a backflow of blood from the atria into the ventricles.

Chamber and Vessel Concordance

Primitive blood vessels begin to appear in the splanchnic mesoderm of the yolk sac on the 17th day. A similar aggregation of cells, also known as blood islands, appear in the embryonic disc on the 18th day. These cells initiate the formation of the embryo's blood vessels which are initially surrounded by a fibronectin rich matrix that is later incorporated into the endothelial lamina. The early development and subsequent reshaping of the endocardial tubes allows a pair of dorsal aortas to attach to their cranial axis and then form the first pair of aortic arches. Four additional aortic arches develop during the fourth and fifth weeks, connecting the rudimentary aortic sac (also known as the truncus arteriosus) to the dorsal aortas, which fuse later to form the median dorsal aorta. This complex network of the aortic arches is eventually remodelled to establish arteries within the upper thorax, neck and head. The dorsal aorta gives rise to three distinctive sets of arterial vessels (Collins, 2008; Schoenwolf et al., 2014):

- The ventral arteries, which supply the gut
- The lateral arteries, which supply the retroperitoneal organs such as the kidneys and the gonads
- The intersegmental arteries, which supply, in part, the head, the neck and body walls

The arteries supplying the gastrointestinal tract are derived from remnants of vitelline arteries and the vitelline duct, which anastomose with the paired dorsal aortae. The dorsal aortae in turn connect to the umbilical arteries, which carry blood from the embryo, and later the fetus, to the placenta.

The primitive venous system consists of three major components:

- The cardinal veins, which drain the head, neck, body walls and limbs
- The vitelline veins, which initially drain the yolk sac
- The umbilical veins, which carry oxygenated blood from the placenta to the embryo/fetus

All three sets of veins initially drain into the right and left sinus horns but their extensive modification shapes the distinctive systemic venous connection with the right atrium. The left sinus horn is eventually transformed into the coronary sinus and the oblique vein of the left atrium. The coronary sinus receives most of the venous blood returning from the coronary vascular bed. The vitelline venous system gives rise to the liver sinusoids and the portal system that transports venous blood from the intestinal tract to the liver. The vitelline system further subdivides within the liver establishing the ductus venosus, a small vessel that directs the embryonic/fetal blood from the umbilical vein directly into the inferior vena cava.

The complex arrangement of the heart is attained by the 55th day of gestation (Schoenwolf et al., 2014). The remaining period of gestation facilitates growth and relative maturation of the cardiovascular structures and corresponding haemodynamic adaptation. Myocardial cells proliferate in conjunction with the rapid accumulation of contractile proteins and metabolic substrates.

READING ACTIVITY

Chapter 12 (Development of the heart, pp 267–303) and Chapter 13 (Development of the vasculature, pp 304–340) in: Schoenwolf, G., Bleyl, S., Brauer, P., Francis-West, P., 2014. Larsen's Human Embryology, fifth ed. Elsevier Churchill Livingstone, Philadelphia.

Buijtendijk, M., F., J., Barnett, P., van den Hoff, M., J., B., 2020. Development of the human heart. Am J Med Genet Part C. 2020; 184C: 7– 22.

Online Resource: Undertake the Intermediate Module on Cardiac Embryology aimed at University students

Hill, M.A., 2018. Embryology. Intermediate Cardiac Embryology. Available from: https://embryology.med.unsw.edu.au/embryology/index.php/Intermediate_Cardiac_Embryology.

REFLECT ON YOUR PRACTICE

- Reflect on the knowledge and understanding you have gained of the embryonic and fetal developments of the cardiovascular system; the key stages of CHD occurrence and changes occurring at birth.
- Do you provide parents with information sheets on cardiovascular developments during pregnancy?
- If yes, are you satisfied with the content of these documents, is the information clear and understandable?
- If no, consider how you would use the knowledge you have gained to produce written information to help parents to enhance their understanding of the causes of CHD.

FETAL CIRCULATION AND CHANGES OCCURRING AT BIRTH

The role of the fetal circulation, functioning from around 3 weeks of fetal life, is to transport blood within the closed circuit of semi-compliant vessels, delivering nutrients, oxygen and metabolic substrates from the placenta to the embryo/fetus and removing fetal metabolic waste products back to the placenta as the fetal lungs and liver are non-functioning. The fetal circulation contains three main shunts/adaptations: the ductus venosus, which takes blood from the left umbilical vein into the inferior vena cava bypassing the liver; the ductus arteriosus, which shunts blood from the pulmonary artery into the aorta, allowing blood to bypass the lungs; and the foramen ovale, a large hole in the atrial septum, which allows blood to flow from the right atrium to the left atrium again diverting blood away from the lungs and instead towards the brain and the body. The right side of the fetal heart is under higher pressure than the left due to pulmonary vasoconstriction, high pulmonary vascular resistance and low systemic vascular resistance. Blood from the right ventricle is directed via the pulmonary artery, 10% flows to the lungs for perfusion for the developing parenchyma in early gestation; the other 90% is directed through the ductus arteriosus into the descending aorta. The flow to the lungs via the branch pulmonary arteries increases from 10% to approximately 20%–25% of the entire cardiac output towards the end of gestation (Rasanen et al., 1996; Davey et al., 2012).

At birth, the fetal circulation needs to adapt to changes in the fetal environment. During the birth increased intrathoracic pressure during the third stage of labour begins to push fluid out of the lungs. After birth the baby will take their first breath, stimulated by changing temperature, light and sound as well as changing gas levels due to cord clamping and hormonal changes in the mother; this fills the opened alveoli with air and inflates the lungs. The increase in circulating oxygen acts on the pulmonary vasculature causing vasodilation and reducing the pulmonary vascular resistance. This drop in pulmonary vascular resistance along with a rise in systemic vascular resistance due to umbilical cord clamping, will cause a change in the atrial pressures, pushing the flexible membranous part of the septum against the less conforming muscular septum closing the foramen ovale and stopping the right to left shunt of blood across the hole. Simultaneously, a change in carbon dioxide levels from the cord clamping, stimulates the respiratory centre in the baby's brain to initiate breathing. Increased oxygen levels and reduced maternal circulating prostaglandins act on the specialised cells of the ductus arteriosus initiating closure of this duct during the first few days to weeks after birth.

Developmental Anatomy and Physiology of the Cardiovascular System

In children, the heart is a small, rounded, three-dimensional pyramid that lies in the mediastinal cavity more horizontally than in adults. The apex of the heart is normally higher and located in the fourth left intercostal space, extending only to the fifth intercostal space by 7 or 8 years of age. The base of the heart lies in an oblique position behind the sternum. It consists of the atria and their respective auricles (small appendages of each atrium). The two ventricles form the inferior aspect of the cardiac silhouette coming together to form the apex.

An individual's heart can generally be calculated by the size of their fist, or 0.5% of the weight of the body (Roberts, 2015), suggesting that an infant weighing 5 kg would have a heart weighing approximately 25 g. A mature heart weighs between 230 and 340 g, and this weight generally reflects the person's body size. However, according to Spratt (2016), this weight is achieved only between 17 and 20 years of age. In children, the normal heart is relatively small, the size varying with age and body surface area. The heart is suspended in a pericardial sac by its attachments to the aorta and the pulmonary artery. This leaves the apex relatively free and allows the ventricles to move the apex forward to strike

against the left side of the chest wall during contraction (systole). This characteristic thrust is best heard as the apex beat on auscultation and is frequently referred to as the point of maximal intensity.

The Normal Cardiovascular System

The normal cardiovascular system can be divided into two functional compartments: the systemic circulation, which is supported by the left ventricle; and the pulmonary circulation, which is supported by the right ventricle. The right and the left ventricles work in relative harmony. This ensures that the systemic circulation transports oxygenated blood and nutrients from the left ventricle through the aorta to the systemic arteries and capillaries. The pulmonary circulation receives its deoxygenated blood from the right ventricle. This blood is then pumped through the pulmonary artery to lungs. Here a complex capillary bed surrounds the alveoli and facilitates gaseous exchange across the capillary-alveolar membranes. This mechanism ensures that oxygenated blood is transported to the left atrium by way of pulmonary venules, which anastomose giving rise to four pulmonary veins, which commonly attach to the posterior wall of the left atrium. The oxygenated blood flows from the left atrium to the left ventricle, which ejects it into the aorta ensuring that the metabolic needs of all organs and tissue are met.

The developed cardiovascular system is an adaptive, but relatively efficient transport network supported by a rhythmically pulsatile four-chambered heart.

The Pericardium

 READING ACTIVITY

Chapter 8 (Blood) and Chapter 9 (The Cardiac System) in Peate & Gormley-Fleming (2015, pp 167–215)
- Name the three anatomically distinctive layers of the heart.
- Give a reasoned account of the functions of these distinctive layers.

The fibrous pericardium encloses, and to some extent protects, the heart. It forms a continuum with the adventitia of the major veins and arteries that communicate with the heart. The serous pericardium is a double-layered membrane that consists of flat secretory epithelium, connective tissue and some adipose tissue, which is present in insignificant quantities in children. The two layers of the serous pericardium form a pericardial cavity, which holds a very small volume of serous fluid that acts as a lubricant preventing the occurrence of friction as the two membranes glide over each other during systole.

The Myocardium

The myocardium, the contractile muscle of the heart, is composed of highly specialised small myocytes rich in specialised contractile proteins, mitochondria and sarcoplasmic reticulum. During embryonic and fetal life the myocardium develops as a result of a gradual increase in myocyte numbers and the intrinsically sustainable contractility. The relatively slow development of myofibrils (contractile elements) within the myocytes throughout fetal life, during infancy and childhood appears to contribute to a characteristic myocyte hypertrophy (i.e. an increase in the size of the myocytes). After birth, in CYP of all ages, the capacity for myocyte hyperplasia may be limited, but myocyte hypertrophy will continue under normal physiological conditions, up to 20 years of age.

The coordinated contraction of myocardium provides the mechanical energy for the transportation of blood throughout the entire vasculature. Both the electrodynamic controls of the heart and the force of myocardial contractility are the consequence of the sophisticated cellular mechanisms that bring about the rhythmic excitation–contraction coupling phenomena. Right ventricular hypertrophy in the neonate is attributed to the workload of the right ventricle and associated physical development of the myocardium during fetal life and can be seen on the neonatal ECG (electrocardiogram) (Dhillon, 2020). However, a clear distinction must be made between the physiological right ventricular hypertrophy and a hypertrophy initiated by some form of pathophysiological change that may affect the competence of the entire cardiovascular and pulmonary systems in neonates and children.

Sources of chemical energy for the fetal and neonatal myocardium. Early studies have indicated that chemical energy production in the fetal heart is largely dependent upon carbohydrates, particularly through glycolysis and lactate oxidation (Fisher, 1984; Lopaschuk and Spafford, 1990). This is partly due to the low oxygen environment, low energy demands and the high levels of lactate and low levels of fatty acids circulating as energy substrates (Lopaschuck et al., 1991). During birth the heart needs to adapt from a fetal to a newborn physiological and hormonal environment, with a significant change from glycolysis to fatty acid β-oxidation as the cardiac energy source (Makinde et al., 1998; Fukushima et al., 2016). There is a slow maturation of glucose oxidation and it is thought that this can result in a reduction of cardiac ATP in the newborn heart (Lopaschuk and Jaswal, 2010). Over the first week of life fatty acid oxidation increases, becoming the main source of cardiac adenosine triphosphate (ATP) production (Lopaschuk et al., 1991; Makinde et al., 1998).

This may be clinically significant in circumstances of hypoglycaemia, which could compromise myocardial contractility and so cardiovascular function in neonates and possibly young children (Gluckman and Heymann, 1996).

The Endocardium

The endocardium is composed of a specialised endothelium and a layer of fibroelastic connective tissue that lines the inner surfaces of the heart including the four cardiac valves. Characteristically, the endocardium is thicker in the atria than the ventricles and this may have a functional significance yet to be determined.

TABLE 12.1 Normal Range of Heart Rates in Children at Rest

Age of the Child	Normal Range (beats/min)	Average (beats/min)
Newborn–6 months of age	90–160	120
6–12 months of age	80–140	110
1–3 years	80–120	100
3–6 years	75–115	90
6–9 years	70–110	90
9–11 years	70–105	85
11–14 years	65–100	80

The faster heart rate in neonates and infants is largely attributed to the smaller size of the ventricular chambers, which are capable of ejecting only a small amount of blood, commonly referred to as the stroke volume, on each ventricular contraction. However, as the child's metabolic demands are high, and these have to be met by an effective cardiac output (the quantity of blood pumped by the left ventricle per minute), the potential deficits created by the small stroke volume are corrected by the higher heart rate. As children grow older, their hearts – and especially the ventricular chambers – evolve, the stroke volume increases, and this contributes to the significant reduction of the heart rate. It is important, however, to appreciate that the normal heart rate and stroke volume in all children fluctuate with activity and crying.

The Cardiac Cycle

The cardiac cycle is defined as the time from the beginning of one heart beat to the beginning of the next. Each cardiac cycle is initiated and governed by an action potential generated within the sinoatrial node and conveyed rapidly to both atria. The fractional delay in the transfer of the impulse from the atria to the ventricles ensures that the atria contract before the ventricles. As a result the blood is pumped by the atria into the ventricles, increasing the ventricular volume, which in turn raises the stroke volume. The four phases of the cardiac cycle are commonly known as:

- Contraction (phase I)
- Ejection or systole (phase II)
- Relaxation (phase III)
- Filling or diastole (phase IV)

Although the rhythmic contraction of the heart is intrinsic (a mechanism frequently referred to as myogenic), the harmonising of the cardiac cycle, in terms of rate, force of contractility and volume output, is accomplished by the autonomic nervous system (Priebe and Skarvan, 2000). The autonomic nervous system has a direct effect on the nodal tissue, the coronary vessels, atrial and ventricular myocardium, and to some extent, augments and supports the adapting cardiac function. Physical activities or crying will also increase the child's heart rates significantly by, among other factors, increasing oxygen demand.

At the onset of ventricular contraction, the atrial and ventricular pressure are fairly equal. However, as the ventricular blood volume increases, the ventricular pressure rises, initiating the closure of the atrioventricular valves. This gives rise to the first heart sound (called 'lub'). Because the pulmonary artery and aortic valves remain closed, the ventricles are said to be in isovolumetric contraction. This raises the ventricular pressure further and causes a bulging of both the semilunar and the atrioventricular valves. The semilunar valves open when the left ventricular pressure exceeds the aortic pressure and the right ventricular pressure exceeds the pulmonary artery pressure. The rapid expulsion of blood during the early phase of systole raises the ventricular pressures further establishing a maximum ejection point. This is followed by the last systole phase, which influences the gradual decline in the ventricular and aortic pressures, and the onset of ventricular diastole or early isovolumetric relaxation, which culminates in the closure of the semilunar valves and the initiation of second heart sound ('dub').

The volume of blood ejected on each ventricular contraction is defined as the stroke volume. The cardiac output is defined as the amount of blood ejected by the heart during each minute (cardiac output = stroke volume × heart rate/min). The cardiac index takes into consideration the child's body surface area and is therefore a measure of the cardiac output per square metre of body surface area. In children, cardiac index values continue to rise to above 4.0 L/min/m^2 up to 10 years of age, and then declines, falling to a new lower normal value of about 2.4 L/min/m^2 (Guyton and Hall, 2006). This phenomenon may be attributed to the normally high metabolic rate in younger children. Exercise and crying will also influence the child's stroke volume, cardiac output and cardiac index, but this is usually transitory in contrast to the factors that have a more definitive effect on cardiac output such as the child's age, size, metabolism and body surface area.

Although the function of the heart shows some degree of adaptability, four constant factors are critical to effective cardiac output and corresponding tissue perfusion. These are the following:

- heart rate
- myocardial contractility
- preload (the volume of blood that returns to and stretches the ventricles prior to contraction)
- afterload (the resistance to the ejection of blood from the ventricle into the great vessels), and total peripheral resistance

Although the heart rate and myocardial contractility are of cardiac origin, both can be augmented by neural and humoral mechanisms. By contrast, the preload and afterload are dependent on blood volume, the size of the heart and the dimension of the blood vessels. There is, however, a cyclical nature to this, in that both preload and afterload are important determinants of cardiac output, which is influenced by the heart rate and myocardial contractility.

CONGENITAL, INHERITED AND ACQUIRED CARDIAC PROBLEMS IN CHILDREN AND YOUNG PEOPLE

Cardiovascular problems, which present in childhood, are commonly classified according to their congenital, inherited or acquired origins.

 ACTIVITY

- Access the companion PowerPoint presentation and define congenital heart disease that occurs in children.
- Distinguish between the common features of acyanotic and cyanotic congenital heart disease that occur in children.
- Distinguish between congenital heart disease, inherited and acquired cardiovascular disease that may occur in children.

Congenital Heart Disease

Antenatal detection of congenital heart disease (CHD) across Great Britain and Ireland occurred in approximately 45% of cases during 2013–14; however, marked regional variations in detection remain (Health Quality Improvement Partnership, 2017). CHD occurs in approximately eight per 1000 live births and can be grouped into two distinctive classifications: acyanotic or cyanotic heart defects.

Acyanotic Heart Defects

The acyanotic heart defects generally include structural problems such as patent ductus arteriosus, atrial septal defect and some ventricular septal defects. In general, children with these defects are initially asymptomatic. If not diagnosed antenatally, the first indication of an underlying cardiovascular problem may be the child's history of recurrent respiratory infection, faltered growth or poor exercise tolerance.

Ventricular septal defects are the most common congenital cardiovascular defects occurring in isolation or in association with more complex cardiovascular anomalies (Townsend et al., 2013) accounting for up to 40% of CHD (Penny and Vick, 2011). These defects are commonly classified according to their size and position in the interventricular septum. Defects are most common in the membranous part of the septum, although they do extend into the muscular part of the septum. A wide range of defects can also occur in the muscular part of the septum. The position, size and complexity of the defect determine the signs and symptoms with which the child presents. For instance, the size of the defect determines the magnitude of the shunting of blood from the left ventricle to the right ventricle. Larger defects tend to have a more profound effect on the right ventricle; consequently infants present early with respiratory difficulties, faltering growth and may present in heart failure. These signs and symptoms are caused by an increase in pulmonary blood flow caused by the amount of blood being shunted from the left ventricle across the defect into the right ventricle. This additional volume of blood is then directed to the lungs, leading to pulmonary plethora, which may compromise normal pulmonary ventilation and gas exchange. In time, the haemodynamic disturbances caused by the abnormal interventricular shunting of blood causes right ventricular hypertrophy and left atrial and ventricular dilatation. This augments the normal shape of the heart, a feature that is observed on the child's chest x-ray (Penny and Vick, 2011).

> ### ▶ REFLECT ON YOUR PRACTICE
>
> A 6-week-old baby is admitted to the cardiac unit with a short history of breathlessness, difficulties with feeding and increasing cyanosis, especially during crying. Following a thorough physical assessment and echocardiogram scan of the baby's heart and greater blood vessels, a diagnosis of ventricular septal defect is made. On arrival to the cardiac unit the baby is found to be in heart failure and will therefore require swift therapeutic intervention and competent nursing care:
>
> - How should this baby's care be managed to maximise the best therapeutic outcome?
> - Give a systematic account of the nursing care that this baby will require.
> - Give a reasoned account of the medical treatment that this baby will require.

Cyanotic Defects

Congenital cardiovascular lesions that cause the baby to be cyanotic from birth account for approximately 25% of all congenital heart defects. Cyanotic defects can be categorised into three groups: right to left shunts (e.g. tricuspid atresia, pulmonary atresia with intact ventricular septum, tetralogy of Fallot); common mixing (e.g. truncus arteriosus); and transposition, although some defects fit into more than one category.

Cyanotic defects are life threatening or life limiting without surgery. If not antenatally diagnosed, cyanotic babies can present in acute heart failure once the foramen ovale and arterial duct close, shortly after birth (Barker et al., 2009). The severity of the cyanosis is determined by the restrictions to pulmonary blood flow, which has a compromising effect on pulmonary gas exchange. Conditions with increased pulmonary blood flow will be less cyanotic, but present in worse heart failure. Diagnosis is not necessary before initiating

immediate interventions to support respiration, administer a prostaglandin infusion, where needed, to maintain arterial duct patency and improve pulmonary blood flow and generally optimise the baby's condition pre-surgery.

Transposition of the great arteries is one of the most common forms of cyanotic congenital cardiac defects that presents in neonates. It occurs more commonly in males than females with a ratio of between 2:1 and 3:1 reported (Blyth et al., 2008). Here the great arteries are transposed, with the aorta arising from the right ventricle and the pulmonary artery arising from the left ventricle. This means that instead of the normal figure of eight circulation, the pulmonary and systemic circulation run as two distinct circulations, which is incompatible with life. In this instance, the baby's survival depends on the presence of other defects, such as a patent ductus arteriosus or atrial or ventricular septal defects, which permit mixing of blood between the pulmonary and systemic circulation. The presence of these associated defects and the degree of mixing between the two bloodstreams also determine the haemodynamic findings.

Inherited Heart Disease

Inherited (or genetic) heart disease is passed on through families, such as inherited cardiomyopathies and inherited arrhythmias (e.g. long QT syndrome, Wolf-Parkinson-White and Brugada syndrome). Often the first indication that there is a problem within a family occurs when someone dies suddenly, because inherited heart disease that is undetected can lead to heart failure and sudden cardiac death.

Acquired Heart Disease

Acquired cardiovascular disease is less common in children than in adults in the developed world. However, the increasing prevalence of obesity and diabetes in CYP has serious implications for their development of cardiovascular disease in the future and the impact of which could be a reversal to the declining death rate for cardiovascular disease that has been seen over the last 50 years in the UK (Townsend et al., 2013).

The acquired cardiovascular diseases can be grouped into those that are caused by:
- infection and inflammation, as in endocarditis, myocarditis and pericarditis; rheumatic disease, Kawasaki disease
- systemic metabolic problems, as in myocardial disease
- heart muscle diseases, as in cardiomyopathy, autoimmune disease
- degenerative, as in neurodegenerative disease and myopathies
- drugs and toxins (e.g. anthracyclines)

Depending on the primary cause, each of these conditions may affect the CYP in very different ways, for instance, the nature and virulence of the pathogen, the magnitude of the metabolic problem or the severity of the abnormal morphological change to the heart. It is therefore important to recognise that CYP affected by any of these problems can present acutely ill, with severe haemodynamic instability, and signs of low cardiac output. Alternatively, some children may experience more subtle forms of ill health and present with faltered growth, reduced exercise tolerance and occasionally cardiac arrhythmias caused by structural changes to the heart muscle in heart failure (Barker et al., 2009) that if untreated may result in sudden death.

The common denominator in the acute and the more long-standing acquired form of heart disease is heart failure, which must be treated in conjunction with any treatment for the underlying cause of the primary disease. However, supportive therapeutic interventions culminating in a successful eradication of the primary disease is not always possible. Surviving CYP with myocardial disease may, in some circumstances, require cardiac transplantation as a means to enhancing their quality of life.

Heart Failure

Heart failure occurs when the heart is unable to pump sufficient amounts of blood to the systemic (and pulmonary) circulation required to meet the metabolic demands of the body. Heart failure is invariably the result of some structural or morphological defects in the cardiovascular system, which in time give rise to characteristic haemodynamic changes that lead to the following:

- Volume overload: commonly caused by left-to-right intracardiac shunts that give rise to right ventricular hypertrophy and increased pulmonary blood flow.
- Pressure overload: commonly caused by obstructive lesions such as coarctation of the aorta and valve stenosis.
- Impaired contractility: caused by factors that affect myocardial contractility, such as cardiomyopathy, myocarditis, hypoglycaemia and low serum potassium, calcium or magnesium.
- High cardiac output demands: caused by such problems as septicaemia, in which peripheral vasodilatation allows an abnormal redistribution of the child's circulating blood volume away from the vital organs.

The pathophysiology of heart failure can be viewed in terms of right ventricular failure and left ventricular failure. Right ventricular failure is characterised by suboptimal ventricular function. This leads to an abnormal rise in end-diastolic pressure, which in turn raises the central venous pressure and causes systemic venous engorgement. The ensuing systemic venous hypertension causes hepatomegaly, and in some instances, dependent tissue oedema. In contrast, left ventricular failure is characterised by abnormal increases in the left ventricular end-diastolic pressure, resulting in haemodynamic changes in the left atrium and the pulmonary veins. As a consequence, the lungs become congested with blood that then raises the pulmonary pressures and contributes to pulmonary oedema. However, because both sides of the heart depend on an adequate function of the other side, failure of one ventricular chamber invariably also causes reciprocal changes in the opposite chamber. This is particularly so in children whose hearts are small and functionally immature. Nevertheless, the cardiovascular system is capable of initiating compensatory mechanisms that result in a sustainable increase in cardiac output in keeping with the metabolic

needs of the body. These compensatory mechanisms include activation of the sympathetic nervous system, increased heart rate, ventricular hypertrophy and dilatation. The failing heart and the compensatory mechanisms are responsible for the clinical features with which the child presents. The four most distinctive features that must be recognised in CYP are:

- impaired myocardial contractility
- pulmonary congestion
- systemic venous congestion
- fluid retention

Each of these features must be critically and methodically evaluated. The intention being to ensure that the:

- severity of heart failure is recognised;
- primary cause is identified;
- best therapeutic and caring interventions are utilised.

 READING ACTIVITY

Roberts, P., Burch, M., 2009. Cardiomyopathy in childhood. Paediatrics and Child Health 19 (1) 15–24.

Panesar, D., Burch, M., 2017. Understanding and treating heart failure in children. Paediatrics and Child Health 27 (2), 43–49.

Barker, J., Williams, C., Tulloh, R., 2009. Understanding and treatment of heart failure. Paediatrics and Child Health 19 (1), 1–8.

 REFLECT ON YOUR PRACTICE

- Reflect on the knowledge and understanding you have gained of congenital, inherited and acquired heart disease and the implications of this for your nursing care

Diagnostic Assessment and Management of the Child

No matter what setting CYP present, nurses have defined responsibilities (Royal College of Nursing [RCN], 2012, 2017). RCN guidance on roles, career pathways, and competence development is available for those caring for CYP and their families with cardiovascular conditions (RCN, 2014), assessment and management being an integral part of the role.

CYP of all ages can present with signs and symptoms that suggest underlying cardiovascular or respiratory problems. Comprehensive history taking and clinical examination are fundamental to evaluating the problem, and identifying the requirement and urgency of further investigations before implementing individualised evidence-based care. Underpinning knowledge of anatomical and physiological problems, as described earlier, serves as a basis for critical analysis of the evidence collected during the cardiac assessment. In general, CYP with acquired heart disease, such as myocarditis, commonly present with symptoms that suggests generalised ill health. In contrast, some CYP with congenital heart disease can be asymptomatic, whereas others present with signs and symptoms that are confined to the cardiovascular and sometimes the respiratory system at a very early stage. The most common features are cyanosis, faltering growth, a cardiac murmur, dysrhythmia and symptoms of heart failure.

Initial Diagnosis

Currently about a quarter of infants with CHD are antenatally diagnosed during fetal ultrasound scans (Health Quality Improvement Partnership, 2017). The percentage of babies with more complex CHD diagnosed antenatally, such as hypoplastic left heart syndrome, is much higher at between 75% and 80% because they are easier to detect by sonographers (Wren et al., 2008; Sharland, 2012; Health Quality Improvement Partnership, 2017). Timing and method of delivery of the baby will be a key factor within the decision-making process, and can influence birth outcome (Landis et al., 2013). Other heart problems may be detected within the first few weeks to months of birth, presentation of which can range from a pattern of faltering weight and repeated respiratory illness, to the manifestation of cyanosis.

Inherited and acquired heart disease may not be detected until later in childhood or even during adult life. For example, cardiac arrhythmias may be diagnosed during fetal life or at any point during growth and development of the child. This can be associated with a structural defect or as an independent manifestation with immediate and long-term treatments tailored accordingly (Premkumar et al., 2016). Irrespective of when the symptoms appear the clinical assessment and management of congenital, inherited or acquired heart problems will require specialist medical, surgical and nursing interventions.

History Taking, Assessment and Investigations

History taking and broader biopsychosocial assessment of the child and their normal daily activities will enable the nurse to identify problems that may require attention. The history must take into consideration the gestational, birth and neonatal history, immunisations, allergies, family and social history, child's cognitive and psychosocial development, achievement of developmental milestones, the child's physical growth, nutritional preferences (to include 'amounts' as well as types of fluid/food dietary intake) and exercise tolerance to normal as well as energetic activity and hobbies.

CHD cannot always be viewed in isolation and co-morbidities may lie with other conditions such as those associated with hepatic or gastric illness. More commonly, CHD can be part of a syndrome such as Down Syndrome; Turners Syndrome; DiGeorge Syndrome; Williams Syndrome and Noonan Syndrome, and are a significant spectrum of associated chromosomal defects (Ko, 2015). The specific needs of such CYP will intertwine with the pathways of treatment and care and it is therefore prudent for the nursing approach to incorporate their additional care requirements though awareness and insight into how the syndromes may present within the field of congenital cardiology (Ko, 2015).

A comprehensive physical examination is normally undertaken by doctors or advanced clinical practitioners, consisting of inspection, palpation and auscultation of the cardiovascular system. However, CYP nurses should be able to undertake a clinical assessment of the cardiovascular system and know when to seek advice for non-normal findings. The subsequent treatment plan will be informed by the evidence collected during holistic assessment, whether during routine monitoring, an emergency situation or derived by critical evaluation of the child's:

- general physical appearance – including posture, activity, demeanour
- cyanotic appearance – peripheral or central
- responsiveness – A.V.P.U. Patient is Alert with full physical and verbal interaction, or responds to Verbal or Painful stimuli, or is Unresponsive
- behaviour – is it normal for this baby, child or young person?
- restfulness and sleep
- vital signs – body temperature, heart rate/rhythm, respiratory rate/effort, blood pressure
- presence of hypoxia – signs include changes to skin colour; confusion; cough; fast heart rate; rapid breathing; shortness of breathing; sweating; wheezing
- state of hydration
- elimination – extent of perspiration, urine output, emesis, faeces

---

👤 ACTIVITY

- Give a reasoned account as to why the above assessments are required.
- Critically evaluate the available evidence and demonstrate how this evidence can be used in the overall management of this child.
- Identify the additional needs of those CYP who have a genetic syndrome in addition to congenital or acquired heart disease. What impact may this have on the family?

Inspection. Whether at birth or later in life inspection of the child's general appearance must include the body size, proportions, growth, skin colour and markings, dysmorphic features, visible pulsations, previous scars and exaggerated shapes to the thorax or spine. Observation of the respiratory rate and pattern will also contribute to a better evaluation of the cardiovascular function. The child's response to stimuli and the surrounding environment will give an indication of the developmental milestones that have been reached and psychosocial functioning.

Palpation. Palpation or touch enables identification of the characteristics of the skin, internal organs and abnormalities and in the case of cardiac examination, the placing of the hand over the precordium allows for the detection of pulsations, heaves or thrills though the anterior chest wall (Ball et al., 2016). A thrill is a vibratory sensation felt on the skin over an area of turbulent blood flow, thus indicating the presence of a significant heart murmur. A heave feels like a 'lifting feeling' under the hand and is a sign of right ventricular enlargement; these are both significant findings and need to be escalated to the medical team. Peripheral pulses can be palpated in superficial arteries such as the brachial, radial, femoral artery and dorsalis pedis. The qualities of the pulse can be described in terms of:

- frequency (rate)
- rhythm (pattern)
- amplitude (volume)

It is important to note that a pulse rate should be counted over a full 1 minute to ensure accuracy of the characteristics assessed. In addition, a marked difference in character between upper and lower limb pulses may indicate significant changes in arterial flow and efficiency of cardiac output.

However, it must be appreciated that pulses may be difficult to feel in neonates and infants because of the relatively low arterial resistance to blood flow generated by the comparative thinness of the tunica media within the walls of the arteries and arterioles. For this reason, in children under 1 year of age, the heart rate should be recorded over the apex of the heart, using a stethoscope rather than by means of palpation of the radial pulse, as it may not be possible to reliably feel the radial pulse. In some cases, it may be advisable to consider auscultation of the apex beat as preferable for children less than 3 years of age, and in older children where their condition dictates (Ball et al., 2016).

The apex beat can also be palpated; the location will change with growth of the chest wall. In children it is found in the fourth left intercostal space in the mid-clavicular line and from the age of approximately 7 years this moves to the fifth left intercostal space in the mid-clavicular line. The apex beat is known as the point of maximal impulse and indicates the pulsation made by the apex of the left ventricle of the heart. Palpation can help further assess heart rate, rhythm and volume.

Auscultation. This involves listening to the heart with a stethoscope to the specific sounds caused by the systematic opening and closing of the atrioventricular valves; semilunar pulmonary artery and aortic valves; or turbulent blood flow within the heart and major blood vessels.

It is not uncommon for neonates and young children to present with a range of heart sounds and murmurs that are not always indicative of an underlying cardiovascular problem. Nevertheless, the presence of cardiac murmurs must be taken into consideration in the overall assessment of the child's cardiovascular system. The two distinguished heart sounds that must be heard are known as S1 and S2. Under normal circumstances, S1 is louder at the apex of the heart in the mitral and tricuspid valve area. Conversely, S2 is best heard near the base of the heart in the pulmonary artery and the aortic valve area. Two further heart sounds, S3 and S4, may be audible. S3 is the result of turbulence during ventricular filling, whilst S4 is generally attributed to a non-compliant left ventricle; both require further cardiovascular assessment.

Cardiac murmurs are important sounds in neonates and young children, and must not be ignored, as they can suggest underlying cardiac or major blood vessel anomalies that will require further systematic screening and critical evaluation. In addition, any murmur identified during common childhood illness (for example during a febrile illness where an increased heart rate can increase turbulence of flow to manifest abnormal sounds) should not be ignored. Referral should be made to a specialist to confirm the presence of either an innocent (benign, functional, physiological) murmur, or pathological (organic) murmur whereby intervention may be required. The Levine Grading Scale, commonly known as the Levine Scale, is a 6-point grading system to define the volume or intensity of a heart murmur heard with a stethoscope (Table 12.2) (Silverman and Wooley, 2008).

Blood pressure. This term generally applies to the arterial pressure in the systemic circulation. Blood pressure (BP) fluctuates with each heartbeat, between a maximum value (systolic pressure) achieved during cardiac systole and a minimum value (diastolic pressure) that reflects the diastolic phase. The physiological adaptation and maintenance of normal blood pressure is principally attributed to baroreceptors, which are present in the carotid and aortic bodies. These receptors augment and sustain the normal systemic BP by reflex. However, in children with hypoxia, fluid retention and heart failure, baroreceptor function compromise will contribute to BP changes.

BP can be measured by invasive methods, such as arterial monitoring; however, BP is commonly measured using an inflatable cuff on the upper arm or the leg (below the knee). It is important to document the location of the child's BP reading on the vital signs recordings chart to ensure accuracy when assessing and evaluating trends in BP measurements. In

---

TABLE 12.2   Grading of Murmurs

The intensity of auscultated sound is graded as follows:
Grade 1. The murmur can only be heard if one listens carefully for some time.
Grade 2. The murmur is faint but can be heard straight away with a stethoscope.
Grade 3. The murmur is moderately loud and can be heard immediately, but there is no palpable thrill or vibration that can be felt.
Grade 4. The murmur is loud and accompanies a palpable thrill.
Grade 5. The murmur accompanies a palpable thrill and is loud enough to be heard with just a slight touch of a stethoscope's rim.
Grade 6. The murmur accompanies a palpable thrill and is so loud that it can be heard before a stethoscope even makes contact with skin.

addition, a marked difference between upper and lower limb BP may indicate significant changes in arterial flow and cardiac output. The accuracy of the measurement is dependent on the size of the cuff and this must be proportional to the length and diameter of the limb (two-thirds of the limb must be covered, e.g. on the upper arm this is two-thirds of the distance between the shoulder and the elbow). Alternatively, a Doppler percutaneous flow probe can measure the systolic and a diastolic pressure to detect cessation of blood flow very accurately. The difference between the systolic and the diastolic pressure values is known as the pulse pressure. The major physiological factors that affect the pulse pressure are the stroke volume, the force of ventricular ejection and the compliance of the arterial vascular network. The greater the stroke volume, the greater the amount of blood that must be accommodated in the arterial network. This produces a rise in the systolic pressure and a fall in the diastolic pressure, which will culminate in a wider pulse pressure.

Wide ranges of factors can influence a child's BP such as maturation of the autonomic nervous system, developments and maturation in the cardiovascular system and corresponding reflex mechanisms. Furthermore, there is some evidence to suggest that the effects of the intrauterine environment, which influences low birth weight along with acceleration of subsequent growth, may also contribute to the development of hypertension in adulthood (Ediriweera et al., 2017). In health, children's BP parameters vary with age, and under normal physiological conditions there should be a gradual increase in the systolic and diastolic pressures according to age (Table 12.3). However, the increase in obesity in the young is a growing concern and extensive therapeutic lifestyle changes need to be implemented to address this in the age group 6–16 years (Brady, 2017). The additional concern is the effect this can have on the development of cardiovascular disease in adulthood and thus the emphasis on promoting physical activity in the young is a prominent public health focus (Andersen et al., 2011).

Temperature. In health, a child's core body temperature is relatively constant at 36.0°C–37.5°C and the peripheral temperature is no lower than 34°C–35°C. However, if the peripheral skin temperature is consistently lower, possible contributing factors need to be considered, such as low environmental temperatures or the child's compromised peripheral perfusion. For CYP with complex cardiovascular disease and underlying poor cardiac output, the risk can be higher, adding to the challenge of identifying sepsis early, which is an increasing national and international concern (Shane et al., 2017; Ansermino et al., 2018). Guidelines on feverish illness in children younger than 5 years are available to support the identification of sepsis within home and health care settings (National Institute for Health and Care Excellence, 2017).

Pulse Oximetry. While pulse oximetry has become common practice within health care since the late 1980s its use has been revolutionary for the assessment and monitoring of CHD (Ewer et al., 2011). In recent years, great efforts have been made to use this measurement for screen duct-dependent CHD in the newborn and across many maternity units the taking of pulse oximetry has been incorporated as a natural element to neonatal assessment screening. Due to this developing clinical approach, improvements have been made to detecting critical CHD soon after birth, which may have been missed previously (Prudhoe et al., 2013).

Chest Radiography

This can determine the position of the heart, its size and shape, chamber and major vessel enlargement or hypoplasia. It depicts the anatomical size and shape of the trachea, the bronchi, and the lungs in relation to the heart. It provides considerable evidence regarding air entry and pulmonary ventilation and demarcates the extent of the pulmonary blood flow and pulmonary venous return. In CYP with cardiac problems such as heart failure, chest radiography will help to establish the extent of the primary anatomical anomalies as well as the severity of pathophysiological problems such as cardiomegaly, pulmonary plethora and pulmonary congestion. In isolation, such evidence may be inconclusive; however, when considered in conjunction with other factors it can contribute to a definitive diagnosis.

Electrocardiography

This records the changes in the electrical potentials during cardiac activity (Table 12.4). Such data also provides information about the anatomical orientation of the heart; the relative size of the chambers of the heart; heart rate, rhythm and origin of excitation; and the spread of the impulse. Disturbances in the normal conduction process can be suggestive of a primary cardiovascular problem. Electrocardiography (ECG) in CYP will also reflect some age-related changes, which must be taken into consideration in the overall evaluation of the child's cardiovascular system.

At birth, the thickness in the right ventricular muscle exceeds the thickness of the left ventricular muscle. This is a physiological phenomenon reflecting the right ventricular workload during fetal life. However, the significant increase

TABLE 12.3	Blood Pressure in Childhood. Readings Are the 50th Centile for Boys	
Age	**Systolic Blood Pressure (mmHg)**	**Diastolic Blood Pressure (mmHg)**
Newborn	73	55
6 months	90	53
1 year	90	56
3 years	92	55
6 years	96	57
9 years	100	61
12 years	107	64
15 years	114	65

Taken from Second Task Force on Blood Pressure Control in Children. 1987. Normal blood pressure readings for boys. In: National Heart. Lung and Blood Institute, Bethesda.

TABLE 12.4	Electrocardiograph Recording of the Function of the Heart as a Pump
Electrocardiographic Event	**Corresponding Physiological Event in the Heart**
P wave	Depolarisation (excitation) of the atria prior to their contraction. The action potential (impulse) is initiated in the sinoatrial node. It spreads through the atrial muscle reaching the atrioventricular node
P-R segment	Atrial depolarisation and conduction of impulses through the atrioventricular node
QRS complex	Depolarisation (excitation) of the ventricles; the repolarisation (relaxation) of the atria is masked by the ventricular depolarisation
S-T segment	End of ventricular depolarisation and the beginning of the ventricular repolarisation
T wave	Repolarisation (relaxation) of the ventricles

in the left ventricular workload, after birth, gradually augments this. Thus, the right ventricular dominance normally seen on ECGs of neonates and young infants is gradually replaced by left ventricular dominance in later childhood (Dhillon, 2020).

The gradual increase in the size of the heart chambers, in conjunction with the ongoing maturation of the myocardium, allows the heart to handle greater quantities of blood volume. In the healthy child this results in increasing ability to alter stroke volume and cardiac output with a lower heart rate. In addition, the increasing chest wall thickness and disease process alteration results in babies and children having large ventricular voltages, particularly in the precordial leads; frontal (rightwards) QRS axes; and faster rates with correspondingly shorter P wave and QRS complex durations and PR and QT intervals. The range of normal at different ages varies significantly (Mehta and Dhillon, 2004).

Some arrhythmias may resolve spontaneously, although more persistent arrhythmias will require definitive therapeutic interventions. For instance, a child with persistent bradycardia caused by conduction problems will require a permanent pacemaker to sustain an acceptable cardiac rhythm. In contrast, CYP with recurrent episodes of profound supraventricular tachycardia may require suitable antiarrhythmic drugs, or if suitable, radiofrequency ablation of the accessory conductive pathways. The primary rationale for these therapeutic interventions is to normalise cardiac rhythm to sustain good cardiac output.

Echocardiography

This technique uses high-frequency sound waves to document detailed images, from which the atria, ventricles, the septal tissue, the atrioventricular and semilunar valves, and the great vessels can be identified, and their dimensions measured. Most CHD and major myocardial changes may be identified using this technique. However, the correct diagnosis and therapeutic intervention is dependent on the precise measurement and critical evaluation of the size and complexity of the cardiovascular problem, although this is better evaluated via invasive assessment though cardiac catheterisation.

Echocardiography cannot be underestimated in its use. It has been effectively used over many years, not only just for fetal and post-delivery diagnosis, but also continuing assessment through stress testing, for transoesophageal views of the heart, tissue Doppler imaging of the heart, and pre- and post-operative monitoring (Khalid and Koenig, 2006).

Cardiac Catheterisation

Apart from open heart surgery, this is the most invasive procedure that a child with a suspected cardiovascular problem may have to undergo. It involves inserting a radio-opaque catheter through a peripheral blood vessel into the respective chambers of the heart. This procedure is usually combined with angiocardiography in which a radio-opaque dye is injected through the catheter into the circulation. Combined, these procedures facilitate the collection of evidence regarding:

- oxygen saturation of the blood within the four chambers of the heart and the greater blood vessels;
- haemodynamic pressure values within the four chambers and the greater blood vessels;
- stroke volume and cardiac output values;
- the position, size and complexity of the cardiovascular defects and anomalies.

In some cases, this procedure can be used to provide treatment such as:

- closing an atrial or ventricular septal defect with a device;
- blocking and eventual closure of blood flow through a patent ductus arteriosus with a device;
- stretching a narrowed vessel, valve, or creating a septal hole via balloon angioplasty to improve blood flow;
- inserting a mesh stent to keep open a narrowed portion of a vessel;
- insertion of a pacemaker via trans-venous access and subcutaneous insertion of the pacing generator;
- radiofrequency ablation of accessory conductive pathways.

Magnetic Resonance Imaging

This is an increasingly popular method for diagnosis and ongoing assessment. With the revolution of high-resolution 3D imaging, MRI scanning is an exciting use of technology, giving detailed views of the heart its vessels and lung fields. In recent years the development of magnetic resonance imaging (MRI) scanning, which allows for a less invasive exploration, has become a very important additional imaging tool in the clinical management of CHD (Helbing and Ouhlous, 2015), and has become increasingly preferential to invasive cardiac catherisation for diagnostic work-up (Heathfield et al., 2013).

Nursing Care Considerations

Complex anatomical defects that present at time of birth will require palliative surgical intervention at the most clinically appropriate time. In some cases, a series of surgical or interventional procedures via cardiac catheterisation are required. The central aim is to re-fashion the heart to provide a circulatory flow that sustains life and provides haemodynamic functioning that promotes growth and development, improves quality of life, while minimising long-term complications. Other problems, such as myocarditis, heart failure and low cardiac output are managed as they arise. In these instances, swift diagnostic and therapeutic interventions consisting of finely balanced hydration, nutrition, inotropic agents and anti-failure drugs, among others, are essential.

For those babies, children and young people who have less severe CHD, treatment may be corrective. For those who acquire heart disease, treatment is aimed at stabilising and minimising the effect while trying to halt the progression of the condition; however, in some instances life sustaining treatments are required such as heart transplantation for cardiomyopathy.

Following holistic assessment of the CYP and a critical review of the clinically significant evidence, therapeutic nursing interventions must be individualised to the pre- and post-operative needs. This may include supporting a child in respiratory distress or heart failure, ensuring that the child's hydration and nutritional intake meets the metabolic demands and psychological support of the child and family. Some of the key nursing priorities are briefly discussed below.

Rest

CYP with established cardiovascular disease, especially heart failure, must be cared for in a manner that will ensure comfort, maximise rest and support cardiac, respiratory, digestive and renal function. Therapeutic nursing interventions must be coordinated to ensure the child's energy expenditure is minimised. Positioning the child to promote comfort, facilitate lung expansion and minimise distress and cardiac workload is an important aspect of nursing. Allowing for frequent rest and sleeping periods will also reduce the workload of the heart; promote the child's scope for healing and restoration of health where this is possible. 'Spoon theory' (Miserandino, 2018) is a contemporary project using spoons to represent energy; it helps CYP explain to others why they lack energy and to think about how they use their energy during the day (Little Hearts Matter, 2018).

Pain

CYP are not always able to communicate verbally their pain, discomfort or distress and every effort must be taken to monitor their emotional, physical and physiological state to ascertain that comforting interventions and appropriate analgesia are administered proactively. For instance, CYP who have undergone surgery may require continuous intravenous infusion of opioids such as morphine sulphate in the immediate post-operative phase and providing the dosages are calculated carefully in relation to the child's body surface area, these drugs are considered as safe and effective in relieving severe forms of pain (Elkomy et al., 2016). However, milder forms of oral analgesia, such as paracetamol, may be given at regular intervals or when required to control less severe forms of pain. For some CYP with chest drains, stronger analgesia such as oral morphine may be required for some time. CYP can experience a significant level of pain following cardiac surgery (Lauridsen et al., 2014); so, appropriate analgesia is paramount, and any related psychological trauma must be recognised and supported.

Providing the CYP is haemodynamically stable, both in the pre- and post-operative phase, provision must be made to encourage active play, socialisation and mobilisation. The involvement of play therapists and youth workers cannot be underestimated for the mental well-being of those who have undergone such a traumatic experience. CYP who are comfortable, pain free and happy are likely to make a quicker recovery in mental and physical health, and levels of pain, anxiety and stress can be reduced (He et al., 2014).

Nutrition and Hydration

Feeding problems after complex cardiac surgery are well documented (Medoff-Cooper and Ravishankar, 2013) and occur at a time when appropriate calorific intake is essential for recovery during a period of critical illness (Justice et al., 2018; Medoff-Cooper et al., 2016; Mitting et al., 2015). Enteral feeding is believed to reduce the systemic inflammatory response experienced by many infants and children admitted to intensive care (Justice et al., 2018). Infants should be offered small but frequent bottle feeds, and where this is not possible, nasogastric tube feeding may have to be considered, especially if the infant manifests respiratory distress or cyanosis. Managing the child's hydration is an important aspect of care and all fluid intake must therefore be monitored carefully to ensure that episodes of overhydration or dehydration are avoided. Working closely with the dietetic team is essential for careful ongoing assessment and management of supplementary nutrition. This could range from increased calorific supplements to a specialist diet as part of a complex treatment pathway.

CYP with heart failure frequently experience problems of systemic fluid retention and hepatomegaly. This may further aggravate the child's respiratory distress and compromise cardiac output and organ perfusion. Digestion and absorption of nutrients and elimination of metabolic by-products may be adversely affected. For some babies, diuretics are required to manage any potential circulatory overload, which is a significant physiological effect of their condition.

Nutritional intake will also be paramount to supporting growth and development, especially if an infant is in an inter-stage period of needing further surgery. This is a potentially vulnerable and fragile time for such babies and can be a very worrying and stressful time for parents and families. Parents are extremely aware of the morbidity and mortality of their offspring and there is a level of caregiver anxiety as they are aware of the need for close monitoring and promotion of good weight gain during inter-stage surgery to underpin overall outcome (Stewart et al., 2015).

ACTIVITY

Read

Justice, L. et al., 2018. Nutrition considerations in the pediatric cardiac intensive care unit patient. World Journal for Pediatric and Congenital Heart Surgery 9 (3), 333–343. doi: 10.1177/2150135118765881.

Reflect on

- The impact of critical illness and cardiac intensive care on the nutrition of children with cardiac problems.
- The impact of systemic fluid retention and hepatomegaly on the child's ability to feed and absorb nutrients.
- Why hepatomegaly could have a compromising effect on the function of the diaphragm and the gastrointestinal tract.
- Why children with CHD may have faltering growth.
- The impact on the parental /caregiver role while striving to promote optimum feeding for fragile infants with functionally univentricular heart conditions, who are in the inter-surgical stage, waiting for their next surgical intervention.

Fluid balance and excretion. Heart failure compromises myocardial contractility and reduces cardiac output. This invariably leads to reduced renal perfusion and activation of the renin-angiotensin-aldosterone system, which causes retention of sodium and water. If unchecked, the persistent retention of sodium and water not only reduces urinary output, but also contributes to the development of pulmonary and systemic oedema. The retention of fluid contributes to weight gain despite the child's reduced nutritional intake and occasional vomiting. It is worth noting that significant fluid retention causes weight gain and tends to mask the child's cachexic state.

 ACTIVITY

- Outline the measures that can be taken to monitor the child's fluid intake and elimination.
- Give a reasoned account as to why the child's blood electrolyte values should be monitored and acted upon.

Wound healing

During critical illness the systemic inflammatory response has been linked to an increased incidence of infection and delayed wound healing; however, as highlighted above, early enteral feeding is believed to have beneficial effects (Justice et al., 2018). The management of sternal or thoracotomy wounds requires minimising pain during routine dressing changes; conformability of the dressing for comfort; a dressing to inhibit introduction of infection and promotion of healthy healing (Morris et al., 2009).

A recent exhibition 'scarred for life' (Somerville Foundation, 2018) has shared the physical and psychological impact of living with a scar for adults who had surgery for CHD as a child. This demonstrates the importance of a supportive approach during re-dressing episodes, aiming to

minimise the psychological trauma that some CYP experience; and the need for ongoing psychological support to encourage coping, adaptation and emotional resilience, especially as many CYP will require further surgical incisions.

Pharmaceutical Interventions

Common medications prescribed for CYP with CHD and specifically for the management of heart failure include: furosemide (a loop diuretic) and spironolactone or amiloride (a potassium-sparing diuretic). In some cases, an angiotensin-converting enzyme (ACE inhibitor) such as captopril or enalapril will be required, as well as digoxin (a cardiac glycoside). CYP who need such medication may also be given potassium supplements to maintain physiologically desirable plasma potassium values.

 READING ACTIVITY

Chapter 18 (The heart pp 246–259) and Chapter 19 (The vascular system pp 265–282) in: Rang et al., 2012. Rang & Dales Pharmacology, seventh ed. Elsevier Churchill Livingston, New York.

National Institute for Clinical Excellence, 2018. British National Formulary for Children. Available from: <https://bnfc.nice.org.uk/>.

 REFLECT ON YOUR PRACTICE

- Explain how the medication used to control heart failure in CYP works. What would be the medications of choice and why?
- Give a reasoned account of the improvements in the CYP health because of the appropriate therapeutic intervention.

Emotional Support and Family Centred Care

Invasive procedures, such as open-heart surgery, are painful and frightening regardless of age. These CYP require emotional and psychological support from their parents, siblings and the practitioners caring for them. Caring for a CYP with congenital or acquired heart disease requires many adaptations of the parental role, so central to the deliverance of care to the CYP are the family and close caregivers. In a recent study, mothers receiving family centred care felt more supported, and adaptation to the stress of parenting a child with CHD was more probable (Bruce et al., 2014).

Parents of infants with minor and complex CHD are at increased risk of experiencing anxiety, stress, depression and post-traumatic stress disorder; this has remained the same for many years regardless of new treatments and improved outcomes (Davis et al., 1998; Pelchat et al., 1999; Brosig et al., 2007; Doherty et al., 2009; Franich-Ray et al., 2013; Fonseca et al., 2013; Fischer et al., 2012). For those families that are coming to terms with having a CYP with a life-long and potentially life-threatening complex disease, a particularly traumatic stage is during infancy, a time of new experiences and thus great adjustment. A programme of psychosocial interventions can have a positive impact on the infant with severe congenital heart disease and also the mother (McCuster et al., 2010).

Within the complex spectrum of congenital heart disease hypoplastic left heart syndrome (HLHS) requires life-saving treatments. Parents experience numerous challenges as they learn to parent a child with complex care requirements and during the child's first year of life there is an appropriate parental response of necessitated vigilant parental control, as parents gain mastery of the skills required to care for their child (Meakins et al., 2015). Along with mastery of complex skills, parents can feel uncertainty about their child's long-term survival and protectiveness develops to help them cope with the managing of their fears, fears that require adequate support (both formal and informal), the lack which can heighten parental vigilance of monitoring and caring for their child with HLHS in order to maintain control (Rempel and Harrison, 2007; Rempel et al., 2012, 2013; Meakins et al., 2015). Parents' experiences can relate to safety and security and the ability to adjust and adapt, so engaging parents and grandparents in the pre-discharge planning is essential to support implementation of patient and family centred care while recognising the differences and preferences of individual family needs (Gaskin, 2017).

In recent years significant attention has been attributed to helping parents of infants with functionally univentricular hearts. The first and significant time of worry and concern within the parenting role is the time of discharge. Here the need to support care within a family centred approach is critical to help parents take on the responsibility of caring for their infant at home. Discharge teaching and planning done throughout the hospital stay allows parents to retain more of the knowledge and skills needed to care for their child at home and continuous teaching along with parental involvement in their child's care before leaving the hospital increases parents' confidence in caring for their child in their transition home (March, 2017). Indeed, this preparedness is something that needs attention as parents are not always adequately prepared for discharge and not equipped with the necessary information to recognise deterioration of their infant following first-stage surgery (Gaskin et al., 2016). This is a crucial time for these infants where the mortality rate during their inter-stage surgical period can be up to 15% (Barron et al., 2009).

Attention to supporting parents following first-stage surgery has gained momentum within the United Kingdom. The development of a Congenital Heart Assessment Tool (CHAT) aims to support parental discharge preparation; vigilance and mastery within the caring role at home; and reassurance and support, thus enabling early identification of a clinical deterioration of an infant (Gaskin et al., 2018). The CHAT provides a traffic light system divided into three columns to assess low risk (green), intermediates risk (amber) and high risk (red), thus enabling the parents to assess the 'normal' behaviour of their child and to assess the development of any clinical concerns and take appropriate action (Gaskin et al., 2016, 2018).

SUMMARY

This chapter has briefly explored the complex cardiovascular problems that impact on the lives of CYP and their families, including:

- review of the embryonic, fetal and developmental anatomy and physiology of the cardiovascular system in children and young people (CYP);

- identifying the causes of congenital, inherited and acquired heart disease in CYP;
- and considering the evidence-based assessment and management of CYP with congenital, inherited and acquired heart disease, adopting a family centred approach to care.

REFERENCES

Andersen, L.B., Riddoch, C., Susi Kriemler, S., Hills, A., 2011. Physical activity and cardiovascular risk factors in children. Br. J. Sports Med. 45 1063–1063.

Ansermino, J.M., Wiens, M.O., Kissoon, N., 2018. We need smarter trigger tools for diagnosing sepsis in children in Canada. CMAJ. 190 (36), E1060–E1061.

Ball, J., Bindler, R., Cowen, K., Shaw, M., 2016. Principles of Pediatric Nursing: Caring for Children, seventh ed. Pearson, Upper Saddle River, NJ. ISBN-13: 978-0-13-425701-3.

Barker, J., Williams, C., Tulloh, R., 2009. Understanding and treatment of heart failure. Paediatr. Child Health 19 (1), 1–8.

Barron, D., Kilby, M., Davis, B., et al., 2009. Hypoplastic left heart syndrome. Lancet 374, 551–564.

Blyth, M., Howe, D., Gnanapragasam, J., Wellesley, D., 2008. The hidden mortality of transposition of the great arteries and survival advantage provided by prenatal diagnosis. BJOG An Int. J. Obstet. Gynaecol. 115 (9), 1096–1100.

Brady, M., 2017. Obesity-related hypertension in children. Front. Pediatr. 5, 197.

British Heart Foundation, 2018. Inherited Heart Conditions. Available from: https://www.bhf.org.uk/informationsupport/support/inherited-heart-conditions.

Brosig, C.L., Whitstone, B.N., Frommelt, M.A., Frisbee, S.J., Leuthner, S.R., 2007. Psychological distress in parents of children with severe congenital heart disease: the impact of prenatal versus postnatal diagnosis. J. Perinatol. 27 (11), 687–692. https://doi.org/10.1038/sj.jp.7211807.

Bruce, E., Lilja, C., Sundin, K., 2014. Mothers' lived experiences of support when living with young children with congenital heart defects. J. Spec. Pediatr. Nurs. (JSPN): J. Spec. Pediatr. Nurs. (JSPN) 19, 54–67. https://doi.org/10.1111/jspn.12049.

Collins, P., 2008. Embryogenesis. In: Standring, S. (Ed.), Gray's Anatomy – The Anatomical Basis of Clinical Practice. Churchill Livingstone, New York.

Davey, B., Szwast, A., Rychik, J., 2012. Diagnosis and management of heart failure in the fetus. Minerva Pediatr. 64 (5), 471–492.

Davis, C.C., Brown, R.T., Bakeman, R., Campbell, R., 1998. Psychological adaptation and adjustment of mothers of children with congenital heart disease: stress, coping, and family functioning. J. Pediatr. Psychol. 23 (4), 219–228. https://doi.org/10.1093/jpepsy/23.4.219.

Dhillon, R., 2020. Paediatric ECGs made easy. Paediatr. Child Health 30 (6), 230–235. https://doi.org/10.1016/j.paed.2020.03.006.

Doherty, N., McCusker, C.G., Molloy, B., Mulholland, C., Rooney, N., Craig, B., Sands, A., Stewart, M., Casey, F., 2009. Predictors of psychological functioning in mothers and fathers of infants born with severe CHD. J. Reprod. Infant Psychol. 27 (4), 390–400.

Ediriweera, D.S., Dilina, N., Perera, U., Flores, F., Samita, S., 2017. Risk of low birth weight on adulthood hypertension–evidence from a tertiary care hospital in a South Asian country, Sri Lanka: a retrospective cohort study. BMC Publ. Health 17, 358.

Elkomy, M.H., Drover, D.R., Glotzbach, K.L., Galinkin, J.L., Frymoyer, A., 2016. Pharmacokinetics of morphine and its metabolites in infants and young children after congenital heart surgery. AAPS. J. 18 (1), 124–133.

Ewer, A.K., Middleton, L.J., Furmston, A.T., Bhoyar, A., Daniels, J.P., Thangaratinam, S., et al., 2011. Pulse oximetry screening for congenital heart defects in newborn infants (PulseOx): a test accuracy study. Lancet 378 (9793), 785–794.

Fischer, A.L., Butz, C., Nicholson, L., Blankenship, A., Dyke, P., Cua, C.L., 2012. Caregiver anxiety upon discharge for neonates with congenital heart disease. Congenit. Heart Dis. 7 (1), 41–45. https://doi.org/10.1111/j.1747-0803.2011.00600.x.

Fisher, D.J., 1984. Oxygenation and metabolism in the developing heart. Semin. Perinatalo. 8, 217–225.

Fonseca, A., Nazare, B., Canavarro, M.C., 2013. Parental psychological distress and confidence after an infant's birth: the role of attachment representations in parents of infants with congenital anomalies and parents of healthy infants. J. Clin. Psychol. Med. Settings 20 (2), 143–155. https://doi.org/10.1007/s10880-012-9329-9.

Franich-Ray, C., Bright, M.A., Anderson, V., et al., 2013. Trauma reactions in mothers and fathers after their infant's cardiac surgery. J. Pediatr. Psychol. 38 (5), 494–505. https://doi.org/10.1093/jpepsy/jst015.

Fukushima, A., Alrob, O.A., Zhang, L., et al., 2016. Acetylation and succinylation contribute to maturational alterations in energy metabolism in the newborn heart. Am. J. Physiol. Heart Circ. Physiol. 311, H347–H363.

Gaskin, K.L., 2017. Patterns of transition experience for parents going home from hospital with their infant after first stage surgery for complex congenital heart disease. J. Pediatr. Nurs. 41, e23–e32.

Gaskin, K., Barron, D., Daniels, A., 2016. Parents' preparedness for their infants' discharge following first-stage cardiac surgery: development of a parental early warning tool. Cardiol. Young 26 (7), 1414–1424.

Gaskin, K.L., Wray, J., Barron, D.J., 2018. Acceptability of a parental early warning tool for parents of infants with complex congenital heart disease: a qualitative feasibility study. Arch. Dis. Child. 103 (9), 880–886.

Gluckman, P., Heymann, M., 1996. Paediatrics and Perinatology: the Scientific Basis. Edward Arnold, London.

Guyton, A., Hall, J., 2006. Textbook of Medical Physiology. WB Saunders, Philadelphia.

He, H.G., Zhu, L., Li, H.C.W., Wang, W., Vehviläinen–Julkunen, K., Chan, W.C.S., 2014. A randomized controlled trial of the effectiveness of a therapeutic play intervention on outcomes of children undergoing inpatient elective surgery: study protocol. J. Adv. Nurs. 70 (2), 431–442.

Health Quality Improvement Partnership, 2017. National Congenital Heart Disease Audit Report 2013–2016. Available from: http://www.ucl.ac.uk/nicor/audits/congenital/documents/annual-reports/National_Congenital_Heart_Disease_2013_16_annual_report.

Heathfield, E., Hussain, T., Qureshi, S., et al., 2013. Cardiovascular magnetic resonance imaging in congenital heart disease as an alternative to diagnostic invasive cardiac catheterization: a single center experience. Congenit. Heart Dis. 8 (4), 322–327.

Helbing, W.A., Ouhlous, M., 2015. Cardiac magnetic resonance imaging in children. Pediatr. Radiol. 45 (1), 20–26.

Hill, M.A., 2018. Embryology. Intermediate Cardiac Embryology. Available from: https://embryology.med.unsw.edu.au/embryology/index.php/Intermediate_Cardiac_Embryology.

Justice, L., et al., 2018. Nutrition considerations in the pediatric cardiac intensive care unit patient. World. J. Pediatr. Congenit. Heart. Surg. 9 (3), 333–343.

Khalid, O., Koenig, P., 2006. The use of echocardiography in congenital heart surgery and intervention. Expert Rev. Cardiovasc. Ther. 4 (2), 263–271.

Ko, J.M., 2015. Genetic syndromes associated with congenital heart disease. Korean. Circ. J. 45 (5), 357–361.

Landis, B.J., Levey, A., Levasseur, S.M., et al., 2013. Prenatal diagnosis of congenital heart disease and birth outcomes. Pediatr. Cardiol. 34 (3), 597–605.

Lauridsen, M.H., Kristensen, A.D., Hjortdal, V.E., Jensen, T.S., Nikolajsen, L., 2014. Chronic pain in children after cardiac surgery via sternotomy. Cardiol. Young 24, 893–899.

Little Hearts Matter (LHM), 2018. The Spoon Theory. Available from: https://www.lhm.org.uk/zipper-zone/lifestyle-information/half-heart-half-energy-2/the-spoon-theory/.

Lopaschuk, G.D., Jaswal, J.S., 2010. Energy metabolic phenotype of the cardiomyocyte during development, differentiation, and postnatal maturation. J. Cardiovasc. Pharmacol. 56, 130–140.

Lopaschuk, G.D., Spafford, M.A., 1990. Energy substrate utilization by isolated working hearts from newborn rabbits. Am. J. Physiol. 258, H1274–H1280.

Lopaschuk, G.D., Spafford, M.A., Marsh, D.R., 1991. Glycolysis is predominant source of myocardial ATP production immediately after birth. Am. J. Physiol. 261, H1698–H1705.

Lynch, T.A., Abel, D.E., 2015. Teratogens and congenital heart disease. J. Diagn. Med. Sonogr. 31 (5), 301–305.

Makinde, A., Kantor, P.F., Lopaschuk, G.D., 1998. Maturation of fatty acid and carbohydrate metabolism in the newborn heart. Mol. Cell. Biochem. 188, 49–56. https://doi.org/10.1023/A:1006860104840.

March, S., 2017. Parents' perceptions during the transition to home for their child with a congenital heart defect: how can we support families of children with hypoplastic left heart syndrome? J. Spec. Pediatr. Nurs. 22 (3), 1–11.

McCusker, C.G., Doherty, N.N., Molloy, B., et al., 2010. A controlled trial of early interventions to promote maternal adjustment and development in infants born with severe congenital heart disease. Child Care Health Dev. 36 (1), 110–117.

Meakins, L., Ray, L., Hegadoren, K., Rogers, L.G., Rempel, G.R., 2015. Parental vigilance in caring for their children with hypoplastic left heart syndrome. Pediatr. Nurs. 41 (1), 31–50.

Medoff-Cooper, B., Ravishankar, C., 2013. Nutrition and growth in congenital heart disease: a challenge in children. Current Opinions in Cardiology 28 (2), 122–129.

Medoff-Cooper, B., Irving, S.Y., Hanlon, A.L., et al., 2016. The association among feeding mode, growth, and developmental outcomes in infants with complex congenital heart disease at 6 and 12 months of age. J. Pediatr. 169, 154–159.

Mehta, C., Dhillon, R., 2004. Understanding paediatric ECGs. Curr. Paediatr. 14 (3), 229–236.

Miserandino, C., 2018. The Spoon Theory. Available from: https://butyoudontlooksick.com/articles/written-by-christine/the-spoon-theory/.

Mitting, R., Marino, L., Macrae, D., et al., 2015. Nutritional status and clinical outcome in post-term neonates undergoing surgery for congenital heart disease. Pediatr. Crit. Care Med. 16 (5), 448–452.

Morris, C., Emsley, P., Marland, E., Meuleneire, F., White, R., 2009. Use of wound dressings with soft silicone adhesive technology. Paediatr. Nurs. 21 (3), 38–43.

National Institute of Clinical Excellence, 2018. British National Formulary for Children. Available from: https://bnfc.nice.org.uk/.

National Institute of Clinical Excellence (CG160), 2017. Fever in Under 5s Assessment and Initial Management. Available from: https://www.nice.org.uk/Guidance/CG160.

Peate, I., Gormley-Flemming, E., 2015. Fundamentals of Children's Anatomy and Physiology: A Textbook for Nursing and Healthcare Students, first ed. Wiley Blackwell.

Pelchat, D., Ricard, N., Bouchard, J.M., et al., 1999. Adaptation of parents in relation to their 6-month-old infant's type of disability. Child Care Health Dev. 25 (5), 377–397.

Penny, D.J., Vick, G.W., 2011. Ventricular septal defect. In: The Lancet, vol. 377. North American Edition, pp. 1103–1112. 9771.

Priebe, H.J., Skarvan, K., 2000. Cardiovascular Physiology Fundamentals of Anaesthesia and Acute Medicine. BMJ Books.

Premkumar, S., Sundararajan, P., Sangaralingam, T., 2016. Clinical profile of cardiac arrhythmias in children attending the out-patient department of a Tertiary Paediatric Care Centre in Chennai. J. Clin. Diagn. Res. 10 (12), SC06–SC08.

Prudhoe, S., Abu-Harb, M., Richmond, S., Wren, C., 2013. Neonatal screening for critical cardiovascular anomalies using pulse oximetry. Archives of Disease in Childhood. Fetal and Neonatal Edition 98 (4), F346–F350.

Rang, H., Dale, M., Ritter, J., Moore, P., 2007. Pharmacology. Churchill Livingstone, Edinburgh.

Rasanen, J., Wood, D.C., Weiner, S., Ludomirski, A., Huhta, J.C., 1996. Role of the pulmonary circulation in the distribution of human fetal cardiac output during the second half of pregnancy. Circulation 94, 1068–1073.

Rempel, G.R., Harrison, M.J., 2007. Safeguarding precarious survival: parenting children who have life-threatening heart disease. Qual. Health Res. 17 (6), 824–837. https://doi.org/10.1177/1049732307303164.

Rempel, G.R., Rogers, L.G., Ravindran, V., Magill-Evans, J., 2012. Facets of parenting a child with hypoplastic left heart syndrome. Nurs. Res. Pract. 1–9, 2019. https://doi.org/10.1155/2012/714178.

Rempel, G.R., Ravindran, V., Rogers, L.G., Magill-Evans, J., 2013. Parenting under pressure: a grounded theory of parenting young children with life-threatening congenital heart disease. J. Adv. Nurs. 69 (3), 619–630. https://doi.org/10.1111/j.1365-2648.2012.06044.x.

Royal College of Nursing, 2012. Core Competences for Nursing Children and Young People. RCN, London. : www.rcn.org/publications.

Royal College of Nursing, 2014. Children and Young People's Cardiac Nursing: RCN Guidance on Roles, Career Pathways and Competence Development. RCN, London. Available from: www.rcn.org/publications.

Royal College of Nursing, 2017. Getting it Right for Children and Young People. Self-Assessment Tool for General Practice Nurses and Other First Contact Settings Providing Care for Children and Young People. Available from: www.rcn.org/publications.

Schoenwolf, G., Bleyl, S., Brauer, P., Francis-West, P., 2014. Larsen's Human Embryology, fifth ed. Elsevier Churchill Livingstone, Philadelphia.

Second Task Force on Blood Pressure Control in Children, 1987. Normal blood pressure readings for boys. National Heart. Lung and. Blood Institute, Bethesda. MD.

Shane, A.L., Sánchez, P.J., Stoll, B.J., 2017. Neonatal sepsis. Lancet 390 (10104), 1770–1780.

Sharland, G., 2012. Fetal cardiac screening and variation in prenatal detection rates of CHD: why bother with screening at all? Future Cardiol. 8 (2), 189–202.

Silverman, M.E., Wooley, C.F., 2008. Samuel A. Levine and the history of grading systolic murmurs. Am. J. Cardiol. 102 (8), 1107–1110.

Somerville Foundation, 2018. Scarred for Life. Available from: https://www.thesf.org.uk/community/scarred-for-life-2.aspx.

Spratt, J.D., 2016. Thorax. In: Standring, S. (Ed.), Gray's Anatomy – the Anatomical Basis of Clinical Practice, Forty-first ed. Elsevier Churchill Livingstone, New York.

Stewart, J., Dempster, R., Allen, R., et al., 2015. Caregiver anxiety due to interstage feeding concerns. Congenit. Heart Dis. 10 (2), E98–E106.

Townsend, N., Bhatnagar, P., Wickramasinghc, K., et al., 2013. Children and Young People Statistics 2013. British Heart Foundation, London.

van der Linde, D., Konings, E.E., Slager, M.A., et al., 2011. Birth prevalence of congenital heart disease worldwide: a systematic review and meta-analysis. J. Am. Coll. Cardiol. 58 (21), 2241–2247. https://doi.org/10.1016/j.jacc.2011.08.025.

Wren, C., Reinhardt, Z., Khawaja, K., 2008. Twenty-year trends in diagnosis of life-threatening neonatal cardiovascular malformations. Arch. Dis. Child. 93, F33–F35.

SUGGESTIONS FOR FURTHER READING

Barker, J., Williams, C., Tulloh, R., 2009. Understanding and treatment of heart failure. Paediatr. Child Health 19 (1), 1–8.

Chien, K., 2000. Genomic circuits and the integrative biology of cardiac diseases. Nature 407, 227–232.

This article explores some of the complex interactions between possible genetic and environmental factors and how these could act as modifiers of human health, particularly cardiovascular disease. Considerable attention is given to the distinctions between the pathogenesis of congenital and that of acquired cardiovascular problem.

Cook, K., Langton, H. (Eds.), 2009. Cardiothoracic Care for Children and Young People: A Multidisciplinary Approach. Wiley Blackwell, Oxford.

A comprehensive and interprofessional guide aimed at all health care professionals working with CYP with CHD. Structured around the timeline of the patient's health care journey.

Panesar, D., Burch, M., 2017. Understanding and treating heart failure in children. Paediatr. Child Health 27 (2), 43–49.

Peate, I., Gormley-Fleming, E. (Eds.), 2015. Fundamentals of Children's Anatomy and Physiology: A Textbook for Nursing and Healthcare Students. John Wiley & Sons.

Roberts, S., 2015. The cardiac system (chapter 9). In: Peate, I., Gormley-Flemming, E. (Eds.), Fundamentals of Children's Anatomy and Physiology: A Textbook for Nursing and Healthcare Students, first ed.

Roberts, P., Burch, M., 2009. Cardiomyopathy in childhood. Paediatr. Child Health 19 (1), 15–24.

A useful resource that easily explains anatomy and physiology related specifically to children and young people.

Ruegger, C., Bucher, H.U., Mieth, R.A., 2010. Pulse oximetry in the newborn: is the left hand pre- or post-ductal? BMC Paediatrics 10 (35).

Seale, A., Shinebourne, E., 2004. Cardiac problems in Down syndrome. Curr. Paediatr. 14 (1), 33–38.

This article provides an excellent account of the spectrum of heart defects, therapeutic interventions and anticipated outcomes in children with Down syndrome.

Srivastava, D., Olson, E., 2000. A genetic blueprint for cardiac development. Nature 407, 221–226.

This article offers an invaluable insight into some of the genetic factors that may influence the development of the embryo's heart.

Sylva, M., van den Hoff, M.J.B., Moorman, A.F.M., 2014. Development of the human heart. Am. J. Med. Genet. 164A, 1347–1371.

http://www.childrenshospital.org/conditions-and-treatments/conditions/a/arrhythmia.

A useful international website to explore along with others such as Cincinnati Children's Hospital and The Royal Children's Hospital Melbourne.

13

Children's Liver Disease

Louise Hair

LEARNING OUTCOMES

- To understand the structure and functions of the liver.
- To understand the concept of and complications related to acute and chronic liver failure.

- To gain insight into the types of liver disease which affect children and young people at different stages of development.
- To understand the indications for and the implications of liver transplantation in children.

GLOSSARY

Bile Yellow-green liquid produced in the liver.
Cholangiocytes Cells which line the bile ducts and transport bile.
Cholestasis Decreased excretion of bile leading to jaundice, itching, fat and vitamin malabsorption.
Cirrhosis Scarring of the liver tissue as a result of longstanding injury to the liver tissue.
Fibrosis The development of fibrous tissue within the liver as a result of injury to the liver tissue, often precedes cirrhosis.
Hepatitis Inflammation of the liver.
Hepatocytes The most numerous liver cells, responsible for the metabolic functions of the liver and production of bile.
Hepatomegaly Enlarged liver, may be palpable below the costal margin.

Hyperbilirubinaemia Elevated levels of bilirubin in the blood causing jaundice.
Kernicterus Neurological damage caused by significantly elevated levels of unconjugated jaundice.
Melaena Dark, tarry, offensive smelling faeces resulting from partly digested blood (indicative of upper gastrointestinal [GI] bleeding).
Pruritus Itch.
Splenomegaly Enlarged spleen, may be palpable below the costal margin.
Steatosis Accumulation of fat in the liver.
Transaminases Enzymes which are produced by hepatocytes (ALT and AST) and cholangiocytes (GGT).

INTRODUCTION

Liver disease in childhood is relatively rare, but before the advent of liver transplantation, was often fatal. During infancy, childhood and adolescence, liver disease may present with acute liver failure, or individuals may develop chronic problems due to an underlying pathology. In neonates and infants, acute liver failure is most likely to be caused by infection or an inherited metabolic disease, whereas chronic liver disease may arise from congenital defects such as biliary atresia. In older children and adolescents, autoimmune liver disease and metabolic conditions such as Wilson disease are more common causes of chronic liver disease. Increasingly, the impact of non-alcoholic fatty liver disease (NAFLD) is also being felt in this age group due to changes in Western diet and lifestyle. More recently, breakthroughs in DNA sequencing and genetic testing have enabled hitherto unexplained childhood liver diseases to be identified and treated earlier with potentially better outcomes. However, in many cases, and in particular for patients presenting with acute liver failure, transplantation remains the only option for long-term survival in childhood liver disease.

DEVELOPMENT, STRUCTURE AND FUNCTIONS OF THE LIVER

In order to fully understand the causes and symptoms of paediatric liver disease, it is essential to have knowledge of the structure and functions of the liver itself (see Fig. 13.1).

The liver is the largest internal organ in the body, situated in the right upper quadrant of the abdomen beneath the diaphragm and above the stomach and intestines.

It begins to appear during weeks 3–4 of embryonic development when a hollow endodermal bud develops from the

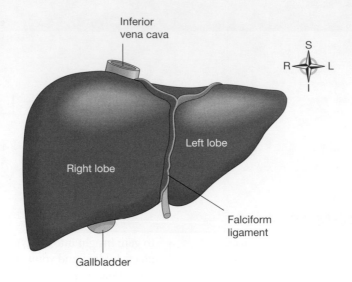

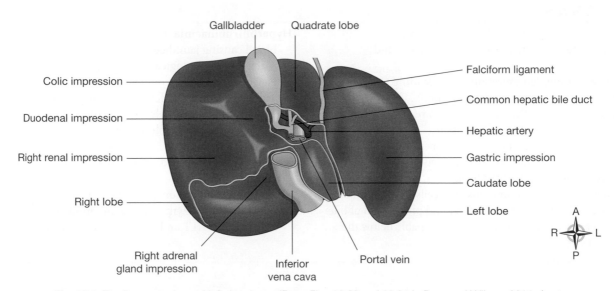

Fig. 13.1 The liver: anterior and inferior views. (From Figs 12.33 and 12.34 in Ross and Wilson, 2014. Anatomy and Physiology in Health and Illness, twelfth ed. Elsevier, p 309.)

foregut (which will become the duodenum) to form the hepatic diverticulum. This will become the liver, gallbladder and pancreas. Cords of endodermal cells extend into the mesenchyme of the septum transversum and the bud divides into two parts – hepatic and biliary. The hepatic part will differentiate into hepatocytes or ductal cells (which will form bile ducts within the liver). The biliary part will form the extrahepatic bile ducts, gallbladder and pancreas (Sandwell, 2005).

Initially two lobes, approximately the same size develop, but the right lobe grows faster than the left, eventually becoming about six times larger. The liver remains covered by a layer of mesenteric tissue, which becomes the connective tissue (Glisson) capsule. The embryonic liver produces blood cells, functioning as a haemopoietic centre, beginning in weeks 4–6 of gestation and peaking between 3–6 months when the bone

marrow begins to take over before stopping at birth (Stringer, 2014). At around 12 weeks' gestation, the hepatocytes begin to produce bile from the breakdown of haemoglobin. The bile is excreted from the cells via the bile ducts into the gallbladder before being released into the gut. By week 13, the bile colours the meconium dark green. The liver plays an important role in the circulation of blood between mother and fetus by means of the umbilical vein, which directs blood from the placenta via the liver into the inferior vena cava. About half enters specialised capillaries (the hepatic sinusoids) and half passes through the ductus venosus and bypasses the liver. At birth, the liver occupies around 40% of the peritoneal cavity and is palpable below the costal margin. It accounts for 4% of the total body weight of infants, dropping to 2% in adults (Stringer, 2014).

The two anatomical lobes of the liver are further divided into four lobes and eight segments, each containing lobules (See Fig. 13.2), which can be described as the 'structural units' of the liver although the 'functional unit' is known as the acinus (Larson and Hauswald, 2014). In contrast to other organs in the body, the liver is unusual in that as well as arterial blood from the hepatic artery, it also receives 75% of its blood supply from the portal vein, which drains blood from the intestinal system and the spleen in order for it to be filtered by the liver. The artery and portal vein along with the main bile duct, lymphatic duct and nerve supply, enter the liver at a region known as the hilum. Venous outflow from the liver is via the hepatic vein into the inferior vena cava.

Each liver lobule is roughly hexagonal in shape and is formed of plates of hepatocytes which radiate out around a central vein. The hepatocytes are in close contact with blood-filled sinusoids and also lie adjacent to ducts or 'canaliculi' into which bile is secreted. Situated around the perimeter of the lobule, clustered together at the six 'corners' are branches of the hepatic artery, hepatic portal vein and bile duct, which together form the portal triad. Blood flows out of the sinusoids into the central vein and is transported out of the liver via the hepatic vein. The sinusoids are lined with phagocytic Kupffer cells, which help eradicate bacteria from the gut, as well as endothelial cells and hepatic stellate cells, which store fat and vitamin A.

The liver performs over 400 functions in the body that can be broadly divided into three categories: metabolic, storage and secretory. These functions include: the metabolism of fat, protein and carbohydrate; the synthesis of blood-clotting factors and inhibitors; detoxification of hormones, drugs and other substances; storage of glycogen, iron and vitamins A, D, E and B_{12}; blood storage and filtration; and bile synthesis and excretion (Box 13.1). The liver plays an important part in maintaining blood glucose levels by storing excess glucose as glycogen and releasing it when required. The hepatocytes also convert non-carbohydrates to glucose (glyconeogenesis) when glycogen stores are depleted. The production of bile salts enables fat in the diet to be emulsified to aid absorption and for further metabolism in the liver. The liver synthesises proteins, predominantly albumin, which is the main plasma protein responsible for maintaining oncotic pressure and transporting substances in the blood. It detoxifies ammonia, produced from the metabolism of amino acids, converting it to urea for elimination via the kidneys. All but one of the proteins and enzymes involved in the clotting cascade are also produced in the liver. The liver also plays a role in the immune system, the Kupffer cells being the first line of defence against

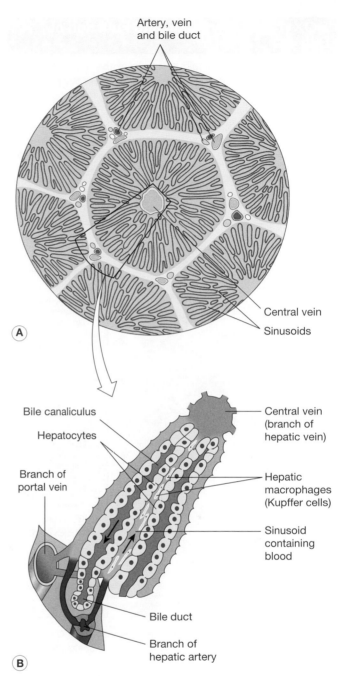

Fig.13.2 A. Magnified transverse section of a liver lobule B. Direction of the flow of blood and bile in a liver lobule. (From Fig. 12.35A in Ross and Wilson, 2014. Anatomy and Physiology in Health and Illness, twelfth ed. Elsevier, p 310.)

pathogens or toxins derived from the gut (Larson and Hauswald, 2014). Despite the hepatocytes' unique ability to regenerate following an insult, any disorders affecting the liver may interfere in these processes due to acute or chronic liver failure.

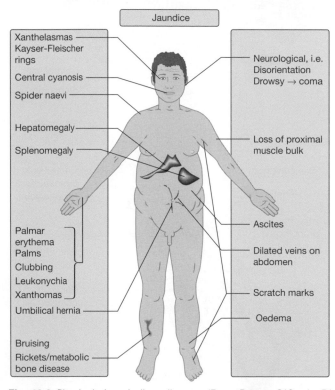

Fig. 13.3 Physical signs in liver disease. (From Bacon, O'Grady, Di Bisceglie, Lake, 2006. Comprehensive Clinical Hepatology, second ed. Elsevier.)

SIGNS AND SYMPTOMS OF LIVER DISEASE

Chronic liver disease develops over time as a result of on-going damage to the liver, whereas acute liver failure is characterised by inflammation and necrosis of the liver tissue. Both may result in jaundice, prolonged clotting, elevated serum transaminases (see Table 13.1) and varying degrees of hepatic encephalopathy. Signs of chronic liver disease also include failure to thrive, metabolic bone disease due to vitamin deficiency, pruritus, portal hypertension and ascites. Additional physical signs which may be seen are shown in Fig. 13.3 although some are less likely to be seen in children. Hypoglycaemia, disturbances in acid-base balance, nausea and vomiting, anorexia and fever and renal dysfunction may also be seen in acute liver failure.

Jaundice

Jaundice (hyperbilirubinaemia) is one of the most common presenting features in liver disease. Raised bilirubin levels (See Table 13.1) result in yellow pigmentation of the skin and the sclera of the eyes due to the inability of the liver to excrete bile properly. Jaundice in liver disease is predominantly due to conjugated hyperbilirubinaemia as opposed to the unconjugated hyperbilirubinaemia, which often presents in the neonatal period. Any infant presenting with jaundice past 2 weeks of age (3 weeks for preterm neonates) must be investigated for prolonged jaundice by carrying out a split bilirubin blood test to determine whether the jaundice is conjugated or unconjugated (see NICE guidance on jaundice in newborn babies under 28 days, 2010). A conjugated fraction of more than 20% of the total is nearly always pathological and a sign of liver disease (Samyn and Mieli-Vergani, 2011). It is important to note that the stools of babies with unconjugated jaundice will be yellow and the urine will be colourless. Conjugated jaundice is often associated with paler stools and yellow urine although this may be difficult to determine without a stool colour chart or if the urine stains the stools and nappy. Conjugated bilirubin in itself is not dangerous as it is water-soluble and therefore cannot cross the blood-brain barrier causing kernicterus, in contrast to high levels of unconjugated hyperbilirubinaemia. However, it is usually a sign of liver disease and therefore children with conjugated jaundice must be referred promptly to a specialist centre for further investigation.

Coagulopathy

The liver is responsible for the synthesis of clotting factors and their inhibitors. Prothrombin time (PT) or international normalised ratio (INR) are used as measures of the liver's synthetic function. Prolonged PT or INR indicate liver failure and the degree to which they are prolonged is related to the severity of the liver failure. In acute liver failure coagulopathy is related to depletion of clotting factors, whereas in chronic liver disease, deficiency in vitamin K, a fat-soluble vitamin, will also result in prolonged clotting due to a reduction in the synthesis of these factors. Checking PT or INR in a child presenting with liver disease is essential and if abnormal, a dose of intravenous vitamin K should be administered and clotting profile checked to assess its response. In children presenting with sepsis, DIC (disseminated intravascular coagulopathy) can also contribute to the coagulopathy (Table 13.1).

Hepatic Encephalopathy

Hepatic encephalopathy (HE) is a reversible neurological disorder resulting from acute or chronic liver failure. Clinical signs range from mild intellectual impairment and sleep disturbances (Grade 1); through to drowsiness, confusion, inappropriate behaviour (Grades 2–3); and coma (Grade 4) (Whitington and Alonso, 2009). Seizures may also occur in acute liver failure and will require appropriate management. Various mechanisms for the development of HE have been proposed and a combination of these theories is the most

TABLE 13.1 Liver Function Tests and Their Meaning

Reference Range	Indication
Total bilirubin 3–20 µmol/L Conjugated bilirubin <20% of total or <7 mmol/L	Raised levels of conjugated bilirubin indicate hepatocyte dysfunction or biliary obstruction.
Transaminases: • Aspartate aminotransferase (AST) 10–50 IU/L	Raised levels may signify hepatocyte inflammation or damage. Significantly raised in acute liver failure, less so in chronic liver disease. Also present in cardiac and muscle tissue, therefore not always specific to liver damage.
• Alanine aminotransferase (ALT) 10–50 IU/L	Raised levels signify hepatocyte inflammation or damage. Significantly raised in acute liver failure, less so in chronic liver disease. More specific to the liver tissue.
• Gamma-glutamyl transpeptidase (GGT) 5–55 IU/L (age dependent)	Raised levels may signify bile duct inflammation or obstruction, non-specific.
Alkaline phosphatase (ALP) <350 IU/L (age dependent)	Raised levels may signify bile duct inflammation or obstruction. Not specific to the liver and may also be raised during normal bone development.
Albumin 35–50 g/L	Reduced levels are found in chronic liver disease or due to poor nutrition or chronic loss from the gut. An indication of the synthetic function of the liver.
Coagulation: • Prothrombin time (PT) 12–15 s	Prolonged may indicate hepatocellular dysfunction or vitamin K deficiency. An indication of the synthetic function of the liver.
• International normalised ratio (INR) 0.9–1.2	
Ammonia <50 mmol/L	Raised levels may indicate abnormal protein catabolism or an inherited metabolic disease.
Glucose >4 mmol/L	Lower levels found in acute or chronic liver failure, metabolic disease or hyperinsulinaemia.

likely cause. The most important mechanism relates to the inability of the liver to detoxify products from the gut resulting in the accumulation of ammonia and other toxins, which then leak into the brain causing neurological impairment (Houlston and O'Neal, 2009).

Diagnosis of HE in children is difficult, particularly in infants although crying, irritability, vomiting and poor feeding may signify encephalopathy due to metabolic conditions. In older children, problems at school and sleep disturbances may indicate lower grade HE. Parents are usually best at picking up early signs of HE such as changes in behaviour.

In acute liver failure, HE may be exacerbated by sepsis, gastrointestinal bleeding, electrolyte disturbances and the use of sedatives. HE can progress rapidly from Grade 1 to Grade 4 and cerebral oedema may develop, ultimately leading to brain stem herniation. This is the most frequent cause of death in acute liver failure (Kelly, 2001).

Treatment of HE involves the avoidance of fasting and sedatives, both of which can precipitate encephalopathy. Lactulose is used to decrease ammonia reabsorption from the gut and antibiotics can suppress the amount of ammonia-forming bacteria in the intestine. Protein restriction, which is standard treatment in adults, is not usually recommended in children as poor nutrition can result. Patients with Grades 1–2 HE should be nursed in a quiet environment with minimal stimuli and monitored regularly for neurological deterioration. Intubation and ventilatory support should be instituted when Grade 3 HE develops or when patients with Grade 1 or 2 HE require sedation, as this may also compromise respiratory effort.

Portal Hypertension

Portal hypertension (PH) in chronic liver disease arises from the development of fibrosis and cirrhosis in the liver. Increased resistance to blood flow forces the portal vein supply to back up into the circulation around the spleen and intestinal system. Spleen size increases and overconsumption of blood cells results in thrombocytopaenia and a fall in white and red cell counts, known as hypersplenism. Blood is diverted into alternative routes in the gastro-oesophageal system, which can lead to the development of thin-walled varices which have the potential to bleed catastrophically. Patients bleeding from oesophageal or gastric varices can present with haematemesis and melaena, whereas signs of red blood loss per rectum is suggestive of bleeding lower down the gastrointestinal tract.

Following a variceal bleed, patients may need fluid resuscitation, red cell transfusions and treatment with intravenous octreotide and ranitidine. They must then be transferred to a specialist centre for upper gastrointestinal endoscopy. Varices can be treated with endoscopic ligation (banding) or endoscopic sclerotherapy in an attempt to force the blood supply into deeper situated veins, which do not bleed (Wong, 2009). Following endoscopy, children with portal hypertension must be monitored for circulatory decompensation, infection, haematemesis and melaena. Pain relief may be required, although non-steroidal anti-inflammatory drugs (NSAIDs) such as ibuprofen are contraindicated. A soft diet is recommended for 24 hours following any intervention. Antibiotics have been shown to improve mortality (Wong, 2009). If portal hypertension is suspected in children with chronic liver disease due to increasing spleen size on ultrasonography and falling blood counts, surveillance endoscopy may be carried out. Repeat endoscopies will then be performed, the frequency depending on the severity of any varices found (Grammatikopoulos et al., 2018).

Other causes of portal hypertension include any obstruction to portal vein flow such as portal vein thrombosis, portal vein cavernoma or compression from a tumour. Impairment or obstruction to venous outflow from the liver via the hepatic veins as seen in a condition called Budd-Chiari syndrome or in patients with decompensated heart disease may also cause PH.

Children with enlarged spleens, which are palpable below the costal margin, are at a higher risk of bleeding if they receive a direct blow to the abdomen. These children should be counselled against participation in contact sports where such an injury is more likely to occur.

Ascites

Portal hypertension and low albumin levels can contribute to the development of ascites – the accumulation of fluid in the peritoneal cavity. Mild ascites may need no treatment or, the use of diuretics such as spironolactone may be effective. However, large volumes of ascites may cause difficulties in breathing, abdominal pain and delayed development in infants due to a grossly enlarged abdomen. Complications such as spontaneous bacterial peritonitis (SBP), hyponatraemia and hepatorenal syndrome are associated with the development of ascites causing significant morbidity and mortality (Sargent, 2009). Management is with diuretics, ascitic taps performed concurrently with a 20% albumin infusion and frusemide, and treatment with broad-spectrum intravenous antibiotics if SBP is diagnosed.

CHILDHOOD LIVER DISEASES

Acute Liver Failure

Acute liver failure (ALF) in children is defined as a multi-system syndrome with the following criteria: prolonged coagulopathy, that is, prothrombin time (PT) >15 s or INR >1.5, which is not corrected by vitamin K, in the presence of clinical hepatic encephalopathy, or a PT 20 s or INR 2.0 regardless of the presence or absence of hepatic encephalopathy. An essential component of the definition in children and adults is the absence of a diagnosed underlying chronic liver disease, but it does differ in adults where hepatic encephalopathy must be present (EASL guidelines on the management of acute liver failure, 2017). These criteria are important when it comes to listing for liver transplantation. Serum transaminase levels are usually high (10 times normal values) and plasma ammonia may be greater than 100 mmol/L (Kelly, 2001).

Other clinical signs of acute liver failure include severe jaundice (although this may be a late feature and is not often seen in metabolic conditions), hypoglycaemia and disturbances in acid-base balance. Uncomplicated acute hepatitis usually resolves spontaneously, but progressive acute liver failure is often fatal with mortality rates of 70% without transplantation (Kelly, 2001). Complications which arise include cerebral oedema, renal failure and sepsis. Multi-system organ failure requires these patients to be nursed in intensive care and referral and transfer to a specialist centre for management of complications and consideration for liver transplant is essential.

Management

Management of ALF involves monitoring and maintenance of serum glucose to more than 4 mmol/L with intravenous glucose, monitoring for infection and prevention of sepsis with prophylactic broad-spectrum antimicrobials, and strict neurological observation. Fluid balance including intravenous and oral intake, and urine output should be carefully monitored with fluids restricted to two-thirds of maintenance requirements unless the patient is dehydrated. Haemodynamic monitoring is essential to detect circulatory compromise and the aim of management is to maintain normal blood pressure. Patients transferred to intensive care for elective ventilation will require management of cerebral oedema with neuroprotective measures including fluid restriction, mannitol or hypertonic saline intravenously and elective hyperventilation. Patients should be nursed with their head elevated at 20–30 degrees and in the midline to improve venous outflow. Intracranial pressure monitoring may be used in children over 2 years of age who are awaiting transplant, but its usefulness is debatable. Inotropes may be required to maintain normal blood pressure and adequate cerebral perfusion pressure. Renal replacement therapy may also be needed if kidney failure develops (Lutfi et al., 2017).

In neonates, sepsis or an inherited metabolic liver disease is the most likely aetiology (see Table 13.2). All neonates should be commenced on intravenous acyclovir until herpes simplex virus infection has been ruled out. Rapid diagnosis of metabolic diseases such as galactosaemia or fructosaemia is important as urgent intervention such as dietary manipulation (e.g. lactose-free formula for galactosaemia) or disease-specific treatment (e.g. NTBC for tyrosinaemia) may be lifesaving (Dhawan, 2008). Gestational alloimmune liver disease (GALD) (previously known as neonatal haemochromatosis) and haemophagocytic lymphohistiocytosis (HLH) also present in the neonatal period, and will require appropriate treatment.

In older children, acute viral hepatitis or drug induced liver failure, particularly following paracetamol overdose is more common. Acetylcysteine must be commenced following paracetamol overdose as ALF following paracetamol toxicity has a 90% survival rate without transplant if treated properly (EASL guidelines on the management of acute liver failure 2017). Undiagnosed chronic liver conditions such as autoimmune liver disease and Wilson disease may also present in this age group with acute liver failure, and again rapid diagnosis and treatment is important. However, if hepatic encephalopathy is present, these patients invariably do not respond to treatment and require urgent liver transplantation (Wang et al., 2016). About 10% of patients will also develop bone marrow failure at the same time or subsequently, and will require bone marrow transplantation (Tung et al., 2000). In around 50% of patients the underlying aetiology is not found and diagnosis is classified as indeterminate or non-A–E hepatitis (Squires, 2008).

TABLE 13.2 Aetiology of Acute Liver Failure

Infection: Viral/Bacterial	Viral hepatitis A, B, C, E; Non-A–E viral hepatitis; Epstein-Barr virus (EBV); cytomegalovirus (CMV); herpes simplex virus (HSV); adenovirus; echovirus; Coxsackie virus leptospirosis; septicaemia; tuberculosis
Metabolic	Tyrosinaemia type 1; galactosaemia; fructosaemia; Niemann-pick type c; mitochondrial disorders; fatty acid oxidation defects; urea cycle defects; Wilson disease
Immune-mediated	Gestational alloimmune liver disease; autoimmune liver disease
Toxin/Drug-induced	Paracetamol overdose; sodium valproate; carbamazepine; halothane; mushroom (*Amanita* sp.) poisoning
Vascular/Ischaemic	Budd-Chiari syndrome; acute circulatory failure; heat stroke; congenital heart disease
Malignancies	Primary and secondary haemophagocytic lymphohistiocytosis (HLH), leukaemia, lymphoma

The prognosis of acute liver failure varies greatly with the underlying aetiology and is worse in children with metabolic disease or indeterminate hepatitis (Dhawan, 2008). PT or INR is the best indicator of survival and is a useful marker of progression. Correction of INR with fresh frozen plasma (FFP) is not indicated unless bleeding is present, or as cover for a procedure where there is risk of bleeding, but intravenous vitamin K should be given regularly. Urgent liver transplantation should be performed if spontaneous recovery is unlikely and before irreversible brain damage caused by cerebral oedema or hypoglycaemia occurs (Kelly, 2001).

REFLECT ON YOUR PRACTICE

How could parents or carers be encouraged to participate in the care of their child in the intensive care environment?

Liver Disease in Infancy

Liver disease in infancy is relatively rare with a reported incidence of approximately 1:2500 live births, but it is associated with high morbidity and mortality (Gottesman et al., 2015). Most causes have a similar presentation with jaundice, pale stools and dark urine, usually within the first 28 days of life. The second most common presentation is spontaneous bleeding, usually secondary to vitamin K deficiency as decreased bile excretion into the intestine results in dietary long-chain fat and fat–soluble vitamin malabsorption (Samyn and Mieli-Vergani, 2011). This may also cause failure to thrive and rickets due to low levels of vitamin D. Hypoglycaemia and hypoalbuminaemia are less common presentations. Infants may be small for gestational age, especially those with Alagille syndrome (see later), metabolic liver disease or intrauterine infection. Dysmorphic features are associated with certain chromosomal abnormalities and congenital infections. Cardiac murmurs or neurological abnormalities may also be associated with specific congenital syndromes. Hepatomegaly and splenomegaly are also common in metabolic conditions.

Fat-soluble vitamins (A, D, E and K) must be prescribed to avoid deficiencies and their complications. Oral supplements may be sufficient but in persisting cholestasis, vitamins may be given intramuscularly to achieve adequate levels. Nutritional requirements are 120%–150% of those of infants without cholestasis due to fat-malabsorption and formulas containing higher concentrations of medium-chain triglycerides (MCT)

TABLE 13.3 Aetiology of Chronic Liver Failure

Cholestatic	Biliary atresia; Alagille syndrome; PFIC; idiopathic neonatal hepatitis
Metabolic	Alpha1-antitrypsin deficiency; Wilson disease; tyrosinaemia type 1; cystic fibrosis
Chronic hepatitis	Autoimmune liver disease; viral hepatitis (B and C); non-alcoholic fatty liver disease; congenital hepatic fibrosis; primary immunodeficiency

should be used. Children with chronic liver disease should be vaccinated against hepatitis A, in addition to the routine childhood vaccinations, and hepatitis B if not already given as part of the normal schedule.

Intrauterine infection, prolonged use of total parenteral nutrition (TPN) and certain endocrine and chromosomal disorders are associated with liver disease in infancy, but the most common causes of cholestatic liver disease are biliary atresia, idiopathic neonatal cholestasis, alpha1-antitrypsin deficiency and progressive familial intrahepatic cholestasis (Table 13.3).

Biliary Atresia

Biliary atresia (BA) is a progressive inflammatory disorder of infancy characterised by the obliteration of a portion of the biliary tree. It affects one in 17,000–19,000 live births in the UK and is more common in east Asian countries with a reported frequency in Taiwan of one in 5000. Without intervention, progressive liver cirrhosis leads to death by 2 years of age (Hartley et al., 2009). Typical presentation is with prolonged (conjugated) jaundice and pale stools in the early weeks after birth although the stools may initially appear pigmented. Stool colour charts are routinely used in Taiwan to aid early recognition of acholic stools (stools which lack pigment due to cholestasis) and biliary atresia. The Children's Liver Disease Foundation (CLDF) also produces these charts in the UK as part of the Yellow Alert Campaign to raise awareness of and improve early diagnosis of liver disease in infants (CLDF Jaundice Protocol, 2018).

There are broadly four different types of BA, which have been described depending on the level of the biliary tree at which obstruction occurs. Type 3 is the most common (>90%) where the most proximal part of the extrahepatic

Type 1 (~5%)

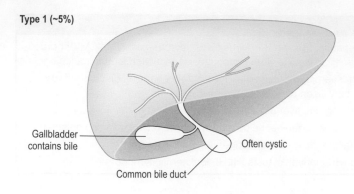

Gallbladder contains bile

Often cystic

Common bile duct

Type 2 (~2%)

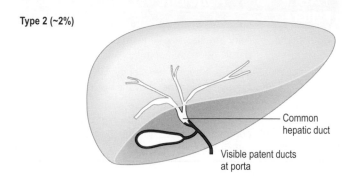

Common hepatic duct

Visible patent ducts at porta

Type 3 (>90%)

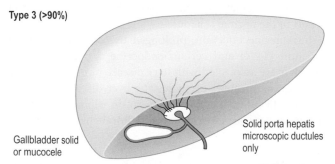

Gallbladder solid or mucocele

Solid porta hepatis microscopic ductules only

Fig. 13.4 Schematic illustration of classification of biliary atresia types 1–3. (From Hartley, J., Davenport, M., Kelly, D., 2009. Biliary atresia. Lancet 374, 1705, Fig. 1.)

biliary tract within the porta hepatis is completely solid (see Fig. 13.4). Although various genetic and environmental factors (infective, inflammatory, toxic) have been implicated, the aetiology remains unknown (Lakshminarayanan and Davenport, 2016). In about 10% of cases, BA is associated with other congenital abnormalities including biliary atresia splenic malformation syndrome (BASM). Polysplenia or asplenia and often situs inversus, intestinal malrotation and vascular anomalies are present. This implies that at least in these cases and in the cystic type (Type 1), BA develops at an earlier point of embryonic development than is thought to be the case with isolated biliary atresia (Lakshminarayanan and Davenport, 2016). Diagnosis is made by liver biopsy, ultrasound scan and exclusion of other common causes of conjugated jaundice.

Management. Infants will undergo a Kasai hepatico-jejunostomy where the entire extrahepatic biliary tree is resected and a loop of bowel (Roux-en-Y) is fashioned to reconnect the small bowel to the remnant of the bile duct with the aim of establishing bile flow. Success of the Kasai procedure is measured by the clearance of jaundice within 6 months of the operation. Some studies have found that the Kasai procedure is more successful if performed before 45 days of age, before progressive liver damage and cirrhosis have occurred, but 70% of infants with successful bile drainage will still develop some degree of fibrosis, portal hypertension and cirrhosis (Feldman and Mack, 2015). Eighty percent of those with a successful Kasai will still survive longer than 10 years with their native liver with good growth and quality of life, but for those who do not clear their jaundice, early transplantation within 6 months to 2 years of age is indicated (Hartley et al., 2009). Biliary atresia is the most common indication for liver transplantation in the paediatric population.

Post–Kasai infants will need to be nursed according to strict guidelines. Pain management and monitoring of fluid balance, electrolytes and blood sugars, and also for signs of infection must be instituted. Some centres use a course of steroids (prednisolone) post-operatively to reduce inflammation, but evidence of their usefulness is limited (Lakshminarayanan and Davenport, 2016). Typical length of hospital stay is 7–10 days following the procedure, during which time infants will return to full enteral feeds and families will be educated around medications and symptoms of chronic liver disease. In the first year after Kasai, 40%–50% of infants will develop cholangitis (infection of the bile ducts) due to the direct communication of the intestine with the intrahepatic bile ducts (Beattie et al., 2009). Presentation can be with pyrexia, recurrence or worsening of jaundice, pale stools and positive blood cultures. Treatment is with appropriate intravenous antibiotics. Cholangitis is less common in older children and those surviving into adulthood with their own liver.

Nutritional input is important in order to maximise growth and development. Specialist formulas with medium chain triglycerides are used, which make it easier to absorb fats when bile flow is compromised. Fat-soluble vitamin supplementation either orally or via intramuscular (IM) injection may be prescribed as well as other medications aimed at improving bile flow. Most infants will have some degree of portal hypertension at the time of Kasai but only 15% will go on to develop bleeding varices, which need intervention (Duche et al., 2010). On-going family support is essential as the course of the disease is unpredictable. Quality of life assessments have shown that children who have survived into adulthood with their own liver (23%–46% at 20 years) have lower scores particularly in emotional and psychosocial areas than their healthy counterparts, but are similar to other chronic conditions. Feldman and Mack (2015) found that 10%–15% of children with BA have significant neurocognitive deficits, 26% will have learning difficulties and up to 40% require special educational support, although there are not enough other studies to support this data and further research is needed.

SCENARIO

A 6-week-old baby boy is admitted to the ward after referral from the GP with prolonged jaundice. A split bilirubin test has determined that this is a conjugated jaundice with a total bilirubin of 152 and a conjugated fraction of 78. On examination of his nappy, the stools are found to be pale with dark urine. A full work up for conjugated jaundice is carried out including blood tests and an ultrasound scan. The ultrasound scan shows an abnormal gallbladder and a liver biopsy is then performed which is consistent with biliary atresia. The baby is referred to the surgeons for a Kasai operation.

Alpha1-Antitrypsin Deficiency

Alpha1-antitrypsin deficiency (A1ATD) is the most common inherited cause of liver disease in infants (Joshi et al., 2017). It is an autosomal co-dominant disorder resulting from a mutation in the *SERPINA1* gene, which codes for alpha1-antitrypsin (A1AT). A1AT is a glycoprotein, which is synthesised in the liver and lungs and acts as a protease inhibitor, protecting the lung tissue from neutrophil elastase which is released by white blood cells in response to infection or environmental irritants. The normal phenotype is PiM, which results in normal levels of A1AT in the blood. The most common mutation found is PiZ resulting in lower levels of A1AT, although many other mutations are also seen, including PiS and Pi null, where no protein is produced. Mutations are most commonly seen in Caucasians particularly of northern European origin. The PiZ mutation results in the production of abnormal A1AT protein, which then accumulates in the hepatocytes leading to a process of chronic inflammation and cell damage. Despite this, only 10%–15% of affected children will develop symptoms of chronic liver disease, requiring supportive treatment, or proceeding to transplantation (Tanash et al., 2015). Research into other factors, which may influence the development of liver disease in these children is ongoing. In adulthood, A1ATD leads to early onset chronic obstructive pulmonary disease (COPD) in most cases but particularly in smokers (Hadzic et al., 2017). In affected infants, presentation is similar to biliary atresia with prolonged jaundice and pale stools and A1ATD must be ruled out as a potential diagnosis before proceeding to a Kasai operation. In older children and young adults, A1ATD may be diagnosed after an incidental finding of elevated transaminases, but a minority will present with advanced cirrhosis and portal hypertension without a history of infantile jaundice (Joshi et al., 2017).

Diagnosis is confirmed by determining the genetic phenotype since serum levels of A1ATD can be misleading and liver histology on biopsy can be similar to that of biliary atresia.

Management. Therapeutic interventions are similar to those for biliary atresia, aimed at maximising growth and development with MCT feeds and fat-soluble vitamins, treating symptoms of chronic liver disease as they arise and considering liver transplantation if required. Family education around the dangers of smoking and passive smoking should be emphasised.

Progressive Familial Intrahepatic Cholestasis

Progressive familial intrahepatic cholestasis (PFIC) disorders are autosomal-recessive conditions, broadly resulting from mutations, which give rise to abnormal membrane transporters involved in bile formation in the hepatocytes. They account for 10%–15% of the causes of cholestasis in children (Jacquemin, 2012). Nomenclature has changed over the years but there is now general acceptance of classification of the disorders according to the transporter or gene involved (Karlsen et al., 2015). Progressive familial intrahepatic cholestasis (PFIC) type 1 (FIC1 protein), BSEP (bile salt export pump protein) deficiency, and MDR3 (multi-drug resistance class 3 protein) deficiency are characterised by chronic cholestasis of varying severity with jaundice, raised serum bile acids and pruritus often being a particular problem. FIC1 and BSEP deficiency present with a low gamma-glutamyl transferase (GGT) cholestasis whereas in MDR3 deficiency, GGT is high. They are usually diagnosed in infancy or early childhood but milder forms of PFIC, also known as benign recurrent intrahepatic cholestasis (BRIC), may present in adolescence and adulthood, with episodes of cholestasis secondary to the use of the oral contraceptive pill, antibiotics or pregnancy (Joshi et al., 2017). Children with PFIC type 1 may also have extrahepatic manifestations of the disease with persistent diarrhoea, pancreatic insufficiency, poor growth leading to short stature, and deafness. BSEP deficiency is also associated with gallstone formation and development of hepatocellular carcinoma in children as young as 1 year and these children must be screened regularly (Jacquemin, 2012). Diagnosis is made by exclusion of other common causes of cholestasis together with ultrasound scanning, liver histology and molecular gene analysis.

Management. Treatment is aimed at enhancing bile acid secretion and inhibiting intestinal reabsorption with ursodeoxycholic acid (UCDA) or cholestyramine, which binds bile acids in the gut. Rifampicin, naltrexone and anti-histamines (used for their sedative effect) are aimed at symptomatic relief of pruritus. Nasobiliary drainage, surgical partial external biliary diversion or ileal exclusion to reduce the amount of circulating bile acids may be beneficial for relieving itch and improving growth in children with FIC1 and common BSEP mutations. As with all chronic liver diseases, aggressive nutritional intervention and fat-soluble vitamin supplementation is also required.

In those patients who develop decompensated cirrhosis, malignancy or have unmanageable pruritus, liver transplantation is the only option (Bull et al., 2018). Transplantation is complicated by the fact that the extrahepatic features seen in PFIC type 1, such as chronic diarrhoea, may worsen. An alloimmune response after transplantation for BSEP deficiency may also lead to the recurrence of the disease in the graft (Hadzic et al., 2017).

Alagille Syndrome

Alagille syndrome is an autosomal dominant condition characterised by a lack of intrahepatic bile ducts, leading to poor bile flow. It is a multi-systemic disorder, which was historically diagnosed when a certain number of additional clinical criteria including cardiac defects, characteristic facies and renal disease were found. More recently however, mutations or deletions in the *JAG 1* (in >95% of cases) and *NOTCH 2* genes have been shown to cause Alagille syndrome (Kamath et al., 2018). Presentation is often with conjugated jaundice, caused by cholestasis and failure to thrive. Initially bile duct proliferation may be seen on biopsy and misdiagnosis with biliary atresia may occur with increased morbidity and mortality following unnecessary hepaticojejunostomy. Cardiac defects with varying severity are common and may have been picked up antenatally. Individuals with Alagille syndrome often have characteristic facies with a prominent forehead, deep-set eyes, low-set ears and a pointed chin. Spinal x-ray may show butterfly shaped vertebrae and on eye examination, posterior embryotoxon, which may aid diagnosis but neither of which cause clinical problems. Renal abnormalities including renal tubular acidosis are also common. The spectrum of liver disease in Alagille syndrome varies greatly with some children being completely asymptomatic through to the development of severe cholestatic liver disease in 20%–30% of cases. This makes the true incidence of Alagille syndrome difficult to ascertain, although one study has estimated it as one in 30,000–50,000 live births (Kamath et al., 2018). The majority of children with cholestasis develop severe pruritus and xanthomas, fat deposits under the skin, due to high cholesterol levels. Unmanageable itch leading to disturbed sleep, impaired cognitive development, low mood and skin trauma from scratching as well as the disfiguring nature of xanthomas may lead to liver transplantation to improve quality of life in these children. However, itch has also been seen to improve in adolescence making medical management, and research into new drugs to relieve pruritus vital, in order to avoid transplantation if possible. Kamath et al. (2010) found that bilirubin levels >111 mmol/L and cholesterol >13.5 mmol/L in children under 5 years were predictive of severe liver disease in later life. For those children with advanced cirrhosis and end-stage liver disease, transplantation is the only option, but outcomes will depend on associated heart and renal disease, which may worsen with the use of immunosuppressive drugs.

Management. Nutritional support with MCT feeds and fat-soluble vitamin supplementation is essential in all children with Alagille syndrome. Nasogastric or gastrostomy feeding may be indicated in children with growth failure as most will not manage to consume the necessary calories orally (Kamath et al., 2010). Severe itch is managed using the same medications as with PFIC, and partial biliary diversion has also been used with varying success (Kronsten et al., 2013). Renal abnormalities should be corrected if possible and renal function must be monitored particularly if nephrotoxic drugs are being used. Renal tubular acidosis can also contribute to poor growth and should be treated with supplemental bicarbonate.

PROFESSIONAL CONVERSATION

James is a third year nursing student.

I was looking after a 3-month-old girl who had been diagnosed with Alagille syndrome. The consultant explained to her parents what the diagnosis meant and possible future implications for her health. After the doctor had gone, her mother asked me whether there was a risk that her other child could also have Alagille syndrome and whether she or her partner might be carriers. I realized that I did not have enough knowledge about the principles of autosomal dominant inheritance to be able to answer her questions.

ACTIVITY

In your student learning group, consider the dilemmas facing parents following a child's diagnosis with an inherited liver disease.

Liver Disease in Older Children and Adolescents
Chronic Viral Hepatitis

Most cases of viral hepatitis will be asymptomatic and resolve spontaneously although some will lead to acute hepatitis and a minority (5%) will progress to acute liver failure (Kelly, 2001). However, hepatitis B and C, which are blood-borne viral infections, can also cause chronic inflammation leading to fibrosis, cirrhosis and hepatocellular carcinoma in older children.

Hepatitis B. Hepatitis B virus (HBV) infection is a global problem with an estimated 2 billion people having been infected and 350 million going on to become chronic carriers of infection (Chen and Chang, 2010). Areas with particularly high prevalence include Southeast Asia, the Pacific and sub-Saharan Africa. In these areas transmission is predominantly perinatal, whereas in areas with low prevalence, such as the USA and western and northern Europe, transmission is usually due to sexual activity or intravenous drug use in adolescence or early adulthood (Shah et al., 2009). Ten genotypes of the hepatitis B virus have been described (A–J), the prevalence of which vary according to geographical region. The HBV virus can also survive more than a week on dry surfaces making infection from bodily fluids amongst household contacts a particular problem. Following transmission of hepatitis B, a portion of the viral genome is incorporated into the DNA of host hepatocytes, which leads to long-term chronic infection (Riehle and Fausto, 2014).

Diagnosis of hepatitis B infection is made on the basis of serum positivity for hepatitis B surface antigen (HBsAg), a protein found on the surface of the hepatitis B virus. Acute infection in children may be symptomatic with anorexia, nausea, vomiting and fever, right upper quadrant pain and hepatomegaly. Jaundice is rare. More commonly however, and particularly in younger children and infants, infection is asymptomatic. Acute infection is usually short lived and marked by seroconversion to hepatitis B surface antibody (anti-HBs) with total recovery of liver damage and the development of immunity to the virus.

Chronic infection is defined as the presence of HBsAg persisting for more than 6 months. In contrast to adults, HBV infection in infancy and early childhood is much more likely to lead to chronic infection. Neonates who develop the virus have a 90% chance of their infection becoming chronic, compared to those who are infected after 6 years of age and have a significantly reduced 6%–10% chance (Chang et al., 1989; Chu et al., 1985, cited by Dumas et al., 2007).

Three phases of chronic infection have been described: immune-tolerant, immune active and inactive. In the immune tolerant phase, high levels of HBsAg, HBV DNA and hepatitis B envelope antigen (a product of the nucleocapsid [envelope] gene of the hepatitis B virus) are found. Despite high levels of viral replication, transaminases remain within normal limits or are only slightly elevated with little evidence of liver damage. This phase can last for years, but at some point when the immune system matures, transaminases become elevated and active inflammation is found. Most patients will undergo HBeAg seroconversion to hepatitis Be antibody (anti-HBe), have lower levels of HBV DNA, a gradual return to normal transaminases and become inactive carriers. However, a minority of children will persist in the active phase or enter a reactivation phase despite HBeAg seroconversion and are at greater risk of developing cirrhosis and hepatocellular carcinoma.

Management. Worldwide universal hepatitis B vaccination remains the goal for eliminating both the hepatitis B infection and its associated complications. The World Health Organization (WHO) called for universal vaccination programmes in 1991 and reported that in 2015 global coverage with the third dose of hepatitis B vaccine had reached 84%, whereas global coverage with the birth dose of hepatitis B vaccine was 39% (WHO, 2018). Countries that have introduced universal hepatitis B vaccination programs have seen a significant reduction in hepatitis B prevalence. The World Health Organization (2018) estimated the prevalence of HBV infection in children under 5 years of age has been reduced to approximately 1.3% from 4.7% prior to its widespread introduction. Babies born on or after 1 August 2017 in England will now also receive the hepatitis B vaccination as part of the routine childhood immunisation schedule. Babies born to HBsAg positive mothers should be given the initial vaccine as soon after birth as possible, and no later than 24 hours after, followed by a more accelerated schedule (Immunisation Against Infectious Disease, Public Health England, 2013). In addition, hepatitis B immunoglobulin (HBIG) should be given to infants of HBsAg and HBeAg positive mothers within 24 hours of birth. However, despite optimum immunoprophylaxis, around 5% of these infants still go on to develop chronic hepatitis B infection. It is of the utmost importance to identify those babies who are at increased risk of developing hepatitis B infection so that the appropriate management can be put in place. All pregnant women should be offered a hepatitis screening test at their pregnancy booking appointment

in their first trimester (NICE, 2017a) so that if they're found to be HBsAg positive they can be referred for specialist advice regarding their own health and the possible consequences to their baby's health. They can also be offered antiviral treatment in their third trimester, if needed, to reduce the risk of the baby becoming infected (NICE, 2014).

The European Society of Pediatric Gastroenterology, Hepatology and Nutrition, (Sokal et al., 2013), highlighted that the clinical care of children with chronic hepatitis B infection is mostly based on the consensus of expert opinion and that evidence-based guidelines on which children to treat, when to treat, and with which medications are needed to improve treatment response and to reduce the risks of antiviral resistance. They also recommended that children with chronic hepatitis B infection should be managed in highly specialist centres, which also forms part of the National Institute of Health and Care Excellence (NICE, 2017b) clinical guideline. NICE (2017b) also outlines the management of children who are HBsAg positive from time of diagnosis to when they are being managed in secondary care. NICE guidance says that in children and young people with an abnormal ALT (on two separate occasions, 3 months apart) and a HBV DNA of more than 2000 IU/mL, a liver biopsy should be performed to assess the level of fibrosis and the potential need for treatment.

Ideally the goal of treatment would be seroconversion to HBeAb and HBsAb positive, and HBeAg and HBsAg negative with an undetectable level of serum HBV DNA. Currently treatment goals are generally limited, outside of clinical trials, because of the lack of availability of licensed medications for children, to halt the progression of liver fibrosis and prevent the development of cirrhosis and hepatocellular carcinoma. Liver health and any progressive liver damage can be monitored through serum transaminases, hepatitis markers and alpha-fetoprotein (AFP), fibrosis on biopsy, liver stiffness on FibroScan and liver texture and appearance on ultrasound.

Current treatments include the use of nucleoside/nucleotide analogues, which tackle the virus at various stages of its replicative cycle either as mono or combination therapy. Pegylated interferon-α 2a may be used to boost the immune response to the virus and is the first line treatment recommended by NICE (2017b) in children and young people with chronic hepatitis B infection and compensated liver disease.

Hepatitis C. Like hepatitis B, chronic infection with hepatitis C virus (HCV) is a worldwide problem with an estimated incidence of 130–170 million people, 11–13 million of these being children under 15 years of age. HCV in children is particularly prevalent in countries such as China, India, Russia, Nigeria, Pakistan and Egypt, and is also predominantly passed on by vertical transmission from mother to child. Maternal intravenous drug use and increasing IV drug use in adolescents in developed countries, as well as contaminated blood products and surgical instruments in lower income countries, are the main sources of infection.

Following maternal transmission of infection, 20% of children will clear the virus without treatment, but the remainder will go on to develop chronic HCV infection.

The majority of children do not have any overt symptoms of hepatitis, with raised transaminases, minimal changes on liver histology and mild hepatomegaly in 10% of cases being the only clinical manifestations (Indolfi et al., 2018). Fibrosis progresses slowly and the severity is related to the duration of the infection. However, by the time they reach adulthood, about 5% of children with chronic hepatitis C will have evidence of hepatic fibrosis and cirrhosis, or have developed hepatocellular carcinoma. Chronic HCV infection is now the main indication for liver transplantation in adults (Abdel-Hady et al., 2014). Diagnosis is by the presence of serum HCV RNA; different genotypes exist, which also respond differently to treatment.

Management. Current treatment in Europe and the USA favours pegylated interferon-α (PEG-IFNα) in combination with ribavirin (RBV) for children between 3 and 12 years. Seventy percent of children achieve a sustained viral response (SVR) rising to more than 90% in those with genotypes 2 and 3. However, the treatment regime involves weekly subcutaneous injections for 24 (genotypes 2 and 3), or 48 (genotypes 1 and 4) weeks and side effects include neutropaenia and depression. Some studies have reported serious neuropsychiatric problems due to treatment, although these are rare. Growth and weight gain may be affected during treatment, but children will usually catch up once finished (Abdel-Hady et al., 2014). Newer combinations of oral antiviral medications with fewer side effects have recently been approved for use in children over 12 years. Sofosbuvir/ledipasvir is used for genotypes 1, 4, and 5 and sofosbuvir in combination with ribavirin for genotypes 2 and 6. These have been shown to have greater efficacy against all genotypes of HCV, but trials are still ongoing before their use may be approved in younger children (Indolfi et al., 2018).

Autoimmune Liver Disease

Autoimmune liver disease is a chronic hepatitis characterised by elevated transaminases, high immunoglobulin G (IgG) levels and autoantibodies in the serum, and characteristic features on liver histology (Mieli-Vergani et al., 2018). Two types of autoimmune hepatitis (AIH) are recognised based on the autoantibody profile: AIH Type 1 is defined by positivity for anti-nuclear antibody (ANA) and/or anti-smooth muscle antibody (SMA) whereas in Type 2, anti-liver kidney microsomal type1 antibody (anti-LKM-1) or anti-liver cytosol type 1 antibody (anti-LC1) is present (Liberal et al., 2016).

AIH is rare with incidences reported of 0.4–3 cases per 100,000 children (Joshi et al., 2017). It typically presents in adolescence, although it can affect children and adults of all ages. AIH is more likely to affect females than males. Nearly 70% of children with AIH will have Type 1 disease, usually presenting in puberty with non-specific symptoms similar to viral hepatitis, including malaise, anorexia, abdominal pain and nausea, followed by jaundice. Younger children are more likely to have Type 2 disease, which is also more likely to present with acute liver failure. Diagnosis can be difficult in ALF as some cases may not have autoantibody positivity at presentation. In both types, more than 50% of

children will have established cirrhosis at the time of diagnosis (Hadzic et al., 2017).

Like many autoimmune diseases, AIH is triggered in genetically susceptible individuals by some unknown environmental factor resulting in a T-cell mediated immune response against liver autoantigens (Liberal et al., 2016). Various viruses such as hepatitis C, B and E, CMV and HSV, and drugs including antibiotics and statins have been proposed as potential triggers for AIH, but a universal cause has not yet been found. AIH may also be associated with other autoimmune conditions including inflammatory bowel disease (IBD).

A similar entity, autoimmune sclerosing cholangitis (ASC), which in addition to the characteristics of AIH, presents with damage to the bile ducts (cholangiopathy), also occurs in children. Prevalence is similar to that of AIH Type 1 with both males and females being equally affected. ASC is more often associated with inflammatory bowel disease and active disease is associated with worsening liver disease (Joshi et al., 2017). Some studies have reported that bile duct disease progresses in 50% of cases leading to end-stage liver disease and the need for transplantation in ASC (Mieli-Vergani et al., 2018) although Rodrigues et al. (2016) found no difference in long-term outcomes between AIH and ASC. Recurrence in the graft after transplantation is seen in both AIH and ASC, but is more common in ASC leading to the need for retransplantation in up to two-thirds of patients (Mieli-Vergani et al., 2018).

Management. The aim of treatment in AIH is to achieve total biochemical remission by suppressing inflammation in the liver and preventing the progression to cirrhosis. This is achieved by the use of immunosuppressive drugs, in particular corticosteroids. Patients are treated with high-dose prednisolone (1–2 mg/kg/day, max. 60 mg in children) and the dose is weaned weekly according to improvement in serum transaminase levels until a lower maintenance dose (2.5–5 mg/day) is reached. Patients may start treatment in the inpatient setting to monitor blood sugars and blood pressure on the initiation of steroids, but further monitoring and blood tests can be done weekly on an outpatient basis if the patient is clinically fit. Patients should be counselled regarding steroid side effects: increased appetite, fluid retention, behavioural changes and worsening of skin conditions, as these can have a negative influence on adherence, particularly in teenagers. Vitamin D and calcium supplementation should be given to promote healthy bone development.

Some patients do not achieve remission on steroid monotherapy or require continued higher doses of prednisolone to maintain normal serum transaminases, putting them at risk of long-term steroid effects. In these patients, second line immunosuppressive therapy is started, usually with azathioprine, at a dose of 1–2 mg/kg/day. Blood tests for Thiopurine S-methyltransferase (TPMT) levels prior to starting therapy and subsequent monitoring for bone marrow suppression should be carried out whilst on azathioprine. For patients intolerant of azathioprine or who fail to respond to treatment, other immunosuppressants can be used. Mycophenolate mofetil (MMF) can be effective and tacrolimus or cyclosporine have also been used with some success although long-term outcomes are not yet known (Liberal et al., 2016). Ursodeoxycholic acid is used in addition in ASC. Children with AIH presenting as acute liver failure, along with hepatic encephalopathy, usually do not respond to any form of immunosuppression and need urgent liver transplantation (Dhawan, 2008).

Withdrawal of treatment may be considered in children who have had 2–3 years of complete biochemical remission and have normal histology on repeat liver biopsy. Some studies have shown 5-year remission rates of up to 40% after withdrawal of immunosuppression, but around 70% of patients will relapse (Joshi et al., 2017). Withdrawal should not be attempted during puberty or when additional autoimmune conditions are present due to the higher likelihood of recurrence of the disease.

 CHILD CONVERSATION

Sarah aged 14 years diagnosed with autoimmune hepatitis.

When I was admitted to the hospital, the doctors told me I had autoimmune liver disease and started me on some tablets. When I went home I started to put on lots of weight and I didn't want to take the tablets especially as I didn't feel unwell. The specialist nurses explained to me what was happening to my liver even though I felt ok. They told me that eventually I would just need to take one tablet every day and I wouldn't get side effects once I was on that dose. Speaking to them made me feel better about taking my medication.

 ACTIVITY

In your student learning group, consider the factors which may influence adherence to treatment in adolescents with autoimmune liver disease.

Wilson Disease

Wilson disease (WD) is an inherited autosomal recessive disorder of copper metabolism caused by mutations in the *ATP7B* gene located on chromosome 13. In general, copper consumption and absorption exceeds our body's daily metabolic needs and the excess is excreted via the hepatobiliary system. In Wilson disease the cellular transport of copper is impaired and it therefore accumulates in body tissues, particularly the liver and brain (see EASL clinical practice guidelines on Wilson disease, 2012). More than 500 mutations in the *ATP7B* gene have been described, with 380 of them causing WD. It commonly presents with liver disease in children aged 6–12 years or with neuropsychiatric problems in adolescents, but WD has been reported in patients as young as 3 years and as old as 60 (Tanner, 2009). Children with liver disease may present with acute liver failure associated with haemolytic anaemia and acute renal failure, and will usually require transplantation. Others may be asymptomatic with only mildly abnormal serum transaminases or will present

with features of advanced cirrhosis including jaundice, portal hypertension and ascites.

Neurological symptoms may be the first clinical sign of WD, may accompany a hepatic presentation, or can develop some years after signs of liver disease. These symptoms may range from a mild tremor to severe disability or psychosis in older patients. Behavioural changes are common and are often misdiagnosed initially.

In older adolescents and adults, diagnosis of WD may be made on the basis of Kayser-Fleischer (KF) (copper) rings in the eyes, on slit lamp examination, together with low serum caeruloplasmin levels. Caeruloplasmin is the major carrier of copper in the blood. However, KF rings are not often found in children presenting with liver disease and caeruloplasmin levels are not always reliable. Twenty-four hour urinary copper collection is helpful, particularly when penicillamine is given and levels are measured pre- and post-administration. Liver biopsy, if not contraindicated due to prolonged clotting, and measurement of liver tissue copper, can also be helpful although levels may be raised, albeit to a lesser degree, in any cholestatic liver disease. Genetic testing can be used for confirmation of diagnosis and screening of asymptomatic siblings, but due to the high number of possible mutations and the length of time it takes, it is not practical for urgent diagnosis in acute liver failure.

Management. Drugs are available for the treatment of Wilson disease but they need to be taken daily and for life. Penicillamine and trientine promote the urinary excretion of copper and also induce other copper chelators, which bind copper and promote its excretion in the urine. Penicillamine is very effective in treating liver disease with recovery of synthetic liver function in 80% of symptomatic patients within 16 months of starting treatment (Socha et al., 2018). Neurological symptoms may take longer to improve, and in some cases, will worsen initially (Tanner, 2009). Side effects of penicillamine include bone marrow suppression, nephrotoxicity and skin changes. Weekly blood counts, blood pressure monitoring and urinalysis for protein and haematuria should be carried out on initiation of therapy. Penicillamine also interferes with pyridoxine (vitamin B_6) action and supplemental pyridoxine should be given. Trientine is often better tolerated in patients who suffer side effects from penicillamine. Zinc may also be used as additional therapy in patients with liver disease or as first-line therapy in asymptomatic patients or patients with neurological symptoms only (Socha et al., 2018). It has a different mechanism of action, interfering with gastrointestinal absorption of copper, but can cause nausea and abdominal pain.

Cystic Fibrosis-Related Liver Disease

The aetiology, diagnosis and management of cystic fibrosis (CF) is covered in chapter 21. However, as children with CF are living longer into adolescence and adulthood due to better respiratory and nutritional management, CF-related liver disease is becoming an increasing problem in this age group. Of patients with CF, 27%–41% have some degree of liver involvement ranging from mildly elevated transaminases to severe portal hypertension and steatosis (Hadzic et al., 2017). The pathogenesis of CF-related liver disease is thought to be multi-factorial with cholestasis due to abnormalities in chloride transport, repeated infections, malnutrition and vascular causes all likely to have a role in the development of fibrosis and cirrhosis.

Management. Management is with ursodeoxycholic acid to improve bile flow, continued nutritional support and monitoring of portal hypertension with surveillance endoscopy and treatment of varices if found. However, some patients will progress to end-stage liver disease and require transplantation. Lung function is an important consideration when transplant is being considered as mortality is higher in patients with less than 50% of predicted forced expiratory volume (PFEV) on lung function testing (Hadzic et al., 2017).

Non-Alcoholic Fatty Liver Disease

Non-alcoholic fatty liver disease (NAFLD) has become the commonest cause of chronic liver disease in children. It is the hepatic manifestation of the metabolic syndrome, closely associated with obesity, insulin resistance and dyslipidaemia, a risk factor for cardiovascular disease in adulthood (Fitzpatrick and Hadzic, 2015). NAFLD is thought to be caused by a combination of environmental factors including high calorie intake, a sedentary lifestyle and lack of exercise, but there is also a genetic predisposition. NAFLD is used to describe the initial pathogenesis, which is characterised by fat accumulation in the liver (steatosis). Secondary factors including oxidative stress and the activation of the immune response may then lead to the more severe phase of the same process, non-alcoholic steatohepatitis (NASH), which is accompanied by inflammation and fibrosis can be differentiated histologically. The disease presents at varying stages in childhood, but generally has the potential to be reversed before progression to cirrhosis and hepatocellular carcinoma. It is likely to become the leading indication for liver transplantation in adulthood.

The incidence of NAFLD is difficult to determine as diagnosis is dependent on liver biopsy, but some studies have put the prevalence in Europe at between 3% and 10% of the paediatric population, rising sharply to more than 70% in obese children (Nobili et al., 2018). Males may be slightly more at risk than females and ethnic variations also exist.

Diagnosis of NAFLD is often due to an incidental finding of elevated transaminases during assessment of obesity or a vague history of abdominal pain and fatigue. Ultrasound will show a fatty liver, but other liver conditions such as Wilson disease, cystic fibrosis and some metabolic conditions can also cause steatosis, and therefore must be ruled out before diagnosis is made (Fitzpatrick and Hadzic, 2015). The commonest phenotype is associated with obesity, which is also a well-recognised risk factor for chronic metabolic, cardiovascular, musculoskeletal and mental health disorders.

Management. The mainstay of management of NAFLD in both children and adults is lifestyle change to include a healthy diet and exercise. A diet low in sugar and, in particular, fructose has been shown to reduce fat in the liver and diets high in protein and low in saturated fat are also thought to be beneficial (Sekkarie et al., 2018). Management of NAFLD

requires a multi-disciplinary approach as lifestyle and dietary changes are difficult to adhere to long-term. Recent studies have shown that less than 10% of children with NAFLD are successful in maintaining weight loss over a 2-year period (Nobili et al., 2018). Input from dietitians, general practitioners, psychologists, schoolteachers and nurses is important to address the issues, which often impact on the implementation of lifestyle changes, including family dynamics and mental health issues. Pharmacological therapies are much needed to support lifestyle changes. Drugs such as metformin have been used to improve insulin resistance in children with NAFLD without type 2 diabetes, but its usefulness is inconclusive. Vitamin E, polyunsaturated fatty acids and probiotics have also been trialled and may have a role in future, but to date no pharmacological intervention has been proven to be effective (Hardy et al., 2015).

 SCENARIO

A 12-year-old girl is admitted to the daycase unit after referral from her local hospital. She had been complaining of mild abdominal pain and feeling tired. Blood tests had shown elevated transaminases and a liver biopsy shows that there is fat in her liver. A full work up excludes autoimmune liver disease, Wilson disease and other causes. She is diagnosed with NAFLD.

REFLECT ON YOUR PRACTICE

How could parents or carers be encouraged to adapt to lifestyle changes following diagnosis of a child with NAFLD?

Liver Tumours

Primary liver tumours are rare in children and account for only 0.5%–2% of all paediatric cancers (Beattie et al., 2009). Benign tumours account for ~25% of these with haemangiomas being the most common. Very rarely teratomas (<1%) in infants and hepatic adenomas (2%) occur in older children. Of the malignant tumours, hepatoblastoma (43%) and hepatocellular carcinoma (23%) are the most common, but occasionally rhabdoid or malignant germ cell tumours occur in the younger age group (<1%) and sarcomas in school age children or adolescents (7%) (Meyers, 2007).

Benign Tumours

Benign tumours include infantile haemangiomata, which are highly vascularised lesions found more commonly in the skin and cutaneous tissue, but which can also occur in the liver. These may be picked up on routine antenatal scans or present with abdominal distension and hepatomegaly after birth. Many will resolve spontaneously but complications can include high-output cardiac failure due to vascular shunting, anaemia, thrombocytopaenia, coagulopathy, cholestasis, failure to thrive and hypothyroidism (Meyers, 2007). Depending on severity, treatment is aimed at supporting cardiac failure with digoxin, diuretics and ACE inhibitors, and encouraging tumour reduction with corticosteroids and chemotherapy.

Surgical ligation or resection of the affected liver lobe may be necessary and liver transplantation is the final option in some cases. Most tumours get bigger before they start to regress.

Mesenchymal hamartoma, which typically appears before 2 years of age, focal nodular hyperplasia (FNH) and inflammatory pseudotumours, which can occur at any age, are other benign tumours, which may require resection. Less common in children is nodular regenerative hyperplasia (NRH), which can involve the whole liver and cause complications such as portal hypertension.

Hepatoblastoma

Hepatoblastoma is an embryonic tumour, which derives from the cells of the fetal liver, primarily epithelial cells, and grows rapidly. It is the most common malignant liver tumour in children and typically presents before 3 years of age. There is a strong link with congenital abnormalities such as trisomy 18/Edwards syndrome and Beckwith-Wiedemann syndrome, which implies a probable genetic influence, but most cases are isolated (Czauderna et al., 2014). Presenting features include abdominal distension and failure to thrive. High alpha fetoprotein (AFP) levels in the blood are a marker of hepatoblastoma and can be used to monitor response to treatment. Computerised tomography (CT) scanning and liver biopsy are used to confirm diagnosis and inform treatment. Management is with a combination of chemotherapy and surgical resection or liver transplant if resection is not possible. Over 60% of tumours are not resectable at presentation and require initial chemotherapy. The PRETEXT system for classifying the PRE-treatment EXTent of the tumour is used worldwide to assess whether the tumour is amenable to resection (Meyers et al., 2014). Metastases do occur via vascular infiltration and often affect the lungs with about 20% of children also having metastatic lung disease at presentation (Meyers, 2007).

⦿ PARENT CONVERSATION

Natalie is the mother of William, aged 2 years.

When they told me my son had a liver tumour, my world fell apart. We were really well supported but there were so many people involved in his care – the oncology team, our local hospital team and the community nursing team. Then we were told we would need to go to a liver transplant centre for surgery and if that didn't work, he would need a liver transplant. It was really hard having even more people involved in his care who didn't know us or what we had been through already.

Hepatocellular Carcinoma

Hepatocellular carcinoma (HCC) is a malignant tumour, which is rarely found in younger children. It commonly affects adolescents, usually with an underlying chronic liver disease such as chronic viral hepatitis (hepatitis B), tyrosinaemia type 1, autoimmune hepatitis or CF–related liver disease. Children with BSEP deficiency are also more likely to develop HCC making early transplantation an important consideration.

HCC is usually multi-focal and highly invasive, causing areas of necrosis and haemorrhage, which makes resection difficult. Presentation is similar to hepatoblastoma, with abdominal distension and a palpable abdominal mass. AFP levels may be raised but not as high as with hepatoblastoma. Lung metastases, intrahepatic vascular and lymphatic dissemination are often already present at time of diagnosis. Again, treatment is with chemotherapy and resection, but as HCC does not respond as well and is often multi-focal, there is a high risk of relapse in the remaining liver. Resection does have a better outcome if the tumour is detected early and is truly localised, but overall prognosis is poor with only 10%–20% long-term survival (Beattie et al., 2009).

Children with malignant liver tumours will have shared care between oncology and transplant centres as well as local community input. Regular communication between the teams is essential to ensure that side-effects of chemotherapy are managed appropriately and the timing for resection or transplantation is optimal.

LIVER TRANSPLANTATION

Liver transplantation has come a long way since the first attempts in the 1960s. Improved surgical techniques, better organ preservation, and new generation immunosuppressive drugs have revolutionised the outcome. Graft survival is now 90%–95% at 1 year and more than 80% at 20 years post-transplant (Kohli et al., 2018). Liver transplantation is now the treatment of choice for patients with acute liver failure or decompensated chronic liver disease and recognition of the impact of chronic liver disease on quality of life and cognitive development has led to transplantation at an earlier age for these children. Transplantation is now also offered for metabolic diseases such as urea cycle defects, organic acidaemias and Crigler-Najjar syndrome, which arise in the liver and can cause severe neurological defects but do not cause liver damage (Bilhartz and Shieck, 2016). However, mitochondrial diseases, which are also manifest outside the liver, are not suitable for transplant due to long-term neurological damage and multi-organ failure (Kelly, 2001). Biliary atresia remains the most common indication for liver transplantation in childhood, followed by acute liver failure (See Table 13.4).

Potential candidates for transplant and their families are assessed in a specialist centre for anatomical, medical, nutritional and psychological fitness for surgery. A multi-disciplinary team approach involving a transplant coordinator, hepatologist, transplant surgeon, anaesthetist, dietitian, psychologist, pharmacist and social worker is vital to ensure any barriers to transplant are identified and support is put in place to address them. Echocardiogram is needed for every patient, as cardiac defects in children with Alagille syndrome or BASM may be a contraindication for transplant or may require surgical correction before transplant can be considered (Bilhartz and Shieck, 2016). Vascular anomalies in children with BASM will also need evaluation with CT scanning. Close monitoring and optimisation of nutrition with nasogastric tube feeding, if necessary, will help recovery following transplant and increase the likelihood of a successful outcome. Renal function must

TABLE 13.4 Characteristics of Paediatric Deceased Donor Liver Transplant Recipients	
Indication	2016/2017
Super urgent	12%
Biliary atresia	37%
Other cholestatic	1%
Metabolic	8%
Other	42%

1 April 2016 to 31 March 2017 Interim Report on Liver Transplantation 2017/2018. NHS Blood and Transplant.

be assessed as results will help inform the best immunosuppression regime, or in rare cases, the need for a combined liver and kidney transplant. Children should be fully immunised if possible prior to transplant as infection risk post-transplant is higher and live vaccines are contraindicated. Accelerated vaccination programmes may be necessary. If there is an expectation that a recipient will have a high chance of survival following transplant with an improved quality of life then transplantation should be offered (Table 13.4).

Candidates deemed suitable for transplant are presented for listing, and if accepted, are placed on the waiting list. Although the organ allocation system for adult recipients has changed recently, for paediatric patients it remains broadly the same. Each paediatric transplant centre in the UK is responsible for maintaining its own waiting list and retrieving organs within a certain geographical area. Organs are allocated according to the following priorities (EASL clinical practice guidelines: liver transplantation 2015):

- Super urgent list – maintained by United Kingdom Transplant (UKT) nationally
- Combined liver and small bowel recipients
- Patients with hepatoblastoma
- Designated geographical retrieval centre
- Other designated UK and Ireland liver transplant centres

If an organ becomes available within a centre's geographical area, which is not required super-urgently, it is offered to those on the waiting list according to blood group. If it is not suitable for any candidates for whatever reason, it will be offered to the other centres on a rotational basis (Littlejohn and Routledge, 2009). Some centres may use the paediatric end-stage liver disease (PELD) scoring system, which looks at five factors: bilirubin, INR, albumin, age and growth as a means of predicting mortality from decompensated liver disease and prioritising children for transplant, although others will rely on clinical expertise (Shepherd, 2009).

 ACTIVITY

In your student learning group, consider some of the moral dilemmas involved in childhood body organ transplant.

Types of Transplant

As with all organ transplants, the demand for donor livers far outstrips the supply available. Conventional liver transplantation involves the resection of the native liver and implantation of a whole liver in its place (orthotopic liver transplantation [OLT]). End to end re-anastomosis of the donor and recipient blood vessels is performed and duct to duct re-anastomosis of the common bile duct or more commonly hepaticojejunostomy is performed to establish biliary drainage (Kohli et al., 2018). In children who have previously had a Kasai hepaticojejunostomy for biliary atresia, the existing roux-en-Y loop may be used. Due to the abdominal size of paediatric patients, paediatric donor livers were initially required for transplantation. However, newer techniques have developed, which involve splitting donor livers into two lobes, graft reduction and living-related donation and these have dramatically increased the size of the donor pool for paediatric patients. In patients with metabolic defects or in acute liver failure, where there is potential for the native liver to recover, auxiliary liver transplantation may be performed. A partial resection (hepatectomy) of the native liver is carried out and a segment of donor liver is then grafted on. This technique is surgically more challenging but has the benefit of being able to withdraw immunosuppression and to allow the graft to die off if the native liver recovers sufficiently. In patients with metabolic defects, which arise in the liver but do not cause cirrhosis, if the auxiliary graft fails, the native liver can still carry out much of the liver function. Hepatocyte transplants have also been used with some success, particularly in neonatal liver failure, to provide a bridge to transplant until a suitable organ becomes available (Kohli et al., 2018).

Surgical complications include primary non-function of the graft which occurs in 1%–2% of patients immediately post-transplant and requires urgent retransplantation (Kohli et al., 2018). Other complications include hepatic artery or portal vein thrombosis, biliary leaks, strictures or obstruction, infection and bleeding. Children are at increased risk of vascular complications because of smaller sized blood vessels and must undergo routine ultrasounds to identify any clots (Bilhartz and Shieck, 2016). Further surgical management may be required as well as post-operative care including fluid management, recognition and treatment of infection, recognition and treatment of rejection and wound care.

Management

Following the immediate post-transplant period where induction with high dose steroids is used, patients will need to be maintained on additional immunosuppressive medications to prevent rejection of the donor liver. The calcineurin inhibitor, tacrolimus has overtaken cyclosporine as the leading primary immunosuppressive medication in paediatric transplantation. Tacrolimus inhibits cytotoxic T-cell generation and allows for the reduction of high dose steroids, which are initially used, to prevent rejection and long-term steroid effects. Side effects of both tacrolimus and cyclosporine are similar and include nephrotoxicity, neurotoxicity, hypertension and GI disturbances, which should all be monitored. However, tacrolimus does not cause excessive hair growth or gingival hyperplasia (gum overgrowth), which are intolerable physical effects of cyclosporine for many patients. Other drugs, which may be used in addition to tacrolimus, include mycophenolate mofetil, which prevents B- and T-cell proliferation, azathioprine and sirolimus. Routine monitoring of liver function tests, immunosuppression levels, white cell counts and renal function is required. Patients on immunosuppressive drugs should also be counselled regarding the use of high factor sunscreen, as the risk of skin cancer is higher.

Despite the use of induction and maintenance immunosuppression, rejection is common post-liver transplantation, occurring in 40%–66% of recipients (Hsu and Reyes, 2014). Acute cellular rejection (ACR) is characterised by rising transaminases and confirmed on liver histology. Severe cases may also present with pyrexia and jaundice. Most cases will respond to pulsing with intravenous high-dose steroids and ensuring maintenance immunosuppression is optimised. Steroid-resistant rejection requires the use of monoclonal antibodies such as antithymocyte globulin (ATG) or Campath. Chronic rejection occurs in 5%–10% of recipients and is characterised by increasing transaminases and cholestasis with resulting jaundice and pruritus (Hsu and Reyes, 2014). Loss of bile ducts is seen on histology and there is little response to increasing immunosuppression. Most patients will go on to need retransplantation at some point although in some cases, the liver will still maintain satisfactory function in the longer term.

Infection following transplantation is common due to immunosuppressive regimes. Following surgery, patients are particularly at risk from bacterial and fungal infections, which require appropriate anti-microbial treatment. Viral infections are also a concern, particularly cytomegalovirus (CMV) and Epstein-Barr virus (EBV). Most paediatric transplant recipients are naïve to these viruses due to their young age, but are often receiving an organ from a positive donor resulting in a primary infection. All recipients who are CMV-negative/donor positive will require IV ganciclovir as prophylaxis against CMV hepatitis. The spectrum of EBV infection ranges from mild flu-like symptoms to the development of post-transplant lymphoproliferative disease (PTLD) and lymphoma. PTLD arises from the proliferation of immature B cells particularly in association with T-cell immunosuppression. Withdrawal of immunosuppression is the first stage of treatment, followed by use of rituximab, a monoclonal antibody, which targets B cells. Patients who develop lymphoma will require chemotherapy. Following transplant, patients must be closely monitored for CMV and EBV infection on blood tests and prompt management with ganciclovir or reduction of immunosuppression is required.

Other viruses which can cause problems are the herpes simplex virus (HSV) and varicella zoster virus (VZV), particularly in children who have not had chicken pox or were unable to be vaccinated prior to transplant. HSV in the form of cold sores requires prompt treatment with oral acyclovir and prophylaxis may be used if close family members suffer regularly, particularly in the first 6 months following transplant. Transplant recipients who are not immune to chicken pox should receive varicella-zoster immune globulin (VZIG) as prophylaxis following a direct contact with a carrier, and IV acyclovir if symptoms of chicken pox develop. Patients and household contacts should also be routinely vaccinated against influenza.

Autoimmune disease may also occur following transplantation, most likely due to a number of factors including genetic susceptibility, exposure to infections and the use of calcineurin inhibitors. This so-called de novo autoimmune hepatitis presents in a similar way to AIH with raised IgG, autoantibody-positivity and elevated transaminases. Treatment is also similar with the use of corticosteroids and secondary immunosuppressive agents such as MMF and azathioprine.

Studies have shown that liver transplantation is a stressful experience for both children and their families with parents reporting psychological symptoms in themselves and their child. Children may experience higher levels of depression and anxiety following transplantation with some studies suggesting that these children score lower than their peers in their emotional well-being, although better than children with chronic illnesses. Ongoing monitoring by the multi-disciplinary team is essential following transplantation to pick up any issues and provide psychosocial support where needed.

Transition

The transition of patients with chronic liver disease or following liver transplantation is increasingly important as more and more of these young people are surviving into adulthood. Non-adherence in the adolescent population is well documented with up to a third of patients not taking their medications or attending clinic appointments (Joshi et al., 2017). This has important implications particularly in liver transplant recipients where non-adherence to immunosuppressive medications is reported to be as high as 50% and a significant cause of graft loss (Dobbels et al., 2005). Centres with dedicated transition services for these patients show an improvement in adherence and engagement with health professionals through a multi-disciplinary approach (Harden, 2012). Education around their liver disease and developing skills in self-management, appropriate to their stage of cognitive development and the individual's physical, emotional and psychosocial needs, is important during the transition period.

Adolescents may become sexually active for the first time during this period and be exposed to smoking, alcohol and drugs. Health promotion advice around appropriate contraception should be given – the progesterone-only pill or depot injection is advocated and immunosuppression may need to be changed if pregnancy occurs. Surveillance and treatment of portal hypertension is particularly important during the second trimester of pregnancy.

Drugs and alcohol may have a significant impact on the liver of patients with established liver disease or transplant and young people should be helped to find strategies to avoid risky behaviours and to resist peer pressure.

◎ EVIDENCE-BASED PRACTICE

The Royal College of Nursing (RCN) has developed a competence framework that 'describes the knowledge, skills and attitudes that are required to deliver patient-centred liver care' (RCN, 2015). There are nine core competencies described, which are designed for all nurses to use, regardless of their area of clinical practice. Competence levels 1–4 can also be used by student nurses to help improve their knowledge, understanding and skill acquisition in caring for people with, or at risk of, liver disease.

SUMMARY

This chapter has provided an overview of the anatomy and physiology of the liver with the aim of providing an understanding of the consequences of paediatric liver disease and the therapeutic interventions necessary to maintain an optimal quality of life when living with chronic liver disease or following liver transplantation. It should be clear that children with liver disease experience varying degrees of symptoms and in some cases will present with liver disease in addition to pre-existing comorbidities. A thorough assessment to identify individual clinical and psychosocial needs is the mainstay of effective nursing care of these children and young people in both the community and tertiary care settings. No matter which health care setting a children's nurse is practising in, they will all have a role to play in the identification of children at risk of developing lifestyle related liver diseases and the implementation of health promotion advice to help tackle these issues.

REFERENCES

Abdel-Hady, M., Bansal, S., Davison, S.M., et al., 2014. Treatment of chronic viral hepatitis C in children and adolescents: UK experience. Arch. Dis. Child. 99 (6), 505–510.

Bacon, B., O'Grady, J., Di Bisceglie, A., Lake, J., 2006. Comprehensive Clinical Hepatology, second ed. St. Louis Elsevier-Mosby Elsevier.

Beattie, M., Dhawan, A., Puntis, J., 2009. Bacterial, Fungal, and Parasitic Infections of the Liver. Paediatric Gastroenterology, Hepatology and Nutrition. Oxford University Press, Oxford.

Bilhartz, J., Shieck, V., 2016. Pediatric liver transplantation. Unique concerns for the critical care team. Crit. Care Nurs. Q. 39 (3), 281–295.

Braccio, S., Irwin, A., Riordan, A., et al., 2017. Acute infectious hepatitis in hospitalised children: a British Paediatric Surveillance Unit study. Arch. Dis. Child. 102, 624–628.

Bull, L., Pawlikowska, L., Strautnieks, S., et al., 2018. Outcomes of surgical management of familial intrahepatic cholestasis 1 and bile salt export protein deficiencies. Hepatol. Commun. 2 (5), 515–528.

Chen, S.-T., Chang, M.-H., 2010. Epidemiology and natural history of hepatitis B in children. In: Jonas, M. (Ed.), Viral Hepatitis in Children: Unique Features and Opportunities. Clinical Gastroenterology New York: Humana Press.

CLDF Yellow Alert Jaundice Protocol, 2018. Early Identification and Referral of Liver Disease in Infants. Children's Liver Disease Foundation, Birmingham.

Czauderna, P., Lopez-Terrada, D., Hiyama, E., Häberle, B., Malogolowkin, M., Meyers, R., 2014. Hepatoblastoma state of the art: pathology, genetics, risk stratification, and chemotherapy. Curr. Opin. Pediatr. 26 (1), 19–28.

Dhawan, A., 2008. Etiology and prognosis of acute liver failure in children. Liver Transplant. 14, S80–S84.

Dobbels, F., Van Damme-Lobaert, R., Vanhaecke, J., De Geest, S., 2005. Growing pains: non-adherence with the immunosuppressive regimen in adolescent transplant recipients. Pediatr. Transplant. 9, 381–390.

Dooley, J., Lok, A., Burroughs, A., Heathcote, J., 2012. Sherlock's Diseases of the Liver and Biliary System. Hoboken Wiley.

Duche, M., Ducot, B., Tournay, E., et al., 2010. Prognostic value of endoscopy in children with biliary atresia at risk for early development of varices and bleeding. Gastroenterology 139 (6), 1952–1960.

Dumas, L., Vergani, D., Mieli-Vergani, G., 2007. Hepatitis B virus: something old, something new. J. Pediatr. Gastroenterol. Nutr. 44 (1), 14–17. Available from: https://journals.lww.com/jpgn/toc/2007/01000.

EASL, 2012. Clinical practice guidelines: Wilson disease. J. Hepatol. 56, 671–685.

EASL, 2015. Clinical practice guidelines: liver transplantation. J. Hepatol. 64(2), 433–485.

EASL, 2017. Clinical Practice Guidelines on the management of acute (fulminant) liver failure. J. Hepatol. 66 (5), 1047–1081.

Feldman, A., Mack, C., 2015. Biliary atresia: clinical lessons learned. J. Pediatr. Gastroenterol. Nutr. 61 (2), 167–175.

Fitzpatrick, E., Hadzic, N., 2015. Paediatric non–alcoholic fatty liver disease: an emerging threat. Paediatr. Today. 11 (1), 9.

Gottesman, L., Del Vecchio, M., Aronoff, S., 2015. Etiologies of conjugated hyperbilirubinemia in infancy: a systematic review of 1692 subjects. BMC Pediatr. 15, 192.

Grammatikopoulos, T., McKiernan, P.J., Dhawan, A., 2018. Portal hypertension and its management in children. Arch. Dis. Child. 103, 186–191.

Hadzic, N., Baumann, U., McKiernan, P., McLin, V., Nobili, V., 2017. Paediatric and adolescent liver disease 1: long-term challenges and perspectives of pre-adolescent liver disease. Lancet Gastroenterol. Hepatol. 2, 435–445.

Harden, P.N., 2012. Bridging the gap: an integrated paediatric to adult clinical service for young adults with kidney failure. BMJ. 344, e3718.

Hardy, T., Anstee, Q.M., Day, C.P., 2015. Non-alcoholic pediatric liver disease: new treatments. Curr. Opin. Gastroenterol. 31 (3), 175–183.

Hartley, J., Davenport, M., Kelly, D., 2009. Biliary atresia. Lancet 374, 1704–1713.

Houlston, C., O'Neal, H., 2009. Hepatic encephalopathy. In: Sargent, S. (Ed.), Liver Diseases: An Essential Guide for Nurses and Health Care Professionals. Chichester: Blackwell Publishing.

Hsu, E., Reyes, J., 2014. In: Murray, K., Horslen, S. (Eds.), 2014. *Diseases of the Liver in Children*: Evaluation and Management. New York: Springer.

Indolfi, G., Thorne, C., El Sayed, M., Giaquinto, C., Gonzalez-Peralta, R., 2017. The challenge of treating children with hepatitis C virus infection. J. Pediatr. Gastroenterol. Nutr. 64, 851–854.

Indolfi, G., Hierro, L., Dezsofi, A., et al., 2018. Treatment of chronic hepatitis C virus infection in children: a position paper by the hepatology committee of European Society of Paediatric Gastroenterology, Hepatology and Nutrition. J. Pediatr. Gastroenterol. Nutr. 66, 505–515.

Jacquemin, E., 2012. Progressive familial intrahepatic cholestasis. Clin. Res. Hepatol. Gastroenterol. 36, S26–S35.

Joshi, D., Gupta, N., Samyn, M., Deheragoda, M., Dobbels, F., Heneghan, M., 2017. The management of childhood liver diseases in adulthood. J. Hepatol. 66, 631–644.

Kamath, B., Loomes, K., Piccoli, D., 2010. Medical management of Alagille syndrome. J. Pediatr. Gastroenterol. Nutr. 50, 580–586.

Kamath, B., Munoz, P., Bab, N., et al., 2010. A longitudinal study to identify laboratory predictors of liver disease outcome in Alagille syndrome. J. Pediatr. Gastroenterol. Nutr. 50 (5), 526–530.

Kamath, B., Baker, A., Houwen, R., Todorova, L., Kerkar, N., 2018. Systematic review: the epidemiology, natural history, and burden of Alagille syndrome. J. Pediatr. Gastroenterol. Nutr. 67 (2), 148–156.

Karlsen, T., Lammert, F., Thompson, R., 2015. Genetics of liver disease: from pathophysiology to clinical practice. J. Hepatol. 62, S6–S14.

Kelly, D., 2001. Managing acute liver failure. Curr. Paediatr. 11 (2), 96–101.

Kelly, D., 2015. Liver and biliary disease in childhood. Medicine 43 (11), 631–635.

Kelly, D., Bucuvalas, J., Alonso, E., et al., 2013. Long-term medical management of the pediatric patient after liver transplantation: 2013 practice guideline by the American Association for the Study of Liver Diseases and the American Society of Transplantation. Liver Transplant. 19, 798–825.

Kohli, R., Cortes, M., Heaton, N., Dhawan, A., 2018. Liver transplantation in children: state of the art and future perspectives. Arch. Dis. Child. 103, 192–198.

Kronsten, V., Fitzpatrick, E., Baker, A., 2013. Management of cholestatic pruritus in paediatric patients with Alagille syndrome: the King's College Hospital experience. J. Pediatr. Gastroenterol. Nutr. 57 (2), 149–154.

Ladhani, S., Flood, J., Amirthalingam, G., et al., 2014. Epidemiology and clinical features of childhood chronic hepatitis B infection diagnosed in England. Pediatr. Infect. Dis. J. 33, 130–135.

Lakshminarayanan, B., Davenport, M., 2016. Biliary atresia: a comprehensive review. J. Autoimmun. 78, 1–9.

Larson, A., Hauswald, M., 2014. Normal Functional Biology of the Liver. Diseases of the Liver in Children: Evaluation and Management. New York: Springer.

Liberal, R., Krawitt, E., Vierling, J.M., Manns, M.P., Mieli-Vergani, G., Vergani, D., 2016. Cutting edge issues in autoimmune hepatitis. J. Autoimmun. 75, 6–19.

Littlejohn, W., Routledge, J., 2009. Liver transplantation. In: Sargent, S. (Ed.), Liver Diseases: An Essential Guide for Nurses and Health Care Professionals. Chichester: Blackwell Publishing.

Lutfi, R., Abulebda, K., Nitu, M., Molleston, J., Bozic, M., Subbarao, G., 2017. Intensive care management of pediatric acute liver failure. J. Pediatr. Gastroenterol. Nutr. 64 (5), 660–670.

Meyers, R., 2007. Tumors of the liver in children. Surg. Oncol. 16, 195–203.

Meyers, R., Tiao, G., de Ville de Goyet, J., Superina, R., Aronson, D., 2014. Hepatoblastoma state of the art: pre-treatment extent of disease, surgical resection guidelines, and the role of liver transplantation. Curr. Opin. Pediatr. 26 (1), 29–36.

Mieli-Vergani, G., Vergani, D., Baumann, U., et al., 2018. Diagnosis and management of pediatric autoimmune liver disease: ESPGHAN Hepatology Committee Position Statement. J. Pediatr. Gastroenterol. Nutr. 66, 345–360.

Murray, K., Horslen, S., (Eds.), 2014. Diseases of the Liver in Children: Evaluation and Management. New York: Springer.

National Institute for Health and Clinical Excellence (NICE), 2010. Jaundice in newborn babies under 28 days. NICE clinical guideline (CG98).

National Institute of Health and Care Excellence (NICE), 2014. Hepatitis B (QS 65).

National Institute of Health and Care Excellence (NICE), 2017a. Antenatal Care for Uncomplicated Pregnancies (CG 62).

National Institute of Health and Care Excellence (NICE), 2017b. Hepatitis B (Chronic) Diagnosis and Management. (CG 165).

Nobili, V., Socha, P., 2018. Pediatric nonalcoholic fatty liver disease: current thinking. J. Pediatr. Gastroenterol. Nutr. 66 (2), 188–192.

Peterson, P., Davenport, M., 2013. Aetiology of biliary atresia: what is actually known? Orphanet J. Rare Dis. 8, 128.

Public Health England, 2017. Hepatitis B. Department of Health. Immunisation against Infectious Disease (Green Book). Department of Health, London.

Riehle, K., Fausto, M., 2014. Mechanisms of liver injury. In: Murray, K., Horslen, S. (Eds.), Diseases of the Liver in Children: Evaluation and Management. New York: Springer.

Royal College of Nursing (RCN), 2015. Caring for People with Liver Disease: A Competence Framework for Nursing Revised Edition. London: RCN.

Rodrigues, A.T., Liu, P.M., Fagundes, E.D., et al., 2016. Clinical characteristics and prognosis in children and adolescents with autoimmune hepatitis and overlap syndrome. J. Pediatr. Gastroenterol. Nutr. 63 (1), 76–81.

Samyn, M., Mieli-Vergani, G., 2011. Liver and biliary disease in infancy. Medicine 39 (10), 565–570.

Sandwell, M. (Eds). Developmental Anatomy and Physiology of Children. A Practical Approach. Elsevier.

Sandwell, M., 2005. The Gastrointestinal tract. In: Chamley, C.A., Carson, P., Randall, D., Sandwell, M. (Eds.), Developmental Anatomy and Physiology of Children. A Practical Approach. Churchill Livingstone, Edinburgh.

Sargent, S. (Ed.), 2009. Liver Diseases: An Essential Guide for Nurses and Health Care Professionals. Chichester: Blackwell Publishing.

Sekkarie, A., Welsh, J., Vos, M., 2018. Carbohydrates and diet patterns in nonalcoholic fatty liver disease in children and adolescents. Curr. Opin. Clin. Nutr. Metab. Care 21 (4), 283–288.

Shah, U., Kelly, D., Chang, M.-H., Fujisawa, T., Heller, S., Gonzalez-Peralta, R.P., Jara, P., Mieli-Vergani, G., Mohan, M., Murray, K., 2009. Management of chronic hepatitis B in Children. J. Pediatr. Gastroenterol. Nutr. 48 (4), 399–404.

Shepherd, R., 2009. Complications and management of chronic liver disease. In: Kelly, D. (Ed.), Diseases of the Liver and Biliary System in Children. Chichester: Blackwell Publishing.

Si-Tayeb, K., Lemaigre, F., Duncan, S., 2010. Organogenesis and development of the liver. Dev. Cell 18, 175–189.

Socha, P., Janczyk, W., Dhawan, A., et al., 2018. Wilson disease in children: a position paper by the Hepatology Committee of the European Society for Paediatric Gastroenterology, Hepatology and Nutrition. J. Pediatr. Gastroenterol. Nutr. 66 (2), 334–344.

Sokal, E.M., Paganeli, M., Wirth, S., et al., 2013. Management of chronic hepatitis B in childhood: ESPGHAN clinical practice guidelines: consensus of an expert panel on behalf of the European Society of Paediatric Gastroenterology, Hepatology and Nutrition. J. Hepatol. 59 (4), 814–829.

Squires, R., 2008. Acute liver failure in children. Semin. Liver Dis. 2, 153–166.

Squires, R., Ng, V., Romero, R., et al., 2014. Evaluation of the pediatric patient for liver transplantation: 2014 practice guideline by the American Association for the Study of Liver

Diseases, American Society of Transplantation and the North American Society for Pediatric Gastroenterology, Hepatology and Nutrition. Hepatology 60 (1), 362–398.

Stringer, M., 2014. Anatomy and Development of the Liver. In: Murray, K., Horslen S. (Eds) Diseases of the Liver in Children: Evaluation and Management. New York: Springer. Diseases of the Liver in Children: Evaluation and Management. Springer.

Tanash, H., Nystedt-Düzakin, M., Montero, L., Sveger, T., Piitulainen, E., 2015. The Swedish α1-Antitrypsin Screening Study: health status and lung and liver function at age 34. Annals of the American Thoracic Society. 12, 807–812.

Tanner, S., 2009. Disorders of copper metabolism. In: Kelly, D. (Ed.), Diseases of the Liver and Biliary System in Children. Chichester: Blackwell Publishing.

Tibbs, C.J., Smith, H.M., 2001. Clinicians' Guide to Viral Hepatitis. Arnold, London.

Tung, J., Hadzic, N., Layton, M., et al., 2000. Bone marrow failure in children with acute liver failure. J. Pediatr. Gastroenterol. Nutr. 31, 557–561.

Waugh, A., Grant, A., 2014. Ross & Wilson Anatomy & Physiology in Health and Illness, twelfth ed. Churchill Livingstone Elsevier.

Wang, Q., Yang, F., Miao, Q., Krawitt, E.L., Gershwin, M.E., Ma, X., 2016. The clinical phenotypes of autoimmune hepatitis: a comprehensive review. J. Autoimmun. 66, 98–107.

Wendon, J., Panel members., Cordoba, J., Dhawan, A., Larsen, F.S., Manns, M., 2017. EASL clinical practical guidelines on the management of acute (fulminant) liver failure. J. Hepatol. 66 (5), 1047–1081.

Whitington, P., Alonso, E., 2009. Acute liver disease. In: Kelly, D. (Ed.), Diseases of the Liver and Biliary System in Children. Chichester: Blackwell Publishing.

Wong, T., 2009. Portal hypertension. In: Sargent, S. (Ed.), Liver Diseases: An Essential Guide for Nurses and Health Care Professionals. Chichester: Blackwell Publishing.

World Health Organization (WHO), 2018. Hepatitis B Factsheet WHO. Available from: http://www.who.int/news-room/fact-sheets/detail/hepatitis-b.

14

Renal Conditions in Childhood

Kathryn Bailey, Karen Tosh

LEARNING OUTCOMES

Discuss common renal conditions with reference to:
- Pathology/pathophysiology
- Signs and symptoms

- Diagnosis
- Treatment/management
- Things to consider

NEPHROTIC SYNDROME

In childhood, several glomerular disorders can present with nephrotic syndrome (NS). It is characterised by the presentation of gross proteinuria, hypoalbuminaemia, oedema and often dyslipidaemia. The most common form, and the focus of this section, is idiopathic NS, which has an incidence of 1.15–16.9 per 100,000 children (Banh et al., 2016). NS is more common in males and pre-school children with significant variance across ethnicity and geographical location. Idiopathic NS has two subtypes: minimal change disease (MCD) and focal segmental glomerulosclerosis (FSGS). The other causes of NS are genetically determined and appear in the first year of life, the most common being Finnish-type, an autosomal recessively inherited disease (Hinkes et al., 2007).

Despite years of study in this area, the pathophysiology of idiopathic NS is not clearly understood, although it is known to be multifactorial. In a normal kidney substances filter from the glomerulus into the nephron through a selective barrier called the basement membrane. Substances move through the barrier on the basis of size and electrical charge. In NS the selectivity of this membrane is impaired by the immune system, and/or genetic mutation, and the glomerulus allows albumin to escape from the blood into the filtrate. Urine therefore tests positive for protein; the condition is characterised by heavy proteinuria, which plays a role in the formation of oedema. The mechanisms involved in the development of oedema in NS are derived from two opposing hypotheses around plasma volume. The first is based on a long held position that plasma leaks into interstitial tissues following a reduction in plasma oncotic pressure as a result of hypoalbuminaemia (underfill). However, the expected decrease in plasma volume is not always present and in some cases it increases. Furthermore, clinical responses to treatment of decreased plasma volume are not always as expected, for example, the signs of remission include a large diuresis and falling proteinuria, but this occurs long before plasma protein levels (and therefore oncotic pressure) normalise

(Teoh et al., 2015). An alternative hypothesis is based on the theory that the epithelial sodium channel is activated by proteases in the glomerular filtrate of children with NS (Kleta and Bockenhauer, 2006). In this instance proteinuria causes primary sodium retention and it is volume expansion (overfill) that contributes to interstitial leakage.

Hypoalbuminaemia is one consequence of NS; dyslipidaemia is another. The levels of cholesterol and triglycerides in the blood rise as a result of increased synthesis by the liver and decreased clearance by the kidneys. Although the exact mechanisms for this are unknown, the potential consequences are a cause for concern. High cholesterol levels have a known association with atherosclerosis and high triglyceride levels may also have atherogenic properties and can cause further renal injury (Vaziri, 2016).

Signs and Symptoms

NS should be suspected when a child presents with oedema and proteinuria. Oedema is a characteristic of NS and it generally appears periorbitally, in the lower extremities and the labia or scrota (Vivarelli et al., 2017). In more serious cases generalised oedema may be present. If the child also has cool peripheries, malaise and abdominal pain it may indicate ascites, pericardial and/or pleural effusions, and potentially cardiovascular shock. Serious infection is an associated morbidity, therefore abdominal pain may also be a result of bacterial peritonitis.

Diagnosis

In the paediatric age group, diagnosis is informed by urinary protein loss of ≥ 40 mg/m^2/h or urinary protein/creatinine ratio ≥ 200 mg/mL or 3+ protein on urinary dipstick and hypoalbuminaemia ≤ 25 g/L (Kidney Disease Improving Global Outcomes [KDIGO], 2012a). Diagnosis is usually made without resorting to biopsy during the initial illness. This approach is taken because the majority of children have idiopathic MCD nephrotic syndrome and biopsies reveal minimal damage to the glomerular epithelial foot processes. A biopsy is therefore reserved for children who have several risk factors or do not respond to treatment. Although most biopsies will reveal MCD (Vivarelli et al., 2017), a few biopsies will identify other microscopic changes that might signify a different approach to treatment and different long-term outlook.

Treatment/Management

Current guidelines recommend corticosteroids in steroid sensitive nephrotic syndrome (SSNS) for a minimum of 12 weeks, then gradual tapering off (Lombel, 2013). This involves starting with a once daily dose of oral prednisone or prednisolone at 2 mg/kg for 4–6 weeks, then 1.5 mg/kg on alternate days for a further 2–5 months. Some children will relapse and require a customised regime depending on the frequency of relapse. The earliest predictor that suggests a relapsing course is the time it takes the child to enter remission after corticosteroid treatment is initiated (Constantinescu et al., 2000). The child on long-term maintenance may receive corticosteroids daily or every second day, depending on frequency of relapse and any active infection (KDIGO, 2012a). There is evidence that alternate day regimes may be more beneficial and produce fewer side effects (Hiraoka et al., 2003). If the child is commenced on long-term maintenance then the parents must be aware of possible side effects such as growth impairment or significant weight gain and cataracts. Parents also have to know about possible psychological side effects such as anxiety, depression and aggression (Mishra et al., 2010).

A small number of children have steroid resistant nephrotic syndrome (SRNS) and others may suffer unacceptable side effects because of prolonged steroid use. There is evidence to support immune dysfunction as a key pathogenic factor in NS (van den Berg, 2004). Treatment therefore includes immunosuppressive or immunomodulator drugs such as calcineurin inhibitors (CNIs), steroid sparing medications such as cyclophosphamide, or rituximab. All these agents are associated with potential adverse effects and there is no consensus as to which is the most appropriate (Downie et al., 2017).

Oedema management includes primary water and salt restriction. Diuretics are reserved for treating substantial oedema, especially if pleural effusions and ascites are impacting lung expansion, as this can cause respiratory distress. Furosemide, a loop diuretic, is commonly prescribed. It is used judiciously because it may result in hypovolaemia, which in turn might increase the likelihood of thrombosis. It should not be used in patients with vomiting or diarrhoea due to the risk of further exacerbating dehydration. Intravenous albumin may also be used in conjunction with furosemide to improve glomerular filtration rate and urinary output (Ghafari et al., 2011).

ACTIVITY

A 10-year-old boy is admitted with significant oedema. His face, abdomen, legs and feet are particularly swollen. He reveals that his scrotum is also oedematous:
- What nursing interventions would you consider appropriate?

As the activity above suggests, caring for a child with oedema is a major focus when the child has nephrotic syndrome. Fluid balance is also important. Fluid intake is normally controlled; the child's input and output the previous day being two of the factors that influence the amount prescribed. Children's body mass index (BMI) and linear growth should be closely monitored. As with chronic kidney disease, carbohydrate intake has to be sufficient to ensure that protein intake can be utilised appropriately and not used for energy purposes (Ko et al., 2017). The child's normal dietary protein requirements should be determined to ensure that these are met. Hyperlipidaemia is not generally a cause for concern during the initial illness. If the child does not respond to treatment and hyperlipidaemia becomes a chronic state, dietary measures such as reduced saturated fat and cholesterol intake are advisable. The value of medications to reduce cholesterol and triglycerides is unclear in children. Finally, because sodium levels may be elevated, dietary sodium has to be controlled (Gallibois et al., 2017). Foods high in sodium should not be consumed and salt should not be added to foods during cooking or at meal times.

Measures must be taken to protect the child from infection and identify it if it occurs. To this end, visitors should be infection free and the number of visitors must be controlled. The child should also be observed for signs of infection such as cough, runny nose and sore ears. Temperature, pulse and respiratory rate should also be recorded regularly.

ACTIVITY

Find resources for supporting children with kidney disease on the National Kidney Federation website:
- https://www.kidney.org.uk/support-for-children-and-young-people

---

Things to Consider

There are a number of issues associated with the disease, including allergic reactions, infection and lymphatic malignancies; how some of these are related is not clear. Upper respiratory tract infection can often precede onset of NS, but peritonitis is the most common complication. Abdominal pain must be carefully assessed with this in mind. The causative organism is usually a pneumococcus and pneumococcal immunisation is recommended for all children; vaccines that are live should be considered carefully (KDIGO, 2012a). Penicillin prophylaxis may be considered for some subgroups (McIntyre and Craig, 1998); however, there have been no randomised controlled trials to test the efficacy of antibiotic prophylaxis in NS (McCaffery et al., 2016). Children on steroids or immunosuppressant therapies are also at risk for viral infections. Chickenpox, in particular, can have devastating effects on an immunosuppressed child. If a child is not immune to varicella-zoster and exposed to chickenpox, then varicella-zoster immune globulin should be administered. Acyclovir prophylaxis should also be administered as an adjunctive (Goldstein et al., 2000; KDIGO, 2012a).

Children with NS are susceptible to venous, and rarely, arterial thrombosis. Disturbances in clotting and fibrinolytic systems occur; antithrombin III levels may be depleted and fibrinogen levels raised. The presence of dehydration, aggressive use of diuretics, immobilisation and indwelling vascular catheters all increase susceptibility to thrombosis. Nurses should be cognizant of the features of deep venous thrombosis. The development of tachypnoea and tachycardia should raise concern as it can indicate pulmonary embolism (Brandão et al., 2011). Thromboembolism requires immediate anticoagulant treatment.

Death caused by NS is rare, but does occur, and is normally attributed to peritonitis and thrombus. Most children over 1 year of age with idiopathic SSNS respond within 4 weeks of treatment. Children with SRNS are likely to relapse after or even during therapy. Parents need to know about the possibility of relapse and be informed to enable them to recognise it. They should monitor the child's weight, test urine for protein and be aware of signs of infection. Children who relapse will require repeated courses of steroids, often for a prolonged period of time. Most will return to normal, although it may take many years.

POSTSTREPTOCOCCAL GLOMERULONEPHRITIS

Glomerulonephritis is an inflammation of the glomeruli of the kidneys. Poststreptococcal glomerulonephritis (PSGN) is a common cause of acute glomerulonephritis in children. However, in developed countries with easy and early access to medical care, the incidence has fallen markedly. This condition develops after a streptococcal infection, the primary site usually being the upper respiratory tract, or skin. There is a latent period between the original infection and the presentation of poststreptococcal glomerulonephritis. If the source of infection is pharyngeal, the period is 1–2 weeks, whereas if the source is the skin, it is 2–4 weeks (Kher et al., 2017). The condition is most often seen in boys and the age of onset is between 2 and 15 years (Eison et al., 2011).

The pathogenesis of poststreptococcal glomerulonephritis is unclear and the involvement of many streptococcal proteins has been proposed. There is evidence that a streptococcal antigen becomes lodged in the glomerular basement membrane (Rodriguez-Iturbe and Batsford, 2007). The hypothesis is that antibodies fix to the antigen, forming an 'in situ' immune complex. The immune complex triggers a second phase, which involves activation of complement. Complement triggers a cascade of events that result in glomerular inflammation. Glomerular capillaries become blocked and glomerular filtering function is impaired resulting in protein and blood being lost in the urine. Consequently, the glomerular filtration rate (GFR) falls and urine output diminishes. GFR is the amount of filtrate that flows into all nephrons in 1 minute. The normal rate in a child is 110–120 mL/min.

The fall in the GFR results in sodium and water retention and the expansion of the blood volume. Body fluid is redistributed and oedema results. Hypertension also occurs. This is partially due to sodium and water retention, but other factors are thought to be involved. In some patients, the reduction in the GFR may be significant and the child may develop acute renal failure.

 ACTIVITY

You can access this helpful video by the Khan academy to review glomerular filtration. Available from:
- https://www.khanacademy.org/science/health-and-medicine/human-anatomy-and-physiology/introduction-to-the-kidneys/v/glomerular-filtration-in-the-nephron

Signs and Symptoms

The clinical severity of poststreptococcal glomerulonephritis is variable, with some children having mild disease and being asymptomatic (Tasic and Polenakovic, 2003). Typical features include haematuria, proteinuria, oliguria, hypertension and periorbital or lower extremity oedema. The degree of oedema varies, it is generally mild, but in some cases it may be severe with accompanying ascites or pleural effusion. Urine assumes a dark colour and output is diminished; some children may present with acute renal failure. Hypertension is common and might be mild but can be severe. If severe, associated symptoms such as headache and visual disturbance occur. The child may present with mild fever, dull abdominal or flank pain and malaise (Eison et al., 2011). Anaemia, uraemia and hypervolaemia contribute to feelings of tiredness.

Diagnosis

Diagnosis is made on history, examination and a number of investigations. Urinalysis reveals blood, protein and high specific gravity. Throat swabs (or skin swabs) may be positive for streptococcal infection. Blood samples are taken and examined for antibody to streptococci and their extracellular products (Lang and Towers, 2001) such as antistreptolysin O (ASO). The normal ASO is less than 166 Todd units; in poststreptococcal glomerulonephritis this is raised. Blood is also examined for evidence of complement activity; a reduction in complement elements C3 and C4 are suggestive of poststreptococcal glomerulonephritis.

Treatment/Management

Appropriate antibiotic therapy should be administered to eliminate any persistent streptococcal infection. This does not alter the course of the condition itself but is important to prevent spread and remove any reservoir of infection. Hospitalisation is not always required, but when hypervolaemia, oedema or hypertension are concerns, the child should be admitted.

Hypervolaemia and the resultant oedema make fluid balance an important focus. Input and output should be accurately documented and the child's weight should be recorded. Hypervolaemia and oedema can be addressed by restricting fluids and sodium intake (Eison et al., 2011). The child's diet should not contain salty foods and salt should not be added to food or during cooking. Dietary manipulation alone may be insufficient to deal with more severe problems and diuretics may be required. Loop diuretics such as furosemide act quickly and effectively.

Hypertension may be mild, moderate or severe. The frequency of recording will differ depending on the circumstance. Dietary measures and administration of diuretics to relieve oedema and hypervolaemia may be all that is required to reduce blood pressure. If hypertension is not alleviated by these means then antihypertensive agents are employed. Severe rises in blood pressure may require intravenous antihypertensive agents.

The prognosis of poststreptococcal glomerulonephritis is excellent; children who develop the condition usually recover, with blood pressure and renal function returning to normal within 6–8 weeks (Rodríguez-Iturbe & Musser, 2008). Less than 1% of children do not recover and go on to develop renal failure resulting in death; however, 97% of these mortalities occur in low-income regions (Carapetis et al., 2005).

WILMS TUMOUR (NEPHROBLASTOMA)

Wilms tumour is the second most common intraabdominal cancer in childhood. It accounts for over 95% of all kidney tumours presenting in children (Pastore et al., 2006). The condition may be bilateral but in the vast majority of cases it is unilateral. It can occur as an isolated problem or may be associated with a congenital syndrome or urogenital anomaly (van den Heuval-Eibrink et al., 2008). Around 75% of cases will present under the age of 5 years, and most commonly, between the ages of 2 and 4 years (Kaste et al., 2008). It affects both boys and girls equally, though females tend to present later (Pritchard-Jones et al., 2012).

Wilms tumour is a malignancy thought to develop in a multi-step process. The classic presentation has a tri-phasic appearance associated with three types of cells, epithelial, blastemal and stromal, which do not all need to be present for diagnosis. During kidney development, renal stem cells differentiate and are responsible for forming the nephrons and connective tissue. In Wilms tumour, some of these stem cells are thought to persist and are referred to as 'nephrogenic rests'. These are present at birth and retain their embryonic differentiation potential and are the precursors of Wilms tumour (Breslow et al., 2006). Wilms tumours are found to contain normal kidney tissue, but they may also contain squamous epithelium, skeletal muscle and cartilage tissue; sometimes the tumours do not contain any of these recognisable cell types. Anaplasia is the presence of uncharacteristic cell types, which present in approximately 5% of cases (Pritchard-Jones et al., 2012). They can be focal or diffuse with diffuse subtypes being more difficult to treat. Wilms tumour invades local structures and spreads via the lymphatic system. The most common sites of metastases are the lungs, followed by regional lymph nodes, liver and, at a late stage, bone.

Genetic Alterations

The genetic mechanisms responsible for Wilms tumour are complex. The majority of cases of Wilms tumour present sporadically, although there are rare cases of inherited presentations (McDonald et al., 1998). Around 10% of presentations occur as part of recognised syndromes such as Denys-Drash, Wilms with aniridia (WAGR syndrome), Beckwith–Weidemann and Perlman syndrome (Scott et al., 2012). A number of genes have been associated with sporadic cases; so far extensive research has implicated chromosomal abnormalities in five loci. The commonest presentation of chromosomal defect in Wilms tumour is found on chromosome 11p15; around 50%–75% of all Wilms tumour cases are characterised by this defect (Scott et al., 2012). The involvement of different genes helps to explain why different areas of the kidney are affected and different cell changes take place. It may also explain why the condition is unilateral or bilateral. It is possible that increasing knowledge about the genetic origins of the disorder may lead to earlier diagnosis or even prevention of the condition in the future.

Signs and Symptoms

The most common initial indication of an isolated Wilms tumour is an abdominal mass (McLorie, 2001). These tumours, often massive, are usually noted by a parent or relative when bathing the child, but may later be identified by the general practitioner (GP). Alternative presenting features include hypertension, which presents in about 25% of cases (Maas et al., 2007), abdominal pain, haematuria and malaise.

Diagnosis

Following identification of the mass, a history is obtained, and an ultrasound is performed. Ultrasound can detect the solid nature of the tumour and distinguish it from other conditions such as hydronephrosis, but it is not definitive. Abdominal computerised tomography and magnetic resonance imaging can help define the position and extent of the tumour, and is used to help plan surgery and confirm the normality of the contralateral kidney.

Treatment/Management

Therapy involves chemotherapy and surgery for all patients. Staging and grading of the tumour is based on surgical and histological findings, and determines the duration of chemotherapy and the specific chemotherapeutic agents. Staging determines the progression and spread of the tumour. Grading is concerned with histology and involves determining the favourable or unfavourable nature of the tumour cells via biopsy. The former demonstrates a tumour composed of recognisable cell types, the latter demonstrates anaplasia and has a poorer prognosis (Pritchard-Jones et al., 2012). Different approaches determine whether preoperative chemotherapy will be undertaken before biopsy and surgery (Kembhavi et al., 2013). Radiotherapy is not usually used but may be required when metastasis is present or following surgery when remnants of the tumour are still present. The International Society of Paediatric Oncology (SIOP) has developed protocols that determine management. When grading and staging are complete, the child commences on pre-nephrectomy therapy. The grading and staging determine the protocol the child embarks on. Cytotoxic therapy generally involves using two or more chemotherapeutic agents. The first-line chemotherapy agents used to treat Wilms tumour include vincristine, actinomycin D and doxorubicin. Pre-nephrectomy chemotherapy induces a dramatic reduction in the size of the tumour (McLorie, 2001). Following chemotherapy, surgery is conducted. In the case of a unilateral tumour surgery is aimed at complete removal of the affected kidney. Bilateral tumours require a different approach. Surgery is carried out to remove the tumour while conserving functional kidney tissue.

Things to Consider

The child may present with an abdominal mass but might not feel ill. The focus of care at this point will be on the parents, who will be devastated when the diagnosis is made. One concern in terms of the child is related to the possibility of metastasis. Unnecessary palpitation of the abdomen should be avoided. The child should be handled carefully. There is a danger that malignant cells could be liberated from the tumour if these measures are not taken. Later nursing interventions will focus on problems associated with chemotherapy. Following chemotherapy, interventions are concerned with the pre- and post-operative care of the child with a nephrectomy. There is a low risk of developing secondary cancers related to treatment. However, the incidence of renal cell carcinoma in the remaining kidney is higher in children who have been treated for Wilms tumour, leading to calls for nephron sparing surgery in primary treatment protocols (Breslow et al., 2010).

There is an overall survival rate of over 90% in localised non-anaplastic cases (Pritchard-Jones et al., 2012). The focus of much current research is achieving similar outcomes in low income regions.

 ACTIVITY

For information about cancers see the Cancer UK Research website. Information on Wilms tumour can be found at:
- http://www.cancerresearchuk.org/about-cancer/childrens-cancer/wilms-tumour?_ga=2.143196599.324555032.1524049373-1619931524.1524049373

ACUTE KIDNEY INJURY

Acute kidney injury (AKI) is the sudden loss of renal function. Failure occurs over a period of hours or days. The kidneys play a major role in maintaining homeostasis. They maintain the body's water, electrolyte and acid–base balance, as well as eliminating waste from the body. In acute renal failure this homeostatic balance is lost and waste is not eliminated effectively. The causes of acute renal failure are traditionally divided into three categories: pre-renal, post-renal and intrinsic.

Pre-renal causes of acute kidney injury are associated with impaired renal blood flow. The kidneys are structurally normal. All types of shock possess the capability to cause acute kidney injury. Shock results in inadequate perfusion pressure and reduction in glomerular filtration rate. Oliguria occurs and the kidneys can no longer maintain their homeostatic functions. If the initiating condition is reversed promptly, kidney damage is prevented. If the initiating condition is not reversed, sympathetic and hormonal activity cause intense renal vasoconstriction and ischaemic renal injury and cell death occurs (Askenazi, 2011).

Intrinsic renal failure is concerned with pathology within the kidney. Glomerulonephritis and nephrotic syndrome are both possible causes. The most common cause, across all age groups, is haemolytic uraemic syndrome (Besbas et al., 2006). This condition is caused by verotoxin-producing *Escherichia coli*, a strain that is carried by cattle. It is thought that meat becomes contaminated during the slaughter process. The organism is destroyed if food is cooked properly, but when a child consumes infected meat, colitis occurs. The verotoxin is then absorbed from the intestinal tract and enters the circulation, where it fixes to receptor sites on renal epithelium. Damage to the glomeruli result in a significant reduction in glomerular filtration thus impairing the kidneys' regulatory functions.

Post-renal causes of acute kidney injury are associated with obstruction. Common conditions that cause obstruction are posterior urethral valves, ureteropelvic obstruction and neurogenic bladder. These conditions impair the flow of urine and back pressure results increasing the pressure in the renal tubules. As filtration depends on the pressure in the glomerulus being higher than that in the tubules, the gradient diminishes, the glomerular filtration rate falls and the kidneys fail (Basile et al., 2012).

Signs and Symptoms

The signs and symptoms of acute kidney injury can be varied and investigations must take place if the child or young person presents with, or is likely to present with chronic kidney disease; heart failure; liver disease; history of acute kidney injury; oliguria (less than 0.5 mL/kg/h); young age or impairment leading to limited fluid intake; hypovolaemia; use of drugs with nephrotoxic potential; symptoms or history of urological obstruction; sepsis; severe diarrhoea; oedema; haematuria; haematological malignancy; hypotension or a deteriorating paediatric early warning score (National Institute for Health and Care Excellence [NICE], 2013).

Diagnosis

To determine acute kidney injury serum creatinine should be measured and compared with the baseline. Imaging studies such as ultrasound may be ordered to determine whether obstruction is a cause (NICE, 2013). Renal biopsy is not routine but may be carried out if diagnosis is unexplained (Kersnik et al., 2001).

Treatment/Management

This is a life-threatening condition and enormous sensitivity is required when dealing with the parents. They should be encouraged to verbalise their feelings. Issues should be discussed with honesty and information provided should be accurate. The parents should be encouraged to participate in care, but only to the degree that they are comfortable with. Parents and carers should be given information about long-term treatment options, monitoring, self-management and support (NICE, 2013).

Urinalysis should be undertaken as soon as acute kidney injury is suspected or detected. Ultrasound scan should be undertaken when pyonephrosis is suspected or the patient is at risk of urinary tract obstruction (NICE, 2013).

Physical management is aimed at eliminating the underlying cause, balancing fluid and electrolytes, controlling acidosis, sustaining nutrition and protecting the child from infection. There may be fluid depletion or overload, thus fluid may have to be replaced or removed. This makes accurate recording of the child's input and output critical. The child's weight is also significant and should be documented twice daily; findings should be documented on an appropriate paediatric early warning scoring tool. If fluid has to be replaced, the cause of the renal failure will influence the choice of fluid used, crystalloid, colloids or blood. In the case of fluid retention, dietary measures can be taken. Sodium and fluid intake can be restricted. Diuretics such as furosemide may be prescribed while the child or young person is awaiting renal replacement therapy or renal function is recovering (NICE, 2013).

Electrolyte balance focuses on sodium and potassium. High sodium levels may occur and are associated with fluid retention and oedema formation and are thus undesirable (KDIGO, 2012b). In the event of hypernatraemia dietary sodium restriction is necessary. High potassium levels are also cause for concern. They may approach dangerous levels due to increased production and decreased elimination.

Hyperkalaemia is life threatening because it disturbs the conductive mechanism of the heart. This may result in dysrhythmia. Cardiac monitoring may be ordered in anticipation of such an event. The goals of acute management are to induce potassium transport into the intracellular space and remove potassium from the body. Initial management involves restricting potassium intake, administration of potassium binding agents, control of acidosis and diuretic therapy aimed at increasing urinary output. Glucose metabolism causes potassium to move into cells. Glucose, insulin or salbutamol may be administered to induce these events (Lehnhardt and Kemper, 2011). Severe hyperkalaemia is one of the reasons for commencing renal replacement therapy.

Acidosis is undesirable for a number of reasons. Prominent among these is its impact on potassium levels. Acidosis promotes the movement of potassium from the intercellular fluid into the extracellular compartment, and thus promotes hyperkalaemia. Acidosis also impacts on cerebral function. Neurological observations are implemented if there is any evidence of confusion or mental impairment. Acidosis may be treated with sodium bicarbonate, glucose and insulin (KDIGO, 2012b).

Acute renal failure is highly catabolic. Parenteral nutrition or enteral feeding may be ordered to meet the child's nutritional requirements (KDIGO, 2012b). The nutritional components are tailored to the child's needs. The amount of energy provided is usually high so that the body does not metabolise body tissues. If body tissue is metabolised for energy, potassium is liberated into an environment where hyperkalaemia may already exist.

The child has to be protected from infection because the immune system is compromised when homeostasis is impaired. Sepsis is a frequent cause of death (Loza et al., 2006). Great care has to be taken to protect the child from nosocomial infections. Hand-washing and protocols designed to eliminate the possibility of cross-infection should be strictly applied. The child should be observed for signs of infection, and antibiotic therapy should be implemented promptly if infection is discovered.

The interventions described above, plus treatment of predisposing causes, may produce the desired response. In the event of continued fluid overload, hyperkalaemia, metabolic acidosis or severe uraemia, renal replacement therapy will be required until renal function returns (KDIGO, 2012b; NICE, 2018). Common modalities include peritoneal dialysis, intermittent haemodialysis and continuous haemofiltration or haemodiafiltration (Flynn, 2002). The choice of modality depends on the child's age, clinical condition and local experience.

Long-term follow-up is required for children and young people beyond puberty to monitor such complications as hypertension, proteinuria and reduced renal function (NICE, 2018). Paediatric patients have a high risk of developing chronic kidney disease and hypertension following acute kidney injury (Basile et al., 2012).

CHRONIC KIDNEY DISEASE

There are numerous causes of chronic kidney disease in children. The most common cause is vesicoureteral reflux (VUR). Other significant causes are the obstructive uropathies such as posterior urethral valves, ureterocele and ureteropelvic junction obstruction. Medical conditions that may result in chronic renal failure are nephrotic syndrome and glomerulonephritis (Kaspar et al., 2016). Chronic renal failure is categorised according to changes in GFR.

Creatinine is a waste product of protein metabolism and serum levels of creatinine can be measured. Creatinine is eliminated from the body by the kidneys. A 24-hour collection of urine is obtained to determine the amount cleared. By comparing serum creatinine to levels cleared in the 24-hour collection, the glomerular filtration rate can be calculated.

Chronic renal failure is regarded as mild, moderate or severe. The criteria are as follows:
- Mild: glomerular filtration rate 60–89 mL/min
- Moderate: glomerular filtration rate 30–59 mL/min
- Severe: glomerular filtration rate less than 15–29 mL/min (Hogg et al., 2003).

Signs and Symptoms

The kidneys are multifunctional. Impairment of these functions produces a variety of clinical features. Common features are poor appetite, stunted growth, anaemia (with associated features), increased or decreased urine output, oedema, hypertension, skin discoloration and pruritus (Becherucci et al., 2016).

Diagnosis

Chronic renal failure diagnosis is based on history, clinical examination, altered laboratory values, various scanning techniques and biopsy. Laboratory values reveal elevated blood urea nitrogen, elevated creatinine, altered calcium/phosphorus ratio, acidosis and electrolyte imbalance. The diagnosis is confirmed by kidney biopsy.

Treatment/Management

There are a number of causes of chronic renal failure and these affect the management. There are also different stages of severity and variable progression. Thus the management described here is generalised.

Growth Impairment

The child's dietary protein intake should be based on the recommended dietary allowances (RDA) for his or her chronological age. Additional increments may be desirable to ensure growth. Increasing dietary protein intake above the RDA has to be balanced against the kidneys' ability to rid the body of waste products of protein metabolism as the renal function will decline with long-term exposure to high dietary protein intake (Ko et al., 2017). The energy portion of the diet has to be high; it is given in the form of fat and carbohydrates. If energy intake is insufficient then protein will be utilised for energy purposes. This will impair the child's growth. Maintaining strict records of intake and output are necessary. Height and weight are also documented.

High sodium levels encourage fluid retention, oedema and also contribute to hypertension (Gallibois et al., 2017). In chronic renal failure, sodium and fluids are usually restricted. Sodium should not be added to cooked food and foods high in salt should be avoided. In some instances, these measures may not suffice and sodium intake may have to be restricted to a specific amount. Elevated potassium levels due to decreased excretion are associated with arrhythmias and cardiac arrest. Foods high in potassium should thus be avoided.

Anaemia

Attempts to curb the onset of anaemia are initially made by encouraging the anorexic child to eat. The diet should be attractive and small portions offered. It should be rich in iron, folic and vitamin B_{12}. These substances may also be given in supplement form. KDIGO (2013) recommend initiating an evaluation for anaemia when haemoglobin levels fall below the age- and sex-specific fifth percentile value. Anaemia is inevitable in chronic kidney disease because of loss of erythropoietin production. As the degree of kidney failure progresses, erythropoietin production fails and anaemia breaks through. Treatment involves administration of erythropoietin. Elimination of anaemia with erythropoietin is very effective (Becherucci et al., 2016).

Hypertension

Hypertension has been linked to the progression of chronic kidney disease (Becherucci et al., 2016). There are a number of mechanisms that may be responsible for hypertension in chronic renal failure. Sodium and fluid retention is one factor. Controlling sodium and fluid intake is therefore employed to control blood pressure. Another mechanism involves the triggering of the renin–angiotensin system (RAS). The mechanism is activated by a falling GFR. Angiotensin II (produced when the renin–angiotensin system is triggered) promotes sodium and water retention and causes widespread vasoconstriction. It also promotes inflammation, fibrosis and scarring of the kidneys (Gallibois et al., 2017). Diuretics and acetylcholinesterase inhibitors are used to counteract the activities of the renin–angiotensin system.

Mineral and Bone Disorder

A precursor of active vitamin D is manufactured in the skin. Another precursor is consumed in the diet and is absorbed from the bowel. Both liver and kidneys modify these precursors and produce biologically active forms. Active vitamin D stimulates the absorption of dietary calcium from the bowel. By doing so, it helps to maintain serum calcium levels. In chronic renal failure the damaged kidneys do not activate the precursors of vitamin D. The result is that calcium absorption from the bowel is impaired and hypocalcaemia results. The problem is compounded by abnormalities in serum phosphorous levels.

Serum phosphorous levels tend to be elevated in chronic renal failure, caused partly by the damaged kidneys, which fail to eliminate the substance. High serum phosphate is undesirable. It binds to calcium and lowers blood levels and also impairs vitamin D action, which also adversely affects calcium levels. Hypocalcaemia stimulates the production of parathyroid hormone that promotes movement of calcium out of bones. Bone demineralisation takes place and the child develops osteodystrophy.

Efforts should be made to maintain calcium levels. Because the damaged kidneys do not activate precursors of vitamin D, an active form should be prescribed. Calcium supplementation may also be provided. Attempts should also made to control serum phosphorous levels. Food high in phosphorous should be avoided and binding agents, such as aluminium hydroxide or calcium carbonate, which prevent phosphorous absorption, should be prescribed. These measures have a positive impact, but as failure progresses bone demineralisation becomes inevitable (Becherucci et al., 2016).

Metabolic Acidosis

Acidosis adversely affects protein metabolism and is strongly implicated in growth delay (Kraut and Madias, 2011). As kidney disease progresses there is a failure to synthesise ammonia (a process necessary to ride the body of hydrogen ions). There is also a failure to effectively reabsorb bicarbonate. These two factors combine to cause acidosis. When serum bicarbonate falls to levels below 22 mmol/L it should be corrected (KDIGO, 2013; National Kidney Foundation, 2000). Sodium citrate or sodium bicarbonate may be administered orally. When a child is on dialysis, the problem can be met by adapting the dialysate solution to include high sodium bicarbonate concentrations.

Dialysis

NICE (2011) note that patients with stage 5 chronic kidney disease should be given information and support in relation to dialysis and pre-emptive transplant. All patients should be offered a choice of peritoneal dialysis or haemodialysis. However, peritoneal dialysis should be the first choice of treatment modality for children under 2 years of age. Children should be offered a choice between Automated Peritoneal Dialysis (APD) and Continuous Ambulatory Peritoneal Dialysis (CAPD). Based on the clinical experience of the NICE guideline development group, children on a liquid diet with a low residual renal function should be offered APD in preference to CAPD (NICE, 2011).

The main advantage in offering APD and CAPD is that the child can pursue his or her normal activities. A catheter is inserted into the child's abdomen and dialysate flows into the abdominal cavity. The catheter lies on one side of the peritoneal membrane and an exchange between dialysate fluid and body fluid on the opposite side of the membrane takes place. In CAPD this process takes around 30 minutes and is undertaken 4 times a day. In APD this process takes place overnight whilst the child is sleeping, with a machine calculating the fluid required to remove the toxins from the blood. Fluid is left in the peritoneal cavity between dialysis in both methods.

Peritonitis is a complication of peritoneal dialysis. Antibiotic treatment is required where peritonitis is identified. Antibiotics can be added to dialysis fluid as well as being taken orally or via the intravenous route. If the peritonitis is severe or happens repeatedly the child may need to convert to haemodialysis. Haemodialysis is much more restrictive; the child has to attend a specialist unit for 3 or 4 hours three times a week.

> ### 🔾 ACTIVITY
>
> For information about treatment options and dialysis for children visit:
> - https://www.infokid.org.uk/treatment

TRANSPLANT

For children who develop end stage renal disease (ESRD), renal transplantation is considered the best option for improved quality and quantity of life. Immunosuppressive strategies have seen significant improvements in graft survival over recent years. Comparatively, there are only a small number of children with ESRD who require renal transplantation, as opposed to adults. However, children can have major medical differences in their response to renal transplantation and tolerance to medication. It is important to recognise that the goals for children's recovery include normal growth and neurological development. To that end there has been a shift towards pre-emptive transplantation to avoid the associated complications of ESRD and long-term dialysis (Saeed, 2012).

SUMMARY

Paediatric nurses are required to care for children with a range of renal conditions. This chapter has attempted to provide an overview of acute kidney injury and chronic renal disease, alongside some more common renal conditions such as Wilms tumour, nephrotic syndrome and poststreptococcal glomerulonephritis as they are the most common disorders associated with the glomerular pathology.

REFERENCES

Askenazi, D., 2011. Evaluation and management of critically ill children with acute kidney injury. Curr. Opin. Pediatr. 23, 201–207.

Banh, T.H., Hussain-Shamsy, N., Patel, V., et al., 2016. Ethnic differences in incidence and outcomes of childhood nephrotic syndrome. Clin. J. Am. Soc. Nephrol. 11, 1760–1768.

Basile, D.P., Anderson, M.D., Sutton, T.A., 2012. Pathology of acute kidney injury. Compr. Physiol. 2 (2), 1303–1353.

Becherucci, F., Roperto, R.M., Materassi, M., Romagnani, P., 2016. Chronic kidney disease in children. Clin. Kidney J. 9 (4), 583–591.

Besbas, N., Karpman, D., Landau, D., et al., 2006. A classification of hemolytic uremic syndrome and thrombotic thrombocytopenic purpura and related disorders. Kidney Int. 70, 423–431.

Brandão, L.R., Labarque, V., Diab, Y., Williams, S., Manson, D.E., 2011. Pulmonary embolism in children. Semin. Thromb. Hemost. 37 (7), 772–785.

Breslow, N.E., Beckwith, J.B., Perlman, E.J., et al., 2006. Age distributions, birth weights, nephrogenic rests, and heterogeneity in the pathogenesis of Wilms tumor. Pediatr. Blood Canc. 47, 260–267.

Breslow, N.E., Lange, J.M., Friedman, D.L., et al., 2010. Secondary malignant neoplasms after Wilms tumor: an international collaborative study. Int. J. Canc. 127 (3), 657–666.

Carapetis, J.R., Steer, A.C., Mulholland, E.K., Weber, M., 2005. The global burden of group A streptococcal diseases. Lancet Infect. Dis. 5, 685–694.

Constantinescu, A.R., Shah, H.B., Foote, E.F., et al., 2000. Predicting first-year relapses in children with nephrotic syndrome. Pediatrics 105 (3 Pt 1), 492–495.

Downie, M.L., Gallibois, C., Parekh, R.S., Noone, D.G., 2017. Nephrotic syndrome in infants and children: pathophysiology and management. Paediatr. Int. Child Health 37 (4), 248–258.

Eison, T.M., Ault, B.H., Jones, D.P., Chesney, R.W., Wyatt, R.J., 2011. Post-streptococcal acute glomerulonephritis in children: clinical features and pathogenesis. Pediatr. Nephrol. 26 (2), 165–180.

Flynn, J.T., 2002. Choice of dialysis modality for management of pediatric acute renal failure. Pediatr. Nephrol. 17 (1), 61–69.

Gallibois, C.M., Jawa, N.A., Noone, D.G., 2017. Hypertension in pediatric patients with chronic kidney disease: management challenges. Int. J. Nephrol. Renovascular Dis. 10, 205–213.

Ghafari, A., Mehdizadeh, A., Alavi-Darazam, I., 2011. Co-administration of albumin-furosemide in patients with the nephrotic syndrome. Saudi. J. Kidney Dis. Transpl. 22, 471–475.

Goldstein, S.L., Somers, M.J., Lande, M.B., et al., 2000. Acyclovir prophylaxis of varicella in children with renal disease receiving steroids. Pediatr. Nephrol. 14 (4), 305–308.

Hinkes, B.G., Mucha, B., Vlangos, C.N., et al., 2007. Nephrotic syndrome in the first year of life: two thirds of cases are caused by mutations in 4 genes (NPHS1, NPHS2, WT1, and LAMB2). Pediatrics 119, e907–e919.

Hiraoka, M., Tsukahara, H., Matsubara, K., et al., 2003. A randomized study of two long-course prednisolone regimens for nephrotic syndrome in children. Am. J. Kidney Dis. 41 (6), 1155–1162.

Hogg, R.J., Furth, S., Lemley, K.V., et al., 2003. National Kidney Foundation's kidney disease outcomes quality initiative clinical practice guidelines for chronic kidney disease in children and adolescents: evaluation, classification and stratification. Pediatrics 111 (6), 416–1422.

Kaspar, C.D.W., Bholah, R., Bunchman, T.E.A., 2016. Review of pediatric chronic kidney disease. Blood Purif. 41, 211–217.

Kaste, S.C., Dome, J.S., Babyn, P.S., et al., 2008. Wilms tumour: prognostic factors, staging, therapy and late effects. Pediatr. Radiol. 38, 2–17.

Kembhavi, S.A., Qureshi, S., Vora, T., 2013. Understanding the principles in management of Wilms' tumour: can imaging assist in patient selection? Clin. Radiol. 68, 646–653.

Kersnik-Levart, T., Kenig, A., Buturovic-Ponikvar, J., 2001. Real-time ultrasound-guided renal biopsy with a biopsy gun in children: safety and efficacy. Acta Paediatr. 90 (12), 1394–1397.

Kher, K., Schnaper, H.W., Greenbaum, L.W. (Eds.), 2017. Clinical Pediatric Nephrology, third ed. Taylor and Francis, Oxford.

Kidney Disease Improving Global Outcomes (KDIGO), 2012a. Clinical practice guidelines for glomerulonephritis. Kidney Int. 2 (2).

Kidney Disease Improving Global Outcomes (KDIGO), 2012b. Clinical practice guidelines for acute kidney injury. Kidney Int. 2 (1).

Kidney Disease Improving Global Outcomes (KDIGO), 2013. Clinical practice guidelines for the evaluation and management of chronic kidney disease. Kidney Int. 3 (1).

Kleta, R., Bockenhauer, D., 2006. Bartter syndromes and other salt-losing tubulopathies. Nephron. Physiol. 104, 73–80.

Ko, G.J., Obi, Y., Tortoricci, A.R., et al., 2017. Dietary protein intake and chronic kidney disease. Curr. Opin. Clin. Nutr. Metabol. Care. 20 (1), 77–85.

Kraut, J.A., Madias, N.E., 2011. Consequences and therapy of the metabolic acidosis of chronic kidney disease. Pediatr. Nephrol. 26, 19–28.

Lang, M.M., Towers, C., 2001. Identifying poststreptococcal glomerulonephritis. Nurse Pract. Am. J. Prim Health Care 26 (8), 34, 37–42, 44–47.

Lehnhardt, A., Kemper, M.J., 2011. Pathogenesis, diagnosis and management of hyperkalemia. Pediatr. Nephrol. 26, 377–384.

Lombel, R.M., Gipson, D.S., Hodson, E.M., et al., 2013. Treatment of steroid-sensitive nephrotic syndrome: new guidelines from KDIGO. Pediatr. Nephrol. 28, 415–426.

Loza, R., Estremadoyro, L., Loza, C., et al., 2006. Pediatric Nephrology. vol. 21, pp. 106–109.

Maas, M.H., Cransberg, K., van Grotel, M., et al., 2007. Renin-induced hypertension in Wilms tumor patients. Pediatr. Blood Canc. 48, 500–503.

McCaffrey, J., Lennon, R., Webb, N.J., 2016. The non-immunosuppressive management of childhood nephrotic syndrome. Pediatr. Nephrol. 31, 1383–1402.

McIntyre, P., Craig, J.C., 1998. Prevention of serious bacterial infection in children with nephrotic syndrome. J. Paediatr. Child Health 34 (4), 314–317.

McDonald, J.M., Douglass, E.C., Fisher, R., et al., 1998. Linkage of familial Wilms' tumor predisposition to chromosome 19 and a two–locus model for the etiology of familial tumors. Canc. Res. 58, 1387–1390.

McLorie, G., 2001. Wilms' tumor (nephroblastoma). Curr. Opin. Urol. 11 (6), 567–570.

Mishra, O.P., Basu, B., Upadhyay, S.K., et al., 2010. Behavioural abnormalities in children with nephrotic syndrome. Nephrol. Dial. Transplant. 25, 2537–2541.

National Kidney Foundation, 2000. Clinical practice guidelines for nutrition in chronic renal failure. Am. J. Kidney Dis. 35 (6) Suppl 2, S1–S140.

National Institute for Health and Care Excellence (NICE), 2011. Chronic Kidney Disease (Stage 5): Peritoneal Dialysis. Clinical Guideline. [CG125].

National Institute for Health and Care Excellence (NICE), 2013. Acute Kidney Injury: Prevention, Detection and Management. Clinical Guideline. [CG169].

National Institute for Health and Care Excellence (NICE), 2018. Renal Replacement Therapy And Conservative Management. Clinical Guidelines.

Pastore, G., Znaor, A., Spreafico, F., et al., 2006. Malignant renal tumours incidence and survival in European children (1978–1997): report from the Automated Childhood Cancer Information System project. Eur. J. Cancer 42, 2103–2114.

Pritchard-Jones, K., Moroz, V., Vujanić, G., on behalf of the Children's Cancer and Leukaemia Group (CCLG) Renal Tumours Group, 2012. Treatment and outcome of Wilms' tumour patients: an analysis of all cases registered in the UKW3 trial. Ann. Oncol. 23 (9), 2457–2463.

Rodriguez-Iturbe, B., Batsford, S., 2007. Pathogenesis of poststreptococcal glomerulonephritis a century after Clemens von Pirquet. Kidney Int. 71 (11), 1094–1104.

Rodríguez-Iturbe, B., Musser, J.M., 2008. The current state of poststreptococcal glomerulonephritis. J. Am. Soc. Nephrol. 19 (10), 1855–1864.

Saeed, B., 2012. Pediatric renal transplantation. Int. J. Organ. Transplant. Med. 3 (2), 62–73.

Scott, R.H., Murray, A., Baskcomb, L., 2012. Stratification of Wilms tumor by genetic and epigenetic analysis. Oncotarget 3 (3), 327–335.

Tasic, V., Polenakovic, M., 2003. Occurrence of subclinical post-streptococcal glomerulonephritis in family contacts. J. Paediatr. Child Health 39 (3), 177–179.

Teoh, C.W., Robinson, L.A., Noone, D., 2015. Perspectives on edema in childhood nephrotic syndrome. Am. J. Physiol. Renal. Physiol. 309, F575–F582.

van den Berg, J.G., Weening, J.J., 2004. Role of the immune system in the pathogenesis of idiopathic nephrotic syndrome. Clin. Sci. 107, 125–136.

van den Heuvel-Eibrink, M.M., Grundy, P., Graf, N., et al., 2008. Characteristics and survival of 750 children diagnosed with a renal tumor in the first seven months of life: a collaborative study by the SIOP/GPOH/SFOP, NWTSG, and UKCCSG Wilms tumor study groups. Pediatr. Blood Canc. 50, 1130–1134.

Vaziri, N.D., 2016. HDL abnormalities in nephrotic syndrome and chronic kidney disease. Nat. Rev. Nephrol. 12, 37–47.

Vivarelli, M., Massella, L., Ruggiero, B., et al., 2017. Minimal change disease. Clin. J. Am. Soc. Nephrol. 12, 332–345.

15

Caring for Children With Non-Malignant Haematological Disorders of Childhood

Kate Khair

LEARNING OUTCOMES

- Demonstrate an understanding of the anatomy and physiology of the haematological system.
- Gain an overview of the common haematological disorders of childhood.

- Understand the role of nurses for caring for children with non-malignant haematological disorders.
- Use relevant contemporary literature to inform the nursing care of children with non-malignant haematological disorders.

INTRODUCTION

There are two aspects of haematology, which form part of the normal haematological system. The first is haematopoiesis (from the Greek, haem = blood and poiesis = to make), which involves the general aspects of blood cell formation in the bone marrow. The second is haemostasis (also from Greek haem = blood and stasis = stagnation), which is the process of blood clotting. Abnormalities within either of these two systems lead to disorders that may cause significant clinical symptoms of bruising, bleeding, anaemia or infection. Some of these conditions can be acute, for example, immune thrombocytopenic purpura (ITP), although the majority, for example, sickle cell disease or haemophilia, are long-term conditions, which used to be fatal in childhood, but with contemporary management can also now be seen as long-term conditions in adolescents and adults. Children with these conditions receive nursing care at home, provided by their parents (Burnes et al., 2008; Vidler, 1999) and themselves, as well as by community paediatric nurses, local general hospitals and tertiary care centres which may be either paediatric, haematological, or both. There are regional haemoglobinopathy centres and haemophilia comprehensive care centres, which provide 24-hour access and advice about treatment of children with these complex conditions.

ANATOMY AND PHYSIOLOGY OF THE HAEMATOLOGICAL SYSTEM

Haemopoiesis

Haemopoiesis occurs from the first few weeks of embryo development predominantly in the liver and spleen. In later fetal life (at about 6–7 months of gestation) the bone marrow takes over, and during childhood and adulthood becomes the source of blood cell production (Hoffbrand et al., 2001). In children the bone marrow in all bones is active in cell production; in adolescence as bone growth ceases cell production occurs only in the sternum, vertebrae, pelvis and ribs. The sternum and pelvis are the sites most commonly used for bone marrow aspiration to establish diagnosis of bone marrow disease/dysfunction.

Haemopoiesis begins with a stem cell, which gives rise to separate lineages developing into a variety of cells, which in turn become erythrocytes (red blood cells [RBC]), leucocytes (white blood cells [WBC]) and thrombocytes (platelets) (Fig. 15.1). The normal ranges for these cells are dependent upon age and sex. The specific actions of these cells are discussed below.

Erythrocytes

Erythrocytes are bi-concave discs, which have a lifespan of approximately 120 days. They transport haemoglobin, which carries oxygen around the body. As the RBC grows old it becomes fragile, the cell ruptures and the haemoglobin is broken down into haemosiderin and bile pigments which are excreted by the liver.

Leucocytes

There are five types of white blood cells (leucocytes): lymphocytes, monocytes, neutrophils, eosinophils and basophils. Each subgroup of white cells plays a different role in immune processes and are involved in inflammation, phagocytosis, allergy and healing. All of these cells have a nucleus, but have a much shorter lifespan than the RBC, being measurable in the blood for a matter of hours; however WBCs leave the blood and move into tissues, where they act as a reservoir to fight infection and then die after a matter of a few days (Campbell et al., 1995, p 610).

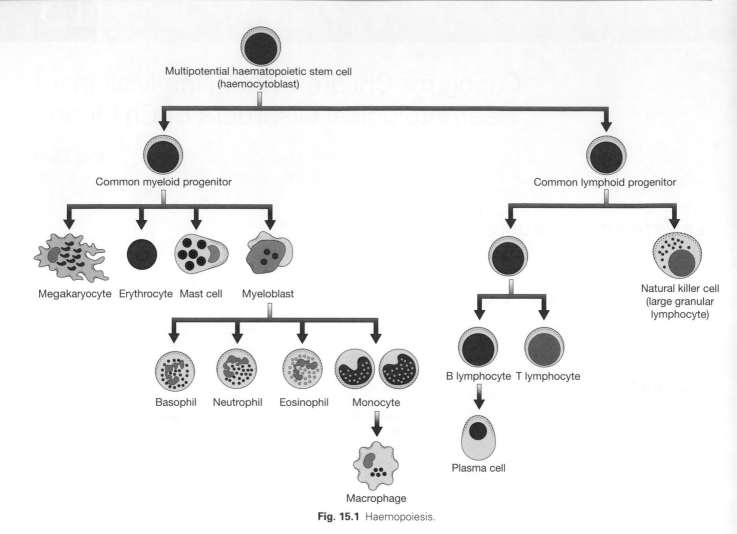

Fig. 15.1 Haemopoiesis.

Thrombocytes

Thrombocytes (platelets) are the smallest cells, originating from megakaryocytes in the bone marrow, and have a life-span of 8–10 days. They are round discs, which are able to change shape due to their structure; they adhere to each other and have coagulation factors that cause a platelet plug at the site of damage to the blood vessel wall. The surface of the platelet is coated with glycoproteins, which are important for adhesion and aggregation and which are fundamental for the formation of the platelet plug.

Coagulation

Coagulation is a complex cascade of actions, involving a variety of mechanisms from blood vessel wall constriction and platelet adhesion to activation of coagulation factors, which adhere to the platelets to form a clot to stop bleeding. If this mechanism was left 'unchecked' thrombosis would occur; to prevent this, coagulation factor inhibitors 'switch off' the coagulation cascade once bleeding has ceased. The coagulation cascade is defined as three interdependent parts: the intrinsic, the extrinsic and the common pathways. The intrinsic pathway begins with 'contact activation' with factor XII becoming activated, this converts factors XI, IX and VIII into their active parts, which work with factor X to initiate clot formation. At the same time the extrinsic pathway generates a 'thrombin burst' when tissue factor is released at the site of injury: activated factor VII circulates in high levels, in turn further activating factor VIII, and factors V and X within the common pathway, where finally thrombin acts to convert fibrinogen to fibrin and a haemostatic plug is formed.

With the exception of von Willebrand factor (which is produced in the endothelium) coagulation factors are produced or synthesised by the liver; therefore liver disease can present with, and be complicated by, coagulation disorders (Fig. 15.2).

INTERPRETATION OF BLOOD RESULTS

Full Blood Count

The full blood count (FBC) is a broad screening test looking at bone marrow cell production, which screens for red cell, white cell and platelet abnormalities. FBC is a relatively easy test to perform, but normal ranges will vary from hospital to hospital. FBC results should be interpreted with knowledge of the normal range of the hospital as well as the child's age, sex and ethnicity. These factors will affect the results, for example, the haemoglobin varies between the sexes and with age.

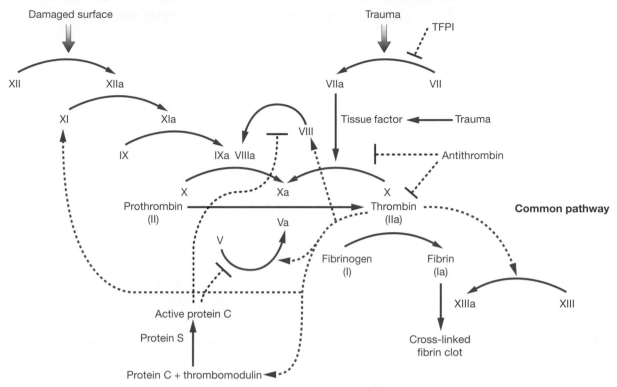

Fig. 15.2 Coagulation cascade.

Bone Marrow Aspiration

Bone marrow aspiration (where the cells of the bone marrow are aspirated in a liquid form into a syringe) and bone marrow trephine (where a core of bone marrow is removed through a large bore needle) are tests to examine the cellular content (aspirate) and the structure (trephine) of the bone marrow. In children, these are most commonly performed under general anaesthesia from the posterior iliac crest (Sepion, 1990) as a diagnostic test when bone marrow failure, leukaemia, metabolic or immunological conditions are suspected. The bone marrow aspirate is spread onto a slide and is easily examined using a microscope; diseases affecting the marrow can be easily diagnosed.

Clotting Screen

The clotting screen is a test of the three aspects of coagulation described above. The activated partial prothrombin test (APTT) is a test of the intrinsic pathway; the prothrombin time (PT) is a test of the extrinsic pathway, whilst the thrombin time (TT) tests the conversion of fibrinogen to fibrin in the common pathway. If the clotting screen suggests that a coagulation disorder may be the cause of bruising/bleeding further investigations are required. Interpretation of an abnormality in the initial coagulation screen and further tests required are detailed in Table 15.1. Not all haematology laboratories will be able to perform all of these tests; referral to a regional paediatric haemophilia centre should be considered if an inherited coagulation disorder is suspected.

NON-MALIGNANT HAEMATOLOGICAL CONDITIONS

Non-malignant haematological conditions lead to a variety of disorders, which present throughout childhood. The majority of these conditions are inherited, for example, sickle cell anaemia and haemophilia, and usually present in infancy and early childhood. Acquired diseases, which may present in later childhood and adolescence, are often severe and may be life-threatening causing problems of infection and bleeding. The commonest non-malignant disorders seen in childhood are discussed in the text to follow; further information on these disorders can be obtained from the paediatric haematology reference books listed in the bibliography.

Bone Marrow Failure Syndromes

Bone marrow failure can be either congenital or acquired. Although extremely rare the commonest form of congenital bone marrow failure is Fanconi anaemia (FA), which is inherited in an autosomal manner and is associated with growth retardation, defects of the skeleton, kidneys or skin, with occasional mental retardation (Hoffbrand et al., 2001, p 91). Children with FA usually show symptoms at around 5–10 years of age with increasing signs of bone marrow failure that may include pancytopenia (reduction in blood count of red and white blood cells and platelets) or leukaemia.

Aplastic anaemia (AA) also presents with pancytopenia, which may be either congenital or acquired. Causes of

TABLE 15.1		Interpretation and Further Investigation of Coagulation Screen Results			
PT	**APTT**	**TT**	**Further Investigations Required**	**Possible Abnormality**	
Prolonged	N	N	Measurement of PT based factors	Factor VII deficiency (extrinsic pathway) Liver disease, vitamin K deficiency	
N	Prolonged	N	Measurement of APTT based factors and vWD screen	Deficiency of factor VIII (haemophilia A/ vWD), factor IX, XI, XII or contact factors (intrinsic pathway)	
			DRVVT	Lupus anticoagulant or other coagulation factor inhibitor	
N	N	Prolonged	Reptilase time and other thrombin time assays	Abnormality of fibrinogen including: Hypofibrinogenaemia, Dysfibrinogenaemia	
Prolonged	Prolonged	N	PT and APTT based factors INR	Deficiency of factor II, V, X (common pathway), Vitamin K deficiency, Liver disease, Massive transfusion, Oral anticoagulants	
N	Prolonged	Prolonged	Reptilase time	Heparin	
Prolonged	Prolonged	Prolonged	D-dimers, Reptilase time	Disseminated intravascular coagulation, Heparin Severe hypofibrinogenaemia or Afibrinogenaemia	
N	N	N	vWD screen, Factor XIII screen/ activity, Platelet function tests	All tests normal but history of bleeding -consider: Mild haemophilia or vWD Factor XIII deficiency, Platelet disorders	

APTT, activated partial thromboplastin time; *DRVVT,* dilute Russell Viper venom time; *INR,* international ratio; *N,* within normal range; *PT,* prothrombin time; *TT,* thrombin time; *vWD,* von Willebrand disease.
Adapted, with permission, from Khair K., Hann I.M., Liesner R., 2003. The investigation of easy bruising. In: David T. (Ed.) Recent Advances in Paediatrics. The Royal Society of Medicine Press, London.

acquired AA include infection, drugs (especially chemotherapy) and exposure to radiation or pesticides.

Kostmann syndrome is rare, also known as severe congenital neutropenia (SCN), and usually detected soon after birth when severe and/or life-threatening infection occurs (Ancliff, 2003).

Osteopetrosis (literally 'stone bone') is a rare inherited disorder where bones harden, becoming brittle. Mild osteopetrosis is usually asymptomatic, but severe forms result in stunted growth, deformity, anaemia from bone marrow failure, blindness and deafness, caused by increased pressure on nerves from bone overgrowth (Hamdan et al., 2006).

Haemoglobinopathy

In infancy children have a variant of haemoglobin known as fetal haemoglobin or HbF. After about 6 months of age they begin to express adult haemoglobin (HbA). Children inherit two sets of haemoglobin genes, one set from each parent. In haemoglobinopathies there is an abnormality in one or both sets of the haemoglobin genes giving rise to an abnormal haemoglobin molecule, which leads to diseases known collectively as haemoglobinopathies.

One of the most significant genetic abnormalities in haemoglobin causes sickle cell anaemia, which is the most common genetic defect in England, affecting 1:2000 births (Dick, 2007); this is most commonly seen in people of Afro-Caribbean descent. The abnormal haemoglobin (HbS) is fragile and unable to carry oxygen effectively, the red cells 'sickle' and break down causing symptoms such as pain, anaemia and

stroke. Children with only one copy of this gene are said to have sickle cell trait (HbAS). Sickle cell disease occurs when two copies of the HbS gene are inherited (HbSS) – one from each parent. See Table 15.2 for a list of haemoglobin gene variants.

Thalassaemia is a group of disorders of the globin genes where one or more of the genes is either missing or is inactive; this is most commonly seen in children of Mediterranean and Asian descent (Modell et al., 2001). There are two subtypes of thalassaemia: α (alpha) and β (beta) thalassaemia. The α subtype causes moderately severe anaemia and splenomegaly, unless two copies of the abnormal α-thalassaemia haemoglobin are inherited, which results in incompatibility with life, often resulting in intrauterine death with hydrops fetalis (Yang and Li, 2009). The β subtype is a much more clinically severe disease presenting in infancy with anaemia, hepatosplenomegaly, bone marrow hyperplasia, infection and osteoporosis (Clarke and Higgins, 2000).

There is a national newborn haemoglobinopathy screening programme in the UK, with all neonates undergoing haemoglobin gene analysis as part of the neonatal screening programme (previously known as the Guthrie test) (NHS, 2006). This has resulted in early diagnosis before children become symptomatic (Bain, 2009).

Bleeding Disorders

The disorders that result in bleeding can be mild to severe, inherited or acquired, as a result of bone marrow abnormalities in platelet production or function, or a reduction or

TABLE 15.2	**Haemoglobin Gene Variants**	
	Haemoglobin Variant	**Clinical Features**
Fetal haemoglobin (HbF)	Normal feature of infancy Switch to adult Hb (HbA) at 6 months of age	Hereditary persistence of HbF caused by genetic abnormalities – leads to anaemia
Haemoglobin A (HbA)	Normal adult haemoglobin	None
Haemoglobin C (HbC)	Most frequently seen in children of west African descent	Mild haemolytic anaemia with splenomegaly
Haemoglobin D (HbD)		No haematological abnormality to mild haemolytic anaemia
Haemoglobin E (HbE)	Most frequently seen in children of southeast Asian descent	Mild hypochromic anaemia
Haemoglobin S (HbS)	Sickle haemoglobin	Sickle cell trait (HbAS) – not usually clinically significant Additional care with anaesthesia Sickle cell disease (HbSS) – severe haemolytic anaemia with sickle cell crises including stroke in young children
Haemoglobin SC (HbSC)		Particular risk of thrombosis and pulmonary embolism
α Thalassaemia	Most commonly seen in children from Mediterranean and Asian descent	Can be mild causing moderately severe hypochromic anaemia but in severe cases is incompatible with life, can cause hydrops fetalis and intrauterine death
β Thalassaemia	Most commonly seen in children of Mediterranean and Asian descent	Severe anaemia from 6 months of age requiring transfusion Hepatosplenomegaly Infections Osteoporosis

absence of any of the coagulation factors. The commonest causes of bleeding are discussed in the following sections as either disorders of platelets or coagulation.

Platelet Disorders

Thrombocytopenia. The full blood count will indicate if there is thrombocytopenia; this should be repeated to confirm this finding. The commonest cause of thrombocytopenia in children is ITP, which often occurs following viral infections (Vora and Makrish, 2001). Although bruising is common, severe bleeding is rare if the platelet count is above 20×10^9/L. If there is persistent thrombocytopenia, referral to a paediatric haematology centre should be considered, aiming to exclude a congenital platelet disorder, leukaemia or a bone marrow failure syndrome. Congenital thrombocytopenias are rare but may present with symptoms of bruising or bleeding soon after birth. Thrombocytopenia with absent radii ('TAR syndrome') is an autosomal recessive disorder characterised by bilateral absence of the radii, which is clinically obvious at birth (Al-Jefri et al., 2000) or may be detected antenatally (Goldmann et al., 2018). Wiskott–Aldrich syndrome is an X-linked immune deficiency disorder associated with bacterial infections and/or eczema (Mullen et al., 1993). Bernard–Soulier syndrome is an autosomal recessive disorder most commonly seen in consanguineous families, which causes mild to severe bleeding in both boys and girls (George et al., 1981).

Functional abnormalities. These are platelet disorders with normal platelet numbers but abnormal function and can be

minor causing bleeding following surgery, or more severe causing life-threatening disorders such as Glanzmann thrombasthenia. Transient abnormalities in platelet function causing easy bruising are common and are often associated with the use of anti-platelet drugs such as non-steroidal anti-inflammatory drugs or aspirin. Other drugs that are known to affect platelet function are listed in Table 15.3.

Inherited platelet function defects are very rare, the most severe of these is Glanzmann's thrombasthenia – an autosomal recessive disorder which results in severe often spontaneous bleeding usually from the mucous membranes, which can be life threatening (Hardisty, 2000). Platelet storage pool disorders, where there is a deficiency in the nucleotide content of the platelet, and platelet release defects, where the nucleotides cannot be released properly, both result in mild to moderate bruising and bleeding following trauma or surgery.

Coagulation Disorders

Von Willebrand disease (vWD) is the commonest inherited bleeding disorder with an incidence of 1:100 to 1:1000. The inheritance varies according to the subtype and affects boys and girls equally. There are three major subtypes of vWD; bleeding in types 1 and 2 is usually mild, but in type 3, which is inherited in an autosomal recessive manner, there is usually severe bleeding, often from mucous membranes from early childhood resulting in mouth and nose bleeds (Mannucci, 2001).

Haemophilia is an X-linked condition in which boys experience bruising and bleeding, which can be severe (Khair et al., 2003). Haemophilia A (classical haemophilia, a deficiency of factor VIII) affects about 1:10,000 boys, whereas haemophilia

TABLE 15.3 Drugs Which May Affect Platelet Function
Cytotoxic therapy
Ethanol
Chloramphenicol
Arsenic
Benzene
Non-steroidal anti-inflammatory drugs
Aspirin
Rifampicin
Penicillin
Sulphonamides
Trimethoprim
Diazepam
Sodium valproate
Carbamazepine
Frusemide
Tolbutamide
Digoxin
Heparin
Warfarin
Methyldopa
Oxyprenolol
Quinine

B (Christmas disease or factor IX deficiency) affects about 1:50,000 boys. The bruising/bleeding is dependent upon the level of factor in the plasma, with the most severe bleeding occurring in those with the lowest factor levels. Although considered an inherited disorder, approximately one in three boys with haemophilia have no previous family history, but have a new genetic mutation in their *FVIII* or *FIX* gene. Girls who are haemophilia carriers may also suffer bruising/bleeding and menorrhagia when in adolescence, as they may also have low factor levels.

SCENARIO 1

John is a 7-year-old boy who has severe haemophilia A. He is accompanied to the ward by his father following a football injury causing an acute knee bleed, which had occurred on the previous day. John usually has prophylaxis every other day and before sport given by his mum who is currently in hospital following the birth of a baby. Dad reports that he had three attempts to treat John after the injury; he only managed to give about half the dose as the needle 'tissued'.

- What framework would you use to assess John's joint?
- What observations do you need to do?
- What do you expect these observations to be?
- Is John's condition mild, moderate or severe?
- Is there anything in the history that would give concern?
- What care would you expect to be initiated?
- What ongoing care does John need?

The other coagulation disorders are very rare compared with haemophilia and vWD; however, they can cause life-threatening bleeding. Deficiency of factor II, V, VII or X can cause significant bleeding when autosomal recessive inheritance has occurred; however, carriers of these disorders can also experience mild bleeding/bruising (Bolton-Maggs et al., 1995). Factor XI deficiency is most commonly seen in children of Ashkenazi Jewish descent; the bleeding tendency is usually mild (Collins et al., 1995). Factor XII deficiency is commonly identified in the laboratory due to prolonged APTT on screening tests, but rarely if ever predisposes to bruising/bleeding. Factor XIII deficiency is an autosomal recessive condition, which presents in the neonatal period with umbilical cord bleeding, delayed cord separation or intracranial haemorrhage (Anwar and Miloszeski, 1999). Disorders of fibrinogen can be both in quantity and/or quality, often presenting in early childhood with bruising and bleeding particularly from the umbilical cord and dysfibrinogenaemia may also cause thrombosis (Lak et al., 1999).

Acquired coagulation disorders are commonly seen in children who are unwell. Vitamin K deficiency is the most common acquired bleeding disorder of childhood being seen in liver disease, gastrointestinal disorders and cystic fibrosis. Neonates who have not received vitamin K prophylaxis at birth can develop haemorrhagic disease of the newborn, which usually presents in the first few days of life (Sutor et al., 1999) and is preventable with the administration of intramuscular (IM) vitamin K at birth. Children with severe liver disease may have abnormal coagulation due to impaired synthesis of coagulation factors. Disseminated intravascular coagulation is uncontrolled activation of coagulation, causing coagulation factor and platelet consumption and usually occurs in children who are critically ill. It is most commonly seen in children in intensive care units.

In summary, the diagnosis of haematological diseases of childhood is predominantly a clinical laboratory test based on sound knowledge of the haematological system and the symptoms produced when this fails. Nursing and medical care is often supportive for what are often life-long and potentially life-threatening diseases.

MANAGEMENT OF CHILDREN WITH HAEMATOLOGICAL DISORDERS

The aims of management of any malignant haematological disease are applicable to all the conditions discussed in this chapter, although there are some disease specific considerations that need to be taken into account. Management aims are:

- to monitor the child's vital signs and overall condition;
- to minimise invasive investigations and treatments;
- to deliver treatments, many of which are intravenous, safely;
- to minimise the risk of side effects and complications of treatment;
- to evaluate the effectiveness of treatment;
- to communicate effectively with the child and family;

TABLE 15.4	Transfusion of Blood Products Including Coagulation Factors	
Procedure	**Process**	**Rationale**
Preparation of child and family	Inform child and family that transfusion is necessary, the reason for the transfusion and what this entails Document consent Ensure venous access is secured	To gain understanding and to document consent To enable transfusion to commence
Prescription	Blood products *must not* be administered unless prescribed by a doctor The prescription should include the infusion rate, volume and infusion time of <4 hours If antihistamine pre-medication is prescribed administer prior to transfusion	Recommendation of British Committee for Haematology Standards in Blood Transfusion Task Force Reduced risk of fluid overload and infection Reduce allergic reactions
Transfusion preparation	Arrange for collection of blood products from blood bank or pharmacy On receipt of blood products onto the ward the collection slip and/or other documentation should be signed Check that the child's details are the same on the blood product, the prescription and the child's wristband	To ensure product on ward in timely manner to be administered to the child To provide audit trail of safe transfusion practice To ensure the correct product is being administered to the correct child
Infusion	Observe the child closely for the first 30 minutes of blood product infusion (not necessary for coagulation factors) Record date and time of start of infusion Monitor vital signs – temperature, pulse, blood pressure as per local (hospital/unit) policy (not necessary in coagulation factors) Monitor infusion site if infusion is being given peripherally	This is when transfusion reactions are most likely to occur To monitor complications such as allergic reactions To monitor for extravasation and phlebitis
Complete transfusion	Remove blood product administration set Dispose of giving set and bag	To reduce risk of infection To ensure safe disposal

Adapted, with permission, from Great Ormond Street Hospital for Children NHS Trust, Clinical Practice Guidelines for Coagulation factors, Cryoprecipitate; Platelet and Red Cell Products transfusion. Available from: www.ich.ucl.ac.uk.

- to provide clear discharge advice;
- to provide ongoing, home/community-based care.

The haematological conditions discussed in this chapter are likely to be life-long, potentially life-threatening disorders, which may be inherited and have genetic implications for the child, their current family and their future family. Children with these conditions are likely to be treated with blood or its constituents; the rationale for this best practice in administration and monitoring are described in Table 15.4. Specific requirements for some children/conditions are addressed later in the chapter.

Bone Marrow Failure

Although rare, the commonest bone marrow (BM) failures syndromes seen in children are listed in Table 15.5. Depending upon the degree of BM failure children will present with a variety of signs and symptoms, which may include anaemia, bleeding and infection. Anaemia in BM failure is caused by low haemoglobin production. Bleeding is due to a thrombocytopenia and/or over production of immature platelets, which do not work effectively, and infection is due to leucopoenia. A combination of low levels of haemoglobin, platelets and white cells is known as pancytopenia.

Characteristics of anaemia
- Pallor

TABLE 15.5	Bone Marrow Failure Syndromes Seen in Children
Aplastic anaemia
Fanconi anaemia
Myelodysplasia syndromes
Schwachman syndrome
Diamond–Blackfan anaemia
Kostmann syndrome
Osteopetrosis
Dyskeratosis congenita

- Hypoxia
- Lack of energy/lethargy
- Shortness of breath – particularly on exercise
Characteristics of thrombocytopenia:
- Petechiae/bruising
- Wet petechiae
- Mouth/nose bleeding
Characteristics of leucopoenia
- Recurrent infection, which may be viral in origin
- Sepsis
- Overwhelming bacterial infection
- Fungal infection

Specific Treatment

The initial management of BM failure is supportive care, including blood product support when red cell and/or platelet transfusions are given. The care of children receiving blood products is detailed in Table 15.4. These should be used to relieve symptoms rather than to treat the FBC – children with BM failure may have a platelet count, which runs in single figures. If there is no bleeding this should be monitored and only treated if they become symptomatic or are to undergo surgery.

Appropriate anti-infective therapy should be used; infection control measures should be strictly adhered to, including avoidance of large groups of other children, who may be carrying viral infections such as chickenpox. Bone marrow transplantation may be used as a cure for these children (see later).

HAEMOGLOBINOPATHY

Sickle Cell Disease

Children with sickle cell disease (SCD) present with a variety of symptoms ranging from painful episodes of 'sickle cell crisis' due to occlusion of blood vessels following sickling of red cells; acute chest syndrome, which may be caused by infection (Vichinsky et al., 2000); liver disease due to gallstones (Bond et al., 1987); leg ulcers; stroke, which most commonly presents between the ages of 2 and 5 years of age (Ohene-Frempong et al., 1998); priapism in adolescent boys and in unvaccinated undiagnosed children; rapid death from pneumococcal sepsis.

Treatment of children with SCD will be individualised and based on their symptoms. All children in the UK are now vaccinated against pneumococcal infection, but it remains of even greater importance that children with SCD are vaccinated against this as well as all routine childhood vaccinations to protect them from infections and reduce the risk of fever and acute chest syndrome. Additionally, children who are (blood) transfusion dependent, should be vaccinated against hepatitis B. Reduced function of the spleen (splenic hypofunction) caused by infarction within the spleen by sickled red cells also leads to increased susceptibility to infection; therefore children with SCD are offered penicillin prophylaxis in an attempt to reduce mortality from sepsis (Gaston et al., 1986).

Children with SCD suffer recurrent painful episodes (crises), which are caused by vasoocclusion; these can vary from mild occlusion with mild to moderate pain, which can be managed at home with mild analgesia such as paracetamol or ibuprofen, through to severe crises, which requires hospitalisation and codeine, pethidine or morphine administration. A child-focused pain score such as the faces pain rating scale (Wong and Baker, 1998) should be used to assess pain and monitor analgesia response. Intravenous fluids should be given if there is dehydration as this will further exacerbate the crisis.

Acute chest syndrome is a potentially fatal complication of SCD, which may present with acute respiratory failure, and may require intensive care and ventilation. On admission to the ward the child should have a full respiratory assessment

(see Chapter 27) including oxygen saturation testing. Sleep studies should be undertaken to observe for obstructive sleep apnoea. An echocardiogram should be undertaken to look for pulmonary hypertension, which is part of chronic sickle lung conditions. If present, a transfusion programme may be initiated. Hydroxyurea, a chemotherapy agent, has been shown to be effective in reducing the recurrence of acute chest syndrome and is used effectively in many children with SCD (Mueller, 2008).

Stroke, which is caused by cerebral ischaemic damage, occurs most often in children aged 2–5 years with as many as 11% of children with SCD suffering clinically evident stroke (Ohene-Frempong et al., 1998). Stroke in SCD is thought to be caused by stenotic lesions in the cerebral arteries, which can be detected as high blood flow abnormalities on transcranial Doppler (TCD) scanning. All children with SCD should undergo annual TCD scanning as there is evidence that exchange transfusion programmes in children with high blood flow abnormalities can prevent stroke. It is now UK practice for children aged over 3 years to have at least annual TCD scanning. Additional risk factors in children with SCD, who have had a stroke, include low haemoglobin levels and obstructive sleep apnoea, both of which lead to hypoxia. Children who have had strokes are most commonly managed on a transfusion programme throughout childhood and adolescence; this can lead to iron overload, which will itself need management (see Thalassaemia section, later). Children with SCD who have suffered a stroke should be assessed in a specialist sickle centre where they can be seen by a paediatric neurologist for initial care. They will require intensive rehabilitation from a multidisciplinary team including nursing, physiotherapy, psychology and occupational therapy.

Priapism is a prolonged (lasting more than 3 hours), painful, unwanted erection, commonly seen in adolescent and young adult males that can be a surgical emergency. Minor attacks can be treated with analgesia, emptying the bladder and taking a warm bath. In severe attacks an urgent urological opinion should be sought. Irrigation of the penis with epinephrine is often an effective treatment, but if this fails emergency venous shunting surgery is necessary.

Liver disease is most commonly caused by gallstones and obstructive jaundice; appropriate surgical intervention should be offered if this becomes problematical.

Characteristics of Sickle Cell Crisis

- Pain
- Respiratory distress with or without fever in chest syndrome
- Acute anaemia
- Priapism
- Stroke

Specific Treatment

- Analgesia
- Keep warm

- Keep well hydrated – including IV fluid administration if necessary
- Full respiratory assessment for children with chest syndrome (see Chapter 27) including:
  - oxygen saturation monitoring and therapy
  - ventilation if indicated
  - overnight sleep studies in non-acute phase of illness
  - pulmonary function testing
- Full neurological assessment for children with stroke
- Transfusion programmes for children with stroke and frequent sickle crises
- Annual transcranial Doppler scanning in all children aged >3 years
- Bone marrow transplantation

👤 SCENARIO 2

Jennifer is a 4-year-old girl who has sickle cell disease. She has been admitted to the ward from the Accident and Emergency (A&E) department with acute chest syndrome and is accompanied by her mum. Jennifer has been 'off colour' for the last 4 days with fever and cough; her brother has similar symptoms though not sickle cell disease.

- What framework would you use to assess Jennifer?
- What observations do you need to do?
- What do you expect these observations to be?
- Is Jennifer's condition mild, moderate or severe?
- Is there anything in the history that would give concern?
- What care would you expect to be initiated?
- What ongoing care does Jennifer need?

THALASSAEMIA

Children with thalassaemia are now surviving into adulthood with good health and are able to lead essentially normal lives (Weatherall and Clegg, 2001). However, thalassaemia remains a severe disease that requires life-long management and care, despite which, complications such as growth failure can occur. Standard treatment of blood transfusions given every 2–3 weeks to correct anaemia enables normal growth and development, limits splenomegaly and the bone marrow expansion, which causes the typical facial bone features of thalassaemia and prevents cardiac failure (United Kingdom Thalassaemia Society [UKTS], 2008).

Treatment of children with thalassaemia will be individualised and based on symptom management. The majority of children are transfusion dependent by the age of 3. This means that they are anaemic, usually with a haemoglobin of less than 7 g/dL without transfusion. This leads to fatigue, poor appetite, developmental delay, failure to thrive and cardiac failure. A transfusion programme that keeps the haemoglobin greater than 10 g/dL is usually successful in alleviating most of these symptoms, although this requires frequent hospital attendances for cross matching and transfusing. A small number of children may be transfused at home following parental training (Madgwick and Yardumian, 1999).

Repeated transfusions lead to iron overload, which can be fatal. Unbound iron that is in the plasma is toxic to cardiac and liver tissue, which can result in cardiomyopathy, cardiac arrhythmia and failure. There can be liver fibrosis leading to liver failure cirrhosis and cancer. There is good evidence that these side effects of transfusion can be overcome through the use of iron chelation therapy where free iron in the plasma is bound to the chelating agent and is excreted via the urine or faeces. The commonest of these chelating therapies is desferoxamine, which is given as an 8–12-hour subcutaneous infusion five to six times per week. This has been shown to be effective in reducing the toxic effects of iron, reducing liver and cardiac toxicity (Brittenham et al., 1994). However, this places a significant burden upon the child and family, with time taken to site needles and infuse products being given as reasons for poor continued adherence to treatment (Telfer et al., 2005). Recent enhancements to improve adherence include 'balloon pumps', which automatically infuse and oral chelation agents, two of which have been licensed for use in children in the UK. Contemporary chelation can be achieved using oral medications (Gomber et al., 2016), which are shown to be both effective and to improve the quality of life of children and their parent/caregiver (Horodniceanu et al., 2017).

Specific Treatment

Blood transfusion
- Pre-arranged transfusions should be given following guidelines in Table 15.5.
- Peripheral cannulation should be undertaken only by experienced staff.
- Central venous access devices may be implanted.

Chelation
- Subcutaneous overnight infusions 5–6 nights per week:
  - subcutaneous infusion needles
  - mechanical pump/infusor
  - monitor treatment success by measuring serum ferritin levels
- Bone marrow transplantation

BLEEDING DISORDERS

Although in itself rare, the commonest significant bleeding disorder is haemophilia, which causes bleeding mainly in the weight-bearing (ankle and knee) joints. Children with haemophilia will present with acutely hot, painful joint swelling (haemarthrosis) usually preceded by trauma. The joint will be flexed (as this reduces pressure within the joint and is less painful) with a limited range of movement. These are treated initially in three ways: by replacement of the missing coagulation factor, by administration of analgesia (avoiding non-steroidal anti-inflammatory drugs as these affect platelet function and worsen bleeding) and implementing physiotherapy guidelines of PRICE (Table 15.6). Recurrent haemarthrosis leads to significant arthritic joint damage; therefore children with

TABLE 15.6	**Management of Soft Tissue Injury/Joint Bleeds With PRICE**
Protection	Use of splints, slings, crutches as applicable. Splints should be individually made, reflecting the degree of swelling and position of the affected joint. Children should be instructed in the use of crutches by an appropriately trained health care professional.
Rest	Use of 'relative rest' or 'controlled activity'. Bed rest is virtually impossible in children with painful, swollen joints, 'sofa rest' while watching television should be encouraged. Controlled activity should be introduced once the joint has settled and normal mobility has been regained.
Ice	Use of cold therapy, either through cold wraps (gel filled refrigerated bandages) or cold compresses where crushed ice can be applied to the affected area for short, timed, periods. The skin should be protected from contact with the ice by use of a towel or pillowcase.
Compression	Use of supportive elastic wraps or bandage, applied loosely so as not to constrict the limb causing more oedema, swelling and pain.
Elevation	Supported elevation (sofa rest for legs, pillows supporting arms) for up to 72 hours following injury. Compression should not be used at same time as elevation.

severe haemophilia, who are most likely to have bleeding are treated with prophylactic factor replacement therapy. This is given as an individualised, tailored dosing/frequency regimen enabling children to participate in sporting activity with reduced risk of bleeding (Khair and Geraghty, 2007).

Nose and mouth bleeds are common in children with coagulation disorders following trauma and occur spontaneously in children with platelet abnormalities. Usual first aid measures for managing nose bleeds (compression of the nose, application of ice packs, sitting with head forward) should be instituted. Mouth bleeds are more difficult as they often fail to respond to first aid measures; however giving an ice lolly may help as this reduces the blood flow to the mouth due to vasoconstriction secondary to cold therapy. In many children this proves ineffective and administration of intranasal or intravenous desmopressin (Khair et al., 2007), tranexamic acid (an anti-fibrinolytic drug, which slows down clot breakdown), clotting factors or platelet transfusions may be necessary. In children with severe platelet disorders, activated recombinant factor VII may be a useful adjunctive therapy and may avoid exposure to blood products (Almeida et al., 2003).

Characteristics of Bleeding Disorders
Joint bleeds
- Pain
- Swollen, hot joint
- Decreased range of movement
- Unable to weight bear
Nose/mouth bleeds
- Last >20 minutes
- Shown no signs of clotting
- Child becoming hypovolaemic:
  - tachycardia
  - hypotensive
  - pale
  - sweaty

Specific Treatment
Joint bleeds
- Use PRICE therapy
- Nurse in position most comfortable to child
- Administer appropriate analgesia
- Administer coagulation factors as prescription
- Monitor range of movement and joint size to ensure bleed has ceased
Mouth bleeds
- Use local first aid measures including cold therapy if possible
- Monitor airway – clots in throat may obstruct airway
- Administer coagulation factors/platelets as prescription
- Continue tranexamic acid for 5 days post-bleed
- Give dietary advice – soft diet until bleeding fully ceased, avoid crisps

BONE MARROW TRANSPLANTATION

Bone marrow transplantation (BMT) has been used as a therapeutic option in children with aplastic anaemia (Myers and Davies, 2009), Fanconi anaemia (Wagner et al., 2007), Glanzmann thrombasthenia (Connor et al., 2008), Bernard–Soulier syndrome (Reiger et al., 2006), thalassaemia (Rajasekar et al., 2009) and sickle cell anaemia (Krishnamurti, 2007). Although this is an encouraging therapeutic option, it is not without long-term sequelae, and is only undertaken in extreme circumstances (Shenoy et al., 2017). Unlike children having BMT for leukaemia, children with the diseases discussed above are unlikely to have experienced prolonged hospitalisation and intensive chemotherapy. Specific attention should be paid to their psychological preparation pre-transplant (Bennett-Rees et al., 2008, p 107). BMT is undertaken in specialist regional paediatric BMT centres and further information on nursing care of children undergoing BMT can be obtained by contacting your local centre.

DISCUSSION OF THE SCENARIOS

Haemophilia Scenario: John

What framework would you use to assess John's joint? Assessment follows the PRICE criteria for assessment and treatment of haemarthrosis – this provides a uniform and rapid assessment tool that can readily be used by nurses. The assessment should therefore include:

- **P**rotection
- **R**est
- **I**ce
- **C**ompression
- **E**levation

What observations do you need to do?

- Pain assessment: asking John and his dad if analgesia has already been given
- The position that the knee is held in
- Can John walk?

What do you expect these observations to be?

- Dad reports that he gave John paracetamol when the injury occurred.
- The knee is held in a flexed position even at rest.
- John is unable to walk, even standing is painful.

Is John's condition mild, moderate or severe?

- John's knee bleed will most likely be assessed as severe as he has had little response to factor VIII given at home by his Dad; he is still unable to weight bear and is still in pain.

Is there anything in the history that would give concern?

- John had substandard treatment of his bleed as his dad couldn't give the factor.
- The factor should have been given before sport and not after the bleed occurred.
- Mum is in hospital with a new baby.

What care would you expect to be initiated?

- Analgesia
- Factor VIII
- PRICE with or without physiotherapy assessment
- Crutches to avoid weight-bearing.

What ongoing care does John need?

- Daily doses of factor VIII until bleed has settled
- Analgesia until knee is no longer painful
- Physiotherapy to achieve pre-bleed range of movement on the knee.

Sickle Scenario: Jennifer

What framework would you use to assess Jennifer?

- Airway
- Breathing
- Circulation

What observations do you need to do?

- Vital signs
- Recession?
- Cough
- O_2
- Pain
- Colour

What do you expect these observations to be?

- Back pain
- Fever
- Pallor

Is Jennifer's condition mild, moderate or severe?

- Severe because of acute chest syndrome

Is there anything in the history that would give concern?

- Brother – who is looking after him?
- Delay in treatment

What care would you expect to be initiated?

- Analgesia
- O_2
- IV fluids
- Bronchodilators
- Physio
- Blood?

What ongoing care does Jennifer need?

- Hydroxyurea
- Referral to respiratory paediatrician
- Pulmonary function
- Parent

REFERENCES

Al-Jefri, A., Bussel, J., Freedman, M., 2000. Thrombocytopenia with absent radii: frequency of marrow megakaryoctye progenitors, proliferative characteristics, and megakaryoctye growth and development factor responsiveness. Pediatr. Hematol. Oncol. 17, 299–306.

Almeida, A.M., Khair, K., Hann, I., et al., 2003. Use of recombinant factor VIIa in children with inherited platelet function disorders. Br. J. Haematol. 3, 477–481.

Ancliff, P., 2003. Congenital neutropenia. Blood. Rev. 4, 209–216.

Anwar, R., Miloszeski, K.J.A., 1999. Factor XIII deficiency. Br. J. Haematol. 107, 468–484.

Bain, B.J., 2009. Neonatal/newborn haemoglobinopathy screening in Europe and Africa. J. Clin. Pathol. 1, 53–56.

Bennett-Rees, N., Hopkins, S., Stone, J., 2008. Preparation for bone marrow transplant. In: Gibson, F., Soanes, L. (Eds.), Cancer in Children and Young People. Wiley, London.

Bolton-Maggs, P.H.B., Hill, F.G.H., 1995. The rarer inherited coagulation disorders: a review. Blood. Rev. 9, 65–76.

Bond, L.R., Hatty, S.R., Horn, M.E., et al., 1987. Gall stones in sickle cell disease in the United Kingdom. Br. Med. J. 295, 234–236.

Brittenham, G.M., Griffith, P.M., Nienhuis, A.W., et al., 1994. Efficacy of desferrioxamine in preventing complications of iron overload in patients with thalassaemia major. N. Engl. J. Med. 331 (9), 567–573.

Burnes, D.P., Antle, B.J., Williams, C.C., et al., 2008. Mothers raising children with sickle cell disease at the intersection of race, gender, and illness stigma. Health. Soc. Work. 3, 211–220.

Campbell, S., Glasper, A.E. (Eds.), 1995. Whaley and Wong's Children's Nursing UK Edition. Times Mirror, London.

Clarke, G.M., Higgins, T.N., 2000. Laboratory investigation of hemoglobinopathies and thalassemias: review and update. Clin. Chem. 46, 1284–1290.

Collins, P.W., Goldman, E., Lilley, P., et al., 1995. Clinical experience of factor XI deficiency: the role of fresh frozen plasma and factor XI concentrate. Haemophilia 1, 227–231.

Connor, P., Khair, K., Liesner, R., et al., 2008. Stem cell transplantation for children with Glanzmann thrombasthenia. Br. J. Haematol. 140, 568–571.

Dick, M., 2007. Sickle Cell Disease in Childhood. Standards and Guidelines for Clinical Care. Detailed Guidance 2007. Available from: www.nhs.uk/sicklandthal.

Gaston, M.H., Verter, J.I., Woods, G., et al., 1986. Prophylaxis with oral penicillin in children with sickle cell anaemia. N. Eng. J. Med. 314, 1593–1599.

George, J.N., Reiman, T.A., Moake, J.L., et al., 1981. Soulier disease: a study of four patients and their parents. Br. J. Haematol. 48 (3), 456–467.

Goldman, B.G., Hehir, M.P., Yambasu, S., et al., 2018. The presentation and management of platelet disorders in pregnancy. Eur. J. Haematol. https://doi.org/10.1111/ejh.13049 (Epub ahead of print).

Gomber, S., Jain, P., Sharma, S., et al., 2016. Comparative efficacy and safety of oral iron chelators and their novel combination in children with thalassemia. Indian. Pediatric. 53 (3), 207–210.

Hamdan, A.L., Nabulsi, M.M., Farhat, F.T., et al., 2006. When bone becomes marble: head and neck manifestations of osteopetrosis. Paediatric. Child. Health 1, 37–40.

Hardisty, R.M., 2000. Platelet function disorders. In: Lilleyman, J., Hann, I., Blanchette, V. (Eds.), Paediatric Hematology. Churchill Livingstone, Edinburgh.

Hoffbrand, A.V., Pettit, J.E., Moss, P.A.H. (Eds.), 2001. Essential Haematology, fourth ed. Blackwell Science, London.

Horodniceanu, E.G., Bal, V., Dhatt, H., Carter, J.A., Huang, V., Lasch, K., 2017. Qualitative modification and development of patient- and caregiver-reported outcome measures for iron chelation therapy. Health. Qual. Life. Outcomes 15 (1), 129.

Khair, K., Baker, K., Mathias, M., et al., 2007. Intranasal desmopressin (Octim): a safe and efficacious treatment option for children with bleeding disorders. Haemophilia 5, 548–551.

Khair, K., Geraghty, S.J., 2007. Haemophilia A: meeting the needs of individual patients. Br. J. Nurs. 16, 987–993.

Khair, K., Hann, I.M., Liesner, R., 2003. The investigation of easy bruising. In: David, T. (Ed.), Recent Advances in Paediatrics. The Royal Society of Medicine Press, London.

Krishnamurti, L., 2007. Haematopoetic cell transplantation: a curative option for sickle cell disease. Pediatr. Hematol. Oncol. 24 (8), 569–575.

Lak, M., Keihani, M., Elahi, F., et al., 1999. Bleeding and thrombosis in 55 patients with inherited afibrinogenaemia. Br. J. Haematol. 107, 204–206.

Madgwick, K.V., Yardumian, A., 1999. A home blood transfusion programme for beta thalassaemia patients. Transfus. Med. 9 (2), 135–138.

Mannucci, P.M., 2001. Treatment of von Willebrand disease. Thromb. Haemostasis 86, 149–153.

Modell, B., Khan, M., Darlison, M., et al., 2001. A national register for surveillance of inherited disorders: beta thalassaemia in the United Kingdom. Bull World Health Organ. 79 (11), 1006–1012.

Mueller, B.U., 2008. When should hydroxyurea be used for children with sickle cell disease? Pediatrics 122, 1365–1366.

Mullen, C., Anderson, K., Blaese, R., 1993. Splenectomy and/or bone marrow transplantation in the management of the Wiskott-Aldrich syndrome: long-term follow-up of 62 cases. Blood 10, 2961–2966.

Myers, K.C., Davies, S.M., 2009. Haematopoietic stem cell transplantation for bone marrow failure syndromes in children. Biol. Blood. Marrow. Transplant. 15, 279–292.

NHS sickle cell and thalassaemia screening programme. London, 2006. Available from: www.screening.nhs.uk/sickleandthal.

Ohene-Frempong, K., Weiner, S.J., Sleeper, L.A., et al., 1998. Cerebrovascular accidents in sickle cell disease: rates and risk factors. Blood 91, 288–294.

Rajesekar, R., Mathews, V., Lakshmi, K.M., et al., 2009. Cellular immune reconstitution and its impact on clinical outcome in children with beta thalassemia undergoing a matched related myeloablative allogeneic bone marrow transplant. Biol. Blood. Marrow. Transplant. 15, 597–609.

Rieger, C., Rank, A., Fiegl, et al., 2006. Allogeneic stem cell transplantation as a new treatment option for patients with Bernard-Soulier syndrome. Thromb. Haemostasis 95, 190–191.

Sepion, B., 2000. Investigations, staging & diagnosis: implications for nurses. In: Thompson, J. (Ed.), The Child with Cancer – Nursing Care. Scutari Press, London.

Shenoy, S., Angelucci, E., Arnold, S.D., et al., 2017. Current results and future research priorities in late effects after hematopoietic stem cell transplantation for children with sickle cell disease and thalassemia: a consensus statement from the Second Pediatric Blood and Marrow Transplant Consortium International Conference on Late Effects after Pediatric Hematopoietic Stem Cell Transplantation. Biol. Blood. Marrow. Transplant. 23 (4), 552–561.

Srivastava A, Santagostino E, Dougall A, Kitchen S, Sutherland M, Pipe SW, Carcao M, Mahlangu J, Ragni MV, Windyga J, Llinás A, Goddard NJ, Mohan R, Poonnoose PM, Feldman BM, Lewis SZ, van den Berg HM, Pierce GF; WFH Guidelines for the Management of Hemophilia panelists and co-authors. WFH Guidelines for the Management of Hemophilia, 3rd edition. Haemophilia. 2020 Aug;26 Suppl 6:1-158. doi: 10.1111/hae.14046. Epub 2020 Aug 3. PMID: 32744769.

Sutor, A.H., von Kries, R., Cornelissen, E.A., et al., 1999. Vitamin K deficiency bleeding (VKDB) in infancy. Thromb. Haemostasis 81, 456–461.

Telfer, P., Constantinidou, G., Andreou, P., et al., 2005. Quality of life in thalassaemia. Ann. N. Y. Acad. Sci. 1054, 273–282.

United Kingdom Thalassaemia Society (UKTS), 2018. Standards for the clinical care of children and adults with thalassaemia in the UK. Available from: www.ukts.org/pdfs/awareness/ukts.

Vichinsky, E., Neumayr, L.D., Earles, A.N., et al., 2000. Causes and outcomes of acute chest syndrome in sickle cell disease. National Acute Chest Syndrome Study Group. N. Engl. J. Med. 342, 1855–1865.

Vora, A.J., Makris, M., 2001. An approach to investigation of easy bruising. Arch. Dis. Childhood 84, 488–491.

Vidler, V., 1999. Teaching parents advanced clinical skills. Haemophilia 5, 349–353.

Wagner, J.E., Eapen, M., MacMillan, M.L., et al., 2007. Unrelated donor bone marrow transplantation for the treatment of Fanconi anemia. Br. J. Haematol. 5, 2256–2262.

Weatherall, D.J., Clegg, J.B., 2001. The Thalassaemia Syndromes, fourth ed. Blackwell Sciences, Oxford.

Wong, D., Baker, C., 1998. Pain in children: comparison of assessment scales. Pediatr. Nurs. 1, 9.

Yang, Y., Li, D.Z., 2009. A survey of pregnancies with Hb Bart's disease in Mainland China. Haemoglobin 2, 132–136.

FURTHER READING

Gibson, F., Soanes, L. (Eds.), 2008. Cancer in Children and Young People. Wiley & Sons, London.

Hoffbrand, A.V., Pettit, J.E., Moss, P.A.H. (Eds.), 2001. Essential Haematology, fourth ed. Blackwell Science, London.

Lilleyman, J., Hann, I., Blanchette, V. (Eds.), 2000. Paediatric Haematology. Churchill Livingstone, Edinburgh.

Provan, D., Singer, C., Baglin, T., et al. (Eds.), 2009. Oxford Handbook of Clinical Haematology, third ed. Oxford University Press, Oxford.

Websites

Aplastic anaemia: www.theaat.org.uk
Fanconi anaemia: www.fanconi.org
Haemophilia: www.haemophilia.org.uk
Sickle cell disease: www.sicklecellsociety.org
Thalassaemia: www.ukts.org

16

Caring for a Child With a Neurological Disorder

Joanna Smith, Catherine Martin

LEARNING OUTCOMES

At the end of reading this chapter you will be able to:
- Describe the overall structure and function of the nervous system.
- Understand the general principles of caring for a child and family, where the child has a neurological disorder.

- Appreciate the range of neurological disorders in childhood and the potential impact for the child and family.
- Describe the common neurological disorders of childhood.

INTRODUCTION

Disorders of the nervous system are an important group of childhood conditions; despite a downward trend, neurological conditions remain a leading cause of mortality and morbidity in children (Moreau et al., 2013). Many hospitalised children have a neurological problem either as the sole or associated complaint. Diseases of the neurological system have a profound impact for the child and family and are probably the most disruptive of all ailments. Caring for the child with any disorder of the nervous system and their families is challenging because the outcome is often uncertain, many conditions are rare and the family will have expert knowledge of the child's needs, which can lead to frustration for parents in seeking support, and feelings of inadequacy for health care professionals. Traditional models of care focusing on the disease process (illness and treatment) are inappropriate. Although key principles can be applied, care must be individually designed, have a developmental focus and be influenced by encouraging the child to reach their full potential.

THE ROLE, STRUCTURE AND FUNCTION OF THE NERVOUS SYSTEM

The nervous and endocrine systems are the main regulatory systems of the body. The nervous system is the most rapid means of maintaining homeostasis, which is achieved by reacting and responding to internal and external stimuli. The nervous system is descriptively divided into the central nervous system (CNS) and the peripheral nervous system (PNS) (Sugerman, 2018). The CNS consists of the brain, the control centre for the entire nervous system and the spinal cord. The PNS consists of the nerve networks, which link the CNS with the periphery.

The PNS has two main subdivisions, the somatic nervous system (SNS) and the autonomic nervous system (ANS). Actions carried out by the SNS are both voluntary and involuntary with sensations being perceived consciously, whereas actions carried out by the ANS are involuntary and not usually perceived consciously. The ANS has sympathetic and parasympathetic divisions and is primarily concerned with the innervation and control of visceral organs, smooth muscles and secretory glands. Where there is both sympathetic and parasympathetic nerve innovation their actions have an antagonistic effect; for example, sympathetic activity increases the force of contraction of cardiac muscle and the heart rate, whereas parasympathetic activity reduces the force of contraction and decreases the heart rate.

Development of the Nervous System

Many neurological problems in infancy occur because of a malformation that has occurred during embryological development (Padgett, 2006). The ectoderm, one of the three primary germ layers present in early embryonic development, forms nervous tissue, the ears, eyes and epidermis. The first obvious sign of nervous system development is during the third week of embryonic life when the dorsal midline of the ectoderm thickens to form the neural plate (Padgett, 2006). The lateral margins of the plate become elevated resulting in a midline depression known as the neural groove. Eventually the neural plate folds and fuses together creating the neural tube. The neural tube is completely closed by the end of the fourth week of embryonic development forming the CNS (Longstaff, 2011). By the fifth week of gestation the rostral portion of the neural tube enlarges and differentiates into the forebrain (cerebrum), midbrain and hindbrain (pons, cerebellum and medulla oblongata) (Fig. 16.1).

In addition to structural developments, the neuroepidermal cells, precursors of supporting (glial) cells and

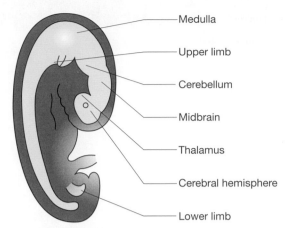

Fig. 16.1 Representation of the brain and spinal cord at 5 weeks' gestation.

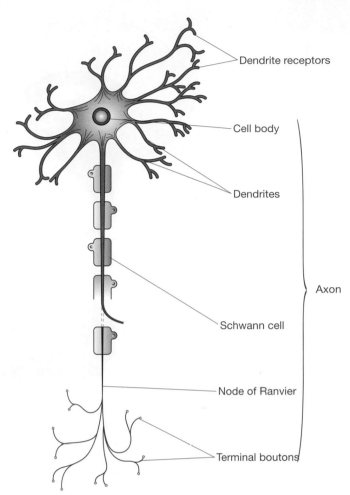

Fig. 16.2 A typical motor neuron.

specialist (nerve) cells, increase in number adding to the expanding cerebral cortex. The cells begin to organise themselves into zones resulting in the typical appearance of the brain: an outer layer of grey matter (cell bodies) and an inner layer of white matter (nerve tracts). During the final stages of specialisation, nerve cells lose the ability to divide, and therefore do not increase in number after birth. Glial cell proliferation and nerve myelination increase the weight and size of the brain, particularly during the first year of life. Nerve myelination occurs from 22 weeks of gestation and is probably not complete until adult life (Padgett, 2006).

Cells of the Nervous System and Their Function

The two cellular components, the neuralgia (glial cells) and the neuron (nerve cells), are unique to the nervous system. Glial cells form the connective tissue of the nervous system; astrocytes provide mechanical support and help maintain the blood–brain barrier; microglia correspond to brain phagocytes; oligodendroglia and Schwann cells form myelin in the CNS and PNS respectively; and ependymal cells form the epithelial linings.

Neurons have a specialised structure that facilitates the transmission of nerve impulses. Based on their function neurons can be sensory, intermediate or motor nerves. Although they have different structure, all nerves have dendrites, a cell body and axon; a typical motor neuron is presented in Fig. 16.2. A stimulus of sufficient strength applied to a dendrite receptor site generates a nerve impulse, which is transmitted along the dendrite to the cell body. The impulse exits via the main axonal process (nerve fibre) ending at the terminal boutons. These contain chemical transmitters capable of stimulating adjacent neurons or affector organs. Generating and conducting a nerve impulse is based on the neuron's ability to maintain a difference in the ion concentration outside and inside the cell membrane. Disruption of the ion concentration causes an ionic current flow, which is conducted along the entire neuron, is independent of any further stimulus and is unidirectional. The speed of the nerve impulse increases if (Longstaff, 2011):

- body temperature increases;
- diameter of the fibre increases;
- myelin is present.

Information passes between neurons at junctions (synapses). When a nerve impulse arrives at the terminal bouton, neurotransmitters such as noradrenaline or acetylcholine are released. These cross the synapse and bind with the receptor site on the adjacent dendrite. Calcium ions are necessary to facilitate this process. Neurotransmitters stimulate or inhibit postsynaptic dendrites, allowing impulses either to proceed or not. Once the neurotransmitter binds with the receptor site it is rapidly deactivated by enzymes in the postsynaptic junction.

Anatomy of the Brain

The brain consists of the cerebrum (two cerebral hemispheres), diencephalon, brainstem and cerebellum (Fig. 16.3). The hemispheres are joined at the base by the corpus callosum, a sheet of nerve fibres, allowing communication between the hemispheres.

The cerebrum is by far the largest part of the brain, and is divided into important functional areas (Fig. 16.4). Specific areas of the cortex perform specific functions (Sugerman, 2018):

- The frontal lobe contains the primary motor cortex responsible for controlling movement, the speech area and higher functions such as personality and behaviour.

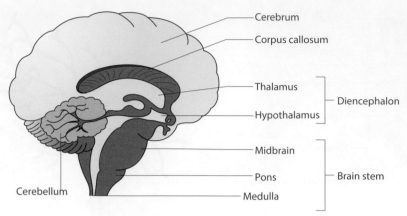

Fig. 16.3 Cross-sectional view of the brain.

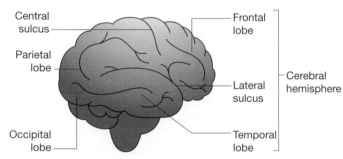

Fig. 16.4 Major subdivisions of the cerebral hemispheres.

- The parietal lobes contain the primary somatosensory cortex where sensations such as touch, pressure, pain and temperature are consciously perceived.
- The occipital lobe contains the visual cortex.
- The temporal lobes contain the auditory cortex, and areas involved in memory and emotions.

Due to the crossover (decussation) of the nerve fibres at the medulla oblongata each hemisphere communicates with the opposite side of the body.

The diencephalon contains several specialist areas, with the two most important being the thalamus and hypothalamus. The thalamus is a relay and integration centre. The hypothalamus coordinates homeostatic mechanisms and has autonomic, neuroendocrine and limbic functions.

The brainstem collectively describes the midbrain, medulla oblongata and the pons. The midbrain contains part of the auditory system. Most nerve fibres from the body transcend the medulla and midbrain, which function as important relay and integration centres. Although anatomically the brain stem is a relatively small component of the brain, its importance cannot be underestimated. It contains many nuclei and tracts that are essential to key vital body functions; for example, the medulla contains nuclei that regulate blood pressure, respiration, maintenance of arousal and initiation of sleep. Like the medulla, the pons contains many functional structures, but primarily acts as a relay centre between the cerebrum and cerebellum.

The cerebellum sits in the base of the cranial cavity in an area known as the posterior fossa. The cerebellum is important in relation to the coordination of motor activity functions such as tone and posture, and operates at an unconscious level. Unlike the cerebral cortex, responses of the cerebellum affect the same side of the body (ipsilateral).

The Ventricular System

The ventricular system is a network of connected chambers or ventricles deep within the brain, which contain cerebrospinal fluid (CSF). There are four chambers: two lateral ventricles situated within the cerebral hemispheres, the third ventricle situated in the diencephalon and the fourth ventricle situated between the brainstem and the cerebellum. The fourth ventricle tapers at its base and becomes the very narrow central canal of the spinal cord.

CSF flows constantly beginning in the lateral ventricles before flowing into the third ventricle, and continuing via the aqueduct of Sylvius to the fourth ventricle. CSF leaves the fourth to circulate around the brain and spinal cord via the subarachnoid space (Fig. 16.5). CSF is reabsorbed into the bloodstream via capillaries on the surface of the cerebral hemispheres.

CSF helps maintain the cerebral chemical environment by supplying nutrients and removing toxic substances, acting as a shock absorber, contributing to maintaining the blood–brain barrier and giving the brain buoyancy. CSF has high sodium, chlorine and bicarbonate levels, low potassium, urea, glucose and amino acid levels, and a negligible protein content (Sugerman, 2018).

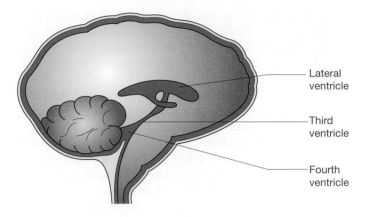

Fig. 16.5 Cerebrospinal fluid flow through the ventricular system.

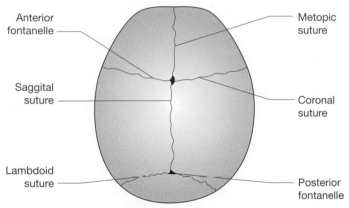

Fig. 16.6 Sutures of the skull.

Blood Supply

The brain requires a continual input of glucose and oxygen, with 20% of the total cardiac output reaching the brain each minute (Sugerman, 2018). The internal vertebral and carotid arteries, and their subsidiaries ensure the brain has a rich blood supply. These vessels form a system of interconnecting arteries in the base of the brain, known as the circle of Willis. The physiological principle behind the circle of Willis is that in the event of damage to one of the arteries supplying the brain there is the potential for compensation from the communicating arteries, thus offering some protection from severe ischaemic damage.

Venous blood primarily returns to the circulation via the superficial veins that drain into the venous sagittal sinus that eventually flows into the internal jugular vein. The deep veins of the cerebral hemispheres drain into the vein of Galen and then into the sagittal sinus.

The composition of the brain's extracellular fluid needs to be regulated because circulatory chemicals can influence the function of neurons. This is achieved by the blood–brain barrier, a complex process that is the consequence of specific characteristics of the cerebral capillaries resulting in a highly selective exchange of substances across their endothelial end plates.

Protection and Coverings

The brain is supported and protected by the skull and the membranous coverings collectively known as the meninges. The bones of the skull are separated at birth, allowing for brain moulding during delivery and rapid growth within the first year of life. Complete ossification occurs at about 8 years of age, and the sutures (Fig. 16.6) cannot be separated even in the presence of raised intracranial pressure after about 12 years of age (Padgett, 2006).

Neuron Regeneration

The traditional approach to neuroanatomy and physiology associates discrete body functions with specific brain structures. However, research has found that latent areas within the brain can in some circumstances undertake the functions of damaged areas (Nudo, 2013). Previously, it was presumed that because neuron cell bodies do not have centrioles and the meiotic spindles that are necessary for cell division, there is little capacity to repair and regain function following damage. However, neurons can survive damage, regenerate new axons and form new synaptic connections (Rose et al., 1997). The process known as reactive synaptogenesis may result in the recovery of function, but can also result in the development of abnormal connections with abnormal recovery.

> ### ACTIVITY
>
> Revisit your knowledge of the nervous system and add more depth by accessing the Evolve website:
> - File Chapter 9 test your knowledge (brain teasers).
> - File Chapter 9 PowerPoint teachings (overview of anatomy and physiology of the brain, embryology and cells of the nervous system).
>   The following textbooks and web sites may be useful:
> - Crossman, A.R., Neary, D., 2015. Neuroanatomy – An Illustrated Colour Text, fifth ed. Churchill Livingstone, Edinburgh.
> - Brain Source; aimed at sharing neuroscience knowledge. Available from: http://www.brainsource.com/
> - Encyclopedia of Life Sciences; comprehensive coverage of a range of topics including neurosciences. Available from: http://www.mrw.interscience.wiley.com/
> - Resting Membrane Potential Explained: Available from: https://www.youtube.com/watch?v=rcacx09VODc

NEUROLOGICAL DISORDERS IN CHILDREN

Neurological disorders in children represent a diverse group of conditions and many children who present with a neurological dysfunction may never have a definitive diagnosis. A lack of diagnosis is particularly difficult and frustrating for the child and family. It is essential for disorders where there is a potential genetic mode of inheritance that the child and family are referred for genetic counselling to assist the parents in decisions relating to planning future children. The outcome of neurological disorders is variable and often unique to the individual child; care must be tailored to meet the specific needs of the child and family. The diversity of neurological conditions is presented in Table 16.1.

> ### 🌐 WWW
>
> Develop your knowledge of these conditions by accessing the following websites:
> - Spina Bifida Hydrocephalus Information Networking Equality. https://www.shinecharity.org.uk
> - Tuberous Sclerosis Association: http://www.tuberous-sclerosis.org
> - Children's Hemiplegia and Stroke Association: https://chasa.org
> - Meningitis Research Foundation: https://www.meningitis.org/
> - SCOPE (focuses on providing supporting for people with disabilities, primarily with cerebral palsy): http://www.scope.org.uk
> - Muscular Dystrophy UK: http://www.musculardystrophyuk.org
> - Child Brain Injury Trust: https://childbraininjurytrust.org.uk
> - Headlines Craniofacial Support: www.headlines.org.uk

Principles of Caring for a Child With a Cerebral Dysfunction

Understanding the principles that underpin the management of the child with both acute and long-term neurological dysfunction is essential if care delivery is to be safe and appropriate. Neurological disorders have a unique effect and care must be based on assessment and meeting individual needs. Therefore the general principles of care need to be adapted to each situation and to the unique needs of the child and family. Seizure management is covered in Chapter 23.

Diagnostic Procedures

Diagnostic procedures are vital in order to assist the clinician to establish, where possible, the correct diagnosis; monitor effects of treatments/interventions; determine the potential prognosis for the child and monitor disease progression.

The child and family require detailed information and preparation prior to investigative procedures. The risks and potential side effects associated with the procedure must be outlined and consent obtained. The type of diagnostic investigations will vary depending on the child's presentation but may include:

- Blood profiling, including urea and electrolytes, metabolic and immunological assays, and genetic screening.
- Lumbar puncture, performed to collect CSF samples in order to detect the presence of bacteria or tumour deposits, and the measurement of CSF pressure. Performing a lumbar puncture in a child with a high intracranial pressure may cause brainstem compression with fatal consequences.
- Neuroimaging: ultrasound, x-rays, computerised axial tomography (CT), magnetic resonance imaging (MRI).
- Specialised physiological imaging techniques such as positron emission tomography (PET) and single-photon

computed emission tomography (SPECT), assist with evaluating cerebral metabolic function and cerebral blood flow.
- Cerebrovascular studies such as angiography, used to identify cerebrovascular abnormalities such as aneurysms and arteriovenous malformations.
- Electroencephalogram (EEG) records the electrical activity of the brain and is primarily used to detect changes in brain activity during seizures. Often used as a continuous monitoring procedure with video recording to correlate a child's presentation with EEG changes (video telemetry).
- Electromyography (EMG) conduction studies are used to measure electrical activity and velocity times in muscle fibres. Particularly useful in assisting in the diagnosis of neuromuscular and peripheral nerve disorders.
- Muscle biopsies measure a range of muscle enzymes. Useful in identifying whether a problem is neurogenic or myogenic in origin, assisting in the diagnosis of neuromuscular conditions.

Some of these procedures, such as PET and SPECT, are only available in specialised centres.

> ### 👤 ACTIVITY
>
> Common imaging techniques are now widely available; therefore all nurses must have appropriate knowledge of these procedures and associated care:
>
> Think about the advantages, disadvantages and care needs of the child who requires an x-ray, CT scan or MRI scan.
>
> What are the risks associated with x-rays, CT scanning or MRI scanning?
>
> What strategies would you use to ensure a 2-year-old child successfully undergoes a CT scan?

Raised Intracranial Pressure

Intracranial pressure (ICP) is the pressure exerted by the cranial contents on the skull. Typical values are 10–15 mmHg in adults, 3–7 mmHg in children and 1.5–6 mmHg in infants (Kukreti et al., 2014). The rigidity of the skull results in the total intracranial volume being fixed. The intracranial contents (brain, CSF and blood) must be maintained in a state of equilibrium. Therefore an increase in volume in one component must be reciprocated by a reduction in volume in another component, known as the Monro–Kellie doctrine (Dunn, 2002), which can be represented by the following equation:

In principle there is little ability of the brain to significantly reduce any of these components and an increase in overall volume results in a rise in ICP (Fig. 16.7). Raised intracranial pressure (RICP) is usually described as an ICP above 20 mmHg sustained for 5 minutes or more (Bratton et al., 2007). Causes include:

$$V \text{ (intracranial vault)} = V \text{ (brain)} + V \text{ (CSF)} + V \text{ (blood)} + V \text{ (other)}$$

Conditions which increase the brain volume:
- space occupying lesions such as tumour, abscess, haematoma;
- cerebral oedema for example following traumatic brain injury or cerebral infection.

TABLE 16.1	**Range of Childhood Neurological Diseases**	
	Features	**Example**
Congenital malformations	Disruption to normal CNS development, usually occurs early in gestational period Often multifactorial genetic transmission	Hydrocephalus Agenesis of the corpus callosum Microcephaly
Neurocutaneous disorders	Errors occurring in early ectodermal cell proliferation results in a group of disorders, which present with combined CNS, ophthalmic and skin abnormalities	Tuberous sclerosis Sturge–Weber syndrome
Vascular disorders	A diverse group of disorders with various aetiologies from structural anomalies to spontaneous intracranial bleeds	Arteriovenous malformations Intracranial arterial aneurysms Moyamoya disease
CNS infections	Common cause of acute neurological disorders Despite improved preventative programmes through vaccination and improved antimicrobial agents CNS infections remain a challenge with significant morbidity	Meningitis Intracranial abscesses Encephalitis (measles, herpes simplex, mumps)
Neoplastic disorders	Most common solid tumours in children Often difficult to treat	Medulloblastoma Astrocytoma Brainstem glioma Craniopharyngioma
Progressive degenerative disorders	Includes the many neurometabolic disorders, which although individually rare, collectively are an important group of disorders Most follow an autosomal recessive inheritance pattern Two major groups are the neuronal storage diseases and the leucodystrophies	Tay–Sachs disease Battens disease Niemann–Pick disease Krabbe disease
Non-progressive brain damage	Persistent disorder as a result of brain insult during early development The underlying problem is static, but subsequent development is affected	Cerebral palsy
Neuromuscular disorders	Normal muscle functioning is dependent upon effective muscle and nerve functioning. Children with this group of disorders present with hypotonia and increasing muscle weakness	Duchenne muscular dystrophy Myasthenia gravis Guillain–Barré
Learning disabilities	A wide range of learning disabilities exist from very specific skill deficiencies to complex disorders affecting the ability to carry out activities of living and achieve independent living Aetiology is often due to hereditary and environmental factors	Fragile-X syndrome Down syndrome Autism Asperger's syndrome

CNS, Central nervous system.

Conditions which increase the blood volume or blood flow:

- obstruction to venous outflow.

Conditions which compromise normal CSF levels:

- blockages within the ventricular system causing hydrocephalus;
- conditions which increase CSF levels are rare, but could include tumours of choroid plexus.

The signs and symptoms of RICP (Eichler and Milonovich, 2013) include:

- alteration in conscious levels; irritability, lethargy, confusion, decreased responsiveness;
- dilated pupils, decreased response to light;
- abnormal motor activity or reflexes;
- increased blood pressure with a compensatory bradycardia sometimes referred to as Cushing's response, bradycardia or apnoea, which are late and ominous signs.

The signs and symptoms of RICP in an infant, prior to fusion of the skull sutures, usually occur late because increased volume forces the membranes between the skull bones to part, accommodating pressure changes. There will be more insidious signs such as irritability, poor feeding, general developmental delay, large and tense anterior fontanelle

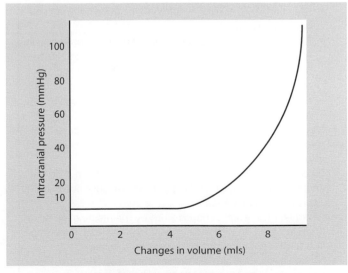

Fig. 16.7 Volume/pressure curve.

even when the infant is in the sitting position, and increased head circumference (Brett and Harding, 1997).

Once the intracranial pressure starts to rise a cycle of events occurs: ICP increases, cerebral blood flow (CBF) decreases, leading to tissue hypoxia resulting in cerebral vasodilation and oedema, causing further increases in ICP. The brain will shift from the area under pressure to an area of less pressure, resulting in compression, traction and shearing of brain structures. Eventually, downward brain shift occurs, resulting in brainstem herniation with vital centres becoming compressed. Management of RICP is based on the need to prevent cerebral ischaemia by maintaining cerebral perfusion pressure (CPP) between 60 and 70 mmHg (Bratton et al., 2007), with care best provided in a children's intensive care unit.

◎ EVIDENCE-BASED PRACTICE

The principles of care for children with RICP, outlined in evidence-based guidelines (Bratton et al., 2007; Adelson et al., 2012), following significant brain injury include:

- Ventilate and maintain oxygenation, aim for a $PaCo_2$ between 30 and 35 mmHg and Pao_2 between 90 and 100 mmHg. Prophylactic hyperventilation is not a recommended treatment for Traumatic Brain Injury but may be of value for brief periods where the $PaCo_2$ is elevated and there is associated acute neurological deterioration, such as acute rises in ICP.
- Minimising the brain's metabolic needs and preventing activities, which normally produce transient rises in ICP, by providing adequate sedation, analgesia and paralysis. No specific evidence is currently available relating to the best sedative, analgesia or neuromuscular blocking agent in the management of head injury. Choice will depend on local guidelines and practices. The use of sedation, analgesia and paralysis will limit the ability to perform full neurological assessments.
- Maintaining an adequate systemic mean arterial pressure to ensure an adequate CPP, above 60 mmHg for children and 50 mmHg for infants. This is achieved by:
  - Appropriate intravenous fluid resuscitation but the administration of fluids must be judicious due to the potential of increasing cerebral oedema if overhydration occurs.
  - Maintaining a normal electrolyte balance with precise fluid management.
  - Maintaining an adequate mean arterial pressure will require the use of inotropic support and the administration of inotropic drugs. Inotropes, such as dopamine or dobutamine (administered by continuous infusion), alter the force or energy of cardiac muscular contractions and are used to treat hypotension.
- Monitor ICP; ICP above 20 mmHg will require active treatment with osmotic diuretics; mannitol is the diuretic of choice.
- Decompression surgery may be indicated if the child has an extremely high ICP and high blood pressure due to generalised cerebral oedema.
- Optimising cerebral venous return by maintaining the head at an angle of 30 degree and position the head in the midline to prevent constriction of the blood vessels.
- Maintain normothermia, prophylactic hypothermia does not have a strong evidence base in relating to improved outcomes.
- Monitor EEG in order to detect seizure activity and ensure prompt treatment of seizures.

CPP, Cerebral perfusion pressure; *EEG,* electroencephalogram; *ICP,* intracranial pressure; *RICP,* raised intracranial pressure.

Neurological Assessment

Accurate neurological assessment and skilled observations are essential if changes in neurological function are to be detected promptly. The purpose of a neurological assessment includes (Hickey, 2014):

- Identifying the child's normal abilities and developmental stage.
- Providing a baseline record of the child's neurological status at the time of admission.
- Identifying the presence and effects of neurological dysfunction.
- Detecting life-threatening situations.
- Identifying changes promptly through serial observations.
- Influencing management decisions by monitoring overall improvements or deteriorations in the child.
- Assisting in the prediction of the eventual outcome of the neurological insult.

▶ REFLECT ON YOUR PRACTICE

Think about the last time you performed neurological observations on a child:

- Why were the observations being undertaken?
- How frequently were the observations being undertaken? Why?
- How and why did you apply a painful stimuli?
- How and why did you act on any changes in the child's condition?

Neurological observations include: assessment of consciousness, pupil reactions, motor functioning and other parameters such as changes to vital signs and seizures. The frequency of undertaking observations will depend on the initial assessment, the stability of the child and the underlying problem. In the acute situation, half hourly to one hourly observations appear to be common practice, as changes in neurological function can occur quickly. Unless a full assessment is carried out, unconsciousness cannot be distinguished from normal sleep.

Assessment of Consciousness

Consciousness is a state of awareness and in general can be thought of as two components – arousal and wakefulness – and is a sensitive indicator of neurological functioning (Hickey, 2014). The first and the most frequently used numerical scale for assessing consciousness, developed in the 1970s in order to reduce subjectivity and ambiguity when assessing a patient's consciousness, is the Glasgow Coma Scale (GCS) (Teasdale and Jennett, 1974). The GCS assesses three parameters, eye opening, verbal response and motor response, with a numerical score given for the best response within each parameter. The GCS has undergone several adaptations for use in children, including the James, Jacobi and Adelaide scales (Kirkham et al., 2008). The scale used should be useful across ages and conditions, clear from ambiguity, and reliable, meaning little variation if different health professionals undertake the assessment. Table 16.2 outlines the components of the GCS scoring system, with the best score being 15.

TABLE 16.2 The Glasgow Coma Scale

Parameter	Score	Components
Eye opening	4	Eyes open spontaneously in response to normal environmental activities
	3	Eyes open in response to direct commands
	2	Eyes open in response to a painful stimulus
	1	Absence of eye opening despite application of a painful stimulus
Verbal response	5	Answers appropriately to questions
	4	Converses but confused
	3	Makes little sense
	2	Incompressible sounds
	1	No verbal response despite the application of a painful stimulus
Motor response	6	Obeys commands
	5	Localisation of a painful stimulus and purposefully moves in an attempt to locate the stimulus and remove it
	4	Withdrawal from the painful stimuli in an attempt to move away from the stimulus, but it is not a purposeful movement
	3	Flexion response to a painful stimulus
	2	Extension to a painful stimulus
	1	Flaccidity, there is no detectable movement or change in tone of the limbs despite repeated and varied stimulation

Teasdale, G., Jennett, B., 1974. Assessment of coma and impaired consciousness – a practical scale. Lancet 2, 81–83.

Spontaneous eye opening in response to normal environmental activities achieves a maximum score of 4, indicating that the arousal mechanisms in the brain stem are functioning. The normal verbal response will depend on the linguistic and cognitive developmental stage of the child, and where possible, should be ascertained from the child or carer prior to undertaking the first assessment. Taking into account the child's developmental stage when assessing verbal response is essential if infants or young children are to achieve the best score possible (Table 16.3). OR When assessing an infant or young child's verbal response their developmental stage must considered to achieve the best score possible. For example, an infant would score a maximum response of 5 if they were alert, babbling or cooing as their normal ability, and an older child would be able to answer age appropriate questions to demonstrate they were orientated. The final component of the GCS assesses the ability of the child to respond to an instruction that requires the child to undertake a motor action. This requires the child to have an appropriate level of understanding in order to interpret and act on the instructions given. In babies or young infants that do not have the cognitive ability to respond to instructions a maximum score of 6 would be recorded if there is normal spontaneous movement.

If a child does not respond to an auditory stimulus or light tactile pressure, and therefore has not achieved the maximum score, the continuation of the assessment requires the application of a painful stimulus. When assessing the motor component of the GCS, it is important to use a central stimulus to ascertain whether the child can locate the site of the stimulus, for example, applying pressure over the supraorbital area (Teasdale and Jennett, 1974). Sternal rub, although a central stimulus, can potentially damage soft tissues (Hickey, 2014). Nail bed pressure may elicit a flexion reflex response and can be misinterpreted as an attempt to localise to pain. Supraorbital pressure is not appropriate to elicit eye opening because it causes grimacing, and simultaneous eye closing. Under 6 months the normal motor response to painful stimulation is flexion (Brett and Kaiser, 1997).

TABLE 16.3 Verbal Component of the Neurological Assessment Adapted for Use in Children (see also Warren 2000)

Score	Verbal Response		
	Infant/Young Child	Older Child/Adult	Grimace – All Ages
5	Alert, babbles, coos/uses words or sentences/usual ability	Orientated	Facial expression and movement usual for the child
4	Less than usual ability or spontaneous irritable cry	Confused	Spontaneous oro-motor activity
3	Cries inappropriately	Inappropriate words	Child grimaces forcefully in response to painful stimulus
2	Occasional whimpers/moans	Inappropriate sounds	Child grimaces slightly in response to painful stimulus
1	No response	No response	No response

Warren, A., 2000. Paediatric coma scoring researched and benchmarked. Paediatr. Nurs. 12 (3), 14–18.

Summation of the three components of the GCS provides a summary of the child's conscious state and can act as a quick reference guide when reviewing the child's condition. The summation ranges in value from 3 to 15, with 15 indicating full consciousness. The score becomes lower as the degree of neurological impairment increases. A score of 8 or less is indicative of significant neurological depression with unfavourable outcomes (Campbell, 2004). Summation of the GCS can conceal the whole picture, and may not be accurate in terms of predicting long-term outcome of the neurological injury, particularly following traumatic brain injury (Reith, 2017). However, in an acute intracranial catastrophe all three components of the GCS are usually depressed.

There are challenges in using the GCS in intensive care settings (Kirkham et al., 2008). Once sedation has been stopped, levels of consciousness should be assessed; the addition of the grimace score to the GCS provides additional information in intensive care settings (Warren, 2000).

Motor Function

Evaluating limb responses can assist in determining the site of brain damage; deficits will correlate to the specific area of the brain injured. Damage to the motor cortex and cerebellum will result in abnormalities in motor function. Assessing *motor function* is not the same as assessing the *motor response* in the GCS. The assessment of motor function aims to provide an overview of the function of each of the four limbs independently, in terms of muscle strength, muscle tone, posture (Peters, 2007). Abnormal posture and movements should be documented, along with the coordination of movements and whether movements are spontaneous or in response to a painful stimulus. The neonate's normal response to stimulation is flexion (Brett and Kaiser, 1997).

Pupil Reactions

Assessment of pupil function provides valuable insights into the physiology of the brainstem. The response of the pupils to light is dependent on intact cranial nerves II and III, which transmit nerve impulses from the retina to the midbrain and from the midbrain to the pupillary muscles, respectively. Assessment of pupils should include size, equality and reactivity to light (Hickey, 2014). The normal response to a direct light stimulus is an immediate brisk constriction of the pupil, and a brisk dilation of the pupil once the light source is removed (Hickey, 2014). Although each eye is examined independently, the response should be observed in both eyes. Light directed into one eye will constrict the pupil in the opposite eye due to the consensual light reflex. The pupil response is graded and recorded descriptively in terms of brisk, sluggish or non-reactive (fixed). The size of the pupil is either recorded as pinpoint, small, moderate or dilated, or on a scale ratio of 1:8. Pupils are usually between 2 and 6 mm in size, but there may be slight discrepancies between the two pupils.

The assessment of the pupil responses is important because:

- Pupil responses can be assessed on patients who are receiving anaesthetic or paralysing agents.

- Extremely small pupils can indicate narcotic overdose or direct lower brain stem compression.
- A large pupil or unequal pupils usually indicate compression of the midbrain and consequently the oculomotor nerve.
- A dilated fixed pupil is an ominous finding and suggestive of a terminal state and should be reported immediately to medical staff.
- An irregular or oval pupil may indicate raised intracranial pressure and be the first sign of oculomotor nerve compression due to transtentorial herniation.
- Drugs that either constrict or dilate the pupils should be accurately recorded.

Vital Signs

Alterations in vital signs can indicate pathophysiological changes within the brain, particularly the brainstem. Cardiovascular observations are particularly important because of the relationship between cerebral haemodynamics and cerebral functioning (Hickey, 2014). Compromise to cerebral blood flow will result in a vasomotor response, with blood being diverted from other body systems to maintain adequate cerebral perfusion; the resultant rise in arterial blood pressure is known as Cushing reflex or response (Hickey, 2014). Tachycardia will initially occur as a result of mild hypoxia, but significant compromises to cerebral blood flow cause further increases in blood pressure, resulting in a compensatory bradycardia. A raise in blood pressure with a compensatory bradycardia suggests an extremely high intracranial pressure and usually denotes an intracranial catastrophe is impending.

Changes in respiratory rate and rhythm can occur with neurological dysfunction. Alterations to normal respirations such as hyperventilation, shallow breathing or irregular breathing should raise concerns. Rapidly expanding lesions such as intracranial haemorrhage, direct medulla damage or brainstem herniation are likely to cause respiratory arrest (Hickey, 2014).

Alterations in body temperature, both hypo- and hyperthermia, can be manifestations of neurological impairments. Hyperthermia is probably more common and can be due to infective and non-infective causes (Hickey, 2014). Central fever due to neurogenic aetiologies are typically associated with brain tumours, trauma and following neurosurgery.

Additional components of the neurological assessment should include observation of the adequacy of the cough and gag reflex, which can become depressed following widespread brain damage. Brain insults resulting in hypoxia have the potential to cause seizures, requiring appropriate monitoring and management and this will compound existing problems.

Care of the Unconscious Child

Unconsciousness is a lack of awareness of one's self, the environment, an impairment of cognitive functioning and an inability to respond to sensory stimuli (Hickey and Elkamand, 2014). Many neurological conditions can result in altered awareness or loss of consciousness, with the depth and duration lasting for seconds, for example, during a short seizure, to months such as following traumatic brain injury.

Children with impaired levels of consciousness and who are unable to maintain their own airway are at risk of hypoxia and hypercarbia, with potential respiratory failure and therefore will require intensive care management (Hazinski et al., 1999). However, many children who have impaired levels of consciousness do not require intensive care facilities, but are dependent on the health care team to meet their needs. The aims of caring for these children include:

- Providing interventions to ensure activities necessary to sustain life are maintained.
- Supporting essential activities of living.
- Preventing complications relating to immobility.
- Maximising the restoration of functions.
- Offering support to the family.

Table 16.4 outlines the needs of the child with impaired conscious levels in relation to maintaining essential activities of daily living and preventing complications.

Nursing Care of the Child Undergoing Neurosurgery

The principles that apply to every child requiring surgery are also important for the child undergoing cranial surgery. The main goals of care are to minimise potential complications of the surgical procedure and the effects of the anaesthetic, by ensuring the child and family are prepared appropriately and safely for surgery, and recovery needs are met. Surgery and anaesthesia disrupt normal functioning and homeostatic mechanisms and are therefore potentially life threatening.

In general there are few specific preoperative requirements prior to cranial surgery. The child will require preoperative blood sampling, including crossmatch, because of the potential for blood loss during surgery. The child and family must be prepared for the immediate postoperative period. This includes the possibility of being nursed in intensive care, the child's appearance including descriptions of the wound/bandages, drains, facial swelling and the range and function of monitoring equipment. It is usual practice to undertake skin preparation and hair removal after induction of the anaesthetic. However, it is essential the child and family are prepared for hair removal.

The postoperative needs of the child following cranial surgery should focus on the prompt detection of complications of both the anaesthesia and the surgical procedure including cerebral haemorrhage, RICP, seizures, cerebrospinal

fluid leakage, pneumocephalus, hydrocephalus, meningitis, metabolic imbalances and a range of neurosurgical deficits (diminished levels of consciousness, communication difficulties, motor and sensory deficits, diminished swallow and gag reflexes, and visual disturbances) (Madden et al., 2014). The immediate postoperative needs of the child following neurosurgery are outlined in Table 16.5.

Pain following neurosurgical procedures occurs as a consequence of muscle and soft tissue damage at the site of the surgical incision. The severity of the pain experienced is linked to the site of surgery; for example, frontal lobe surgery is associated with lower pain intensity compared with occipital and posterior fossa approaches (Thibault et al., 2007). Clinical practice guidelines relating to acute pain in children are available, and applicable for children undergoing neurosurgical procedures, for example the Royal College of Nursing (2009) guidelines on the recognition and assessment of acute pain in children. Children with neurological problems may have communication difficulties, an inability to express pain because of nerve and/or muscle damage, and associated cognitive, behavioural and emotional difficulties (Hunt et al., 2003). Pain assessment may be more challenging and these children are likely to receive less analgesia than their able counterpart; therefore a robust assessment considering the individual response to pain and tailored interventions is essential (Twycross et al., 1999). Despite morphine being used widely in the majority of surgical specialties, its use following major neurosurgery is variable, probably because of concerns of respiratory depression (Roberts, 2005). Side effects such as respiratory depression can be detected early if the child is assessed regularly and oxygen saturation levels are monitored continuously, because respiratory slowing occurs well before respiratory arrest.

Neurological deficits that occur as a result of surgery may require the child's care to shift in focus from managing acute surgical needs to a programme of rehabilitation.

Preparing the child and family for discharge must include: advice relating to the specific neurosurgical procedure; support, education and assessment of competency if the family are to take responsibility for ongoing care and interventions; contact details of services and professionals involved in ongoing care and if appropriate the details of the child's named key health professional.

Neurodisability

Traditional models of care focusing on disease and treatments are not always appropriate for a child with a neurological

TABLE 16.4 Caring for the Unconscious Child

Actual/Potential Problems	Nursing Interventions
Altered neurological functioning due to cerebral dysfunction	Monitor neurological functioning through regular assessment Manage alterations in sleep patterns and periods of irritability through structuring activities appropriately, having planned rest periods, using relaxation techniques such as aromatherapy and massage Drugs such as melatonin may be prescribed for sleep disturbances – review their use regularly Ensure stimulation activities are planned and appropriate for the child's age and condition Assess and manage pain appropriately
Risk of altered respiratory function due to underlying cerebral dysfunction, inability to maintain airway and immobility Potential problem of atelectasis and chest infection	Assess respiratory function and identify risk of airway obstruction, ensure position does not compromise the airway, use airway aids and suctioning as appropriate Appropriate monitoring such as respiratory rate and effort, colour, peripheral perfusion and pulse oximetry Assess gag and swallow reflexes, in conjunction with a speech and language therapist, keep the child 'nil by mouth' until these reflexes have returned Ensure regular chest physiotherapy, ensure position changes and passive movements are incorporated into care activities Monitoring for signs of chest infection by recording temperature and changes in the amount and colour of secretions
Unable to maintain nutrition and hydration Potential problems of malnutrition, anaemia, electrolyte disturbances and gastric ulcers	Assess nutritional status, including monitoring of the child's weight Provide a good nutritional intake by appropriate methods that meet the needs of the child; enteral feeding via a nasogastric/jejunal tube may be necessary. A gastrostomy tube may be more appropriate if long-term enteral feeding is required Ensure nutritional intake reflects increased calorific intake, liaise with the dietician to ensure the correct composition and volume of feed Monitoring intake and output, observing for signs of under/over-nourishment and dehydration If gag and swallow reflex have been assessed to be adequate and there are no other contraindications oral food and fluids should be encouraged. The re-introduction of oral feeding may need to be supplemented by enteral feeding because neurological problems may result in oral-motor difficulties, reduced alertness and increased fatigability contributing to inadequate nutritional intake Consider the child's needs in relation to positioning and supportive seating, taste and textures, likes and dislikes, choice of utensils, and effective age appropriate communication
Unable to maintain self-care needs	Ensure care is appropriate in meeting individual needs and consider usual family practices in relation to maintaining hygiene needs There needs to be particular emphasis on the assessment of the mucous membranes of the eyes and oral cavity for dryness; take appropriate action to keep clean and moist: • corneal dryness will require instillation of artificial tear drops or gels such as hypromellose drops • protecting the eyes by the use of patching if the child is unable to completely close the eyes. Assessing oral hygiene needs and involvement of dental hygienist/dentist as appropriate, ensure frequent teeth brushing; consider the need to use suction techniques to prevent aspiration
Potential Complications of Immobility	
1. Skin breakdown	Assess pressure areas using a recognised child-appropriate assessment tool. Implement preventative measure based on the assessment to ensure the integrity of the skin is maintained
2. Muscular skeletal deformities; muscle wasting, muscle contractures, peripheral nerve impairment and poor muscle tone	Liaise with the therapy team to establish individual positioning regimens. Principles include maintaining the child's head in neutral position, with the spine and hips positioned in alignment with the head, maintaining flexion of the limbs and preventing extension of the ankles Ensure staff and child safety by used appropriate moving and handling equipment and techniques Ensure correct positioning is used at all times and use splints where appropriate
3. Poor circulation and inadequate lung functioning	Undertake passive exercises and regular position changes in order to improve circulation, relieve pressure, facilitate lung expansion, prevent urinary stasis, improve gut mobility and minimise muscle atrophy Anti-coagulant therapy and anti-embolism stockings will be necessary in older children
4. Infections, particularly chest and urine infections	Ensure regular chest physiotherapy, ensure position changes and passive movements are incorporated into care activities Monitor for signs of chest infection by recording temperature and changes in the amount and colour of secretions Minimise the risk of urine infection; where appropriate nurse the infant child in nappies and older child in pads; ensure meticulous skin care. An indwelling catheter is a potential sources of infection; if required maintain local policies in relation to the care of indwelling catheters and apply the principles of universal infection precautions Assess for the risk of infection by observing colour, smell and concentration of urine and measurement of body temperature
5. Constipation	Monitor bowel motions and manage constipation appropriately including high-fibre diet or supplements, adequate hydration and use of suppositories as necessary

TABLE 16.5 Immediate Post-Operative Care Following Cranial Surgery

Actual/Potential Problems	Nursing Interventions
Potential airway obstruction and inadequate oxygenation due to depressed conscious levels and the effects of prolonged anaesthesia	Maintain the child's airway by positioning in the recovery position/use airway aids Assess and monitor respiratory effort and oxygen saturation levels Maintain oxygen therapy; ventilatory support may be necessary Assess the child's neurological status
Potential cardiac and respiratory instability due to neurological depression and effect of prolonged anaesthetic, particularly following surgery to the posterior fossa area, which contains vital control centres	Assess and monitor the child's respiratory effort, oxygen saturation levels and vital signs Ventilatory support and invasive blood pressure monitoring may be necessary Assess and report changes in the child's neurological status
Altered neurological functioning due to potential risk of intracranial pressure (ICP) increases as a result of generalised cerebral oedema and haemorrhage	Regular neurological assessment in order to detect neurological changes, which may indicate a rise in ICP Management of RICP Monitor for signs of haemorrhage including observing wound bandages and drains, if present, for excessive blood loss, changes in conscious levels, raised pulse, falling blood pressure, changes in peripheral perfusion The child may require blood transfusion therapy and/or surgical control of bleeding/removal of haematoma if bleeding is excessive The position of the child's head is important and usually dependent on the procedure and surgeon's preference. In general nursing a child with the head elevated at 30°C and head in the midline is the norm, which facilitates good venous return. However, in some surgical procedures for example certain types of shunts, nursing the child upright may result in the development of a subdural haematoma due to rapid drainage of the cerebrospinal fluid
Potential fluid and electrolyte disturbances due to an inability to take oral fluids	The child's fluid intake and output must be monitored In the early post-operative period the child will have an intravenous infusion Unless there is potential damage to the ninth and tenth cranial nerves, which may affect swallowing, the child may begin oral fluids as soon as consciousness is regained. It may be necessary for the child to undergo assessment by a speech and language therapist prior to commencing oral fluids
Maintaining fluid and electrolytes in children who have undergone cranial surgery is a balance between ensuring adequate circulatory blood volume in order to maintain good cerebral perfusion and preventing over-hydration, which will add to cerebral oedema	The management of fluids will be influenced by the type of surgery and tolerance of oral fluids, with the type and amount of fluids administered specific to each child's needs and urea and electrolyte profile Where prolonged intravenous fluid are required the child will need regular blood sampling (including serum osmolality) and circulatory assessment (pulse, blood pressure, capillary refill, temperature gradient difference between core and periphery)
Potential problem of inappropriate antidiuretic secretion or diabetes insipidus following surgery to the posterior fossa area	Measure and monitor urine output, test and record specific gravity Samples will be required in order to measure urine and blood osmolarity
Potential inability to maintain normal thermoregulation	Monitor the child's temperature regularly
Hyperpyrexia can be a result of hypothalamus dysfunction and/or irritation of cerebral tissues, for example, the direct contact of blood with cerebral tissues	Manage pyrexia appropriately because any increase in core temperature increases cerebral metabolic rate, increases cerebral perfusion and potentially adds to any rises in intracranial pressure
Vomiting, as a direct result of RICP and potential side effects of anaesthetic agents	Administer anti-emetics. If vomiting persists the child will require continuation of intravenous fluids and a detailed nutritional assessment Omeprazole may be prescribed to prevent gastric irritation
Pain as a result of wound incision, positioning in theatre, stretching of the meninges and raised intracranial pressure (RICP)	Assess pain and administer regular analgesia Intravenous opioids may further compromise respiratory effort; oral or rectal codeine may be a suitable alternative Unresolved pain may hinder the ability to undertake an effective neurological assessment
Potential for the development of seizures due to cerebral inflammation/irritation	Observe the child for signs of seizure activity In the unconscious child this may require continuous electroencephalogram (EEG) monitoring Follow seizure management guidelines
Promote wound healing following surgical incision Potential wound infection	Maintain universal infection control measures Wound bandages are usually present for the first 24–48 hours and assist in reducing swelling at the wound site and help secure any drains that may be present Prophylactic antibiotics are rarely recommended Observe wound for redness, hardness and presence of exudate, which may indicate presence of infection and leakage of cerebrospinal fluid (CSF) Monitor the child's temperature Clips are often used to secure the wound and usually removed 7–10 days post-operatively

problem, where there can be uncertainty about the impact of treatments on functional outcomes (Rosenbaum and Gorter, 2012). Furthermore, neurological conditions that result in disabilities significantly impact on the child's developmental trajectory. The focus of care is to maximise the child's function, and facilitate the family, and child where appropriate, to be involved in the child's care and care decisions. The environment, and the role of friends and friendships in providing opportunities for the child to develop peer connections is important in relation to the child's social development (Rosenbaum and Gorter, 2012).

Along with the demands of delivering care interventions, living with a child with a neurodisability can result in financial, social and emotional challenges for the child and family. It is essential that in addition to meeting the child's physical needs, the psychosocial needs of the child and family are addressed to ensure family well-being. Programmes of care must be individually designed and aimed at encouraging the child to reach his or her full potential, working within a developmental context, to ensure the child is integrated into their community. This can only be achieved through integrated services, where different professionals will take the lead in meeting the needs of the child and family, at different points in the illness trajectory (National Confidential Enquiry into Patient Outcome and Death, 2018). Clear leadership through the role of a key worker is essential with effective communication between the multidisciplinary team, who must have common goals and adopt a child- and family-orientated approach to care.

Nurses are key members of the multidisciplinary team and their roles include: assessment of the child, particularly identifying actual or potential problems relating to activities of living; co-ordination of care and maintaining effective links with all team members; providing technical and physical care; integrating therapies initiated by other professionals into the child's daily routines; providing emotional support; and involving the family in care (Long et al., 2002).

SEMINAR DISCUSSION TOPIC

Donna is a third-year nursing student undertaking a specialist placement on a neurosciences ward. She has been learning to care for children with complex needs, particularly enhancing her practical skills in areas such as tracheostomy and gastrostomy care.

Donna has been caring for Amy, 14 months old, who has a progressive degenerative disease. Amy's development has always been delayed and she did not achieve independent sitting. Recently, her condition has deteriorated, with a loss of abilities, daily seizures and increased spasticity.

Donna feels able to care for Amy in relation to ensuring her physical needs are met. However, she is finding it difficult to accept that Amy has an undiagnosed condition, with a short life expectancy. She finds it hard to communicate with Amy's parents.

- What issues do you think are important to discuss in relation to this scenario within Donna's learning set?

Emotional and Psychological Needs of the Child and Family

Living with a child with a long-term condition can result in challenges above usual parenting; parents have to adapt and cope to being responsible for their child's health condition. Furthermore, family life can be disrupted because of the unpredictability of the child's condition, the frequency of acute hospital admissions and the need to accompany the child for therapies and clinic appointments (Smith et al., 2015a). The diagnosis of a neurological disorder can be devastating for the child and family, with ongoing uncertainty associated with the unpredictable nature of their child's condition, and balancing meeting the specific needs of the child and the whole family (Smith et al., 2015b). For children with neurological disorders the impact of the disorder can have far-reaching effects that can potentially impact on the child's physical, cognitive and affective (behaviour, personality) functions. Poor psychological adjustment, such as emotional and behavioural problems, are higher in children with neurological disorders than other long-term conditions (Hysing et al., 2009). Changes in cognitive and affective functions can be particularly difficult for the family, having the potential to alter all dimensions of family life and changing the anticipated expectations parents may have for their child. It is essential that the emotional and psychological needs of the child and family are identified early, to ensure that the child and family are offered appropriate support (Hysing et al., 2009).

The family will have many questions in relation to the child's condition, why and how it has happened, and they may be experiencing feelings of guilt. These feelings may be compounded in situations when there is no definitive diagnosis or the child's condition is life threatening; parents my feel frustrated and isolated. Extensive investigations and unpleasant treatments will add to the general despair. The family may be angry that vague signs and symptoms have gone unnoticed. There will be fears in relation to the prognosis and long-term outcomes. The family may be experiencing difficulty in accepting the changes in their child and grieving for the child they know, love and who has been an integral part of their lives. These emotions will affect the family's ability to comprehend information given to them.

It is essential to establish the usual coping strategies and support systems used by the child and family. Long-term support should be aimed at supporting and developing existing mechanisms. Nursing interventions, which form an integral part of everyday practice in supporting the emotional and psychological needs of the child and family, include:

- Ensuring the family is given enough opportunity to ask questions and that responses are clear, accurate and honest.
- Providing and reinforcing information regularly, keeping the family updated. Essential information should be communicated effectively between the whole multidisciplinary team, to ensure a consistent approach to care.
- Including the child in discussions at a level appropriate to their age and stage of development.
- Providing support by listening to the family's anxieties and concerns.
- Ensuring a non-judgemental approach to care, respecting the cultural, religious and spiritual beliefs of the family.

- Assisting the family to make realistic goals in relation to their child's care.
- Ensuring care is child and family centred, all aspects of care are discussed and care planning is negotiated with family, and child where appropriate.
- Recognising that if a child requires care in different settings, this can result in anxiety for the child and family; ensuring that systems facilitate smooth transfers can alleviate some of this anxiety.
- Interdisciplinary team working is essential to ensure the child and family's needs are met.

Overview and Principles of Managing Selected Neurological Conditions in Childhood

This section will provide an overview of selected neurological conditions. Meningitis is covered in Chapter 40, development conditions including cerebral palsy in Chapter 24 and learning disabilities, including Down syndrome, in Chapter 47.

Brain Tumours

Brain tumours are the most common solid tumour and the second most common cancer in children and young people, with leukaemia being more prevalent (Philips and Philips, 2018). In the UK, approximately 300 young people are diagnosed annually with a brain tumour, with both genders affected equally (Cancer Research UK, 2013). While improved treatment and management of childhood cancers has reduced the overall mortality and morbidity, differences exist across tumour types, with poorer outcomes reported for brain tumours (Johnston et al., 2010); brain tumours account for 40% of deaths due to cancer in children (Philips and Philips, 2018). Tumours in general are divided into malignant or benign, referring to the ability of the tumour to spread and the sensitivity to treatment. With brain tumours, factors that determine outcomes are less clear and influenced by the anatomical position of the tumour and age at presentation. The accessibility of the tumour for surgical treatment influences management options, therefore potential outcomes.

Aetiology

The causes of brain tumours are unclear; contributing factors may include (Johnson et al., 2014):
- Genetic factors and family history of cancers including brain tumours.
- Disorders of the immune systems including allergic conditions; there is a potential link to exposure to infectious agents in certain age groups.
- Congenital anomalies.
- Environmental exposures such as radiation and pesticides, and tentative links to medications, alcohol, smoking and the diet during pregnancy.

Epidemiology of Common Brain Tumours in Children (Johnson et al., 2014)

- Gliomas are the most common type of brain tumour, and develop from glial cells; incidence and outcomes depend on the location and histology of the tumor. Astrocytomas are found throughout the brain, developing from glial astrocytes and have a tendency to form large cysts. Astrocytomas are graded from I to IV, with grade I tumours being benign and slow growing and grade IV highly malignant and commonly referred to as glioblastoma. The majority of astrocytomas in children are graded I or II.
  - Brainstem gliomas have varied histology and a definitive diagnosis is not always achieved for it is not always possible to perform a biopsy because of the position of the tumour within the brainstem. Most brainstem gliomas are high-grade astrocytomas, that are fast growing, diffuse and highly malignant, with extensive branching and a poor response to treatment.
- Medulloblastomas are the most common of a group of embryonic tumours collectively known as primitive neuroectodermal tumours (PNET). PNET develop from neuroepithelial cells and usually occur within the posterior fossa. The tumour cells have no clear line of demarcation from normal tissue and often permeate along the CSF pathways resulting in tumour deposits in the spinal cord.
- Ependymomas originate in the ependymal tissue within the ventricular system and range from benign through to highly malignant tumours. Ependymomas have many similarities with medulloblastomas, including a tendency to metastasise along the CSF pathways.
- Craniopharyngiomas are benign, slow-growing tumours arising from epithelial cells within the pituitary gland. Diagnosis can be time consuming and often delayed because signs and symptoms are vague and insidious. Craniopharyngiomas are difficult to treat due to the anatomical location and the tumour adhering to surrounding tissues, with associated endocrine dysfunctions.

Fig. 16.8 shows the anatomical position of the common brain tumours in children.

Presentation

The signs and symptoms of brain tumours are variable, and depend on the age of the child, type of tumour and position in the brain. Symptoms developing quickly are suggestive of a rapidly growing or aggressive tumour and occur because of raised intracranial pressure, with gradual symptoms more likely to be caused by a low grade or benign tumour. While signs and symptoms are similar to many childhood illnesses, typically children present with headaches particularly on waking, persistent nausea and vomiting, behaviour changes/irritability, abnormal eye movements and changes in vision, motor symptoms, seizures, and increased head circumference in young children (Children's Brain Tumour Research Centre, 2017). In addition, there will be specific symptoms related to compression of structures within the direct vicinity of the tumour. Children with a medulloblastoma, cerebellar astrocytoma or brainstem ependymoma typically present with cerebellar signs such as ataxia, poor coordination and altered gait. Tumours within the posterior fossa can obstruct CSF flow resulting in hydrocephalus, causing a rise in intracranial pressure. Tumours compressing the spinal cord may cause neck stiffness. The symptoms of craniopharyngiomas

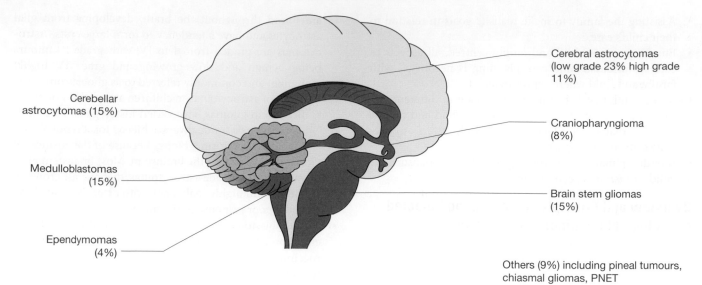

Fig. 16.8 Common brain tumours: position and frequency. *PNET,* Primitive neuroectodermal tumours.

are insidious, and include visual field defects as a result of compression on the optic nerve discs and disruption to pituitary functioning causing growth and endocrine abnormalities such as lethargy, delayed growth and sexual maturation, and diabetes insipidus.

Diagnosis

Diagnosing brain tumors can be difficult because the presenting symptoms can be vague and non-specific or similar to those of more common childhood illnesses. It is essential to take a detailed history of the child's signs and symptoms. Delayed diagnosis has been associated with a range of factors such as attributing headaches to childhood migraine, persistent vomiting to infections and failure to measure head circumference in infants or assessing visual problems in uncooperative children (Children's Brain Tumour Research Centre, 2017). A child suspected of having a brain tumour must be referred to a paediatric neurologist for immediate assessment (National Institute for Clinical Excellence [NICE], 2015). Diagnosis will be made following a detailed neurological examination and confirmed by a MRI or CT scan. Children with medulloblastoma will require imaging of the spinal cord to determine spinal metastasis and a lumbar puncture may be performed to identify the presence of tumour cells within the CSF.

Treatment and Management of Children With Brain Tumours

The outcomes for children with brain tumours have improved with advancements in imaging, radiotherapy, neurosurgical techniques and chemotherapy. Developments in genomic technologies are resulting in the emergence of novel approaches that will influence the future management of brain tumours (Gajjar et al., 2015). While surgery is usually the definitive treatment for brain tumours (Turini and Redaelli, 2001) many children will require multimodal therapy: surgery, radiotherapy, chemotherapy and symptom management. Surgery aims to:

- Remove the tumour and provide a cure wherever possible.
- Remove as much tumour as possible.
- If removal is not possible, obtain a biopsy to make a definitive diagnosis.

The general care of the child requiring neurosurgery has been outlined earlier within this chapter, and applies to children requiring surgery to remove a brain tumour. In addition to complications associated with neurosurgery, posterior fossa syndrome is a potential complication following posterior fossa tumour resection, with the symptoms particularly distressing for the child and family. The syndrome is characterised by mutism that usually presents 48 hours after surgery, but a broad range of symptom can develop including ataxia, facial nerve palsies, dysphagia, loss of tone, motor weakness and apathy/emotional liability (Gadgil et al., 2016).

Radiotherapy targets and disrupts the action of deoxyribonucleic acid, which is essential for cell division. Radiation primarily affects cells during division; therefore rapidly growing tumour cells are especially sensitive to radiation exposure. Radiotherapy contributes to the poor neurocognitive outcome for children with brain tumours; the aim is to deliver therapeutic doses of radiation that cause tumour cell destruction and inhibit cell division, but minimise the effects to surrounding healthy tissue (Ajithkumar et al., 2017). Radiotherapy techniques have evolved with widespread use of image-guided radiotherapy, photon therapy and functional imaging ensuring more precise delivery to the tumour site (Ajithkumar et al., 2017). Radiotherapy is not recommended for children less than 3 years of age because of the high susceptibility of the immature developing brain to radiation damage impacting on growth and cognitive development (Ajithkumar et al., 2017).

Radiotherapy is typically administered five times a week for approximately 6 weeks, 2–3 weeks following surgery or diagnosis (Turini and Redaelli, 2001) and is used for:

- Inoperable tumours;
- Tumours only partially removed at surgery;

- Destroying any remaining tumour seeds post-surgery;
- Reducing the tumour size in order to manage acute symptoms prior to surgery;
- Secondary brain metastasis.

Radiotherapy can be physically and emotionally difficult for children; therefore it is essential to ensure the child and family is fully prepared for the procedure (Grissom et al., 2016). The child will be required to remain in a precise position throughout the treatment to ensure the radiation is delivered to the exact site of the tumor. An individually constructed mould ensures consistent positioning of the treatment area during every radiotherapy session. Children with posterior fossa tumours will be required to lie in a prone position to allow the radiation to be directed to the posterior base of the skull. The psychological needs of the child are important and for young children sedation or general anaesthesia may be necessary. However, daily sedation/anaesthesia have potential risks such as respiratory depression and aspiration, and delayed recovery from the procedure. Play therapists are invaluable in preparing and supporting the child during radiotherapy and may negate the need for sedation (Grissom et al., 2016).

Acute toxicity can occur during or immediately following radiotherapy as a result of inflammation at the tumour site (Cox et al., 2015). Headaches, nausea and vomiting typically occur within the first week after therapy because of a rise in ICP as result of cerebral oedema, requiring the child's neurological status to be monitored. Other side effects include loss of appetite, fluid and electrolyte disturbances, localised skin irritation, and depending on the dose, permanent hair loss at the site of the radiotherapy (Cox et al., 2015). Children receiving radiotherapy are at risk of developing radiotherapy somnolence weeks to months after the completion of treatment. This is usually self-limiting and characterised by general malaise and excessive lethargy, up to 20 hours a day.

Chemotherapy is not a definitive treatment for brain tumours because drugs administered systemically are not effectively transported across the blood–brain barrier due to the tight junction between capillary endothelial cells in the brain (Wu et al., 2014). However, chemotherapy is an important adjunct therapy, for example, in young children as it offers an opportunity to limit tumour expansion until radiotherapy can be delivered, thus increasing the long-term survival rates of these children. The difficulty of chemotherapy for the treatment of brain tumours can be overcome by (Wu et al., 2014):

- multidrug combinations;
- administrating chemotherapy drugs directly into the brain or spinal cord (intrathecal administration);
- disruption of the junctions of the capillary endothelial cells by using drugs such as mannitol to transiently open the junctions.

Children receiving chemotherapy should be cared for in a dedicated children's cancer centre. In these centres inter-disciplinary teams have the expertise in caring for children with cancers treatment protocols are adapted to incorporate the current evidence, and outcomes are monitored (NICE, 2016). Nurses are an essential member of the inter-disciplinary team

and in the case of nurse-led chemotherapy services, nurses implement treatment plans, assessing and adjusting treatments and monitoring side effects (Roe and Lennan, 2014). Good communication between professionals in order to meet the physiological and psychological needs of the child with a brain tumour and their family is essential. Nurses have an essential role in identifying and managing the side effects of chemotherapy. Side effects vary depending on the chemotherapy agent and dose, but include neutropenic sepsis, chemotherapy induced nausea and vomiting and diarrhoea, stomatitis, fatigue, drug hypersensitivity and alopecia (Roe and Lennan, 2014).

Corticosteroids, primarily dexamethasone, usually prescribed as a short course of treatment, may reduce cerebral swelling and provide temporary relief from symptoms at diagnosis and where there is acute radiotherapy-induced inflammatory response (Schiff et al., 2015). Low-dose steroids may help to reduce the symptoms of radiotherapy somnolence. Persistent symptomatic hydrocephalus may require the insertion of a ventricular shunt.

Long-Term Outcomes

Many children and young people who have had a brain tumour will require rehabilitation, and for some for the rest of their lives (NICE, 2016). The health-related quality of life for people who have survived childhood brain tumours tends to be poor, with many survivors unable to live independently. While outcomes are variable, the effect of the tumour and treatments can result in permanent motor and sensory disabilities, cognitive deficits, visual and hearing loss and chronic endocrine problems. Radiotherapy, in particular, has been linked to long-term developmental delay because of subcortical white-matter degeneration and can cause ophthalmic and auditory damage (Ajithkumar et al., 2017). Many children will require special educational assistance because of changes to cognitive functioning. Endocrine dysfunction, particularly growth hormone deficiency and hypothyroidism, requires hormone replacement therapy and occurs as a result of pituitary and hypothalamic damage following irradiation to the posterior fossa area (Cullen et al., 2002). Children and young people with cancer may have future fertility problems (NICE, 2016).

Neurological disabilities, as a result of the effects of the tumour and/or treatments, will require the child to have access to a dedicated neuro-rehabilitation team, enabling children and young people to become independent adults (NICE, 2016). It is vital that the emotional and psychological needs of the child and family are met.

Craniosynostosis

Craniosynostosis is a complex condition of premature fusion (synostosis) of one or more of the cranial sutures (Garrocho-Rangel et al., 2018). Synostosis of a single suture occurs in about one in 2000 births with fusion of the sagittal suture the most common type of craniosynostosis occurring in about 50% of cases (see Fig. 16.6; Greenwood et al., 2014).

In about 10% of children, craniosynostosis occurs as part of a syndrome, Apert and Crouzon being the most well-known, where typically one or more sutures are fused and there are changes to the facial skeleton. In Apert syndrome there is also fusion of the fingers and toes (Greenwood et al., 2014).

Aetiology

Most cases of craniosynostosis are sporadic and the cause unknown. However, craniosynostosis syndromes probably have a genetic mode of inheritance (Greenwood et al., 2014):

- Non-syndromic craniosynostosis may be due to a single gene defect.
- If a parent and child have craniosynostosis, or two siblings have craniosynostosis with unaffected parents, the risk of another child developing craniosynostosis increases.
- There may be an X-linked mode of inheritance, particularly with sagittal, metopic and lambdoid synostosis, which is more common in boys.

While there is possible genetic link, the cause of craniosynostosis is probably multifactorial (Garrocho-Rangel et al., 2018; Greenwood et al., 2014), and has been linked to:

- multiple births/intrauterine compression/birth complications;
- low birth weight babies;
- older maternal and/or paternal age;
- Caucasian ethnic groups;
- drug teratogenicity, particularly anticonvulsants such as sodium valproate and phenytoin;
- environmental factors such as pesticides.

Presentation

In the newborn the cranial sutures are separated by a membranous space, which facilitates rapid cranial growth as part of normal development (see Fig. 16.6). Premature closure of one of the cranial sutures inhibits normal perpendicular brain growth and the skull is forced to grow in a direction parallel to the fused suture (Garrocho-Rangel et al., 2018). The cranial bones remain small and underdeveloped at the site of fusion, while the unaffected bones enlarge to accommodate brain growth, distorting the normal shape of the skull. The characteristic head shape is related to the suture or sutures fused (Fig. 16.9). Craniosynostosis may be apparent at birth, but the deformity is usually diagnosed in early infancy when the abnormal head shape becomes more pronounced (Panchal and Uttchin, 2003). Diagnosis is usually made by visual inspection of the skull, palpitation of the sutures, and cranial anthropometric measurements (Garrocho-Rangel et al., 2018), with a CT scan performed to identify the extent of cranial involvement and the presence of other intracranial abnormities (Buchanan et al., 2017). Children suspected of having craniosynostosis must be referred to a specialist craniofacial centre for assessment and treatment planning (Buchanan et al., 2017).

Premature closure of all the cranial sutures can occur, referred to as craniostenosis or oxycephaly, causing significant neurological problems including impaired cognitive and motor functions, optic nerve atrophy and death because total

Type of synostosis	Characteristic skull shape
Sagittal synostosis: - fusion of the sagittal suture - most common form of craniosynostosis - accounts for 50%–55% of cases	Scaphocephaly 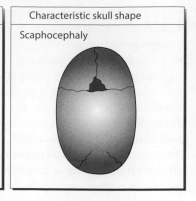
Coronal synostosis: - fusion of one or both of the coronal sutures - accounts for 20%–25% of cases	Brachycephaly 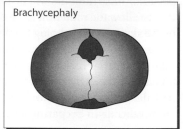
Metopic synostosis: - fusion of the metopic suture - accounts for approximately 10% of cases	Trigoncephaly 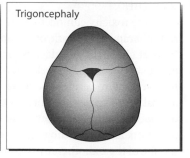
Lambdoid synostosis: - fusion of one or both of the lambdoid suture - rare, accounting for 3%–5% of cases	Plagiocephaly 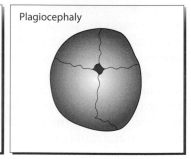

Fig. 16.9 Types of craniosynostosis and characteristic features.

brain growth is restricted and increased intracranial pressure is likely.

Treatment and Management Options

Craniosynostosis is treated surgically; the aim is to prevent progression of the deformity and a rise in intracranial pressure. Surgery is usually performed at about 8–12 months of age depending on the sutures involved (Garrocho-Rangel et al., 2018; Buchanan et al., 2017), as within this time frame the deformity will not have progressed, the bones will be more malleable and following surgery the growing brain will promote a normal head shape, resulting in better cosmetic results. Early treatment potentially minimises later complications such as visual, nasal, phonetic and dental problems, psychological issues and learning disabilities (Greenwood et al., 2014; Panchal and Uttchin, 2003). Prior to surgery, neurodevelopmental assessment is necessary to establish if there are any developmental problems; this can assist in predicting the long-term outcomes and will enable the craniofacial team to offer realistic expectations (Buchanan et al., 2017). The family must be provided with comprehensive information about the condition, prognosis, and treatment options, and psychological support to enable them to make an informed choice about whether to proceed with surgery (Kluba et al., 2016). Surgery can range from excision of the fused suture, for example in sagittal synostosis, to complex craniofacial surgery involving the repositioning and reshaping of the skull and facial bones. Children may be required to wear a molding helmet post-operatively to encourage the head to develop into a normal shape. Correction of craniofacial syndromes requires surgery throughout childhood, with future procedures determined by alterations to cranial-facial structures as the child grows (Panchal and Uttchin, 2003). Surgery and the management of children with craniosynostosis must occur within a designated centre, with care delivered by an experienced inter-disciplinary team (Buchanan et al., 2017).

There may be significant post-operative swelling and the child should be positioned at a 45-degree head tilt to reduce cerebral oedema. Parents should be given realistic expectations of their child's appearance post-surgery and be informed that the child may not be able to open his or her eyes. Blood loss may be significant and the child must be monitored for cardiac instability. The amount of blood loss and circulating fluid volumes need to be regularly assessed through repeated blood sampling to monitor full blood count, urea and electrolytes, clotting factors and serum osmolality. The child must be monitored for signs of haemorrhage including observing bandages and drains for excessive blood loss, changes in conscious levels, raised pulse, falling blood pressure and changes in peripheral perfusion. An elevated temperature could indicate a wound infection; however, hyperpyrexia is common during the first 3–4 days post-operatively, usually as a result of irritation of cerebral tissues by the presence of blood (Panchal and Uttchin, 2003). Parents will require support and advice in positioning and handling their child post-surgery.

Long-Term Outcomes

The extent of the child's long-term care needs and resultant deficits depends on a range of factors including:

- the presence of an associated syndrome;
- the severity of craniosynostosis and sutures involved;
- damage caused by raised intracranial pressure;
- shunt related complications, if hydrocephalus develops (outlined later in this chapter).

Children with sagittal craniosynostosis have the most favourable outcomes with fewer associated problems compared to other single suture craniosynostosis (Greenwood et al., 2014). Children with syndromic craniosynostosis will have a range of associated problems including visual and hearing problems, palate abnormalities, mental health issues and learning difficulties. For many children and their families, body image is a significant

issue and the child and family will require psychological support to assist and support them in managing emotional distress. The follow-up care for children with craniosynostosis will vary depending on the extent of the individual child's needs, but for children with complex needs this is life long.

Epilepsy

An epileptic seizure is abnormal, excessive or synchronous neuronal activity in the brain that interrupts cerebral function. Epilepsy is a disorder where there is a predisposition to generate epileptic seizures. A diagnosis of epilepsy is considered if a child has at least two unprovoked seizures occurring less than 24 hours apart or one unprovoked seizure with at least a 60% probability of further similar seizures occurring over the next 10 years or has an epilepsy syndrome (Fisher et al., 2014). Epilepsy can be thought of as being resolved for individuals who either had an age dependent epilepsy syndrome or who have remained seizure free for 10 or 5 years without medication (Fisher et al., 2014). Epilepsy can be thought of as an umbrella term used to describe a range of conditions characterised by recurrent, unprovoked seizures.

Epilepsy is one of the most common neurological conditions in both adults and children. Approximately 1 person in 2500 is diagnosed with epilepsy each year, with a worldwide prevalence rate of between 4 and 10 per 1000 people (de Boer et al., 2008). Approximately 1 in every 150 children is diagnosed with epilepsy, with the highest incidence rates occurring within the first year of life (Camfield and Camfield, 2015).

Aetiology

Epilepsy in children can be due to genetic conditions such as neurodegenerative disorders and congenital malformations that occur during cerebral development, and irreversible brain damage such as traumatic brain injury, CNS infections, perinatal hypoxia, perinatal intraventricular haemorrhage and brain tumours (de Boer et al., 2008). Many children with epilepsy have associated neurological disorders. However, for about 50% of children with epilepsy there is no known cause (Camfield and Camfield, 2015). A family history of epilepsy increases the risk of a child developing epilepsy, suggesting a genetic link. Epilepsy is more prevalent in families who are socioeconomically disadvantaged (Heaney et al., 2002).

Classification

The current classification of epilepsy is based on the 2017 International League Against Epilepsy (ILAE) system based on seizure type (Fisher et al., 2017):

- Focal onset: where seizure activity is generated within a localised area of the brain and seizure presentation depends on the specific function at the site of the abnormal activity, there may be awareness or impaired awareness at the time of the seizure.
- Generalised onset: where there is widespread nervous disruption across both hemispheres that can result in a range of seizure manifestations.
- Unknown onset.
- Unclassified.

In addition, many epileptic syndromes exist, which have characteristic seizure patterns, signs and symptoms; examples include infantile spasms (West syndrome), Lennox–Gaustaut syndrome and juvenile myoclonic epilepsy. Rare types of epilepsy include sleep seizures and photosensitive epilepsies. Prolonged seizures can result in status epilepticus, which is a medical emergency.

Presentation and Diagnosis

A diagnosis of epilepsy is usually only made after two or more seizures (Fisher et al., 2014). Accurate diagnosis is dependent on a good history and detailed description of the seizure activity. In order to classify the type of epilepsy it is essential to consider the age of onset of the first seizure, the types of seizure activity, presence of underlying neurological problems, family history and EEG findings. In children, video or ambulatory EEG recording is appropriate where diagnosis is difficult after clinical assessment and standard EEG is inconclusive (NICE, 2018). Neuroimaging is appropriate in infants to identify structural abnormalities. Neuropsychological assessment should be considered in children in order to identify learning disabilities and cognitive dysfunction.

Epilepsy can result in a range of seizure presentations (Fisher et al., 2017); the common descriptors include:

- Absence: sudden and usually brief loss of awareness of the surroundings and the child may appear to be staring or have rapid eye blinking.
- Atonic: sudden and brief loss of muscle tone resulting in the child falling to the ground, often referred to as a drop attack.
- Aura: abnormal sensations as a result of stimulation of a specific area within the brain, such as visual hallucinations or illusions, auditory, taste or smell hallucinations; may precede other seizure types.
- Automatism: involuntary repetitive motor activity such as lip smacking.
- Clonic: limb jerking caused by the muscles contracting and relaxing in quick succession.
- Myoclonic: a sudden contraction of the muscles that can affect the trunk or be restricted to one or both arms or legs.
- Tonic: increased muscle tone resulting in stiffness.
- Tonic-clonic: increased muscle tone that results in rigidity followed by the clonic phase where there are rhythmical jerking movements. Jerking movements can last for a variable period of time and there may be reflux emptying of the bladder and bowels. The tonic-clonic phase may be preceded by an aura; there may be confusion and lethargy once the seizure activity has ceased.
- Versive movements: tonic or clonic head and eye deviations, which are involuntary and result in sustained unnatural positioning of the head and eyes.

Treatment and Management Options

Treatment plans should be individualised and based on the seizure type/epilepsy syndrome, co-medication and co-morbidity, and developed in conjunction with the young person and child, as appropriate, and their family. The first-line treatment for epilepsy is antiepileptic drugs, with a single antiepileptic drugs (monotherapy) used wherever possible NICE, (2018); the aim is to use a single drug in the lowest possible dose to control seizures, while minimising side effects. A wide range of antiepileptic drugs are available and choice will depend on the type of seizures and underlying diagnosis, with monotherapy being successful in the majority of children (Marson et al., 2007a,b). First-line treatment recommended by NICE (2018) includes: carbamazepine or lamotrigine for focal onset seizures; sodium valproate for generalised onset seizure. However, sodium valproate must not be used in pregnancy because of the risk of malformations and developmental abnormalities in the baby. Combination/adjunctive therapy should only be considered when monotherapy is unsuccessful. Children with complex or refractory epilepsy must be managed in specialist tertiary services. Caution is needed when changing medications or drug manufacturers because some antiepileptic drug preparations can vary in pharmacokinetics properties.

Antiepileptic drugs can, for the majority of children with epilepsy, result in the child being seizure free (Sillanpää and Schmidt, 2009). However, adherence to treatment is essential (NICE, 2018) and can be optimised by:

- Educating children, young people and their families about their condition and the importance of taking medication as prescribed.
- Sharing care decisions and simplifying medication regimens.
- Reducing the stigma associated with epilepsy.
- Facilitating positive relationships with the child or young person with epilepsy and their family.

Parents, and children, as appropriate, need to understand the action of the drugs, side effects, drug toxicity monitoring and possible drug interactions (including over-the-counter drugs). Epilepsy specialist nurses should be an integral part of the care team and in addition to supporting the child and family, have a vital role in educating others about epilepsy, including schools and the wider communities.

👤 ACTIVITY

Martin, a young person of 16 years, has been diagnosed as having juvenile myoclonic epilepsy within the last 12 months. He has frequent absence seizures where he loses consciousness for between 5 and 30 seconds from which he recovers spontaneously, and is able to continue previous activities. He also has occasional generalised (tonic-clonic) seizures, lasting between 2 and 5 minutes.

How would you assist Martin if you witnessed him having a generalised seizure at school?

- You may wish to check your answer on the Epilepsy Action website: Available from: http://www.epilepsy.org.uk, and search for first aid for seizures.

Two-thirds of people with epilepsy seizures respond well to antiepileptic drugs, leaving one-third of people with uncontrolled seizures (Laxer et al., 2014). Because of uncontrolled seizures, refractory or intractable epilepsy is more likely to occur if there is a high seizure frequency in the early stages following diagnosis, additional neurological disorders or structural brain abnormalities and is difficult to manage even with multiple drug therapy (Laxer et al., 2014). Additional treatment options, which may offer opportunity to reduce seizure activities in children with refractory epilepsy (NICE, 2018) include:

- Psychological interventions such as relaxation and cognitive behaviour therapy: psychological interventions may be used as adjunctive therapy, especially when children and young people have drug-resistant focal epilepsy.
- Ketogenic diet: a diet high in fat but low in carbohydrate. Using fat as the main energy source rather than glucose results in the production of ketones, which are thought to have antiepileptic properties.
- Surgery: corpus callosotomy is a palliative procedure, where the corpus callosum is divided, which aims to prevent seizure activity affecting both hemispheres; cerebral resections (focal or unilateral hemispherectomy) aim to remove the site of the seizure activity in uncontrolled localised epilepsy. Surgery requires accurate diagnosis and a focal site for seizure activity.
- Vagal nerve stimulation: a stimulator is surgically placed under the skin in the left upper chest. It is connected to the vagal nerve by electrodes, which are then programmed to stimulate the nerve. The exact reasons for a reduction in seizure activity remain unclear.

There is no reliable evidence to support these treatments, but they appear successful for some children (NICE, 2018).

◎ EVIDENCE-BASED PRACTICE

The Cochrane Library has a range of systematic reviews relating to treatment options for epilepsy. The Cochrane Library can be accessed at the following:

- http://www.cochrane.co.uk

  The National Institute for Clinical Excellence has a range of evidence-based guidelines relating to epilepsy in children and adults, search for epilepsy:

- http://www.nice.org.uk

Care of the child with epilepsy involves supporting the child and family during diagnosis and in the management and understanding treatment modalities. Children and young people with epilepsy should be empowered to manage their condition. Health professionals have a key role in promoting the self-management of epilepsy, which may be best achieved through active child specific interventions, for example by joining support groups and participating in workshops (NICE, 2018). Parents, children as appropriate, and young people should be provided with information on sudden unexpected death associated with seizures and the importance of preventing seizures. Information must be tailored to the child's relative risk of sudden unexpected death associated with seizures (NICE, 2018). The child and young person with epilepsy, and their family should know how to contact a named individual when information is needed.

Increased metabolism during frequent seizures and disruption to normal eating patterns may place the child at risk of undernourishment. Children with epilepsy are at risk of injury; parents, carers and teachers need the skills required to maintain the child's safety during a seizure and ensure a safe environment without placing undue restrictions on the child. Health care advice will need to be tailored to the individual child.

The normal challenges of adolescence will be increased for the young person with epilepsy. The young person will need support and advice about lifestyle choices such as independent living, career opportunities, learning to drive, insurance issues, the need to continue medication, contraception and planning a family (NICE, 2018). Children, young people and adults with epilepsy should be given appropriate information before they make important decisions, for example, seeking employment and planning to start a family.

⊕ WWW

A wealth of lifestyle and practical advice relating to epilepsy is readily available on the following web site:

- Epilepsy Action: http://www.epilepsy.org.uk

  The International League Against Epilepsy's mission is to ensure that health professionals, patients, care providers, governments, and the public have the educational and research resources that are essential in understanding, diagnosing and treating people with epilepsy. Information about the association can be found by accessing the link below.

- International League Against Epilepsy: https://www.ilae.org

---

Long-Term Outcomes

The long-term outcome for children with epilepsy is variable; some types of epilepsy progress with increased seizure frequency over time, while others remain static or improve with age (Laxer et al., 2014). Outcome is dependent on the cause of the epilepsy and in general worse when there is high seizure frequency (Laxer et al., 2014). The risk of premature death is higher for people with epilepsy compared to the general population, with the most common reason being sudden unexpected death associated with seizures (Laxer et al., 2014). The effectiveness of antiepileptic drugs achieves protracted remission in 70% of people with epilepsy; the remaining 30% will have an intractable and disabling condition (Hanna et al., 2002; Sillanpää and Schmidt, 2009). For children with refractory epilepsy the family may require additional support in relation to supporting their child with daily living activities and to promote social, motor and cognitive function of the child in order to maximise their potential.

Hydrocephalus

Hydrocephalus comprises of a highly diverse group of disorders that have little in common except an increased volume of CSF within the intracranial fluid spaces. Hydrocephalus is one of the most common brain disorders in children; the overall incidence is 79–123 per 100,000 births, with the lower incidence reflecting high-income countries (Dewan et al., 2018).

Aetiology

The majority of children with hydrocephalus have an identifiable cause, typically a result of congenital malformations, for example, aqueduct stenosis, Arnold–Chiari malformations and Dandy-Walker syndrome (Tully and Dobyns, 2014). Other causes of hydrocephalus include:

- Tumours that obstruct the flow of CSF.
- Infections such as meningitis can cause adhesion between the epithelial linings of the CSF spaces, obstructing CSF flow.
- Intraventricular haemorrhage in premature infants causing an initial blockage within the ventricles and secondary obstruction due to scarring.
- Associated with neural tube defects.
- Rare causes include arteriovenous malformations, obstruction of venous sinuses (intracranial hypertension), craniosynostosis or hypersecretion of CSF.

Presentation

The presentation of hydrocephalus depends on the age of onset, cause and whether there is rapid rise in ICP (Lotfinia, 2017). In newborn babies and infants the skull is expandable and the skull sutures have not yet fused; therefore increases in CSF levels will not cause a rapid rise in ICP compared to older children and adolescents, when the skull sutures are rigid. Hydrocephalus in an infant will result in a rapidly increasing head circumference, tense anterior fontanelle, widening of the skull sutures, scalp vein distension, loss of upward gaze and neck rigidity (Lotfinia, 2017). The infant often has a characteristic appearance with a small face in comparison to head size and the eyes have a typical sun-setting appearance (the sclera is not visible below the iris). Nystagmus, poor feeding, vomiting and irritability are important additional symptoms. Older children may present with more classic signs of an increase in ICP, outlined earlier in this chapter. The causes of hydrocephalus are different across the age span, which influences management options and functional outcomes (Lotfinia, 2017; Mazzola et al., 2014).

Diagnosis

Congenital hydrocephalus can be diagnosed by ultrasound scan, where ventricular enlargement can be detected and measured, as early as the 13th week of gestation. However, accurate diagnosis will require amniocentesis in order to obtain samples for alpha-fetoprotein levels and to identify chromosomal abnormalities. Post-natal diagnosis is usually made following neurological examination, and an increase in head circumference in infants, with CT and/or MRI scans confirming the diagnosis.

Treatment and Management

The management of hydrocephalus will depend on the cause, associated brain abnormalities and whether ICP is rising rapidly. If severe brain damage is suspected and hydrocephalus is diagnosed early in pregnancy, termination may be offered. Although very rarely hydrocephalus can subside of its own accord, the risk of delaying treatment must be balanced with

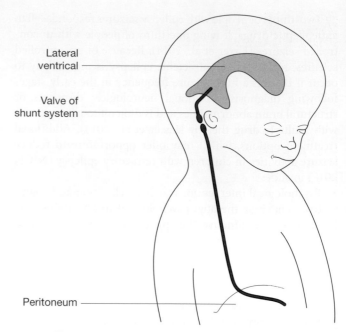

Fig. 16.10 Position of a ventriculoperitoneal shunt.

the potential of compromising normal brain development. Conservative management is rarely a long-term option and is generally reserved for the premature infant post-intraventricular haemorrhage (Chumas et al., 2001). Conservative management includes use of diuretics (acetazolamide and furosemide), intraventricular thrombolytic agents (tissue plasminogen activator, urokinase, or streptokinase) or serial lumbar punctures to remove small volumes of CSF; however, these measures are associated with increased neurological morbidity (Lotfinia, 2017; Mazzola et al., 2014). Ventricular shunts, the main treatment for hydrocephalus, are difficult to insert in acutely ill premature infants and often become dysfunctional (possibly due to high CSF protein levels) and infections are common.

The two main surgical procedures used to treat hydrocephalus are endoscopic third ventriculostomy, where an opening is made through the third ventricle and chiasmatic cistern, facilitating cerebrospinal fluid drainage, and the insertion of a ventricular shunt. Endoscopic third ventriculostomy has an advantage in that unlike ventricular shunts there is no need for a permanent device (Lotfinia, 2017). Success rates following third ventriculostomy are variable because there may be associated problems contributing to the hydrocephalus, such as poor CSF absorption, and is only suitable where there is certainty the CFS obstruction is in the third or fourth ventricles (Chumas et al., 2001; Lotfinia 2017).

The vast majority of children with hydrocephalus are managed by the surgical insertion of a shunt that diverts excess CSF from the ventricles into another body cavity. A catheter is inserted into the ventricles (the proximal catheter) through a burr hole made in the temporal bone of the skull, just behind the ear. This catheter is attached to a unidirectional valve system situated over the skull. The valve is attached to a second catheter (the distal catheter), which is placed into a body cavity such as the peritoneum (ventriculoperitoneal shunts) or the left atrium (ventriculoatrial shunts). Ventriculoperitoneal shunts (Fig. 16.10) are usually the first choice because they are

TABLE 16.6 Main Complications of Ventricular Shunts

Complication	Examples
Infection causes colonisation of the shunt system by bacteria causing blockage	Meningitis Wound infection Peritonitis (ventriculoperitoneal shunts) Septicaemia (ventriculoatrial shunts)
Mechanical failure can result in malfunction or blockage of system	Proximal obstruction: the catheter becomes lodged in tissue such as choroid plexus, brain tissue Distal obstruction: the development of intra-abdominal cysts, cerebrospinal fluid (CSF) ascites Catheter misplacement: intracranial, intra-abdominal, intravascular Fractures and disconnections of the catheter Migration of catheter into hollow viscera such as bladder or inguinal canal
Functional failure	Over-drainage Under-drainage
Miscellaneous problems affecting shunt function	Intracranial hypotension Post-shunt pericerebral collections Slit ventricle syndrome

easier to insert, catheters can be of sufficient length to allow for growth, good absorption of CSF occurs across the peritoneum and there is not the added potential of septicaemia, bacterial endocarditis and shunt nephritis, associated with ventriculoatrial shunts (Lotfinia, 2017).

All shunts operate on the same principle; the valve has a threshold pressure, below which the valve remains closed and above which the valve opens allowing CSF to flow through the shunt system. Different valve systems have different resistant pressures: low pressure (5 cmH$_2$O), medium pressure (10 cmH$_2$O) and high pressure (15 cmH$_2$O) (Lotfinia, 2017). One of the major functional problems with shunt valves is CSF flow increases when the child is upright due to the effects of gravity resulting in over drainage of the ventricles. This occurs because when in an upright position a larger pressure differential exists between the head and abdomen, resulting in CSF flowing at a higher rate than when a child is lying flat.

A trouble-free shunt is a desirable but elusive goal and there are numerous potential complications with intraventricular shunts (Chumas et al., 2001). Shunt failure is a major issue, with reported failure rates of 50% during the 2 years following insertion (Lotfinia, 2017). Complications can be broadly divided into three groups: infection, mechanical failure and functional problems (Table 16.6). Shunt failure must be recognised and treated promptly because increased pressure in the brain can result in loss of consciousness, brain damage and death (Iskandar et al., 1998). Recognising shunt malfunction is problematic because symptoms are highly variable and often unique to each child (Barnes et al., 2002). Although the combination of vomiting, drowsiness and headache are highly predictive of shunt malfunction, these are the same presenting symptoms of many childhood illnesses, particularly viral infections.

The immediate care of the infant or child and family following diagnosis of hydrocephalus must include providing clear and timely information, and offer support to parents who will experience a range of emotions at the time of diagnosis (Smith et al., 2015b). Parents will require support while their child is waiting for surgery (Spina Bifida and Hydrocephalus Information Networking and Equality charity offer valuable resources and support), and advice particularly for the infant on ways to comfort an irritable child, assisting with feeding and positioning techniques.

The principles of care for the child requiring surgery for hydrocephalus, whether endoscopic third ventriculostomy or insertion/revision of a shunt, are the same as any neurosurgical procedure and have been described earlier in the chapter. A sudden rise in intracranial pressure due to rapidly increasing CSF levels within the ventricles has the risk of cerebral herniation and life-threatening consequences; these children must be monitored and managed appropriately. In addition, care will be primarily aimed at preparing the child for investigations (CT scan) and theatre in an organised and structured manner. The child who has been vomiting as a result of RICP will require intravenous fluids to correct dehydration.

The immediate potential post-operative complications following insertion of a shunt include intraventricular haemorrhage, blockage of the shunt and subdural haemorrhage, due to rapid overdrainage of the ventricles. Positioning of the child is an important consideration and will be influenced by the type of shunt inserted; nurses must ensure they have clear post-operative instructions.

There is no specific care relating to the shunt once inserted; avoiding lying on the shunt site may prevent skin breakdown, particularly in the immediate post-operative period. The child and family will require detailed advice and support in relation to detecting signs and symptoms of shunt failure, and who to contact if they are concerned about the shunt. Parents living with a child with a shunt usually become attuned to changes in their child and should be involved in care decisions (Smith et al., 2015c).

WWW

The Spina Bifida and Hydrocephalus Information Networking and Equality charity provides support for families across the UK. A wealth of lifestyle and practical advice relating to hydrocephalus is available on their website:

- Spina Bifida and Hydrocephalus Information Networking and Equality (SHINE): Available from: https://www.shinecharity.org.uk

  The Journal of Neurosurgery (2014), special edition on hydrocephalus has a wealth of information on the treatment of hydrocephalus and management of shunts; all articles are open access and can be accessed at the following link:

- https://thejns.org/pediatrics/view/journals/j-neurosurg-pediatr/14/Supplement_1/j-neurosurg-pediatr.14.issue-Supplement_1.xml

Long-Term Outcomes

The child's long-term care needs depend on the reasons for the hydrocephalus, duration of symptoms before treatment and treatment complications, and the presence of associated conditions (Lotfinia, 2017). Epilepsy is an important predictor of poor intellectual outcome in children with hydrocephalus (Bourgeois et al., 2018). The majority of children with hydrocephalus will attend mainstream school; however, 40%–60% of children will have neurological deficits such as physical, cognitive and behavioural difficulties. These children will require appropriate multidisciplinary team input to ensure they reach their full potential. The quality of life for children with hydrocephalus is lower when compared to children with other long-term conditions (Kulkarni, 2010). Physical disabilities for children with hydrocephalus and spina bifida have lower quality of life scores in domains related to self-care, continence and mobility, and children with hydrocephalus alone have lower scores in relation to school performance and communication difficulties (Kulkarni et al., 2010).

Living with a child with hydrocephalus impacts on the family's quality of life because meeting the ongoing care needs for their child increases the pressure on family relationships (Smith et al., 2015a,b). The uncertainty and potential life-threatening nature associated with shunt malfunction is an ongoing and often overwhelming concern for families (Smith et al., 2015b).

Traumatic Brain Injury

Acquired brain injury can result from both traumatic and non-traumatic insults to the brain. Trauma due to an external force, which may produce a diminished or altered state of consciousness is the main cause. Traumatic brain injury is the leading cause of mortality and morbidity in children: the annual incidence of brain injuries worldwide is 691 in 100,000 children accounting for 4 in 100,000 hospital admissions, and 9 in 100,000 deaths (Thurman, 2016). Boys under 10 years have a 1.4-times greater risk of injury than girls, which rises to 2.2 times in boys over 10 years (Thurman, 2016). The survival rate following traumatic brain injury has increased due to medical and technological advances.

Aetiology

The increase in the number of children sustaining a head injury over the last 30 years is primarily due to increased road traffic use; however, falls are the main cause in developing countries (Dewan et al., 2016). Causes of traumatic brain injury in children and associated factors (Dewan et al., 2016; Nguyen et al., 2016; Parslow et al., 2005; Thurman, 2016) include:

- Road traffic accidents: accounting for 40%–60% of head injuries, with the majority resulting from a child pedestrian hit by a moving car. Road traffic accidents are the leading cause of injury in young people over 15 years of age.
- Falls: the leading cause of injury in children aged less than 5 years of age and account for 20%–30% of head injuries; severe head trauma is rare in home accidents.

- Non-accidental injury: the most common cause of severe head injury in children under 1 year.
- A higher incidence in boys because they develop distance and spatial interpretation later than girls and are more likely to participate in risk-taking behaviours.
- Seasonal variations, with the peak incidence occurring during spring and summer and between 2 pm and 10 pm.
- Other variables that influence a child's vulnerability to traumatic brain injury include the presence of visual or hearing impairments, learning deficits, low socioeconomic status, urban residence and previous head injury.

Classification

Traumatic brain injury is usually defined as an insult to the brain, not of a degenerative or congenital nature, caused by an external force that results in a diminished or altered state of consciousness (Brain Injury Association of America, 2005). Most traumatic brain injuries are mild with a GCS of 13 or above on initial assessment, with only about 10% of injuries requiring medical intervention (Dewan et al., 2016; Nguyen et al., 2016).

Presentation

Minor traumatic brain injury results in transient symptoms such as concussion, no abnormal neurological signs, GCS above 13, dizziness, confusion, headaches and vomiting (Satz et al., 2001). Major traumatic brain injury results in unconsciousness, potentially compromising vital functions and an inability to maintain the airway, which threatens life.

Major traumatic brain injury can be described as having two phases:

Primary injury occurring at the time of injury and can result in:

- Closed head injury due to rapid acceleration or deceleration forces.
- Diffuse axonal brain injury as a result of stretching, twisting and tearing of nerve fibres.
- Shearing and compression of tissues on the bony ridges inside the skull can result in damage to arteries and veins causing haemorrhage.
- Rotational forces add to the shearing effect, particularly where structures are mobile such as the brainstem and corpus callosum – common in shaken babies.
- Open or penetrating injuries involve the brain becoming exposed and damaged.
- Skull fractures can be linear, comminuted and depressed. Basal skull fractures are particularly important due to the danger of secondary CSF infection.
- Localised contusions often occur on the crest of the gyri of the cerebral cortex, and although they may produce dramatic focal neurological signs, tend to have a good overall progress, scarring may result in post-traumatic seizures.

Secondary injury occurs after the initial impact as a result of:

- Cerebral hypoxia and ischaemic damage.

- Ongoing haemorrhage.
- Oedema, which usually peaks 24–48 hours after the injury.
- Seizures and the development of CNS infection further may compound secondary injury.

Treatment and Management

Minor head injury is common in children and admission to hospital is not always necessary, but is often a precaution if there has been a seizure, a skull fracture, an unstable GCS or the cause is suggestive of serious injuries, and to manage persistent symptoms such as vomiting (NICE, 2017). Care focuses on the detection of neurological changes by undertaking a thorough assessment and ongoing neurological observations. The child and family will require appropriate support and detailed discharge advice.

👤 ACTIVITY

Danny is 2 years old and has fallen in the playground at nursery. He vomited twice and is irritable. He is currently in the emergency department with his mother. His Glasgow Coma Score is 15 and after a thorough examination he is able to go home. His mother is happy with the decision, but is anxious about the possible consequences of Danny's fall.

What advice would you give her in relation to observing Danny over the following 48 hours and long-term complications?

Identify the potential long-term complications.
- You may wish to check your answer by referring to NICE, (2017) guidelines: head injury: assessment and early management of head injury in infants, children and adults. Available on the NICE website: http://www.nice.org.uk.

The NICE, (2017) guidelines relating to the assessment and early management of head injury in infants, children and adults outlines the initial priorities of care as: assessment and stabilisation of the airway, breathing and circulation, assessment of neurological status and ascertaining the degree of injury to initiate appropriate levels of care. All children with a GCS less than 8 after stabilisation will require transfer to a tertiary paediatric intensive care facility. Once the child has been stabilised, the child and family must be supported through the phases of recovery or adapt to permanent changes in their child (Singer, 1996):
- Traumatic brain injury is a sudden unwanted event and potentially life-threatening with immediate disruption to family life and an unpredictable outcome. The aim of initial care is to stabilise the child, prevent secondary ischaemic damage, begin the rehabilitation process, support the child and family, and manage increases in ICP, outlined earlier in this chapter.
- Intensive management and dependence on life-support systems is variable, with fluctuating responses and ongoing uncertainty. The agitated child is often difficult to manage and may be distressing for parents. Parents may feel hopeless.

- As the child's level of awareness returns and motor and cognitive recovery begins, the full extent of injuries becomes more apparent and the enormity of the changes, particularly emotional and behaviour changes, can be overwhelming for the child and family.
- Discharge from hospital and transition to community care needs to be well planned if the child and family are to adjust to the effects of the injury. Issues relating to the child's future education require detailed assessment and advanced planning. After major traumatic brain injury, children require detailed continual assessment to monitor development because later milestones may not be achieved or the child may grow into deficits.

🌐 WWW

Practical advice relating to head injury is available on the Headway National Head Injuries Association website:
- http://www.headway.org.uk

◎ EVIDENCE-BASED PRACTICE

The NICE, (2017) guidelines relating the assessment and early management of head injury in infants, children and adults are found on the NICE website:
- http://www.nice.org.uk

Long-Term Outcomes

The outcome following minor head injury is favourable and in general there are no long-term effects in relation to cognitive and psychosocial functioning (Satz et al., 1997). Deficits associated with mild to moderate head injury include social disinhibition, intellectual impairment, psychiatric disorders, perceptual distortion, learning problems, sensory impairment, neuromotor deficits and severe economic implications. However, long-term psychological and mental health problems are more likely if the injury was severe enough to require hospital admission, when there are multiple previous head injuries or pre-existing mental health problems (Emery et al., 2016).

It is estimated that about 20% of children and young people who have sustained a major traumatic brain injury have long-term disabilities (Thurman, 2016) and includes difficulties in relation to performing daily living skills, poor communication skills and general adaptation (Keenan et al., 2018; Polinder et al., 2015). Cognitive, behavioural and psychological recovery (and future development) may not necessarily correlate with physical improvements. Overall, the health-related quality of life in relation to mental and general health is poor for children who have suffered a severe TBI (Polinder et al., 2015). Factors affecting the outcome of major traumatic brain injury include: age (with the poorest outcome in infancy, possibly due to age-specific response to trauma), severity and type of injury, extent of secondary damage, disruption of normal development and pre-existing conditions (Keenan et al., 2018).

SUMMARY

Caring for the child and family where the child has a neurological problem can be particularly challenging, but highly rewarding. The challenges relate to a lack of exposure to caring for children with rare disorders, the uncertain outcome of many conditions, and the potential of many conditions to cause dramatic changes in function for the child, both cognitively and physically. This chapter has outlined the nervous system and general principles of care required for a child with a neurological problem. It is not a comprehensive guide to the management of the wide range of neurological conditions of childhood, but does provide insight into the common conditions. There has been an emphasis on an interdisciplinary approach to care delivery, and the need to ensure care delivery is individually designed and strongly influenced by encouraging the child to reach their full potential. Links have been made with other chapters where appropriate.

REFERENCES

Adelson, P.D., Bratton, P.D., Carney, N.A., et al., 2012. Guidelines for the acute medical management of severe traumatic brain injury in infants, children and adolescents - second edition. Pediatr. Crit. Care Med. 13 (1), S1–S82.

Ajithkumar, T., Price, S., Horan, G., et al., 2017. Prevention of radiotherapy-induced neurocognitive dysfunction in survivors of paediatric brain tumours: the potential role of modern imaging and radiotherapy techniques. Lancet Oncol. 18 (2), e91–e100.

Barakat, L.P., Li, Y., Hobbie, W.L., et al., 2014. Health-related quality of life of adolescent and young adult survivors of childhood brain tumors. Psycho Oncol. 24 (7), 804–811.

Barnes, N.P., Jones, S.J., Hayward, R.D., et al., 2002. Ventriculo-peritoneal shunt blockage: what are the best predictive clinical indicators? Arch. Dis. Child. 87, 198–201.

Bourgeois, M., Sainte-Rose, C., Cinalli, G., et al., 2018. Epilepsy in childhood shunted hydrocephalus. In: Cinalli, G., Ozek, M., Sainte-Rose, C. (Eds.), Pediatric Hydrocephalus. Springer, New York.

Brain Injury Association of America, 2005. Facts about Traumatic Brain Injury. www.biausa.org.

Bratton, S.L., Chestnut, R.M., Gajar, J., et al., 2007. Guidelines for the management of severe traumatic brain injury. VIII. J. Neurotrauma 24 (suppl. 1), S55–S58.

Brett, E.M., Harding, B.N., 1997. Hydrocephalus and congenital anomalies of the nervous system other than myelomeningocele. In: Brett, E.M. (Ed.), Paediatric Neurology, third ed. Churchill Livingstone, London.

Brett, E.M., Kaiser, A.M., 1997. Neurology of the newborn. In: Brett, E.M. (Ed.), Paediatric Neurology, third ed. Churchill Livingstone, London.

Buchanan, E.P., Xue, Y., Xue, A.S., et al., 2017. Multidisciplinary care of craniosynostosis. J. Multidiscip. Healthc. 10, 263–270.

Camfield, P., Camfield, C., 2015. Incidence, prevalence and aetiology of seizures and epilepsy in children. Epileptic Disord. 17, 117–123.

Campbell, C.G.N., Kuehn, S.M., Richards, P.M.P., et al., 2004. Medical and cognitive outcome in children with traumatic brain injury. Can. J. Neurol. Sci. 31 (2), 213–219.

Cancer Research UK, 2013. Cancer Statistics Data Table: Teenage and Young Adult Cancer Incidence, UK, 2000–2009. Available from: https://www.cancerresearchuk.org/sites/default/files/cs_dt_tya.pdf.

Children's Brain Tumour Research Centre, 2017. The Brain Pathways Guideline: A Guideline to Assist Healthcare Professionals in the Assessment of Children Who May Have a Brain Tumour. Children's Brain Tumour Research Centre, Nottingham.

Chumas, P., Tyagi, A., Livingston, J., 2001. Hydrocephalus–what's new? Arch. Dis. Child. Fetal Neonatal Ed. 85 (3), 149–154.

Cox, M.C., Kusters, J.M., Gidding, C.E., et al., 2015. Acute toxicity profile of craniospinal irradiation with intensity-modulated radiation therapy in children with medulloblastoma: a prospective analysis. Radiat. Oncol. 10 (241), e1–e9.

Cullen, P.M., Derrickson, J.D., Potter, J.A., 2002. Radiation therapy. In: Baggott, C.R., Kelly, K.P., Fochtman, et al. (Eds.), Association of Pediatric Oncology Nurses. Nursing Care of Children and Adolescents with Cancer, third ed. WB Saunders, Philadelphia.

de Boer, H.M., Mula, M., Sander, W.J., 2008. The global burden and stigma of epilepsy. Epilepsy Behav. 12, 540–546.

Dewan, M.C., Rattani, A., Mekary, R.A., et al., 2018. Global hydrocephalus epidemiology and incidence: systematic review and meta-analysis. J. Neurosurg. 1, 1–15.

Dewan, M.C., Mummareddy, N., Wellons, J.C., Bonfield, C.M., 2016. Epidemiology of global pediatric traumatic brain injury: qualitative review. World Neurosurg 91, 497–509.

Dunn, L.T., 2002. Raised intracranial pressure. J. Neurol. Neurosurg. Psychiatry 73 (suppl. 1), i23–i27.

Eghwrudjakpor, P.O., Allison, A.B., 2010. Decompressive craniectomy following brain injury: factors important to patient outcome. Libyan J. Med. 5, 1–6.

Eichler, V.F., Milonovich, L.M., 2013. Neurological disorders. In: Hazinski, M.F. (Ed.), Nursing Care of the Critically Ill Child, third ed. Mosby, St Louis.

Emery, C.A., Barlow, K.M., Brooks, B.L., et al., 2016. A systematic review of psychiatric, psychological, and behavioural outcomes following mild traumatic brain injury in children and adolescents. Can. J. Psychiatr. 61 (5), 259–269.

Fisher, R.S., Acevedo, C., Arzimanoglou, A., et al., 2014. A practical clinical definition of epilepsy. Epilepsia 55 (4), 475–482.

Fisher, R.S., Cross, J.H., D'Souza, C., et al., 2017. Instruction manual for the ILAE 2017 operational classification of seizure types. Epilepsia 58 (4), 531–542.

Gadgil, N., Hansen, D., Barry, J., et al., 2016. Posterior fossa syndrome in children following tumor resection: knowledge update. Surg. Neurol. Int. 7 (suppl. 6), S179–S183.

Gajjar, A., Bowers, D.C., Karajannis, M.A., et al., 2015. Pediatric brain tumors: innovative genomic information is transforming the diagnostic and clinical landscape. J. Clin. Oncol. 33 (27), 2986–2998.

Garrocho-Rangel, A., Manríquez-Olmos, L., Flores-Velázquez, J., et al., 2018. Non-syndromic craniosynostosis in children: scoping review. Oral Med. and Pathol. 23 (4), 421–428.

Greenwood, J., Flodman, P., Osann, K., et al., 2014. Familial incidence and associated symptoms in a population of individuals with non-syndromic craniosynostosis. Genet. Med. 16 (4), 302–310.

Grissom, S., Boles, J., Bailey, K., et al., 2016. Play-based procedural preparation and support intervention for cranial radiation. Supportive Care 24 (6), 2421–2427.

Hanna, N.J., Black, M., Sander, J.W.S., et al., 2002. The National Sentinel Clinical Audit of Epilepsy-Related Deaths. Epilepsy - Death in the Shadows. The Stationery Office, London.

Hazinski, M.F., Headrick, C., Bruce, D., 1999. Neurological disorders. In: Hazinski, M.F. (Ed.), Manual of Pediatric Critical Care. Mosby, St Louis.

Heaney, D.C., MacDonald, B.K., Everitt, A., et al., 2002. Socioeconomic variation in incidence of epilepsy: a prospective community based study in southeast England. Br. Med. J. 325, 1013–1016.

Hickey, J.V., 2014. Neurological assessment. In: Hickey, J.V. (Ed.), The Clinical Practice of Neurological and Neurosurgical Nursing, seventh ed. Lippincott, Philadelphia.

Hickey, J.V., Elkamand, B., 2014. Management of patients with depressed levels of consciousness. In: Hickey, J.V. (Ed.), The Clinical Practice of Neurological and Neurosurgical Nursing, seventh ed. Lippincott, Philadelphia.

Hunt, A., Mastroyannopoulou, K., Goldman, A., et al., 2003. Not knowing - the problem of pain in children with severe neurological impairment. Int. J. Nurs. Stud. 40, 171–183.

Hysing, M., Elgen, I., Gillberg, C., et al., 2009. Emotional and behavioural problems in subgroups of children with chronic illness: results from a large-scale population study. Child Care Health Dev. 35, 527–533.

Iskandar, B.J., Tubbs, S., Mapstone, T.B., et al., 1998. Death in shunted hydrocephalic children in the 1990's. Pediatr. Neurosurg. 28, 173–176.

Johnson, K.J., Jennifer Cullen, J., Barnholtz-Sloan, J.S., et al., 2014. Childhood brain tumor epidemiology: a brain tumor epidemiology consortium review. Cancer Epidemiology Biomarkers 23 (12), 2716–2736.

Johnston, W.T., Lightfoot, T.J., Simpson, J., et al., 2010. Childhood cancer survival: a report from the United Kingdom Childhood Cancer Study. Cancer Epidemiology 34 (6), 659–666.

Keenan, H.T., Clark, A.E., Richard Holubkov, R., et al., 2018. Psychosocial and executive function recovery trajectories one year after pediatric traumatic brain injury: the influence of age and injury severity. J. Neurotrauma 35, 286–296.

Kirkham, F.J., Newton, C., Whitehouse, W., 2008. Paediatric coma scales. Dev. Med. Child Neurol. 50 (4), 267–274.

Kluba, S., Rohleder, M., Wolff, K., et al., 2016. Krimmel: parental perception of treatment and medical care in children with craniosynostosis. Int. J. Oral Maxillofac. Surg. 45, 1341–1346.

Kukreti, V., Mohseni-Bod, H., Drake, J., 2014. Management of raised intracranial pressure in children with traumatic brain injury. J. Pediatr. Neurosci. 9 (3), 207–215.

Kulkarni, A.V., 2010. Quality of life in childhood hydrocephalus: a review. Childs Nerv. Syst. 26, 737–743.

Laxer, K.D., Trinka, E., Hirsch, L.J., et al., 2014. The consequences of refractory epilepsy and its treatment. Epilepsy Behav. 37, 59–70.

Long, A.F., Kneafsey, R., Ryan, J., et al., 2002. The role of the nurse within the multi-professional rehabilitation team. J. Adv. Nurs. 37 (1), 70–78.

Longstaff, A., 2011. Instant Notes – Neuroscience, third ed. Taylor and Francis, Abingdon.

Lotfinia, I.A., 2017. Review in pediatric hydrocephalus: physiology, classification, clinical presentation, imaging and treatment. JSM Pediatric Neurology 1 (1), 1002.

Madden, L.K., Than, P.K., Shahlaie, K., 2014. Management of patients undergoing neurosurgical procedures. In: Hickey, J.V. (Ed.), The Clinical Practice of Neurological and Neurosurgical Nursing, seventh ed. Lippincott, Philadelphia.

Marson, A.G., Al-Kharusi, Alwaidh, M., et al., 2007a. The SANAD study of effectiveness of valproate, lamotrigine or topiramate for generalised and unclassifiable epilepsy: an unblinded randomised controlled trial. Lancet 369, 1016–1026.

Marson, A.G., Al-Kharusi, A.M., Alwaidh, M., et al., 2007b. The SANAD study of effectiveness of carbamazepine, gabapentin, lamotrigine, oxcarbazepine or topiramate for the treatment of partial epilepsy: an unblinded randomised controlled trial. Lancet 369, 1000–1015.

Mazzola, C.A., Choudhri, A.F., Auguste, K.I., et al., 2014. Pediatric hydrocephalus: systematic literature review and evidence-based guidelines. Part 2: management of posthemorrhagic hydrocephalus in premature infants. J. Neurosurg. Pediatr. 14 (suppl. l), 8–23.

Moreau, J.F., Fink, E.L., Hartman, M.E., et al., 2013. Hospitalizations of children with neurological disorders in the United States. Pediatr. Crit. Care Med. 14 (8), 801–810.

National Confidential Enquiry into Patient Outcome and Death (NCEPOD), 2018. Chronic Neurodisability: Each and Every Need. NCEPOD, London.

National Institute for Clinical Excellence (NICE), 2015. Suspected Cancer: Recognition and Referral. NICE, London (NG 12).

National Institute for Clinical Excellence (NICE), 2016. Cancer Services for Children and Young People: Recognition and Referral. NICE, London (QS55).

National Institute for Clinical Excellence (NICE), 2017. Head Injury: Assessment and Early Management of Head Injury in Infants, Children and Adults. NICE, London (NICE guideline CG 176).

National Institute for Clinical Excellence (NICE), 2018. Epilepsies: Diagnosis and Management. NICE, London (NICE guideline CG 137).

Nguyen, R., Fiest, K., McChesney, J., et al., 2016. The international incidence of traumatic brain injury: a systematic review and meta-analysis. Can. J. Neurol. Sci. 43 (6), 774–785.

Nudo, R.J., 2013. Recovery after brain injury: mechanisms and principles. Front. Hum. Neurosci. 7, 887.

Padgett, K., 2006. Alterations of neurological function in children. In: McCance, K.L., Huether, S.E. (Eds.), Pathophysiology: The Biological Basis for Disease in Adults and Children, fifth ed. Mosby, St Louis.

Panchal, J., Uttchin, V., 2003. Management of craniosynostosis. Plast. Reconstr. Surg. 111 (6), 2032–2049.

Parslow, R.C., Morris, K.P., Tasker, R.C., et al., 2005. Epidemiology of traumatic brain injury in children receiving intensive care in the UK. Arch. Dis. Child. 90, 1182–1187.

Peters, A., 2007. Neurological observations. In: Glasper, E.A., McEwing, G., Richardson, J. (Eds.), Oxford Handbook of Children's and Young Peoples Nursing. Oxford University Press, Oxford.

Philips, A., Philips, J., 2018. Cancer in children and young people 1: incidence. Available from: https://www.powerwatch.org.uk/library/downloads/child-cancer-1-incidence-2018-08.pdf.

Polinder, S., Haagsma, J.A., van Klaveren, D., et al., 2015. Health-related quality of life after TBI: a systematic review of study design, instruments, measurement properties, and outcome. Popul. Health Metrics 13 (4), 1–12.

Reith, F.C., Lingsma, H.F., Gabbe, J., et al., 2017. Differential effects of the Glasgow Coma Scale score and its components: an analysis of 54,069 patients with traumatic brain injury. Injury 48 (9), 1932–1943.

Roberts, G.C., 2005. Post-craniotomy analgesia: current practices in British neurosurgical centres – a survey of post-craniotomy analgesic practices. Eur. J. Anaesthesiol. 22, 328–332.

Roe, H., Lennan, E., 2014. Role of nurses in the assessment and management of chemotherapy-related side effects in cancer patients. Nurs. Res. Rev. 4, 103–115.

Rose, F.D., Johnson, D.A., Attree, E.A., 1997. Rehabilitation of the head injured child: basic research and new technology. Pediatr. Rehabil. 1 (1), 3–7.

Rosenbaum, P., Gorter, J.W., 2012. The "f-words" in childhood disability: I swear this is how we should think! Child Care Health Dev. 38, 457–463.

Royal College of Nursing (RCN), 2009. Updated Full Guidelines: The Recognition and Assessment of Acute Pain in Children. RCN, London.

Satz, P., Zaucher, K., McCleary, et al., 1997. Mild head injury in children and adolescents: a review of studies 1970–1995. Psychol. Bull. 122 (2), 107–131.

Schiff, D., Lee, E.Q., Nayak, L., et al., 2015. Medical management of brain tumors and the sequelae of treatment. Neuro Oncol. 17 (4), 488–504.

Sillanpää, M., Schmidt, D., 2009. Early seizure frequency and aetiology predict long-term medical outcome in childhood-onset epilepsy. Brain 132 (4), 989–998.

Singer, G.H.S., 1996. Constructing supports. In: Singer, G.H.S., Glang, A., Williams, J.M. (Eds.), Children with Acquired Brain Injury. Paul H Brookes Publishing, Baltimore.

Smith, J., Cheater, F., Bekker, H., 2015a. Parents' experiences of living with a child with a long-term condition: a rapid structured review of the literature. Health Expect. 18 (4), 452–474.

Smith, J., Cheater, F., Bekker, H., 2015b. Parents' experiences of living with a child with hydrocephalus: a cross-sectional interview based study. Health Expect. 18 (5), 1709–1720.

Smith, J., Cheater, F., Bekker, H., Chatwin, J., 2015c. Are parents and professionals making shared decisions about a child's care on presentation of a suspected shunt malfunction: a mixed method study? Health Expect. 18 (5), 1299–1315.

Sugerman, R.A., 2018. Structure and function of the neurological system. In: McCance, K.L., Huether, S.E. (Eds.), Pathophysiology: The Biological Basis for Disease in Adults and Children, eighth ed. Mosby, St Louis.

Teasdale, G., Jennett, B., 1974. Assessment of coma and impaired consciousness - a practical scale. Lancet 2, 81–83.

Thibault, M., Girard, F., Moumdjian, R., et al., 2007. Craniotomy site influences post-operative pain following neurosurgical procedures: a retrospective study. Can. J. Anaesth. 54 (7), 544–548.

Thurman, D.J., 2016. The epidemiology of traumatic brain injury in children and youths: a review of research since 1990. J. Child Neurol. 31 (1), 20–27.

Tully, H.M., Dobyns, W.B., 2014. Infantile hydrocephalus: a review of epidemiology, classification and causes. Eur. J. Med. Genet. 57 (8), 359–368.

Turini, M., Redaelli, A., 2001. Primary brain tumours: a review of research and management. Int. J. Clin. Pract. 55 (7), 471–475.

Twycross, A., Mayfield, C., Savory, J., 1999. Pain management for children with special needs: a neglected area? Paediatr. Nurs. 11 (6), 43–45.

Warren, A., 2000. Paediatric coma scoring researched and benchmarked. Paediatr. Nurs. 12 (3), 14–18.

Wu, L., Li, X., Janagam, D.R., Lowe, T.L., 2014. Overcoming the blood-brain barrier in chemotherapy treatment of pediatric brain tumors. Pharmaceut. Res. 31 (3), 531–540.

17

Children and Young People With Complex Motor Disability

Jackie Parkes, Sonya Clarke

LEARNING OUTCOMES

- Appreciate the perspectives of individual level and population-based approaches to assessment and planning care for the Children and young people (CYP) with complex motor disability.
- Describe the leading causes of complex motor disability in childhood.
- Recognise the relative contribution to be made by the medical and social models of disability.
- Be able to locate and interpret information (routine and other) on children and young people with complex motor disability in the United Kingdom (UK).

- Recognise children and young people as rights holders and active service users of health care.
- Recognise the central role of parents as experts in the management of children with complex disability.
- Understand the role of the CYP nurse in identifying unmet need through competent nursing assessment of the CYP with complex motor disability and their family.
- Be able to critically apply proposed outlines for nursing assessment in the care of the CYP with complex motor disability and their families.

INTRODUCTION

The aim of this chapter is to focus on the care of the CYP with complex motor disability, and on the issues their families face, in the context of community and hospital. The chapter uses both an individual-level and a population-based perspective to explore both the needs of the CYP with complex motor disability and the needs of their families. An individual level approach focuses on the needs and unique experiences of an individual – a child, young person, their parents and siblings. This perspective is important in developing an individualised assessment of need and tailored plan of nursing care. It contrasts with a population-based approach, which considers the needs and experiences of groups of CYP and their families with similar conditions and usually living in the same geographic area (e.g. in a Health and Social Services Trust or one region of the UK). This perspective is important for prevention of disease, health promotion and planning and targeting services to those in greatest need. The CYP nurse has a role to play at both levels of assessment and intervention in relation to CYP health and more specifically with regard to children and young people with complex motor disability.

DEFINITIONS, NUMBERS, NEEDS AND SERVICES

Definition of Complex Motor Disability

The term 'complex motor disability' is interpreted here to mean a person with cerebral palsy who has a permanent disorder of posture and movement caused by disturbances in the developing brain. Cerebral palsy (CP) is the term for a range of movement difficulties. It is caused when parts of the brain that control movement and posture are damaged during pregnancy

or shortly after birth. The changes in the brain are permanent, but how the body is affected can change as the child grows and develops. The impact of cerebral palsy can vary greatly, from mild activity limitations to severe restrictions of activity and participation (Northern Ireland Cerebral Palsy Register [NICPR], 2018). Cerebral palsy is the most common cause of physical disability in childhood, with a prevalence of approximately 2.0 per thousand live births (Cans et al., 2008). The Northern Ireland cerebral palsy register (2018) reports:
- two in five children with CP are born premature
- three in five children with CP are born at normal birthweight (2500 g or more)

People with cerebral palsy may also have problems with speech, vision and hearing, intellectual difficulties and epilepsy (Imms et al., 2015). The motor disorders of cerebral palsy are often accompanied by disturbances of sensation, perception, cognition, communication and behaviour and by secondary musculoskeletal problems (Rosenbaum et al., 2007). Cerebral palsy is a good example of such a condition with most having at least one additional associated impairment in conjunction with problems related to movement. CP is classified depending on the type of movement disorder and the parts of the body affected. Movement disorders include:
- Dyskinetic: 5% disorganised movement patterns with varying muscle tone
- Ataxic: 2.5% low muscle tone associated with short and jerky movements
- Spastic: 92% increase in muscle tone related to speed of movement
  - Bilateral spastic CP: 52% – quadriplegia or diplegia
  - Unilateral spastic CP: 40% – hemiplegia

Cerebral palsy can be severe: approximately one in three children are unable to walk and one in four has no useful arm or hand function (Parkes et al., 2001a). The impact of disability experienced is further increased by the presence of other severe associated impairments: one in four children with cerebral palsy have severe learning disability (IQ < 50) and one in ten have no useful vision (Parkes et al., 2001a).

In addition, some children with complex motor disability will depend on technology to sustain their lives, for example, requiring assisted ventilation, artificial feeding, or care associated with having a colostomy, ileostomy, urostomy or catheterisation (Glendinning et al., 2001). It should be noted that the terms 'complex motor disability', 'complex health care needs' and 'technology-dependent children' are not interchangeable, although many of the same children are common to all three groups.

 ACTIVITY

Consider what constitutes cerebral palsy in the 21st century? Review the paper by Smithers-Sheedy et al. (2014). Available from:
- https://onlinelibrary.wiley.com/doi/full/10.1111/dmcn.12262

Leading Causes of Motor Disability

Due to advances in medical technology, there are increasing numbers of children with complex health needs (CWCHN) (Welsh et al., 2014). McConkey et al. (2001, p 13) define CWCHN as 'children primarily with physical care needs, such as those who are technologically dependent, have a life-limiting or life-threatening condition, acquired brain injury resulting in significant impairment and/or children with multiple impairments from birth'. Caring for a CWCHN is an enormous, often overwhelming task for families and can have detrimental effects on the carer's mental and physical health. Cerebral palsy is up to 80 times more common among babies born too soon or too small and the number of tiny babies surviving continues to increase (NICPR, 2018). Also, interventions like chemotherapy and ventilation, now available in the community, have improved the life span of children with degenerative conditions.

Although it is important for the children's nurse to appreciate the underlying medical diagnoses and pathology of complex motor disabilities, medical diagnosis alone does not predict service needs (Gordon et al., 2000; World Health Organization [WHO], 2001). For this reason, only a short overview of medical causes is presented here.

The leading causes of complex motor disability that may give rise to complex needs in children include cerebral palsy, spina bifida, Duchenne muscular dystrophy and other degenerative and neuromuscular conditions like spinal muscular atrophy. Cerebral palsy is the leading cause of physical disability in childhood (Parkes et al., 2001a; Surveillance of Cerebral Palsy in Europe [SCPE], 2000) and has been defined as 'an umbrella term covering a group of non-progressive, but often changing motor impairment syndromes,

secondary to lesions or anomalies of the brain arising in the early stages of its development' (Mutch et al., 1992, p 549). A number of rare metabolic disorders (e.g. Lesch–Nyhan syndrome) and genetic syndromes (e.g. Turner syndrome) can also result in neuromotor impairments and disability. For some children, the underlying medical diagnoses remain uncertain.

Some of these conditions will invariably lead to premature death (e.g. Duchenne muscular dystrophy), whereas others are likely to mean the child and family will have a lifetime of disability requiring specialist help and support (e.g. cerebral palsy). Although conditions like cerebral palsy and spina bifida are not fatal per se, premature death is associated with more severe forms (Crichton et al., 1995; Hutton et al., 1994). It has been estimated that of those with the most severe disabling cerebral palsy (unable to walk, no useful arm or hand function and with intellectual impairment): 70% will survive to age 10; 50% will survive to age 20; and 40% will survive to 30 years (Hutton and Pharoah, 1998).

Medical and Social Models of Disability

As children's nurses we need to be aware and appreciate the 'larger' issues around disability as a political, social and emerging academic discipline in its own right. Generally speaking, we are taught and tend to assume the 'medical model' in assessing and intervening in the care of children with disability and their families. The medical model supposes that disability is the result of pathology and impairment, resulting in deficit of function and rendering the person disabled and unable to participate fully in 'normal' life. Our interventions are aimed at the level of the individual and include pre- and post-operative surgical care, medication, rehabilitation and the provision of aids and appliances to help the individual adapt and 'fit into' mainstream society. Although it could be argued that this perspective is at least partially appropriate, the contrasting social model of disability has gained increasing validity and recognition.

The social model of disability conceives that impairments do not make a person disabled but rather that it is society who disables people by failing to accommodate their differences (Priestley, 2003). The manifestation of this 'failure to accommodate' means that people with disabilities are excluded from mainstream life through segregated education, few and poorly paid employment opportunities, and difficulty gaining access to buildings and using public transport, among other things (Priestley, 2003). In the social model of disability, the level of intervention is aimed at changing societal attitudes and societal behaviour towards people with disability.

The distinction between these models is not merely an academic one, because how we think about disability will influence our nursing practice. The children's nurse has a clear responsibility to provide nursing care and meet the immediate physical and psychological needs of the child and family. We also have a wider role to play.

The World Health Organization and Disability

In 1980 the World Health Organization (WHO) published the much-cited International Classification of Impairments, Disabilities and Handicaps (ICIDH). This defined impairment as 'any loss or abnormality of psychological, physiological or anatomical structure or function'; disability as 'any restriction or lack (resulting from impairment) of ability to perform an activity in the manner within the range considered normal for a human being'; and handicap as 'a disadvantage for a given individual, resulting from an impairment or a disability, that limits or prevents fulfilment of a role that is normal'.

This framework has now been revised to form a more positive 'components of health' classification called the International Classification of Functioning, Disability and Health (or ICF; WHO, 2002). Previously, the ICIDH was a 'consequences of disease' classification that focused on the impact of disease on the individual (WHO, 1980). By contrast, the ICF focuses on health and measuring function regardless of the reason for the impairment (WHO, 2002). The terms and concepts of 'disability' and 'handicap' have now been replaced by the terms 'activity limitations' and 'participation restrictions', respectively.

 ACTIVITY

Read a beginner's guide to the ICF called 'Towards a common language for functioning, disability and health' at:
• http://www.who.int/classifications/icf/icfbeginnersguide.pdf

The ICF provides a conceptual framework for the 'definition, measurement and policy formulations for health and disability' (WHO, 2002, p 2) for use in health care and at the levels of individual, institution and population. Finally, one of the additional unique features of the ICF is recognition and classification of the environmental factors (such as social attitudes and social structures), which are derived from the social model of disability. Assessment of these features is necessary to complete the 'picture' of health and disability.

In the context of children's nursing it is important to appreciate the ICF because it is relevant and could be used in nursing practice in the following ways (adapted from WHO, 2002):

• To provide standardised descriptions and a conceptual framework of health and health-related states for individual children and their families. For example, it could be used in relation to assessing and planning care for children with complex motor disability.

• Use of standardised language to promote interdisciplinary communication (with physiotherapists, occupational therapists, paediatricians, for example) and make comparisons about health, health care and health outcomes in children with complex needs within geographic areas and between geographic areas.

• More generally, to provide reliable summary measures of population health for surveillance purposes and monitoring health outcomes.

• The ICF promotes assessment of the 'contextual factors' or barriers that limit the participation of individual children with complex motor disability or populations of children with complex motor disability and their families.

• It provides a systematic coding scheme for health care information systems.

 REFLECT ON YOUR PRACTICE

What would be the advantages and disadvantages of including the ICF as part of routine nursing assessment in the care of children with complex motor disability?

SOURCES OF INFORMATION ON CHILDREN WITH COMPLEX MOTOR DISABILITY

Information about the numbers of children with complex motor disability or other forms of disability have been described as 'invisible' from the routine statistics published by government (Gordon et al., 2000). Most regions within the UK have a formal, computer-based system for monitoring child health – a child health surveillance system. The sorts of information recorded on child health surveillance systems include birth notifications, immunisations, preschool health checks and the identification of any special needs. These systems tend to be orientated towards provision of services and have limited use as complete sources of information on specific conditions like cerebral palsy (Parkes et al., 1998). Furthermore, these routine information systems could, but generally do not, publish information on children with complex needs as part of routine statistics.

Some of the gaps in the routine information about children with special and complex needs have been filled by ad hoc ('one-off') surveys carried out in Great Britain and Northern Ireland. In Great Britain, the Office of Population Censuses and Surveys conducted surveys of childhood disability in 1985 and 1988 (Bone and Meltzer, 1989), which were subsequently reanalysed by Gordon et al. (2000). Glendinning et al. (1999, 2001) also reported on the numbers of technology-dependent children living in the UK; Beresford (1995) on the numbers of parents caring for a severely disabled child at home (in England) and Roberts and Lawton (2001) on severely disabled children whose families have accessed the Family Fund.

In Northern Ireland, sister Office of Population Censuses and Surveys (OPCS) surveys were conducted by the Policy, Planning and Research Unit in 1989 and 1990 (Duffy, 1995; Smith et al., 1992). A survey was undertaken in Scotland to identify the numbers and service needs of children with motor impairment and their families (Gough et al., 1993). The results of these surveys are summarised in Table 17.1. Some caution must be used in the interpretation of Table 17.1 because differences between surveys will be partly due to differences in the way 'disability' and 'severe disability' have been defined. It should be noted that the impact of disability may increase with age and studies of disability need to take this into account.

> **ACTIVITY**
>
> The Family Fund Trust is an independent organisation that provides financial support and information services to families caring for a severely disabled or ill child (less than 16 years of age). The Family Fund Trust is government funded. Read more about the Family Fund at:
> * https://www.familyfund.org.uk/

Some longitudinal studies of childhood motor disability do exist in the form of dedicated case registers of children with cerebral palsy. Currently, five such registers are actively recording cases in Northern Ireland, parts of England and Scotland. These registers fulfil an important function in providing unique information about the prevalence, severity and survival of children and young adults with cerebral palsy in the UK. The registers are also used to monitor trends over time and between areas and act as a sampling frame for research into causation and services. Table 17.2 summarises some of the literature on the numbers and prevalence of children with cerebral palsy in different parts of the UK, including information from the five registers referred to above.

Cerebral Palsy Registers

Cerebral palsy registers have been established to actively record cases of CP. These registers fulfil an important function in providing unique information about the prevalence, severity and survival of children and young adults with cerebral palsy in the UK. The registers are also used to monitor trends over time and between areas and act as a sampling frame for research into causation and services. World Cerebral Palsy Day occurs annually on 6 October.

For example, the aim of the Northern Ireland Cerebral Palsy Register (NICPR) is to establish a systematic approach to the surveillance of CP among children in Northern Ireland (NI), to support research and audits into the condition; covering causes, treatment, assessment and health and social care service provision.

The NICPR in 2018:
* is a confidential record of children with cerebral palsy in Northern Ireland;

TABLE 17.1 Summary of Surveys of Childhood Disability and Technology-Dependent Children in the United Kingdom

Author and Year	Geographical Area	Definition Used	Numbers and Proportions of Children With a Disability (Including Children With Severe/Multiple Problems Where Known)
OPCS Bone & Meltzer, 1989	England, Wales, Scotland	'Disabled' as defined by the ICDIH (WHO); aged 0–15 years	360,000 disabled children (3.2% of the child population in the UK); 327,000 disabled children in England & Wales
OPCS Gordon et al., 2000	As above	Reanalysed OPCS data and redefined disability and identified clusters of disability	45,000 children with the most severe and multiple disabilities
PPRU Smith et al., 1992; Duffy, 1995	Northern Ireland	'Disabled' as defined by the ICDIH (WHO); aged 0–15 years	14,600 disabled children (3.5% of the child population in NI); 2600 'severely disabled'
Gough et al., 1993	Scotland	Motor impairment of central origin born 1985–1986 and resident in Scotland 1991–1992	244 children with a motor impairment of central origin (0.3% of child population in Scotland). Two-thirds had moderate–severe disability in relation to personal care; more than half had severe learning disability
Beresford, 1995	UK (using the Family Fund database)	Been helped by the Family Fund and been in recent contact with the Family Fund; children <16 years	Collected data on 1100 families caring for a severely disabled child. Estimates 150,000 families are caring for a severely disabled child
Glendinning et al., 2001	UK	Technology-dependent children	Estimates 6000 technology-dependent children in the UK (although some double counting may have occurred); 2800 children receiving artificial feeding (British Artificial Nutrition Survey cited by Glendinning et al.)

ICDIH, International Classification of Impairments, Disabilities, and Handicaps; *OPCS,* Office of Population Censuses and Surveys; *WHO,* the World Health Organization.

TABLE 17.2	Studies of Children and Young People With Cerebral Palsy					
Reference (Alphabetical)	Geographical Area	Method	Birth Years	Number of Children	Rate per 1000 Live Births	
Colver and Mackie, 1998	North East of England	Case register	1991–1993	287	2.4	
Edmond et al., 1989	Great Britain	British Perinatal Mortality & Birth Survey	1958, 1970	40, 41	2.5	
Ingram, 1955	Edinburgh	Ad hoc survey	1938–1952	208	1.9	
Jarvis et al., 1985	North East of England	Case register	1960–1975	421	1.6	
Johnson and King, 1998	Oxford	Case register	1984–1991	697	2.5	
MacGillivray and Campbell, 1995	Avon	Taken from a handicap register	1969–1988	489	2.1	
Parkes et al., 2001b	Northern Ireland	Case register	1981–1993	784	2.2	
Pharoah et al., 1990	Mersey	Case register	1980–1984	309	1.9	
Pharoah et al., 1998	Mersey, Oxford & Scotland	Case registers	1984–1989	1649	2.1	
Williams et al., 1996	North East Thames	Case register	1980–1986	672	1.6	

- has collected data on CP for 40 birth years (1977–2017);
- has the support of 110 clinicians across Northern Ireland who report cases of CP;
- is held at the School of Nursing and Midwifery, Queen's University Belfast;
- is one of 24 active registers in Europe that contribute information to the Surveillance of Cerebral Palsy in Europe collaboration.

For more information please visit: www.qub.ac.uk/research-centres/nicpr.

Although it could be argued that disability and complex motor disability remains relatively rare, the following extract written by a parent clearly highlights the impact on the child and family and their need for ongoing, intensive support to cope.

The Impact of Having a Child With Complex Motor Disability

The following 'real life scenario' written by a parent provides a unique and special insight into the parent's feelings and experiences of having a child with complex needs. It is strikingly similar to other accounts by parents who have reiterated many of the same messages (Beresford, 1994; Kingdom and Mayfield, 2001).

In the account presented here, the parent does not elaborate on the precise 'medical equipment' she uses. However Beresford (1995) identified the following equipment being used by 1100 families for a severely disabled child at home: nasal feeding tubes (18%), suction equipment (16%), nebulisers and inhalers (10%), gastric feeding tubes (12%), a feeding pump (12%), catheters (7%), oxygen (9%), ventilators (7%), other things (14%). Clearly, parents have to develop advanced clinical skills to look after their child at home. The children's nurse has a clear role to play in teaching families these skills, sourcing and providing equipment, anticipating and preventing potential problems and supporting parents at home to provide the highest quality care.

SCENARIO

Real-Life Scenario by a Parent of a Child With Complex Motor Disability

My son Daniel [a pseudonym] was born in 1998 and what should have been a wonderful event became a tragedy. Daniel has athetoid cerebral palsy. He is now 4 ½-years-old and is a 24-hour job. Apart from physical exhaustion looking after a handicapped child, the mental torment is nearly worse. Watching your child day to day and wondering if he will see another one or if the next illness will be the last and you have to say 'goodbye'.

The needs of the child are great and this can be where health services mainly focus. However, the needs of the parent often fall by the wayside. Practical help is required from the start in the form of advice, supplies and respite care. I 'fell' through the net and did not receive any real help until my son was 2 ½-years-old. Daniel was then assigned a community nurse who realised our plight and set out to help. She organised all supplies, including nappies and medical equipment. Something as simple as this eased the load and was something less to worry about. She was excellent for advice on Disability Living Allowance and Motability transport. She also arranged hospice and respite care, which are wonderful, and tried to make life that little bit easier.

Too many parents are struggling on their own with limited information and resources as all too often one parent has to give up work to be the carer. This is what happened to me. There are few day-care facilities who can deal with a child with a nasogastric tube, a tracheostomy and epilepsy.

Emotional support is rare. It does not have to be an expensive organisation. Someone to talk to, have a coffee with and who does not mind if you have a good cry to get things off your chest, is often all that is required, but it is not out there. If it does exist, many parents are not told.

This might all sound like 'me, me, me', however to give Daniel a good life, I have to be strong mentally as well as physically. To put Daniel in care if I have a breakdown would cost approximately £700 per week. Me caring for my son is free.

I cannot describe the mental torture of knowing my son will die. Only a mother who walks a day in my shoes could possibly understand the constant struggle for help and advice. The situation has not improved a great deal in the last 20 years.

Aim of Services

In 1991 the UK government ratified the United Nations Convention on the Rights of the Child (United Nations General Assembly, 1989) and by doing so undertook to commit to the principles laid out by the Convention. Several articles within the Convention are relevant to children with disabilities (Articles 2, 3 and 12). More specifically, Article 23 states:

> ... *a mentally or physically disabled child should enjoy a full and decent life, in conditions which ensure dignity, promote self-reliance, and facilitate the child's active participation in the community.*

Article 23 should form the basis for providing services and interventions to the child with complex motor disability and his or her family. The overall aim of services to children with complex motor disability must also include early detection (and prevention where possible), early intervention and family support. The ultimate aim for all children with health or special needs must be to help them achieve the maximum potential and the best quality of life possible:

Children with profound and multiple disabilities and/or complex and continuing health care needs should enjoy the highest quality of life possible, receiving quality health, social and educational services which meet their needs and the needs of those who care for them, and respect their lifestyle and culture (Ward et al., 2003).

SEMINAR DISCUSSION TOPIC

Use the real-life scenario presented earlier and the account provided by Kingdom and Mayfield (2001):

- What issues or 'patient' problems can you identify? Distinguish between child-centred problems and parent-centred problems.
- To what extent do the parents' experiences and perceptions match the aims of services for children with disability specified above?
- Discuss the role of the children's nurse in addressing each of the issues or problems identified.
- What other professionals might the children's nurse interact with to help ensure the needs of this child and family are met?

FAMILIES' EXPERIENCES OF SERVICES

As we have already heard from parents, help and support is available from a wide range of services and professionals, some of whom focus directly on helping the child, whereas others concentrate on assisting the parents and family. Sloper and Turner (1992) found that parents of severely disabled children were in contact with a large number of professionals, as many as 10 in any 1 year, with a range of 5–17. Similarly, in a study of children with moderate to severe cerebral palsy, Parkes et al. (2002) also found that families were in contact with an average of seven service providers in a 6-month interval, with a range of 1–13. Not surprisingly, parents of children

with disability have reported problems related to coordination of services and fragmentation of care. Bamford et al. (1997) described this as 'deficiencies in the total care concept'.

Sloper and Turner (1992) found that many parents reported that they had encountered problems in finding and coordinating services, particularly in the early days after diagnosis, as reported elsewhere (Bamford et al., 1991; Haylock et al., 1993; Watson et al., 2002). In particular, parents have reported that professionals often duplicate work and seem unable to detect where the gaps in services are (Rees, 1983). Haylock et al. (1993) found school (i.e. special education) offered families a form of integration of care that they very much appreciated; again, this has been reported elsewhere (McConachie et al., 1999).

The inadequacies of respite care for families with a child with special needs, both in terms of quantity and quality of services available, have been repeatedly identified in the literature (Beresford, 1994, 1995; McConkey and Adams, 2000; Stalker, 1990). The children's nurse has a particular role to play here in terms of finding respite facilities, giving families good information and helping and preparing them psychologically to avail of services (Miller, 2002; Ross and Parkes, 2004). Families with a child with complex problems that require nursing care (e.g. problems with active seizures requiring medication) may find it more difficult to find respite from both the formal and informal sector because of their child's specialist requirements and the level of responsibility required of carers (Beale, 2002; Parkes, 1998). Families of children with severe and complex needs are at higher risk of stress and feelings of being unable to cope (Sloper and Turner, 1993).

ACTIVITY

Read about a model of good practice in relation to providing holistic care for children with complex health care needs and their families. See the following sections:
- News and Blogs
- Real stories
- Events
  Visit: http://www.thechildrenstrust.org.uk/

There are many examples of good practice in the care of children with complex motor disability both in the literature and in our local communities. Ross and Parkes (2004) outlined a model of good practice for the children's community nurse in relation to the care of a child with complex motor disability and the child's family. This paper highlights the unique role that the children's nurse can play in coordinating a multidisciplinary response that helps to 'cut down' excessive visits by numerous professionals, while at the same time tailoring services to meet with the child and family's individual needs.

A number of 'care interfaces' and transitional phases may exist for the child with complex motor disability and their family, which the children's nurse must be aware of and anticipate. These interfaces exist where the child and family 'move' from one service arrangement to another, for example from community to hospital or from child to adult services, as a result of changing need or developmental stage. These interfaces and transitional phases are times when the child and family may need extra help and support to cope and where service providers are 'at risk' of failing due to inadequate planning, poor cooperation or coordination between multiagencies.

The children's nurse in collaboration with the child's paediatrician, the family and other members of the multidisciplinary team, can act as coordinator of health and social care services and ensure that adequate advance planning takes place before discharge from hospital or transfer to another setting. Children with complex needs often receive hospital services at a number of hospital locations (McConachie, 1997) and this highlights the importance of children's nurses communicating with one another across institutional boundaries.

What Families Want From Services

The introduction of the key worker or lead professional role to support children with disabilities and complex health needs has been advocated in a succession of social policy guidance going back more than 20 years (Department of Health [DoH], 2004; Department for Children, Schools and Families, 2007; Children and Young People's Health Outcomes Forum, 2012).

EVIDENCE-BASED PRACTICE

Based on a recent study by Whiting (2014) which investigates the experiences of parents of children with complex health needs in relation to the help and support they receive when caring for their child. A series of in-depth semi-structured interviews were undertaken with the parents of 34 children (33 families) with a disability or a complex health need. Families were categorised into one of three subgroups:
- Children with a disability.
- Children with a life-limiting or life-threatening illness.
- Children with technology dependence.

Findings in relation to parental experience of the need for help and support, two major categories were identified, namely 'people', and 'processes and resources', as well as a series of subcategories. Areas were multiagency support, key working, advocacy, emotional and psychological support and respite. Respite care was identified as the greatest unmet need.

Conclusion drawn from the study reports parents to identify a range of helping behaviours among key professional staff involved in support provision.

Helpful characteristics and behaviours displayed by professional staff by Whiting (2014) were as follows:
- Establishment of trust in the relationship, including valuing and recognising parental instinct.
- Valuing relationships with families that were long lasting.
- Being prepared to 'go the extra mile' or 'work beyond the job description'.

- Responding positively.
- Availability of out-of-hours contact, not necessarily being face-to-face, but on the end of a telephone.
- Providing emotional and psychological support.
- Practical problem solving.
- Being knowledgeable about the child's condition and needs.

IMPLICATIONS FOR PRACTICE

- Respite may give parents the resilience to continue caring for their child. Many do not receive any respite and others find it difficult to accept help.
- Open access to the local children's ward should be provided wherever possible because it can be a great source of out-of-hours support.
- It is important to establish a trusting relationship with the child's parents, to help them solve problems, know about the child's conditions and needs, and provide emotional and psychological support.

Setting Standards: the Children's National Service Framework

In 1998 the government launched a programme of National Service Frameworks (NSFs) for a number of key patient groups with the aim of 'driving the modernisation agenda' within the NHS. The aims of the NSFs are to set national standards for key interventions, develop strategies to support the implementation of interventions and to increase quality and decrease variation in service provision. An outline of the development of the Children's NSF is provided by Smith (2003). The Standards for Hospital Services is the first part of the Children's NSF and is available online.

ACTIVITY

Find the latest information on the development of the Children's National Service Framework, including a downloadable copy of the Standards for Hospital Services:
- https://www.gov.uk/government/publications/national-service-framework-children-young-people-and-maternity-services

There is also a Children's NSF Disabled Children and Young People and those with Complex Health Needs which is available at theme www site.

ACTIVITY

Access the draft document at:
- https://www.gov.uk/government/publications/national-service-framework-children-young-people-and-maternity-services

For earlier work on the development of a charter for children with disabilities and their families, see Milner et al. (1996).

NURSING ASSESSMENT AND INTERVENTIONS

This section addresses a small number of activities of living that should be assessed by the children's nurse involved in the care of a child with complex motor disability – at home in the community, or on admission to hospital. Reasons for hospitalisation can include orthopaedic surgery, nutritional management including surgery, and other medical reasons such as management of a chest infection or pneumonia and respite care. The issues discussed here include mobility, eating and drinking and communication. These areas have been identified as the subject of specialist referrals in the literature (Cass et al., 1999) and as relevant on the basis of our own clinical and research experience. Other problems not mentioned here, but addressed elsewhere in this book, include the management of the child with seizures, sensory impairments and pain management.

Many of the problems encountered by children with complex motor disability are interrelated and require complex analyses by the children's nurse to understand the relationship between patient problems and their underlying causes. Cass et al. (1999) identified a useful hierarchy of assessment involving consideration of six levels. This model proposes that problem solving 'high'-level functions, like communication, depends on the resolution of lower-level functions affecting communication (e.g. head control). Sensory impairments can affect the ability to communicate; the presence of active seizures may impact on the child's general alertness and motivation, and can affect eating and drinking. These examples underline the importance of taking a holistic approach to assessing and planning care for children with complex motor disability and listening carefully to parents and carers. They also highlight the importance of undertaking an assessment in a multidisciplinary environment where joint planning can be undertaken (Cass et al., 1999).

In the context of children's nursing, the Roy adaptation model (1976) has much to offer the assessment of children with complex problems. This model focuses on the responses of the 'adaptive' person to a constantly changing environment (Fawcett, 1995). Roy's nursing assessment comprises two stages:

1. Stage one: identification of 'adaptive' and 'maladaptive' behaviours in relation to four domains:
   - physiological mode
   - self-concept mode
   - role function mode
   - interdependence
2. Stage two: identification of the stimuli that are thought to be responsible for the maladaptive behaviours. These stimuli are grouped into:
   - *Focal stimulus:* the one most directly and immediately confronting the patient (as defined by nurse, child [where possible] and family)
   - *Contextual stimuli:* all other stimuli present that influence the behaviour being observed

- *Residual stimuli:* the wider influences the patient may experience related to parent and family knowledge, beliefs, motivations, confidence and abilities

The principles of competent nursing assessment include use of an appropriate model in which to frame: the assessment; the involvement of the parents and the child, where possible; use of positive language about what the child is able to do, as well as what they are unable to do; and regular review of the assessment undertaken. The emphasis within assessment will change according to the child's age and developmental stage and the family's needs (Cogher et al., 1992). However, we propose core elements for consideration under the problems 'mobility', 'eating and drinking' and 'communication'.

Parents are increasingly being recognised for the experts that they are in the care and the management of their child with disability (Beresford, 1994, 1995; de Geeter et al., 2002; NSF, 2003; Taanila et al., 2002). It is vital that nursing assessment takes place in meaningful dialogue with the parent. Assessment will involve observation of the parent–child interaction and of the child alone and against developmental milestones, as well as through nursing interventions (e.g. taking vital signs).

The principles of competent nursing intervention with the child with complex motor disability include establishing a meaningful, working partnership with the child and family; meeting the child's prioritised needs for nursing care; identifying and meeting the child and family's information needs and promoting their adaptation to the environment in which they are being cared for. Communicating with and coordinating other service providers is vital to avoid duplication or the opposite – opening a new gap in the family's support network. In the case of hospitalisation, preparation for discharge should be begin on the day of admission.

 ACTIVITY

Review Northern Ireland's 2009 Developing Services to Children and Young People with Complex Physical Healthcare Needs at:
- https://www.health-ni.gov.uk/sites/default/files/publications/dhssps/developing-services-children09_1.pdf

Mobility

Complex motor impairment involves dysfunction of postural control, especially in children with cerebral palsy (Brogan et al., 1998; Westcott et al., 1997). Posture will be significantly affected in children with other conditions affecting truncal control and muscle strength (e.g. spina bifida, spinal muscular atrophy). Posture has been defined as the ability to maintain or control the centre of mass in relation to the base support (Westcott et al., 1997). A sitting position is defined as a static balance, in comparison to a dynamic balance, which relates to walking. Attaining static balance is a prerequisite of dynamic balance.

In the long-term management of the child with complex motor disability, specialist physiotherapists and occupational therapists jointly oversee the assessment and planning of

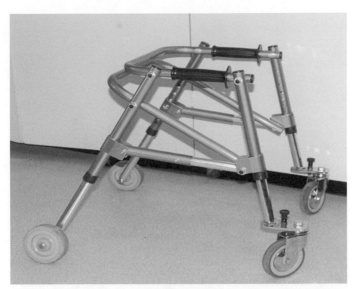

Fig. 17.1 Postural control walker. This walker or rollator can be pushed or pulled (in reverse). It encourages the child to adopt a good posture, with the shoulders back, upright posture and leg extension.

mobility (Fig. 17.1) and seating arrangements. This service is usually run in conjunction with the skill and expertise of specialist technicians in seating, aids and appliances. These professionals aim to optimise the child's posture and comfort, which will then enhance the child's respiration, eating, drinking, digestion, ability to communicate and help with moving and handling by the child's parents and carers. Physiotherapy services tend to be arranged, as might be expected, to provide the most intense levels of treatment to those most severely affected (Gough et al., 1993; Haylock et al., 1993; Parkes et al., 2002). The aims of the physiotherapy for the child with complex motor disability are likely to be conservative and directed towards preventing further complications, as well as advising and supporting families to continue with 'good practice' at home.

The physiotherapist is the most common professional seen by the population of children with cerebral palsy (Parkes et al., 2002), but is likely to be only one of the many key providers for children with complex problems. The children's nurse has a responsibility to liaise closely with the child's physiotherapist and occupational therapist to ensure good practice in relation to mobility, seating and positioning; and to adopt strategies aimed at preventing contractures or pressure areas and ensure these are incorporated in the plan of nursing care. Also, any new developing problems, for example, hip pain or dislocation, need to be identified and appropriate nursing interventions taken as early as possible. In the absence of independent walking, useful arm and hand function becomes particularly important to achieve independent mobility as a wheelchair user.

Bottos et al. (2001) found that the introduction of powered wheelchairs (Fig. 17.2) for children with severe motor disability, including those with coexisting severe learning disability, enabled 21 of 27 children to move around independently and led to improved socialisation, but interestingly not to overall quality of life. The majority of parents in this study were not in favour of the introduction of powered wheelchairs at the beginning of the study but 23 of 25 expressed positive feelings at the end of the study.

There is evidence that the mobility of children with cerebral palsy is also affected by the environment or setting (Palisano et al., 2003), which should be taken into consideration by the children's nurse when undertaking assessment of the child and family. Palisano et al. (2003) found there was increased independence at school or in the community with wheelchair use, although few children self-propelled or used powered wheelchairs. However, this independence diminished at home for the most severely affected children, 39% of whom were carried about by a parent. Capturing information about the child's functional abilities in different settings (Figs 17.3 and 17.4) is therefore very important and should include a description of abilities at home, in school and in the community.

Orthopaedic surgery can lead to improvements in the day-to-day management of children in relation to personal hygiene, dressing and mobility. More specifically, the aims of orthopaedic surgery for the child with complex motor disability includes improving function, preventing pain, improving hygiene and appearance (Cogher et al., 1992). Innovative treatments such as botulinum toxin also have a role in assisting management of limbs and joints affected by spasticity. Botulinum toxin is injected in minute amounts into targeted muscles and creates a temporary paralysis (see Korman et al. [2003] for guidelines on the use of botulinum toxin injections for spasticity associated with cerebral palsy in children).

Nursing Assessment of Mobility

In relation to assessment of the child's mobility and seating, we suggest the criteria in Box 17.1 are considered as part of good practice to ensure a complete and accurate assessment

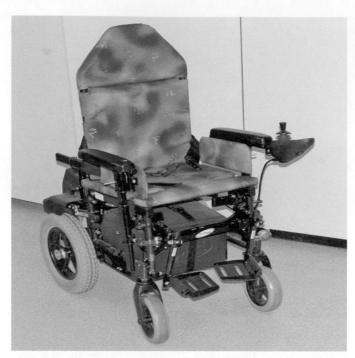

Fig. 17.2 Powered wheelchair. This chair has a child-operated control panel to give the child more independence. This example is suitable for a child with head control, although a head rest can also be added, and should be for all children during transport. Note the seat belt and foot plates to ensure good positioning and safety. An electric battery sits under the seat and must be charged regularly.

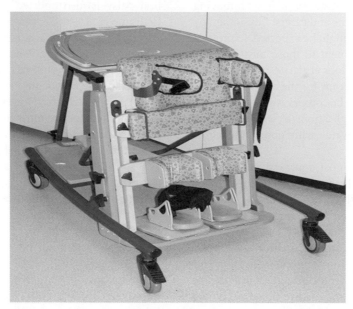

Fig. 17.3 Prone stander. A prone stander offers an alternative position to help prevent deformities. It offers optimum hip symmetry and ensures a prolonged, passive stretch at the hips, knees and feet and ankles. This stander can also promote alertness and has an adjustable work surface to help prevent the child drooping forward.

of need is conducted. Some of these suggestions are derived from an assessment form developed by Evans et al. (1989), aimed at standardising the description of children with motor impairment of central origin. We have adapted the content of the box to reflect an assessment form using the Roper et al. (1990, p 56) model for nursing practice and this template is used throughout.

Nursing Interventions in Mobility

The children's nurse, and particularly those with specialist orthopaedic training, has much to offer the child with complex motor disability and their family in terms of skill and knowledge in relation to mobility.

Adaptive seating can prevent or delay musculoskeletal deformities, enhanced postural control, upper limb control

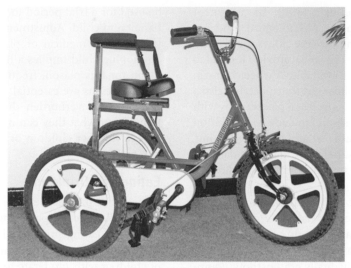

Fig. 17.4 Adapted tricycle. This tricycle comes with a seat belt and foot plates with straps. Riding the tricycle encourages good positioning, postural control and muscle strength. It is suitable for children who are non-ambulant. It promotes reciprocal movement by breaking total body synergy associated with involuntary movements.

BOX 17.1   Proposed Nursing Assessment of Mobility for Children With Complex Motor Problems

Therapy History
- Take a brief physiotherapy history.
- Who usually treats the child? Where? How often?
- Do the parents conduct any regimes at home?
- Describe usual parental practice.
- Discuss any preventive strategies with the parents, e.g. does the child wear splints at night?
- Check when and how these are applied.

Type of Motor Impairment
- Describe the nature of the motor impairment.
- Is there altered tone? If yes, is it increased or decreased?
- Are there abnormal or involuntary movements?

Extent of Motor Impairment
- Describe the distribution of the impairment.
- How many limbs are affected?
- Is one side of the body more affected than the other?
- Are the legs more affected than the arms?
- Are the arms more affected than the legs?

Head, Neck and Trunk Control
- Describe the distribution of the impairment.
- Is the child able to hold their head up? For how long?
- If not, what is the most comfortable way to support the child's head?
- Can the child sit unsupported? For how long?
- If not, what is the best way to support the child in a sitting position?
- Is there any evidence of curvature of the spine?

Leg Function
- Assess the level of motor independence.
- Is the child able to walk 15 steps unaided?
- How far can the child walk (give approximate distance)?
- Comment on the use of aids for walking (e.g. crutches, sticks, rollator).
- If the child uses a wheelchair, can he or she mobilise independently? How far?

Arm Function
- Assess the level of motor independence.
- Does the child have any self-care or self-mobilising skills?
- Does the child require assistance with dressing? If yes, how much assistance?
- Does the child require any help with eating or drinking? If yes, how much?

Aids and Appliances
- Assess and describe good handling and posture regimes for the child: include seating, standing and mobility.
- Describe any other appliances used, e.g. night splints.

Complications
- Assess if any complications exist.
- Describe any contractures that are present and describe position, severity and impact on child's ability. Check ankles, knees, hips, elbows and wrists.
- Describe the child's feet and footwear noting any abnormalities of posture (e.g. valgus) or problems related to comfort.
- Note the presence of scoliosis or kyphosis because this may have important implications for positioning and comfort.

and oral motor control (Roxborough, 1995). The treatment can also increase comfort, improve physiological function, enhance function abilities and increase the child's social interaction. Cogher et al. (1992, pp 152–166) provide a detailed description of the types of seating available. A wheelchair can offer not only independent mobility and transport, but also a position for eating and drinking, as well as a place to play with toys. Arranging suitable seating should include consideration of body posture, head control, and feet and limb positioning. Restraining straps, cushion requirements and material type are also vital in assuring the safe transport, tissue viability and hygiene needs of the child.

Providing equipment for mobility and positioning, especially if spinal curvature is present or has undergone correction, will often involve a dedicated orthotic team. Specialist technicians whose purpose is to maximise function, comfort and social acceptability will individually craft orthotic equipment (Fig. 17.5). Standard equipment will be adjusted to meet the needs of the individual. The parent will also require easy storage of equipment at home and during transportation, with ease of assembly and disassembly a high priority. If the equipment is static, consideration of space within the home is an important factor.

A main intervention in relation to seating and mobility is teaching parents about safe lifting and handling of the child, about continuing therapy routines at home and about safe use and storage of the equipment. The equipment can then be used for a trial period to review its effectiveness for both parent and child. Adjustments are often required, especially if the child's medical or physical status has changed. The developing child implies a limited life span for such equipment; for this reason, frequent check-ups and adjustments by technicians are essential for optimum use. Care must be taken not to 'overburden' the family with too high expectations about what they can manage at home, given that they may have other children or family commitments, and may also work.

Eating and Drinking

An association between severe neurodevelopmental conditions like cerebral palsy and impaired oromotor function leading to eating problems has been identified (Gisel and Alphonce, 1995). Samson-Fang et al. (2003) cited that 27% of children with moderate to severe cerebral palsy included in a North American follow-up study were found to be malnourished (as measured by skin-fold thickness). Problems with eating and drinking vary from mild problems related to control of salvia or chewing ability, to severe problems with disturbances of gut motility, reflux and vomiting.

One of the most important assessment indicators of health in children is growth and a primary reason for intervening in eating and drinking is concern about the adequacy of nutrition as evidenced by poor growth. Children with severe oromotor impairment can take from 2 to 12 times

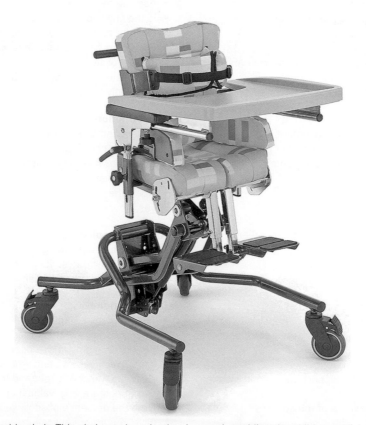

Fig. 17.5 Adaptable chair. This chair can be raised or lowered, enabling the child to participate in different activities that take place at different heights – eating, playing or working at a desk. Note the knee blocks to help maintain hip position. The chair also has trunk and lateral supports with adjustable foot plates.

longer to manipulate and swallow a standard amount of pureed food, and 1–15 times longer to chew and swallow solid food (Gisel and Patrick, 1988). These children are at higher risk of experiencing poor growth and weight gain, although artificial feeding techniques have been found to be effective in helping to establish weight gain. Furthermore, persistent feeding problems in young children with cerebral palsy have been identified as a marker for poor feeding, growth and developmental outcome later in childhood, and could be used to identify those children with cerebral palsy who might benefit from gastrostomy feeding (Motion et al., 2002). Given the complexity of the problems, a team approach to assessment is most effective and usually consists of parents, teacher, speech and language specialist, occupational therapist, physiotherapist, dietician, paediatrician and children's nurse.

Nursing Assessment in Eating and Drinking

The severely affected child is assessed for his or her ability to coordinate sucking and breathing during feeds, with evidence of problems recognised during weaning. An inability to gain weight and the deterioration to low-weight-for-age-specific percentiles within the first year of life are characteristic. The assessment of eating and drinking impairment is based on measures of growth and eating skills: eating efficiency and oral motor skills (Gisel and Alphonce, 1995). To make a detailed eating and drinking assessment, knowledge of what happens at meal times along with aspects of proposed change

by the parent/carer is necessary. A profile of contributing factors is also required as part of the assessment and planning prior to professional intervention.

A second component that relates to the assessment and planning of eating and drinking is drooling. This problem is again often associated with cerebral palsy children with poor oromotor function. Intensive drooling leads to negative social interactions, schooling issues and physical effects: chapped and sore lips and chin, sodden clothes and often an unpleasant smell (Lloyd Faulconbridge et al., 2001). The multidisciplinary team assesses such drooling along with individual planning and intervention.

In relation to assessment of the child's eating and drinking, the criteria in Box 17.2 are considered part of good practice to ensure that a complete and accurate assessment of need is conducted. Some of the suggestions in the box are derived from Evans et al. (1989) and Cogher et al. (1992).

Nursing Interventions in Eating and Drinking

If it is apparent that adequate nutrition is being achieved, parents may just need reassurance, especially if eating is very messy. Simple alterations to posture and seating can prove very effective in enhancing dietary intake. Oral fluid intake may be altered through a thickening agent; a thicker consistency prevents reflux, choking and aspiration. This approach can also encourage a higher fluid intake and prevent dehydration. Food consistency may also be changed, for example, from mashed to puréed textures. A change in equipment – spoons

---

BOX 17.2 Proposed Nursing Assessment of Eating and Drinking for Children With Complex Motor Problems

Adequacy of Nutrition
- Assess growth: height, weight.
- Assess rate of growth.
- Compare parent and professional assessment of growth and nutritional status.
- Take feeding history: length of time to complete a meal; assess daily intake and daily loss (vomiting).
- Describe amount and type of food intake.

History
- Find out about early feeding habits.
- Seek and include histories of dietetic and speech and language therapy input.
- Assess if any referrals might be necessary.

Oral Skills
- Note dentition, any structural problems that might make eating or breathing while eating difficult.
- Observe and comment on ability to chew, swallow, clear palate, control saliva.
- Look for drooling.

Tolerance
- Assess if the child is prone to choking, coughing, spluttering, vomiting. Record frequency.

- Cogher et al. (1992) emphasise the importance of assessing tolerance through behaviours – turning away, refusing to eat, crying, grimacing, gagging or vomiting.

Food Preferences
- Describe the child's food preferences.
- Also describe the preferred texture (lumpy, solid, puréed); preferred feeding utensils.

Feeding Technique
- Describe breathing pattern while eating and assess the risk of aspiration as far as possible.
- Describe the parents' technique.
- How do the parents position the child for eating and drinking?
- What special utensils do they have, or are preferred?

Digestion and Elimination
- Is there any evidence of pain and discomfort on eating and drinking?
- Is there any history of constipation or other gastrointestinal problems: reflux, obstruction, rupture?

Parents' Attitudes
- Find out about parents' feelings towards their child's nutrition, and eating and drinking: are these associated with stress?

(Fig. 17.6) and cups (Fig. 17.7) – often works in harmony with feeding techniques, which again reduce the risk of choking and aspiration. Cogher et al. (1992) also suggest desensitising the child's face and mouth before eating by the use of touch, if behaviour intolerance or an excess of involuntary movements are present.

Alternatively, a period of hospitalisation may be necessary often for the insertion and parental education of a nasogastric tube feeding. Failure of such a system due to either non-compliance or tube insertion issues may lead to a long-term option, that of a gastrostomy feeding system. Gastrostomy is not without risk, although the benefits of adequate nutrition usually outweigh the risks of complications. Gastrostomy feeding has been associated with improved growth and quality of life in children with cerebral palsy (Smith et al., 1999). This system, established by insertion of a tube through the abdominal wall into the stomach, is for long-term use. Regardless of the feeding method utilised, oral hygiene of the mouth is essential to reduce tooth decay and other related medical problems. Support and trouble-shooting for all feeding interventions can be sought within the community from a variety of health care professionals and at relevant hospital clinics.

◎ EVIDENCE-BASED PRACTICE

The American Academy for Cerebral Palsy and Developmental Medicine (AACPDM) undertook a systematic review of the outcomes of gastrostomy feeding in children with cerebral palsy (Samson-Fang et al., 2003). The findings of the systematic review are summarised below:

- Ten studies met all the inclusion criteria and were included in the review. The 10 studies contain results on a total of 281 individuals.
- All the studies were described by Samson-Fang et al. (2003) as comprising 'very low levels of evidence' when evaluated against the AACPDM quality rating scheme.
- Overall, however, there was consistency in the results, which favoured gastrostomy feeding.

This systematic review provides an excellent example of how to investigate the evidence base for practice in a rigorous way and could be used as the 'gold standard' in assessing the evidence for children's nursing.

Feeding and language-related problems often go together in children with severe cerebral palsy, even though speech production does not inevitably correlate with earlier oral-motor patterns (Dormans and Pellegrino, 1998). The next section considers the related area of communication.

More recently, Parkes et al. (2010) report the prevalence, clinical associations, and trends over time of oromotor dysfunction and communication impairments in children with cerebral palsy. Multiple sources of ascertainment were used and children followed up with a standardised assessment including motor speech problems, swallowing/chewing difficulties, excessive drooling and communication impairments at age 5 years.

Of the total, 1357 children born between 1980 and 2001 were studied (781 males, 576 females; median age 5 years 11

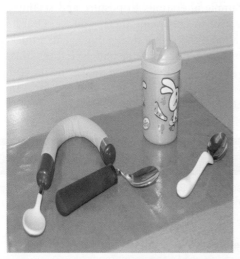

Fig. 17.6 Spoons. Flexi-spoons are available to help children feed more easily and independently.

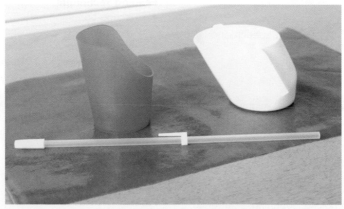

Fig. 17.7 Cups and straws. A cup with an angled rim means that the child does not have to throw the head back if self-feeding. If being fed from these cups, the feeder has extra control in the amount of liquid the child receives. The straw has a non-return valve that helps children with poor sucking ability. Note the non-slip mat to prevent spillages.

months, interquartile range 3–9 years; unilateral spastic CP, n = 447; bilateral spastic CP, n = 496; other, n = 112; Gross Motor Function Classification System [GMFCS] level: I, 181; II, 563; III, 123; IV, 82; V, 276). Of those with 'early-onset' CP (n = 1268), 36% had motor speech problems, 21% had swallowing/chewing difficulties, 22% had excessive drooling, and 42% had communication impairments (excluding articulation defects). All impairments were significantly related to poorer gross motor function and intellectual impairment. In addition, motor speech problems were related to clinical subtype; swallowing/chewing problems and communication impairments to early mortality; and communication impairments to the presence of seizures. Of those with CP in GMFCS levels IV–V, a significant proportion showed a decline in the rate of motor speech impairment (p = 0.008) and excessive drooling (p = 0.009) over time. In summary, these impairments are common in children with CP and are associated with poorer gross motor function and intellectual impairment.

What this paper adds
- Half the population of children with CP will have one or more impairments of oromotor function, or communication or both.
- The risk of these impairments increases with declining gross motor function and intellectual impairment.
- Motor speech impairment and excessive drooling have significantly declined in the non-ambulant CP population over time.

Communication

Speech and language facilitate learning and regulate behaviour; they are also critical developmental tasks that form the basis for all social interactions. The ability to communicate is fundamental to expressing personal need or opinion. Children will often use their natural modes of communication, such as vocalisation, eye-pointing, gesture and body movements. Play can also enhance communication through motivation, imagination and the development of social skills. Several examples of good practice exist in the literature (Brodin, 1999; Crawford and Raven, 2002) and make useful suggestions to strengthen play opportunities for this group. Children restricted by physical and cognitive limitations, who are not given adequate opportunities for free play, are being further disadvantaged.

Children with significant neuromotor impairments may experience problems related to articulation of speech and language and/or problems related to intellectual ability and the ability to communicate and express themselves. Pennington and McConachie (1999) studied the interaction between non-verbal children with severe motor impairment and their carers. The findings indicated that the adults took control of conversations, instigated topics, asked questions and issued commands. The children provided the required responses, using a restricted range of communicative functions. This highlights the importance of children's nurses understanding how to communicate with non-verbal children. However, work conducted by Beail (1985) found that nurses had

low-level and poor-quality interactions with children with multiple disabilities; it is to be hoped that awareness and practice have changed since then.

Nursing Assessment in Communication

In relation to the assessment of a child's communication abilities, the criteria in Box 17.3 are considered part of good practice to ensure a complete and accurate assessment of need is conducted. Some of the suggestions are derived from Evans et al. (1989) and Cogher et al. (1992).

BOX 17.3 Proposed Nursing Assessment of Communication for Children With Complex Motor Problems

Oromotor Abilities
- Are problems related to articulation of speech apparent (dysarthria)?
- Record history of speech and language therapy.

Social Interaction
- What motivates the child to communicate: happy? sad? hunger? pain? Assess in conjunction with parents.
- Describe child's experiences and knowledge of play.
- Is the child able to participate in symbolic play?

Means of Expression
- Describe means of expression: verbal or non-verbal.
- Alternative methods of communication: eye pointing? sounds?
- Formalised systems such as Makaton?
- Describe if any involuntary facial expressions are apparent – these can sometimes be misleading.

Non-Verbal Skills
- Describe non-verbal skills, especially if the child is unable to speak.
- Describe eye contact, vocalisation, body movements (head control, unwanted movements, facial grimacing).
- Describe if the child is able to 'take turns' in any interaction, assess attention span.

Comprehension
- Is there a reliable yes/no response: to nurse, to parents, to others?
- Ask parents level of understanding.
- Also record type of school attended; psychologist's reports.

Use of Expressive Language
- Describe use of expressive language: range and depth of vocabulary. Age appropriate?

Phonology
- Describe how the words sound: accurate?

Family Communication
- Describe any child and family communication strategies that might exist, in particular the role of play, particular games.
- Describe how the parents and siblings communicate with the child.

Nursing Interventions in Communication

Effective assessment is imperative to optimise a child's communication and development potential. Impairments, including hearing, visual, cognitive (learning disability), attention deficits, respiratory problems, orthopaedic anomalies and other medical conditions (e.g. seizures, respiratory problems, gastroesophageal reflux), may all affect the child's ability to communicate (Cass et al., 1999). The key interventions to facilitate communication in the child with complex motor problems, as described by Cogher et al. (1992), should focus on good positioning – to maximise eye contact and minimise involuntary movements and facilitated expression through constructive play and augmented communication systems (Figs 17.8 and 17.9).

To maximise the successful use of augmentative communication systems, the child should be introduced to the system as early as possible; professionals and parents need to be trained to facilitate the child and there needs to be planning and cooperation between the professional multi agencies (Ko et al., 1998). During a period of hospitalisation, it is essential that the children's nurse supports the child to continue to use and develop his or her skills in augmentative communication systems as far as possible.

Ineffective communication can lead to frustration, which is sometimes interpreted as 'bad behaviour' in the child. Frustration can be expressed through non-compliance to care with rigid or thrashing torso and high vocalisation. The child may be expressing a need to change position or to resolve hunger, toiletry needs or pain. Free play can help alleviate such communication difficulties through development of the whole child. Behavioural cues may be misleading so parents and health professionals must be cautious in their assessment and planning. Facial impressions can be misunderstood due to low muscle tone, and vocalisations can be misinterpreted due to increased laryngeal spasticity.

Promoting function requires the building of skills as well as developing compensatory mechanisms to help the child best function within the limits of his or her motor and cognitive abilities. Once a child's communication deficits and potential have been established, the specialist team of speech therapist and medical consultant must implement a phase of planning. Such planning will be shared within a larger team,

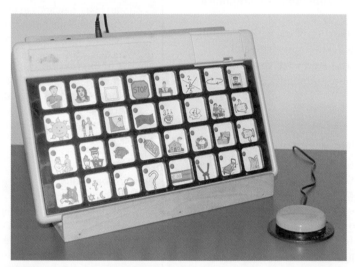

Fig. 17.8 Symbols for communication. Picture symbols can be used to communicate. This communications board is activated by a switch. The child practises controlling the switch through work and play.

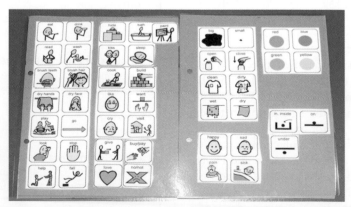

Fig. 17.9 More symbols. This Makaton system is another example of symbols for communication. It is based on picture symbols. The child points at the words, and with practice, can build up relatively sophisticated communication. A booklet can be customised for each individual child.

to include the paediatric nurse, health visitor, teacher, physiotherapist and occupational therapist. The aim is to develop all areas that will facilitate optimum communication for the child. If speech is not an available option, alternative skills such as pointing, picture boards, and non-verbal cues will be developed to ensure the child's needs are met. If the child is visually and hearing impaired, non-verbal responses such as body language along with the positive communication of a familiar parent/carer is vital for effective child communication.

SUMMARY

This chapter has brought together a number of perspectives in the consideration of children with complex motor disability. Although complex motor disability is relatively rare, as are the conditions that give rise to it, the level of need and support required by children and their families is high and lifelong. Multiple agencies are involved in the provision of care and services to these children and care must be taken not to overburden families with too many professionals, but at the same time ensure their needs are met. Parents caring for a child with complex motor disability are experts in their own right and a valued partner for the children's nurse. This chapter considered a small number of predominant problems experienced by children with complex needs. In particular, detailed consideration was given to what the children's nurse should assess and how they should intervene in the areas of mobility, eating and drinking and communication.

ACKNOWLEDGEMENTS

We would like to thank Daniel's Mum for her frank and honest account of her experiences caring for her son. We would also like to thank Mrs Sheila McNeill, Paediatric Physiotherapist, and Mrs Julia Maskery, Paediatric Occupational Therapist, for advice on the use of aids and adaptations as featured in the photographs and accompanying text; and Mrs Doris Corkin, Nurse Lecturer, for reading and commenting on an earlier draft.

REFERENCES

Bamford, D., Griffith, H., Kernohan, G., 1991. I Felt Like Running Away: The Social and Emotional Implications of Cerebral Palsy. Boys' and Girls' Welfare Society, London.

Bamford, D., Griffith, H., Kernohan, G., 1997. Analysis of consumer satisfaction with cerebral palsy care. Br. J. Soc. Work 27, 605–614.

Beail, N., 1985. The nature of interactions between nursing staff and profoundly multiply handicapped children. Child Care Health Dev. 11, 113–129.

Beale, H., 2002. Respite care for technology-dependent children and their families. Paediatr. Nurs. 14, 18–19.

Beresford, B., 1994. Positively Parents. Caring for a Severely Disabled Child. Social Policy Research Unit. HMSO, London.

Beresford, B., 1995. Expert Opinions. A National Survey of Families Caring for a Severely Disabled Child. Policy Press, Bristol.

Bone, M., Meltzer, H., 1989. The Prevalence of Disability Among Children. HMSO, London.

Bottos, M., Bolcati, C., Sciuto, L., et al., 2001. Powered wheelchairs and independence in young children with tetraplegia. Dev. Med. Child Neurol. 43, 769–777.

Brodin, J., 1999. Play in children with severe multiple disabilities: play with toys – a review. Inte. J. Dis. Dev. Edu. 46, 25–34.

Brogan, E., Hadders-Algra, M., Forssberg, H., 1998. Postural control in sitting children with cerebral palsy. Neurosci. Behav. Rev. 22, 591–596.

Cans, C., De-la-Cruz, J., Mermet, M.A., 2008. Epidemiology of cerebral palsy. Paediatr. Child. Health 18 (9), 393–398.

Cass, H., Price, K., Reilly, S., et al., 1999. A model for the assessment and management of children with multiple disabilities. Child. Care. Health. Dev. 25, 191–211.

Children and Young People's Health Outcomes Forum, 2012. Report of Children and Young People's Health Outcomes Forum. England: Children and Young People's Health Outcomes Forum Available at https://assets.publishing.service.gov.uk/government/uploads/system/uploads/attachment_data/file/216852/CYP-report.pdf.

Cogher, L., Savage, E., Smith, M.F., 1992. Cerebral Palsy. The Child and Young Person. Chapman & Hall Medical, London.

Colver, A.F., Mackie, P., 1998. North of England collaborative cerebral palsy survey. Ann. Rep.

Crawford, C., Raven, K., 2002. Play preparation for children with special needs. Paediatr. Nurs. 14, 27–29.

Crichton, J.U., MacKinnon, M., White, C.P., 1995. The life expectancy of person with cerebral palsy. Dev. Med. Child Neurol. 37, 567–576.

de Geeter, K.I., Poppes, P., Vlaskamp, C., 2002. Parents as experts: the position of parents of children with profound multiple disabilities. Child. Care. Health. Dev. 28, 443–453.

Dormans, J.P., Pellegrino, L. (Eds.), 1998. Caring for Children with Cerebral Palsy: A Team Approach. Brookes Publishing, London.

Duffy, B., 1995. PPRU Surveys of Disability Report 5: Disabled Children in Northern Ireland: Services, Transport and Education. Policy Planning and Research Unit, Belfast.

Edmond, A., Golding, J., Peckham, C., 1989. Cerebral palsy in two national cohort studies. Arch. Dis. Child. 60, 1113–1121.

Evans, P.M., Evans, S.J.W., Alberman, E., 1989. A standard form for recording clinical findings in children with a motor deficit of central origin (letter). Dev. Med. Child Neurol. 31, 121–127.

Fawcett, J., 1995. Analysis and Evaluation of Conceptual Models of Nursing, third ed. FA Davis, Philadelphia.

Gisel, E.G., Alphonce, E., 1995. Classification of eating impairments based on eating efficiency in children with cerebral palsy. Dysphagia 10, 268–274.

Gisel, E.G., Patrick, J., 1988. Identification of children with cerebral palsy unable to maintain a normal nutritional state. Lancet 1, 283–286.

Glendinning, C., Kirk, S., Guiffridda, A., et al., 1999. The Community Based Care of Technology Dependent Children in the UK: Definitions, Numbers and Costs. National Primary Care Research and Development Centre. University of Manchester, Manchester.

Glendinning, C., Kirk, S., Guiffridda, A., et al., 2001. Technology-dependent children in the community: definitions, numbers and costs. Child. Care. Health. Dev. 27, 321–334.

Gordon, D., Parker, R., Loughran, F., et al., 2000. Disabled Children in Britain. A Re-Analysis of the OPCS Disability Survey. The Stationery Office, London.

Gough, D., Li, L., Wroblewska, A., 1993. Services for Children With a Motor Impairment and Their Families in Scotland. Public Health Research Unit. University of Glasgow.

Haylock, C., Johnson, A.M., Harpin, V.A., 1993. Parents' views of community care for children with motor disabilities. Child. Care. Health. Dev. 19, 209–220.

Hutton, J., Cook, T., Pharoah, P.O.D., 1994. Life expectancy in children with cerebral palsy. Br. Med. J. 309, 431–435.

Hutton, J., Pharoah, P.O.D., 1998. Life expectancy in people with cerebral palsy. Abstract from an annual meeting. In: Colver, A., Mackie, P. (Eds.), North of England Collaborative Cerebral Palsy Survey. Annual Report November 19–25.

Imms, C., Novak, I., Kerr, C., et al., 2015. Improving allied health professionals' research implementation behaviours for children with cerebral palsy: protocol for a before-after study. Implement. Sci. 10 (16), 2–8.

Ingram, T.T.S., 1955. A study of cerebral palsy in the childhood population of Edinburgh. Arch. Dis. Child. 60, 1113–1121.

Jarvis, S.N., Holloway, J.S., Hey, E.N., 1985. Increase in cerebral palsy in normal birthweight babies. Arch. Dis. Child. 60, 1113–1121.

Johnson, A., King, R., 1998. Oxford Register of Early Childhood Impairments. Annual Report 1997. National Perinatal Epidemiology Unit, Oxford.

Kingdom, S., Mayfield, C., 2001. Complex disabilities: parents preparing professionals. Paediatr. Nurs. 13 (7), 34–38.

Ko, M.L.B., McConachie, H., Jolieff, N., 1998. Outcome of recommendations for augmentative communication in children. Child. Care. Health. Dev. 24, 195–205.

Korman, L.A., Paterson Smith, B., Ballrishnan, R., 2003. Spasticity associated with cerebral palsy in children. Pediatr. Drugs 5, 11–23.

Lloyd Faulconbridge, R.V., Tranter, R.M., Moffat, V., et al., 2001. Review of management of drooling problems in neurologically impaired children: a review of methods and results over 6 years at Chailey Heritage Clinical Services. Clin. Otolaryngol. 26, 76–81.

MacGillivray, I., Campbell, D., 1995. The changing pattern of cerebral palsy in Avon. Paediatr. Perinat. Epidemiol. 9, 146–155.

McConachie, H., 1997. Organization of child disability services. Guest editorial. Child Care Health Dev. 23, 3–9.

McConachie, H., Salt, A., Chadury, Y., et al., 1999. How do child development teams work? Findings from a UK national survey. Child. Care. Health. Dev. 25, 157–168.

McConkey, R., Adams, L., 2001. Matching short break services for children with learning disabilities to family needs and preferences. Child. Care. Health. Dev. 26, 429–443.

Miller, S., 2002. Respite care for children who have complex healthcare needs. Paediatr. Nurs. 14, 33–37.

Milner, J., Bungay, C., Jellinek, D., et al., 1996. Needs of disabled children and their families. Arch. Dis. Child. 75, 399–404.

Motion, S., Northstone, K., Emond, A., et al., 2002. Early feeding problems in children with cerebral palsy: weight and neurodevelopmental outcomes. Dev. Med. Child Neurol. 44, 40–43.

Mutch, L., Alberman, E., Hagberg, G., et al., 1992. Cerebral palsy epidemiology: where have we been and where are we going? (Annotation). Dev. Med. Child Neurol. 34, 547–551.

National Service Framework (NSF), 2003. Online. Available at http://www.doh.gov.uk/nsf.

Northern Ireland Cerebral Palsy Register (NICPR), 2018. Available at https://www.qub.ac.uk/research-centres/NorthernIrelandCerebralPalsyRegister/.

Palisano, R.J., Tieman, B.L., Walter, S.D., et al., 2003. Effect of environmental setting on mobility methods of children with cerebral palsy. Dev. Med. Child Neurol. 45, 113–120.

Parkes, J., 1998. Children with cerebral palsy in Northern Ireland: needs and services. In: Unpublished PhD Thesis. Queen's University, Belfast.

Parkes, J., Dolk, H., Hill, A.E., 1998. Does the child health computing system adequately identify children with cerebral palsy? J. Publ. Health Med. 20 (1), 102–104.

Parkes, J., Donnelly, M., Hill, N., 2001a. Focusing on Cerebral Palsy: Reviewing and Communicating Needs for Services. Scope, London.

Parkes, J., Dolk, H., Hill, N., et al., 2001b. Epidemiology of cerebral palsy in Northern Ireland: 1981–1993. Paediatr. Perinat. Epidemiol. 15, 278–286.

Parkes, J., Donnelly, M., Dolk, H., et al., 2002. Use of physiotherapy and alternatives by children with cerebral palsy: a population study. Child. Care. Health. Dev. 28 (6), 469–477.

Parkes, J., Hill, N., Platt, M.J., et al., 2010. Developmental medicine and child Neurology. London 52 (12), 1113–1119.

Pennington, L., McConachie, H., 1999. Mother–child interaction revisited: communication with non-speaking physically disabled children. Int. J. Lang. Commun. Disord. 345, 391–416.

Pharoah, P.O.D., Cooke, T., Cooke, R.W.I., et al., 1990. Birthweight-specific trends in cerebral palsy. Arch. Dis. Child. 65, 602–606.

Pharoah, P.O.D., Cooke, T., Johnson, A., et al., 1998. Epidemiology of cerebral palsy in England and Scotland 1984–1989. Arch. Dis. Child. Fetal Neonatal Ed. 79 (1), F21–F25.

Priestley, M., 2003. Disability. A Life Course Approach. Polity Press, Cambridge.

Rees, S.J., 1983. Families' perceptions of services for handicapped children. Int. J. Rehabil. Res. 6, 475–476.

Roberts, K., Lawton, D., 2001. Acknowledging the extra care parents give their disabled children. Child. Care. Health. Dev. 27, 307–319.

Roper, N., Logan, W.W., Tierney, A.J., 1990. The Elements of Nursing. Churchill Livingstone, Edinburgh.

Rosenbaum, P., Paneth, N., Leviton, A., et al., 2007. The definition and classification of cerebral palsy. Dev. Med. Child Neurol. 49, 1–44.

Ross, A., Parkes, J., 2004. Making doors open: the role of the children's community nurse in caring for a child with severe cerebral palsy. Paediatr. Nurs. 16(5), 14–8.

Roxborough, L., 1995. Review of the efficacy and effectiveness of adaptive seating for children with cerebral palsy. Assist. Technol. 7, 17–25.

Roy, C., 1976. Introduction to Nursing: An Adaptation Model. Prentice-Hall, Englewood Cliffs, NJ.

Samson-Fang, L., Butler, C., O'Donnell, M., 2003. Effects of gastrostomy feeding in children with cerebral palsy: an AACPDM evidence report. Dev. Med. Child Neurol. 45, 415–426.

Sloper, P., 1999. Models of service support for parents of disabled children. What do we know? What do we need to know? Child. Care. Health. Dev. 25, 85–99.

Sloper, P., Turner, S., 1992. Service needs of families of children with severe physical disability. Child. Care. Health. Dev. 18, 259–282.

Sloper, P., Turner, S., 1993. Risk and resistance factors in the adaptation of parents of children with severe physical disability. JCPP (J. Child Psychol. Psychiatry) 34, 167–188.

Smith, F., 2003. 'Getting the right start': the children's national service framework. Paediatr. Nurs. 15, 20–21.

Smith, M., Robinson, P., Duffy, P., 1992. PPRU surveys of disability report 2: the prevalence of disability among children in Northern Ireland. In: Policy. Planning and Research Unit, Belfast.

Smith, S.W., Camfield, C., Camfield, P., 1999. Living with cerebral palsy and tube feeding: a population-based follow-up study. J. Pediatr. 135, 307–310.

Smithers–Sheedy, H., Badawi, N., Blair, E., et al., 2014. What constitutes cerebral palsy in the twenty–first century? Dev. Med. Child Neurol. 56, 323–328.

Stalker, K., 1990. Share the Care: An Evaluation of Family-Based Respite Care. Jessica Kingsley, London.

Surveillance of Cerebral Palsy in Europe (SCPE), 2000. Surveillance of cerebral palsy in Europe: a collaboration of cerebral palsy surveys and registers. Dev. Med. Child Neurol. 42, 816–824.

Taanila, A., Syrjala, L., Kokkonen, J., et al., 2002. Coping of parents with physically and/or intellectually disabled children. Child. Care. Health. Dev. 28, 73–86.

United Nations General Assembly, 1989. Convention on the Rights of the Child. UNICEF, Geneva.

Ward, T., Worswikc, J., Inglis, A., et al., 2003. Children with complex, continuing health needs and/or life-limiting conditions. Report of the Task Group. Children's National Service Framework: Disabled Children External Working Group. Online. Available from: http://www.doh.gov.uk/nsf/children.

Watson, D., Townsley, R., Abbot, D., 2002. Exploring multi-agency working in services to disabled children with complex healthcare needs and their families. J. Clin. Nurs. 11, 367–375.

Welsh, R., Dyer, S., Evans, D., et al., 2014. Welsh identifying benefits and barriers to respite for carers of children with complex health needs: a qualitative study. Contemp. Nurse 48 (1), 98–108.

Westcott, S.L., Lowes, L.P., Richardson, P.K., 1997. Evaluation of postural stability in children: current theories and assessment tools. Phys. Ther. 77, 629–645.

Whiting, M., 2014. Support requirements of parents caring for the child with disability and complex health needs. Nurs. Child. Young People 26 (4), 24–27.

Williams, K., Hennessey, E., Alberman, E., 1996. Cerebral palsy: effects of twinning birthweight and gestational age. Arch. Dis. Child. 75, F178–F182.

World Health Organization (WHO), 1980. International Classification of Impairments, Disability and Handicap (ICIDH). World Health Organization, Geneva.

World Health Organization (WHO), 2001. Beginner's Guide. Towards a Common Language for Functioning, Disability and Health (ICF). World Health Organization, Geneva.

World Health Organization (WHO), 2002. International Classification of Functioning, Disability and Health. World Health Organization, Geneva.

Caring for Children and Young People With Orthopaedic Disorders

Sonya Clarke

BONE BIOLOGY

The Function of the Skeletal System

The musculoskeletal system consists of 206 bones with their surrounding muscles. The main functions of the bones of the skeleton are to support and give shape to the body, to protect vital organs and to provide a system of levers that enables the body to make movements. In addition, bone serves as storage sites for certain minerals such as calcium and is also responsible for the production of red and white blood cells, a function performed by the red bone marrow. Yellow bone marrow acts as a storage site for lipids.

 ACTIVITY

Using a suitable anatomy and physiology textbook or suitable online source, identify and name the different bones of the body. Examine the relative significance of each bone in relation to its main function and location within the human skeleton.

Bone Structure

Bones are extremely strong and can withstand considerable forces. Bone is very resilient and can return to its normal shape after the removal of the force that caused it to become

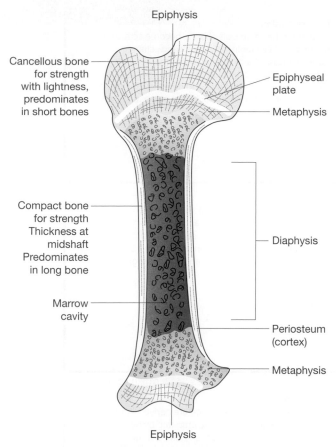

Fig. 18.1 Cross-section of bone.

misshapen. This tensile strength and resilience is due to the framework of interwoven fibres within bone called *collagen*, which is a tough, white, slightly flexible material. Bones are made up of two types of tissue (Fig. 18.1):

- Compact or cortical bone: the dense and hard part of the bone that gives the bone its shape and strength. It is made up of many rods, known as the Haversian system. These have a central canal, which contains blood vessels and nerve fibres, and is surrounded by several sheets of bone tissue called lamellae. The Haversian canals branch and interweave, giving bone great strength along lines of stress.
- Cancellous or spongy bone: composed of fine bars of bony tissue that interlace with one another to give a honeycomb appearance. These bars of tissue are known as the trabecular bone and are strong, light and provide an excellent structure to absorb stress. The space within the trabeculae is filled by the red blood marrow.

All bones are covered by a layer of fibrous tissue called periosteum, which protects the bone and allows the circumference of the bone to grow.

Bone Growth, Formation and Resorption

- Bone repair and remodelling occurs throughout life (Wright, 2014) (Fig. 18.2). Bone remodelling is a continuous metabolic process within the body which involves the breakdown and renewal of bone by specialised cells. This process secures skeletal integrity and blood mineral

homeostasis throughout the life course; imbalances in bone remodelling can result in bone conditions. Clarke and Santy-Tomlinson (2014, p 30) report the function of osteoclasts developed from circulating monocytes and located around the surface of the bone is around 'the resorption of bone which is important in the development, growth, maintenance and repair of bone'. The specialist process by 'osteoclasts' cells takes around 2 weeks followed by cell death. Osteoblasts which have no mitotic potential and located on the surface of bone are reported to be involved in 'bone formation by secreting organic compounds and minerals' (Clarke and Santy-Tomlinson 2014, p 30). The specialist process by 'osteoblasts' cells over time, that is, 2–3 months, create the new layered bone which becomes denser and with some of the osteoblasts become osteocytes when trapped within the new bone. Their function is then to maintain the daily cellular activities of bone. From infancy through to adolescence, bones are actively growing in length, width and density (Table. 18.1). Bone remodelling is regulated by several factors including: Mechanical loads arising from muscle forces regulate the process of bone formation and resorption. For example, a tennis player's racket arm is typically stronger and wider than a non-player's arm because the remodelling bone has adapted to the increased daily strain and loading experienced when serving the ball.

- Calcium: this is the most abundant mineral found within the body. It is arranged around the matrix of collagen, which gives bone its strength and rigidity. Calcium is stored in the bone and released when serum calcium levels are low. A normal serum calcium level is required to allow adequate muscle contraction, transmission of impulses across nerve cells, activities of some enzymes and the building of strong bones.
- Parathyroid hormone (PTH): controls distribution of calcium. When serum calcium concentrations are low the hormone causes increased calcium absorption from the intestines, calcium reabsorption by the kidneys and increased bone resorption. Parathyroid hormone also regulates the synthesis of the active metabolites of vitamin D, which also enhance absorption of calcium from the intestine.
- Sex hormones: oestrogen and testosterone provide a 'control' over bone resorption and keeps bone remodelling in homeostasis.

Fracture Repair and Bone Healing

The fractured ends of the bone bleed and form a clot. The inflammatory healing process commences and the dead tissue and clot is removed by macrophages. The initial strands from the blood clot begin to change into osteoid tissue, which develops and forms callus around the fracture site; osteoclasts remove necrotic bone and osteoblasts develop new bone (Clarke and Santy-Tomlinson, 2014). Between 6 and 12 weeks, as the callus hardens, the bone regains some mechanical strength. Further callus maturity occurs between 12 and 26 weeks. By 1–2 years bone remodelling has occurred (see Fig. 18.2) and normal bone shape has been restored. As children

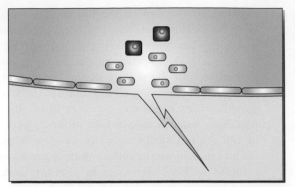

Bone resorption
At random the lining cells of bone become activated by substances including PTH & calcitriol, change from a pancake shape to a cuboid shape. The cells then secrete ODF (osteoclast differentiating factor) which allows the cells to fuse and differentiate into mature multinucleated osteoclasts (bone eating cells).

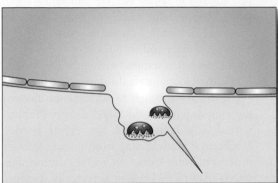

The osteoclast resorb (munch) away at the bone. New osteoclasts are activated and start resorption as the remodelling moves across the area of bone requiring repair. This resorption lasts around 2 weeks, then the osteoclasts undergo apoptosis (programmed cell death).

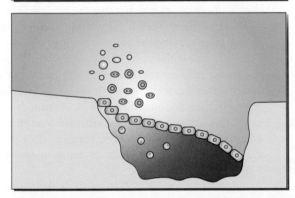

Bone formation
Osteoblasts (bone forming cells) are derived from marrow stromal cells. They are attracted by bone derived growth factors and the remains of the self-destructed osteoclasts.

The secreting osteoblasts then make layers of osteoid and slowly refill the cavity. The osteoblasts secrete a range of growth factors including osteocalcin and other proteins. The osteiod mineralises as the cavity fills.

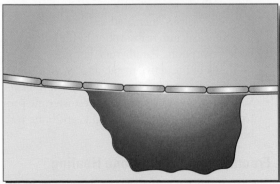

Over a period of around 3–4 months the crystals of mineral become closely packed together and the density of the new bone increases. The final osteoblasts turn into lining cells which participate in the release of calcium from the bone. Some osteoblasts turns into osteocytes (bone cell) which remain in the new bone and are connected by long cell processes which can sense mechanical stresses to the bones

Fig. 18.2 Bone remodelling. *PTH,* Parathyroid hormone. (Reproduced with permission from Silverwood, 2003.)

have a growing skeleton fracture healing is faster than in adults (Wright, 2014). It is also acceptable for the fracture fragments not to be in true alignment and/or have a degree of angulation. It is however key to know the child's age and injury.

Joints

A joint or articulation is where two or more bones are in close contact with each other. Joints are classified according to their mobility and structure into fibrous, cartilaginous or synovial. Fibrous joints exist between bone and cartilage. The surfaces are simply joined by fibrous tissue and there is little or no movement. Cartilaginous joints allow a small degree of movement and are covered by layers of cartilage linked by a thick pad of tissue, for example, between vertebral bones. Synovial joints, which include all limb joints, permit a great deal of movement and are the most common type of joint. Hyaline cartilage covers the articulating surfaces to prevent friction and a fibrous capsule encloses the joint and helps hold the bones in place. A synovial membrane lines the capsule, which secretes synovial fluid to lubricate the structure.

 ACTIVITY

Identify the differing types of joint within the human skeleton and justify the joint type in relation to its function and location.

Skeletal Muscle

The skeletal muscles are known as voluntary muscles because they produce movement under voluntary control. These muscles are composed of large elongated cells known as muscle fibres, which are bound together by connective tissue into small bundles and are further bound into larger bundles forming the muscle. Each muscle is enveloped in a sheet of fibrous tissue known as the fascia, which is continuous with the tendon. Tendons are composed of bands of fibrous tissue, which attach muscles to bones.

Muscle activity is coordinated and most muscles work in pairs or groups; muscle tissue is capable of contraction and relaxation and may be stimulated by nervous, chemical, electrical or thermal stimulation.

FRACTURES

A fracture is quite simply a break in the continuity of bone. Most fractures are diagnosed from the description of the injury and the physical appearance of the limb, confirmed by plain x-ray. Physical signs and symptoms of a fracture may include (Clarke and Santy-Tomlinson, 2014):
- pain, which may be throbbing or localised: the pain is often aggravated by active or passive movement;

- impaired, or loss of, function due to pain and the nature of the fracture;
- swelling at the fracture site caused by oedema/haematoma formation; usually increases in the first 12–24 hours following injury;
- a deformity may be seen or felt (palpate);
- abnormal movement in a particular limb due to movement at the fracture site;
- tenderness and/or bruising at the fracture site;
- crepitus (grating) heard or felt when the ends of the broken bone are un-deliberately rubbed together.

Types of Fracture

There are many descriptions of fractures, depending on the nature of the injury and the force that causes the fracture (Fig. 18.3). In children, a fracture through the epiphyseal (growth) plate may result in interference or complete cessation of bone growth of that long bone, which will produce a limb-length discrepancy. These fractures are known as epiphyseal fractures and are classified into five types (Fig. 18.4).

Other Descriptions of Fractures

A fracture may be displaced or undisplaced. An undisplaced fracture is one in which the bone ends are lined up, whereas in a displaced fracture the bone ends or fracture fragments are out of alignment and will require correction.

Open (compound) fractures are fractures in which the soft tissue and skin envelope have been disrupted by, for example, the acute angulation of the fracture which breaks through the skin. Such fractures are in immediate danger of infection and risk development of osteomyelitis. Most fractures do not break through the skin and are called closed fractures.

Intra-articular fractures may present where the fracture involves the joint surface. If there is a step or gap in the joint surface this may need surgery to correct it.

TABLE 18.1	Skeletal Development	
Infancy	Rapid growth in proportion and size as calcium is added to cartilage-like bones	
	Calcium content in relation to body size increases faster than any other stage of life	
Childhood	Growth continues	
	Bone density and thickness increase	
	Bone formation outpaces resorption	
Adolescence/young people	Growth accelerates	
	Bone growth peaks around ages 12–17 years in boys and ages 11–15 years in girls	
	Bone density and thickness increase	
	Bone formation outpaces resorption	
Age 20	90% of peak bone mass achieved	
Age 35	Peak bone mass achieved	
	Note: Peak bone mass is about 30% higher in men than women	
Age 40	Bone resorption begins to outpace formation	
	Adult bone loss occurs at a rate of 6%–8% per decade	

Gallo, Agatha M. "Building strong bones in childhood and adolescence: reducing the risk of fractures in later life." *Pediatric Nursing,* vol. 22, no. 5, Sept.-Oct. 1996, p. 369-374.

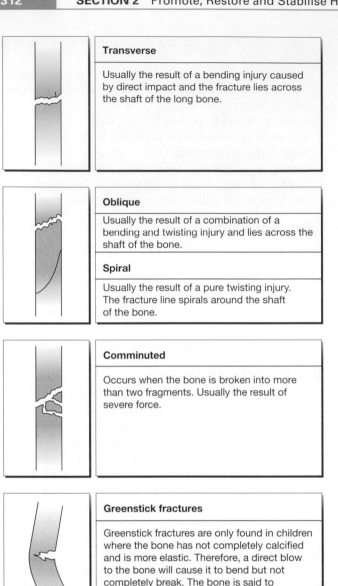

Transverse

Usually the result of a bending injury caused by direct impact and the fracture lies across the shaft of the long bone.

Oblique

Usually the result of a combination of a bending and twisting injury and lies across the shaft of the bone.

Spiral

Usually the result of a pure twisting injury. The fracture line spirals around the shaft of the bone.

Comminuted

Occurs when the bone is broken into more than two fragments. Usually the result of severe force.

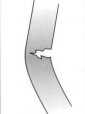

Greenstick fractures

Greenstick fractures are only found in children where the bone has not completely calcified and is more elastic. Therefore, a direct blow to the bone will cause it to bend but not completely break. The bone is said to resemble a green twig which never breaks cleanly.

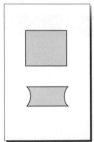

Crush fractures

Examples of crush fractures may be seen when the bone is pathologically weak due to disease. For example, children with moderate/severe osteogenesis imperfecta will have several crush fractured vertebrae.

Fig. 18.3 Types of fracture.

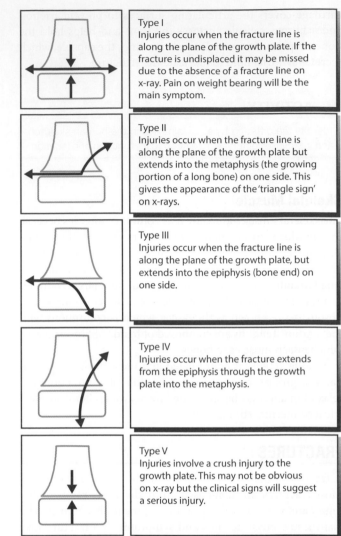

Type I
Injuries occur when the fracture line is along the plane of the growth plate. If the fracture is undisplaced it may be missed due to the absence of a fracture line on x-ray. Pain on weight bearing will be the main symptom.

Type II
Injuries occur when the fracture line is along the plane of the growth plate but extends into the metaphysis (the growing portion of a long bone) on one side. This gives the appearance of the 'triangle sign' on x-rays.

Type III
Injuries occur when the fracture line is along the plane of the growth plate, but extends into the epiphysis (bone end) on one side.

Type IV
Injuries occur when the fracture extends from the epiphysis through the growth plate into the metaphysis.

Type V
Injuries involve a crush injury to the growth plate. This may not be obvious on x-ray but the clinical signs will suggest a serious injury.

Fig. 18.4 Epiphyseal fractures.

Fracture Complications

There are many potential associated complications with fractures including the following:

- Infection: in open fractures, a wound infection may spread from the skin and soft tissues and infect the underlying bone. Children are often at increased risk due to the activity at the time of fracture, which may involve dirt, grit or grass. The child with an open wound should have the wound cleaned and be commenced on systemic antibiotic therapy. If the wound is very dirty it will be left open, dressed appropriately and then closed later on.
- Malunion: this occurs when the fracture heals in the wrong position/alignment. This may be due to poor reduction or the result of an unstable fracture that slips following reduction. It is important that all children with fractures are seen afterwards as frequently as needed to ensure the bone heals in the right position.
- Delayed union: this complication occurs for a variety of reasons. It may be because the blood supply to the fracture is poor or the fracture is inadequately immobilised. The fracture heals but takes longer than expected.
- Non-union: the fracture fails to heal. This may be due to infection, trapped soft tissues or local bone necrosis.

- Avascular necrosis: the blood supply becomes disturbed to the bone fragments causing failure to heal. It may not present until some time following the injury.
- Fat embolism: a fat deposit originating from the bone marrow at the fracture site may enter the blood stream and block a blood vessel. This may have potentially fatal consequences if the blockage is caused in a major organ, for example, the lungs.
- Damage to structures: in severe fractures other structures may be affected, for example, ischaemia to blood vessels, nerves, organs.
- Compartment syndrome: the fascial compartments within the upper and lower limbs are at risk when bleeding occurs into them from the fracture. The closed non-elastic space fills with blood and increases the pressure on the venous drainage, thereby raising the pressure in the compartment. This starves the muscle cells of oxygen and they die. The circulation can also be disturbed by a bone fragment or very tight plaster cast. The signs and symptoms of compartment syndrome in an upper limb may include:
  - painful clawing of the fingers with increasing pain on passive extension of the fingers
  - altered sensation, including a burning sensation or patchy loss of sensation
  - the pulse is weak, intermittent or absent
  - the fingers are cold and bluish
  - weak ability to flex the fingers

Many texts have described the signs of compartment syndrome as the five Ps:
- pallor
- paraesthesia
- paralysis
- pain
- pulselessness

However, the main symptom to note is pain, which is out of proportion to the injury and which is intractable (Royal College of Nursing [RCN], 2014). This condition needs to be recognised early because it is limb-threatening and prompt surgical attention can save the limb. The completion of compartment pressures can also be a key part of the assessment. For further information, review: https://www.ncbi.nlm.nih.gov/books/NBK448124/.

Neurovascular Observations

When a child enters the hospital with a fracture, the neurovascular status should be assessed initially. The Royal College of Nursing (RCN) and British Orthopaedic Association (BOA) co-developed an observation chart designed to help monitor patients who may have or be at risk of developing acute limb compartment syndrome: https://www.rcn.org.uk/professional-development/publications/pub-005457. The chart was developed for adults and children – any alteration of these observations should be reported immediately to the orthopaedic team and the clock reset.

🔧 PROFESSIONAL CONVERSATION

Rebecca is a Newly Qualified Registered Children's Nurse on Part 1 of the NMC Register

Yesterday we had a young boy who had a supracondylar fracture to his left elbow. I observed when checking neurovascular observations that his fingers were very dusky and when I tried to extend his fingers he was screaming out in pain. I was very concerned but didn't really feel very confident so I went to ask the ward manager but she was busy with a parent. I remembered what my preceptor had told me so I contacted the orthopaedic registrar. He came to the ward immediately and within 20 minutes the child was being escorted to theatre for a fasciotomy to release the pressure on his brachial artery. Later the registrar came and thanked me. He said I had probably saved the boy from developing Volkmann ischaemia or losing his arm. I am really glad I listened to my preceptor and now really do realise the importance of neurovascular observations.

Failure to recognise a compartment syndrome of the forearm may result in the child developing Volkmann ischaemic contracture caused by progressive muscle necrosis. The muscle is replaced by scar tissue leading to flexion contractures and clawing of the fingers. The result of this condition involves operations to release forearm flexors, muscle slide and tendon lengthening. Prevention through diagnosis would be attained by restoration of blood flow through reduction of compartmental pressure.

Treatment of Fractures

The five Rs summarise the five main aims of fracture treatment:

1. Resuscitation: the child with a fracture should rarely require fluid resuscitation, but the nurse should be aware of the signs and treatment necessary for shock. In fractures, shock may be related to pain and blood loss.
2. Reduction: describes the realignment of the fractured bone ends. The best reduction will take place under general anaesthesia where the surgeon can manipulate the bone and observe the correction using an image intensifier. This is especially relevant to children in whom it would not be acceptable to attempt reduction using sedation in the casualty department. Alignment may be acceptable in children with greenstick fractures.
3. Restriction: after the fracture has been manipulated into a good position it needs to be held until bony union occurs (usually 6 weeks in children). The methods used to hold the fracture will depend on the bone affected and the nature of the injury and will include one of:
   - plaster cast
   - traction
   - internal or external fixation

   The aim of restriction is to prevent any deformity and allow bone growth to proceed normally.
4. Restoration: when a limb is immobilised, there is a risk that the muscles and joints will stiffen and lose some function.

Therefore it is important that the child is encouraged to exercise all joints and muscles except those affected by the injury. For example, a child with a fractured distal radius who has an above-elbow cast can be encouraged to exercise all digits, which keeps the fingers nimble, encourages the muscle to move within the cast and promotes venous return.

5. Rehabilitation: when the method of restriction has been removed the limb must be exercised to restore normal ranges of movement. Children are generally quick to return to normal activity but may require the help of a physiotherapist.

 ACTIVITY

A child presents with head injury and an open fractured femur following a road traffic accident.
- What immediate nursing and medical approach should be taken to resuscitate this 7-year-old child who has deteriorating consciousness and is in hypovolaemic shock?
- Prioritise and analyse each intervention in relation to how it will stabilise the child's condition.

Methods of Holding Fractures
Plaster Casts

Plaster casts hold a number of advantages for the child with a fracture, including:
- allowing the child to mobilise and perform most activities of daily living
- low cost and readily available
- light and porous, which allows the skin to breathe
- relatively easy to use and apply
- strong, providing protection
- permeable to x-rays
  Disadvantages include:
- it may cause discomfort including itching and feel heavy and warm and a child will be tempted to push toys and small objects down the cast leading to pressure sores
- it may hide developing problems:
  - a poorly applied cast may cause pressure on the skin and encourage the development of a pressure ulcer
  - a surgical wound following an open reduction may develop sepsis
- it is not waterproof

REFLECT ON YOUR PRACTICE

Consider what education and skills you need to be competent in the application of a plaster cast.
   In what way does this relate to your professional accountability and the recommendations of the British Orthopaedic Association (BOA)?

Plaster casts – nursing care. Wright (2014) considered the following when caring for an inpatient with a plaster cast:
- Care should be taken not to apply pressure to the cast during the drying period to avoid causing dents in the cast (plaster of Paris takes 24–48 hours to dry; synthetic, fibreglass casts take around 30–60 minutes). The limb should be supported on a pillow to provide even pressure along the cast which prevents undue pressure on bony prominences.
- Elevation of the limb may be necessary to help reduce the amount of swelling which, within a cast, may cause constriction and neurovascular impairment.
  Plaster casts – observations.
- The cast should be observed regularly for cracking, softening or breakdown.
- If a child has had an open reduction, the cast should be observed for blood loss, which will stain the cast. A line drawn around the cast illustrates any further blood loss.
- Neurovascular observations should be performed – including regular pain assessment.
- When the child has recovered and appears stable the cast may need trimming to improve comfort. Hip spica casts will need protection around the edges to prevent contamination by urine and faeces.

Before a child is discharged home, the parent and child should receive advice regarding care of the plaster (sample discharge advice in companion PowerPoint presentation). See 358-359 for nursing and discharge care for a hip spica cast.

 ACTIVITY

Examine your hospital's plaster care advice sheet given to the patient on discharge.
- Can you think of ways of improving the information provided and could it be made more child friendly?

Plaster casts – cast bracing. Cast bracing is commonly used following internal fixation of a femoral or tibial fracture. The cast brace comprises plaster casts on the upper and lower limb, which are connected by hinges. These allow a greater degree of mobility to help prevent joint stiffness and allow the child to mobilise with partial weight-bearing, which encourages bone healing.

TRACTION

The Royal College of Nursing (RCN) published guidance in 2015 on the principles and application of traction commonly used today. Traction is a pulling force. It is used to reduce and maintain alignment of fractures, to immobilise inflamed or injured joints, relieve pain, correct mild deformities and reduce muscle spasm. Traction is either fixed or balanced:
- Fixed traction is achieved by exerting a pulling force on the point splinted between two fixed points.

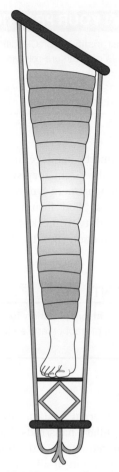

Fig. 18.5 Thomas splint traction.

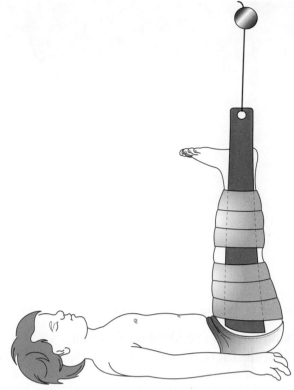

Fig. 18.6 Gallows traction.

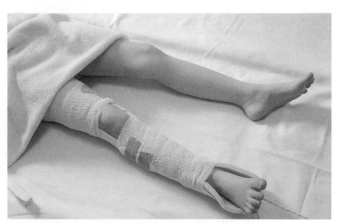

Fig. 18.7 Simple skin traction.

- Balanced traction exerts a pulling force on the part held between two mobile points, and works by using the patient's weight against the applied load.

Common forms of balanced and skin traction used with children include:

- Thomas splint traction: fixed traction that works against the force of the body (Fig. 18.5). It is used in the treatment of femoral fractures usually as a means to hold and pull the fracture until the swelling subsides before internal or external fixation.
- Gallows traction: works by the body's weight being balanced by an applied load. It is frequently used in babies and infants with femoral fractures to allow the swelling to subside prior to the application of a hip spica (Fig. 18.6). It may also be used as part of the conservative treatment for the child with developmental dysplasia of the hip (DDH).
- Simple skin traction (Fig. 18.7): commonly used to rest the affected limb or joint prior to surgery and to reduce pain/muscle spasm. It involves applying adhesive or non-adhesive strips of material to either side of the affected limb. The limb is then bandaged, taking care to leave the knee free. The cord allows a pull to be exerted on the strips, which is transmitted from the material and skin to the underlying tissues and bone. Only a moderate amount of pull can be exerted using weights and the bed end is then elevated to provide counter traction.

- Skeletal traction: now rarely used in children because of the advances in surgical techniques. It may be used if the alignment of the fracture is difficult to achieve and maintain and internal fixation is not possible. It involves the insertion of a sterile pin through an area of strong bone, such as the femoral condyles, tibial tuberosity or calcaneum. A metal stirrup is then attached to the pin ends and cord fastened to it. Weights are attached to the stirrup and hang over a pulley; they are then left free hanging over the elevated bed end. Skeletal traction is also used following trauma, such as when the integrity of the skin is damaged and the application of skin traction would be difficult.
- Slings traction: used for children with hip conditions who require a combination of bed rest and allows the

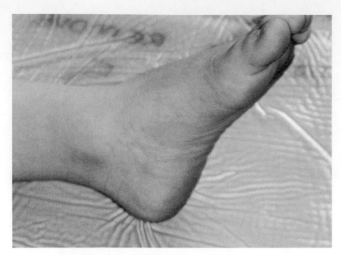

Fig. 18.8 Polymer gel pad.

physiotherapist to teach the child a range of exercises performed on the hip and lower limbs.

Nursing Care of the Child on Traction

Once traction has been applied, the child's pain and discomfort is usually relieved, but analgesia may still be required. The nurse should be aware of the following observations and care when nursing children on traction.

The Position of the Patient

The position required for successful traction will often cause difficulty with the activities of daily living including eating, drinking, washing, elimination and learning. Assistance with these activities is essential, as well as maintaining the privacy and independence of the patient.

Once over the initial discomfort of an injury, the child will become frustrated and bored due to loss of mobility. The school-age child may display poor behaviour. This should be dealt with sensitively but firmly to prevent general disruption to the ward. The nurse should employ the full skills of the play specialist and ward teacher, and encourage full parental participation in their child's care. Once adjustment has been made, the child will quickly establish a rapport with the ward team.

The child is at risk from the usual complications of bed rest:

- Pressure ulcers: bony prominences, including the buttocks and heels, are at risk of pressure ulcers as the result of the constant pressure between the skin surface and the hard mattress. Frequent cleansing, minor alterations in position and the use of pressure-reducing mattresses or polymer gel pads (Fig. 18.8) will lessen the risk of pressure sore development.
- Kidneys: urinary stasis may result in kidney stones or a urinary tract infection leading to difficulty passing urine; therefore the child should be encouraged to drink plenty of fluids.
- Bowel: significantly reduced exercise and the decrease of roughage can lead to constipation; therefore the child's diet should include increased fibre and fluid. Laxatives may be prescribed.

Bandages

Constriction of the limb by bandages used with traction may cause disturbance to the circulatory system, muscles, joints and nerve supply. Compartment syndrome may also develop. Bandages should be applied firmly, but not tightly, and removed each span of duty to check skin integrity/sensitivity due to adhesive skin traction (Box 18.1).

Internal Fixation

The many types of internal fixation devices include plates, screws and intramedullary nails/rods. Internal fixation (Fig. 18.9) allows accurate reduction of the fracture and stabilisation of the reduced position. It allows the child to mobilise and avoids joint stiffness by encouraging prompt rehabilitation. It encourages good bone union and reduces the time spent in hospital. Complications include the risks associated with a general anaesthetic, the potential of infection and other postoperative complications. Further surgery is required to remove the device. When possible, the surgeon will remove the fixation device at 6–12 months, although removal may not always be possible and the device may be safely left in situ.

External Fixation

A fracture may be held by transfixing screws, which pass through the bone above and below the fracture. The screws are held together with a rigid frame or lockable sliding bar. External fixation is particularly useful for fractures with severe soft tissue damage, fractures with nerve or blood vessel damage, unstable comminuted fractures that can be held to length until bone healing occurs and infected fractures where internal fixation may be unwise (Clarke and Santy-Tomlinson 2014). The fixation device is left in place until bone healing occurs. Older children may remove the screws themselves by using Entonox in outpatients (Pickup and Pagdin, 2000), avoiding further general anaesthesia. Complications occurring from external fixation are pin-site infections and occasionally delayed union. Occasionally a stress fracture may occur at the site of one of the screws following removal. External devices (Fig. 18.10) are used in limb reconstruction and leg-lengthening treatments throughout the UK.

◎ EVIDENCE-BASED PRACTICE

Skeletal Pin Site Care

There remains little consensus regarding the correct management of skeletal pin sites; however, UK practice is generally guided by the most recent Cochrane review. Surgical literature tends to focus on the prevalence of pin site infections, whereas nursing literature usually describes pin care techniques as measures to minimise complications. Until evidence-based practice based on a significant multicentre trial is published, individual centres should review the literature themselves to reach local multidisciplinary consensus. A Cochrane review is expected in 2019 – two pertinent publications include Timms (2013) which provides a fresh consensus for pin site care in the UK and a good summary of the 2010 Pin Site consensus guidelines. This paper includes the most recent Cochrane review by Lethaby et al. (2008), and the eight factors chosen from this to formulate the guidelines, and to provide a good overview. Secondly, Georgiades (2018) provides a more recent and valuable review of the studies on pin site crust retention, and it does show that crust retention does reduce the incidence of pin site infection and should only be removed when infection is present to allow drainage.

BOX 18.1 Application of Skin Traction

- Check for allergies.
- Skin traction can be a painful procedure for a child and careful preparation must therefore be given, including a detailed explanation and appropriate analgesia before the procedure is commenced, to gain the child's cooperation and trust.
- Privacy should be maintained throughout the procedure.
- The limb should be cleaned prior to applying the adhesive skin traction, to prevent the risk of infection.
- The ankle joint is kept free allowing normal movement of that joint.
- The patella is left free and the leg placed in slight flexion, thus preventing deformity and stiffness.
- Pressure on bony prominence should be avoided or pressure sores may occur.
- Folds and creases in the strapping should be avoided to prevent discomfort or sores.
- The temperature and colour of the limb is checked to ensure the tension of strapping is correct.

Silverwood, B., 2006. Practice 34: Traction. In: Twigg, E. & Mohammed, T. (Eds.), Practices in Children's Nursing: Guidelines for Hospital and Community, second ed. Churchill Livingstone, Edinburgh, pp. 411–420.

▮ SCENARIO

Charlotte is a second-year adult branch student nurse who is on allocation within the local general hospital emergency department (ED).

A 4-year-old boy is brought to the ED department by emergency ambulance and is taken immediately to the resuscitation room. The child appeared pale, was immobilised with a hard collar around the neck and had a splint around his leg with a large blood-stained dressing.

Later, after the child is transferred to the nearest children's hospital, Charlotte asks her mentor why aspects of the child's assessment and stabilisation were different and why the child was rushed to another hospital when all the 'hard work' had been done. The mentor responded by explaining how the management of polytrauma (multiple injuries) is different between children and adults.

POLYTRAUMA

Trauma is the most common cause of death in childhood. The most common causes of multiple trauma in children include road traffic accidents, falls from height and physical child abuse. Initial assessment and management of children with multiple injuries should be carried out within a dedicated resuscitation room according to the guidelines of advanced paediatric life support (APLS) and advanced trauma life support (ATLS) as recommended by the Royal College of Surgeons. Initial stabilisation should be followed by transfer to a specialist paediatric centre with the necessary paediatric intensive care unit, specialist neurological, anaesthetic, orthopaedic, radiological and medical teams.

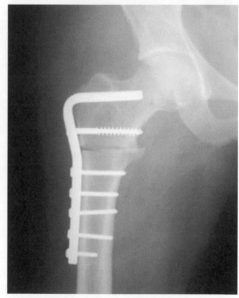

Fig. 18.9 Internal fixation.

Within an adult-orientated centre it is important to remember that during initial assessment children present specific anatomical differences from the adult:

- The head and tongue are large whereas the face and oral cavity are small. This may present difficulties with endotracheal intubation and the large head increases the risk of cervical spine injuries during the time of the accident.
- Regarding the airway, infants are obligate nose breathers, nasal passages are narrow and therefore easily obstructed and children between the ages of 3 and 8 years commonly present with adenotonsillar hypertrophy. The differences in

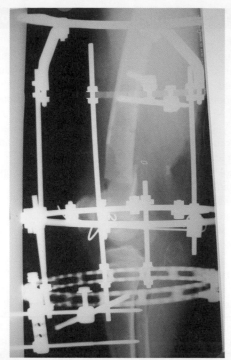

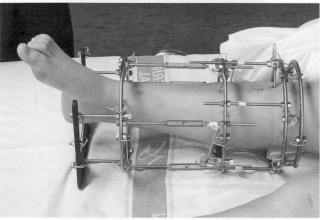

Fig. 18.10 External fixation (Ilizarov frame).

the anatomy of the epiglottis and larynx require a different intubation technique. Ribs are more horizontal in appearance, elastic in structure and breathing diaphragmatic, leading to considerable lung injury without fracture.

- Blood volume varies according to age. Bearing in mind the smaller circulating blood volume in relation to age and size a femoral fracture may produce enough blood loss to lead to haemorrhagic shock/cardiac decompensation. The pulse rate of children is higher and blood pressure lower and is more prone to the effects of anxiety. Cardiac output is largely dependent on the heart rate as the stroke volume is small and fixed meaning bradycardia is poorly tolerated.
- Abdominal organs are more vulnerable as the abdominal wall is thin and the diaphragm more horizontal.

- Children's bones have growth plates, injury to which may cause permanent growth arrest of that bone leading to short limbs.

Structured APLS and ATLS Approach

On arrival in the casualty department, ATLS advises four steps in the management of the child presenting with polytrauma:

1. Initial assessment
2. Resuscitation
3. Secondary survey
4. Definitive care

Steps 1 and 2 are performed simultaneously.

Initial Assessment (Primary Survey) and Resuscitation

Assesses vital functions and consists of five steps:

A = Airway patency and cervical spine control: if the gag reflex is absent or in doubt the child's airway will be maintained by utilising an oropharyngeal (Guedel) airway or endotracheal intubation. The trauma team will assume that cervical spine injury will have occurred so a rigid collar will be applied.

B = Breathing adequately to maintain oxygenation: assessment will be made of reduced respiratory effort and for potential life-threatening emergencies such as tension pneumothorax, haemopneumothorax and pericardial tamponade.

C = Circulation and control of bleeding: the aim here is to detect the presence of circulatory shock (Table 18.2) and sites of blood loss which, where possible, should be controlled. Intravenous access is paramount; however, access is often difficult in children due to peripheral shutdown. Intraosseous needles (special needles designed to be screwed into the lumen of the bone) may be used until a central line is accessed later. Shock is managed by rapid fluid bolus/replacement and administration of high concentration oxygen through bag and mask or reservoir mask.

D = Disability (neurological assessment): the central nervous system is examined only after completion of ABC and resuscitation. Initial assessment will determine if the child is:
- A = alert
- V = responds to voice
- P = responds to pain
- U = unresponsive

During the secondary survey the child will be scored using the Glasgow Coma Score.

E = Exposure: to fully examine front and back; secondary survey.

Secondary Survey

Following the initial assessment and resuscitation, strong analgesia such as morphine will be considered to lessen pain. The child will undergo radiological examination of the cervical spine, pelvis and chest (other x-rays may depend

TABLE 18.2 Recognition of Stages of Shock

Sign	ASSESSMENT OF % BLOOD LOSS		
	<25	25–40	>40
Heart rate	Tachycardia	Tachycardia	Tachycardia or bradycardia
Systolic blood pressure	Normal	Normal or decreasing	Decreasing
Pulse volume	Normal/reduced	Reduced	Reduced
Capillary refill time (normal <2 s)	Normal/increased	Increased	Increased
Skin	Cool, pale	Cold, mottled	Cold, pale
Respiratory rate	Tachypnoea	Tachypnoea	Sighing
Mental state	Mild agitation	Lethargic, uncooperative	Reacts only to pain

on the history and initial assessment) and a thorough head to toe, front and back examination. Vital signs of ABCDE will be continually checked and interventions made to deal with other, less life-threatening injuries. For example, a nasogastric tube may be passed to relieve gastric dilatation and a urinary catheter passed to prevent urinary retention and allow accurate recording of fluid balance. The secondary survey may take place within the secure environment of a paediatric intensive care unit where definitive care will commence.

Orthopaedic Definitive Care in Polytrauma

- Bone is more elastic in children than in adults; pelvic fractures require increased high-energy trauma to occur. Most pelvic fractures rarely cause difficulties and unite well with minimal intervention.
- Children are at increased risk of spinal cord injury. The cervical spine area must be protected with a hard collar and the child log-rolled until detailed examination and investigation has ruled out spinal cord injury.
- Fractures of the long bones should be stabilised as soon as possible. In the short term, a femoral fracture will be stabilised using splintage; however, it is preferable to stabilise all long bone fractures through internal or external fixation (see Fig. 18.10) because it aids nursing care and provides secure stabilisation. Neurovascular assessment should take place as soon as the child's initial resuscitation is completed, as the risk of compartment syndrome is increased in children with multiple injuries.
- Most compound or open fractures are caused by high-energy road traffic accidents. The presence of an open fracture often suggests other injuries. Open fractures are classified as shown in Table 18.3.

Open fractures may require immediate intervention through an operative procedure to stabilise, clean and close the wound to prevent the development of sepsis. The injury will require copious irrigation to clean the wound. Vascular repair may be performed immediately following stabilisation of the fracture. A plastic surgeon may be required to perform complex free flap skin grafts in the most serious cases. The child will be commenced on broad-spectrum intravenous antibiotics.

Advances in paediatric medical and surgical management ensure the child with multiple injuries often makes a full recovery. However, every attempt should be made to reduce the risk of potential fatal injury through education, car safety, traffic calming and suitable children's play areas.

  WWW

Visit the Resuscitation Council UK for the latest advanced paediatric resuscitation guidelines at:
- http://www.resus.org.uk

OSTEOGENESIS IMPERFECTA

Description

Osteogenesis imperfecta (OI), commonly known as 'brittle bone disease', is a genetic skeletal dysplasia in which the skeleton is osteoporotic (Cole, 2002) – the bones break easily. It is also associated with weak teeth due to poor dentine, blue sclerae (a bluish tint to the whites of the eyes), kyphosis (forward curvature) and scoliosis (sideways curvature) of the spine, easy bruising and bleeding, hypermobility, weak muscles, and progressive hearing loss. Bone deformities may lead to chronic pain. The defective gene affects the body's collagen in one of two ways: underproduction of otherwise normal collagen fibres (mild OI; type I) or abnormal or 'bent' collagen fibres, giving more severe forms. The defect interferes with bone turnover, leading to an inability to accumulate bone as healthy children would (Hill et al., 2003). The characteristic features of osteogenesis imperfecta vary immensely between each child. The classification now in general use was proposed by Sillence et al., in 1979 and is based on genetic, clinical and radiological features (Table 18.4).

Overall OI is rare, being found in about 6 per 100,000 people; which means there are likely 3000–4000 people in the UK with the condition (https://brittlebone.org/what-is-oi/about-oi/). Children with severe osteogenesis imperfecta may be diagnosed in utero using ultrasound, or at birth when the baby presents

TABLE 18.3   Classification of Open Fractures

Type I	An open fracture with a wound <1 cm long and clean
Type II	An open fracture with a laceration >1 cm long without excessive soft tissue damage, flaps or avulsions
Type III	Massive soft tissue damage, compromised vascularity, severe wound contamination, marked fracture instability
Type IIIA	Adequate soft tissue coverage of a fractured bone despite extensive soft tissue laceration or flaps or high-energy trauma irrespective of the size of the wound
Type IIIB	Extensive soft tissue injury loss with periosteal stripping and bone exposure; usually associated with massive contamination
Type IIIC	Open fracture associated with arterial injury requiring repair

Bell, 2002.

TABLE 18.4   Classification of Osteogenesis Imperfecta (OI)

Type	Description
I	Most common and mildest form of OI
	Fractures occur occasionally, especially before puberty
	Normal or near normal stature
	Sclera often blue
	Bone deformity is minimal or absent
	Brittle teeth (dentinogenesis imperfecta); hearing loss
	Collagen structure is normal but the amount is less than normal
II	Most severe form
	Lethal at birth, or shortly following birth, due to complex respiratory problems
	Growth retardation in utero
	Numerous fractures, long bones crumpled and bowed, ribs appear beaded
	Collagen abnormal
III	Bones fracture easily. Fractures often present at birth, plain x-rays may show partially healed fractures
	Several crush fractured vertebrae
	Short stature
	Sclera may be blue, but may lighten with age
	Brittle teeth and hearing loss common
	Barrel shaped rib cage. Respiratory problems possible
	Triangular face
	Bone deformity severe. Spinal curvature present
	Collagen abnormal
IV	Bones fracture easily, especially in infants and children
	Shorter than average stature. Crush fractured vertebrae
	May have bowing of long bones and develop spinal curvature
	White sclera. Brittle teeth and hearing loss possible
	Collagen abnormal

with 'classic' features including a triangular face and several new and healing fractures of long bones. However, children with milder forms may face a long road towards diagnosis. Many parents have to endure investigation by the authorities of suspected child abuse (Mahoney, 2000).

Treatment

The management of OI focuses on minimising fractures and maximising function and independence. This is achieved through a combination of coordinated surgical and medical management with physiotherapy and occupational therapy.

Medical Management

This includes the administration of a bisphosphonate. This is based on the chemical structure of a naturally occurring substance within the body called pyrophosphate (Wright, 2014) which binds very strongly to bone, reducing the actions of osteoclasts. The beneficial effects of pamidronate include:

• a substantial increase in bone mass
• a reduction in fracture frequency
• increase in height of previous crush-fractured vertebrae
• a reduction of chronic bone pain and fatigue

- improved mobility and reduced dependence on mobility aids
- increase in thickness in the tube walls of long bones

The treatment is given in combination with multidisciplinary care. The physiotherapist deals with improving mobility and physical function and the occupational therapist maximises the child's independence of performing the activities of daily living.

Surgical Management

The mainstay of surgical management is intramedullary rod fixation. The aim of rodding long bones is to correct and prevent bony disorders. Rods are either fixed length or expanding. Expanding rods are telescopic and expand as the bone grows in length. These hold a number of advantages over fixed rods, because the child requires less frequent change of the rod and only when the rod requires revision; only the expanding part of the rod is changed (Stockley et al., 1989). Complications may include infection, migration or separation of the rod and a bent rod following fracture (Wilkinson et al., 1998). Although the operation may appear complicated, the average length of the admission lasts only 3–4 days. The perioperative period lasts around 1–2 hours, the child returns to the ward with an intravenous infusion (until diet and fluids are re-established) and a patient-controlled analgesia (PCA) to ensure adequate pain control. A lightweight cast or a cotton/crepe bandage will protect the limb for 4–6 weeks.

Nursing Care

The nursing care of osteogenesis imperfecta is outlined in Table 18.5.

 WWW

For further information regarding osteogenesis imperfecta visit:
- http://www.oif.org

DEVELOPMENTAL DYSPLASIA OF THE HIP

Description

Developmental dysplasia of the hip (DDH) is a recent term used to describe a dislocation of the hip joint occurring at birth (congenital) or during the first year of life (Judd, 2014). The head (ball) of the femur does not sit true in the acetabulum (socket). There are varying degrees of dislocation including the following:

- Unstable: the shape of the head of the femur and acetabulum are normal or near normal. Using manipulation, the head of the femur may be moved in and out of the acetabulum.
- Subluxed: the head of the femur is only in partial contact with the acetabulum. The acetabulum is not of a normal shape.

- Dislocated: the head of the femur lies completely out of the joint. Usually the shape and size of the joint is abnormal and will deteriorate further if left out of the joint.

DDH may affect one or both hips, but it's more common in the left hip. It's also more common in girls and firstborn children. About one or two in every 1000 babies have DDH that needs treating (www.nhs.uk/conditions/developmental-dysplasia-of-the-hip/). The cause of DDH is unclear but it is believed that there may be a genetic factor because it tends to run in families. Other examples of contributory factors include lax ligaments, which is caused by increased levels of oestrogen during pregnancy, overdue pregnancies and breech deliveries. Environmental causative factors have been shown in the North American Indian and Eskimo population where babies are carried with their legs straight.

The classic signs of DDH may include the paediatrician observing a 'hip click' during routine postnatal checks. Other signs may include: the thigh showing a partial lateral rotation, flexion and abduction, asymmetry of the hips and a flattening of the buttock. The baby will be referred to a paediatric orthopaedic surgeon who will perform ultrasound scanning to establish the severity of the condition.

Treatment

Treatment will depend on the time of diagnosis, but may be divided into conservative and surgical treatments.

Conservative

The aim is to hold the legs abducted and flexed so that the head of the femur falls naturally into the acetabulum. The constant pressure of the ball of the femur helps to mould the acetabulum and therefore stabilise the hip. This may be achieved in a young baby by the wearing of double nappies or the wearing of a special splint shaped in the form of an 'X' or 'H'. This fits around the thighs of the legs and wraps over the shoulders to maintain position. Examples include the Cambridge splint, Pavlik harness and von Rosen splint. The splint will be worn constantly for a minimum of 12 weeks and is removed only for examination.

Traction was, until a few years ago, the treatment of choice for babies whose treatment had failed with splints or for a baby diagnosed later. The hip is reduced by gradually abducting the hips over a 4- to 6-week period before being held in plaster. A popular example was the Japanese frame. Plaster fixation is commonly used following manipulation of the hips under anaesthesia. The types of plaster casts used include a double hip spica or a frog plaster. The baby is reviewed in clinic at 6 weeks where the hips are reassessed for hip stability. Plaster treatment may last for 6–9 months, and the family requires support and advice during this period.

Surgical

Surgical treatments are used when either the conservative method has failed or the diagnosis is made late. Common procedures include the following:

- Tenotomy: the groin tendon is lengthened. This releases a tight tendon that had prevented satisfactory reduction of the hip.

TABLE 18.5	**Nursing Care of Osteogenesis Imperfecta (OI)**
Parents	Listen to what the parents have to say about the handling of their child. Regard them as colleagues because they are experts in their child's routine care.
Babies and infants	Toys should be soft and easy to handle.
Lifting	Head, trunks and buttocks should be evenly supported when the baby is lifted. Make your movements slow, methodical and gentle.
Changing nappies	Avoid lifting by the ankles. Change the nappy by lifting under the buttocks and place the nappy with the other hand.
Dressing	May suffer excessive sweating. Use cotton clothing. Position/set out clothes next to the baby. Openings should be generous. Slip your hand up the sleeve and pull the baby's arm through.
Positioning	Babies with OI can develop flattening of the head. Reposition frequently on alternate sides and supine. Support the position with soft rolled sheets.
Feeding	Often a poor feeder. Small, frequent feeds. Hold the child to give comfort, utilising a soft pillow.
Constipation	Ensure adequate hydration. Advice on diet, including fibre and fruit.
Transporting around hospital	Traditional methods, i.e. in the cot, are satisfactory. Consider using a car seat, which provides a comfortable protective environment.
Older children	Very independent. Regarded as above normal intelligence (Wacaster, 1996) and appreciate normal adult conversation.

- Open reduction: allows the femoral head to be surgically placed in the acetabulum. The position is maintained by plaster cast.
- Femoral derotation osteotomy: a surgical break of the bone used to return the femur to a normal anatomical position following open reduction of the hip. The break is held in place by a blade plate until bone healing has occurred and the plate is removed between 6 and 12 months. A hip spica cast is used to maintain position during the first 6–8 weeks.
- Salter osteotomy: may be performed in a late diagnosis where poor development of the acetabulum has occurred. This involves surgical reconstruction of the acetabulum to prevent further dislocation.

NURSING CARE OF A CHILD WITH A HIP SPICA CAST

The age and developmental stage of the child is important when planning care. Hip spicas are cumbersome and uncomfortable for the child and parents, who have to carry a largely immobile child in a heavy cast, although young children soon learn to drag themselves around the floor despite the hip spica. Parents must be taught how to lift and carry the child before discharge. Parents should be made aware of the signs of wound infection under the plaster – usually identified by an unpleasant smell from the plaster combined with a pyrexia. If this occurs, or if the cast cracks or softens, the parent should contact the hospital promptly.

Hygiene

The plaster edges must be examined for rough edges, which can cause skin breakdown. A daily sponge-down replaces bathing. Talcum powder should be used sparingly around the plaster because it can cause excessive irritation to the skin under the cast. Hair washing can be a problem and usually requires two people, one to hold the child over the bath, the other to wash. Nappy care requires some thought. A smaller disposable nappy is usually required as it does need to be changed more frequently; nappy tapes are removed prior to tucking in the nappy.

Sleeping

Younger children are less likely to be affected by the plaster, although wind can be troublesome, therefore winding after feeding is important. The younger child is more vulnerable and should not be positioned on their tummy when sleeping and preferably to sleep in the parent's room. Children in casts may sleep for only short periods and often become restless. Disturbed nights can result from itching and an inability to turn over. A child in a spica takes up much more room than one without, therefore the width of the bed may require thought; placing the mattress on the floor can be useful and also removes the fear of the child falling out of bed. Supporting the child in a comfortable position can be done with foam or pillows but care must be taken to prevent pressure points or strain on the cast. The child may require fewer bed clothes – the plaster acts as insulation.

Transport

This is often a major problem for the family with a child in a hip spica cast but the ability to get out of the home is important for the parent and child. Smaller babies will often fit into a push chair with some extra support from pillows. Transporting a child in a cast by car is difficult; however, specialists do exist within the UK who can safely secure a child in a car seat. An occupational therapist will advise the parent regarding safe transport.

Eating and Drinking

Some children are able to eat and drink lying on their tummies; others require support in an upright position either strapped in a normal high chair or using a bean bag. There are also designs available of specific 'hip spica' chairs. A closed cup or straw is the best method of drinking and preventing too many accidents.

Clothing

Usually larger sizes are required; these can be split and then applied using tapes, poppers, Velcro or zips.

Play

Play and activity should be encouraged as much possible to allow the child to develop as normal and to provide him or her with a means of releasing the tension experienced while in plaster. Physical and very active play will be almost impossible. The child will have to rely on imaginative or 'craft' types of play. A child in a plaster can become isolated from friends and peers. Contact should therefore be encouraged, although games should not be allowed to become too boisterous.

 ACTIVITY

Devise some play activities for the following children on the ward:
- A 10-month-old on gallows traction.
- Two 8-year-old boys with Thomas splint traction.
- A 14-year-old girl on bilateral skin traction.

TALIPES (CLUBFOOT)

Description

Congenital (present at birth) talipes (ankle and foot) equino-varus (pointing downwards and inwards) is the most common congenital abnormality of the feet, which are malformed and irregularly positioned. It varies in type and severity. The cause is unknown, although there may be a hereditary or genetic component. It has been associated with other congenital conditions and it may be caused by the position of the foot in utero. Incidence is one per 1000 births (Catteral, 2002). Diagnosis is usually made at birth but is increasingly diagnosed through prenatal ultrasound scanning. The aims of treatment are to have a functional, pain free, plantigrade foot and able to get into normal footwear.

Treatment
Conservative Treatment

This includes physiotherapy on newborn babies: the parent is taught to stretch the ligaments and tendons. Adhesive strapping is applied around the foot, up the sides of the legs and anchored around the knee in an overcorrected position. Plaster cast fixation involves the foot being manipulated by the surgeon into an overcorrected position, with the knee flexed to prevent the cast slipping off. The cast is changed regularly due to the rapid growth of the baby and the foot is re-manipulated. This acts by stretching the soft tissues. The Ponseti technique appears to be the current treatment of choice – it involves serial progressive casting with tendo-achilles tenotomy (Judd, 2014).

Surgical Treatments

These vary widely in type and will depend on the severity of the talipes and the child's age. Surgical intervention is usually started at 9 months, with the aim of achieving correction in time for walking. Examples include soft tissue releases followed by a period in plaster through to bony procedures of the foot. A resistant foot may be corrected by using an external circular frame (Ilizarov frame), which allows the position of the foot to be altered slowly by both stretching the soft tissues and distracting osteotomies in the bones of the foot. When a normal position is achieved the frame is 'locked' until bone healing has occurred. The whole period of treatment may take around 6 months followed by a period in plaster.

PERTHES DISEASE

Perthes disease, also known as Legg–Calvé–Perthes disease, after Legg (an American), Calvé (a Frenchman) and Perthes (a German), was first described around 1910. It is characterised by a loss of circulation to the head of the femur leading to avascular necrosis. This is followed by a period of revascularisation lasting 18 months to 2 years. During this period the bone is soft and revascularisation often results in fracture and or collapse of the femoral head. The resulting non-spherical shape causes the child to have stiffness and pain. The cause of Perthes' disease is unknown; statistics show that it is more common in boys than girls around ages 3–8 years.

The child often presents with an acutely painful hip due to inflammation of the hip joint. There is often a painful obvious limp that has appeared merely over a few hours. The condition is usually diagnosed through x-ray following other investigations to rule out conditions that cause similar symptoms, for example, epiphyseal dysplasia.

Treatment
Conservative/Surgical Treatment

Traditionally, these children were placed on periods of prolonged bed rest and non-weight-bearing on the affected hip because it was thought weight bearing caused the head to collapse. Treatment approaches now suggest maintaining the head within the acetabulum. This may be achieved conservatively by using a non-steroidal anti-inflammatory drug (NSAID) for pain relief and traction, that is, skin traction or slings and springs which enable the hip to rest alongside physiotherapy and hydrotherapy which keeps the hip moving. Surgical options include arthrodiastasis which aims to protect the femoral head and preserve its height during the early fragmentation stage of the condition – this involves application of an external fixator (Judd, 2014). Alternative options include a femoral rotational osteotomy or pelvic osteotomy. If the hip shows tightness on examination the child may already have flattening of the femoral head and the outcome will be less favourable. In such cases a period of traction and physiotherapy is given to release tightness usually followed by surgical hip adductor releases.

It is known that diagnosis before the age of 4 years leads to a good outcome, irrespective of treatment, and in all ages at least 70% of affected children do well with no long-term disability.

DISCHARGE PLANNING

Effective discharge planning for the child who undergoes orthopaedic surgery should begin at the preadmission clinic or on admission to the ward. The family should receive information about care of a plaster cast and or the importance of cleansing pin sites for external fixators. They need to be able to recognise potential complications of surgery, including the signs of infection and the difference between 'routine' discomfort and severe pain. Parents should be encouraged to follow the exercises given by the physiotherapist to maintain joint mobility. The children's nurse must act as the coordinator to ensure the child and family receives multidisciplinary ongoing care in the community, including the community nursing team, social services, occupational therapy and physiotherapy. For example, an older child going home with a spica cast may require home assessment by the occupational therapist, who will need to arrange for the child to have a urinal, bed pan or even a hoist to enable transfer from the bed to a wheelchair. A number of support groups supply advice, support and information for families of children with specific conditions.

 WWW

For further information about support groups, visit:
• http://www.steps-charity.org.uk/

It is outside the scope of this chapter to provide a detailed review of the many childhood orthopaedic conditions. Review the references and further reading sections of this chapter or use the many online sources.

REFERENCES

Catteral, A., 2002. Early assessment and management of the club foot. In: Benson, M.K.D., et al. (Ed.), Children's Orthopaedics and Fractures, second ed. Churchill Livingstone, Edinburgh, pp. 464–477.

Clarke, S., Santy-Tomlinson, J., 2014. Orthopaedic and Trauma Nursing: An Evidence-Based Approach to Musculoskeletal Care. Wiley Blackwell, London.

Cole, W., 2002. Bone, cartilage and fibrous tissue disorders. In: Benson, M.K.D., et al. (Ed.), Children's Orthopaedics and Fractures, second ed. Churchill Livingstone, Edinburgh, pp. 359–383.

Georgiades, D., 2018. A systematic integrative review of pin site crusts. Orthopaedic. Nurs. 37 (1), 6–42.

Hill, C., Hampshire, D., Silverwood, B., Bishop, N.J., 2003. Recent advances in the management of osteogenesis imperfecta. Curr. Paediatr. 13, 151–157.

Judd, J., 2014. Chapter 22. Common childhood orthopaedic conditions, their care and management. In: Clarke, S., Santy-Tomlinson, J. (Eds.), Orthopaedic and Trauma Nursing: An Evidence-Based Approach to Musculoskeletal Care. Wiley Blackwell, London, pp. 290–308.

Lethaby, A., Temple, J., Santy, J., 2008. Pin site care for preventing infections associated with external bone fixators and pins. Cochrane Database Syst. Rev. (4), CD004551, John Wiley and Sons, Oxford.

Mahoney, C., 2000. Handle with care. Nursing Times 96, 1 24–26.

Pickup, S., Pagdin, J., 2000. Procedural pain: Entonox can help. Paediatric. Nurs. 12 (10), 33–36.

Prior, M.A., Miles, S., 1999. Casting: part one. Nurs. Stand. 13 (28), 49–53.

Royal College of Nursing (RCN), 2011. Guidance on Pin Site Care. Report and Recommendations for 2010 Consensus Project on Pin Site Care. RCN, London.

Royal College of Nursing (RCN), 2015. Traction: Principles and Application. RCN, London.

Royal College of Nursing (RCN) and British Orthopaedic Association (BOA), 2014. Peripheral Neurovascular Observations for Acute Limb Compartment Syndrome. RCN, London.

Sillence, D.O., Senn, A., Danks, D.M., 1979. Genetic heterogeneity in osteogenesis imperfecta. J. Med. Gen. 16, 101–116.

Stockley, I., Bell, M.J., Sharrard, W.I., 1989. The Role of Expanding Intermeduallry Rods in Osteogenesis Imperfecta. Bone Joint Surgical British vol. 71 (3), 422–427.

Timms, A., 2013. A fresh consensus for pin site care in the UK. Int. J. Orthopaedic. Trauma. Nurs. 17, 19–28.

Wilkinson, J.M., Scott, B.W., Clarke, A.M., et al., 2006. Surgical stabilisation of the lower limb in osteogenesis imperfecta using the Silverwood B. Practice 34: Traction. In: Twigg, E. Mohammed, T. (Eds.), Practices in Children's Nursing: Guidelines for Hospital and Community, second ed. Churchill Livingstone, Edinburgh, pp. 411–420.

Wacaster, P., 1996. Managing Osteogenesis Imperfecta: A Medical Manual. Osteogenesis Imperfecta Foundation, Gaithersburg, USA.

Wilkinson, J.M., Scott, A.M., Clarke, M.J., 2006. Surgical stabilization of the lower limb in osteogenesis imperfecta using the Sheffield telescopic intramedullary rod system. J. Bone Joint Surg. 80 -B, 6.

Wright, E., 2014. Chapter 23. Fracture management in the infant, child and young person. In: Clarke, S., Santy-Tomlinson, J. (Eds.), Orthopaedic and Trauma Nursing: An Evidence-Based Approach to Musculoskeletal Care. Wiley Blackwell, London, pp. 309–322.

ADDITIONAL RESOURCES

British Orthopaedic Assocation, 2015. National casting standards. Available from: https://www.boa.ac.uk/wp-content/uploads/2015/12/BOA-National-Casting-Standards.pdf.

British Orthopaedic Assocation, 2019. Orthopodcasts. Available from: https://www.boa.ac.uk/training-education/orthopodcasts/.

Jester, R., Santy, J., Roger, J., 2011. Oxford Handbook of Orthopaedic and Trauma Nursing. University Press, Oxford.

RCN publications: https://www.rcn.org.uk/library/subject-guides/orthopaedic-and-trauma-nursing.

19

Caring for Children With Infection and Altered Immune Responses

Alison Mosenthal, Deborah Martin

LEARNING OUTCOMES

- To understand the different phases of the immune response.
- To describe the defence mechanisms the body has to prevent infection occurring.
- To differentiate between innate and adaptive immunity.

- To consider the normal and abnormal pathophysiology changes that can occur during the immune response.
- To apply knowledge of the immune system to principles of nursing practice, in relation to the care of a child with an infection.
- To outline the assessment of a child with acute infection.

INTRODUCTION

From birth a baby is immediately exposed to a variety of potentially harmful microbes such as bacteria, viruses, fungi and parasites. The immune system is a collection of specialised cells and tissues that provide resistance to infection and it is the coordinated response of these cells that provides the immune response and protection from the pathological effects of infectious diseases (Abbas et al., 2016). In this chapter the two types of immunity that provide host defence against infection will be discussed:

- The innate immune system, which provides the immediate nonspecific protection and the first line of defence against an invading organism.
- The adaptive immune response, which provides specific protection against a known pathogen.

As part of the response to infection the innate and adaptive immune systems initiate the inflammatory response and this will be considered in relation to assessing the child with an infection and providing appropriate nursing care.

THE IMMUNE SYSTEM AND DEFENCE AGAINST INFECTION

At birth the immune system of the newborn infant is immature, but protection is provided initially by immunity passed by the mother to the fetus in utero. During the first year of life the baby's immune system will develop to provide protection as the maternal immunity reduces and the baby is exposed to infectious organisms.

For all individuals the immune system is constantly challenged by exposure to numerous microorganisms in the environment and infectious agents from affected individuals. Organisms that cause disease are called pathogens and the main classes are:

- viruses
- bacteria

- protozoa
- worms

The nature of these pathogens is to invade the host, reproduce and to infect other hosts and they will use different mechanisms to achieve this (MacPherson and Austyn, 2012). Many bacterial pathogens will live and replicate within the extracellular cavities of the body or on the epithelial surfaces that line the body cavities. However, pathogens such as viruses that live intracellularly will cause disease by damaging and invading the cells (Murphy and Weaver, 2016). The host defence to prevent infection by pathogens is provided by the immune system of the individual.

REFLECTION ON YOUR PRACTICE

Identify the names of some of the infective organisms that were the cause of infections in children that you have nursed and differentiate between those that were bacterial and viral infections.

An individual's ability to protect themselves against infection is provided by the specialised cells and tissues of their immune system whose function is to prevent and eliminate infections. The age of the child and any deficiency in, or abnormal development of, the immune system may compromise this protective ability, and this can result in serious or life-threatening illness.

Innate immunity is sometimes termed natural immunity and is nonspecific, preventing the entry of microbes and enabling their removal before they enter the host tissues (Abbas et al., 2016). It is a very rapid response and is normally effective within minutes or hours.

The adaptive immune response takes longer and may take several days but includes a feature which supports rapid future responses – immunological memory. This occurs when there is a specific response to a known foreign protein

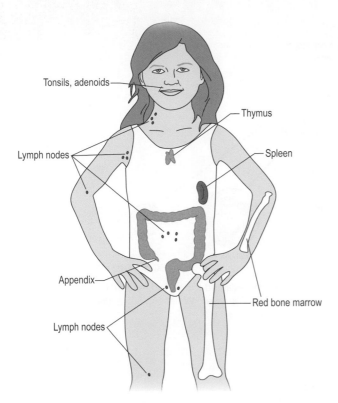

Fig. 19.1 Diagram to show organs and tissues of the immune system.

(antigen). Subsequently if the antigen is encountered again during a second infection the response can be mounted very quickly.

The organs, tissues, cells and molecules that make up the immune system are connected by the blood and lymphatic systems (Fig. 19.1) and it is the white blood cells that are primarily involved in both the innate and adaptive immune responses.

The white blood cells that are predominately involved in the innate response are:

- Tissue macrophages and monocytes – some of which are already present in the lymph tissues and others that can be recruited to the sites of infection and develop into mature macrophages from the circulating monocytes. These cells play an important part in initiating the innate immune response and display phagocytic properties where the invading microbe will be engulfed, ingested and destroyed.
- Granulocytes also known as polymorphonuclear leukocytes (PMN) – these are the most abundant of circulating white cells and the most significant of these are the neutrophils (70% of circulating white cells) which have phagocytic properties and are actively involved in destroying invading microbes with the macrophages.
- Mast cells resident in mucosal and connective tissue containing histamine and cytokines (chemical messengers) which will trigger an inflammatory response in the presence of infection.
- Natural killer cells which play an important part in the destruction of virally infected cells.

The white blood cells that are involved in the adaptive immune system are the lymphocytes and these are divided into two main groups: B and T cell lymphocytes. Both types of cells are produced in the bone marrow, but the B cell lymphocytes will mature there before circulating in the blood whereas immature T cells migrate to the thymus gland situated in the upper anterior thorax above the heart where they will undergo a maturation process. Both B and T cell lymphocytes will migrate to the peripheral lymphoid organs where they will be activated by foreign antigens (Murphy and Weaver, 2016).

- B cell lymphocytes have receptors on the surface of the cells that respond to a known antigen or foreign protein and once exposed to this antigen will grow and multiply rapidly to produce two types of mature cells – plasma cells which secrete soluble proteins called antibodies and memory cells which when they come into contact again with the antigen will rapidly divide to produce plasma cells which when exposed to the same antigen at a later time will rapidly divide to produce mature plasma cells to provide a faster response to the infection. This response is manipulated in the vaccination process to provide protection from childhood diseases (Public Health, 2019).
- T cell lymphocytes having undergone the maturation process in the thymus gland, differentiate into different types of cells – some will become regulator and coordinator cells as part of the adaptive immune system and others will become cytotoxic cells that can kill cells which are infected with viruses and other infective organisms. An important feature of these cells is that they also learn to differentiate between self and non-self to recognise the body's own cells, which is an important factor in the control of the immune response (Fig. 19.2).

Innate Immune System

The innate immune system provides the first line of defence against infection from pathogenic organisms and consists of natural barriers and a range of nonspecific mechanisms which initiate the inflammatory response. The natural barriers are present from birth and are there to protect the baby from environmental and pathogenic organisms. They include the skin and the mucosal surfaces of the respiratory, gastrointestinal and urogenital tracts, providing physical, biochemical and mechanical barriers to invading pathogens on the body surfaces (Rote, 2019). If these barriers are breached, then a sequence of events occurs involving biochemical and cellular responses and this activates the inflammatory response to limit the extent of tissue damage from infection. During this process, which is nonspecific in terms of the invading pathogen, the adaptive immune system will be activated. This will start the process of providing specific immunity with the formation of antibodies against the pathogen should the individual encounter this microorganism again. The natural barriers and inflammation will now be discussed in relation to their protective function as part of the innate system and related to the assessment and nursing care of the infant and child (Fig. 19.3).

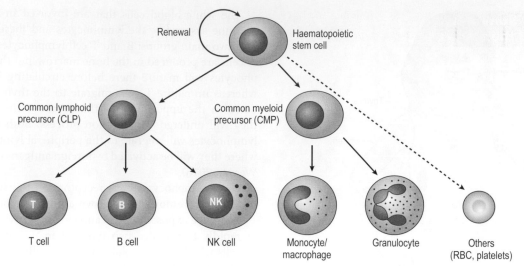

Fig. 19.2 Diagram to show white blood cells involved in immune function. (Adapted from MacPherson, G., Austyn, J.M., 2012. Exploring Immunology Concepts and Evidence. Wiley-Blackwell, Weinheim.) This diagram is also in Peate and Gormley-Fleming (2015)

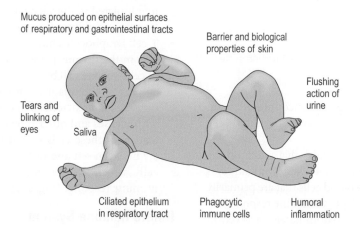

Fig. 19.3 The key features of innate immunity.

The Skin

The skin is the largest organ in the young baby and it provides an intact, dry surface that is resistant to the penetration of microorganisms. At birth the skin is sterile but rapidly becomes colonised by microorganisms many of which are harmless and are called commensal. These commensal organisms help to protect the skin from colonisation by potential pathogenic organisms, and skin-to-skin contact with the mother after delivery provides contact with her commensal organisms to initiate this process. However, hospital acquired infections also known as nosocomial infections can be transmitted from the skin of health care workers to patients with the result that effective hand hygiene when carrying out any care procedure is now a key feature of infection control policy (National Institute of Clinical Excellence [NICE], 2017a).

The skin protects against injury and infection using the keratin layers on the outer surface of the skin to prevent penetration of the skin by microorganisms. There are also dendritic cells and macrophages within the dermis and the role of

these cells is to recognise, ingest and destroy microorganisms. These cells also play a part in the adaptive immune response by presenting the antigens and activating T cells for future recognition of the antigen (Box 19.1).

In the preterm infant the skin is more permeable with a thinner epidermis and immature stratum cornea which makes the skin more permeable and therefore more susceptible to infection as the barrier function of the skin is compromised. The skin of the preterm infant is also more fragile and vulnerable to skin tears from the use of probes and dressings and the handling by parents and health care staff. This can lead to infection once the protective barrier function of the skin has been breached (Bedford Russell, 2010). The use of skin film dressings and tapes with antiseptic cleaning agents and skin assessment tools can help to promote skin integrity when caring for the preterm and sick infant (Silva et al., 2018).

If the epidermal layers of the skin are breached with a wound or burn, then infective organisms can enter the subcutaneous tissues where they can rapidly multiply and cause

BOX 19.1 Summary of Protective Functions of the Skin

- Intact skin resistant to microorganisms
- Presence of commensal organisms
- Skin secretions such as sweat and sebum
- Thickness of skin
- Sloughing off of old skin cells and rapid replacement of new skin cells
- Presence of immune cells within the dermis of skin
- Presence of immune proteins such as antibodies and complement

BOX 19.2 Summary of Protective Functions of the Gastrointestinal Tract

- Presence of mucus
- Huge numbers of innate immune cells such as macrophages and dendritic cells
- Large quantities of IgA and IgG produced from B cells
- Gut-associated-lymphoid tissue (GALT)
- Saliva
- Protection from breast-feeding
- Hydrochloric acid in stomach
- Commensal bacteria
- Movement of faeces

serious infections. This is a feature in infected atopic dermatitis and is discussed in the scenario below.

 SCENARIO

Khaleda has been admitted with infected atopic dermatitis and microbiology reports indicate that her skin is infected with MRSA (methicillin-resistant *Staphylococcus aureus*).

- From your understanding of the barrier properties of innate immunity, identify why she is more prone to developing an infection in her skin.
- Discuss how you will manage her care. To inform your discussion these are topics you may wish to consider
  - infection control procedures
  - risk factors for developing MRSA
  - the rationale behind presenting symptoms
  - treatment strategies
  - the evidence base for treatment

Mucosal Surfaces

The mucosal epithelial surfaces of the respiratory, gastrointestinal and genitourinary tracts provide both mechanical and chemical barriers to infective organisms. The epithelial cells provide tight interconnected junctions that prevent microorganisms passing through to the cells and tissues below. These epithelial surfaces also secrete mucus which lubricates the surfaces and prevents microorganisms adhering to the surface. Tears, perspiration and sweat also contain lysozyme which is an antibacterial enzyme that can break down bacterial walls and provide an acidic environment in which most bacteria are unable to survive (Rote, 2019).

Respiratory Tract

In the respiratory tract the mucus produced by the goblet cells trap the invading microorganisms and the upper respiratory tract is lined with ciliated epithelial cells. These cilia move the mucus towards the mouth and nose where it is expelled by coughing and sneezing. In children where there is impaired mucus production such as cystic fibrosis the secretions are very viscous and the child is unable to remove them, which leads to recurrent respiratory infections. There is also evidence to indicate that there is reduced immunological activity in the pulmonary mucosa of the newborn infant which makes them particularly susceptible to respiratory infections (Drajac

et al., 2017) with respiratory syncytial virus (RSV) the most predominant viral infection that causes bronchiolitis in children under the age of 2 years (Public Health England, 2017).

Gastrointestinal Tract

In the gastrointestinal tract goblet cells secrete mucus, which not only has barrier functions, but also provides lubrication for peristalsis where the contents of the gastrointestinal tract are moved towards the anus. There are also specialised cells within the epithelium which produce antimicrobial peptides as another protective function (MacPherson and Austyn, 2012).

At birth the gut is relatively sterile but rapidly becomes colonised with bacteria, and during the first year of life these increase progressively to develop the immune system and assist with digestive and absorption processes. The introduction of breast milk in the preterm infant helps to facilitate this, and the earlier that enteral feeds are established helps to prevent infections from occurring (Bedford Russell, 2015). The use of antibiotics can affect the commensal bacteria in the gastrointestinal tract and this may result in pathogenic organisms replacing them which will subsequently cause infections.

Apart from providing a physical barrier the mucosal surfaces also provide chemical substances that are antimicrobial. Gastric secretions contain hydrochloric acid and again this low pH, in conjunction with bile salts and digestive enzymes, helps to destroy ingested pathogens. An inability to secrete gastric acid may make a child more susceptible to gastrointestinal infections such as *Salmonella* (MacPherson and Austyn, 2012; Helbert, 2017) (Box 19.2).

 EVIDENCE-BASED PRACTICE

Access the National Institute of Clinical Excellence (NICE, 2019) pathway on fluid and nutritional management in children with diarrhoea and vomiting at:

https://pathways.nice.org.uk/pathways/diarrhoea-and-vomiting-in-children

From the information presented consider:

- What advice would be given to a parent in managing the fluid requirements for their child?
- What clinical signs would indicate the child is dehydrated?
- When should parents seek further medical advice?

Urogenital Tract

The urinary tract is protected against microorganisms by the passing of sterile urine but the most common infective organisms in urinary tract infections *Escherichia coli* (*E. coli*) are found in the gut and perineal areas suggesting that bacteria ascend the urinary tract (Prajaparti, 2018). The virulence of the organism is also a factor and once in the bladder the infective organism will adhere to the bladder epithelium and initiate an inflammatory response (Jadresic, 2013).

Children under the age of two who have poor toilet hygiene, those who have congenital and structural abnormalities of the urogenital tract, or problems with voiding the bladder resulting in stasis of urine, are most at risk of developing urinary tract infections.

Obtaining an uncontaminated specimen of urine in babies and young children can be problematic, but it is important to identify the causative organism and further investigation may be required if a positive result is obtained. A clean catch specimen can be obtained followed by thorough skin cleaning and if this is not possible may need to be obtained by catheterisation or by suprapubic catheterisation.

 EVIDENCE-BASED PRACTICE

Access the NICE guidelines scenario on urinary tract infections in children at:

https://cks.nice.org.uk/urinary-tract-infection-children

Plan the nursing care of an infant and child with a urinary tract infection. In your plan consider the following:
- the age of the child
- what nursing observations are required
- what investigations may be required and what nursing interventions would support them
- what treatment may be prescribed

INFLAMMATION

The innate immune system will initiate the second line of defence if these mechanical and biochemical barriers of the body are breached by microorganisms by the process of inflammation.

Inflammation is the body's nonspecific response to tissue damage or injury and is an essential part of the innate immune system. The role of inflammation is to localise and minimise tissue damage and to ensure that the specialised cells and proteins that are required are transported to the site of infection (MacPherson and Austyn, 2012).

The cells and proteins that are involved in this process are:
- **Mast cells** which are found in the connective tissue and release the inflammatory mediators, histamine and serotonin, at the site of tissue damage that occurs from infection by pathogenic organisms or injury. These act on the blood vessels causing vasodilation which increases the blood flow to the affected area, and this allows for transport of cells and plasma proteins

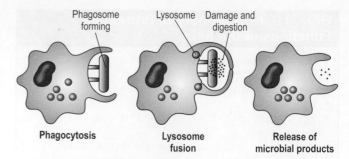

Fig. 19.4 The action of neutrophils.

and also provides oxygen and nutrients for the cellular activity that is taking place. This increase in blood flow causes heat and redness in the affected area. The inflammatory mediators also make the blood vessels more permeable and with the increased blood flow fluid from the plasma will leak out of the surrounding capillaries into the surrounding tissues. The presence of plasma proteins, clotting factors and antibodies in this fluid increases the osmotic pressure and draws more fluid out of the blood vessels. This results in swelling within the tissues causing the oedema that is associated with inflammation.

- **White blood cells** are monocytes and neutrophils and provide the body's first line of cellular defence. The monocytes develop into macrophages once they enter the tissue and these cells have receptors that can distinguish between invading pathogens such as bacteria, fungi and viruses. Neutrophils have receptors that recognise bacteria and other pathogens and are essential for the defence against pyogenic (pus forming) bacteria such as *Streptococcus pyogenes* and *Staphylococcus aureus*.

The neutrophils which are produced in the bone marrow and have a short life span of 1–2 days are not normally present in the tissues but once infection is detected they migrate quickly to the site of the infection by a process of chemotaxis (release of chemicals to attract them). There is also an increase in the production of neutrophils within the bone marrow by stimulation from the colony stimulating factors released by the tissue macrophages. In conjunction with the tissue macrophages the neutrophils will destroy the invading microorganisms by phagocytosis where they engulf, ingest and destroy the organism intracellularly by releasing antimicrobial substances contained within granules in the cytoplasm of the cell (Fig. 19.4). These cells are effective in removing bacteria, small parasites such as protozoa, damaged and dead cells, and provide an important mechanism in the defence against infection by eliminating infectious microorganisms before they become pathogenic. During the inflammatory process dead tissue and phagocytes will accumulate and this production of fluid and cells is known as pus. If the pus is not able to drain from the affected area, then it will collect and form an abscess.

Once phagocytosis has occurred, further enzyme pathways are activated, and this provides an oxidative burst which produces toxic molecules that will damage the pathogens. Children who have a rare immune deficiency called *chronic granulomatous disease* are unable to initiate this oxidative process, and although they have normal levels of neutrophils which migrate to the site of infection and commence phagocytosis, they are unable to kill the invading bacteria. These children will present with fungal and staphylococcal and streptococcal infections such as abscesses, ear, nose and throat infections and pneumonia (Helbert, 2017).

Infection and inflammation will result in an increase in the number of circulating neutrophils within the body and can be estimated in a blood test for full blood count (FBC). The number of neutrophils in childhood varies according to age. At birth a full term baby will have a high neutrophil count, which will rise within the first 2 weeks of life and then fall to within the normal range for an adult, rising to a normal adult range by the age of 4 years (Huether et al., 2019). However, a neonate born preterm will have lower circulating neutrophils and babies born small for gestational age or born to mothers with hypertension associated with pregnancy will also generally have lower neutrophil counts so that infection in the neonate may be associated with neutropaenia (low neutrophil count) (Bedford Russell, 2015). In addition, children born with congenital neutropaenia and those who have neutropaenia because of oncology treatments are at significant risk of bacterial infections and require extremely prompt treatment if presenting with pyrexia.

- **Plasma proteins** are also activated during the inflammatory process and include kinins, the complement system and clotting factors. The kinins increase the permeability of the blood vessels and increase the vasodilation of the blood vessels in the affected area. In addition, bradykinin is produced and with prostaglandins produced by the mast cells, stimulate pain nerve endings which can contribute to the pain associated with inflammation.

Complement consists of soluble proteins which are proteolytic enzymes that are present in circulating blood and become activated when in contact with foreign cells such as bacteria and fungi. The complement system acts as a cascade with one component activating the next with different triggers initiating this cascade. The effect of this process is to increase the vasodilation of the blood vessels and to attract the phagocytic cells (macrophages and neutrophils) to the affected site by the process of chemotaxis. In addition, the complement will enhance the process of phagocytosis by the process of opsonisation where the microbes are coated with complement and directed to the specialised receptors on the phagocytes where they will be engulfed and destroyed particularly against pus forming bacteria such as *S. pyogenes* and *S. aureus*. Complement levels are decreased in the neonate but rapidly increase to near adult levels within weeks of birth. However, children who have a genetic defect in their ability to produce

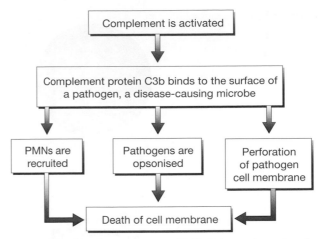

Fig. 19.5 The role of complement. *PMN,* Polymorphonuclear Leukocytes.

complement are very susceptible to these infections and complement deficiency may also contribute to autoimmune conditions such as systemic lupus erythematosus and other immune disorders (Abbas et al., 2016; Helbert, 2017) (Fig. 19.5).

The clotting factors are also stimulated to arrive at the site of inflammation and migrate through the permeable walls of the blood vessel where they start to produce fibrin which forms an insoluble mesh. This helps to localise the infection by trapping bacteria and preventing the spread of infection.

Systemic Effects of Inflammation

Generally, this inflammatory process will contain the infection within a localised area and this can be seen, for example, with tonsillitis where the tonsils look red and swollen and may have white spots present indicating the presence of pus. The child will have a painful sore throat and may have difficulty in swallowing but eventually the body will get rid of the pus that has been formed by drainage into the lymph system and tissue macrophages in the affected area (Fig. 19.6).

In addition, the child may also have a systemic response and can feel unwell with a fever, malaise, muscle pains and loss of appetite. This systemic response is due to the release of cytokines which are proteins that act as chemical messengers affecting the immune cells. Some of them will stimulate the inflammatory response whereas others will act on:

- the bone marrow to stimulate the production of blood cells and enhance the phagocytic activity of the neutrophils;
- the liver to stimulate the production of plasma proteins such as C Reactive Protein (CRP);
- the hypothalamus where the temperature regulating centre is affected to produce the temperature associated with fever (Helbert, 2017).

The main cytokines that are involved in this process are interleukin (IL)-1 and IL-6 and the tumour necrosis factor (TNF), and they are sometimes referred to as *endogenous*

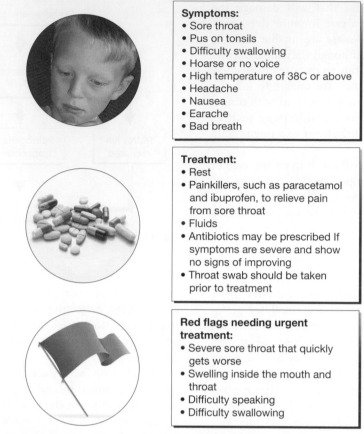

Symptoms:
- Sore throat
- Pus on tonsils
- Difficulty swallowing
- Hoarse or no voice
- High temperature of 38C or above
- Headache
- Nausea
- Earache
- Bad breath

Treatment:
- Rest
- Painkillers, such as paracetamol and ibuprofen, to relieve pain from sore throat
- Fluids
- Antibiotics may be prescribed If symptoms are severe and show no signs of improving
- Throat swab should be taken prior to treatment

Red flags needing urgent treatment:
- Severe sore throat that quickly gets worse
- Swelling inside the mouth and throat
- Difficulty speaking
- Difficulty swallowing

Fig. 19.6 Symptoms and treatment of tonsillitis. Original picture had arrows to the three pictures from picture of inflamed tonsils.

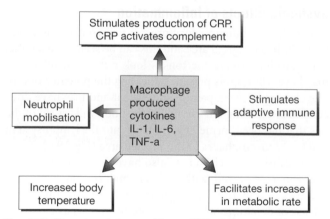

Fig. 19.7 The role of the cytokines. *CRP, C* Reactive Protein; *IL,* Interleukin; *TNF,* tumour necrosis factor.

pyrogens (fever producing substances). The increased temperature will inhibit the action of invading pathogens (Murphy and Weaver, 2016).

As part of the inflammatory process prostaglandins are released by the mast cells and these act upon the sympathetic nervous system, which raises the metabolic rate within the body to deal with the inflammatory processes. There is a resulting increase in oxygen requirements so that when observing a child with fever a rise in pulse and respiratory

rate is noted. There is also an increase in peripheral vasoconstriction which helps to conserve heat within the body and decreases the activity of the digestive tract, so the child may appear pale and lethargic with decreased appetite (Fig. 19.7).

Feverish illnesses are very common in children particularly in the under-5 age group and are the most common reason for parents to seek medical advice. It is important to carry out a thorough assessment of the child as it may be indicative of a more serious bacterial infection such as meningitis, pneumonia or a urinary tract infection (Mosenthal 2019). To assess the child, guidelines in the form of a traffic light system are used so that a consistent approach is made, and appropriate treatment is provided (NICE, 2017b).

Sepsis

The normal response to an infection is to localise and control the infection but in severe infections toxins from the infective organism are released into the blood providing an overwhelming response from the innate immune system. This can be life threatening. The response of the inflammatory mediators and cytokines in high concentrations can cause vasodilation and increased permeability of the blood vessels causing low blood pressure (hypotension) and poor perfusion of the tissues, which if not treated quickly can result in multi-organ failure, known as septic shock.

LEARNING ACTIVITY

Mesenteric adenitis is a condition where the lymph glands in the abdomen become swollen and painful, usually associated with a viral infection. It is common in young children who complain of abdominal pain which is generalised or located in the lower right quadrant of the abdomen and is sometimes mistaken for appendicitis (Fig. 19.8).

Using your knowledge of inflammation:
- Identify the possible symptoms that the child may present with.
- What observations and investigations should be carried out to assist with the diagnosis of this condition?
- Write an information leaflet for parents and carers to assist them in caring for the child.

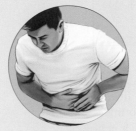

Abdominal pain usually caused by a viral infection following a respiratory infection but may also be bacterial.

Mesenteric lymphadenitis

The name comes from the mesentery which is the tissue that connects intestines to the wall of the abdomen and has lymph nodes contained within it

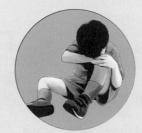

Self-limiting infection lasting few days to 4 weeks.

Occurs mainly in boys during childhood but common in age group 5–8

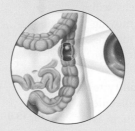

Lymph glands swell and become inflamed in the mesentery. Causes abdominal pain in the right lower quadrant of the abdomen (illac fossa)

Other symptoms include
- Pyrexia
- Tachycardia
- Nausea, vomiting and diarrhoea

Fig. 19.8 Mesenteric adenitis.

The risk factors for the onset of sepsis in children are as identified by NICE (2016):
- Age of the child – children under the age of one and preterm babies are at significant risk because of their immature immune system
- Impaired immune function because of medication, illness of the child, such as a child on long-term steroid treatment, or the child with cancer who has had his/her immune system suppressed as part of oncology treatment
- The child with a critical illness or injury
- The presence of indwelling central venous catheters
- Invasive procedures such as cannulation
- Surgical procedures
- Breaches to skin integrity such as wounds and burns

It is important that any child presenting with suspected sepsis is assessed following the NICE (2016) guidelines adapted from fever management and using the age-related algorithms and risk stratification tools. Assessment of the child should include the following:
- Temperature – in a baby under 3 months a temperature of 38°C is a concern, but temperature may be under 36°C

- Heart rate
- Respiratory rate – observing for tachypnoea and signs of respiratory distress
- Level of consciousness – observing for change in behaviour and response using the Glasgow coma scale AVPU (alert, verbal, pain, unresponsive)
- Capillary refill – to assess the level of peripheral perfusion
- Oxygen saturation
- Blood pressure (if there is appropriate equipment and a correct cuff size)

Children who are very unwell, unrousable or with a marked change in behaviour with very poor colour and signs of respiratory distress should be investigated urgently by a medical practitioner. The use of paediatric early warning scores (PEWS) facilitates the early detection of deterioration in the child's condition, and in addition the UK Sepsis Trust (2019) has identified screening tools which use a red flag system based on observations of vital signs to trigger interventions within the community and in hospital settings.

THE ADAPTIVE IMMUNE SYSTEM

The adaptive immune system provides the third line of defence for individuals by responding specifically to infective organisms (the innate immune system provides a generalised response). This specific response is by the B and T cell lymphocytes found in the lymph tissue such as lymph nodes, the spleen and the specialised mucosal lymphoid tissue found within the respiratory and gastrointestinal tracts such as the tonsils and adenoids, Peyer patches and the appendix (see Fig. 19.1).

Immature B and T cell lymphocytes along with other blood cells are produced in the liver, spleen and bone marrow in a fetus. After birth children produce blood cells and therefore lymphocytes within the bone marrow. These cells will migrate into the circulation with immature T cells moving to the thymus gland to undergo maturation before moving to the lymph tissues with the B cell lymphocytes, which have matured within the bone marrow.

The B and T cell lymphocytes both have the ability to recognise a specific antigen which is a foreign molecule found on the surfaces of pathogenic organisms such as bacteria, viruses and fungi. These molecules are also found on toxins produced by bacteria such as tetanus and diphtheria, cancer cells, transplanted tissue, transfused blood cells and environmental agents such as food and pollens (Rote and McCance, 2019).

One of the features of the adaptive immune system is that both the B and T cell lymphocytes will only respond to one specific antigen which gives the specificity of the adaptive immune system. Prior to the initial contact with the antigen the B and T cell lymphocytes are described as immunocompetent because they can respond to a specific antigen but have not yet encountered it. After the initial encounter the lymphocytes will respond much faster when meeting the antigen again. This demonstrates the memory function of the immune system and provides protection against future exposure to the same specific foreign organism.

The immunity provided by B cell lymphocytes is known as humoral immunity and the immunity provided by the T cell lymphocytes is known as cell mediated immunity.

Humoral Immunity

B cell lymphocytes are produced in the bone marrow and mature there before being released into the blood system. As

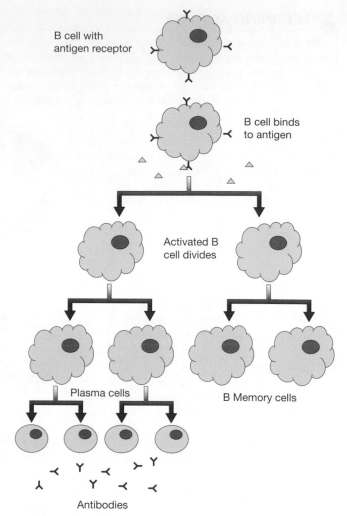

Fig. 19.9 Diagram to show development of B cell lymphocytes.

discussed earlier, the B cell lymphocytes have specific surface receptors to antigens and when exposed to the antigen the B cell lymphocytes are stimulated to grow and multiply rapidly. This production of similar cells from the same cell is called cloning and two types of mature cells are produced – plasma cells and memory cells. The plasma cells secrete antibodies which are also known as immunoglobulins, and these are soluble proteins which will bind with the specific antigens. The memory cells will circulate within the blood so that when the antigen is encountered again, they rapidly start to divide to produce mature plasma cells (Fig. 19.9).

Antibodies or immunoglobulins will bind with the specific antigen using a lock and key analogy, that is, only one receptor site will bind with that specific antigen. This links to the specificity discussed above. There are five classes of immunoglobulins (Ig) which vary in molecular size and function:

- IgG
- IgA
- IgM
- IgE
- IgD

Immunoglobulin G (IgG) is the most abundant of all the antibodies accounting for 75%–80% of total serum immunoglobulin and provides most of the protection against infection. It passes through the placenta providing maternal protection to the newborn infant for the first few months of life. This occurs mainly in the last trimester of the pregnancy, so a premature infant will have insufficient protection and is significantly at risk of infection in the newborn period. Infection is the leading cause of mortality and morbidity in the newborn and the risk increases with low birth weight and prematurity of the infant (Bedford Russell, 2015). Nursing care of the preterm infant requires extreme vigilance with hand hygiene, infection control practices and with the interventions required to support these babies with invasive procedures (the insertion of cannulas, the presence of indwelling catheters and parenteral nutrition).

Immunoglobulin A (IgA) is found in the body's secretions such as saliva, tears, breast milk and nasal secretions and within the mucous membranes of the respiratory and gastrointestinal tracts. This provides localised protection to potentially harmful microbes that are ingested and inhaled. The newborn infant acquires further maternal protection from the mother's colostrum and breast milk where the presence of IgA will provide mucosal immune protection. Introduction of breast milk to premature babies will help to facilitate the gut being colonised with the normal commensal bacteria which are tolerated by the immune system. Children who have a deficiency in IgA (the most common immune deficiency occurring in 1:300–1:400 of the population) may have an increased susceptibility to respiratory and gastrointestinal infections and this can result in recurrent ear and chest infections in early childhood.

Immunoglobulin M (IgM) is the largest of the antibodies in molecular weight and is found in both blood and lymph. It is the most predominate antibody in the early phase of the immune response and has an important role in the agglutination of microbes and activation of complement (Helbert, 2017).

Children who are born with a genetic defect in the immune system that results in immunodeficiency and present with recurrent and unusual infections that may be life-threatening, are likely to have low serum levels of one or more of these antibodies which form part of the diagnostic tests for the condition.

Immunoglobulin E (IgE) is found on the surfaces of mast cells and the blood cells basophils and differs from the other antibodies as it is found predominately within the tissues. When it binds with an antigen the release of chemical mediators from the mast cells such as histamine can cause an acute inflammatory response and trigger an allergic reaction (Helbert 2017). Antigens that trigger this response are known as allergens, and children who are atopic with an increase susceptibility to conditions such as eczema and asthma can have high serum levels of IgE, whereas normally it accounts for less than 0.01% of serum antibodies. In diagnostic tests for allergy the serum level of IgE against a specific allergen can be determined.

Immunoglobulin D (IgD) is found on the surfaces of B cell lymphocytes and plays an important part in the activation of these cells.

Cellular Immunity

Immature T cell lymphocytes undergo maturation within the thymus gland and during this process they learn to recognise the body's own cells and differentiate between self and non-self, recognising antigens such as pathogens, cancer cells and transplanted cells. The immature T cells need to be initially exposed to the foreign proteins on the cell membrane of the antigen to recognise that specific antigen on future contact. by specific T cell receptors (TCR) Following maturation, the T cells will migrate to the spleen and lymph tissue, and when they are exposed to the antigen presenting cells that have been activated by the innate immune response they will be stimulated to react to the known antigen. There are four classes of T cells and their functions are summarised below:

- Cytotoxic T cells – these cells destroy and kill abnormal cells such as virus infected cells, cancer cells and cells of transplanted tissue.
- Helper T cells – these cells, when activated, act on both the innate immune system and the adaptive immune system. They release cytokines which will stimulate the production of B cells and cytotoxic T cells and they also recruit phagocytic cells and neutrophils to the site of infection.
- Regulatory T cells – these cells suppress the immune response of the B and T cells once the antigen has been destroyed and is an important feature of the immune system as it helps to prevent overactivity of the immune system.
- Memory T cells – these cells reactivate antigen specific T cells when the antigen is next encountered. This allows for a more rapid production of the antigen specific T cells so that the body can respond more quickly to future infections by the same pathogen.

Fig. 19.10 illustrates the humoral and cellular components of the adaptive immune system.

Primary and Secondary Response to Infection

When the body encounters a pathogen for the first time there is an initial delay as the T cells are activated to stimulate the production of the B cell lymphocytes and this is called the primary response to the infection. As discussed above, one of the features of the adaptive immune system is the ability to respond more quickly to future infections of the same pathogen due to the presence of memory B and T cell lymphocytes and this is known as immunological memory. On a subsequent exposure to the same antigen the response will be much faster and more powerful to ensure that the antigen is destroyed effectively, and this is known as the secondary response to infection (Fig. 19.11).

Immunity can be acquired either actively by the individual responding to the antigen and producing antibodies or passively when the individual has the antibodies transferred to them.

Natural acquired immunity is the body's normal response to infection whereas artificial acquired immunity is by the process of vaccination when the body develops immunological memory without a primary infection (Helbert, 2017). Vaccines contain small amounts of the infective organism that are either inactivated (killed) or attenuated (weakened) so that they will not cause an overwhelming infection but will allow the body to develop the memory cells for any further

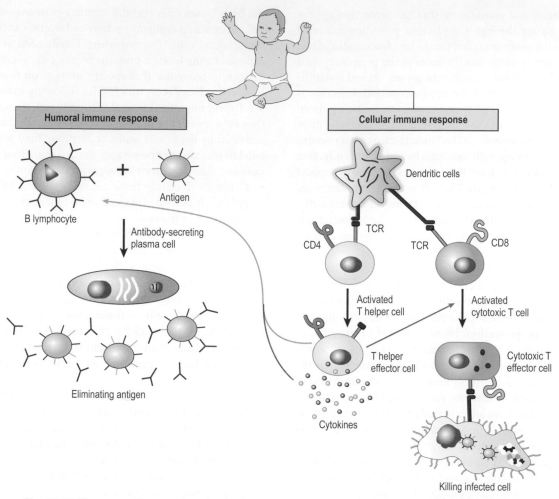

Fig. 19.10 Diagram to illustrate the adaptive immune system. *CD4,* helper T cells; *CD8,* cytotoxic T cells; *TCR,* T cell receptor. (Available from: https://en.wikibooks.org/wiki/Structural_Biochemistry/Genetic_code/Immune_System.)

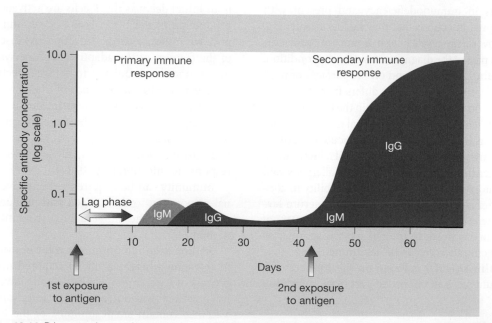

Fig. 19.11 Primary and secondary response to infection. *Ig,* Immunoglobulin. (Peate and Gormley Fleming 2015)

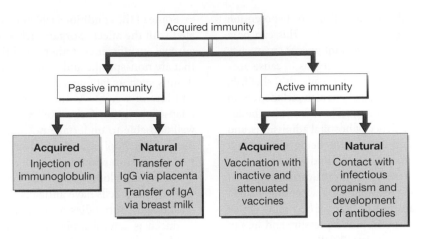

Fig. 19.12 Active and passive immunity. *Ig,* Immunoglobulin.

encounters. Vaccination against communicable diseases provides an essential public health initiative and children should receive their vaccinations in-line with the current vaccination schedule (Public Health England, 2019).

Natural passive immunity is the immunity that a newborn baby acquires by the transfer of maternal IgG through the placenta and IgA from the colostrum and breast milk. Artificial passive immunity occurs when the child with an immunodeficiency (deficiency in the immune system) receives an infusion or an injection of antibodies from pooled plasma donations (Fig. 19.12).

Alterations in the Immune Response

From the overview above it is apparent that the immune system provides a complex network of mechanisms to protect the individual from foreign antigens particularly infectious organisms. At times this ability to protect the individual is compromised and there may be an inappropriate immune response, which can result in serious or life-threatening reactions. This may be because of a deficiency of the immune system or an excessive immune response which is described as a hypersensitivity reaction (Helbert, 2017).

• **Immune deficiency** is a defect or deficiency in components of the immune system which can result in an increased susceptibility to infection.

• **Primary immune deficiency (PID)** or congenital immunodeficiency is caused by a genetic abnormality resulting in rare but life-threatening conditions. A history of

parental consanguinity, or a family history of unexplained death of children within the family, may indicate an inherited familial disease, but in some cases it will be due to a spontaneous genetic mutation.

Diagnostic tests for PID will take place when a child is admitted with a serious life-threatening infection or presents with recurrent infections that are persistent, severe or unusual. It is normal for a child in the first two years of life to have upper respiratory tract infections as their immature immune system develops, but it is unusual for a child to have recurrent continuous respiratory infections or episodes of pneumonia and this requires further investigation.

Treatment for immune deficiency will be determined by the severity and type of antibody deficiency. Children with a mild antibody deficiency may require prophylactic antibiotics, with early intervention of an alternative antibiotic therapy in the event of an infection. For those children who have a severe antibody deficiency replacement antibody treatment may be required, which is administered either intravenously or subcutaneously providing protection against a wide range of pathogenic organisms. This is life-long treatment and administration of the treatment will range from weekly to monthly depending on the age of the child and route of administration.

• **Secondary immune deficiency** is acquired immune deficiency caused by factors such as infection, medical treatments, exposure to environmental toxins and nutritional defects.

• **Hypersensitivity reactions** are excessive immune responses by the adaptive immune system to an antigen after previous exposure to it.

• **Allergy (Type I hypersensitivity)** is an immediate hypersensitivity reaction triggered by antigens known as allergens mediated by IgE. On exposure to the allergen there is a rapid increase in the production of IgE which binds to the mast cells found predominantly in the gastrointestinal tract, respiratory tract and the skin. Release of histamine from the mast cells causes constriction of smooth muscle, vasodilation and vascular permeability.

Anaphylaxis is the most severe Type I hypersensitivity where a systemic reaction occurs. This causes angioedema resulting in airway obstruction if the larynx is affected, hypoxia, bronchoconstriction, vasodilation resulting in hypotension and collapse of the patient. (Mosenthal 2019) This can be a life-threatening situation and it is important to seek emergency medical treatment. The most common allergens to cause anaphylaxis are foods that include nuts, milk, eggs, fish, shellfish, fruits and legumes. However other allergens also include venom from insect stings, latex and some drugs. Children under the age of 4 years have the highest incidence of hospital admissions, and symptoms often present when the child is being weaned and new foods are introduced into the diet. A child who has had an anaphylactic reaction may present with an urticarial rash, facial swelling, difficulty in speaking or swallowing, wheezing, nausea and vomiting, abdominal pain, feeling dizzy or becoming floppy and unresponsive due to a drop in blood pressure and loss of consciousness (Anaphylaxis Campaign, 2019).

The incidence of allergy in the UK is high as approximately 20% of the population are affected with conditions such as allergic rhinitis, asthma, eczema and food allergies. Allergy conditions usually present in early childhood and diagnosis and treatment of the conditions can have a considerable impact on families. Advice on the avoidance of the allergen, and an individualised care plan for the child outlining the severity of the allergic reaction with appropriate treatment is required. For those children who have had an anaphylactic reaction intramuscular epinephrine will be prescribed and parents and carers will need support and education to administer this. Children should carry their anaphylaxis treatment with them at all times and staff in nurseries and schools will also require support and guidance to manage this.

👤 SCENARIO

Emily, aged 18 months, has been diagnosed with peanut allergy following an anaphylactic reaction when she ate a peanut butter sandwich. She required epinephrine in the Accident and Emergency department and developed asthma-like symptoms but has now made a full recovery.

- What advice would you give Emily's parents about avoiding future contact with nuts?
- What medication is Emily likely to be prescribed?
- What factors should the nurse consider when planning an individualised care plan for Emily to support her family when she is discharged home?

- **Autoimmune disease** occurs when the adaptive immune system loses its ability to distinguish self from self and the immune system starts to attack the body's own cells. They are rare conditions and can be difficult to diagnose and include conditions such as:
  - Juvenile idiopathic arthritis affecting joints, skin and sometimes the lungs
  - Crohn disease and coeliac disease affecting the gastrointestinal tract
  - Type 1 diabetes mellitus affecting the pancreas and production of insulin
  - Addison disease affecting the adrenal glands and production of adrenal hormones

Some of the conditions will have specific symptoms associated with the affected organ such as symptoms of diabetes or adrenal insufficiency. Other conditions will have symptoms that are non-specific and characteristic of other medical conditions such as fatigue, recurrent fevers, unexplained rashes and loss of weight. At times the child may have periods of relapse when they feel unwell; and remission, when they feel well and able to undertake normal activities. This can affect the child's schooling and social activities.

- **Transfusion reactions** occur when an individual receives the wrong blood group based on the ABO blood groups. Red blood cells have antigens on the surface of their cells and IgM antibodies against these cell antigens are produced as natural antibodies. This means that a person with blood group A has anti-B antibodies, group B has anti-A antibodies and group O has both anti-A and anti-B antibodies. If a person inadvertently receives the wrong blood group, for example, blood group A receives blood from a blood group B donor, who has antibodies to group A, then an acute hypersensitivity reaction will occur. IgM antibodies are very effective at activating complement and haemolysis (destruction of the red blood cells) will occur (Helbert, 2017). This can be an extremely rapid reaction which can cause shock and is potentially fatal.

The Rhesus (Rh) D factor is the classification of individuals as positive or negative depending on whether they express the Rh system antigen on the cell surface of the red blood cells. This can cause specific problems when a Rhesus negative mother and a Rhesus positive father produce a Rhesus positive fetus. During delivery there may be a mixing of maternal and fetal blood and the mother is exposed to a foreign antigen and will produce IgG anti-Rh antibody. In a subsequent pregnancy this IgG antibody will cross the placenta and destroy fetal red blood cells causing death of the fetus in utero or haemolytic disease of the newborn (MacPherson and Austyn, 2012). This can be prevented by giving the mother an injection of anti-D antibody prior to delivery so that any Rh positive antigens that may enter the mother's blood are destroyed before the mother is able to make anti- Rh antibodies (Helbert, 2017).

🔖 REFLECTION ON PRACTICE

Consider a patient that you have nursed who has required a blood transfusion:

- What checks are required to ensure the safe administration of blood to a patient?
- What observations of vital signs would you carry out for your patient?
- What advice and support would you give to the parent while their child is receiving a transfusion?

The Immune System and Transplantation

Transplantation of tissue and cells plays an important part in the treatment of children with cancer, conditions requiring organ transplant such as heart or lung transplant, and primary immune deficiency. The introduction of foreign tissue and cells causes an immune response by the adaptive immune system and will result in the rejection of the transplanted tissue. The T cell lymphocytes of the recipient will be activated by the antigens of the donor cells, which are called transplant antigens. Tissue typing of the donor and recipient is carried out to ensure the greatest level of compatibility and where possible using a related donor – there is a 1:4 chance that a sibling will provide an identical match on testing.

Immunosuppressive (anti-rejection) treatment is administered prior to organ and stem cell transplants to prevent graft versus host disease. The suppression of the bone marrow means that the child is at significant risk of infection and should be nursed in isolation in a single room during their stay in hospital with specific precautions taken to ensure that the child is not exposed to potential risks of infection. Once the child is discharged home the child and family will require continuing care to monitor their recovery. Parents are advised to seek urgent medical care if the child becomes unwell with a temperature or has been in contact with a communicable disease such as chicken pox or measles.

CONCLUSION

This introduction to the immune system has provided an overview of the innate and the adaptive immune system and the essential role that they provide in protecting the individual from infection. There has been an emphasis on how this relates specifically to the development of the immune system in childhood and how alterations in the immune system can affect the infant and child and how this relates to the care of the child and family.

REFERENCES

Abbas, A.K., Lichtman, A.H., Pillai, S., 2016. Basic Immunology, fifth ed. Elsevier, St Louis.

Anaphylaxis Campaign, 2019. Signs and symptoms. Available from: https://www.anaphylaxis.org.uk/what-is-anaphylaxis/patient-signs-and-symptoms/.

Bedford Russell, A., 2010. Infection in the term and preterm infant. In: Meeks, M., Hallsworth, M., Yeo, H. (Eds.), Nursing the Neonate, second ed. John Wiley & Sons Ltd., Chichester.

Bedford Russell, A., 2015. Neonatal sepsis. Paediatr. Child. Health. 25 (6), 271–276.

Drajac, C., Laubreton, D., Riffault, S., et al., 2017. Pulmonary susceptibility of neonates to respiratory syncytial virus infection: a problem of innate immunity? J. Immunol. Res. 2017, 8734504. Available from: https://doi.org/10.1155/2017/8734504.

Helbert, M., 2017. Immunology for Medical Students, third ed. Elsevier Ltd., Philadelphia.

Huether, S., Rote, S.N., McCance, K., 2019. Structure and function of the hematologic system. In: McCance, K.L., Huether, S.E. (Eds.), Pathophysiology: The Biologic Basis for Disease in Adults and Children, eighth ed. Elsevier, St Louis, pp. 890–1017.

Jadresic, L., 2013. Urinary tract infection in children. Paediatr. Child Health 24 (7), 289–292.

MacPherson, G., Austyn, J.M., 2012. Exploring Immunology Concepts and Evidence. Wiley-Blackwell, Weinheim.

Mosenthal, A. 2019 Inflammation, immune response and healing. In Gormley Fleming, E. Peate, I (Eds),Fundamentals of Children's Applied Pathophysiology. John Wiley & Sons Ltd. Chichester.

Murphy, K., Weaver, C., 2016. Janeway's Immunobiology, ninth ed. Garland Science, New York.

National Institute of Clinical Excellence (NICE), 2016. Sepsis: recognition diagnosis and early management. Available from: https://www.nice.org.uk/guidance/NG51 [accessed 30 March 2017].

National Institute for Clinical Excellence (NICE), 2017a. Healthcare-associated infections: prevention and control in primary and community care. Available from: https://www.nice.org.uk/guidance/cg139/chapter/1-guidance.

National Institute of Clinical Excellence (NICE), 2017b. Fever in under 5s: assessment and clinical management. Available from: https://www.nice.org.uk/guidance/cg160.

National Institute of Clinical Excellence (NICE), 2019. Urinary tract infection – children. Available from: https://cks.nice.org.uk/urinary-tract-infection-children.

NHS Improvement, 2018. SBAR communication tool- situation, background, assessment, recommendation. Available from: https://improvement.nhs.uk/resources/sbar-communication-tool/.

Prajaparti, H., 2018. Urinary tract infection in children. Paediatr. Child Health 28 (7), 318–323.

Public Health England, 2017. Respiratory syncytial virus (RSV): guidance, data and analysis. Available from: https://www.gov.uk/government/collections/respiratory-syncytial-virus-rsv-guidance-data-and-analysis.

Peate, I. & Gormley Fleming, E. 2015 Fundamentals of Children's Anatomy and Physiology. John Wiley & Sons Ltd., Chichester.

Public Health England, 2019. Complete immunisation schedule. Available from: https://www.gov.uk/government/publications/the-complete-routine-immunisation-schedule.

Rote, S.N., 2019. Innate immunity: inflammation and wound healing. In: McCance, K.L., Huether, S.E. (Eds.), Pathophysiology: The Biologic Basis for Disease in Adults and Children, eighth ed. Elsevier, St Louis, pp. 190–219.

Rote, S.N., McCance, K.L., 2019. Adaptive immunity. In: McCance, K.L., Huether, S.E. (Eds.), Pathophysiology: The Biologic Basis for Disease in Adults and Children, eighth ed. Elsevier, St Louis, pp. 220–255.

Silva, E., Oude-Reimer, M., Frauenfelder, O., et al., 2018. Skin care of newborn infants in European standards of care for newborn infants. Available from: https://newborn-health-standards.org/skin-care-infants/.

UK Sepsis Trust, 2019. Professional guidelines. Available from: https://sepsistrust.org/professional-resources/clinical/.

20

Caring for Children With Diabetes and Other Endocrine Disorders

Liz Gormley-Fleming

LEARNING OUTCOMES

- Describe the key function of the endocrine system.
- Appreciate how disordered function of the endocrine system presents and affects the child.
- Understand the care requirements of the child and family in relation to specific endocrine disorders.

- Understand the specialist nature of caring for a child with diabetes.
- Recognise the importance of continuing care and support required by the child and family with an endocrine disorder.

ENDOCRINE SYSTEM

The endocrine system is a chemical communication system that provides the means to control a number of physiological processes within the body. As it is a communication network, the endocrine system contains transmitters, signals and receivers that are called hormone-producing cells, hormones and receptors. The endocrine system consists of a number of distinct glands and some tissues in other organs. The endocrine glands (Fig.20.1) are:

- pituitary gland
- thyroid gland
- four parathyroid glands
- two adrenal glands
- pancreatic islets (also known as the islets of Langerhans)
- pineal gland
- thymus gland
- two ovaries in the female
- two testes in the male

Endocrine glands secrete hormones directly into the bloodstream, whereas exocrine glands pass their secretions directly into body cavities. The hormones released by endocrine glands are carried in the bloodstream to their target organ, where they are active. The activity of a number of endocrine glands is regulated through the activity of the hypothalamus.

The Hypothalamus

The hypothalamus is the central control unit that stimulates a number of key body functions: thermoregulation, thirst, hunger and stress response. Located in the midbrain, below the thalamus, it controls the pituitary gland directly and exerts its influence indirectly over other glands (Waugh and Grant, 2018). The hypothalamus communicates directly with the pituitary gland via a portal system. This enables the rapid delivery of hormones from the hypothalamus to the pituitary gland.

At birth the hypothalamus is immature. This can impact on a number of physiological functions, for example, thermoregulation in the newborn as the newborn is at risk of heat loss (Peate and Gormley-Fleming, 2015). Non-shivering thermogenesis occurs as a result of hormone release and serves a vital function in the early life of the newborn baby.

The hypothalamic hormones that either stimulate or inhibit the release of anterior and posterior hormones are secreted by the neurosecretory cells. These hormones are formed in the median eminence of the hypothalamus (the area that is connected to the pituitary gland by the pituitary stalk). Nine separate hormones are secreted (Table 20.1).

▶ POWERPOINT

Access the companion PowerPoint presentation and revise your knowledge in relation to hormone structure, action of hormones, regulation, synthesis, metabolism and excretion of hormones.

Access the companion PowerPoint presentation and look at the discussion on hypopituitarism and hyperpituitarism including pituitary tumours to enhance your knowledge.

You are also advised to revise the section on growth hormone production, regulation and synthesis before proceeding to the next section of this chapter on growth hormone deficiencies.

Pituitary Gland

Also known as the hypophysis, the pituitary gland develops from the merging of different tissues (Fig. 20.2). This small pea-like gland is located in a small depression in the sphenoid bone: the sella tursica. It has two independent

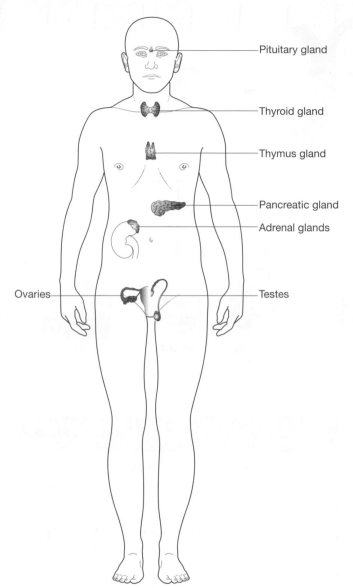

Fig. 20.1 The glands within the body.

Pituitary gland
Thyroid gland
Thymus gland
Pancreatic gland
Adrenal glands
Ovaries
Testes

TABLE 20.1	The Hypothalamic Hormones	
Hypothalamus		
Synthesis of posterior pituitary hormones and transport via nerve axons	Hypothalamic hormones carried in hypothalamohypophyseal portal system	
Pituitary gland		
Posterior pituitary (neurohypophysis)	*Middle lobe*	*Anterior lobe (adenohypophysis)*
Oxytocin	Melanocyte-stimulating hormones	Trophic hormones: ACTH, adrenal cortex hormone
Vasopressin (antidiuretic hormone)		
Thyroid stimulating hormone (TSH)		
Growth hormone (GH)		
Follicle stimulating hormone (FSH)		
Luteinising hormone (LH)		
Prolactin (PRL)		

segments: the anterior pituitary gland and the posterior pituitary gland.

Anterior Pituitary Gland

The anterior pituitary gland is the true gland as it originates from an upgrowth of glandular epithelium from the pharynx and is known as the adenohypophysis. This is only linked to the brain via the venous hypothalamohypophyseal portal system. This network transports blood from the hypothalamus to the anterior pituitary, thereby transporting releasing and inhibiting hormones secreted by the hypothalamus. These hormones influence secretion and release of other hormones formed in the anterior pituitary (see Table 20.3); growth hormone is the most abundant hormone that is synthesised by the anterior pituitary gland.

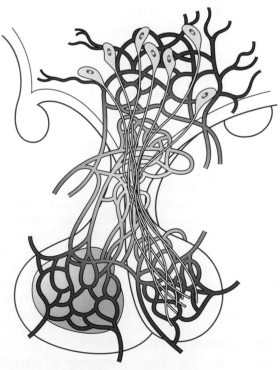

Fig. 20.2 The pituitary gland.

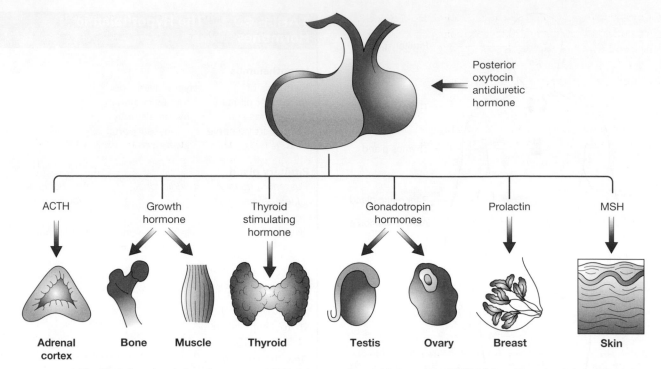

Fig. 20.3 Anterior pituitary hormones. *ACTH*, Adrenocorticotrophic hormone; *MSH*, Melanocyte stimulating hormone.

Hormones of the Anterior Pituitary

Corticotrophin-releasing hormone: controls release of tropic hormones, such as adrenocorticotrophic hormone (ACTH)

Thyrotrophin-releasing hormone (also known as thyroid-stimulating hormone [TSH])

Growth-hormone-releasing factor TSH inhibition

Gonadotrophin-releasing hormone

Somatostatin-releasing hormone (also known as growth-hormone [GH] somatotrophin-release inhibiting factor)

Prolactin-lactogenic hormone (PRL)

Follicle stimulating hormone (FSH)

Luteinising hormone (LH)

Melanocyte-stimulating hormone (MSH)

Posterior Pituitary Gland

This is derived from a downgrowth of nervous tissue from the base of the brain and is known as the neurohypophysis. It has nervous connections with the hypothalamus, down which the antidiuretic hormone (ADH) and oxytocin pass. ADH and oxytocin are synthesised in the nerve cell bodies of the hypothalamus, transported along the axons, and then stored and secreted by vesicles within the axon terminals. Their release is triggered by nerve impulses from the hypothalamus.

Disorders Affecting the Pituitary Gland

Disorders affecting the pituitary gland result in disruption in regulation of hormone secretion. Symptoms vary depending on the location of the disorder, and are related to a disturbance in

TABLE 20.2 Disorders of Pituitary Hormones	
Hypopituitarism	**Hyperpituitarism**
Growth hormone: somatic growth retardation	Somatic growth acceleration Adrenal hyperfunction
Adrenocorticotrophic hormone (ACTH): adrenal hypofunction	Hyperthyroidism Precocious puberty/retarded sexual development
Thyroid hormone: hypothyroidism	
Follicle stimulating and luteinising hormone: absence/regression of secondary sexual characteristics	Prolactin: stops menstruation
Prolactin	

production of a specific hormone or group of hormones, and relate to the role they play in maintaining health and development.

Hypopituitarism

This term denotes subnormal pituitary hormone production. It is generally a result of disorders of the anterior pituitary and may involve one or more of the hormones produced (Table 20.2). Deficiencies of anterior hormone production are due to primary disease or a disorder of the anterior pituitary. There is either an inadequate production or an insufficient supply of hypothalamic releasing hormone. The typical presentation of a child with hypopituitarism is a low target hormone level, and a low or inappropriate normal level of the corresponding tropic hormone level (Corenblum, 2016). The end result of this is eventual secondary failure of the target gland (Kim, 2015). Secondary hypopituitarism, which is attributed to dysfunction of the hypothalamus, affects the synthesis and release of releasing hormones and release inhibiting hormones.

The child with hypopituitarism will initially present with low target hormone levels. The function of the pituitary is assessed by the target gland function hormone levels. Diagnosis is based on hormone profile, duration of onset and other physiological presentations such as height and weight increase or decrease. An example of conditions that are caused by hypopituitarism are diabetes insipidus, tumours of the pituitary gland and disorders of growth.

POWERPOINT

Access the companion PowerPoint presentation and refer to the discussion on growth hormone for detailed information on assessment and diagnosis in relation to family history, child's history, radiographic and imaging findings, and laboratory findings.

Factors contributing to pituitary hyposecretion include congenital hypopituitarism due to genetic abnormalities or other developmental defects. Congenital hypopituitarism is mainly related to growth hormone deficiency. Disordered pituitary hormone secretion that develops after birth is referred to as acquired hypopituitarism This may have resulted from central nervous system trauma, meningitis or encephalitis, vascular abnormalities or haemorrhage, brain tumours, pituitary tumours and/or radiation therapy.

Hyperpituitarism

Hyperpituitarism is a disorder in which excessive secretion of growth hormone increases the growth rate. Pituitary tumours that secrete hormones produce characteristic symptoms of excessive hormone levels. This is rare in children. Symptoms may range from complaints such as listlessness or restlessness to more severe symptoms such as headaches, vomiting or dizziness. In addition, problems due to an increase in any of the hormones produced may give rise to growth, adrenal or sexual dysfunction (see Table 20.2).

Hormonal abnormalities occurring as a result of pituitary tumours or defects will be discussed under specific headings. Oversecretion of growth hormone is usually caused by a pituitary adenoma.

Precocious Puberty

Precocious puberty is defined as the onset of secondary sex characteristics by the age of 8.5 years in females and 9.5 years in males (Rudolf et al., 2011). It is either gonadotrophin dependent or gonadotrophin independent. It is more likely to occur in females and may be idiopathic in origin or likely due to the premature onset of normal puberty. It is recognised today that pubertal development has started to occur earlier due to improvements in nutrition and socioeconomic conditions. Although it is rare in males, it is far more likely to be due to organic causes. The causes of precocious puberty may be:
- idiopathic/familial tendency
- CNS abnormalities

- acquired – following surgery, trauma, irradiation
- congenital abnormalities – hydrocephalus
- tumours
- adrenal – congenital adrenal hyperplasia, tumours
- ovarian tumours
- testicular tumours
- exogenous sex steroids
- hypothyroidism

Diagnosis. Diagnosis is based on physical examination, blood analysis, bone age measurements, ultrasonography and radiological imaging – magnetic resonance imaging (MRI) or computed tomography (CT) scanning.

Treatment. This is dependent on the cause and may necessitate surgery, chemotherapy or irritation if a tumour is diagnosed. For the female with idiopathic precocious puberty, treatment will depend on the age of diagnosis. Monitoring of growth patterns is essential. Treatment is usually administration of gonadotrophin releasing hormone subcutaneously, intramuscularly or intranasally for those cases that are gonadotrophin dependent.

Role of the nurse. The aim of nursing care should focus on the education of the child and parent about the condition, medication administration and to provide emotional support for the family. There may be psychological and behavioural difficulties associated with the early progression into puberty. It must be emphasised to the family that the child is achieving their other developmental milestones – cognition, emotional development and social development – according to their chronological age even if their physical development and appearance is advanced. The challenge for the child and family is having to cope with the physical and emotional changes at an age that cognitive development has not yet reached, and secondly, the future height of the child will be impacted upon due to premature fusion of the bones.

Growth Hormone Deficiencies. Growth hormone deficiency exists when growth hormone is absent or is produced in inadequate amounts to support normal growth. If growth hormone deficiency occurs in combination with one or more other pituitary hormone deficiencies, the condition is related to hypopituitarism, as described earlier.

Growth hormone deficiency can be congenital, resulting from deficiency of hypothalamic growth hormone releasing hormone that may be associated with defects such as septo-optic dysplasia, or primary pituitary disorders such as defects in the growth hormone gene. Most congenital cases of growth hormone deficiency are currently considered idiopathic (Cuttler, 2002), which is the most common form, accounting for approximately 50%–70% of cases (National Institute for Health and Care Excellence [NICE], 2010).

Fetal growth is growth hormone independent and therefore infants with congenital growth hormone deficiency are born a normal size and weight. However, growth hormone deficiency may present in the newborn period with hypoglycaemia, and prolonged jaundice. These symptoms are often significant early diagnostic features. Growth hormone deficiency becomes evident only during the first years of life, when linear growth begins to slow and is the third percentile or less by the age of 1 year.

Acquired growth hormone deficiency may be the result of injury, infection, inflammatory and granulomatous disease, radiation or tumours of the pituitary gland and/or the

TABLE 20.3 Nursing Care and Management of Growth Hormone Deficiencies

Characteristics of Child With Growth Hormone Deficiency	Nursing Considerations
Short stature	Accurate assessment and monitoring of height and weight
Delayed growth of all body parts	Accurate recording/plotting height and weight on appropriate growth chart
Delayed skeletal maturation	Early recognition of deviation in height and weight pattern
Immature facial appearance	Accurate detailed assessment of child's health and health problems
Increased subcutaneous fat	Assessment of family history
In prolonged growth failure the child will be shorter than children of the same age	Referral for medical consultation and assisting and supporting the child/family during medical examination, radiological surveys and endocrine studies
Hypoglycaemia may be present particularly in young children	

hypothalamus; it may become evident during infancy or childhood. Failure to grow normally may also be a key feature of other underlying medical conditions, for example, chronic renal insufficiency, Turner syndrome, Prader–Willi syndrome, Down syndrome, neurofibromatosis, and as a result of chronic disease. Among children who are of very short stature (i.e. at least 3 standard deviations below the population mean), 25% have growth hormone deficiency (NICE, 2010).

Principles of nursing care and management. Care and management will be based on the assessment of individual needs of the child and in collaboration with the child and family (Table 20.3). The deficiency is identified by serum analysis of growth hormones. MRI is also required to identify underlying pathology. DEXA scans may be required to determine bone age. A detailed history of the child's physical status and social situation needs to be ascertained. The child's growth is in proportion although they may look younger than their age due to the effect of growth hormone and the storage of body fat.

In children with growth hormone insufficiency, exogenous (biosynthetic) growth hormone (somatropin) is administered by subcutaneous injection; the dose is increased during the period of adolescence. It is continued until the child attains their final height (Rudolf et al., 2011). Treatment must always be initiated and monitored under the guidance of a paediatrician who specialises in growth disorders of childhood. The recommended dose varies according to the child's condition and is self-administered at home six to seven times a week. Biosynthetic human growth hormone has been licensed for use in the UK for long-term treatment of children who have growth failure due to inadequate secretion of normal endogenous growth hormone (NICE, 2010). A variety of growth

hormone preparations and devices are available, knowledge of which is important if the nurse is to help the child and family choose the most suitable product and device. Although treatment enables many children to reach their adult height potential, this may mean many years of treatment for the child.

Establishing a partnership with the child and family is essential to achieve the optimum impact of therapy. Treatment that takes place over a long period of time may be extremely challenging for many families (Ball and Bindler, 2006). The initial and ongoing education of the child and family and the monitoring and maintenance of long-term compliance to achieve the best possible outcomes are important aspects within the role of the children's nurse. In the presence of secondary growth hormone deficiencies, the underlying lesion needs to be treated and prognosis is related to the underlying lesion.

Side effects of growth hormone therapy are rare but can include headache, visual problems, nausea and vomiting, fluid retention (peripheral oedema), arthralgia, myalgia, paraesthesia, antibody formation, hypothyroidism and reactions at injection site. Particular attention should be paid to treating children with risk factors associated with diabetes mellitus and slipped capital epiphyses.

Storage and preparation of medication, as well as choosing and alternating the injection site are important aspects of the education process. Timing of administration of growth hormone may be dependent on family routines. The evening is usually the recommended time as this mimic the pattern of normal production of growth hormone (Hockenberry et al., 2003). Compliance to treatment may be enhanced by enabling the child to take control over administration of growth hormone, which may be achieved by the use of the pen injector. The best results are seen in those that are treated early before psychological effects occur.

▶ REFLECT ON YOUR PRACTICE

- Explain to a parent the technique required to administer a subcutaneous injection.

 ### ACTIVITY

Children and parents need to understand the importance of complying with treatment regimens and to be competent in administration. This requires that the child and family are educated regarding the rationale for treatment and adverse effects. What would be your learning outcomes for the child and family if you had to prepare an educational package?

 ### ACTIVITY

Review a growth chart for a boy and a girl from birth to 18 years. Identify the nurse's responsibilities in relation to the assessment of the following:
- weight
- standing height
- supine length
- head circumference
  Review the PowerPoint presentation for measurement technique for standing height.

TABLE 20.4 Normal Growth Rates for Height in Children

Age	Growth in Height (cm/year)
0–6 months	18–26
6–12 months	15–28
1–2 years	10–13
2–3 years	7–10
3–4 years	5–8
4–5 years	5

Child and family resources. Raising awareness of the guidance on the use of human growth hormone in children with growth failure (NICE, 2010; website: https://www.nice.org.uk/guidance/ta188) and encouraging parents to discuss this guidance with their doctor will provide further encouragement to comply with treatment.

The Human Growth Foundation is a national organisation of parents who provide education and guidance on the physical, psychological and social development of children with growth problems. This resource may be beneficial in providing parents and children with additional support and advice. Good nutrition and adequate rest are vital when promoting growth. A well-balanced diet with appropriate calorie and protein intake needs to be encouraged.

Children's nurses have a significant role in the routine monitoring of growth and the assessment of growth disorders. The development of good history-taking skills and an accurate, repeatable measurement are central to the success of growth assessment and evaluation. Measuring height needs to be precise, but it is subject to error because of poor technique and inappropriate equipment. The child should be measured by the same observer using the same measuring instrument if possible, to maintain accuracy and consistency (Gormley-Fleming, 2010). Parental height should also be measured with the mid-parental centile and target height plotted on the percentile chart (Drake and Kelnar, 2006).

During therapy, the child's growth needs to be monitored against expected growth on standard growth charts to assess ongoing response to treatment (Table 20.4). Explain to the parents that developmental expectations are the same for a child with growth hormone deficiencies as they are for a child who is developing normally. Expected growth may be based on parental height. It is recommended that treatment should be discontinued if the child's growth velocity is less than 50% from baseline in the first year of therapy, that is, if extra height gain is not at least half the height gain in the year before treatment began. Persistent problems with adherence to treatment should also be considered as part of the re-evaluation process (NICE, 2010). Height is greatest on getting up in the morning – up to 2 cm can be lost over the whole day. Measurements made at different times of the day can significantly affect the measured height and the estimated rate of growth.

Recognition of the complexity of problems experienced by the child and family in relation to growth deficiency and/or short stature is necessary if physical and psychosocial dilemmas are to be overcome. Children who are small for their age may have problems with friends, teachers and parents, who tend to treat them as though they are younger and have reduced expectations of them.

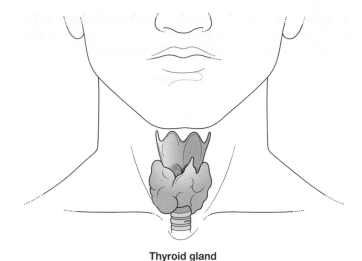

Thyroid gland

Fig. 20.4 The thyroid gland.

In turn, children may not act their age because it is not expected from them, and thus experience problems with self-esteem and ability to interact appropriately with others. The child or young person should be encouraged to dress age appropriate rather than size and treated in an age-appropriate manner. Those involved in the care of these children should be aware of the importance of emphasising abilities and strengths rather than physical size.

> **POWERPOINT**
>
> Access the companion PowerPoint presentation and revise your knowledge on the production and regulation of secretion of the thyroid hormones before proceeding to the next section of this chapter on disorders of thyroid function.

Disorders of Thyroid Function

The function of the thyroid gland is to regulate the cellular metabolism. Thyroxine T4, triiodothyronine T3 and calcitonin are hormones secreted by the thyroid. These hormones are responsible for normal development of the muscular, skeletal and nervous systems. Disturbance in the secretory pathway of the thyroid hormones may result in an increase or decrease in production. Some of the most common endocrine disorders are disorders of the thyroid gland. The two main disorders are hypothyroidism and hyperthyroidism.

Hypothyroidism

Hypothyroidism is either congenital or acquired (juvenile hypothyroidism-Hashimoto syndrome). It is due to a deficiency in the secretion of thyroid hormones. Congenital hypothyroidism is relatively common and occurs in approximately one in 4000 births (Lissauer and Clayden, 2011). Early detection is imperative as this is one of the few preventable causes of severe learning difficulties. This is achieved by neonatal screening. Treatment is lifelong with oral replacement of thyroxine. Cause of congenital hypothyroidism are:

- aplasia or hypoplasia of the thyroid gland (Fig. 20.4);
- hereditary defects in thyroid hormone synthesis that may be associated with maternal administration of antithyroid drugs during pregnancy;

- iodine deficiency – common worldwide but rare in the UK; preventable by iodination of salt in the maternal diet;
- thyroid stimulating hormone (TSH) deficiency.

Acquired Juvenile Hypothyroidism

Juvenile hypothyroidism may be primary or secondary. This is more common in females (Ball and Bindler, 2006). Primary causes include:

- defective hormone synthesis resulting from acute thyroiditis caused by bacterial infection;
- subacute non-bacterial inflammation associated with viral infections;
- autoimmune (circulating antithyroid antibodies) thyroiditis occurring as a result of Hashimoto disease is the most common cause of juvenile hypothyroidism in children (Lissauer and Clayden, 2011);
- an endemic of iodine deficiency or antithyroid drugs, or loss of thyroid tissue can be contributory factors in hypothyroidism.

Secondary hypothyroidism is due to insufficient stimulation of the thyroid gland by thyroid stimulating hormone as a result of hypothalamic or pituitary disorders.

Other autoimmune disorders may develop, for example, type 1 diabetes mellitus. This is more common in children with Down and Turner syndromes. Addison's disease may also occur in some families (Lissauer and Clayden, 2011).

Nursing assessment and diagnosis. Routine neonatal biochemical screening, blood spot test, must be performed on all infants either prior to discharge from hospital or in the community. Congenital hypothyroidism (CHT) is one of the disorders included in this screening. Current guidance screen for nine conditions as listed below:

- cystic fibrosis
- sickle cell disease
- congenital hypothyroidism (CHT)
- inherited metabolic diseases (IMDs). These are genetic diseases that affect the metabolism.
  - phenylketonuria (PKU)
  - medium-chain acyl-CoA dehydrogenase deficiency (MCADD)
  - maple syrup urine disease (MSUD)
  - isovaleric acidaemia (IVA)
  - glutaric aciduria type 1 (GA1)
  - homocystinuria (HCU)

This will identify most infants that are affected by these disorders.

In children under the age of two the symptoms may not be as clear as those associated with hypothyroidism, therefore nursing assessment and ongoing monitoring of the neonate with presenting problems is vital to ensure early diagnosis of the condition. Serial measurement of weight, length and head circumference is an important aspect of assessment. Presenting symptoms depend on extent of dysfunction and age at onset. However, if undetected and left untreated in early childhood, permanent defects can arise, for example, mental retardation, deafness, deceleration in growth and other nervous system disorders. At birth there may be difficulty in identifying hypothyroidism. Hypothermia, delay in passing meconium and neonatal jaundice may be significant signs and require immediate investigation.

Clinical manifestations of hypothyroidism may not be evident until after 4 months of age. Signs and symptoms may include:

- failure to thrive and feeding problems;
- a hoarse cry and protruding tongue caused by myxoedema of oral tissue and vocal cords;
- the child may present with constipation and abdominal distension due to hypotonia of abdominal muscles;
- umbilical hernia may also be present;
- a subnormal temperature, excessive sleeping, slow pulse and a cold, mottled skin may be present;
- puffy eyes and loss of the eyebrows may be present.

Often the baby is seen as being a 'good' baby, as the baby is often quiet. Skeletal growth may be decelerated due to impaired synthesis of protein, poor absorption of nutrients and lack of bone mineralisation. Enlargement of the thyroid gland, known as goitre, may be evident, particularly in older children. Puberty may be delayed and obesity is often present. If the condition remains undiagnosed and untreated, the child will be dwarfed with short limbs (cretinism) as well as presenting with delayed intellectual development.

Transient hypothyroidism is rare in children but not unknown. It may result as secondary to maternal medication, for example, carbimazole or maternal antibodies that cross the placenta.

Care and management. Once diagnosis is confirmed, treatment is replacement therapy, which is prescribed according to the child's hormonal levels. Treatment is required on a lifelong basis. Regular estimates of hormone levels are essential to prevent development of hyperthyroidism. In addition, regular monitoring of growth is necessary throughout childhood. Assessment of cognitive development should also be undertaken. Education for both parents and the child (depending on their age) is essential as they need to demonstrate an understanding of the disorder and treatment required.

 SCENARIO

Kate, a 12-year-old school girl, has been referred to the assessment unit by her GP. She has a history of weight loss, anxiety and has not been sleeping. Her mum has reported that Kate's hands are shaking and when you examine her you notice that this is a fine tremor.

- When undertaking Kate's nursing assessment, what specific information would you be required to obtain?
- What specific requirements would need to be considered when planning Kate's care?

Kate's dad asks you what you think could be wrong. What do you think you would say?

A discussion of this scenario appears at the end of the chapter.

WWW

More information on the neonatal blood spot screening programme can be found on:

- https://www.gov.uk/guidance/newborn-blood-spot-screening-programme-overview

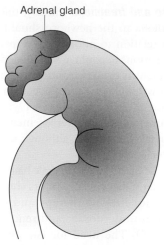

Adrenal gland

Fig. 20.5 The adrenal gland.

TABLE 20.5	Disorders of Adrenal Function	
Hyperfunction of Adrenal Cortex	**Hypofunction**	
Cushing syndrome: increased levels of circulating cortisol	Acute adrenocortical insufficiency	
	Chronic adrenocortical insufficiency: Addison's disease	
Congenital adrenal hyperplasia: increased secretion of adrenal androgens and oestrogens leading to virilisation or feminisation Primary hyperaldosteronism Hyperfunction of adrenal medulla Phaeochromocytoma: increased secretion of catecholamines		

 POWERPOINT

Access the companion PowerPoint presentation and review regulation of adrenal and renal function before proceeding with the next section of this chapter on disorders of adrenal function.

Hyperthyroidism

Hyperthyroidism is a condition in which the thyroid hormones exert greater than normal responses. Thyrotoxicosis may also be used to identify the raised level of thyroid hormone. Generally, there is excess secretion of thyroid hormones, which might be associated with acute, subacute or chronic thyroiditis, tumours of the thyroid, or other tumours of the pituitary (which secretes thyroid-stimulating hormone). This leads to an increase in basal metabolic rate, cardiac function, gastrointestinal function, weight loss, and metabolism of fats, proteins and carbohydrates. While rare in childhood it is most common in teenage girls. Specific diseases that cause hyperthyroidism include Graves' disease and toxic multinodular goitre. Graves' disease is an autoimmune disease and is the most common form (Cappa et al., 2011).

Congenital hyperthyroidism may occur in infants of mothers who have Graves' disease as a result of transplacental transfer of immunoglobulins (Ball and Bindler, 2006)

Assessment and diagnosis. Hyperthyroidism is four times more common in girls than boys and most frequently presents in childhood between ages of 12 and 14 years. The condition usually presents with a history of deterioration in school performance.

The other clinical features of hypothyroidism will vary according to the amount and length of hypersecretion. The onset is subtle, thus diagnosis may not be reached for a length of time. Weight loss, diarrhoea, rapid growth in height, tachycardia, tremors, increase in appetite, anxiety, learning difficulties/behaviour problems and goitre may be present. Eye signs are uncommon in children, but exophthalmos may

be evident if diagnosis is delayed (Lissaeur and Clayden, 2011).

Diagnosis is achieved by laboratory analysis of thyroxine and triiodothyronine levels. A thyroid scan will also be performed. Antithyroid antibodies may also be identified in laboratory analysis.

The aim of treatment is to inhibit excessive secretion of the thyroid hormones. First-line treatment is oral medication, and this is generally for a 2-year period. Adjunct therapy may also be required, for example, beta-blockers. Radioiodine treatment may follow oral medication. Surgery may also be considered if other treatment modalities are unsuccessful. However, if too much thyroid tissue is removed it may lead to underactivity necessitating the need for thyroxine medication long term. Ongoing monitoring will be required to assure the T4 level is maintained within normal parameters.

Nursing care. The aim of nursing care of the child with hyperthyroidism should focus on the education of the child and their parents. They need to be aware of the need to promote rest, the importance of compliance with treatment to avoid relapse and to provide emotional support. Pre- and post-operative care for the child undergoing subtotal or total thyroidectomy is very specific, but the general principles of pre- and post-operative care still apply.

Disorders of Adrenal Function

Disorders of the adrenal cortex (Fig. 20.5) are related to either hyperfunction or hypofunction (Table 20.5).

Congenital Adrenal Hyperplasia

This is a group of disorders of adrenal steroid synthesis. Excessive secretion of androgens by the adrenal cortex may occur as a result of a number of conditions of the adrenal gland. However, the most common disorder affecting children is congenital adrenogenital hyperplasia, an inborn deficiency of various enzymes (21-hydroxylase) necessary for the biosynthesis of adrenal steroidogenesis (Hockenberry et al., 2003). It is an autosomal recessive disorder. Interference with the biosynthesis of glucocorticoids in fetal life results in cortisol secretion being diminished and an increased production of adrenocorticotrophic hormone, which stimulates hyperplasia of the adrenal gland. There is an increased production of various adrenal hormone precursors, including androgens. Deficiency of enzymes necessary for biosynthesis of mineralocorticoids may result in diminished secretion of aldosterone.

In its severe form, excess adrenal androgen production beginning in the first trimester of fetal development results in virilisation of the female infant and life-threatening hypovolaemic and hyponatraemic shock (adrenal crisis) in the newborn.

In females with severe form congenital adrenal hyperplasia (CAH) they will present with ambiguous genitalia at birth due to excess adrenal androgen, which has been produced in utero. In mild cases 21-hydroxylase deficiency may not be diagnosed until early childhood and precocious pubic hair develops along with clitoromegaly.

In males the diagnosis may be later due to the presence of normal genitalia. Failure to thrive, recurrent vomiting, hyponatraemia, hyperkalaemia and eventually shock will occur as a result of salt-wasting adrenal hyperplasia.

Assessment and diagnosis. Due to the block in the adrenal production of corticosteroids a build up of androgenic precursors occurs and this may lead to ambiguous genitalia in the newborn baby. This is rare. In the female with potentially normal ovaries and uterus, virilisation occurs and sexual development is therefore along heterosexual lines. The abnormality of the external genitalia may vary from mild enlargement of the clitoris to complete fusion of the labioscrotal folds, forming a scrotum, a penile urethra, a penile shaft and enlargement of the clitoris to form a normal-sized gland.

Signs of adrenal insufficiency (salt loss) may be present during the first days of life. This is an acute presentation with hyponatraemia, hyperkalaemia, hypoglycaemia, dehydration, hypotension and circulatory collapse. In the older child presentation usually occurs when the enzyme defect is milder; salt loss may not occur – this accounts for approximately 25% of cases (Ball and Bindler, 2006). If untreated, growth rate and skeletal maturation are accelerated. Pubic hair appears early, acne may be excessive, and voice may deepen. Excessive pigmentation may develop as a result of melanocyte stimulation by excessive production of adrenocorticotrophic hormone (Kappy et al., 2003).

In males, sexual development proceeds normally. Male infants may appear normal at birth but present with salt-losing crisis in the first 2–4 weeks. The infant may present with vomiting, poor weight gain, poor feeding and electrolyte imbalance. The older male child who was not losing sodium may present with rapid growth and precocious sexual development.

Hormonal studies are essential for accurate diagnosis. Adrenal ultrasonography, CT scanning, and MRI may define pelvic anatomy or enlarged adrenals or indicate the presence of an adrenal tumour. Pelvic ultrasonography may help in delineating the internal anatomy of a newborn with ambiguous genitalia.

Nursing care and treatment. Initially, the recognition of ambiguous genitalia in the newborn should be attended to immediately in relation to informing the parents and commencing investigations to confirm sexual identity. Early diagnosis and treatment is crucial. Aims of treatment consist of normalising growth velocity and skeletal maturation using the smallest dose of glucocorticoids that will suppress adrenal function. Mineralocorticoid replacement helps to sustain normal electrolyte homeostasis, although excessive use may result in hypertension.

Patient education is necessary as has been described for other endocrine disorders. Parents should understand the child's need for lifelong therapy and the side effects, as well as signs of underdosage and requirements during illness Petty (2015). The need for compliance should be stressed and the importance of the child carrying appropriate identification. Surgical intervention may be necessary for reconstruction of the female genitalia as soon as possible during infancy in an effort to support ongoing physical and psychological development. Multiple surgical procedures may be necessary, which will require ongoing psychological support for the child and parents. They require ongoing support as they come to terms with the sex of the baby and decisions that they may have to make regarding the need for surgical interventions. Reassurance regarding surgical interventions and the future care and treatment, which will be a lifelong commitment, need to be discussed.

Ambiguity in relation to the sex of the newborn can have a devastating effect on parents and other siblings. At this time, anticipation of parental reaction, which may be likened to the process of bereavement and loss, may enhance the nurse's ability to engage in a more therapeutic way at this time. Parents need to have information in relation to the infant's condition reinforced, while at the same time being provided with the opportunity to express their own sorrow, loss and disappointment. A decision regarding gender should only be made once all investigations are completed and naming the baby should also be delayed until gender determination is made. Their beliefs and values on gender need to be explored. The health care professional should avoid referring to the baby as 'your son' or 'your daughter' and instead refer to the baby as 'your baby'. Genetic counselling should be provided for the child when they reach adolescence and supportive counselling should be organised for the parents along with genetic screening for any future pregnancies.

As the hereditary form of adrenogenital hyperplasia is an autosomal-recessive disorder, parents should be referred for genetic counselling.

👤 ACTIVITY

What would be your key priorities when planning care for a child who is being admitted to your ward with a known diagnosis of Addison's disease who is vomiting?

Chronic Adrenocortical Insufficiency (Addison's Disease)

Primary adrenal cortical insufficiency is rare in children and is due to the inability to produce enough steroid hormone. Adrenal insufficiency (Table 20.6) is a reduction in the release of the glucocorticoids and or mineralocorticoids. This may be the result of:

- hereditary enzymatic defects (congenital adrenal hyperplasia)
- loss of adrenal function due to autoimmune destruction of the gland (Addison's disease)
- pituitary hypothalamic tumours
- irradiation of the hypothalamus
- haemorrhage/infraction – neonatal, meningococcal septicaemia
- adrenoleukodystrophy – a neurodegenerative disorder
- tuberculosis

POWERPOINT

Access the companion PowerPoint presentation and review regulation of adrenal and renal function before proceeding with the next section of this chapter on disorders of adrenal function.

Acute Adrenocortical Insufficiency (Adrenal Crisis)

Acute adrenal insufficiency (adrenal crisis) is most common in the child with undiagnosed chronic adrenal insufficiency, who is exposed to additional severe stress such as major illness, trauma or surgery. Some of the aetiological factors include haemorrhage into the gland from trauma, which may be caused by a prolonged, difficult labour; fulminating infections, such as meningococcaemia, which results in haemorrhage; and necrosis (Waterhouse–Friderichsen syndrome).

Other factors include abrupt withdrawal of exogenous sources of cortisone, or failure to increase dosage during stress such as surgery or burns and during stressful periods, injury or cold, for example (Ball and Bindler, 2006).

This condition is rapid in onset. All symptoms as identified in chronic adrenocortical insufficiency are exaggerated. The child may present with circulation collapse, confusion or coma and therefore require emergency interventions. Nursing care is focused on:

- fluid and electrolyte resuscitation
- intravenous administration of glucocorticoids until oral therapy becomes possible
- administration of mineralocorticoids when oral intake is tolerated
- treatment of the underlying illness

Prolonged care and treatment, as for the child with chronic adrenocortical insufficiency, will be required.

Cushing Syndrome

Cushing syndrome results from prolonged exposure of the tissues to glucocorticoids. It may be caused by primary dysfunction as a result of neoplasm or adenoma of the adrenal cortex, or by hypersecretion of adrenocorticotrophic hormone as a result of a pituitary tumour. In addition, Cushing-like syndrome may be an adverse effect from long-term exogenous administration of cortisone used in the treatment of allergic, autoimmune, neoplastic, haematologic, skin and other diseases.

Clinical manifestations. Cushing syndrome is extremely rare in children and young people (Rudolf et al., 2011). However, the resulting hypercortisol causes considerable morbidity in childhood and adolescence (Storr et al., 2003). The earliest and most common signs in almost all presenting with the condition are:

TABLE 20.6 Causes of Adrenal Insufficiency

Characteristics of Glucocorticoid Deficiency	Characteristics of Mineralocorticoid Deficiency	Nursing Considerations
Poor weight gain, weight loss, anorexia	Hyponatraemia	Assessment of dietary intake to avoid obesity
Hypoglycaemia	Hyperkalaemia	Prevent episodes of hypoglycaemia
Weakness/fatigue	Nausea	Ensure additional sodium intake (as in table
Increased levels of adrenocorticotrophic hormone and melanocyte stimulating hormone give rise to hyperpigmentation of skin and mucous membrane	Gastrointestinal complaints Hypotension Tachycardia	salt) – increase intake in event of sweating, vomiting, diarrhoea
		Assessment and ongoing monitoring of cardiovascular status
		Frequent monitoring of vital signs, blood pressure
		Monitor compliance to treatment of replacement therapy of glucocorticoid and mineralocorticoids on long-term basis
		Assessment and monitoring for signs of over-treatment:
		• monitor growth and development and observe for signs of Cushingoid features
		• regular follow-up and provision of ongoing support and education
		• encourage child to wear medic alert bracelet

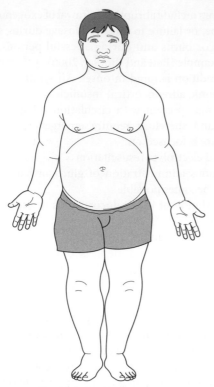

Fig. 20.6 Cushing syndrome.

• Generalised obesity, which is characterised by facial rounding (moon face) and 'buffalo hump' (Fig. 20.6). These result from accumulation of adipose tissue in the trunk, facial and cervical areas.

• Transient weight gain from sodium and water retention may occur due to the mineralocorticoid effects of cortisol.

• Growth retardation or complete arrest of growth is present in all but 10% of affected children (Chrousos, 2002).

• Other clinical manifestations include sleep disturbance, irritability and depression.

• Muscle weakness and fatigue, due to protein wasting is caused by the catabolic effects of cortisol.

• Loss of protein matrix leads to osteoporosis, with pathological fractures.

• Loss of collagen also causes weakening and thinning of the skin through which capillaries become visible. These changes, together with fluid retention, account for the characteristic purple striae.

• Loss of collagenous support makes blood vessels more susceptible to rupture, leading to bruising. Thin atrophied skin is easily damaged and leads to skin breaks and ulceration (McCance and Huether, 2014).

• Hyperpigmentation is associated with high serum levels of adrenocorticotrophic hormone, which is thought to increase melanotropic activity. Thus skin, mucous membranes and hair acquire a characteristic bronze colour.

• Hypertension due to increased vascular sensitivity to catecholamines, which are increased as a result of increased levels of cortisol.

• Elevated levels of cortisol also cause suppression of the immune system, which increases the child's susceptibility to infection and poor wound healing.

• Amenorrhoea, advancement or arrest of pubertal development may be encountered.

Glucose intolerance occurs because of cortisol-induced insulin resistance and increased gluconeogenesis and glycogen in the liver. As childhood obesity is now considered a public health concern, potential endocrine causes should be considered. Obesity may occur secondary to damage to the hypothalamus, disruption of the hormone leptin production or more obvious, some of the classic endocrine disorders are associated with weight gain (Crocker and Yanovski, 2009).

Assessment and diagnosis. Diagnosis is confirmed through blood sampling and urine testing. Excess cortisol levels may be obtained indirectly by ascertaining fasting blood glucose levels for hyperglycaemia. Serum electrolyte levels for hypokalaemia and alkalosis will also be measured. The levels of urinary free cortisol and plasma cortisol will be elevated. Ideally this urine sample should be obtained in the evening (Ball and Bindler, 2006).

A dexamethasone (cortisone) test may be used to confirm the diagnosis and confirm the cause. Administration of exogenous cortisone normally suppresses production of adrenocorticotrophic hormone. Cortisol levels remain elevated in children with Cushing syndrome. This helps differentiate between children who are obese and those who appear to have Cushingoid features (Rudolf et al., 2011).

CT scanning or MRI may be carried out when an adrenocorticotrophic hormone-secreting adenoma of the pituitary is suspected.

Care and management. Treatment is specific according to the cause for hyperadrenocorticosteroid levels. Therefore differentiation among pituitary, adrenal and other causes is essential for effective treatment. For adrenal and pituitary causes, treatment generally involves surgical, irradiation and post-operative replacement of cortical hormones.

When Cushingoid features are a result of steroid therapy, the effects may be lessened by administration of the drug in the morning, as this maintains the normal diurnal pattern of cortisol secretion. Also, an alternate day schedule allows the anterior pituitary an opportunity to maintain more normal hypothalamic–pituitary–adrenal control mechanisms (Ball and Bindler, 2006)

Primary Hyperaldosteronism

Primary hyperaldosteronism may be caused by a benign adrenal tumour or by adrenal hyperplasia. This condition results in increased sodium levels with water retention, and potassium depletion. The condition is characterised by paraesthesia, tetany, weakness, polyuria, nocturnal enuresis, periodic paralysis, low serum potassium, elevated sodium levels, hypertension, metabolic acidosis and production of a large volume of urine with a low specific gravity. Plasma and aldosterone levels are elevated, but other steroid levels are variable.

Treatment is with glucocorticoids or spironolactone, which blocks the effects of aldosterone, thereby promoting the excretion of sodium and water and preserving potassium (Hockenberry et al., 2003). Subtotal or total adrenalectomy for hyperplasia may be necessary, and surgical removal of a tumour, if present.

The role of the nurse in relation to providing holistic care and treatment from the stage of diagnosis to long-term management of primary hyperaldosteronism is similar to that for other endocrine disorders. When surgery is indicated then involvement in pre- and post-operative care becomes the priority.

Phaeochromocytoma

Phaeochromocytoma is a tumour of the adrenal medulla but may be located wherever chromaffin tissue is present, for example, sympathetic ganglia and carotid body. In the majority of cases it is benign and treatable. Approximately 10% are malignant (National Health Service [NHS], 2018). Physical manifestations are generally caused by excess secretion of catecholamines. Symptoms may include:

- increased anxiety, such as perspiration and headaches, palpitations, tachycardia, hypertension and hyperglycaemia;
- dizziness, weakness, nausea and vomiting with diarrhoea;
- weight loss and anorexia;
- pallor;
- blurring of vision and dilated pupils;
- papilloedema, retinopathy and enlargement of the heart;
- in severe cases, signs of congestive heart failure may be evident nervousness, excitability and overactivity.

Nursing assessment and diagnosis. Diagnosis can be challenging. A careful history of the onset of symptoms and association with stressful events is helpful in distinguishing between an organic and a psychological cause for the problem (Ball and Bindler, 2006). The symptoms occur intermittently as the catecholamines are released intermittently from the tumour. Therefore serum catecholamines are elevated, particularly when the child is symptomatic. Urinary excretion of catecholamines parallels serum levels. The tumour may be identified on CT scan or MRI.

Nursing care and management. Nursing care is primarily supportive. Surgical removal of the tumour is the treatment of choice. Prior to surgery, the child's physical condition must be adequately stabilised. Manipulation of the tumour may cause sudden and profound, potentially fatal changes in blood pressure. Hypertension with associated tachycardia may be the result of excessive release of catecholamines during removal of the tumour. Hypotension may occur as a result of catecholamine withdrawal. A pre-operative preparation requirement involves the administration of medication, aimed at inhibiting the effects of catecholamines. The major group of drugs used is the adrenergic blocking agents. Beta-adrenergic blocking agents may be required when α-adrenergic blocking agents are ineffective in controlling release of catecholamines alone. The wanted effect of pre-operative drug administration is to lower the blood pressure and minimise the symptoms the child has previously presented with.

During the pre-operative period, frequent recordings of clinical observations are required to monitor blood pressure and heart and respiratory rate in an effort to detect hypertensive episodes and observe for signs of congestive heart failure. Daily blood glucose monitoring is required to observe for signs of hyperglycaemia.

The child is likely to remain in hospital in the weeks prior to surgery because of the necessary pre-operative preparation and monitoring. The effects of prolonged hospitalisation may increase emotional distress for the child and thus aggravate symptoms. Parental presence and involvement in the child's care must be encouraged. Parents must be fully informed about the child's condition so that they can promote an environment for the child that is as restful and as stress free as possible. They require detailed information regarding the child's surgery and complications that may arise as a result. The child may require admission to the intensive care unit following surgery until the condition is stable post-operatively.

The Gonads: Ovaries and Testes

A variety of abnormalities in chromosomal distribution, gonadal differentiation, gonadal function, testosterone synthesis and action, or adrenal function can lead to aberrant development of internal or external genital structures as described under the section congenital adrenal hyperplasia.

 POWERPOINT

Access the companion PowerPoint presentation and review:
- abnormalities in female pubertal development and ovarian function.

  Before proceeding with the next section of this chapter, on diabetes mellitus, review:
- endocrine regulation of blood glucose.

DIABETES MELLITUS

Diabetes mellitus refers to a group of metabolic disorders characterised by hyperglycaemia. As a long-term condition, it can have a major impact on the life of both the child and their family. It is the result of a lack of the hormone insulin and/or an inability to respond to endogenous insulin. This interference has varying degrees of disruption of carbohydrate and fat metabolism and storage, excessive gluconeogenesis from protein catabolism, water and electrolyte imbalance. As a result of an autoimmune response within the body, damage to the beta cells in the pancreas occurs.

In childhood, the incidence of type 1 diabetes is greater than type 2 diabetes. Type 1 diabetes occurs in 1:500 children (Diabetes UK, 2018). The incidence of type 2 is increasing in all age groups and across races and may now account for between one-fifth and one-third of all new cases of diabetes.

Type 2 diabetes occurs as a result of body's resistance to insulin (Beckwith, 2010). The general care required for both type 1 and type 2 diabetes is similar apart from the initial care at the point of diagnosis (NICE, 2015).

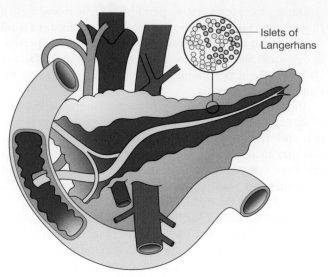

Fig. 20.7 The pancreas.

Monogenic diabetes accounts for a small percentage of diabetes in children and results from the inheritance of mutation or mutations in a single gene most often those that regulate beta cell function. Monogenic or mitochondrial diabetes should be considered other than type 1 or type 2 diabetes if:

- diabetes presents in the first year of life;
- ketonaemia is absent or rare during episodes of hyperglycaemia;
- presence of optic atrophy, retinitis pigmentosa, deafness, systemic illness or another syndrome (NICE, 2015).

Pathophysiology

Insulin is a hormone secreted by the beta cells located in the islets of Langerhans within the pancreas. It functions to maintain homeostasis and is secreted in response to a rise in the blood glucose level. Insulin acts on cell membranes stimulating the uptake of glucose, amino acids and fats. In addition, it is associated with conversion of glucose to glycogen in the liver and muscles, storage of fat in adipose tissue and prevention of gluconeogenesis and the breakdown of protein and fat.

Glucagon is secreted in the alpha cells of the islets of Langerhans and is released when the blood glucose level is low, causing the liver to convert stored glycogen into glucose and release into the blood stream. Insulin and glucagon influence the blood glucose level, each balancing the effects of the other maintaining normoglycaemia (blood glucose levels of 4–8 mmol/L).

In the diabetic patient, the diminishing level of insulin secretion (type 1 diabetes) or when insulin secretion is inadequate to meet the increasing demand posed by insulin resistance (type 2 diabetes), an inability to utilise available glucose causes elevated blood glucose levels and catabolic breakdown of fat with the ensuing production of ketones.

TYPE 1 DIABETES

Type 1 diabetes is characterised by an absolute insulin deficiency resulting in hyperglycaemia and the possible development of diabetic ketoacidosis. Most cases result from a cell-mediated autoimmune response of the insulin producing cells of the pancreatic islets (Fig. 20.7). This response results in recruitment of cytotoxic lymphocytes and production of anti-insulin and anti-islet cell antibodies, which progressively destroy the beta cells of the islets of Langerhans in the pancreas. Susceptibility to immunological damage has been associated with strong genetic determinants in combination with environmental factors. Environmental triggers of this immune process that have been proposed include viruses, cows' milk proteins and chemical toxins. Signs and symptoms are:

- polyuria
- dehydration
- polydipsia
- weight loss
- excessive tiredness
  Late characteristics include:
- vomiting due to the ketonaemia
- abdominal pain
- hypovolaemic shock
- hyperventilation due to acidosis
- drowsiness and coma

Diagnosis

Onset may be acute, precipitated by the stress of an acute illness or insidious over weeks and months. The classic presenting symptoms are thirst, polydipsia, polyuria, weight loss and a recent history of recurrent infections. Diagnosis is made in the symptomatic child by a random plasma glucose level greater than 11.1 mmol/L (NICE, 2015; World Health Organization [WHO], 2006). Urine testing may also be undertaken for the presence of glucose and ketones. Confirmation of diagnosis can be made on elevated blood glucose alone (Rudolf, Lee and Levene, 2011). However, the oral glucose tolerance test (OGTT) may be required to determine diagnosis if a fasting plasma level of 6.1–6.9 mmol/L is reported. Children suspected of type 1 diabetes should be referred to a multidisciplinary paediatric diabetes team immediately for assessment.

Initial Care and Management

The initial management will depend on the child's clinical condition. Those in advanced diabetic ketoacidosis require urgent hospitalisation for emergency treatment. Most newly presenting children can be managed on subcutaneous insulin, but intravenous fluids and an insulin infusion is required if the child is vomiting or dehydrated. Newly presenting children not requiring intravenous therapy should have the choice of in-patient management or home-based care depending on clinical need and in consideration of the family's preference. A child presenting with moderate hyperglycaemia without acidaemia, who is clinically stable and is tolerating oral fluids, may be successfully managed at home with the support of medical and nursing diabetes specialists.

The goals of treatment in diabetes, as with any chronic condition, are to enable the child and family to live a normal life. The goals are:

- good metabolic control to avoid variation in blood glucose level and maintain it within as normal parameters as possible;

- education for the child and family in how to competently manage their diabetes;
- achieve normal growth and development with full participation in school and social activities;
- good general health and well-being;
- normal socialisation with peer groups;
- minimisation of long-term complications.

The goal of insulin therapy is to administer as sufficient a dose of insulin as needed to achieve a serum level that equals physiological insulin secretion levels (Rudolf et al., 2011). Establishing the correct dosage of daily insulin requires adjustments to be made based on food intake and forthcoming exercise in addition to blood glucose levels. In adolescence, due to insulin resistance, insulin requirements increase. These higher doses are reduced at the end of growth and puberty.

The choice of insulin regimen is determined in consideration of the child's age, family circumstances, lifestyle and individual preferences. Twice daily injection therapy consists of a mixture of long-acting and fast-acting insulin administered before breakfast and evening meal. Premixed pens are available in different percentage ratios of long-acting to rapid-acting insulin. Children on multiple daily injection therapy (MDI) administer a dose of fast-acting insulin before each meal based on the carbohydrate content of the meal and a long-acting insulin, generally given before bed. Continuous subcutaneous insulin infusion (CSII) or an insulin pump may be used if multiple injections are not appropriate. Insulin therapy is part of the care package given to families at diagnosis, which also includes:

- on-going education and management strategies;
- practical instruction in injection therapy and blood glucose monitoring;
- dietary management;
- liaison with nurseries, schools and other secondary care settings;
- psychosocial support.

Children with type 1 diabetes should have their injection sites reviewed at each clinic visit. Suitable containers for collecting sharps must be provided and arrangements for collection and disposal of these containers should be available (NICE, 2015).

Diet

Nutritional recommendations are the same for all healthy children with or without diabetes. Children with diabetes need sufficient calories to satisfy the requirements for growth and development, as well as achieving the best possible blood glucose control. The intake of calories and nutrients needs to be balanced with the amount of insulin given at a particular time and in consideration of the amount of activity undertaken during the day. NICE (2015) recommends level 3 carbohydrate-counting education from diagnosis to all children with type 1 diabetes. Level 3 carbohydrate counting is carbohydrate counting with the adjustment of insulin dosage according to an insulin:carbohydrate ratio. A low glycaemic index diet will help to improve blood glucose control and reduce the risk of hyperglycaemic episodes.

The type of insulin regime will affect the advice given. It is essential to consider the whole family's customary food habits.

Asking the child or parents to keep a food diary for a week is a useful way of understanding meal routines, content and food combinations. Dietetic input is an integral part of diabetes management and review of personal eating patterns, likes and dislikes, different cultures and religions need to be discussed on an individual basis.

A twice daily insulin regimen requires a regular meal pattern of consistent content interspersed with snacks to prevent blood glucose levels dropping between meals. This regime does not respond well to high glucose foods, which should be kept to a minimum as they will generate swinging blood glucose levels. More flexible meal planning is an option for those receiving multiple injections or on insulin pump therapy.

Exercise

Exercise should be encouraged for all children as it is known to reduce the risk of cardiovascular disease. Having type 1 diabetes should not be a barrier to exercise. The child and family will require advice on insulin and dietary management prior to exercise. Williams et al. (2011) identified that children with type 1 diabetes had lower cardiorespiratory fitness and this could possibly be attributed to levels of activity or the physiological impact of having type 1 diabetes. The child and family will need to understand the effects of exercise on blood glucose levels and devise strategies to prevent hypo- and hyperglycaemic episodes. The effects of exercise are as follows:

- The uptake of glucose to the muscles will increase without increasing the need for insulin.
- Absorption of insulin will be accelerated if an active part of the body is used for the injection site prior to exercise.
- Insulin must be available during exercise, however, or the uptake of blood glucose will be impeded. In the absence of adequate circulating insulin there will be a lack of glucose inside the cells resulting in an exaggerated response from counter-regulatory hormones leading to hyperglycaemia and the likelihood of ketosis (Williams et al., 2011).
- Hypoglycaemia may become evident hours afterwards as the liver replenishes its stores of glycogen.

Exercise needs both glucose and insulin. If there is insufficient glucose available for the muscles cells, there is an increased risk of hypoglycaemia during exercise. If there is too little circulating insulin, then the available glucose cannot be transported to the muscles and is likely to result in elevated blood glucose levels and the risk of developing ketoacidosis. After exercise the muscles are more sensitive to circulating insulin as glycogen stores within the muscle cells are replenished, leading to an increased risk of hypoglycaemia 8–10 hours after the event (Rodbard, 2008).

The child and family will need to:

- Adjust their insulin and food intake as necessary. Carbohydrates are required if glucose level is <7 mmol/L before exercise.
- Learn how their blood glucose responds to different exercise activities.
- Be aware of exercise induced hypoglycaemia.
- Be aware of the delayed onset of hypoglycaemia: 8–10 hours post-exercise (NICE, 2015).

POWERPOINT

Access the companion PowerPoint presentation and review the section on insulin therapy: requirements of new-onset diabetes for more detailed information.

Careful monitoring is advised pre- and post-exercise including a review of insulin requirements. During prolonged episodes of vigorous activity, additional carbohydrate is needed to replenish energy stores. Individual exercise plans are useful for the serious athlete and can be tailored to the type of energy expenditure and duration of exercise being undertaken.

Needle Phobia

Newly diagnosed children and young people are often fearful of the injection process. Once a routine is established in the home environment, most children settle into the pattern of diabetes management and accept that it is a necessary procedure. However, a few can present with symptoms of needle phobia. If not resolved, it may affect treatment and diabetes control as the child or young person may adopt strategies such as insufficient blood glucose monitoring or omitting insulin injections, in an attempt to minimise the number of invasive procedures they might have in day. Identifying needle phobia as distinct from objecting to injections is difficult. Close observation of the injection process, looking for signs of extreme anxiety in the child, will alert the children's nurse to needle phobia that may need the support of a clinical psychologist.

Blood Glucose Monitoring

Self-monitoring of blood glucose (SMBG) is one of the main management tools used to optimise diabetes control. It gives insight into the child's immediate blood glucose status and an opportunity to treat as well as avoid out-of-range values. In type 1 diabetic patients, frequent blood glucose monitoring is associated with an improved HbA1c and is linked to better insulin adjustment for food and a more rapid response to elevated blood glucose levels being treated with additional insulin. The aims of self-monitoring blood glucose are to:

- monitor daily blood glucose fluctuations.
- assist with daily insulin dose adjustments.
- identify hypoglycaemia and monitor during recovery.
- identify hyperglycaemia and monitor during resolution.
  The optimal targets for blood glucose control are:
- fasting plasma glucose level of 4–7 mmol/L in the morning when waking.
- a plasma glucose level of 4–7 mmol/L before meals and at other times during the day.
- a plasma glucose level of 5–9 mmol/L after meals.
- a plasma glucose level of 5 mmol/L when driving (NICE, 2015)

Children and young people are encouraged to perform regular blood glucose monitoring; five capillary blood glucose tests per day should become an established part of the

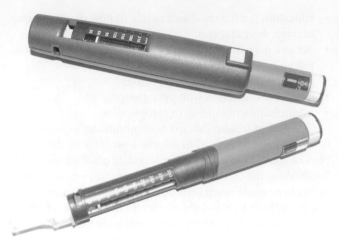

Fig. 20.8 The Penmate *(top)* with needle hidden; the NovoPen *(bottom)* has a 6-mm needle.

child's routine (NICE, 2015). Ideally this should be before meals. There is a wide variety of excellent blood glucose meters available for home use.

Real-time continuous glucose monitoring is becoming increasingly popular. This sensor-based blood glucose monitoring provides continuous data of blood glucose level as opposed to snapshots obtained through SMBG. The advantage of this is that readings can be performed as often as needed and it automatically stores glucose data every 15 minutes. A second advantage is that sensor-based devices alarm so are advantageous for children who have frequent hypoglycaemia, impaired awareness of hypoglycaemia, or who have the inability to communicate or recognise symptoms of hypoglycaemia. The use of sensor-based monitoring devices has demonstrated enhanced control of glucose levels (Edge et al., 2017). Real-time continuous glucose monitoring should be considered for use with neonates and young children as opposed to SMBG, and children who engage in high levels of physical activity, children who have comorbidities, for example, anorexia nervosa, or who require medication that can make blood glucose control labile.

The diabetes care team will give advice on the most suitable monitors available and give education in how to use and interpret results.

 EVIDENCE-BASED PRACTICE

To ensure the most reliable and consistent absorption of insulin, injections should be made into subcutaneous adipose tissue. The angle of the needle can be either 45 or 90 degrees, as preferred by the child (Gormley-Fleming and Martin, 2018). There is a difference in absorption rate and duration of different insulins when injected into subcutaneous fat and muscle. Intramuscular injection speeds up absorption and can lead to unexpected hypoglycaemia. It is also more painful for the child if given IM.

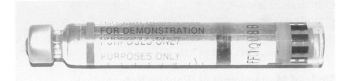

Fig. 20.9 An insulin cartridge.

Additional testing at different times during the day is advised:

- In association with exercise to optimise insulin to carbohydrate adjustment.
- During bouts of illness when blood glucose levels are fluctuating, and additional doses of insulin are required to prevent hyperglycaemia and the risk of developing diabetic ketoacidosis (DKA).
- To confirm hypoglycaemia and monitor recovery.
- During periods of rapid growth when insulin requirement is increasing.

It is important to reassure the child or young person that SMBG is a positive tool in managing their diabetes whatever the blood glucose results may be. Each result is just a piece of information that can be used to improve overall control and is not a reflection of them as an individual (Hanas, 2007).

HbA1c

During the life cycle of the red blood cell (approximately 120 days) glucose becomes attached to the haemoglobin molecule and forms glycated haemoglobin, which is represented as a percentage or as mmol/mol (International Federation of Clinical Chemistry [IFCC] unit of reporting). Known as the HbA1c, it reflects the general blood glucose levels in the previous 2–3 months. Ideally the test is carried out during an outpatient consultation so that it might be used to inform ongoing management.

NICE (2015) recommends the target for HbA1c level should be 6.5% (48 mmol/mol) or lower to minimise long-term complications. The child's individual management plan for diabetes should aim to achieve this.

Urinary and Blood Ketone Testing

Urinary ketone testing is advocated during periods of uncontrolled hyperglycaemia, insulin deficiency and during bouts of illness. Their early identification will alert the child or parent to the heightened risk of developing diabetic ketoacidosis. Urinary ketone test strips are available on prescription. The presence of moderate or large urinary ketones associated with hyperglycaemia reflects insulin deficiency and the risk of ketoacidosis.

Blood ketone testing meters are available for home monitoring. They should be offered to children to test for ketonaemia for when they are ill or if they have hyperglycaemia (NICE, 2015).

Diabetic Ketoacidosis

DKA is caused by a relative or absolute deficiency of insulin. It is a medical emergency requiring immediate treatment in

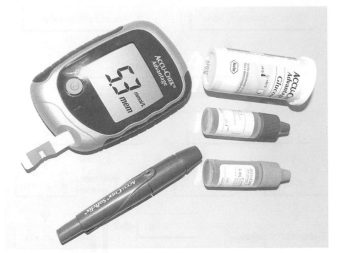

Fig. 20.10 Blood glucose monitoring equipment.

hospital with intravenous rehydration and insulin infusion. It is associated with significant morbidity and mortality. Up to 80% of newly diagnosed diabetics worldwide will present in DKA (de Vries et al., 2013). There are a number of risk factors for the potential development of DKA:

- The newly diagnosed. An improvement in the recognition of symptoms within primary care services has led to a reduction of DKA, though this is variable from one country to another.
- Infection/trauma. Infection or trauma can result in acute stress producing an elevation in counter-regulatory hormones that increase levels of circulating glucose.
- Growth spurt/puberty. The demand for insulin during a growth spurt or puberty requires a corresponding increase in insulin doses.
- Poor control/missed injections. Missed insulin injections coupled with dietary indiscretions will increase the risk of developing DKA and in consequence, recurrent episodes of DKA may be a reflection of mismanagement and will need psychological support to break the cycle of repetition.
- Insulin pump therapy. Insulin pump therapy uses only rapid- or short-acting insulin and therefore the reserve of circulating insulin is small when compared to injection therapy. If delivery of insulin is interrupted from the pump, DKA can develop very quickly.

It is important to establish the cause of DKA so that strategies can be employed to reduce the risk of further episodes. An understanding of the altered physiology that occurs when insulin is insufficient is required by the nurse and this is outlined in Fig. 20.11.

Characteristics of Diabetic Ketoacidosis

Presenting signs and symptoms include:

- hyperglycaemia
- polyuria
- polydipsia
- abdominal pain

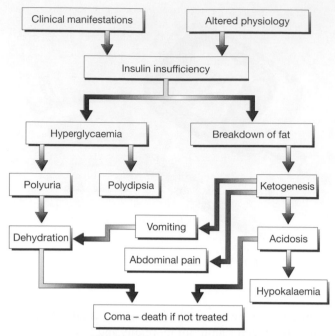

Fig. 20.11 Diabetic ketoacidosis.

- nausea and vomiting
- general weakness
- reduced level of consciousness
- weight loss
- Kussmaul breathing (deep sighing respirations)
- acetone smell on breath
  However, not all these symptoms may be present.

Diagnosis of Diabetic Ketoacidosis

Diagnosis is based on presenting signs and symptoms, clinical assessment of dehydration, abdominal pain/vomiting and neurological status. Hyperglycaemia is found: plasma glucose level >11 mmol/L, on bedside blood glucose testing initially and acidosis confirmed by venous/arterial blood gas analysis. Ketonuria is detected by urine dipstick testing. In a child who is not diagnosed with type 1 diabetes and presents with a plasma glucose >11 mmol/L and any symptoms that may indicate DKA, they need to be referred to an acute paediatric facility immediately. Children who are taking insulin for their diabetes may develop DKA even with a normal blood glucose level (NICE, 2015).

A diagnosis of DKA will be confirmed by:
- acidosis (blood pH below 7.3)
- ketonaemia (blood beta-hydroxybutyrate above 3 mmol/L) or ketonuria (++ and above on testing strip)
- severe DKA will be diagnosed if blood pH is below 7.1

Initial Management of DKA

Senior clinical staff must be informed immediately of diagnosis. Initial assessment will include:
- level of consciousness
- vital signs: temperature, heart rate, blood pressure, respiratory rate and note any Kussmaul breathing
- history of nausea or vomiting

- hydration status
- body weight
- plasma sodium, potassium, urea and creatinine, plasma bicarbonate, pH and pCo2

Goals of Management of Diabetic Ketoacidosis

- Restoration of fluid volume. Fluid boluses should only be given on the orders of a senior paediatrician. The aim is to replace the fluid deficit gradually over 48 hours as rapid fluid replacement has been indicated as a risk factor for cerebral oedema. Sodium chloride 0.9% with added glucose will be administered intravenously to rehydrate and maintain fluid until the glucose concentration is below 14 mmol/L (NICE, 2015). Potassium chloride will added to the infusion.
- Inhibition of lipolysis. Intravenous insulin is given to suppress the production of ketone bodies and restore normal glucose utilisation and resolve acidosis. This is commenced 1–2 hours after the intravenous fluids (IV) have been commenced. If the child is a known diabetic and receiving insulin via an insulin pump this will need to be discontinued prior to starting the IV insulin.
- Replacement of electrolytes. As potassium is drawn out of the cells by hypertonicity and lost through osmotic diuresis, there is a substantial depletion of total body potassium. Once circulatory function has been restored, it must be replaced by adding to the intravenous infusion. However, potassium replacement should be delayed until urinary output is documented.

The extent of specific deficits in each patient determines the severity of the ketoacidosis.

Nursing Care

Nursing care requires ongoing assessment and the child should be cared for on a High Dependency Unit or with one to one nursing if they are less than 2 years of age or have severe DKA (a blood pH of <7.1). When caring for any child with DKA, continuously assess with particular attention to:
- maintaining accurate fluid balance
- maintain insulin therapy
- all urine samples being tested for presence of ketones
- hourly BP and observations as indicated by condition and PEWS
- hourly or more frequent neurological observations for signs and symptoms of cerebral oedema
- hourly blood glucose measurements (using bedside blood glucose meter)
- levels of consciousness using Glasgow Coma Scale
- cardiac monitoring: presence of a flat T-wave may indicate hypokalaemia

Oral fluids/feeds should not be given to a child with DKA who is receiving intravenous therapy unless their ketosis is resolving, they are alert, and they are not nauseated or vomiting.

The child's condition should be monitored until blood glucose returns to normal, ketonuria is resolving and oral feeding has been re-established. The child might require a nasogastric tube if they have an altered level of consciousness to prevent aspiration. All nursing interventions must be accurately reported on and recorded. All interventions should be explained to the child and family as they will need support and reassurance during both the acute and recovery phase of management.

Cerebral Oedema

Cerebral oedema is a complication of diabetic ketoacidosis and is the most common cause of death in children with type 1 diabetes (Lissauer and Clayden, 2011). Children's nurses need to be alert for the signs and symptoms of cerebral oedema and report immediately to a senior medical clinician if the patient reports a headache or shows signs of confusion, irritability or reduced level of consciousness, increase in their blood pressure, decreased heart rate or indeed any change in their neurological status. Prompt recognition and treatment may prevent long-term neurological problems.

 WWW

Review the education and management required for children and young people with type 1 and type 2 in the guidelines produced by NICE, 2015 (sections 1.2 and 1.3). Available from: https://www.nice.org.uk/guidance/ng18.

Hypoglycaemia

Hypoglycaemia is an acute complication of diabetes. The blood glucose level drops resulting in decreased energy production for the cells. This may be due to a mismatch between insulin administered, food consumed and recent exercise. Medication, alcohol and drug use may also cause hypoglycaemia. It may be defined as mild if the episode is self-treated and resolves, or severe if the intervention of a third party is required. Left untreated it has the potential to be life changing.

Signs and Symptoms

The symptoms vary but common symptoms include: hunger, dizziness, feeling shaky, sweating, headache, tingling around the mouth, difficulty paying attention, confusion, behavioural changes, feeling angry, pallor. With the drive to achieve tight glycaemic control, the incidence of hypoglycaemia is almost inevitable.

Hypoglycaemia is generally accompanied by signs and symptoms that are in response to the body's attempt to raise the blood glucose level known as autonomic activation, and symptoms originating in the brain related to glucose deficiency in the nervous system referred to as neurological dysfunction (neuroglycopenia). Hypoglycaemia is considered to be a recorded plasma blood glucose level of ≤3.9 mmol/L.

The aim is to restore blood glucose level to within normal limits (4–8 mmol/L) aiming to reach 5.6 mmol/L. This may be referred to as the '15 rule'.

- Take immediate action and give a fast-acting carbohydrate, such as dextrose tablets or a glucose drink (e.g. 10–20 g) by mouth. Biscuits, milk, cake and fruit are not suitable food to treat hypoglycaemia as the glucose will be absorbed too slowly and the blood glucose may continue to drop.

TABLE 20.7	Characteristics of Hypoglycaemia
Characteristics	**Nursing Considerations**
Blood glucose <3.9 mmol/L	Requires immediate administration of fast-acting sugar to raise blood glucose 10–20 g of dextrose
Hunger, weakness, shaking, sweating	Check blood glucose level after 15 minutes
Drowsiness at unusual times	Assess the need for additional carbohydrate or possibility of hyperglycaemia
Headache, behavioural changes	If child presents with seizure or in a coma administer intramuscular glucagon as directed – may cause nausea and vomiting so need to administer oral carbohydrate when child is awake
Loss of consciousness	Check consistency in routine
Convulsions	Check that correct insulin dosage is being administered
	Encourage regular blood glucose monitoring
	Encourage controlled snacking
	Encourage child/family compliance
	Ensure all involved with the child on a daily basis are educated and trained in recognition and treatment of hypoglycaemia

- The blood glucose level should start to rise, and symptoms improve in 10–15 minutes. Re-test blood glucose level to confirm return of normoglycaemia after 15 minutes.
- With normoglycaemia restored a long-acting carbohydrate should be given to maintain blood glucose level.
- If the child has regular hypoglycaemia episodes a review by the diabetic team should be considered.

NB: Patients using insulin pump therapy do not require an additional long-acting carbohydrate after a hypoglycaemic episode.

Treatment of Mild/Moderate Hypoglycaemia

For severe hypoglycaemia, urgent treatment is required. Oral glucose solution should not be administered if the level of consciousness is reduced (NICE, 2015). If the child is unconscious administer IM glucagon. There should be a response within 10 minutes. The child should be transferred to hospital as there is a further risk of hypoglycaemia. Review by a paediatrician is required. If recovery is inadequate, IV glucose 10% may be required to be administered. Hypoglycaemic events should be evaluated and the cause determined in an effort to avoid similar episodes.

TYPE 2 DIABETES

The incidence of type 2 diabetes is rising in children as the prevalence of childhood obesity continues to rise. It is associated with obesity, insulin resistance and metabolic syndrome and is seen in both the paediatric and adolescent population (Lissauer and Clayden, 2011). Type 2 diabetes occurs when there is insufficient insulin secretion to meet the demand created by insulin resistance. A lack of exercise and a sedentary lifestyle, coupled

TABLE 20.8 Signs and Symptoms of Hypoglycaemia

Autonomic Signs and Symptoms of Hypoglycaemia	Neuroglycopenic Signs and Symptoms of Hypoglycaemia
Irritability	Weakness, dizziness
Trembling	Odd behaviour, poor judgment
Heart palpitation	Unsteady gait
Pallor	Difficulty concentrating
Feeling hungry	Difficulty hearing
Cold sweatiness	Blurred vision
	Loss of consciousness
	Seizures

TABLE 20.9 Treatment of Hypoglycaemia

Mild/Moderate Hypoglycaemia	Severe Hypoglycaemia
The child or parent/caregiver is aware of hypoglycaemic episode and is able to take appropriate action to resolve	Symptoms of hypoglycaemia temporarily disable the child and assistance is required by parent or caregiver Oral glucose is given providing swallow reflex is present; an injection of intramuscular glucagon if no swallow reflex In the hospital setting, intravenous glucose

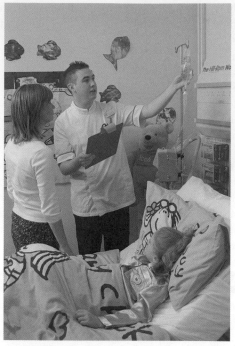

Fig. 20.12 Intravenous therapy in progress.

with excessive calorie intake, are recognised risk factors for obesity and type 2 diabetes. This presents society with a major public health issue with profound implications for the health of future generations and will inevitably place a significant financial burden on our health care system (Rodbard, 2008). Although there is limited data on the future health outcomes in children with type 2 diabetes, it is expected that the progressive nature of the condition will mirror that seen in the adult population, but occur at a much younger age.

Clinical findings may be similar to type 1 diabetes in childhood presenting as milder symptoms that develop slowly; however, the presence of insulin resistance is a strong indicator of type 2 diabetes. A diagnosis of type 2 diabetes is made when the presence of elevated plasma blood glucose levels are not thought to be type 1 diabetes or monogenic diabetes or any other underlying cause of hyperglycaemia; however, the levels are sufficient to put the individual at risk of cardiovascular complications. Diagnosis is confirmed if fasting blood glucose concentrations are >7.0 mmol/L on two separate days, or if random glucose concentrations of 11.1 mmol/L or above on two separate occasions (Rosenbloom et al., 2009).

Management Strategies

The goals of treatment are:
- to encourage weight loss
- to increase physical activity
- to achieve normoglycaemia
- to adopt a healthier lifestyle
- reduction in the rate of complications

A child with type 2 diabetes is likely to have a one in five chance of having a parent with type 2 diabetes. This is particularly challenging for health care professionals as it requires a greater emphasis on changing behaviour and eating patterns that are often deep seated in the child's lifestyle, and success is dependent on the whole family's ability to modify their way of life and eating practices.

The target HbA1c is 48 mmol/mol (6.5%) for children with type 2 diabetes. It is important that the child and family understand the benefit of achieving this target in preventing long-term complications. The HbA1c level will be measured every 3 months.

Standard release metformin should be offered to children diagnosed with type 2 diabetes (NICE, 2015). The aim is to reduce insulin resistance, increase the secretion of endogenous insulin or slow post-prandial glucose absorption.

Monogenic Diabetes

Monogenic diabetes results from one or more mutations in a single gene which may be dominantly or recessively inherited, or may simply be a spontaneous occurrence. The clinical spectrum is broad, ranging from asymptomatic hyperglycaemia to a severe acute presentation. Monogenic diabetes has been reported in all races and ethnicities. The characteristics of monogenic diabetes are:
- presentation of diabetes before 6 months of age;
- it can run in families through several generations;
- children don't produce enough insulin – which differs from type 2 diabetes, where the individual produces sufficient insulin but are unable to utilise it;

TABLE 20.10	Clinical Characteristics Between Type 1 and Type 2 Diabetes	
Characteristics	Type 1 Diabetes Mellitus	Type 2 Diabetes Mellitus
Age	Throughout child-hood	Usually pubertal, however becoming more common in childhood
Onset	Often acute	Insidious
Obesity	Not typically present, often thin	Typically present
Family history of type 2 diabetes	Uncommon	Common
Polyuria	Symptomatic	Mild or absent
Polydipsia	Symptomatic	Mild or absent
Tiredness	Common	Common
Ketonuria	Common	Rare

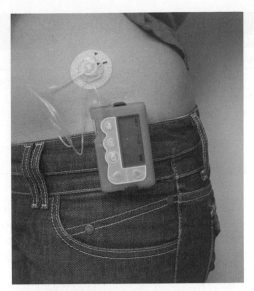

Fig. 20.13 Insulin pump therapy.

- children with monogenic diabetes may not need insulin treatment and can often be treated with oral glycaemic therapy or diet modification alone.

In children, most cases of monogenic diabetes are associated with mutations in genes that regulate β-cell function (Carmody et al., 2016). Diagnosis is based on molecular genetics. Often incorrectly diagnosed initially, type 2 diabetes may be diagnosed instead of monogenic diabetes. A diagnosis of monogenic diabetes will have implications for other family members who may have been misdiagnosed with type 1 or type 2 diabetes.

Insulin Pump Therapy

Insulin pump therapy also known as continuous subcutaneous insulin infusion (CSII) is now readily available in the UK. It has been successfully used in all age groups and offers a more flexible approach to diabetes management. The advantage of insulin pump therapy is its ability to mimic physiological insulin release by continuously delivering rapid (or short) insulin into subcutaneous tissue (Fig. 20.13).

The pump has a refillable reservoir connected via tubing to a subcutaneously placed catheter that is changed every few days. The pump is programmed to deliver a basal (background) rate of insulin throughout the day and calculated bolus doses are given at the push of a button for meal carbohydrate intake. Current pump technology allows for variable hourly rates of insulin that are set according to the individual child's basal requirement and mealtime bolus insulin doses can be adjusted in speed and duration of delivery based on the composition of a meal and its anticipated glycaemic effects.

Suitability for Continuous Subcutaneous Insulin Infusion

For patients with type 1 diabetes who are:
- unable to achieve target HbA1c and who experience disabling hypoglycaemia despite multiple daily injection therapy, OR
- have elevated HbA1c (8.5% or above) on multiple daily injections despite high levels of motivation.

In addition:
- for children under 12 years of age CSII may be a treatment option for type 1 diabetes provided MDI is impractical or inappropriate. However, a trial of injection therapy would be expected during teenage years (NICE, 2010).

The child's basal requirement and mealtime bolus insulin doses can be adjusted in speed and duration of delivery based on the composition of a meal and its anticipated glycaemic affects. Initiation of therapy should be carried out by trained professionals in CSII and ongoing care by a diabetes team experienced in pump therapy.

CSII is expensive compared to conventional therapy and its use in the UK is dependent on clinical need. Comparative studies between the efficacy of CSII and MDI from a clinical perspective are inconclusive; however, of note is the reduction in frequency and severity of hypoglycaemic episodes reported in patients using CSII. Families describe high levels of satisfaction, a more spontaneous approach to food, fewer glycaemic excursions and increased independence for the older child and adolescent (Plotnick et al., 2003).

Insulin injections are commonly given via an insulin pen, although using a syringe and needle is still a practice used in some areas when specific combinations of long- and short-acting insulins are not available as a pre-mixture. Before mixing insulin in the same syringe, there is a need to establish that this procedure does not change the pharmacokinetics of both types of insulin, otherwise the practice should be avoided.

Long-Term Complications of Type 1 Diabetes Mellitus

There are four major long-term complications associated with type 1 diabetes:
- Retinopathy
- Nephropathy
- Neuropathy
- Cardiac disease

TABLE 20.11	Long-Term Vascular Complications	
Complications	**Outcomes**
Retinopathy	Visual impairment – cataracts, blindness
Nephropathy	Renal failure, hypertension
Neuropathy	Pain, paraesthesia, muscle weakness, autonomic dysfunction
Cardiac disease	Atherosclerosis, hypertension, cardio-vascular disease

The outcomes from these are presented in Table 20.11. While these complications are uncommon in childhood and may not be clinically visible, early functional and structural abnormalities may be evident in the microvascular systems after a few years following diagnosis. Evidence has indicated that meticulous treatment and control of type 1 diabetes will reduce the risk of microvascular complication significantly (NICE, 2015).

Retinopathy is the commonest cause of blindness in developed countries. The prevalence of microvascular disease is high in young people with type 1 diabetes and this may rapidly progress towards visual impairment (Holman et al., 2015). Hence, annual screening is imperative to detect the early stages of retinopathy. Other complications of type 1 diabetes include:

- delayed growth
- delayed onset of puberty
- associated autoimmune conditions – coeliac disease, hypothyroidism, hyperthyroidism, vitiligo and primary adrenal insufficiency
- lipohypertrophy
- skin ulceration
- limited joint mobility

Monitoring of growth and development is essential. There may be an increase in height at the time of diagnosis, however, poor weight gain, decrease in the attainment of height and late pubertal development have been reported in those who have poor glycaemic control (Kordonouri et al., 2007). After the initial diagnosis and the child's weight is satisfactory they need to be monitored for excessive weight gain. This may occur due to a high energy intake and excessive exogenous insulin. It is more common during puberty, especially in females, thus necessitating a reduction in their insulin dose towards the end of puberty (Lissauer and Clayden, 2011). Obesity will also increase the risk of cardiovascular defects. Girls with type 1 diabetes are more at risk of being obese and developing eating disorders along with the risk of having polycystic ovary syndrome.

Foot problems are the most frequent problem of diabetic neuropathy leading eventually to lower limb amputation for up to 15% of the associated diabetic population. As glycaemic control is difficult to maintain around and during puberty, it has been recognised that this is when microvascular problems are likely to occur (Shaw and Cummings, 2012). Compliance with treatment and monitoring is not always congruent with the adolescent lifestyle, hence the need for early education of the parents and the child. NICE (2015) guidelines advise examination of the feet on diagnosis and then annually. Education is also required about correctly fitting shoes and socks, and toenail cutting.

To minimise the long-term impact of type 1 diabetes and with a view to maximisation of the quality of life of the child, regular surveillance for, and the effective management of complications needs to occur. Screening should be carried out in accordance with recommendations from NICE (2015). This advises that the child with type 1 diabetes should:

- attend diabetes clinic four times a year
- have regular dental examinations
- be monitored for hypertension annually from the age of 12 years
- have an eye examination for diabetic retinopathy annually
- be monitored for thyroid disease annually
- carry or wear a medi-alert bracelet
- have their annual immunisation against influenza if over 6 months of age
- be immunised against pneumococcal infection

Children with type 1 diabetes are more at risk of psychological and social issues resulting in emotional and behavioural difficulties. Emotional support should be tailor made to reflect their social, cultural and age needs. The lack of adequate psychosocial support has been identified as impacting negatively on the child with type 1 diabetes. Behavioural intervention therapy should be considered when there are concerns about psychological well-being (NICE, 2015).

Young People and Type I Diabetes

Normal physical, psychosexual and developmental maturation in the young person is affected by diabetes (Lissauer and Clayden, 2011). During this phase of development, the child will move from dependence to a more autonomous lifestyle and are expected to take increasing responsibility for their care and health needs. Cognitive changes occur: concrete thinking moves to more abstract thinking. Young people are unable to comprehend the long-term and unseen consequences of their actions. The health care professional must be alert to the health needs and social issues that may affect the adolescent during this developmental phase.

In addition, diabetes is often more difficult to control due to hormonal changes of puberty as well as the emotional difficulties associated with this phase of development (Shaw and Cummings, 2012). For some, this stage of development will present with behavioural changes such as denial, indifference or depression about their illness. In addition, there may be an unwillingness to conform to treatment regimes, which may give rise to conflict with family and health professionals. There may be a tendency to avoid aspects of their diabetic management, for example, omit insulin injections or manipulate the regime, and ignore dietary needs. Blood glucose monitoring may not be carried out or results may be falsified. Many teenage girls experiment with crash diets at some time, which is likely to cause major problems in diabetic control. Low adherence rates increase mortality and morbidity, thus affecting quality of life in the long-term and may necessitate additional health care resources.

This is a time when the young person should be encouraged to take increasing control for their diabetes. Compliance has been defined as to the extent that medical advice is followed to achieve therapeutic goals (Royal College of Paediatrics and Child Health [RCPCH], 2015). Evaluation of adherence is an essential role of the health care practitioner and this is best achieved by asking the young person about their management of their diabetes. Low adherence rates may also test the limits of acceptable behaviour. It may be helpful to identify short-term goals for them and ensure that effort to improve their control is communicated promptly and enthusiastically. Parental influence has been shown to positively improve compliance, particularly the strength of the parent–child relationship (Drew et al., 2010; Mlynarczyk, 2013). A united team approach, with agreement on the essentials they wish to promote, and clear, unambiguous guidelines for health and diabetic management is necessary.

Repeated information has been identified as a method of improving adherence (Osterberg and Blaschke, 2005). Consideration must also be given to the appropriate management of any mental-health issues if adherence to treatment is to be achieved. Behaviour intervention therapy is recommended (NICE, 2015).

Peer group pressure may be utilised to promote health, especially in relation to smoking and alcohol consumption. However, peer influence has limited effect on compliance (Drew et al., 2010). Online support groups and holiday camps provide opportunities for young diabetics to meet and learn about their diabetic management.

Mental Health and Diabetes

Mental health has been identified as a significant co-morbidity in type 1 diabetes (NHS, 2016). A strong correlation between high HbA1c, missed appointments and psychosocial issues has been identified (Garvey et al., 2013).

Diabetes has been linked to an increased risk of eating disorders (Philpott, 2013). This may include manipulation of insulin or hypoglycaemic agents to manage body weight. Screening tools should be employed so risk can be identified, and the young person supported as required.

Ongoing, timely access to mental health professionals should be an integral aspect of the transition provision for young people and their families as they move from one service to another.

Transition to Adult Services

The young person with type 1 diabetes should experience a smooth transition of care from children's diabetic services to adult diabetic services. Transition should consider the broader changes that the young person may be experiencing during this phase of their life. The transition between services should not be another challenge.

Transition is a multifaceted process and it must acknowledge the medical, psychosocial and educational needs of the young person – it is a purposeful and planned process. Best practice advocates that transition from children's service to adult services is best undertaken during a period of stability and is planned on an individual basis. Best practice advocates that services for young people with diabetes will require engagement with both paediatric and adult diabetic services (National Health Service, 2016). The young person and their families must be provided with knowledge, skills and confidence about the transition process and the services they will be accessing in the future. Transition should be based on the emotional development of the individual and not on chronological age. Local protocols for transition to adult services should be in place (NICE, 2015). The practical aspects of transition of care for young people with diabetes needs to be made clear to them, such as the glycaemic levels required, screening process and any unfamiliar terminology. Continued engagement with the multidisciplinary team has been identified as having a positive impact on HbA1c level following transition, preventing episodes of DKA and reduced length of stay (Farrell et al., 2018).

Child and Family Education

The primary goal in caring for children and young people with diabetes is to enable them and their families to manage their own lifestyle and condition, by providing support and structured education as well as drugs and treatment. Therefore a coordinated, multidisciplinary team approach to care and management in partnership with the child and family is essential if the following long-term outcomes are to be achieved:

- normal growth and development;
- maintaining as normal a home and school life as possible;
- good diabetic control, appropriate knowledge, good technique and self-reliance;
- avoidance of hypoglycaemia;
- prevention of long-term complications.

This will be reflected in the child's personal record that contains the clinical record of care, treatment and management. A personal diabetes record should include the following:

- an agreed care plan, including education and the personal goals of the child and family in relation to care and treatment;
- information as to how the child's diabetes is to be managed until the next review to foster greater understanding and ownership of the goals of diabetes care;
- identification of social and educational needs, how they will be met and who will be responsible;
- identification of the named contact.

Central Role of the Nurse

Care of the child with type 1 diabetes requires a multidisciplinary approach through collaboration with paediatricians, endocrinologist, general practitioners, dieticians, psychology services and education providers. It has been shown that children from deprived or Black and Minority Ethnic backgrounds (BAME) backgrounds have poorer control of their diabetes (RCPCH, 2018). The nurse, particularly the community children nurse, plays a central role in the assessment and planning

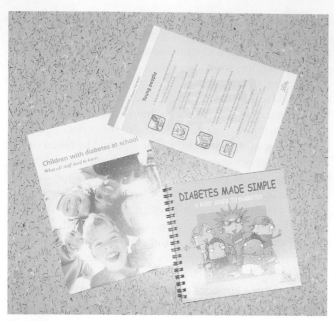

Fig. 20.14 Examples of information available for child, family and others.

of care for the child and family. The management of diabetes is a complex process and the aim of nursing care should be to meet the holistic needs of the child and family from diagnosis through to the long-term care required with a view to maintaining a good quality of life. The lifestyle changes are probably greater for the child and family with diabetes than other long-term conditions. Good facilitation of the child's and families care needs will enable a family centred care approach to be adopted. Effective management of diabetes increases life expectancy and reduces the risk of complications developing (Diabetes UK, 2018). As this is a lifelong condition, the nurse must consider what the developmental stage the child is at when planning care. The timing and giving of information are very important in the initial period after diagnosis and it should be remembered that this will need revisiting at a later time.

Initial education for the child and parents/carers is crucial. This will focus on the skills necessary for discharge from hospital, injection technique, home glucose monitoring, recognition of hypoglycaemic episode and hyperglycaemia, dietary management, exercise and recording of information. The child and parents/carer should also be informed of what action to take during normal expected illnesses.

Ongoing nursing assessment is required with the focus on the child's physiological status, psychological state and family's response to diagnosis and treatment constantly being revisited. This will necessitate the nurse accessing other members of the multidisciplinary team as required to support the child and family. The nurse is the central contact point for accessing the multidisciplinary team on behalf of the child and family. Parental guilt may be present at the time of diagnosis and for a period of time after diagnosis. Education requirements should be planned to suit the needs of the child and family and delivered to meet their needs.

Coping mechanisms need to be assessed and understood by the nurse so that the plan of care for the child and parents

will correctly reflect their educational needs. Individual plans of care should be developed by the child, parent, diabetic nurse and team to address their specific needs in terms of normal life activities, that is, school and social clubs.

Home management at the time of diagnosis provides immediate opportunities for the children's nurse to educate the child, parents and others in relation to diabetes. Books, teaching aids and website addresses might enhance the learning process and provide guidance for child and parent in the absence of the nurse (Fig. 20.14). Opportunities should be made for child and family to explore their perceptions of the impact of diabetes on their lives and the implications of care required by the child, and the immediate problems they envisage. Meeting with other parents and children with diabetes may provide additional support.

Parents need to understand the positive support their child will need throughout childhood and into adolescence to optimise physical, psychological, intellectual, educational and social development. As diabetes is a long-term condition, the child needs to take on the responsibility and develop the confidence to be self-caring (Rudolf et al., 2011).

This chapter has identified the common childhood endocrine disorders and considered the physiology, signs and symptoms, nursing care and educational requirements of the child and family.

DISCUSSION OF THE SCENARIOS

Kate: Graves' Disease

Observations necessary to assess Kate's need to plan her nursing interventions include:

- vital signs of temperature, pulse and blood pressure may be elevated, and Kate may complain of palpitations due to hyperthyroid state;
- observation of skin for warmth, moistness and flushed appearance;
- respiratory difficulties may present as a result of hypervascularity and enlargement of the thyroid gland;
- enlargement of the thyroid gland may be evident;
- enlargement and protrusion of the eye balls leading to irritation, pain, lacrimation, photophobia and blurred vision;
- monitoring of height may indicate a degree of accelerated growth and development;
- monitoring weight may indicate a loss despite having an increased appetite;
- Kate may complain of excessive weakness and lack of ability to engage in usual activities;
- observation of her emotional state, nervous excitability and mood stability is necessary as there may be associated hyperactivity of the sympathetic division of the autonomic nervous system.

Kate's Specific Care Requirements

The symptoms of hyperthyroidism may fluctuate with spontaneous remissions and exacerbations. Mild cases may require no treatment. The condition is generally treated with medical interventions and/or radiation therapy.

Bedrest is advisable at the beginning of medical treatment. This treatment is aimed at controlling symptoms of nervous instability, tachycardia and hypertension that may require the administration of β-adrenergic blocking agents (propranolol, atenolol). Continual monitoring of vital signs is necessary to evaluate effectiveness of interventions and monitor for early signs of complications.

Drugs that interfere with thyroid hormone synthesis, namely carbimazole or propylthiouracil, may be prescribed according to the individual needs of the child. Treatment with antithyroid drugs must be continued for at least 2–3 years, with the smallest drug dosage that will produce a symptom-free state in the child.

When response to medical treatment is not achieved then radiation therapy with radioactive iodine may be considered. In some cases, radioiodine is considered the initial treatment of choice (Kappy et al., 2003).

In hypothyroidism and hyperthyroidism, the aim of care is to achieve an optimal level of thyroxine that will enable growth and development, including enhancement of intellectual ability. Kate and her parents need to understand the nature of the condition, the aims and different types of treatment, including dosages of prescribed medication and repeat prescriptions, as well as the signs of under- and over-treatment The consequences of non-compliance needs to be discussed. As with all other conditions the provision of literature and appropriate website addresses as identified may enhance understanding.

Attendance at clinics is essential to:

- monitor Kate's response to medication;
- assess growth and development;
- provide the opportunity for Kate and her family to discuss their fears or problems associated with the care and management of the condition;
- enable them to meet other families who have been caring for their children with similar problems, which for some may prove beneficial.

The children's nurse can remain as the named contact person and through assessment in collaboration and negotiation with the child and family can plan the education and ongoing support required.

SUMMARY

This chapter has provided an overview of the common childhood endocrine disorders and considered the physiology, signs and symptoms, nursing care and educational requirements of the child and family.

Development of knowledge and understanding has been enhanced through active participation and the companion PowerPoint presentation.

REFERENCES

Ball, J.W., Bindler, R.C., 2006. Child Health Nursing: Partnering With Children and Families. Prentice Hall, Englewood Cliffs, NJ.

Beckwith, S., 2010. Diagnosing Type 2 diabetes in children and young people. Br. J. Sch. Nurs. 5 (1), 15–19.

Cappa, M., Bizzarri, C., Crea, F., 2011. Autoimmune thyroid diseases in children. J. Thyroid Res. 2011, 675703.

Carmody, D., Stoy, J., Greenley, et al., 2016. A Clinical guide to monogenic diabetes. In: Weiss, R.E., Refetoff, S. (Eds.), Genetic Diagnosis of Endocrine Disorders, second ed. Elsevier, Philadelphia, PA, pp. 21–30.

Chrousos, G.P., 2002. Chapter 264. Cushing syndrome and cushing disease. In: Finberg, L., Kleinman, R. (Eds.), Saunders Manual of Pediatric Practice, second ed. WB Saunders Co, Philadelphia, pp. 909–911.

Corenblum, B., 2016. Hypopituitarism (panhypopituitarism). Medscape. Available from: https://emedicine.medscape.com/article/122287-overview.

Crocker, M.K., Yanovski, J.A., 2009. Paediatric obesity: etiology and treatment. Endocrin. Metab. Clin. 38 (3), 525–548.

Cuttler, L., 2002. In: Finberg, L., Kleinman, R.E. (Eds.), Saunders Manual of Pediatric Practice, second cd. WB Saunders, London.

de Vries, L., Oren, L., Lazar, L., et al., 2013. Factors associated with diabetic ketoacidosis at onset of Type 1 diabetes in children and adolescents. Diabet. Med. 30, 1360–1366.

Diabetes UK, 2018. Your child and diabetes. Available from: https://www.diabetes.org.uk/guide-to-diabetes/your-child-and-diabetes.

Drake, A., Kelnar, C., 2006. The evaluation of growth and the identification of hormone deficiency. Arch. Dis. Child. 91, 61–67.

Drew, L.M., Berg, C., Wiebe, J., 2010. The mediating role of extreme peer orientation in the relationship between adolescent-parent relationship and diabetes management. J. Fam. Psychol. 24 (3), 299–306.

Edge, J., Acerini, C., Campbell, F., et al., 2017. An alternative sensor-based method for glucose monitoring in children and young people with diabetes. Arch. Dis. Child. 102 (6), 543–549.

Farrell, K., Fernandez, R., Salamonson, Y., et al., 2018. Health outcomes for youth with Type 1 diabetes at 18 months and 30 months post transition from pediatric to adult care. Diabetes Res. Clin. Pract. 139, 163–169.

Garvey, K.C., Wolpert, H.A., Finklestein, J.A., 2013. Health care transition in young adults with type 1 diabetes: barriers to timely establishment of adult diabetes care. Endocr. Pract. 19 (6), 946–952.

Gormley-Fleming, E., 2010. Assessing and vital signs – a comprehensive review. In: Glasper, E.A., Aylott, M., Batterick, C. (Eds.), Developing Skills for Children's and Young People's Nursing. Elsevier.

Gormley-Fleming, E., Martin, D., 2018. Children's and Young People's Nursing Skills at a Glance. Wiley, Blackwell.

Hanas, R., 2007. Type 1 Diabetes in Children, Adolescents and Young Adults, third ed. Class Publishing, London.

Hockenberry, M.J., et al., 2003. Wong's Nursing Care of Infants and Children, seventh ed. Mosby, London.

Holman, N., et al., 2015. Microvascular Disease in Children's and Young People in England and Wales. RCPCH, London.

Kappy, M.S., et al., 2003. In: Hay, W.W., Hayward, A.R., Levin, M.J., Sondheimer, J.M. (Eds.), Current Pediatric Diagnosis and Treatment, sixteenth ed. McGraw-Hill, London.

Kim, S.Y., 2015. Diagnosis and treatment of hypopituitarism. Endrcrinol. Metab. 30 (4), 443–455.

Kordonouri, O., Maguire, A., Knip, M., et al., 2007. Other complications and associated conditions. Pediatr. Diabetes 8, 171–176.

Lissauer, T., Clayden, G., 2011. Illustrated Textbook of Paediatrics, fourth ed. Mosby, Edinburgh.

McCance, A., Huether, B., 2014. Pathophysiology: The Biological Basis for Disease in Adults and Children, seventh ed. Mosby, St Louis.

Mlynarczyk, S., 2013. Adolescents perspectives of parental practices influence diabetic adherence and quality of life. Pediatr. Nurs. 39 (4), 181–189.

National Health Service (NHS), 2016. Diabetes Transition Service Specification. NHS, Leeds.

National Health Service (NHS), 2018. Phaeochromocytoma. Available from: https://www.nhs.uk/conditions/phaeochromocytoma/.

National Institute for Health and Care Excellence (NICE), 2010. Guidance on the Use of Human Growth Hormone (Somatropin) in Children with Growth Failure. NICE, London. Available from: https://www.nice.org.uk/guidance/ta188.

National Institute for Health and Care Excellence (NICE), 2015. Diabetes (Type 1 and Type 2) in Children and Young People: Diagnosis and Management. NICE, London. Available from: https://www.nice.org.uk/guidance/ng18.

Osterberg, L., Blaschke, T., 2005. Adherence to medication. N. Engl. J. Med. 353, 487–497.

Peate, I., Gormley-Fleming, E., 2015. Fundamentals of Children's Anatomy and Physiology. A Textbook for Nurses and Healthcare Students. Wiley Blackwell, Oxford.

Petty, J., 2015. Endocrine disorders. In: Peate, I., Gormley-Fleming, E. (Eds.), Fundamentals of Children's Anatomy and Physiology. A Textbook for Nurses and Healthcare Students. 2015 Wiley Blackwell, Oxford.

Philpott, U., 2013. Eating disorders in young people: development, diagnosis and management. J. Diabetes Nurs. 17 (6), 228–232.

Plotnick, L.P., et al., 2003. Safety and effectiveness of insulin pump therapy in children and adolescents with type 1 diabetes. Diabetes Care 26 (4), 1142–1146.

Roberts, R., Walsh, J., 2006. Pumping Insulin, fourth ed. Torrey Pines Press, California.

Rodbard, H., 2008. Diabetes screening, diagnosis and therapy in paediatrics patients with type 2 diabetes. Diabetes Care 10 (8), 184.

Rosenbloom, A.L., Silverstein, J.H., Amemiya, S., et al., 2009. ISPAD clinical practice consensus guidelines 2009 compendium. Type 2 diabetes in children and adolescents. Pediatr. Diabetes 10 (Suppl. 12), 17–32.

Royal College of Paediatrics and Child Health (RCPCH), 2015. National Diabetes Project Audit Report. RCPCH, London.

Royal College of Paediatrics and Child Health (RCPCH), 2018. State of Child Health 6. RCPCH, London.

Rudolf, M., Lee, T., Levene, M., 2011. Paediatrics and Child Health, third ed. Wiley Blackwell Publishing, Oxford.

Shaw, K.M., Cummings, M.H., 2012. Diabetes: Chronic Complications, third ed. Wiley-Blackwell, Chichester.

Storr, H.L., Plowman, P.N., Caroll, P.V., et al., 2003. Clinical and endocrine responses to pituitary radiotherapy in paediatric Cushing's disease. An effective second line treatment. J. Clin. Endocrinol. Metab. 88 (1), 34–37.

Waugh, A., Grant, A., 2018. Ross and Wilson. Anatomy and Physiology in Health and Illness, thirteenth ed. Elsevier, Edinburgh.

Williams, B.K., et al., 2011. Lower cardiorespiratory fitness in children with Type 1 diabetes. Diabet. Med. 28, 1005–1007.

World Health Organization (WHO), 2006. Definition and Diagnosis of Diabetes Mellitus and Intermediate Hyperglycaemia. Report of a WHO/IDF Consultation. WHO, Department of Noncommunicable Disease Surveillance, Geneva.

USEFUL WEBSITES

British Society of Paediatric Endocrinology and Diabetes. Available from: http://www.bsped.org.uk.

Diabetes UK. Available from: http://www.diabetes.org.uk.

21

Caring for Children With Gastrointestinal Problems

Julia Winter

LEARNING OUTCOMES

- Consider the factors which contribute to gut health in infants and children.
- Identify the causes and management of vomiting in infants and children.
- Identify the causes of acute and chronic diarrhoea in infants and children.
- Recognise and distinguish between presentation of acute and chronic disorders.

- Identify the causes of sudden acute gastrointestinal problems requiring surgery.
- Consider the management of both acute and chronic gastrointestinal disorders, adopting a family-centred approach to care.
- Review the changes in incidence in chronic gastrointestinal disorders, considering causes and implications for health care practice.

GLOSSARY

Anal stenosis Narrowing or stricture of the anal canal and sphincter.

Atresia Absence or closure or a natural passage or channel, imperforation.

Bulimia An eating disorder, which is characterised by self-induced vomiting after eating.

Haemolytic uraemic syndrome A pathological condition which involves the rupture (haemolysis) of red blood cells, subsequent anaemia, low platelet count and kidney failure.

Hirschsprung's disease Congenital aganglionosis of the colon leading to loss of gut motility.

Imperforate anus A congenital obstruction of the anal opening.

Intussusception Telescoping of one portion of the intestine into another.

Malrotation Failure during normal embryonic development of normal rotation of all or part of an organ.

Meconium ileus Obstructed bowel due to impacted, tenacious meconium.

Microbiome The microorganism complement within a particular environment.

Myopathies Disease of muscles.

Neurofibromatosis Growth of neurofibromas (smooth soft or firm tumours) anywhere in the myelinated nervous system (autosomal inheritance).

Organic causes A disease that occurs as a result of anatomical or physiological abnormality.

Pyloric stenosis A congenital disorder in which the pylorus is thickened causing obstruction of the gastric outlet.

Scleroderma Hardening of skin.

Systemic lupus erythematosus A chronic autoimmune disease.

Villous atrophy Wasting or flattening of the villi.

🌐 WWW

Use this site, or similar, to look up terms you are not sure of:
- https://www.online-medical-dictionary.org/

VOMITING

Vomiting in infants and children is a common problem and therefore likely to be experienced by the majority of families and all children's nurses. Causes of vomiting are diverse and are summarised in Table 21.1. This table shows that causes of vomiting differ between infants and older children. Some are associated with anatomical dysfunction requiring surgery. Other causes of vomiting can be medically managed, such as gastro-oesophageal reflux.

👤 ACTIVITY

Choose one of the problems requiring surgery:
- Using a systematic approach, plan the care the child would require before and after surgery.
- How could you make sure you adopted a family-centred approach?

  You can check principles of pre- and post-operative care on the companion PowerPoint presentation.

Gastro-Oesophageal Reflux

Gastro-oesophageal reflux (refluxing of stomach contents into the oesophagus) is frequently seen, to varying degrees, in infants.

TABLE 21.1   Causes of Vomiting

Infant	Older Child
Overfeeding (>200 mL/kg/day)	Gastroenteritis
Gastrointestinal obstruction	Systemic infection
Pyloric stenosis and other sphincter disorders	Raised intracranial pressure
Duodenal or ileal atresia	Cyclic vomiting (abdominal migraine)
Congenital malrotation	Migraine
Hirschsprung's disease	Bulimia
Meconium ileus (in cystic fibrosis)	Poisoning
Intussusception	Pregnancy
Gastro-oesophageal reflux	
Whooping cough	
Systemic infection (e.g. urinary tract)	

Aetiology

The most common cause is functional immaturity of the gastro-oesophageal sphincter. It is more frequently seen in children with complex neuro disabilities (National Institute for Health and Care Excellence [NICE], 2015a) such as cerebral palsy, and also in children with Down syndrome. Whereas mild reflux (possetting) is generally harmless, it becomes problematic when associated with faltering growth or complications develop. In an extended integrative review Puccini and Berretin-Felix (2015) suggest that although functional reflux in early infancy with no obvious mechanical cause may be benign, reflux of physiological origin can lead to altered pathology, which is a threat to infant growth, development and respiratory function. These include oesophageal scarring, due to refluxing of gastric acid, which can lead to strictures. There is also the risk of aspiration and potentially apnoea. Diagnostic investigations aim to assess any aspiration risk, degree of severity and structural abnormality such as hiatus hernia.

 WWW

Use the internet to find a diagram of the stomach showing the pyloric and gastro-oesophageal sphincters, located at the top and bottom of the stomach. The affected sphincter is the gastro-oesophageal.

Diagnosis

Diagnostic investigations include:

- contrast studies: show degree of reflux, strictures, altered anatomy of oesophageal junction;
- 24-hour pH probe studies: detect presence of gastric acid in oesophagus;
- ultrasound of gastro-oesophageal junction: can demonstrate reflux but no other anatomical defects;
- radionuclide salivagram: aspiration (NICE, 2015a).

Management

Management centres mainly on thickening feeds, for example, with carob gum–based products and nursing the infant in a more upright position. In more severe cases, drugs to increase gut motility and speed stomach emptying have been used. The condition is viewed by some as a normal physiological variant (NICE, 2015a) which will resolve spontaneously between age 6 months to 1 year. Only those infants whose condition is complicated, for example by aspiration, need further medical or surgical intervention.

It is important that an accurate medical and nursing assessment is made of infants and children presenting with vomiting to identify and treat quickly any significant underlying medical problems and 'red flags' (red flag meaning a symptom that may denote a serious condition). Key points to consider are:

- The overall state of the child, including level of consciousness, circulatory and respiratory function. Does the child need urgent resuscitation?
- Feeding history: the child who is being overfed, and vomiting the excess, will seem happy and thriving, as will a child with some minor regurgitation. However, other more serious causes of vomiting will lead to weight loss, faltering growth, and in more severe cases, potentially dehydration and death.
- Pattern of vomiting, for example, projectile vomiting presenting from 3 to 6 weeks may indicate pyloric stenosis. Bile-stained vomiting is suggestive of obstruction and needs further investigation as a matter of urgency.
- Haematemesis.
- Vomiting following paroxysms of coughing is suggestive of whooping cough: check immunisation status.
- Access to poisons such as medication, alcohol and other chemicals.
- Febrile: infection both within and outside of the gastrointestinal systems can cause vomiting. If diarrhoea is present, gastroenteritis is likely. If not, it is useful to consider urinary tract infection, meningitis and middle ear infection (NICE, 2015a).

Key investigations are summarised in Table 21.2.

DIARRHOEA: ACUTE AND CHRONIC

As with vomiting, diarrhoea is also a common childhood problem and may be experienced in conjunction with vomiting or on its own. Causes of diarrhoea can be broadly categorised as infectious, inflammatory/allergy mediated or due to malabsorption.

Acute Infectious Diarrhoea

Acute infectious diarrhoea is a common medical problem of childhood accounting for significant numbers of hospital admissions. Although most cases are an unpleasant and debilitating experience, poor management – particularly in the vulnerable young child, the immune compromised, or in severe cases – can lead to life-threatening dehydration and complications including haemorrhagic septicaemia. It is a major cause of morbidity and mortality in developing countries.

Causative Organisms

These can be both viral and bacterial, with trends in seasonal causes seen and a correlation between age group and vulnerability to type of organisms. A summary is shown in Table 21.3.

TABLE 21.2 **Key Investigations for Vomiting**	
Investigation	**Significance**
History	Offers 80% of diagnostic information
Urea and electrolytes	Imbalance in gastroenteritis and pyloric stenosis
Chloride	Depleted in pyloric stenosis
pH and bicarbonate	Metabolic alkalosis common in pyloric stenosis
Toxicology	If poisoning suspected or to exclude
pH monitoring and barium swallow	To show gastro-oesophageal reflux
Presence of gastric peristalsis during feeding and presence of pyloric tumour on palpation	Indicate pyloric stenosis
Bile-stained vomit	Intestinal obstruction
Urine for culture	Presence of infection
Imaging studies	Obstruction

Miall, R., Rudolph, M., Levene, M., 2007. Pediatrics at a Glance, second ed. Blackwell, Oxford; Moreno-Villares, J., Polanco, I., 2009. Vomiting in Paediatric Gastroenterology: An Atlas of Investigation and Management. Clinical Publishing, an Imprint of Atlas Medical Publishing Ltd., Oxford.

👤 ACTIVITY

Other less common bacterial causes of diarrhoea include *Yersinia enterocolitica, Aeromonas, Plesiomonas.*
What can you find out about these organisms?

As most acute episodes of gastroenteritis are self-limiting, management focuses primarily on assessment of the degree of dehydration and replacing fluid loss. This is successfully achieved in most cases with the use of oral rehydration solution (ORS). Other factors to consider from a nursing perspective include enabling family management of the child with an acute attack at home and education to minimise the risk of further episodes that might be caused, for example, by poor food handling and preparation techniques. If the child is admitted, minimising the risk of infection to other patients is also of considerable importance.

Although acute gastroenteritis is the most common cause of diarrhoea, particularly in the preschool child, other causes of diarrhoea could be considered.

↪ REFLECT ON YOUR PRACTICE

- What nursing interventions can you implement to reduce the risk of infection to others in the ward environment?
- How can you ensure that a resident family is not posing an infection threat?
- Using Paediatric Early Warning Scoring Systems (Gold et al., 2014), what signs would alert you to a deteriorating child?

You will find additional guidance in the Royal College of Nursing (RCN) publication *Essential Practice for Infection Prevention and Control* (RCN, 2017).

MALABSORPTION AND FOOD ALLERGIES

Causes of malabsorption are multiple and include allergy, auto immune dysfunction, pathophysiology leading to functional absorption problems such as cystic fibrosis and short bowel syndrome. Untreated these will lead to chronic diarrhoea and faltering growth (failure to thrive).

Cystic Fibrosis
Aetiology

Cystic fibrosis (CF) is an autosomal recessive inherited disorder. It is more common in the Caucasian population, and currently affects 1:2500 live births in the UK (Taylor-Robinson et al., 2018). The gene responsible is the cystic fibrosis transmembrane regulator *(CFTR)* gene located on the long arm of chromosome 7, with ΔF508 being the most common mutation, although 2000 other variations are known at the time of writing (Cystic Fibrosis Trust, 2018; National Human Genome Research Institute, 2013); 1 in 25 individuals is likely to be a carrier.

Nearly 2000 mutations have been reported in the *CFTR* gene to date; however, only 127 are known to be disease causing. A Canadian study found of these mutations, only 15 occur with an overall frequency greater than 1%, but there is variation in the regional prevalence of specific mutations across Canada (Quon and Wilcox 2015).

The CTFR fault affects the movement of salt and water out of cells and the disease primarily affects the exocrine glands, with normal mucous replaced by thick stick secretions (Paranjape and Zeitlin, 2008). Sufferers do not have normal life expectancy, although this is improving with treatment advances.

👤 ACTIVITY

Check your understanding of autosomal recessive inheritance. Draw a diagram to illustrate this and check if you are correct by checking on the companion PowerPoint presentation.

Exocrine glands regulate production of both sweat and mucous. Children affected by cystic fibrosis, regardless of symptom severity, have increased sodium and chloride levels in saliva and sweat. As they are unable to effectively reabsorb sodium and chloride this leads to increased losses, particularly in warmer conditions and creates an increased risk of dehydration, hypochloraemia and hyponatremia (Martiniano et al., 2016). The production of viscous mucous accumulates, obstructing the mucous-secreting glands in affected organs. There is also obstruction of small passages, namely the bronchioles of the lungs, pancreatic and biliary ducts. Affected individuals therefore may present with varying symptoms, dependent on the degree of severity.

TABLE 21.3	Summary of the Causative Organisms of Diarrhoea	
Organism	**Epidemiology/Pathology**	**Symptoms**
Rotavirus	Most common causative organism in UK. Particularly affecting the under 2s More common in cooler times of year Damages mucosa with severe inflammatory changes Incubation 1–3 days Transmission: faecal/oral	Fever >38°C for approx. 48 hours Vomiting, profuse watery diarrhoea, may last up to a week
Norwalk virus	Similar pathology to rotavirus Transmission: faecal/oral, contaminated water	Affects all ages. Duration 2–3 days Resembled food poisoning Diarrhoea and vomiting and abdominal cramps
Giardia (protozoan)	Most common cause of non-bacterial diarrhoea in North America Favours cool moist conditions More common in children May be asymptomatic carriers Pathophysiology not proven – suspect either produces toxin or causes mechanical obstruction of the absorptive surface of intestine Incubation up to 1 week Transmission: contaminated food, water sources, person to person	Diarrhoea average 1 week May be longer and may be transient or persistent disaccharide intolerance
Escherichia coli	More common in summer Produces toxins, which bind to mucosal villi and cause profuse secretion of water and electrolytes Can also invade and destroy epithelium Incubation variable Transmission: contaminated and undercooked food, person to person	Common in nursery (child care) populations and travellers Fever, green watery and explosive diarrhoea, abdominal distension Usually settles 3–10 days Note: *E. coli* 157 also causes abdominal cramps, haemorrhagic colitis and haemolytic uraemic syndrome
Salmonella typhi	Produces fever Incubation period 7–14 days; can be up to 30 days Becomes systemic illness with septicaemia and requirement for antibiotics	Abdominal pain, nausea Fever, systemically unwell Lower incidence in developed countries
Shigella	More common in toddler age groups More common in late summer Causes enterotoxin production – see earlier Incubation 1–7 days Transmission: person to person or fomites	Sudden high fever Abdominal cramps Watery diarrhoea with mucus and blood May also have headache, neck stiffness and potential for convulsions with fever
Campylobacter jejuni	More common in toddler age groups and young adults More common in late summer Enterotoxin production and loss of absorptive surface from villi Incubation 1–7 days Transmission: birds are most common host. Carried on foods and milk	Fever, watery or sticky diarrhoea, may be blood and leucocytes Vomiting Usually self-limiting, rarely leads to complications such as haemolytic uraemic syndrome, septicaemia Infectivity can be limited with erythromycin

Baker, R.A., Mondozzi, M., Hockenbery, M., 2011. Conditions that produce fluid imbalance. In: Hockenberry, M., Wilson, D. (Eds.), Wong's Nursing Care of Infants and Children, ninth ed. Elsevier, Missouri.

Symptoms commonly include digestive and respiratory problems, for example:
- shortness of breath
- persistent cough
- hyperhidrosis (excessive sweating)
- limited lung capacity
- 'salty' skin
- wheezing
- abdominal pain
- pneumonia
- excessive appetite but little weight gain
- large, foul-smelling stools
- diarrhoea
- impaired fertility
- reduced bone mass

Respiratory Function

Failure to expectorate bronchial secretions by normal ciliary movement results in accumulation of secretions, which then create a medium for infection. Lung damage is progressive over time as continued obstruction causes atelectasis and emphysema.

The focus however in this chapter is on gastrointestinal function.

Gastrointestinal Function

Gastrointestinal problems are due to occlusion of the pancreatic ducts with mucous concretions. Outflow of pancreatic enzymes is obstructed, resulting in impaired digestion and absorption of nutrients, particularly fats and proteins. Over time, fibrosing of the pancreas occurs, which may account for the increased incidence of insulin-dependent diabetes in cystic fibrosis sufferers.

Diagnosis

Newborn 'heel prick' screening was introduced in the UK in 2007, so the majority of diagnoses are made in early infancy. Later diagnosis is supported by presence of the symptoms described earlier, but is confirmed by a 'sweat test'. This is achieved by collection of sweat and measuring the quantity of sodium chloride contained within. Many parents of infants with cystic fibrosis will remark that their child 'tastes salty'. Sweat chloride concentration of ≥60 mmol/L is thought to be indicative of CF. Levels lower than 29 mmol/L in the child aged up to 6 months of age and ≤39 mmol/L for older patients are thought to be normal (Traeger et al., 2014).

Other diagnostic tests include (Cystic Fibrosis Trust, 2018):
- prenatal chorionic villous sampling
- meconium ileus in neonatal period
- genotyping

Management

The human genome project is enabling the development of both personalised medicine not only in the treatment of diseases such as cystic fibrosis, but also precision medicine (National Human Genome Research Institute [NHGRI], 2016).

Personalised medicine refers to planning disease management as it presents for the individual, informed by the patient's own clinical characteristics, including their genetic profile, lifestyle, environment, disease severity and symptoms.

Although CF therapies have historically focused on symptom management arising from the genetic errors, treatment advances now include drug compounds which can address defects in *CFTR* structure. Marson et al. (2017) offer an example of CF oriented personalised medicine as adjusting the dosage of pancreatic enzyme replacement according to response, food intake and individual size and weight, so the greater determinants are the presentation and context; whereas precision medicine considers these factors plus the genotype and the outcomes of clinical testing.

Whatever the treatment approach, the aim of gastrointestinal management of cystic fibrosis is to ensure the child achieves adequate nutrition for optimal growth with minimal gastrointestinal symptoms. The mainstay of treatment is pancreatic enzyme replacement (pancreatin), which contains the enzymes protease, lipase and amylase that assist in the digestion of protein, fats and starch, respectively. Supplements are given orally to children with exocrine pancreatic insufficiency. Pancreatin is inactivated by gastric acid and heat; therefore supplements are most effective in an enteric-coated form and given immediately prior to or with meals and snacks. Pancreatin can cause perioral and buccal mucosa irritation,

so children should be taught to swallow quickly and not retain it in the mouth. Large doses may cause perianal irritation. Pancreatin is usually porcine in origin so this factor should be considered in relation to the child and family's religious beliefs. The dosage required is variable and it should be noted there is an identified association between high-dosage pancreatin and fibrosing colonopathy, a condition that can lead to pain and intestinal obstruction (NICE, 2018).

As absorption of nutrients from the small intestine is reduced in children with cystic fibrosis, their carbohydrate, fat and protein calorie requirements are in excess of the norms for their age, if optimal height and weight is to be maintained. It is recommended that overall calorie requirements are between 120% and 140% of the recommended daily allowance (RDA), with 40% of intake provided by fats. However, studies continue to show that within both preschool and school-age groups, significant numbers of children do not meet the recommended calorie and fat intakes (Powers et al., 2002; Filigno et al., 2017).

Optimal calorie intake may be supported by supplemental feeding including enteral tube feeding (NICE, 2017).

Achieving optimal nutritional management in a family-managed setting requires focused education. Although there is sometimes the belief among health professionals that the child and family with a chronic illness become 'experts', families benefit from clear supportive information. The nutritional status of a child with CF at the age of 3 has been shown to be a predictor of later lung function and survival (Pitts et al., 2008; Stephenson et al., 2015). Dodge and Turck (2010) remind us that grappling with the nutritional demands of a healthy child in infancy can be challenging without the additional demands of CF. Interprofessional management should support optimal nutrition in the infant and growing child. Given the impact of chronic disease on the child and family as an integrated unit, adopting a family-focused approach is good practice. Clear communication and agreed care strategies should be developed between the acute and ambulatory care settings. Consideration should be given to the financial support the child and family might need.

There are indicators that children with cystic fibrosis have an altered perception of body image, and societal pressure in terms of ideal body image may influence nutritional behaviours. Male adolescents and young men may experience stress being unable to achieve a well-developed physique, whereas adolescent females may favour being more petite and not engage with adequate nutrition. So young people with CF are vulnerable to body image dissatisfaction, but in dissimilar ways to unaffected individuals (Helms et al., 2017).

Coeliac Disease
Aetiology and Pathophysiology

Coeliac disease (gluten-sensitive enteropathy), although characterised by problems with absorption, is an autoimmune disorder triggered in the affected individuals by exposure to gluten containing foods. There is an association with other autoimmune disorders, and coeliac disease is a well-recognised co-morbidity with diabetes (Denham and Hill, 2013).

Coeliac UK (2018) suggest that 1% of the UK population have coeliac disease and it affects all major ethnicities. Those affected have a permanent intolerance to the α-gliadin protein that is found in wheat, barley and rye, and in hybrids of these. The mechanisms and origins of the abnormal allergic response to gluten are not fully understood, although some individuals have a genetic predisposition, which is dependent on specific alleles of the human leucocyte antigen (HLA) system, the DQ2 (90% of Caucasian people with coeliac disease), and less frequently, the DQ8 (Bodis et al., 2018).

On ingestion of gluten-containing cereals, first of all wheat and secondly barley and rye, traces of gluten-derived peptides come in contact with the antigen-presenting cells (APC) located in the lamina propria of the intestinal mucosa. In DQ2- or DQ8-positive subjects, this activates an abnormal immune response leading to the typical coeliac enteropathy – intestinal villous atrophy with crypt hyperplasia (Kagnoff, 2007).

The villous atrophy decreases the absorptive surface of the gut wall and the amount of enzymes usually available on the villous surface.

 ACTIVITY

Using online sources look up the term 'crypt hyperplasia', 'villous atrophy' and view histology images.

The result is passage of partly undigested food through the intestinal tract, leading commonly to diarrhoea or other abdominal symptoms such as cramping and bloating. Due to the presence of large amounts of undigested fat, bulky, foul-smelling pale stools 'steatorrhoea' may be present. Over time the ability to absorb proteins, carbohydrates, calcium, folic acid, iron and some vitamins also decreases and the child presents with weight loss, including both fat and muscle wasting. Symptoms may be noted from infancy as weaning introduces gluten-containing foods, but progresses until symptoms become noticeable. Increasingly diagnosis may occur at any life stage. Other symptoms are associated with poor nutrition and include fatigue, anaemia and susceptibility to infection. There are also known associations with neurological symptoms such as neuropathies. It should be noted that coeliac disease is increasingly being identified in asymptomatic patients or with atypical presentation (Goebel, 2018). This is particularly relevant in children who have related or associated disorders, as discussed later.

Diagnosis

Diagnosis is made on history and presentation as described above. Familial trend is also a characteristic of coeliac disease. Initial blood tests for tissue transglutaminase with findings confirmed by the presence of α-gliadin antibodies (present in response to gluten), and anti-reticulin and anti-endomysial antibodies (which are present when the gut mucosa is damaged) may be made (Parzanese et al., 2017). Definitive diagnosis is made by duodenal biopsy and microscopic examination of the structure of the villi. Additionally, children

(and adults) with coeliac disease will demonstrate clinical remission of signs when given a gluten-free diet.

Management

The mainstay of management still centres on diet, and complete remission of gut changes is seen with a gluten-free diet. The diet is a lifetime requirement. Recent research is exploring the role of immunotherapy, drugs which block gluten transfer across the epithelium of the gut and supplemental therapy with gluten degrading enzymes and vaccines. These are not yet mainstream treatment and remain at the stage of clinical research (Parzanese et al., 2017).

Managing the diet consistently poses challenges for the child and family. Obvious gluten-containing foods such as bread, biscuits and cakes can be replaced and the range and palatability of products has increased in response to the increasing prevalence and consumer demand. Gluten also appears under many guises within foods and examples include thickeners for commercially prepared meals, and desserts and flavourings in processed snack foods. Food labelling has improved and gluten is an identified allergen which must be identified on food labelling in the UK (Food Standards Agency, 2015). Support groups such as Coeliac UK advise on gluten-free commercial products, recipes and special dietary products. Major supermarket chains are steadily increasing their range of specialist dietary products. Referral to a paediatric dietician is useful.

 ACTIVITY

Think of an average menu for a birthday tea party for a 4-year-old. How much of it is likely to contain gluten?

How could you advise a parent to manage the normal social activity of party invitations?

Useful family focused resources:
- Coeliac UK
  Available from: https://www.coeliac.org.uk/healthcare-professionals/resources/

Complications/Related Problems

It is known that coeliac disease coexists in children with other conditions; they may be asymptomatic. As the potential complications of untreated coeliac disease include reduced fertility, reduced bone density and gastrointestinal malignancy, routine screening for coeliac disease may be considered for children with:

- Down syndrome (prevalence of coeliac disease = 4%–17%)
- Insulin-dependent diabetes (prevalence of coeliac disease = up to 8%
- Ulcerative colitis and Crohn's disease
  ‣ Autoimmune thyroiditis (~15%)
  ‣ Autoimmune liver disease
  ‣ Unexplained raised transaminases without known liver disease
  ‣ Intussusception
  ‣ Dermatitis herpetiformis
  ‣ Relatives of coeliac patient (Murch et al., 2013)

The common factor with some of the above seems to be the existence of autoimmune problems. Coeliac disease is also associated with other complications or disorders (not mentioned above) including:

- an increased lifetime risk of some cancers
- dental problems
- infertility

Food Allergies Versus Intolerance

Food allergies have gained recent media coverage as poor food labelling has resulted in fatalities (BBC News, 2018). Food allergies at their worst will provoke an anaphylactic reaction or more commonly create milder gastrointestinal symptoms and in infants and children, faltering growth. The terms 'allergy' is also often misused and misunderstood by the public and in terms of the impact on health; the distinction should be better understood. The following section will explore the distinction between allergy and intolerance in relation to dairy products.

Cow's Milk Allergy

Cow's milk allergy is primarily a disease of childhood and it has been suggested affects 7% of bottle-fed infants and 0.5% of breast-fed babies, the latter being due to maternal transference (Caffarelli et al., 2010; Vandenplas et al., 2007; NICE, 2015b). Incidence is highest in children under 5 years, and in Caucasian populations. One study showed 55.5% incidence in Caucasian children compared to 16.6% in African American and 4.7% in Asian children, respectively (Warren et al., 2013). There is an increased prevalence in infants in whom there is history of prematurity, atopy or other gastrointestinal disorders (NICE, 2015b).

Cow's milk protein is made up of two major elements – casein and whey – in a proportion of approximately 80:20. Casein and the β-lactoglobulin component of whey are the most allergenic. The most hypersensitive children can react not only to ingested dietary milk proteins but also if there is skin contact.

Aetiology

A hypersensitivity to cow's milk protein has two main immunologically mediated routes:

1. Immunoglobulin E (IgE)-mediated cows' milk protein allergy results from the release of histamine and other inflammatory mediators from mast cells and basophils in response to cows' milk protein. This type of reaction is seen as the most immediate response.
2. Non-IgE-mediated cows' milk protein allergy is thought to be caused by T cells (NICE, 2015b).

Diagnosis

Assessment is primarily based on history and will seek to distinguish between IgE or T cell mediated allergy. Of interest in the assessment will be history of other allergy mediated disorders such as asthma and eczema. Presenting symptoms differ between IgE and T cell mediated reactions. IgE reactions tend to be a more severe with a rapid onset post-ingestion. Gastrointestinal symptoms can include angioedema,

colic, and diarrhoea. In addition, there may be other systemic symptoms such as skin reactions and respiratory compromise and anaphylaxis. T cell mediated reactions and have a slower onset, which can be delayed for a number of days. Symptoms are similar and can include colic, constipation, reflux, loose stools. There may be respiratory symptoms and growth delay if diagnosis is delayed (NICE, 2015b).

Blood tests for IgE antibodies are helpful in confirming diagnosis. Differential diagnosis should also be excluded, for example, including lactose intolerance or inflammatory bowel disorders.

Management

Management can be achieved with replacement feeding, removing the allergen. Some children will tolerate hydrolysed formulas, in which the cow's milk proteins are broken down into smaller molecules, but some require total exclusion of milk proteins and replacement feeds.

Soya based replacement feeds are no longer recommended for infants under 6 months as mineral absorption is less than optimal and there can be an increase in serum oestrogens associated with their use (NICE, 2015b).

The majority of children will 'grow out' of milk allergies over the course of their childhood.

Lactose Intolerance

Whereas cow's milk allergy is an immunologically mediated reaction to cow's milk proteins, cow's milk intolerance refers to problems with the digestion, absorption or metabolism of components of cow's milk, which are due to a deficiency of the enzyme lactase. Although milk allergy primarily affects infants and younger children with a good chance that the condition will resolve as the child matures, lactose intolerance usually presents later in childhood and tends to persist. Transient lactose intolerance can also occur post-gastrointestinal infection and secondary persistent lactose intolerance can be associated with other disorders which compromise the small bowel, for example coeliac disease or inflammatory bowel disease. Primary early onset lactose intolerance occurs more in communities where dairy products are not a dietary staple (Misselwitz et al., 2013).

Pathophysiology

Lactose is a disaccharide found in milk and also 'hidden' in some pre-prepared foodstuffs. Absorption requires a process of hydrolysis and conversion to a monosaccharide. In the absence of the enzyme lactase, this process is incomplete. Persistence of lactose in the small intestine creates an osmotic pull of fluid dilating the gut; transit time then decreases leading to incomplete digestion. Persistence of lactose in the large intestine results in bacterial fermentation, a by-product of which is hydrogen gas. The increase in fluid and the presence of gas leads to bloating, loose stools and associated malabsorption.

Diagnosis

Various tests support diagnosis, including blood glucose monitoring post-ingestion of a measured 'dose' of lactose.

Hydrogen produced in the colon is excreted via the lungs, so exhaled hydrogen can be measured.

Management

Management centres on diet and the replacement of lactose containing milk and milk formulas with alternates. Live yogurt and fermented products such as cheeses are better tolerated than regular milk as the presence of lactobacilli supports digestion. Prehydrolysed milk products and plant-based products can be used, but for young children these can result in nutritional deficiencies. In secondary lactose intolerance treatment is directed at the cause.

Inflammatory Bowel Disease

Inflammatory bowel disease (IBD) has been described as an 'expanding global health problem' (M'Koma, 2013). IBD has become increasingly prevalent in children and young people. IBD encompasses both ulcerative colitis and Crohn's disease; the incidence of each in the UK is around 10 per 100,000 people every year with a prevalence of around 240 per 100,000 and up to one-third of diagnoses are made before the age of 21 (NICE, 2015c, 2017).

Aetiology

Research to date is unable to offer any definitive causes for IBD. There appears to be a genetic predisposition with 'susceptibility' genes being located and therefore familial history. Our developing understanding of the gut microbiome offers insight into how there may be an interplay of susceptibility and risk causing gut flora, such as an increased load of enteroinvasive *Escherichia coli*. The hygiene hypothesis, first proposed by Strachan in 1989 (Brookes and Cheng, 2015) in relation to childhood allergic rhinitis, asthma and atopy is also useful to consider in relation to IBD. Cholapranee and Ananthakrishnan (2016) and Oliveira and Monteiro (2017) identify from a meta-analysis a relationship between lack of early challenge to the immune system and incidence of IBD. Studies show smoking offers protection against ulcerative colitis but not Crohn's disease. In affected individuals, immunologically mediated inflammatory responses in the intestinal mucosa are exaggerated (Zhang and Li, 2014).

⊚ EVIDENCE-BASED PRACTICE

In 1990s studies were published which suggested a link between the Measles, Mumps, Rubella (MMR) vaccine and the development of autism and IBD; these were subsequently discounted.
- Identify what these studies were and what their impact might have been on the wider child public health agenda.
- Consider how you can ensure that children and their families can be helped to make decisions about their care and treatment, based on accurate interpretation of the evidence available.

Diagnosis

Ulcerative colitis and Crohn's disease are distinguished in their pathophysiological presentation. Although ulcerative colitis is confined to the colon, Crohn's disease can affect the whole of the gastrointestinal tract from mouth to anus. Childhood onset of the disease (IBD) is associated with a more extensive and less easily managed form of disease in comparison to adult onset (Oliveira and Monteiro, 2017).

Some symptoms are shared between Crohn's disease and ulcerative colitis but there are differences. In children ulcerative colitis commonly presents with abdominal pain and bloody diarrhoea. There might be a similar presentation for Crohn's disease, but symptoms can be more subtle, for example, diarrhoea, weight loss and anaemia. Crohn's disease is more often associated with extraintestinal symptoms than colitis, including uveitis, arthritis and primary sclerosing cholangitis. Crohn's disease, unlike colitis, is also associated with short stature, although sustained nutritional impairment will affect growth (Oliveira and Monteiro, 2017).

Diagnosis is made on the basis of specific inflammatory and serological markers and confirmed and distinguished with endoscopy and histology (Oliveira and Monteiro, 2017; NICE, 2017). A differential diagnosis of coeliac disease should also be excluded.

Management

Management approaches have evolved in response to understanding developing from genome studies and pharmaceutical advances. In common with diseases such as cystic fibrosis personalised medicine is also becoming a treatment feature, focusing on identifying likelihood of response to treatment regimen and disease progression, subject to the patient profile (Flamant and Roblin, 2018).

Physiological management approaches differ, to some extent, between ulcerative colitis and Crohn's disease, although the aims are shared, including the need to induce and maintain remission, secure a reduction in symptoms, and promote normal physical, social and emotional growth and development.

Pharmacological interventions include the use of 5-aminosalicylates (5-ASAs) used to support remission induction in mild to moderate ulcerative colitis and in mild Crohn's disease. Corticosteroids are used for more moderately severe disease, but their long-term use as a maintenance therapy is contraindicated due to side effects. Other therapies used in more severe or unresponsive disease include anti-tumour necrosis factor monoclonal antibodies, for example infliximab and adalimumab. These are recommended to induce remission in severe childhood IBD (Oliveira and Monteiro, 2017). Surgery is an option, but is more successful where disease is localised, as found in ulcerative colitis.

🧍 ACTIVITY

Using either web-based resources or pharmacology texts:
- Identify the different actions of each of the groups of drugs listed in the above text.
- How would you explain their actions to an 11-year-old child?

Some children may develop perianal lesions or proctitis, both of which are difficult to treat. Rectal water-soluble steroids or 5-ASA drugs may be used successfully for management of proctitis.

Emergency care is required for the child who develops severe colitis, including administration of intravenous fluids, electrolytes, antibiotics and steroids. Perforation is a risk and surgery may be required.

Arguably, physical care and management is clearly described, with specific protocols to follow. However, the potential impact of inflammatory bowel disease on the child and family, both socially and mentally, is worthy of consideration within nursing strategies. Some studies suggest that young adults who developed IBD as children have problems with self-esteem. The average age at diagnosis coincides with onset of puberty and adolescence.

▶ REFLECT ON YOUR PRACTICE

How might the adolescent child with inflammatory bowel disease be supported, using a multi-disciplinary approach, to minimise the threat to self-esteem?

Constipation

Constipation, which can be defined as delay or difficulty in defecation, is a common paediatric problem. Normal frequency of bowel movements varies from child to child, ranging from more than once per day to none for several days, and infrequency alone is not necessarily a problem. Causes of constipation are broadly differentiated into organic and non-organic. Organic causes are shown in Table 21.4.

However, for the majority of children presenting with constipation problems, the cause is non-organic or idiopathic (functional) constipation. Non-organic causes include poor dietary management, including insufficient fibre, dehydration, developmental problems that complicate toilet training, emotional abuse, depression and also inappropriate/punitive toilet training practices in the younger child. There are also those who have a familial tendency and sedentary lifestyle.

In early years the most common cause of constipation is functional – meaning it exists in the absence of obvious cause. It is thought to commonly develop in response to the child having unpleasant emotional experiences or pain associated with defecation. This results in the child deliberately holding faeces. This results in retention of faeces in the colon, fluid is reabsorbed and the faecal mass becomes impacted (large dry and hard). Consequently, liquid faeces leak around the impacted mass, causing involuntary soiling (encopresis). The problem is progressive as the child becomes frightened, anticipating that the experience of defecation will be painful and difficult. Soiling is unpleasant and may create tension in the home, nursery or school, which can lead to social isolation and feelings of poor self-worth.

Diagnosis

Idiopathic (functional) non-organic constipation is diagnosed on the basis of medical and psychosocial history taking

TABLE 21.4	**Organic Causes of Constipation**
Cause	**Examples**
Anatomic malformations	Imperforate anus Anal stenosis Pelvic mass
Metabolic and gastrointestinal	Cystic fibrosis Diabetes mellitus Coeliac disease Hypothyroidism
Neuropathic	Spinal cord problem Neurofibromatosis
Intestinal nerve or muscle disorders	Hirschsprung disease Visceral myopathies and neuropathies
Abnormalities of abdominal muscles	Prune belly syndrome Gastroschisis Down syndrome
Connective tissue disorders	Systemic lupus erythematosus Scleroderma
Drugs	Opiates Phenobarbitone Antihypertensives Antidepressants
Miscellaneous	Lead poisoning Vitamin D overdose

Auth, M., Vora, M., Farrelly, P., et al., 2012. Childhood constipation. BMJ 345, 7309. Available from: https://www.ncbi.nlm.nih.gov/pubmed/23150472 (accessed January 2019); Singh, H., Connor, F., 2018. Paediatric constipation: an approach and evidence-based treatment regimen, Aust. J. Gen. Pract. 47 (5), 273–277. Available from: https://www1.racgp.org.au/ajgp/2018/may/paediatric-constipation (accessed February 2019).

and physical examination. Initially, organic causes need to be excluded. Indicators of organic causes would include general malaise or other systemic signs such as weight loss, nausea/vomiting, and blood in the stools or abdominal distension. Rectal examination allows the size of the rectum to be assessed and also amount and type of stool. The perineum and perianal area can be examined at the same time to assess for signs of trauma. If there is nothing of note and there is a history of toileting difficulties and stool-withholding behaviour, it is likely that the cause is functional. The most commonly used defining criteria for functional constipation are 'Rome III' (The Rome Foundation, 2007, cited by Lacy et al., 2016). If it is inappropriate to conduct a rectal examination, for example if the child refuses or abuse is suspected, abdominal x-ray can be used to determine whether impacted faeces are present.

▶ REFLECT ON YOUR PRACTICE

Consider the kind of questions that might be asked to establish the state of a child's bowel function (colour, shape, frequency, size, associated with pain):
* How might some children and families find this interview?
* How can it be facilitated to be more comfortable?

Management

NICE (2015c) clinical knowledge summaries suggest a staged approach to management. This is described as follows:

1. Exclude other serious differential diagnoses through consideration of red flags.
2. Determine if there are impacted faeces.
3. Remove/resolve impaction.
4. Maintenance: using education, support, diet and medications.
5. Follow-up.

Successful and complete disimpaction achieved using oral and/or rectal medication is arguably a precursor to successful ongoing management.

Oral medications include electrolyte solutions, either alone or in combination with high-dose laxatives, for example lactulose or senna. Ideally, stool softeners, such as lactulose, should be used before stimulants to minimise the pain of passing a large, hard stool. Rectal preparations can also be used, including saline and phosphate enemas, and some success has been achieved using glycerol suppositories.

Following disimpaction, management moves to maintenance using a 'whole child' approach. This includes laxative therapy, dietary, and behaviour modification, focusing on making bowel evacuation a non-stressful experience.

Dietary changes aim to increase fluids and include fruit, fibre and non-absorbable carbohydrates. Laxatives can include an osmotic laxative, such as lactulose, docusate sodium and polyethylene glycol (Movicol). Softeners are combined with bowel stimulants, which include senna and sodium picosulphate. Rectal medication may be used, but with caution, given the associated unpleasant experiences it may engender.

During the treatment and management phases, close family support and education is required. Families need to understand the origins of the problem and where additional problems such as soiling have developed, making it clear that this is likely to be non-intentional. Families may need support to set realistic objectives, in terms of outcomes over time, and to develop the ability to manage behaviour reinforcement using positive learning approaches. Education and encouragement to change the family diet to one that is more balanced may also be required.

 WWW

The following website offers further reading and management guidelines. Available from:

- http://www.eric.org.uk

You could consider to what extent guidelines are consistent between organisations and care teams.

SUMMARY

This chapter has offered an overview of some of the major gastrointestinal problems likely to be encountered by children's nurses. Additional information can also be found on the Evolve website. Generally, acute problems can be managed effectively, with positive outcomes expected in most cases. However, there is an increase in the incidence of chronic illnesses in child health, some of which have been explored in this chapter. This is creating a need to focus on long-term family centred care and to continue to develop strong links between ambulatory and acute care settings. Continuing to strengthen multi-professional cooperation in care commissioning and delivery remains a child health professional responsibility. It is envisaged that this will continue to be a key challenge in child health care for the foreseeable future.

REFERENCES

Auth, M., Vora, M., Farrelly, P., et al., 2012. Childhood constipation. BMJ 345, 7309. Available from: https://www.ncbi.nlm.nih.gov/pubmed/23150472 (accessed January 2019).

Baker, R.A., Mondozzi, M., Hockenbery, M., 2011. Conditions that produce fluid imbalance. In: Hockenberry, M., Wilson, D. (Eds.), Wong's Nursing Care of Infants and Children, ninth ed. Elsevier, Missouri.

BBC News, 2018. Pret a Manger to label products after allergy death. Available from: https://www.bbc.co.uk/news/business-45731201 (accessed December 2018).

Bodis, G., Victoria Toth, V., Schwarting, A., 2018. Role of human leukocyte antigens (HLA) in autoimmune diseases. Rheumatol. Ther. 5 (1), 5–20.

Brookes, L., Cheng, L.E., 2015. The hygiene hypothesis – redefine, rename, or just clean it up? Available from: https://www.medscape.com/viewarticle/842500_0.

Caffarelli, C., Baldi, F., Bendandi, B., 2010. Cow's milk protein allergy in children: a practical guide. Ital. J. Pediat. 36, 5. Available from: https://cks.nice.org.uk/cows-milk-protein-allergy-in-children.

Coeliac UK., 2020. About coeliac disease Available at: https://www.coeliac.org.uk/information-and-support/coeliac-disease/about-coeliac-disease/ (Accessed Jan 2021).

Cholapranee, A., Ananthakrishnan, A.N., 2016. Environmental hygiene and risk of inflammatory bowel diseases: a systematic review and meta-analysis. Inflamm. Bowel Dis. 22, 2191–2199. https://doi.org/10.1097/MIB.0000000000000852.

Cystic Fibrosis Trust, 2018. What are the causes of cystic fibrosis? Available from: https://www.cysticfibrosis.org.uk/what-is-cystic-fibrosis/what-causes-cystic-fibrosis (accessed December 2018).

Denham, J., Hill, D., 2013. Celiac disease and autoimmunity: review and controversies. Curr. Allergy Asthma Rep. 13 (4), 347–353.

Dodge, J., Turck, D., 2010. Cystic fibrosis: nutritional consequences and management. Best Pract. Res. Clin. Gastroenterol. 20 (3), 531–546.

Flamant, M., Roblin, X., 2018. Inflammatory bowel disease: towards a personalized medicine. Therap. Adv. Gastroenterol. 11, 1756283X17745029. Available from: https://www.ncbi.nlm.nih.gov/pmc/articles/PMC5784543/ (accessed January 2019).

Filigno, S., Robson, S., Szczesniak, R., et al., 2017. Macronutrient intake in preschoolers with cystic fibrosis and the relationship between macronutrients and growth. J. Cyst. Fibros. 16 (4), 519–524.

Food Standards Agency, 2015. Food Allergen Labelling and InformaRequirements Under the EU Food Information for Consumers; Regulation No. 1169/2011. Technical Guidance FSA, UK.

Goebel, S., 2018. Celiac Disease (Sprue). Available from: https://emedicine.medscape.com/article/171805-overview (accessed December 2018).

Gold, D., Mihalov, L., Cohen, D., 2014. Evaluating the pediatric early warning score (PEWS) system for admitted patients in the pediatric emergency department. Acad. Emerg. Med. 21 (11), 1249–1256.

Helms, S., Christon, L., Dellon, E., et al., 2017. Patient and provider perspectives on communication about body image with adolescents and young adults with cystic fibrosis. J. Pediatr. Psychol. 42 (9), 1040–1050.

Kagnoff, M., 2007. Celiac disease: pathogenesis of a model immunogenetic disease. J. Clin. Invest. 117 (1), 41–49.

Lacy, B., Mearin, F., Chang, L., Chey, W., Lembo, A., Simren, M., Spiller, R., 2016. Bowel Disorders. Gastroenterology 2016 150, 1393–1407. Available at: https://theromefoundation.org/wp-content/uploads/bowel-disorders.pdf. (accessed January 2021).

Marson, F., Bertuzzo, C., Ribeiro, J., 2017. Personalized or precision medicine? The example of cystic fibrosis. Front. Pharmacol. 8, 390. Available from: https://www.ncbi.nlm.nih.gov/pmc/articles/PMC5476708/ (accessed December 2018).

Martiniano, S., Sagel, S., Zemanick, E., 2016. Cystic fibrosis: a model system for precision medicine. Curr. Opin. Pediatr. 28 (3), 312–317.

Miall, R., Rudolph, M., Levene, M., 2007. Pediatrics at a Glance, second ed. Blackwell, Oxford.

Misselwitz, B., Pohl, D., Frühauf, H., et al., 2013. Lactose malabsorption and intolerance: pathogenesis, diagnosis and treatment. United European Gastroenterol. J. 1 (3), 151–159.

M'Koma, A., 2013. Inflammatory bowel disease: an expanding global health problem. Clin. Med. Insights Gastroenterol. 14 (6), 33–47.

Moreno-Villares, J., Segovia, M., 2009. Vomiting in paediatric gastroenterology: an atlas of investigation and management. Clinical Publishing, an Imprint of Atlas Medical Publishing Ltd., Oxford.

Murch, S., Jenkins, H., Auth, M., et al., 2013. Joint BSPGHAN and Coeliac UK guidelines for the diagnosis and management of coeliac disease in children. Arch. Dis. Child. 98, 806–811.

National Human Genome Research Institute (NHGRI), 2016. An overview of the Human Genome Project. Available from: https://www.genome.gov/12011238/an-overview-of-the-human-genome-project/ (accessed December 2018).

National Institute for Health and Care Excellence (NICE), 2015a. Gastro-oesophageal reflux disease in children and young people: diagnosis and management. Available from: https://www.nice.org.uk/guidance/ng1 (accessed December 2018).

National Institute for Health and Care Excellence (NICE), 2015b. Cows' milk protein allergy in children: summary. Available from: https://cks.nice.org.uk/cows-milk-protein-allergy-in-children (accessed December 2018).

National Institute for Health and Care Excellence (NICE), 2015c. Clinical knowledge summary: ulcerative colitis. Available from: https://cks.nice.org.uk/ulcerative-colitis (accessed February 2019).

National Institute for Health and Care Excellence (NICE), 2017. Clinical knowledge summary: Crohn's disease. Available from: https://cks.nice.org.uk/crohns-disease. (accessed February 2019).

National Institute for Health and Care Excellence (NICE), 2018. Exocrine pancreatic insufficiency. Available from: https://bnf.nice.org.uk/treatment-summary/exocrine-pancreatic-insufficiency.html (accessed December 2018).

Oliveira, S., Monteiro, I., 2017. Diagnosis and management of inflammatory bowel disease in children. BMJ 31, 357: j2083. Available at: https://www.ncbi.nlm.nih.gov/pmc/articles/PMC6888256/. (accessed January 2021).

Paranjape, S., Zeitlin, P., 2008. Atypical cystic fibrosis and CFTR-related diseases. Clin. Rev. Allergy Immunol. 35 (3), 116–123.

Parzanese, I., Qehajaj, D., Patrinicola, F., et al., 2017. Celiac disease: from pathophysiology to treatment. World J. Gastrointest. Pathophysiol. 8 (2), 27–38.

Pitts, J., Flack, J., Goodfellow, J., 2008. Improving nutrition in the cystic fibrosis patient. J. Pediatr. Health Care 22 (2), 137–140.

Powers, S., Patton, S., Byars, K., et al., 2002. Caloric intake and eating behavior in infants and toddlers with cystic fibrosis. Pediatrics 109 (95), 75–79.

Puccini, F., Berretin-Felix, G., 2015. Gastroesophageal reflux and swallowing in newborns and infants: integrative review of literature. Rev. CEFAC. 2015 17 (5), 1664–1673 Available at: (accessed January 2021).

Quon, B., Wilcox, P., 2015. A new era of personalized medicine for cystic fibrosis – at last! Can. Respir. J. 22 (5), 257–260.

Royal College of Nursing (RCN), 2017. Essential Practice for Infection Prevention and Control Guidance for Nursing Staff. RCN, London. Available from: https://www.rcn.org.uk/professional-development/publications/pub-005940 (accessed December 2018).

Singh, H., Connor, F., 2018. Paediatric constipation. An approach and evidence-based treatment regimen. AJGP 47 (5), 273–277. Available from: https://www1.racgp.org.au/ajgp/2018/may/paediatric-constipation (accessed February 2019).

Stephenson, A., Tom, M., Berthiaume, Y., et al., 2015. A contemporary survival analysis of individuals with cystic fibrosis: a cohort study. Eur. Respir. J. 45 (3), 670–679.

Taylor-Robinson, Archangelidi, O., Carr, S., et al., 2018. Data resource profile: the UK Cystic Fibrosis Registry. Int. J. Epidemiol. 47 (1), 9e–10e. Available from: https://www.ncbi.nlm.nih.gov/pmc/articles/PMC5837577/ (accessed October 2018).

Traeger, N., Shi, Q., Dozor, 2014. A relationship between sweat chloride, sodium, and age in clinically obtained samples. J. Cyst. Fibros. 13 (1), 10–14.

Vandenplas, Y., Koletzko, S., Isolauri, E., et al., 2007. Guidelines for the diagnosis and management of cow's milk protein allergy in infants. Arch. Dis. Child. 92, 902–908. Available at: https://adc.bmj.com/content/archdischild/92/10/902.full.pdf. (accessed January 2021).

Warren, C., Jhaveri, S., Warrier, M., et al., 2013. The epidemiology of milk allergy in US children. Ann. Allergy Asthma Immunol. 110 (5), 370–374.

Zhang, Y.Z., Li, Y.L., 2014. Inflammatory bowel disease: pathogenesis. World J. Gastroenterol. 20 (1), 91–99. Available from: https://www.ncbi.nlm.nih.gov/pmc/articles/PMC3886036/ (accessed January 2019).

22

Caring for Children With Genitourinary Problems

Karen Tosh, Kathryn Bailey

LEARNING OUTCOMES

Discuss common genitourinary tract conditions with reference to:
- pathology/pathophysiology
- signs and symptoms
- diagnosis
- treatment/management
- things to consider

URINARY TRACT INFECTIONS

The term 'urinary tract infection' (UTI) refers to a common bacterial infection involving the lower urinary tract (cystitis) and or the upper urinary tract (pyelonephritis) (Goilav, 2017).

UTIs initially occur more in boys. In the 0- to 3-month category 20% of uncircumcised males are likely to have a UTI; in females the figure is 7.5%. In the 6- to 12-month category UTIs are more prevalent in females (Shaikh et al., 2008). Frumkin's study (2014) showed more positive cultures in females at 2 years of age. In children over 3 years the prevalence is higher in girls than boys (O'Brien, 2013).

It is convenient to categorise UTIs into two groups. Upper urinary tract infections and lower urinary tract infections. An infant or child with a temperature over 38°C and bacteriuria, or lower than 38°C with bacteriuria and loin pain should be considered to have acute pyelonephritis/upper urinary tract infection. Infants and children with no systemic signs or symptoms, but have bacteriuria should be considered to have cystitis/lower urinary tract infection (National Institute for Health and Care Excellence [NICE], 2007).
- Cystitis involves the bladder and urethra and tends not to be associated with long-term sequelae.
- Acute pyelonephritis involves the ureters and kidneys and can be associated with arterial hypertension and chronic kidney disease. However, with improvements in antibiotic therapies such risks have recently been questioned (Morello et al., 2016).

The most common causative organism associated with UTI is *Escherichia coli* (*E. coli*). This organism is responsible for 80% of infections (Kocak et al., 2016). *E. coli* is normally found in the large bowel, where it is involved in vitamin K production. The bacteria enter the urethra via the perineum. The cell membrane of the *E. coli* bacterium contains protein structures called adhesions, which facilitate bacterial adhesion to the surface of urogenital cells. This adhesion prevents the bacteria from being washed away during micturition. The infection ascends the urethra and enters the bladder, where the bacteria adhere to the cells that line the internal surface.

Susceptibility to Urinary Tract Infection

Some children are more susceptible than others to urinary tract infection. Uncircumcised boys under 1 year old are more prone than circumcised boys; the short female urethra increases susceptibility in girls. Constipation is linked to repeated urinary tract infection. Constipation impairs voiding by compressing the urethra or the bladder neck leading to a high urine residual. This creates the conditions in which bacteria can flourish. Treatment of constipation may result in the resolution of urinary tract infection (Loening-Baucke, 2007). More recently, obesity has been identified as a risk factor for urinary tract infections in girls; there was no significant increased risk for boys (Grier et al., 2016). Ultimately, congenital abnormality of the renal tract places the child at risk. Vesicoureteric reflux is the most common congenital abnormality of the genitourinary tract. Obstructive uropathies are also significant causes of urinary tract infection (Roth et al., 2002).

> **ACTIVITY**
>
> Find further information on a number of common genitourinary issues on 'Great Ormond Street Hospital's' web page under 'conditions we treat'. https://www.gosh.nhs.uk/conditions-and-treatments/conditions-we-treat

Signs and Symptoms of a Urinary Tract Infection

Signs and symptoms presented will depend on the age of the infant or child and whether or not they can verbalise their symptoms. Infants under 3 months will commonly display symptoms of irritability, lethargy, vomiting and fever. Carers may note poor feeding and failure to thrive. In some cases they may display abdominal pain on palpation, have offensive urine and/or display signs of haematuria and jaundice. Infants and children over 3 months will display fever, abdominal pain and loin tenderness, vomiting and poor feeding; less common are lethargy, irritability, haematuria, offensive cloudy urine and general malaise. In the verbal child they may note frequency, dysuria and changes to their continence (NICE, 2007).

Diagnosis

Urinary tract infection in children is problematic because it is not always obvious. In addition, when it is identified it may be difficult to distinguish between a lower and upper urinary tract infection. The younger the child, the more likely these problems are to occur.

Collecting Urine

Undertaking a clean catch urine sample is the preferred method of urine collection (NICE, 2007). In children who are able to stop and start the stream of urine, a midstream specimen can be collected. The logic underpinning the collection of a midstream specimen is that the initial passage of urine flushes bacteria from the urethral orifice and thus reduces the likelihood of contamination. For infants who are too young to undertake such a collection or children unable to cooperate, a clean catch specimen should be obtained. This can be achieved by positioning the infant over a sterile container and waiting for voiding to occur. It can be helpful for the child's carers to assist with this process as it can be time consuming, and for the child to be given fluid to drink to encourage urination. For the older child the carers should assist the child to void into the sterile container.

If a clean catch urine is not obtainable, urine should be collected by other non-invasive methods such as urine collection pads placed inside nappies. The pads are checked every 10 minutes until the child is found wet. A syringe is then used to aspirate urine from the pad. Although pad specimens are still prone to contamination, there is some evidence that they are more effective than bag specimens (Feasey, 1999) and that urine from a urine collection pad can provide clinically reliable results (MacFarlane et al., 2005). There is also evidence that parents prefer to use the pad method when home collection is required (Liaw et al., 2000). It should be noted that cotton wool balls, gauze or sanitary towels must not be used to collect urine.

The use of U-bags is controversial. Collections made by this method are notorious for becoming contaminated; as many as one-third of specimens taken in this way yield false-positive results (Li et al., 2002). Uncircumcised boys are particularly at risk. U-bags are commonly used for non-toilet trained children but should not be used in high-risk cases (Al-Orifi, 2000). If it has not been possible or practical to collect urine using a non-invasive method, urine should be collected by a catheter sample or suprapubic aspiration. Suprapubic aspiration should not be performed prior to confirmation of urine in the bladder by ultrasound (NICE, 2007).

Irrespective of the method of obtaining urine for culture, the specimen should be transferred to a specimen bottle immediately. It should be transferred to the laboratory within 30 minutes. It can then be stored in a fridge at 4°C until processing.

ACTIVITY

Reflect on your practice.
- What methods of urine collection are you familiar with?

Urine Testing

False results can occur in all tests. Clinicians should use clinical criteria for treating their patients if urine testing is not supportive of the findings. Suspected urinary tract infections in infants under 3 months should always be referred to a paediatrician and a urine sample obtained for microscopy and culture (NICE, 2007).

Nursing and medical staff should undertake a dipstick test for infants and children over 3 months but under 3 years. The nurse should be alert to the amount of urine that is produced; it may be diminished in urinary tract infection. The colour is also significant. Healthy urine will lie somewhere between clear and straw coloured. Infected urine is commonly cloudy. The smell of urine is traditionally thought to be a significant factor, but it appears not to be a reliable indication of urinary tract infection in children (Struthers et al., 2003).

Dipstick testing may prove positive for blood and/or protein. These substances are not particularly predictive of a urinary tract infection; they may be present but equally they may not. Much more predictive is the presence of nitrite and leucocyte esterase. Nitrate is a substance that is normally found in urine. Most bacteria convert nitrate to nitrite; it takes them around 4 hours to do this. This is why morning testing for nitrite is a good idea. A dipstick can also be used to detect the presence of leucocyte esterase. This is an enzyme produced by white blood cells; its presence indicates infection. A urine sample that is positive for leucocyte esterase and nitrites strongly suggests urinary tract infection. If leukocyte esterase or nitrite, or both are present the urine should be sent for culture and antibiotic therapy should commence. If they are both negative there is no need to send the sample for culture unless there is a suspicion of pyelonephritis, the infant is under 3 months of age, the infant or child is suffering from recurrent urine infections, the clinical symptoms and dipstick do not correlate, or there is a high risk of serious illness (NICE, 2007).

Treatment/Management

When an infant under 3 months of age is suspected of having a UTI they should be referred to a paediatrician. Treatment should commence in line with the NICE fever guidelines for under 5s by giving parenteral antibiotics to infants under 1 month old with a fever, and all infants 1–3 months with a fever who appear unwell and/or have a low white blood cell count (NICE, 2013).

Children over 3 months with an upper respiratory tract infection should be treated with oral antibiotics for 7–10 days. Intravenous antibiotics given for 2–4 days followed by oral antibiotics for a duration of 10 days is also advised if the infant/child has symptoms such as fever, rigors, vomiting or dehydration. Most small children who are febrile with a UTI do not develop renal damage; however one-fifth of children will do so, therefore rapid treatment is required (Swerkersson et al., 2017; NICE, 2007).

Infants or children over 3 months who are considered to have a lower urinary tract infection should be prescribed oral antibiotics for 3 days such as trimethoprim, nitrofurantoin, cephalosporin or amoxicillin. If the child remains unwell after 24–48 hours they should be reassessed (NICE, 2007).

Nursing Considerations

Assessment must include pain, hydration, stasis and temperature. Assess the type of pain and if the location varies. Pain may occur only on micturition. Bladder spasms may occur. Loin pain may be present. Non-pharmacological methods such as distraction and heat pads should be considered. Analgesia should be prescribed and administered as required. The child may be dehydrated because of reduced intake and increased insensible loss. It is necessary to observe for signs of dehydration and record input and output. The child's weight should also be recorded. Older children can be encouraged to consume adequate fluids, but younger children might require intravenous support. Temperature control may be necessary. Children with lower urinary tract infections may have a mild temperature rise. Those with upper urinary tract infections may have more substantial temperature rises. Cooling measures should be implemented and antipyretics administered as per the NICE guidelines on fever in the under 5s (NICE, 2013).

Investigations

Imaging is used during the acute illness and later to identify any damage to the kidneys and any predisposing causes of UTI. The diagnostic imaging methods that are usually considered include ultrasonography, dimercaptosuccinic acid scanning (DMSA) and voiding cystourethrogram (VCUG).

Ultrasonography is a non-invasive test that provides information about the structure of the renal tract and dilation of the collecting system. It can identify dilated or duplicated ureters, ureteroceles and horseshoe kidneys. The test is limited because it cannot identify acute pyelonephritis or subsequent renal scarring. It may also fail to detect hydronephrosis. NICE (2007) recommend that ultrasound be undertaken during acute infection to identify abnormalities of the urinary tract for all infants and children with atypical UTI. Ultrasound should be carried out within 6 weeks of a UTI for infants younger than 6 months with a first UTI. It is not necessary to perform ultrasound on infants and children who have had a lower urinary tract infection unless they are younger than 6 months or had recurrent infections.

DMSA scanning can be used during an acute UTI when an upper urinary tract infection is suspected. It can detect inflammation of the kidney substance and confirms the diagnosis of acute pyelonephritis. However, NICE guidelines note that DMSA scan should be undertaken within 4 to 6 months following an acute infection, with the scan being brought forward if the infant or child experiences a subsequent UTI whilst waiting for a DMSA scan. Later DMSA scanning can be used to determine the presence of any scarring. Ehsanipour et al.'s (2012) study noted more than one-half of the children with acute pyelonephritis had one or more renal scars.

Micturating cystourethrogram (MCUG) provides information about the bladder and flow of urine. It identifies the presence of vesicoureteric reflux and the grade of reflux. A MCUG can be carried out before or after the child has completed their initial antibiotic course (Mahant et al., 2001). The procedure involves catheterisation and instillation of contrast media. Preparing the child and family before investigation can reduce the distress associated with the procedure. Storytelling and play have both been found to be effective (Phillips et al., 1998).

Things to Consider

Children who have had one UTI are at risk of further infections. It is therefore imperative that parents and carers are given appropriate education and guidance to both prevent and manage UTIs and the treatments required (NICE, 2007). There are ways of limiting the likelihood of a second infection. Detailed discussion concerning these interventions must take place. Information given to parents (and children) should be verbal and reinforced on paper.

 ACTIVITY

Reflect on your practice.
- Do you provide parents/carers with information sheets on prevention of urinary tract infection?
- Are you satisfied with the clarity of these documents?
- Is the information comprehensive and accurate?

Parents and children should be taught the gross anatomy of the urinary tract and the nature of ascending infection. From this point they can then appreciate the recommended hygiene habits that must be practised. If a child is in nappies, these should be changed as soon as possible after soiling. Perineal hygiene is important in girls; wiping away from the urethra is recommended. Cotton underwear is advisable because synthetic materials may increase heat and sweating and encourage bacterial growth. Bubble baths should not be added to bath water and perfumed soaps are inadvisable. Using bubble baths and perfumed soaps may disturb the urethral flora and encourage bacteria to ascend.

Stasis of urine should be avoided so the child should drink frequently and also be given the opportunity to void every hour or two. It is also necessary to teach parents to look for the features of a urinary tract infection. They may also have to learn how to obtain specimens and test them for nitrite and leucocyte esterase. Finally, the importance of complying with antibiotic therapy should be discussed and the necessity to attend follow-up clinic appointments and investigations should be stressed.

VESICOURETERIC REFLUX

Vesicoureteric reflux (VUR) is the abnormal back flow of urine from the bladder into the ureter or into the ureter and kidneys. The condition may be unilateral or bilateral. VUR is usually a primary disorder caused by an anatomical defect at the junction between the ureter and the bladder. There is solid evidence that VUR has a familial basis (Noe et al., 1992), although it is not well understood due to the multi-factorial genetic penetrance (Lee et al., 2017). Primary VUR is thought to be an autosomal dominant disorder with incomplete penetrance and variable expression.

The ureters enter the bladder at an oblique angle on the posterior right and left lateral surface. The oblique course is continued through the bladder wall. Each ureter terminates in a ureteral orifice found at both sides of the upper level of the trigone. When the intravesical pressure is increased during micturition the detrusor muscle contracts and the intravesical section of the ureters are passively compressed. This valvular mechanism normally prevents reflux. The effectiveness of this mechanism is dependent on an adequate length of intravesical ureter (Belman, 1997). A study by Magoma et al. (2013) has shown that the morphology of the pelvic ureter length between males and females differ. Boys are more likely than girls to have VUR (Tekgul et al., 2012).

VUR predisposes to urinary tract infection because urine that is refluxed into the ureter(s) trickles back into the bladder producing an increased urine residual, which provides the conditions for an infection to take place. Reflux then provides a route by which the infection can reach the kidney. Urinary tract infection with VUR is associated with renal scarring and is an important cause of hypertension and renal failure. It is therefore important in the management of these children that they are kept free from infection, for reflux without infection will not damage the kidney (Tekgul et al., 2012).

Diagnosis

Children are not routinely screened for VUR, but screening should take place following a UTI where there is a family history of VUR (NICE, 2007). One of the mainstays in the diagnosis of VUR is micturating cystourethrogram/voiding cystourethrogram. A MCUG provides precise anatomic detail and allows grading of the VUR. MCUG testing will grade the severity of reflux from grade 1 to grade 5. Grade 1 is the least severe, where urine flows back up the ureters but does not reach the renal pelvis. Grade 5 is the most severe, where a lot of urine reaches the kidney causing swelling of the ureter and kidney. Grading by the international scale remains the major means of categorising patients and determining treatments (Tekgul et al., 2012). It is important to remember that MCUG is an invasive procedure involving the trauma of catheterisation, the potential for infection and exposure to radioactivity; however, it remains the gold standard.

DMSA scanning is best to visualise cortical tissue and kidney function and to monitor renal scarring. Infants with a prenatal diagnosis of hydronephrosis will undergo ultrasonography of the kidney and bladder. This procedure is non-invasive and provides reliable information regarding the kidney structure (Tekgul et al., 2012).

Treatment/Management

The objective of medical management is to keep the urine infection-free while waiting for spontaneous resolution. This is an effective treatment and can work in all grades of reflux, but the higher the grade the less likely spontaneous resolution is. Resolution is nearly 80% in VUR grades I–II, and 30% to 50% in VUR grades III–V within 4–5 years of follow-up.

Medical management involves the prescription of intermittent or continuous prophylactic antibiotics. Circumcision during early infancy may be considered (Tekgul et al., 2012). Management also emphasises the importance of measures designed to minimise the likelihood of UTI. The parent/child is taught the importance of adequate fluid intake, appropriate wiping action, regular toileting, double voiding to expel refluxed urine, and avoidance of constipation.

Surgical management of VUR is not routinely recommended (NICE, 2007). However, surgery is considered for patients with grades IV and V reflux as spontaneous resolution is less likely. Surgery is also considered when prophylaxis fails to prevent urinary tract infection or further renal damage. Open surgery involves lengthening the intramural part of the ureter by re-implantation of the offending ureter or ureters by submucosal embedding. The aim of re-implantation is to create an adequate intravesical tunnel, to allow compression of the ureter against the detrusor muscle (Tekgul et al., 2012).

Subureteral injection of bulking materials has become increasingly popular because it is minimally invasive and performed as a day case. Endoscopic injection therapy involves using a standard operating cystoscope to visualise the ureteric orifice. A substance is then injected below the epithelial layer, just inside the edge of the orifice. This narrows the lumen preventing reflux of urine into the ureter. The technique takes about 15 minutes (Tekgul et al., 2012). Teflon was the original injected substance but concerns arose concerning particle migration to lymph, liver and lungs. Other substances such as collagen, autologous fat, silicone and more recently Deflux, a copolymer of dextranomer microspheres and hyaluronic acid, have been used. Trials have shown Deflux to be effective in treating reflux (Lightner, 2002).

Follow-Up

Children who are being treated prophylactically have to attend clinics on a regular basis, usually every 3 months. They have their urine checked for infection, and undergo blood pressure and growth monitoring. Clinic appointments also provide the opportunity to reinforce the importance of compliance with medication. Further radiological studies may be necessary to ensure that reflux has not worsened, or more hopefully, that it has actually resolved. If the child has been treated surgically, follow-up continues to be important but the nature of the surveillance changes with fewer specimens required and fewer radiological studies.

HYPOSPADIAS

Hypospadias is a congenital anomaly of the male genitalia. There are conflicting estimates regarding worldwide prevalence of hypospadias, with the majority of studies reporting a prevalence of 5–50 per 10,000 male births. A higher incidence has been reported in European countries and North America (Springer et al., 2016). In hypospadias, the urethral meatus is abnormally located on the ventral side of the penis, anywhere from the glans to the perineum. Around 70% of cases will present distally and in these situations the meatus is positioned in the glans.

Mid-shaft and proximal hypospadias, though less prevalent are more serious, particularly proximal hypospadias, which may be penoscrotal, scrotal or perineal (Holmes, 2012). The condition may present in isolation or may be associated with other genitourinary abnormalities. These include inguinal hernia, cryptorchidism, bifid scrotum and vesicoureteral reflux (Shih and Graham, 2014). Chordee, or curvature of the penis, frequently accompanies hypospadias, as does a lack skin on the ventrum of the penis and an excess on the dorsum resulting in a hooded appearance (Mouriquand et al., 2009). Less common features include penoscrotal transposition and urethral hypoplasia; however, both are indicative of greater complexity.

Urethral development takes place between 8- and 20-weeks' gestation. Before 8 weeks, male and female external genitalia appear identical. The action of androgens (e.g. testosterone, androsterone) trigger the development of the male genitalia. Hypospadias results when the embryological urethral groove fails to close. Partial androgen receptor insensitivity is a recognised cause of hypospadias. Another related cause is 5-alpha-reductase deficiency. Testosterone has to be transformed by 5-alpha-reductase so that it can activate androgen receptors. A deficiency of 5-alpha-reductase impairs testosterone action; hypospadias is one of a number of possible consequences.

Diagnosis

Hypospadias is generally identified on physical exam at birth or soon after when an abnormal urine stream is noted; however, there are improvements in antenatal identification with fetal ultrasound scanning. Hypospadias is a feature of several chromosomal and miscellaneous genetic abnormalities as well as some endocrine anomalies, so a complete genetic and endocrine work-up should be performed if cryptochordism is present or if the genitalia are ambiguous. It is so frequently associated with some syndromes, such as Smith-Lemli-Opitz syndrome and Mowat-Wilson syndrome, that its presence can help support diagnosis of these conditions (Shih and Graham, 2014).

Treatment/Management

Surgical correction is ideally carried out within the second 6 months of life; numerous procedures have been developed to achieve this. A Mathieu repair or a variant of the Snodgrass procedure are common approaches to distal hypospadias (Buschel and Carroll, 2018). A one-stage repair may also be sufficient to reverse proximal hypospadias but a two-stage procedure, such as the staged Bracka repair, is more common. Irrespective of the number of stages required, the objective is the same: to bring the urethral meatus to the tip of the penis, correct any chordee, and create a functional and cosmetically acceptable glans and penile shaft.

Postoperative Care

Pain is one of the major problems in the immediate postoperative period. Penile block, caudal or epidural analgesia

are employed to minimise this. Postoperative pain assessment and regular analgesia are required. Because different techniques are used, there are variations in the use of catheters and stents; some techniques employ them and others do not (Buschel and Carroll, 2018). There is also disagreement about wound dressings; different types have been utilised and some argue that they do not offer any advantage (McLorie et al., 2001; van Savage et al., 2000). Sanders (2003) suggests that a barrier film can be applied before a dressing is attached to ease removal. Alternative modes of dressings that promote ease of removal have been suggested. Essentially arguments for dressings suggest they provide support, protection and minimise discomfort; arguments against dressings include pain, necrosis and distress when they require removal (Pfeil and Lindsay, 2010). Irrespective of whether these adjuncts are used, the assessment of adequate urinary output is essential and the nurse should attempt to ensure that the child does not tamper with dressings, stents or catheters.

When dressings are used, removal is a source of anxiety for parents and is painful and upsetting for the child. Before removal of the dressing, the child is given analgesia. It is common practice to then place the child in a bath to soften the dressing material. Despite this, the dressing is often still difficult to remove without upsetting the child. Distraction techniques can be employed and parent participation encouraged as a means of reducing distress.

Things to Consider

Postoperative complications include infection, retention and fistula formation; stenosis, strictures and diverticulum formations may also occur. Antibiotics are prescribed to minimise the likelihood of infection. The nurse must still be alert for signs of infection such as elevated temperature, discharge from the wound and foul-smelling urine. Retention may be anatomical or drug induced. All children, irrespective of the surgical technique employed, should be observed for this complication. Fistula may occur in the week following surgery and urine leaks may appear from a point along the reconstructed tract. Spontaneous closure is rare and further surgery is required in this case.

Studies have identified a high level of satisfaction with the outcome of distal hypospadias surgery, but long-term results are not as good for boys with more complicated hypospadias. Long-term problems concern micturition difficulties and problems with sexual function. Micturition difficulties are generally caused by stricture. Urethral dilation may be necessary and in some cases open urethroplasty may be required. Sexual function problems, such as erection and ejaculation difficulties, have been reported following repair of severe hypospadias.

⚲ ACTIVITY

For further information go to the 'Hypospadias UK' website here: https://www.hypospadiasuk.co.uk.

CRYPTORCHIDISM

Cryptorchidism (undescended testis) is when one or both testes are not contained within the scrotal sac. It is one of the commonest congenital malformations, but can also be acquired; causes are multi-factorial. The incidence of congenital cryptorchidism in full-term males at birth is 1% to 4.6% and can be up to 45% in preterm males (Radmayr et al., 2016). In early fetal development the testes are located within the abdominal cavity. Mediated by hormonal and mechanical factors, the testes descend into the scrotum in two phases. The first stage occurs trans-abdominally between 7 and 12 weeks' gestation, then during the second stage, which occurs after 18 weeks' gestation, the testes move through the inguinal canal adopting their final scrotal position in the two months before birth (Patni et al., 2017). Sometimes one or both testes fail to descend; the former is more common. If one or both fail to descend, they may still fall within the first year; this is particularly true in the case of premature babies. Orchidopexy is normally required if the testes remain undescended by 6 months of age (corrected for gestational age) and completed no later than 18 months of age to prevent negative sequelae (Radmayr et al., 2016). Cryptorchidism may also be acquired. In this situation the testes are in a normal scrotal position initially but one or both become undescended later. The pathogenesis of acquired cryptorchidism is unknown, although possible causal factors such as failure of the spermatic cord to elongate have been proposed. Because cryptorchidism can be diagnosed during infancy (congenital) and later childhood (acquired), boys undergo the operation at different ages.

Diagnosis

Examination of the genitalia and documenting the absence or presence of the testes, as part of normal screening in the neonatal period, helps to differentiate between congenital or acquired presentations. History taking for the older child is important, especially if there has been previous surgical intervention.

Treatment/Management

Management will be determined by the classification of the undescended testes based on presence, location and whether they are palpable or non-palpable. When testes are palpable, orchidopexy and orchidolysis procedures can be carried out using a scrotal or inguinal approach (Novaes et al., 2013). The operation is often carried out as a day case procedure and involves mobilising the testes, spermatic cord and blood supply. The testes or testicle is then brought down into the scrotum and secured by suture. The presence of non-palpable testes should be determined by diagnostic laparoscopy; if present, the appropriateness of removal versus repositioning should be determined.

On return from theatre a dry dressing may be in place. It is removed prior to, or during, a shower the following day. The stitches dissolve a week later. Initially there is considerable swelling and bruising of the scrotum. This will cause discomfort and moderate pain relief will be required. Quiet play should be encouraged. Energetic play/exercise should be avoided for 10–14 days, especially straddling activities such as cycling. There are complications associated with the procedure; however, these are rare. They include wound infection, haematoma or dehiscence. Damage can also occur to the blood supply or spermatic cord during the operation, resulting in testicular atrophy and loss of testicular function (Penson et al., 2013).

Things to Consider

If a newborn male presents with bilateral undescended or non-palpable testes and any other features indicative of disorders of sex development (DSD), concomitant hypospadias in particular, then full genetic and endocrine screening is essential.

Children with cryptorchidism are at risk from a number of undesirable consequences. Compared with other males they have a greater risk of testicular torsion. This occurs when the testicle twists on the spermatic cord and results in disturbance of blood flow, ischaemia and infarction of the testicle. Emergency surgery is required to save the testicle.

The condition is also associated with infertility. If bilateral cryptorchidism remains untreated the adult male will be infertile. However, surgery does not ensure fertility. The treated male may be fertile, sub-fertile or infertile (Goel et al., 2015). A successful outcome appears to be related to the position of the testes before operation, the age at operation and an adequate blood supply to the testes following surgery. There is disagreement on the potential for hormone treatment to improve fertility in adulthood, but current European guidelines suggest its use to preserve fertility potential for boys with bilateral undescended testes (Radmayr et al., 2016)

Cryptorchidism is an established risk factor for testicular cancer. It is possible that hormonal conditions cause both cryptorchidism and testicular cancer. Another possibility is that the higher temperature, to which the undescended testicle is exposed, promotes tumour formation. There appears to be a relationship between the age at which the male undergoes orchidopexy and the likelihood of testicular cancer (Walsh et al., 2007). Early orchidopexy appears to be associated with a more positive outcome. The risk of testicular cancer is still present even though orchidopexy has been carried out. All males should carry out testicular examination at regular periods. Those who have had cryptorchidism have added reason to do so.

 ACTIVITY

There is some debate about what age it is appropriate to educate boys on testicular health and self-examination. How would you approach this conversation with the parents of a child who is high risk?

PHIMOSIS AND CIRCUMCISION

Phimosis refers to a partial or complete non-retractable foreskin. In almost all male infants there is a normal physiological adhesion between the prepuce and the glans which protects the glans and keeps it soft and moist. By age 3 years retraction becomes possible for around 90% of infants. Persistent or pathological phimosis can cause meatal stenosis, dysuria and inflammation; it has also been linked to penile carcinoma. Lichen sclerosis (previously termed balanitis xerotica obliterans [BXO]) is an inflammatory disorder that affects the prepuce and glans and is the commonest cause of true pathological phimosis.

Circumcision refers to excision of the prepuce, the outer portion of the foreskin covering the penis. Circumcision may be carried out for cultural reasons, prophylactic reasons or for phimosis. The commonest medical indicators for circumcision are pathological phimosis, recurrent episodes of urinary tract infection and/or balanoposthitis, an acute inflammation of the foreskin and glans (Royal College of Surgeons [RCS], 2016). There is some evidence that topical steroids to treat phimosis may be an effective alternative to circumcision in some cases (Moreno et al., 2014).

Cultural Circumcision

The most common reason for circumcision is cultural or religious. Circumcision is a sacred ritual for Muslims and Jewish people. The timing differs for each religion. Jewish babies are circumcised on the eighth day of life. Muslim children are circumcised between the seventh day following birth and up to puberty.

Prophylaxis

Circumcision which is not medically indicated is extremely contentious. Arguments in favour of routine circumcision for prophylactic reasons focus on a number of conditions. Urinary tract infection is one. The literature suggests that there is a greater risk of urinary tract infection in the uncircumcised child in the first year of life (Morris and Wiswell, 2013). Human papillomavirus (HPV) is another condition in which circumcision may be beneficial. HPV is a sexually transmitted disease and strains of the virus are linked to cancer of the cervix. Wawer et al. (2011) present evidence that male circumcision is associated with reduced risks of penile HPV infection and cervical cancer in female partners.

Circumcision may also have a positive impact on the transmission of human immunodeficiency virus (HIV). Szabo and Short (2000) explain that the inner lining of the foreskin, the mucosal layer, contains Langerhans cells. These cells are targets for HIV. The authors suggest that during heterosexual intercourse the foreskin is pulled back leaving the vagina exposed to an area rich in virus. Circumcision, it is thus argued, would reduce the likelihood of HIV transmission. In sub-Saharan Africa, where HIV is extensive, circumcision as a means of prevention of HIV is being advocated as an additional HIV prevention strategy (Rain-Taljaard, 2003; World Health Organization [WHO], 2015). This position is not without its critics. Others argue that it is not acceptable, citing medical, ethical and legal reasons (Hill and Denniston, 2003).

Treatment/Management

No matter what the reason for circumcision, there are risks attached. Bleeding, infection, meatal stenosis, injury to the glans or urethra and negative cosmetic or sensory consequences are all possible, albeit rare complications (RCS, 2016). On return from theatre the wound may be exposed or a dressing such as Vaseline gauze may be in place. The penis will look swollen and possibly bruised; child and parents should be prepared for this. The wound can be cleaned with moistened cotton balls. It should be observed for infection and bleeding. If bleeding does occur it is usually minor and self-limiting; severe bleeding is uncommon. A white/yellowish exudate forms after 48 hours; this should not be confused with pus. It is granulation tissue and part of the healing process. Pus has a thicker consistency and smells malodorous. Infection is a rare occurrence but if it does occur the wound is cleansed regularly and antibiotic therapy commenced.

 ACTIVITY

For further information and myth-busting discussion, go to the Circumcision Facts web page here: http://circfacts.org/.

SUMMARY

Paediatric nurses are required to care for children with congenital and acquired anomalies of the genitourinary tract. This chapter has attempted to offer an insight into some of the more common anomalies. Nurses caring for children must have a well-developed knowledge of UTI, because it is very common and because of its association with impaired renal function, hypertension and end-stage renal disease. VUR was given prominence in this chapter because it is intrinsically linked to UTI and is the most common congenital abnormality of the renal tract. Children are commonly subject to surgical procedures involving the genitourinary tract. To this end, hypospadias, cryptorchidism, phimosis and circumcision were included.

REFERENCES

Al-Orifi, F., McGillivray, D., Tange, S., et al., 2000. Urine culture from bag specimens in young children: are the risks too high? Canada. J. Pediatr. 137 (2), 221–226.

Belman, A.B., 1997. Vesicoureteral reflux. Pediatr. Clin. 44 (5), 1171–1190.

Buschel, H., Carroll, D., 2018. Hypospadias. Paediatr. Child Health 28 (5), 218–221.

Ehsanipour, F., Gharouni, M., Rafati, A.H., et al., 2012. Risk factors of renal scars in children with acute pyelonephritis. Braz. J. Infect. Dis. 16 (1), 15–18.

Feasey, S., 1999. Are Newcastle urine collection pads suitable as a means of collecting specimens from infants? Paediatr. Nur. 11 (9), 17–21.

Frumkin, K., 2014. Bacteriology of urinary tract infections in emergency patients aged 0–36 months. J. Emerg. Med. 48 (4), 405–415.

Goel, P., Rawat, J.D., Wakhlu, A., et al., 2015. Undescended testicle: an update on fertility in cryptorchid men. Indian J. Med. Res. 141 (2), 163–171.

Goilav, B., 2017. Urinary tract infections in children. BMJ Best Practice. Online. Available from: https://bestpractice.bmj.com/topics/en-gb/789. (accessed 31 July 2018).

Grier, W.R., et al., 2016. Obesity as a risk factor for urinary tract infections in children. Clin. Pediatr. 55 (10), 952–956.

Hill, G., Denniston, G., 2003. HIV and circumcision: new factors to consider. Sex. Transm. Infect. 79 (6), 495–496.

Holmes, L.B., 2012. Common Malformations. Oxford University Press, Oxford.

Kocak, M., Buyukkaragoz, A., Celebi Tayfur, K.A., et al., 2016. Causative pathogens and antibiotic resistance in children hospitalized for urinary tract infections. Pediatr. Int. 58, 467–471.

Lee, K.H., Gee, H.Y., Shin, J.I., 2017. Genetics of vesicoureteral reflux and congenital anomalies of the kidney and urinary tract. Investig. Clin. Urol. 58 (Suppl. 1), S4–S13.

Li, P.S., Ma, L.C., Wong, S.N., 2002. Is bag urine culture useful in monitoring urinary tract infection in infants? J. Paediatr. Child Health 38 (4), 377–381.

Liaw, L.C., Nayar, D.M., Pedler, S.J., et al., 2000. Home collection of urine for culture from infants by three methods: survey of parents' preferences and bacterial contamination rates. BMJ 320 (7245), 1312–1313.

Lightner, D.J., 2002. Review of the available urethral bulking agents. Curr. Opin. Urol. 12 (4), 333–338.

Loening-Baucke, V., 2007. Prevalence rates for constipation and faecal and urinary incontinence. Arch. Dis. Child. 92 (6), 486–489.

Macfarlane, P.I., Ellis, R., Hughes, C., et al., 2005. Urine collection pads: are samples reliable for urine biochemistry and microscopy? Pediatr. Nephrol. 20, 170–179.

Magoma, G., Ogeng'o, J.A., Awori, K., 2013. Morphometry of the pelvic ureter. J. Morphol. Sci. 30 (2), 73–76.

Mahant, S., To, T., Friedman, J., 2001. Timing of voiding cystourethrogram in the investigation of urinary tract infections in children. J. Pediatr. 139 (4), 568–571.

McLorie, G., Joyner, B., Herz, D., et al., 2001. A prospective randomized clinical trial to evaluate methods of postoperative care of hypospadias. J. Urol. 165 (5), 1669–1672.

Morello, W., La Scola, C., Alberici, I., et al., 2016. Acute pyelonephritis in children. Pediatr. Nephrol. 31 (8), 1253–1265.

Moreno, G., Corbalán, J., Peñaloza, B., et al., 2014. Topical corticosteroids for treating phimosis in boys. Cochrane Database Syst. Rev. 2 (9), CD008973.

Morris, B., Wiswell, T., 2013. Circumcision and lifetime risk of urinary tract infection: a systematic review and meta-analysis. J. Urol. 189 (6), 2118–2124.

Mouriquand, P., Demede, D., Gorduza, D., et al., 2009. Hypospadias. In: Gearhart, J., Rink, R., Mouriquand, P. (Eds.), Pediatric Urology, second ed. Saunders and Elsevier, Philadelphia, pp. 526–543.

National Institute for Health and Care Excellence (NICE), 2007. Urinary Tract Infection in Under 16s: Diagnosis and Management. Clinical Guideline [CG54]. Published date: August 2007. Last updated: September 2017.

National Institute for Health and Care Excellence (NICE), 2013. Fever in Under 5s: Assessment and Initial Management. Clinical Guideline [CG 160]. Published date: May 2013. Last updated: August 2017.

Noe, H.N., Wyatt, R.J., Peeden Jr J.N., et al., 1992. The transmission of vesicoureteral reflux from parent to child. J. Urol. 148 (6), 1869–1871.

Novaes, H.F., Carneiro Neto, J.A., Macedo, A., et al., 2013. Single scrotal incision orchidopexy – a systematic review. Int. Braz J. Urol. 39 (3), 305–311.

O'Brien, K., 2013. The prevalence of urinary tract infections (UTI) in children under five years old presenting with an acute illness in UK general practice. PhD Thesis. Cardiff University.

Patni, P., Mohanty, S.K., Singh, R., 2017. Embryonic development of the testis. In: Singh, R., Singh, K. (Eds.), Male Infertility: Understanding, Causes and Treatments. Springer, Singapore, pp. 13–24.

Penson, D., Krishnaswami, S., Jules, A., et al., 2013. Effectiveness of hormonal and surgical therapies for cryptorchidism: a systematic review. Pediatrics 131 (6), e1897–e1907.

Pfeil, M., Lindsay, B., 2010. Hypospadias repair: an overview. Int. J. Urol. Nurs. 4 (1), 4–12.

Phillips, D.A., Watson, A.R., MacKinlay, D., 1998. Distress and the micturating cystourethrogram: does preparation help? Acta Paediatr. 87 (2), 175–179.

Radmayr, C., Dogan, H.S., Hoebeke, P., et al., 2016. Management of undescended testes: European Association of Urology/European Society for Paediatric Urology guidelines. J. Pediatr. Urol. 12, 335–343.

Rain-Taljaard, R., Lagarde, E., Taljaard, D., et al., 2003. Potential for an intervention based on male circumcision in a South African town with high levels of HIV infection. AIDS Care 15 (3), 315–327.

Roth, K., Koo, H.P., Spottswood, S.E., et al., 2002. Obstructive uropathy: an important cause of chronic renal failure in children. Clin. Pediatr. 41 (5), 309–314.

Royal College of Surgeons (RCS), 2016. Commissioning Guide: Foreskin Conditions. Royal College of Surgeons, England.

Sanders, C., 2003. Comparison of dressing removal following hypospadias repair. Br. J. Nurs. 12 (Suppl. 15), S21–S28.

Shaikh, N., Morone, N., Bost, J.E., et al., 2008. Prevalence of urinary tract infection in childhood: a meta-analysis. Pediatr. Infect. Dis. J. 27 (4), 302–308.

Shih, E.M., Graham, J.M., 2014. Review of genetic and environmental factors leading to hypospadias. Eur. J. Med. Genet. 57 (8), 453–463.

Springer, A., van den Heijkant, M., Baumann, S., 2016. Worldwide prevalence of hypospadias. J. Pediatr. Urol. 12 (3), 152.e1–152.e7.

Struthers, S., Scanlon, J., Parker, K., et al., 2003. Parental reporting of smelly urine and urinary tract infection. Arch. Dis. Child. 88 (3), 250–252.

Swerkersson, S., Jodal, U., Sixt, R., et al., 2017. Urinary tract infection in small children: the evolution of renal damage over time. Pediatr. Nephrol. 32 (10), 1907–1913.

Szabo, R., Short, R.V., 2000. How does male circumcision protect against HIV infection? BMJ 320 (7249), 1592–1594.

Tekgul, S., Riedmiller, H., Hoebeke, P., et al., 2012. EAU guidelines on vesicoureteral reflux in children. Eur. Urol. 62 (3), 534–542.

van Savage, J., Palanca, L., Slaughenhoupt, B., 2000. A prospective randomized trial of dressings versus no dressings for hypospadias repair. J. Urol. 164 (3 Pt 2), 981–983.

Walsh, T.J., Dall'Era, M.A., Croughan, M.S., et al., 2007. Prepubertal orchidopexy for cryptorchidism may be associated with lower risk of testicular cancer. J. Urol. 178 (4 Pt 1), 1440–1446.

Wawer, M.J., Tobian, A.A., Kigozi, G., et al., 2011. Effect of circumcision of HIV-negative men on transmission of human papillomavirus to HIV-negative women: a randomised trial in Rakai, Uganda. Lancet 377 (9761), 209–218.

World Health Organization (WHO), 2015. Male circumcision for HIV prevention. Online. Available from: http://www.who.int/hiv/topics/malecircumcision/en. (accessed 31 July 2018).

23

Skin Disease in Children and Young People

Jean Robinson

LEARNING OUTCOMES

- Demonstrate an understanding of the anatomy and physiology of skin.
- Show ability to assess and describe skin disease and lesions using appropriate terminology.
- Gain an overview of the common skin conditions in children and young people.
- Have an appreciation of the potential psychological effects of skin disease on children and young people and their families' quality of life.
- Understand the importance of the role of the nurse in caring for children with skin disease and the specific skills required.
- Understand the importance of educating children, young people and their families and carers in the practical aspects of the treatment and management of their skin disease.

ⓔ For images of the conditions discussed in this chapter please see http://evolve.elsevier.com. See inside cover for access details.

INTRODUCTION

Skin disease is very common accounting for 10% of primary care workload. In 2006 nearly a quarter of the population in England and Wales went to their general practitioner (GP) with a skin problem – the most common of which were skin infections and eczema. Different disorders are associated with different times of life, for example, eczema is most common in babies and young children, acne is most common in adolescents and psoriasis has its peak in the second and third decades of life. Impetigo, hand, foot and mouth disease, chicken pox, molluscum contagiosum and haemangiomas are all commonly seen in paediatric dermatology practice. Collodion babies, some genetic ichthyotic disorders and some variants of epidermolysis bullosa present at birth (Gawkrodger and Ardern-Jones, 2017), and offer nurses great challenges in supporting their care needs.

BIOLOGY OF THE SKIN

The skin is one of the body's largest organs with a surface area of nearly 2 m² and making up about 16% of body weight. Its most important function is to act as a barrier to protect the body from external factors and keep the internal structure intact. Other functions include preventing loss of body fluids, reduction of ultraviolet (UV) penetration, regulation of body temperature, acting as a sensory organ and affording a gripping surface, a role in vitamin D production, acting as an outpost for immune surveillance and communication and cosmetic appearance. It is capable of failure and the results

of this can be physically and psychologically debilitating and potentially lethal (Gawkrodger and Arden-Jones, 2017).

Structure

The skin is made up of three layers: the epidermis, dermis and subcutis.

Epidermis

This is the outer layer coming into contact with the external environment. It is about 0.1 mm thick although it is thicker on the palms and soles and its main job is protective. The main cells of the epidermis are keratinocytes producing proteins called keratins, which are the major constituents of the stratum corneum, nails and hair. The epidermis is divided into four layers: stratum basale or basal cell layer, stratum spinosum (prickle cell layer), stratum granulosum (granular cell layer) and stratum corneum (horny layer).

Basal Cell Layer (Stratum Basale)

This is mainly made up of keratinocytes of which a small proportion is stem cells and constantly divide. Five percent to 10% of the basal cell population are melanocytes which make melanin. Melanin gives colour to skin and hair and protection from UV radiation. Basal keratinocytes also synthesise antimicrobial peptides which are important in defence against bacteria.

Prickle Cell Layer (Stratum Spinosum)

Keratinocytes migrate upwards and are interconnected by desmosomes (the prickles). Langerhans cells which are immunologically active cells are found in this layer.

Granular Cell Layer (Stratum Granulosum)

Cells become flattened in this layer.

Horny Layer (Stratum Corneum)

This is the uppermost layer of the epidermis and made up of layers of flattened dead cells called corneocytes. These contain keratin filaments. The corneocytes also contain a natural moisturising factor (NMF), which helps to attract and hold water in the cells. Between the corneocytes is a complex mixture of lipids known as lipid lamellae. The skin barrier is often referred to as a brick wall with the corneocytes as the bricks and the lipid lamellae the matrix (Cork et al., 2009). The lipid lamellae forms the main pathway for substances to travel across the skin barrier (Agner et al., 2016). Filaggrin protein (FLG) is important for the structural integrity of the stratum corneum by aggregating keratin filaments inside corneocytes and then helping to make a cornefied envelope around the corneocytes, as well as helping to maintain pH and the water holding capacity of the stratum corneum (McAleer et al., 2013).

Dermis

This is a tough supportive connective tissue matrix which contains specialist structures of varying thickness from 0.6 to 3.0 mm. It contains fibroblasts, which synthesise collagens that are major structural proteins, elastin and other connective tissue and components such as proteoglycans that absorb water.

Subcutaneous Layer

This is loose connective tissue and fat and usually 1–3 cm thick on the abdomen.

Embryology of the Skin

The epidermis starts to develop at 4 weeks of gestational age (GA), nails at 7 weeks and the dermis at 11 weeks. The stratum corneum starts to develop at 15 weeks of GA and is not complete until about 34 weeks GA (Kusari et al., 2019). The stratum corneum is 30% thinner and the overall epidermis 20% thinner in babies (Stamatas et al., 2010) so caution should be exercised when recommending oils for neonatal skin as a recent study of olive and sunflower oils in neonates showed better hydration but changes to the lipid structure, which are currently of unknown clinical significance (Cooke et al., 2016).

Derivatives of Skin

Hair, nails, sebaceous glands and sweat glands are all derivatives of skin. Skin also has a good supply of nerves with the highest density of these being found in areas such as the hands, face and genitals. There is also a rich blood supply and lymphatic drainage is also important.

Terminology

Dermatology has its own unique vocabulary which it is helpful to know in order to describe skin disease (Table 23.1).

TABLE 23.1	Terminology
Term	**Description**
Annular	Ring-shaped
Bulla	Similar to vesicle but larger >5 mm diameter
Confluent	Joined up
Cyst	Nodule with epithelial–lined cavity filled with fluid or semisolid material
Erythema	Redness of skin
Erythroderma	Uncommon but important dermatological emergency–infection, hypothermia and cardiac failure are all complications
	Generalised exfoliative dermatitis >80% of skin is red–secondary process representing spread of a dermatosis or systemic disease throughout skin
Excoriation	Superficial abrasion, often linear resulting from scratching
Exudate	Leakage of fluid from blood vessels into surrounding tissue
Flexural	Bend in structure as in inner elbow
Folliculitis	Inflammation of hair follicles
Generalised	Total body area, widespread
Guttate	Small drop-like lesions distributed in a shower
Hyperkeratosis	Thickening of stratum corneum
Hyperpigmentation	Increase in pigment
Hypopigmentation	Decrease in pigment
Lesion	Area of disease, usually small
Lichenification	Chronic thickening of the skin with increased skin markings
Linear	In a line
Localised	Limited areas of involvement which are clearly defined
Macule	Localised area of colour
Nodule	Larger than papule >5 mm diameter
Papule	Small solid elevation <5 mm diameter, can be flat topped or dome shaped
Plaque	Palpable elevation of skin usually >2 cm in diameter
Pustule	Visible collection of free pus in a blister
Rash or eruption	More widespread skin involvement, usually several lesions
Scale	Accumulation of thickened readily detached fragments of keratin – can be fine or large
Ulcer	Circumscribed area of skin extending through epidermis into dermis. Usually result of impaired blood or nutrient supply to the skin
Vesicle	Small blister <5 mm in diameter filled with clear fluid

Peters, 2001; Gawkrodger, D.J., Arden-Jones, M.R., 2017. Dermatology: An Illustrated Colour Text. Elsevier, London.

Examination of the Skin

The whole of the skin should be examined in good, preferably natural, light. The distribution, location and colour of any lesions should be noted along with their shape and size. Touch is often very helpful. Note whether lesions are unilateral or bilateral and check the oral mucosa, hair and nails too (Gawkrodger and Arden-Jones, 2017).

COMMON SKIN INFECTIONS

When the skin barrier fails or is penetrated infections can lead to disease. Skin infections are a common problem and can be bacterial, fungal or viral in origin often exacerbating underlying conditions, for example, eczema.

Impetigo

Impetigo or skin infection is a very common superficial bacterial infection with two classic forms which occur in about 1% of children (Oranje et al., 2015). It occurs most commonly on the face and extremities, but can occur anywhere on the body and lasts about 1–3 weeks. The causative organisms have changed over the years but currently are mostly due to *Staphylococcus aureus (S. aureus)* and less commonly *Streptococcus* or sometimes by a combination of both organisms.

Non-bullous Secondary Impetigo

This is more common in children over 2 years of age and accounts for over 70% of cases (Burr, 2003). The lesions usually form in areas where the skin has been injured in some way, for example, minor grazes or cuts, insect bites and eczema. Initially blisters develop, which then develop into the classic golden-crusted lesions that can coalesce and spread all over the body. Most of these are due to *S. aureus* with the rest due to a mixed growth of *Staphylococcus* and *Streptococcus*.

Bullous Impetigo

This form is more common in babies and those under 2 years of age (Koning et al., 2012). It is characterised by vesicles and bullae (which don't break very easily and can persist for several days). It favours warm and humid environments and in neonates usually develops on the buttocks and in the inguinal areas. It is nearly always caused by *Staphylococci,* where localised toxin production leads to lesions which develop on intact skin.

Diagnosis

Bacterial skin swabs should be taken especially if the impetigo is recurrent to ensure the causative bacteria is correctly identified and adequately treated. To take a swab moisten the tip of the swab, apply to the affected skin and rotate to the swab between the fingers to pick up debris before putting into appropriate transport medium (RCN/BDNG, 2008).

Management

There is no standard therapy. Neonates with bullous impetigo should have systemic antibiotic therapy, which may be needed intravenously as it can be a life-threatening condition in the very young. The main goal of treatment is to clear the causative bacteria. In children with limited and uncomplicated impetigo topical mupirocin or fusidic acid have been shown to be equally as effective as oral antibiotics. It is generally agreed that the use of systemic antibiotics for extensive disease is practical and appropriate (Yeoh et al., 2016).

Impetigo is contagious so children in hospital should be nursed in a cubicle with appropriate precautions. Families need advice about good hygiene measures and hand washing with the use of separate flannels and towels. There is no good evidence to support disinfection measures (Koning et al., 2012). Children should stay away from nursery or school until no new lesions develop or until 48 hours after antibiotic treatment has been started (Public Health England, 2019). Children should be discouraged from picking their scabs. Bacteria can be harboured in nasal passages, so carriage should be considered in children with recurrent episodes of impetigo, swabs taken from the child and parents and nasal antibiotics given as appropriate.

It is also crucial that any underlying skin condition, for example, eczema (Charman and Lawton, 2006), and tinea or cold sores are also treated. This is vitally important for children with eczema where infection will act as a driver.

Panton Valentine Leucocidin *Staphylococcus aureus* Skin Infection

Panton-Valentine Leucocidin *S. aureus* (PVL-SA) is an increasing problem in primary care and dermatology practice (British Association of Dermatologists [BAD], 2019a)) and illustrates very well the importance of keeping abreast with developments in nursing and medicine. PVL-SA is a toxin produced by less than 2% of *S. aureus* and has been linked to the much better recognised community onset methicillin-resistant *S. aureus* (MRSA). PVL toxins are consistently associated with skin and soft tissue infections, for example, boils, carbuncles, cellulitis and folliculitis, and are relatively rare in invasive disease (Shallcross et al., 2013), but do lead to pain and erythema which are out of proportion to the severity and size of the lesions. It should always be considered where more than one family member has boils, or a child or young person has recurrent boils or skin infections.

The five risk factors are:
1. Contaminated articles shared, for example, towels
2. Close contact, for example, family life
3. Crowding
4. Cleanliness and poor hygiene
5. Cuts and compromised skin integrity, for example, eczema (Health Protection Agency, 2008)

Management

Bacterial skin swabs should be taken and the possibility of PVL raised with the microbiology laboratory so PVL gene testing can be performed. The appropriate antibiotic therapy can then be given. To reduce spread, families should wash their hands frequently with liquid soap, change towels and bedding daily, stay away from gyms and swimming pools until the infection has cleared and cover infected areas with plasters. Families should also all receive decolonisation treatment with topical antiseptics for showers and hair washing and nasal antibiotic therapy for 5 days according to local policies (BAD, 2019a).

Staphylococcal Scalded Skin Syndrome

This is an acute painful toxic illness usually of infants or young children. The skin is affected but mucous membranes are spared. It is caused by *S. aureus* which produces a toxin leading to damage of a key protein called desmoglein, which binds skin cells together (Gawkrodger and Arden-Jones, 2017). This damage leads to sheets of superficial parts of the epidermis shedding leaving denuded erythematous areas which resemble a scald, hence the name of the condition (BAD, 2019b).

Management

Infants and children should be admitted to hospital for treatment with systemic antibiotics after a skin swab for bacterial culture has been taken and supportive treatment. Skin should be gently cleaned with a suitable soap substitute and an ointment-based emollient, for example, White soft paraffin/liquid paraffin 50:50 (WSP/LP 50/50) should be applied liberally to all areas, but especially the denuded areas which will be painful. The ointment will provide a barrier as well as preventing the skin from sticking to sheets and clothing. Careful attention should be paid to fluid and electrolyte balance.

FUNGAL INFECTIONS

Fungal nail infections are rare in children but infections of the scalp and skin are common and all too often misdiagnosed and incorrectly treated (Ferguson and Fuller, 2017)

Tinea Capitis

Tinea capitis or scalp ringworm is now endemic in the UK and is caused by a specialist group of fungi which depend on their host or environment for survival. The host can be an animal (zoophilic), human (anthropophilic) or they can live in soil (geophilic). In the past in the UK *Microsporum canis* which is zoophilic was dominant. Although still seen in rural UK this is no longer the case in inner city cosmopolitan communities where *Trichophyton tonsurans*, an anthropophilic dermatophyte, accounts for about 50%–90% of cases. *T. tonsurans* has an endothrix pattern of infection where the fungus penetrates inside the hair shaft so topical treatment will not work and systemic treatment must be given. Hair loss in an inner city child should always be considered as tinea capitis until proven otherwise (Ferguson and Fuller, 2017). It mostly occurs in 3–8 year olds and is more common in type V1 skin, but is seen in children from all ethnic backgrounds who very rarely have any underlying immune deficit (Fuller et al., 2003).

Presentation includes some or all of the following symptoms:

- mild flaking and scale on the scalp
- areas of patchy hair loss

- pustules
- local lymphadenopathy

Kerions

These are boggy, painful inflammatory masses with areas of potentially permanent hair loss and the result of a severe inflammatory reaction to the dermatophyte. They are quite often mistaken for bacterial abscesses (Feltham and Sargant, 2016). Surgical intervention is inappropriate.

Diagnosis

Swabs are of little value. Skin scrapings and hair samples for mycology need to be taken using a blunt scalpel or similar instrument. Infected hair root stumps are helpful but plucking does not produce the best samples. Samples should be collected into folded dark paper squares and not refrigerated. Culture can take 4–6 weeks.

Management

Treatment should be started immediately especially for children with kerions. Kerions are often incorrectly diagnosed as bacterial scalp infections and antibiotics or inappropriate surgical interventions undertaken may result in delayed treatment. Topical antifungals are of little value and systemic treatment is essential (Chen et al., 2016). Shampoos such as selenium sulphide may be used as an adjunct.

Oral antifungal choice depends on the causative dermatophyte. Griseofulvin at 15–20 mg/kg daily for 6–8 weeks remains the only licensed formulation for tinea capitis in the UK. Recent guidelines advise using terbinafine as it has been shown that this is more effective in the treatment of *T. tonsurans* than griseofulvin. Dosage is weight related for 2–4 weeks. Itraconazole oral suspension (for 4 weeks) is safe, cost effective and widely used. Unfortunately, terbinafine is not available in suspension and tablets need to be crushed. This may be a cause of treatment failure. All formulations have reasonable safety profiles (Chen et al., 2016). Id reactions, which are localised or generalised popular eruptions, can occur 1–2 weeks after starting treatment and are sometimes thought to be drug reactions. It is important not to stop the treatment as the reaction will resolve as the infection is treated (Ferguson and Fuller, 2017).

Practical Advice

There is no need for children to miss school or nursery once they are on treatment (Health Protection Agency, 2007). Screening should be considered for the whole family as other family members (especially children) may be affected. Children's hair brushes and combs should be cleaned with simple bleach. Barbers should disinfect multi-use equipment.

VIRAL INFECTIONS

Molluscum Contagiosum

Molluscum contagiosum is a common skin condition caused by a pox virus which affects 40% of children (Oranje et al., 2015). It is responsible for many consultations in primary care and causes enormous parental anxiety. The condition is self-limiting and relatively harmless but can at times be itchy and uncomfortable. It usually presents as single or multiple umbilicated smooth, flesh coloured dome shaped lesions, which usually last up to 18–24 months (Olsen and Gallagher, 2014). They resolve spontaneously, often becoming inflamed before resolution. They leave no scars unless picked or squeezed.

Treatment

Treatments aim to speed up the healing process but none have been shown to be convincingly effective. Cryotherapy or imiquimod cream are used by some practitioners, but the natural resolution of molluscum contagiosum remains a strong reason for not intervening (van der Wouden et al., 2017).

Herpes Simplex

Herpes simplex (HSV) is a very common acute, self-limiting vesicular eruption. There are two types – HSV 1 and HSV 2. Type 1 is usually facial or non-genital and type 2 is genital due to sexual contact but some cross over is seen (Gawkrodger and Arden-Jones, 2017). It is very contagious and spread by direct contact. The virus penetrates the epidermis and replicates in the epithelial cells. The latent virus will travel down to the dorsal root ganglion where it can lie dormant until in response to some trigger (e.g. colds, strong sunlight, stress, menstruation [Docherty, 2001]). In the future it can reactivate and travel back down the sensory nerve and re-infect the epithelial cells at the nerve ending. This ability to recur is a hallmark of HSV infection.

Primary infection usually occurs in children but can be sub-clinical so go unrecognised. Symptoms include: inflammation of the gums and mouth (gingivostomatitis), rapidly eroding and painful vesicles on the lips (cold sores) and mucous membranes (Chi et al., 2015). Children may be miserable and pyrexial and some can have problems eating and drinking. In severe cases intravenous fluids may be needed. Some children may present with a localised painful vesicle on a finger (herpetic whitlow).

Complications

* These are rare but serious (Gawkrodger and Arden-Jones, 2017). Secondary bacterial infection is usually due to *S. aureus.*
* Eczema herpeticum, where widespread HSV infection occurs in children with eczema is a dermatology emergency requiring urgent input.
* Disseminated HSV in neonates or immunosuppressed children is also serious.
* Herpes encephalitis may not always be accompanied by skin lesions.
* Erythema multiforme (EM) HSV is the most common cause of recurrent EM – an immune-mediated disease characterised by target lesions (lesions named for their resemblance to the bull's eye of a shooting target) on the hands and feet.

Management

Mild HSV may not need any treatment at all.

Children with more severe disease will need symptomatic management with oral fluids and paracetamol. Topical or systemic aciclovir may be needed for severe attacks in the neonate, the immunocompromised or children with eczema herpeticum. Prophylaxis may need to be used in some cases.

Anogenital Warts

Warts in the anogenital region can be harmless and transfer can happen at delivery or from a parent when handling and caring for the child. However perianal warts can be an indicator of sexual abuse and it is sensible to seek advice from a paediatrician when treating genital warts in children.

Hand, Foot and Mouth Disease

This occurs in epidemics amongst young children. It is commonly due to Coxsackie A16 virus or less commonly Enterovirus 71. Children usually present with fevers, general malaise, oral blisters or ulcers and red-edged vesicles on the hands and feet (Gawkrodger and Arden-Jones, 2017). These symptoms usually appear about 3–6 days after exposure to the virus and will generally resolve within a week. Children require supportive measures, for example, ibuprofen and or paracetamol and encouragement with oral fluids. Hand washing may prevent spread, and children should stay away from nursery or school until clear.

Chickenpox (Varicella Zoster)

Varicella is an acute, highly infectious disease common in children under the age of 10 (Macartney and McIntyre, 2008). It is caused by the varicella-zoster virus (VZV) which also causes shingles and has an incubation period of 7–21 days. It is infectious from 5 days before the rash develops until 6 days after. It is characterised by a widespread maculopapular rash which turns into vesicles. It often starts on the trunk and then moves to the limbs. Some children will have only a few spots but some will have very widespread disease. Lesions are often seen at multiple stages of development at once – vesicles, papules and crusted lesions. Fever and general malaise are also usually present.

Management

This is a serious disease in neonates, and pregnant women, children and adults who are immunocompromised. In these groups exposure to the virus may require varicella-zoster immunoglobulin (VZIG), and in those who develop the disease treatment with systemic aciclovir.

* For most healthy children the disease is self-limiting and treatment is supportive.
* Paracetamol and ibuprofen should be given for pyrexia.
* Traditionally lotions, for example, calamine are used although there is limited evidence to support their use (Tebrugge et al., 2006) or the use of systemic antihistamines.
* Lukewarm baths may provide some relief.
* Scabs should not be picked off but left to fall off naturally.
* Oral fluids should be encouraged – a small number of children with sores in their mouths may require intravenous fluids.

Complications

The most common is secondary bacterial infection (Macartney and McIntyre, 2008). More serious are pneumonia, encephalitis, dehydration, hepatitis and ataxia. Women who contract varicella in the first 20 weeks of pregnancy have a 2% risk of the fetus developing congenital varicella syndrome and women in the last trimester have an increased risk of pneumonia.

VZV does remain dormant in the dorsal ganglia and can reactivate to cause herpes zoster (shingles). Primary infection usually provides lifelong immunity but secondary infections can occur.

INFESTATIONS

Scabies

Scabies is an itchy parasitic infection of the skin caused by the scabies mite, *Sarcoptes scabiei*, and spread through skin-to-skin contact or more rarely contact with infested fomites, for example, clothing and towels (Gawkrodger and Arden-Jones, 2017). The mites burrow into the epidermis and the female lays eggs, which hatch and develop into adults in 2 weeks. They have a life cycle of 6 weeks. The mites and their products, for example, eggs, faeces and dead parasites cause an immediate or delayed hypersensitivity reaction, usually about 3 to 6 weeks after the first infestation.

The condition leads to intense itching, which is often worse at night, and disseminated inflammatory papules around the umbilicus, genitals, waist, breasts, buttocks, axillary folds, wrists, interdigital spaces and fingers (Strong and Johnstone, 2007). Babies may also have papules on the scalp, trunk, palms and soles. Secondary bacterial infection can occur.

Diagnosis

Usually made on clinical findings and examination.

Treatment

Treatment options vary worldwide. Where treatment is required for mass populations oral ivermectin is usually given, but in Europe topical treatments such 5% permethrin cream or less commonly malathion liquid (Strong and Johnstone, 2007) are usually used. Treatment must be given and used simultaneously by the affected child and all other family members including any other close contacts. Failure to achieve these, results in ongoing issues and is a common problem.

Treatment should be applied to dry skin. Baths should not be taken before the applications as this will increase absorption of the treatment. Treatment should be applied to all skin (not just the itchy parts) from the neck down including groins and axillae, finger and toe webs and under nails after which clean clothes should be put on. Children under the age of 2 years should also have their heads treated, taking care not to get the treatment in the eyes or mouth. Treatment is left on overnight for 8–12 hours, repeating application if hands are washed during this period. A shower or bath should then be undertaken. The whole treatment should be repeated after 7 days.

Clothing, bedding, towels and any other items should all be machine washed at 50 degrees or higher, dry cleaned or sealed and stored in a plastic bag for one week (BAD, 2020a).

Scratching should subside but can continue for up to 6 weeks and a topical steroid can be used for any persistent papular areas. Treatment failure is usually due to incorrect application of treatment or failure to treat a close contact, so clear verbal and written explanation should be given to parents and carers.

ECZEMA

Atopic eczema (atopic dermatitis) is a chronic inflammatory itchy, dry skin condition (National Institute for Health and Care Excellence [NICE], 2007) with increased transepidermal water loss. It is an episodic disease of exacerbations and remissions. Atopy defines those who have an inherited tendency to develop asthma, allergic rhinitis or eczema (Gawkrodger and Arden-Jones, 2017). *A-topos* is the Greek for alien (or out of place) and eczema means to boil out. It is episodic and marked by flares and remissions affecting up to 15%–20% of children by the age of two, clearing in most by teenage years with reported rates of 65% by age seven and 74% by sixteen (Williams and Strachan, 1998).

The causes of eczema are not completely understood but progress has been made and it is thought to result from a weakened skin barrier and a predisposition towards allergic inflammation (Agner et al., 2016). Although whether the primary issue is defects in the skin barrier leading to increased allergen exposure and subsequent IgE sensitisation, or the immune system is the primary issue and the skin barrier becomes dysfunctional secondary to the IgE sensitisation, is not clear (Elias et al., 2009). Skin barrier function can be affected by loss or reduced function of filaggrin protein (*FLG*), increased protease activity affecting skin pH and impaired lipid processing (Bolognia et al., 2017). A loss-of-function mutation of the *FLG* gene is the strongest genetic risk factor for atopic eczema. There is also a deficit in the amount of certain types of lipids along with some compositional changes and a reduction in the total amount of lipids. This leads to impaired skin barrier function allowing for entry of allergens into the skin and the release of proinflammatory cytokines (a large group of small proteins secreted by specific immune cells and important in cell signalling) which cause inflammation of the skin (Ager et al., 2016). At the same time Th2 cytokine IL-4 and IL-1 down regulate the expression of *FLG* so causing further damage to the skin barrier.

The publication of guidelines (NICE, 2007), and the Royal College of Paediatrics and Child Health (RCPCH) in 2011 on the management of eczema recognised the importance of giving professionals a structured and stepped approach tailored to the severity of the eczema to work on, while also emphasising the need for professionals to adopt a family-centred, holistic approach, and emphasising the importance of meeting the educational needs of children and their parents and carers. Despite this, many parents feel that health professionals fail to take the condition seriously, and they are subjected to a 'trial and error' approach as well as experiencing a great deal of conflicting advice (Santer et al., 2012).

Diagnostic criteria for atopic dermatitis/eczema

- Evidence of an itchy skin condition (or reported scratching or rubbing in a child) plus three or more of the following:
- History of flexural involvement or the cheeks in children under 4 years
- History of asthma or hay fever (or in a first-degree relative in children under 4 years of age)
- History of generalised dry skin in the past year
- Visible flexural eczema (or eczema affecting the cheeks and forehead and outer limbs in children under 4 years
- Onset under 2 years of age (not always diagnostic if child is less than 4 years of age)

McHenry PM, Williams HC, Bingham EA 1995 Management of atopic eczema. British Medical Journal 310:843-847.

Lichenfication or thickening, extensor surface rather than flexural eczema and discoid, follicular and papular patterns of eczema are all more commonly seen in children of Black and Minority Ethnic groups, (Atherton 1995).

Assessment of eczema severity

Eczema can and does have significant physical, psychological and financial effects on families lives, (Beattie and Lewis 2006; Yang et al 2009). Sleep disturbance in particular may have a long term effect ton children and their day time functioning, (Camfferman et al 2010) and a marked impact on parental sleep patterns (Moore et al 2006).

Severity of eczema varies from clear and mild through moderate to severe where clear skin will have no impact on quality of life through to severe where eczema will be widespread with incessant itching, thickened and dry skin and severe limitations on everyday life and activities and nightly sleep disturbance.

NICE (2007) stresses the need for holistic assessment at each consultation generally based on:

- Clinical signs associated with disease activity
- Extent of disease
- Symptoms such as itch and sleep disturbance
- Quantities and strength of treatments required
- Impact of disease on the child and family's quality of life and functioning.

This assessment can be done using several objective tools which include the infant and children's dermatology life quality indices, (Lewis-Jones 1995) as well as visual analogue scales and the patient orientated eczema measure (POEM).

Triggers

Triggers include irritants, for example, soaps and detergents, infections, and allergens including contact, food and aeroallergens, nylon clothing, house dust mite and animal dander. The role of factors such as stress, humidity or temperature extremes is not clear (Ersser and van Onselen, 2010).

Treatment

There is currently no cure for eczema but there are many treatments available and the aim is to use them to control the condition. Treatments should be tailored to the severity of the eczema in a stepped approach (NICE, 2007), with emollients as a basis, and other treatments, for example, topical corticosteroids being added or stopped as the eczema flares or remits. The main cause of treatment failure is parents/carers not using prescribed topical treatments (Bewley et al., 2008; Santer et al., 2013). Factors which have been identified by families for this are: lack of knowledge, complicated treatment regimes, not knowing how much or when to use treatments, dissatisfaction with treatment strategies, infrequent follow-up, 'steroid phobia' and the use of complementary therapies (Sokolova & Smith, 2015), conflicting advice (Santer and Burgess, 2012, 2013), and sometimes difficulty accepting the 'control not cure' strategy offered by health professionals (Smith et al., 2010; Santer et al., 2013).

Many parents struggle with the physical and emotional burden of caring for a child with eczema (Eliott and Luker, 1997; Santer et al., 2012, 2013). Parents feel exhausted and stressed out, and many report child resistance to treatments resulting in 'cream wars'. Health professionals need to address these issues and offer parents and carers realistic regimes, (Lawton, 2014) in conjunction with balanced and consistent information about treatment plans. These should be delivered verbally, via demonstration, and in writing and reiterated on further consultations (Santer and Burgess, 2013).

Emollients

Emollients which increase hydration in the stratum corneum (Voegeli, 2011) are the mainstay of managing eczema but are often underused. They should be used even when there is no active disease. They are available as bath oils, soap substitutes and lotions, gels, sprays, creams and ointments. In general, the drier the child's skin, the greasier the leave-on emollient should be, but it is also recognised that the most effective emollient is one that the child and family like and will therefore use (Carr, 2009; Voegeli, 2011).

The value of bath oils has been controversial for some time (DTB, 2007; Tarr and Iheanacho, 2013). The BATHE trial (Santer et al., 2018), which looked at the use of bath emollients in children aged 1 to 11 years with parents reporting moderately severe eczema, found no clinical evidence of clinical benefit from the inclusion of emollient bath additives in the standard management of eczema in children. However, babies and children with severe eczema may well benefit from their use and this needs more research (Flohr and Ahmed, 2018). There is consensus that all children will require the use of a soap substitute. The use of water softeners has not been found to reduce eczema severity (Thomas et al., 2011). Chronic use of diluted bleach has been shown to decrease the clinical severity of eczema in children with clinical signs of secondary infection and is used in some centres (Huang et al., 2009; Guys' and St Thomas' NHS Trust, 2016).

Practical demonstrations on how to apply emollients should be carried out. They should be applied in the direction of hair growth to discourage folliculitis and allowed to 'sink

TABLE 23.2	Examples of Emollients			
Lotions	**Creams and Gels**	**Ointments**	**Bath Additives**	**Sprays**
Eucerin intensive (10% urea)	Balneum plus (contains urea and anti-pruritic lauro-macrogals)	50% White soft paraffin 50% liquid paraffin (50:50)	Balneum bath oil	Dermamist
E45 Lotion	Unguentum M	White soft paraffin	Balneum plus bath oil (soya oil with anti-pruritic lauromacrogals)	Emollin
Dermol 500 lotion	Doublebase	Emulsifying ointment	Oilatum junior (fragrance free)	
Aveeno lotion	E45 cream	Yellow soft paraffin	Oilatum shower gel	
Keri lotion	Eucerin intensive cream (10% urea)	Diprobase ointment	Oilatum bath formula	
	Diprobase cream	Hydrous ointment	Oilatum Plus (with benzalkonium chloride and triclosan)	
	Dermol cream (contains antiseptic)	Epaderm ointment	E45 bath additive	
	Cetraben cream	Hydromol ointment	Alpha keri bath	
	Epaderm cream		Dermalo	
	Aveeno cream		Diprobath	
	Calmurid (contains urea)		Hydromol emollient	
	Hydromol cream		Doublebase emollient shower	
	Aqueous cream (soap substitute)		QV bath oil	
	QV cream		Dermol 600 bath emollient (with benzalkonium chloride)	
	Oilatum cream		Dermol 200 shower emollient	

(British Dermatological Nursing Group (BDNG), 2012. Best practice emollient therapy: a statement for healthcare professionals. Dermatol. Nurs. 11 (4), s1–s19.)

in'. They should not be mixed with topical corticosteroids as this is likely to dilute the steroid and they are probably best applied at least 20 minutes before emollients (Voegeli, 2011). Frequency of application will depend on the severity of the child's eczema but for many will need to be done at least twice a day and more often if the child's skin is very dry (Charman and Lawton, 2006) including at school. It is also essential that sufficient quantities are prescribed for the child. NICE (2007) recommends at least 250 g per child per week. If ointments are used there is an increased risk of contamination and it is advisable to use a spatula or clean spoon to decant from the pot to avoid contamination (Lawton, 2014). Parents should be advised to take moisturiser with them when out. The use of olive oil should be discouraged due to its adverse effects on the integrity of the stratum corneum and mineral based emollients should be used instead (Danby et al., 2013) (Table 23.2).

Topical Corticosteroids

Topical corticosteroids (TCS) are widely agreed to be very important in the treatment of children's eczema for many years. They inhibit the production and action of inflammatory mediators in the skin and thus reduce inflammation and itch. When used appropriately they are safe and effective with rare side effects enabling children to achieve maximum clinical benefit. Unfortunately many children worldwide have undertreated eczema due to steroid phobia mainly related to belief about skin thinning, which is often generated and reinforced by health professionals who also exhibit steroid

phobia similar to parents, and affect parental perspectives and TCS adherence in a negative way (Bewley, 2008; Mooney et al., 2015; Bos et al., 2019). Contrary to popular belief TCS do not cause atrophy, hypopigmentation, hypertrichosis, osteoporosis, purpura or telangiectasia when used appropriately (Mooney et al., 2015). Striae, short-term hypothalamic pituitary axis alteration and ophthalmological disease are rare and usually follow prolonged and excessive use of TCS. It is essential that health professionals offer balanced, consistent and informed advice about their use in conjunction with practical demonstration of their use.

How to use TCS

- Use only when the eczema is not controlled by emollients, and apply only to active areas of eczema (red, itchy, inflamed, lichenified or thickened) and on open areas of eczema, but not on open areas of skin due to cuts or surgical wounds, and stop when there is no active disease.
- Avoid the advice to 'use sparingly' (Bewley, 2008; Carr, 2009; Smith et al., 2016) because it sends out a message that TCS are inherently dangerous and is likely to discourage their use.
- Apply a sufficient amount to the eczema to make the skin shiny rather than the 'fingertip unit' method advocated by many health care professionals, which is difficult and confusing for parents and children to calculate (Carr, 2009).
- Apply no more than once to twice daily as indicated on prescription.
- Ointments are generally more effective than cream formulations (except on very wet infected eczema).

TABLE 23.3	Topical Corticosteroids and Their Potencies	
Potency	**Formulation**	**Proprietary Name**
Mild	Hydrocortisone 0.1%–2.5%	*Dioderm, Efcortelan*
	Hydrocortisone with antimicrobials	*Canesten HC, Daktacort, Fucidn H*
Moderately potent	0.05% clobetasone butyrate	*Eumovate*
	0.05% aclometasone dipropionate	*Modrasone*
	0.05% clobetasone butyrate with antimicrobials	*Trimovate*
Potent	0.1% bethamethasone valerate	*Betnovate*
	fluticasone propionate	*Cutivate*
	mometasone furoate	*Elocon*
	0.1% betamethasone valerate with antimicrobials	*Fucibet, Betnovate C*
Very potent	clobetasol propionate	*Dermovate*

- Combination antibiotic steroid preparation should only be used for 14 days as longer use can encourage bacterial resistance.
- In general, potent and very potent steroids should be avoided for children unless prescribed by a dermatology specialist (Table 23.3).

Additional Management Options

Calcineurin Inhibitors

Tacrolimus and pimecrolimus are useful second-line treatments for moderate to severe atopic eczema (NICE, 2004). They have anti-inflammatory properties but are not TCS so do not cause skin atrophy and are safe for use on the face and around the eyes. There may be an initial burning or stinging sensation when applied but this usually wears off. There is no reliable data demonstrating an increased risk of skin cancer as was initially identified (Burr, 2003). It is recommended that treatment with these products is only initiated by physicians with experience in dermatology.

Antihistamines

There is no support for the routine use of antihistamines but a trial of non-sedating antihistamines for a month in children with severe itching or urticarial may be offered (NICE, 2007). Disease control is crucial in improving sleep (Patel et al., 2018), but short-term use of sedating antihistamines to help children to sleep may be helpful coupled with behavioural techniques.

Silk Garments

The use of these garments is unlikely to be cost effective for health providers even if the small observed benefits in a recent study were genuine (Thomas and Bradshaw, 2017).

Complementary Therapy

Many parents are keen to make use of complementary therapies, often due to concerns about using topical corticosteroids. Several herbal medicines, for example, Wau wa cream, Abido, OSAS and Magic cream have all been found to contain potent or super potent TCS (National Eczema Society, 2015). Homeopathy is frequently suggested but there is no evidence to suggest it is an efficacious treatment for eczema (Ernst, 2012). There is also no convincing evidence of any benefit from dietary supplements, for example, evening primrose oil, borage or fish oil (Bath-Hextall et al., 2012).

Skin Infections

Bacteria and viruses can all worsen eczema and are probably the most common reasons for children with eczema to be in hospital. Bacterial infections are the most common and should always be considered where adequate use of a mild or moderately potent topical steroid and emollients have not controlled a child's eczema within 7 to 14 days. The signs and symptoms of bacterial infection (NICE, 2007) with *S. aureus* and/or *Streptococcus* include weeping, pustules, and crusts, atopic eczema failing to respond to therapy, rapidly worsening atopic eczema, fever and malaise. A bacterial skin swab should be taken if organisms other than *S. aureus* are suspected or if antibiotic resistance is relevant.

Eczema herpeticum caused by herpes simplex is much less common but can spread very quickly and potentially be very serious (Charman and Lawton, 2006). Signs of this infection are:

1. Areas of rapidly worsening atopic eczema.
2. Clustered blisters consistent with early stage cold sores.
3. Punched out erosions (circular, depressed, ulcerated lesions) usually 1–3 mm that are uniform in appearance but may coalesce to form larger areas of erosion with crusting.
4. Possible fever, lethargy or distress (NICE, 2007).

Children with this infection will need treatment with aciclovir and appropriate systemic antibiotics if secondary bacterial infection is suspected or present. They should be referred for same day specialist dermatological advice, and in some children with involvement of the skin around the eyes ophthalmologic advice may be indicated. Some children will require hospital admission.

Food Allergies and Dietary Management

Food allergy is more common in children with eczema. It is an immune-mediated hypersensitivity reaction to food and can be divided into immunoglobulin E (IgE), mediated (immediate onset) reactions and non-IgE mediated (delayed) reaction affecting respiratory, skin and gastrointestinal systems (RCPCH, 2011). The risk of food allergy is greatest among those with early onset and severe eczema (Martin et al., 2014). Cows' milk protein, egg, peanut, wheat and soy are the most common allergens. Symptoms of non-mediated allergy in infants include gastro-oesophageal reflux, loose or frequent stools, blood or mucus in stools, colic, poor feeding and faltering growth. Management will involve allergy-specific advice with avoidance of relevant allergens, prevention and treatment of further reactions and dietetic support. Care does need to be taken to ensure that only foods relevant to the causality of eczema are removed to avoid the risk of unnecessary nutritional compromise (Rancé 2008). A heightened awareness of food allergy risk amongst health care practitioners treating infants with eczema, especially if early onset and severe, is warranted.

There is currently not enough evidence to recommend using probiotics for the treatment of eczema (Boyle et al., 2008).

School

The difficulties faced at nursery and school by children with eczema are often underestimated. Eczema can cause practical problems, for example, need for emollients, hand writing, hand washing, physical education (PE), swimming and exams as well as issues with self-esteem. Children should have a health care plan outlining their needs. They should be able (with appropriate help and supervision) to use soap substitutes and apply their emollients in an appropriate private space. Children may need extra time before and after swimming lessons to apply emollients and shower. Small children will need distraction if itchy. Other pupils may need information about eczema (National Eczema Society, 2017) and staff may need to be alert to any difficulties children with eczema experience with other pupils.

Severe Eczema

Some children with widespread or difficult to treat severe disease where topical treatments are ineffective may require treatment with phototherapy or systemic treatments: ciclosporin, methotrexate and less commonly azathioprine or a short course of oral prednisolone. These all need careful monitoring of the child and should only be prescribed by a dermatology specialist. Children with recurrently infected eczema as well as those whose quality of life is markedly affected should be referred to specialist dermatology services (NICE, 2007).

Education and Information

Treatments will not work unless the child and their parents and carers understand how and when to apply and use them as lack of information, strain, helplessness and lack of confidence in medical treatments all lead to suboptimal treatment (Smith et al., 2010). Health professionals need to make sure that they spend time educating children and their parents on how often and how much of the treatments to use, how to step treatments up or down and how to deal with infected eczema

(NICE, 2007). This should involve practical demonstrations (Lawton, 2014). It is also important that information is clear and unambiguous (Lewis-Jones, 1995) and in language which parents can understand, if necessary, making use of health advocates or interpreters (Kell and Hawkins, 2005). There are storybooks available, although these are aimed more at the younger child and tend to focus on the use of emollients (Tappel, 2018). All information should be reinforced at every consultation, addressing any factors which could affect adherence (NICE, 2007). Written information should be supplied as appropriate as this can help with adherence (Edwards and Titman, 2010).

Resources
National Eczema Society

Formed in 1975, The National Eczema Society has two principal aims: first, to provide people with independent and practical advice about treating and managing eczema; secondly, to raise awareness of the needs of those with eczema with health care professionals, teachers and the government.
Hill House Highgate Hill London N19 5NA
www.eczema.org.uk
0207 281 3553
Eczema information helpline 0870 241 3604

PSORIASIS

Psoriasis is a relatively common chronic non-infectious immune-mediated inflammatory skin condition affecting about 1% of children worldwide, about a third of whom have a strong family history of the disease. At least nine possible chromosomal loci for genes linked to psoriasis have been found (Gawkrodger and Arden-Jones, 2017). There is no cure. It is now widely recognised as a systemic immune-mediated disorder associated with metabolic diseases which can impact on life expectancy (Reich, 2012). Children with psoriasis have higher rates of obesity, hyperlipidaemia, hypertension, diabetes, metabolic syndrome, polycystic ovarian syndrome, non-alcoholic liver disease and elevated liver function enzyme levels than children who do not have psoriasis. Children with psoriasis are also at increased risk of developing these comorbidities irrespective of obesity status. These increased metabolic risks warrant early monitoring and lifestyle modification (Paller et al., 2013; Tollefson et al., 2018).

Psoriasis is characterised by an over proliferation of keratinocytes replicating too quickly. The number of cycling epidermal cells is increased seven-fold but the cell cycle time is not reduced (Gawkrodger and Arden-Jones, 2017). This is driven by the activation of certain helper T cells producing interleukin (IL)-17, IL-22 and tumour necrosis factor (TNF) which orchestrate the inflammation in the skin resulting in the proliferation of keratinocytes and endothelial cells. A further key cytokine with potent IL-17 and IL-22 promoting properties is IL-23 (Eberle et al., 2016; Eichenfeld et al., 2018). Understanding of these pathways is fundamental to understanding the role of biologic treatments which aim to directly neutralise IL-23 or IL-17.

The incidence and prevalence of psoriasis in childhood are steadily increasing and it is recognised that it has the potential for significant medical, social, financial and psychological burdens with a significant impact on affected children and their families and carers (Shah t al., 2015; Tollefson et al., 2018; Eichenfeld et al., 2018).

Presentation

Psoriasis varies in severity from mild to widespread and life threatening. Some children will have scalp involvement and some also nail changes.

See Table 23.4 for presentations.

Management
Topical

This will vary dependent on severity but may include topical corticosteroids, emollients, vitamin D analogues (calcipotriol), mixes of steroid and vitamin D analogues, calcineurin inhibitors and dithranol. As with eczema management children and parents and carers will need education in their use and application. These will all be used in conjunction with emollients.

Phototherapy

Phototherapy, particularly narrow band ultraviolet B, is widely used, safe and effective, but does have a cumulative effect and requires two to three visits per week. This may not be practical for some families (Eichenfeld et al., 2018).

TABLE 23.4 Presentation Patterns of Psoriasis

Presentation Pattern	
Plaque	Well-defined, disc shaped plaques involving knees, elbows, scalp, hair margin or sacrum
	Plaques usually red, covered in scale
	Sometimes itchy
Guttate	Acute symmetrical eruption
	Raindrop-like pattern
	Usually trunk and limbs
	May follow streptococcal throat infection
Generalised pustular	Rare but serious
	Sheets of small yellowish pustules on erythematous background
	Spread rapidly
	Child unwell with fever and malaise
Nail	Thimble pitting most common
Scalp	Generally quite well demarcated and scale thickened
Napkin psoriasis	Well-defined psoriasiform eruption in the nappy area of infants. Few go on to develop true psoriasis

(Gawkrodger, D.J., Arden-Jones, M.R., 2017. Dermatology: An Illustrated Colour Text. Elsevier, London.)

Conventional Systemic Therapy

Methotrexate, acitretin and ciclosporin are all systemic agents which can be used to treat children with severe disease but they require specialist input and monitoring.

Biologics

Targeted therapy for psoriasis has dramatically altered the treatment landscape for adults with psoriasis. These target cytokines in the inflammatory cascade and are slowly being added to the therapy options for children.

Psychological

The psychological impact of psoriasis on children and their parents is well recognised (Tollefson et al., 2018; Eichenfeld et al., 2018) and development of support strategies for families is recommended.

Psoriasis Association
Dick Coles House 2 Queensbridge Northampton NN4 7BF
01604 251 620
mail@psoriasis-asociation.org.uk

ACNE VULGARIS

Acne is one of the most common skin conditions affecting most adolescents. It usually starts at puberty but can also occur in young children. It can run in families but most cases are sporadic and occur for unknown reasons. It is characterised by open comedones (blackheads) and closed comedones (whiteheads), pustules, papules, cysts and scars. It varies in severity from a few spots on the face, neck, back or chest to much more significant problems which can result in scarring. It can also impact on a young person's self-confidence and psychological well-being (Halvorsen et al., 2011) (BAD, 2020b).

Acne results from:
- Increased sebum secretion by the sebaceous glands due to hyper-responsiveness to circulating hormones – mostly androgens.
- Pilosebaceous duct hyperkeratosis and comedone formation.
- Colonisation of the duct with *Propionibacterium acnes*.
- Release of inflammatory mediators.
- Some medications, for example, contraceptive injection or pills or potent topical steroids inappropriately used on the face can trigger acne.

(Gawkrodger and Arden-Jones, 2017)

Management

There is currently no cure for acne but treatments can be very effective in preventing the formation of new spots and scarring. Treatment depends on the type and severity of the acne and the young person's psychological state. Young people will often have tried over-the-counter products before seeking further help and it is important that nurses understand the use of these so they can support young people to use them effectively and appropriately. It is very important that patients understand that there are really no quick treatment option and results from treatments will only be seen over a prolonged period of weeks to months. Most patients will also need a combination of treatments tackling different elements of the disease process and patients often need further explanations.

Acne treatment falls into the following categories:

1. Topical treatments
2. Oral antibiotics
3. Oral contraceptive
4. Isotretinoin capsules

Topical Treatments

These usually work well for those with mild acne and are usually also needed in addition to systemic treatments for those with more severe acne. There are a variety of these, for example, benzoyl peroxide, antibiotics (e.g. erythromycin, tetracycline and clindamycin), retinoids (e.g. tretinoin, isotretinoin and adapalene), azelaic acid and nicotinamide. These should all be applied to the whole affected area and not just to individual spots, usually at night or sometimes twice daily depending on the treatment. Some can be irritating to the skin so it may be advised that the treatment is initially used on just a small area of skin for a few applications before being applied to the whole area. Patients are sometimes then advised to start using the treatment once or twice daily before gradually building up to regular daily use (Penzer, 2010).

Oral Antibiotics

Antibiotics may be prescribed and are usually erythromycin or a type of tetracycline. Tetracycline should not be given to children under 12 years because deposition of tetracycline in growing bones and teeth through binding with calcium causes staining, and in some cases, hypodontia (BNF, 2019). The antibiotics need to be given for at least 2 months and often up to 6 months. Some should not be taken at the same time as food.

Hormonal Therapies

The combined oral contraceptive pill containing both oestrogen and progesterone has been found to be effective in reducing acne lesions in females with moderate to severe acne. They are less suitable for young teenage girls in whom ovulation is less well established. These treatments do increase the risk of deep vein thrombosis particularly in patients who smoke, are overweight or have a family history of this.

Isotretinoin

Isotretinoin belongs to a group of drugs closely related to vitamin A (BAD, 2019c) and is a very effective treatment for severe acne. It can only be prescribed if patients are under the care of a dermatologist in the UK. While not a cure most patients see a significant improvement in their acne. It works by reducing sebum excretion, inhibiting *P. acnes* and also has an anti-inflammatory effect. Dosage is weight based. A course lasts for 4–6 months dependent on how well the patient can tolerate the drug and will generally be continued until there are no new spots. It is better absorbed when taken after a meal or snack containing some fat. Alcohol is best avoided.

Side effects. Side effects are significant and require detailed discussion with patients (Penzer, 2010).

Side effects include dry sensitive skin, chapped lips, dry eyes and sometimes dry nose and nose bleeds if the inside of the nose is very dry. Patients should carry a lip balm or Vaseline with them at all times, and if they are a contact lens user they should use soft lenses or wear glasses. Patients should be advised to avoid waxing, epilation and dermabrasion whilst taking isotretinoin and for at least 6 months afterwards.

Side effects include the following:

- Increased sensitivity to the sun so sun exposure should be avoided and if necessary, a high factor sun protection product should be used.
- Muscle and joint aches especially after exercise.
- Temporary hair thinning.
- Vision can be affected, especially night vision.
- Increased serum lipid levels and mild liver inflammation so these should be monitored during treatment.
- Peanut or soy allergy.

Isotretinoin contains soya oil and occasionally patients with soya allergy may react to trace levels and rarely patients with peanut allergy may cross-react to soya proteins in the oil.

Rare and more serious side effects

Psychological impact. Isotretinoin can lead to changes in mood and/or behaviour and there have been reports of suicide. Acne in itself can lead to patients feeling low and any patients who have ever had low mood, suicidal ideations, depression or any other mental health problem may need assessment by a psychiatrist before starting isotretinoin. Patients should also be advised that if family or friends are concerned at all about their behaviour or mood changes while they are taking isotretinoin, they should see their doctor and stop taking it immediately.

Teratogenic effect. Isotretinoin is teratogenic so pregnancy prevention is key while taking isotretinoin and for a month afterwards for female patients. Young people need to be sensitively assessed on their sexual activity before starting. If not sexually active they may opt out of the pregnancy prevention programme. If sexually active a pregnancy test must be undertaken before starting treatment and at monthly intervals during the course before further prescriptions are issued. Females must use one or ideally two forms of contraception for a month before starting treatment and continue until 5 weeks after treatment to allow for the drug to be completely excreted from the body (BAD, 2019c).

General Advice for Skin Care (BAD, 2020b)

There is very little evidence that any foods cause acne. Diet can influence acne. High glycaemic index (GI) diets e.g. sugar and sugary foods, white bread, potatoes, white rice etc) have been shown to cause or aggravate acne so switching to a low GI diet may help. There is also some evidence that consuming milk and dairy products may trigger acne in some people but this hasn't been studied yet in much detail.

- Wash gently with oil-free soaps and washes.
- Try to avoid squeezing spots but this can be difficult (Penzer, 2010), so if squeezing pustules, stretch the skin on either side with a tissue rather than nails. Whiteheads should not be squeezed.

- Foundation and cover up can make acne worse, but try and use non-comedogenic products which are probably less troublesome.
- There is very little evidence that any foods cause acne.
- Acne is a distressing disease for young people to cope with and manage and nursing support and education may help to ensure treatments are used appropriately and effectively.

WWW

www.acnesupport.org.uk

INFANTILE HAEMANGIOMAS

Infantile haemangiomas (Greek for blood-vessel growth; BAD, 2017) are the most common vascular tumours of infancy affecting about 4% of infants. They are sometimes called 'strawberry marks' because the surface of some look similar to a strawberry. The pathogenesis is still not fully understood but endothelial cells start to overgrow either when in utero or soon after birth. They can be superficial or deep in the skin and affect other organs, most commonly the liver. Haemangiomas are more common in premature and low-birth-weight infants, twin/multiple pregnancies, females and Caucasians, and placental anomalies are an important risk factor. Most affect the face but any part of the skin or organs can be affected. If an infant has more than 5–10 haemangiomas, an abdominal ultrasound should be carried out to look for haemangiomas deeper in the body.

Haemangiomas usually appear in the first few weeks of life as a small red mark or swelling and grow rapidly for the first few months, but can continue to grow slowly for the following 6–12 months. Most haemangiomas then spontaneously shrink in size for up to 10 years, but some don't grow much at all and some don't shrink. Most leave no visible mark but some resolve with residual blood vessels visible and some may leave a scar, a pale area of skin or an area of loose or thickened tissue. These require no treatment at all.

About 10%–15% of haemangiomas need intervention due to ulceration, functional impairment, or a risk of disfigurement (Hoeger et al., 2015; Solman et al., 2018). Since 2008 oral propranolol has radically changed the treatment of infantile haemangiomas and is the first line therapeutic agent although its exact mechanism is still not completely understood.

Ulceration

Ulceration is the most common problem in 15% of patients, mostly in the first 4 months. Approximately 50% involve the lower lip and perineum. These can be very painful and often result in scarring.

Functional Impairment

Vision

Periocular haemangiomas need treatment if causing or likely to cause visual impairment by occluding the visual axis, compressing the globe or expanding into the retrobulbar space. Up to 80% of children with untreated periocular haemangiomas will have complications such as amblyopia, refractive errors and strabismus. These children also need ophthalmology review.

Breathing

Haemangiomas which block the nostril can impact on feeding as well as breathing. Airway haemangiomas can develop in babies who do not have skin lesions. The risk of airway haemangiomas is higher with segmental haemangiomas found in a 'beard distribution'. These babies must be assessed for respiratory symptoms such as hoarseness and stridor and need to be managed in conjunction with an ENT specialist.

Feeding

Haemangiomas of the lip can adversely affect feeding, especially if ulcerated and nursing care of the ulceration is very important.

Ear

If a haemangioma is causing symptomatic obstruction of the ear canal, which usually results in recurrent ear infections, treatment is also warranted.

Disfigurement

This can result from haemangiomas located in central areas of the face, particularly nose, lip, forehead and cheek and on the ears.

Management

Ultrasound and magnetic resonance imaging (MRI) scanning may be required for large subcutaneous or multiple haemangiomas.

Topical beta-blockers can be used on smaller areas. These block beta-adrenergic receptor making the blood vessels narrower and reducing the amount of blood flowing through them. These are dropped on to the haemangioma and spread carefully with a clean finger to cover the surface (Great Ormond Street for Children NHS Foundation Trust, 2014).

Oral Propranolol

This has revolutionised the management of haemangiomas. Its use should be initiated in clinical settings equipped for the safe and immediate management of any adverse event, in particular cardiovascular events. Baseline heart rate and blood pressure are required and baseline glucose levels, in small for dates babies, preterm babies and those with faltering growth or history of hypoglycaemia. Admission is generally recommended for babies under 2 months of age as well as those with the previously listed issues for monitoring of heart rate and blood pressure. Dosage is generally 2–3 mg/kg/day and treatment is usually for at least 6 months or until it is felt the haemangioma will not show any further growth. The response rate is 96%–98%.

Side effects: these are reversible and, in most cases, benign.

Very common: bronchitis, sleep disorders, and diarrhoea and vomiting

Common: bronchiolitis, bronchospasm, slightly decreased blood pressure, nightmares, irritability, somnolence, constipation, cold extremities

Uncommon: AV-block decreased heart rate

Unknown frequency: bradycardia, symptomatic hypotension vasoconstriction, Raynaud phenomenon, hypoglycaemic seizures

EPIDERMOLYSIS BULLOSA

Epidermolysis bullosa (EB) comprises a group of rare inherited diseases resulting from mutations in a large variety of skin genes (Fine et al., 2008). One in 17,000 live births will be an infant with a form of EB (Debra). EB is characterised by fragility and blistering of skin and mucous membranes. This is due to the layers of skin not adhering normally to each other leading to splits between the layers. There are four major types, each with several subtypes, based on the site of blister formation. The disease course is variable dependent on type. Skin biopsy will be needed to classify individual cases. In severe EB generalised blistering, chronic ulcerations and resultant scarring leads to multi-organ involvement, major morbidity and life-threatening complications. There is no cure and multidisciplinary management is based on protecting the skin, avoiding trauma, and reducing the likelihood of infection along with symptomatic treatment of skin and other organ manifestations and complications (El Hachem et al., 2014). The condition carries an enormous family and parental burden (Dufresne et al., 2015). Due to the rarity of EB in the UK care is led from nationally funded centres of expertise (Table 23.5).

TABLE 23.5	Classification of Inherited epidermolysis bullosa (EB)				
Type of EB	**Genetic inheritance**	**Level of cleavage**	**Subtype**	**Location of blisters**	**Disease course**
EB simplex Affects about 70% of EB sufferers	Autosomal dominant	Basal cells of epidermis	Generalised	Areas of friction or trauma	Intense levels of blistering from neonate which heal without scarring
			Weber-Cockayne	Trauma related to hands and feet	
			Dowling-Meara	Generalised severe form Blisters at birth on face, trunk and limbs	As above but can present in adolescence or adulthood
				Can involve mouth GI tract and respiratory tracts	Very rare May be fatal in infants but may subside as child grows up
Junctional (JEB) Affects about 10% of those with EB Generalised severe (previously Herlitz JEB) Affects about 50% of those with JEB	Autosomal recessive	Basement membrane zone		Widespread including mouth and GI and respiratory tracts	From birth Blisters and large eroded areas and pain Scarring Usually fatal in infancy with few surviving to 2nd or 3rd year of life Death usually due to malnutrition, electrolyte imbalance, infection or obstructive airway issues
Junctional Generalised intermediate (previously non Herlitz JEB)	Autosomal recessive	Basement membrane zone		Widespread or localised	As for Junctional severe but less life restrictions
Dystrophic (DEB) About 20% of EB	Autosomal recessive	Subepidermal		Widespread including mouth, pharynx and eyes	Severity variable Blisters appear from trauma or spontaneously and heal with scarring and fusion of fingers and toes Can be problems with eating Abnormal teeth and nails
	Autosomal dominant			Smaller blisters on limbs and areas of trauma	Those with recessive DEB have a high risk of developing a squamous cell carcinoma before the age of 30 years Less serious than recessive but does scar and blistering life long

(Fine, J.D., Eady, R., et al., 2008. The classification of inherited epidermolysis bullosa (EB): report of the Third International Consensus Meeting on Diagnosis and Classification of EB. J. Am. Acad. Dermatol. 58, 931–950; Gawkrodger, D.J., Arden-Jones, M.R., 2017. Dermatology: An Illustrated Colour Text. Elsevier, London.)

Care of the EB Newborn and Infant

The baby with EB will generally stay in hospital until they are clinically stable and the parents feel confident enough to take the baby home and manage the care there with support. In addition to the skin care required, nutritional and feeding issues will need to be addressed, and a precise diagnosis will need to be made through a skin biopsy (El Hachem et al., 2014). The newborn baby with EB will need to have changes made to the way they are fed, handled and have their nappies changed with additional blister and skin care. Babies remain in their hospital of birth and the specialist EB nurses will come to them as the skin of a baby with EB may be extraordinarily sensitive and unnecessary trauma from transportation can thus be avoided. The genetic implications must be clarified and discussed with the parents. Children's community nursing teams and community paediatricians and social care will need to be involved before discharge.

Care:

- Nurse in a cot rather than an incubator if possible as heat and humidity can encourage blisters.
- Remove cord clamp and replace with a ligature to avoid skin damage.
- If needed intravenous access should be via an umbilical venous catheter. Silicone based tape (Mepitac) should be used to secure any lines.
- Naso and pharyngeal suction should be avoided – if needed use a soft catheter and minimal suction.
- Use clip sensors for oximetry.
- If electrodes needed cut off the adhesive ring and use Mepitac.
- Silicone medical adhesive remover, for example, Appeel should be used to remove any dressings, electrodes, clothing or dressing adhered to wounds.
- Apply padding before applying a blood pressure cuff.
- Name bands should not be used.
- Dress babies as they are often irritable and unsettled and will rub and damage their skin if left naked. Once the correct dressings are in place the babies are usually more comfortable and to some extent shielded from trauma. Dress in normal clothes turned inside out so seams can't rub.
- Nappies – the elastic round the legs of nappies will rub so a cotton wipe should be inserted into the nappy and left to cover the elasticated legs. Rather than using water to clean the babies, WSP/LP 50:50 should be used.

(El Hachem et al., 2014).

Feeding

In less severely affected babies breast-feeding may be possible. Soft paraffin should be applied to the nipple and breast and the baby's face and lips to reduce friction.

Bottle fed babies should have the softest teats available. Commercially available teats should be softened with warm boiled water. The teat holes can be enlarged. Haberman teats may be useful as the teat is long and the baby's nose doesn't come into contact with the plastic bottle, and the valve enables the baby to feed with less effort so even babies with oral ulceration can feed. Some babies may find it easier to feed from a spoon.

Nasogastric feeding – a few babies may not be able to fed orally. A small soft polyurethane tube fixed for a few weeks will minimise internal damage and reduce trauma.

Handling

The baby should not be picked up by pushing the hands underneath. Instead they should be rolled away and then back on to the hands and lifted. Never lift under the arms. Handling by parents should be encouraged as early as possible once the correct technique has been learned.

Baths can be done in warm water and then the baby should be patted not rubbed dry with a soft non-fluffy towel or sheet.

Dressings – the baby may need an opioid prior to the procedure. Individual dressings may vary with time but will aim to protect skin from further damage, encourage healing of blistered areas and not stick to wounds. Mepitel is a suitable dressing as it is a silicone mesh which is easily removed with no pain or trauma. A secondary dressing, for example, Mepilex has a similar silicone surface as well as a foam backing to provide protection and absorption from exudative erosive areas. The dressing is then secured with a suitable tubular stretch bandage. These are usually changed about twice a week although if there is a lot of exudate the Mepilex can be changed more often and the Mepitel left in situ. Parents should be educated in their use while in hospital but will need education and support to do so. They will also need practical input and support from their local community children's nursing team as well as ongoing specialist liaison and support from the specialist nurses attached to the national supra-regional centres.

Where fingers or toes are involved, the digits should all be separated by cutting dressings into strips to work between each digit. The first finger should be carefully kept extended and separated from the rest of the hand.

Blisters – puncture new ones as they arise with a sterile needle but leave the roof intact.

Topical antibiotics – these should be used with caution as adverse effects may be systemic as a result of percutaneous absorption.

These children will require long-term input from the multi-disciplinary team. The infants and children will need support in the following areas:

Chronic Issues

- Presence of chronic wounds susceptible to infection
- Chronic itching
- Anaemia and malnutrition secondary to oral and gastrointestinal involvement and chronic wounds
- Psychological problems related to disease acceptance and social relationships (nursery, school, etc.)

(El Hachem et al., 2014; Lynne and James, 2018).

Patient Support Organisation

Debra (Dystrophic EB Research Association)
13 Wellington Business Park

Dukes Ride
Crowthorne
Berkshire RG45 6LS
Tel. 01344 771961
Debra@debra.org.uk
www.debra.org.uk

THE ICHTHYOSES

Ichthyoses are inherited disorders of keratinisation and epidermal differentiation. They are characterised by dry scaly skin and vary from mild to life threatening. Inherited ichthyoses have now been classified into syndromic and non-syndromic; in the latter the disorder is expressed only in the skin. Non-syndromic ichthyoses include autosomal recessive congenital ichthyosis (ARCI), harlequin ichthyosis, lamellar ichthyosis, self-healing collodion baby and congenital ichthyosiform erythroderma. Recently a lot of progress has been made in understanding pathomechanisms, and more genes causing ARCI have been identified (Takeichi and Akiyama, 2016). Emollients are the mainstay of treatment. Urea containing emollients may be used at certain times and sometimes treatment with oral acitretin may be required. These children benefit from specialist dermatology input.

Collodion Baby

This term is applied to a baby's appearance at birth when they are born covered with a parchment-like yellow shiny and tight membrane which can look a bit like a sausage skin. The term is thus a phenotype rather than a disease entity (van Gysel et al., 2002). Facial features may be distorted and the baby's mouth may look as if it is being held open (eclabium) because of the tightness of the skin, which can make sucking and feeding difficult. The eyelids may be everted with exposure of the mucosal membranes (ectropion). The skin is much thicker and less flexible and as a result the fingers and joints can be contracted (Shwayder and Akland, 2005). Constriction bands can also result in reduced blood supply and swelling of the limbs. If the membrane is tight over the chest there can be problems with hypoventilation. As the baby starts to breathe and inflate their chest the membrane will start to tear. The collodion membrane can be complete or localised and usually breaks up over the first 1–2 weeks of life and sheds. It is associated with some risks during the neonatal period, but overall prognosis has improved and current mortality should be negligible. Some of these babies are born prematurely or of low birth weight and some will be the children of consanguineous parents. About 10% of these babies eventually develop normal skin (self-healing collodion baby) (van Gysel et al., 2002) but the rest will go on to develop a form of autosomal recessive congenital ichthyosis (ARCI), lamellar, non-bullous ichthyosiform erythroderma or bathing suit ichthyosis. There is currently no way to predict the final diagnosis. Dermatology and genetic follow-up will be needed. This is clearly a very upsetting time for parents and they will need support and information and education on how to look after their baby's skin.

Classification (see Table 23.6)

Management of Newborn Collodion Baby and Harlequin Ichthyosis

Management is supportive and for many of these babies is best delivered in a neonatal unit with multi-disciplinary input (see Table 23.7).

TABLE 23.6 Classification		
Disorder	**Inheritance**	**Clinical Features**
Harlequin ichthyosis (HI)	Autosomal recessive Due to *ABCA12* mutation	Severe. Three babies born annually in UK and 50% will die during neonatal period. Born encased in 'armour' of thick scale plates separated by deep fissures. Hyperkeratosis. Ectropion and eclabium. Constricting bands around extremities can restrict movement. Prone to sepsis, dehydration and impaired thermoregulation (Rajpopat et al., 2011). Treatment with oral acitretin encourages shedding of the thickened skin. Babies will need care similar to collodion babies during the neonatal period. Multi-disciplinary care will be needed. Babies who survive into infancy and beyond develop skin changes resembling severe congenital ichthyosiform erythroderma, NBCIE.
Lamellar ichthyosis	Autosomal recessive Eight causative genes identified, *TGM1* most common	Variable severity. Characteristic scales are large, thickened and dark grey or brown. Does not usually involve erythroderma.
Congenital ichthyosiform erythroderma	Autosomal receive Nine causative genes identified	Frequently born as collodion baby. After membrane shed, erythroderma and scale appear. Scales typically fine and white or grey. If severe, erythroderma persists, but in milder cases it improves with time.

TABLE 23.7 Nursing care of Newborn Collodion baby and Harlequin ichthyosis	
Right Care	
Respiration – can be limited by the collodion membrane or thickened plaques in Harlequin ichthyosis (HI), also by pain and discomfort as they tear and shed.	Monitoring of respiratory function and effort. Oral retinoids not usually required in collodion babies but in HI survival rates are higher in those who received acitretin (Rajpopat et al., 2011) although not clear if it is this or improved neonatal care.
Increased trans-epidermal water loss (TEWL) due to incompletely differentiated epidermis and cracks and fissures in skin –may be six or seven times that of a normal newborn baby and increases proportionally with prematurity. Electrolyte imbalance. Thermodysregulation with possible hypothermia.	Nurse in enclosed humidified (60%–80%) incubator to minimise heat loss. Fluid administered intravenously if needed. Maintain baby's temperature at 36.5°C–37°C – incubator too hot and baby may become erythematous and associated pyrexia mistaken for infection; too cold and baby may become cold. Weigh daily and record fluid balance. Daily baths with added medicated bath oil and soap substitute. Application of ointment-based emollients every 2–4 hours to all areas. Urea based products should be avoided as abnormal absorption.
Potential infection from skin.	Monitor vital signs. Do not attempt to remove membrane with scissors – allow to split and shed spontaneously. Avoid invasive procedures as much as possible.
Ectropion (if present).	Immediate ophthalmology input. Eye care with gentle cleaning. Lubricating eye ointments to lids and surrounding skin to trap moisture.
Feeding – can be difficult if respiratory compromise and also due to eclabium if present.	Monitor weight. Consider input from speech and language therapy and appropriate choice of teat if bottle feeding. Support for mother in breast feeding. Supplementary feeding via nasogastric tube may be needed.
Growth failure occurs in some ichthyosis probably due to increased TEWL and impaired skin barrier. Pain due to cracking and splits in membrane.	Dietetic input. Calorie supplementation. Monitor pain. Give appropriate analgesia, which may include opioids especially before procedures such as bathing.
Profound impact on quality of life of child and family relating to physical health, daily life and interactions with others.	Communication of diagnosis should be offered as soon as possible. Genetic counselling. Psychological support strongly recommended. Encourage mother-baby bonding. Organise support in primary care before discharge – health visitor and community children's nursing team.

(Mazereeuw-Hautier, J., Vahlquist, A., Traupe, H., et al., 2019a. Management of congenital ichthyoses: European guidelines of care, part one. Br. J. Dermatol. 180 (2), 272–281; Mazereeuw-Hautier, J., Hernandez-Martin, A., O'Toole, E.A., et al., 2019b. Management of congenital ichthyoses: European guidelines of care, part two. Br. J. Dermatol. 180 (3), 484–495.)

Ichthyosis Support Group

PO BOX 1242 Yateley GU47 7FL

Tel. 0845 6029202

www.ichthyosis.org.uk

PSYCHOLOGICAL EFFECTS OF SKIN DISEASE ON CHILDREN AND THEIR FAMILIES

The number of children and young people affected by mental health problems is rising; with children from low-income families and those who are looked after or adopted, care leavers or victims of abuse are more likely to develop problems. In addition, children and young people with disabilities or long-term conditions are also particularly vulnerable. This includes children and young people with skin disease, for example. Nurses need to consider the psychological context and recognise situations which might impact on parents' and children's ability to implement care regimes and successfully manage disease so that interventions can be put in place to address them.

REFERENCES

Agner, T. (Ed.), 2016. Skin Barrier Function. Current Problems in Dermatology, Karger, Basel, vol. 49, pp 144-151.

Atherton, D.J., 1995. Eczema in Childhood the Facts. Oxford University Press.

Bath-Hextall, F.J., et al., 2012. Dietary supplements for established eczema. Cochrane. Database. Sys. Rev. 15 (2), CD005205. https://doi.org/10.1002/14651858.CD005205.pub3.

Beattie, P.E., Lewis-Jones, M.S., 2006. A comparative study of impairment of quality of life in children with skin disease and children with other chronic childhood diseases. Br. J. Dermatol. 155, 145–151.

Bewley, A., 2008. Expert consensus: time for a change in the way we advise our patients to use topical steroids. Br. J. Dermatol. 158, 917–920.

Bolognia, J.L., Schaffer, J.V., et al., 2017. Dermatology, vol. 2. fourth ed. Elsevier, London.

Bos, B.M.B., Antonescu, M.B., Osinga, H., et al., 2019. Corticosteroid phobia (corticophobia) in parents of young children with atopic dermatitis and their health care providers. Pedriatr. Dermatol. 36, 100–104.

Boyle, R.J., Bath-Hextall, F.J., Leonardi-Bee, J., et al., 2008. Probiotics for treating eczema. Cochrane. Database. Sys. Rev. 8 (4), CD006135. https://doi.org/10.1002/14651858.CD006135.pub2.

British Association of Dermatologists (BAD), 2019a. Panton Valentine Leukocidin *Staphylococcus Aureus* (PVL-SA) Skin Infection Patient Leaflet. www.bad.org.uk.

British Association of Dermatologists (BAD), 2019b. Staphylococcal Scalded Skin Syndrome. Patient Leaflet. www.bad.org.uk.

British Association of Dermatologists (BAD), 2020b. Acne Patient Leaflet. www.bad.org.uk.

British Association of Dermatologists (BAD), 2020a. Scabies Patient Leaflet. www.bad.org.uk.

British Association of Dermatologists (BAD), 2018a. Propranolol for Haemangiomas of Infancy. Patient Leaflet. www.bad.org.uk.

British Association of Dermatologists (BAD), 2019c. Isotretinoin Patient Leaflet. www.bad.org.uk.

British Dermatological Nursing Group (BDNG), 2012. Best practice emollient therapy: a statement for healthcare professionals. Dermatol. Nur. 11 (4), s1–s19.

British National Formulary, 2019. British National Formulary (BNF). Pharmaceutical Press.

Burr, S., 2003. Impetigo. In: Barnes, K. (Ed.), Paediatrics: A Clinical Guide for Nurse Practitioners. Elsevier Science, London, pp. 70–72.

Camfferrman, D., Kennedy, J., et al., 2010. Eczema and sleep and its relationship to daytime functioning in children. Sleep. Med. Rev. 14(6), 359–369.

Carr, J., 2009. Evidence-based management of atopic eczema. Br. J. Nur. 18 (10), 603–610.

Charman, C., Lawton, S., 2006. Eczema: What Really Works? Robinson, London.

Chen, X., Jiang, K., Yang, M., et al., 2016. Systemic antifungal therapy for tinea capitis in children. Cochrane. Database. Syst. Rev. CD004685. https://doi.org/10.1002/14651858.CD004685.pub3.

Chi, C.C., Wang, S.H., Delamere, F.M., et al., 2015. Interventions for prevention of herpes simplex labialis (cold sores on the lips). Cochrane. Database. Syst. Rev. 7 (8), CD010095. https://doi.org/10.1002/14651858.CD010095.pub2.

Cooke, A., Cork, M.J., et al., 2016. Olive Oil, sunflower oil or no oil for baby dry skin or massage: a pilot, assessor-blinded, randomized controlled trial (the Oil in Baby SkincaRE (OBSeRvE) Study). Acta Derm. Venereol. 96, 323–330.

Cork, M.J., Danby, S., 2009. Skin barrier breakdown: a renaissance in emollient therapy. Br. J. Comm. Nurs. 13 (6), 250–257.

Danby, S.G., Al Enezi, T., Sultan, A., et al., 2013. Effect of olive and sunflower seed oil on the adult skin barrier. Pedriat. Dermatol. 30 (1), 42–50.

Docherty, C., 2001. Infections and infestations. In: Hughes, E., van Onselen, J. (Eds.), Dermatology Nursing: A Practical Guide. Churchill Livingstone, London.

Drugs, Therapeutics Bulletin (DTB), 2007. Bath emollients for eczema. Why use them? 45 (10), 73–76.

Dufresne, H., Hadj-Rabia, S., Taieb, C., et al., 2015. Development and validation of an epidermolysis bullosa family/parental burden score. Br. J. Dermatol. 173 (6), 1405–1410.

Eberle, F.C., Jurgen, B., et al., 2016. Recent advances in understanding psoriasis. F100Research, vol. 5, London.https://doi.org/10.1.12688/f1000research.7927.1.

Edwards, M., Titman, P., 2010. Promoting Psychological Well-Being in Children with Acute and Chronic Illness. Jessica Kingsley, Washington, DC.

Eichenfeld, L.F., Paller, A.S., 2018. Pediatric psoriasis: evolving perspectives. Pedriatr. Dermatol. 35, 170–181.

El Hachem, M., Zambruno, G.Z., Bourdon-Lanoy, E., et al., 2014. Multicentre consensus recommendations for skin care in inherited epidermolysis bullosa. Orphanet. J. Rare Dis. 9 (1), 76.

Elias, P.M., Schmuth, M., 2009. Abnormal skin barrier in the aetiopathogenesis of atopic dermatitis. Cur. Opin. Alle. Clin. Immunol. 9 (5), 437–446.

Elliott, B., Luker, K., 1997. The experiences of mothers caring for a child with severe atopic eczema. J. Clin. Nurs. 6 (3), 241–247.

Ernst, E., 2012. Homeopathy for eczema: a systematic review of controlled clinical trials. Br. J. Dermatol. 139 (1), 73–76.

Ersser, S.J., van, O., 2010. Eczema. In: Penzer, R., Ersser, S.J. (Eds.), Principles of Skincare. Wiley-Blackwell.

Feltham, J.E., Sargant, N., 2016. Kerion celsi: a misdiagnosed scalp infection. Arch. Dis. Childhood. 101, 503.

Ferguson, L., Fuller, L.C., 2017. Spectrum and burden of dermatophytes in children. J. Infect. 74 (Suppl. 1), S54–S60.

Fine, J.D., Eady, R., Bauer, E.A., et al., 2008. The classification of inherited epidermolysis bullosa (EB): report of the Third International Consensus Meeting on Diagnosis and Classification of EB. J. Am. Acad. Dermatol. 58, 931–950.

Flohr, C., Ahmed, A., 2018. New evidence challenges use of bath emollients for children with eczema. BMJ. 3 (361), k1791. https://doi.org/10.1136/bmj.k1791.

Fuller, L.C., Child, F.C., et al., 2003. Scalp ringworm in south-east London and an analysis of a cohort of patients from a paediatric dermatology department. Br. J. Dermatol. 148 (5), 985–988.

Gawkrodger, D.J., Arden-Jones, M.R., 2017. Dermatology: An Illustrated Colour Text. Elsevier, London.

Great Ormond Street for Children NHS Foundation Trust (GOSH NHS Foundation Trust), 2014. Treating Small Infantile Haemangiomas with Topical Timolol Information Sheet.

Guy's and S.T.' NHS Trust, 2016. The use of Milton baths in dermatology. Patient Information Leaflet. Leaflet number: 4303/VER2.

Halvorsen, J.A., Stern, R.S., Dalgard, F., et al., 2011. Suicidal ideation, mental health problems and social impairment are increased in adolescents with acne: a population based study. J. Invest. Dermatol. 131 (2), 363–370.

Health Protection Agency (HPA), 2007. Tinea Capitis in the United Kingdom. A Report on its Diagnosis, Management and Prevention. Health Protection Agency, London.

Health Protection Agency (HPA), 2008. Guidance on the Diagnosis and Management of PVL-Associated *Staphylococcus aureus* Infection (PVL-SA) in England. HPA.

Hoeger, P.H., Harper, J.L., Baselga, E., et al., 2015. Treatment of infantile haemangiomas: recommendations of a European expert group. Eur. J. Pediatr. 174 (7), 855–865.

Huang, J.T., Abrams, M., et al., 2009. Treatment of *Staphylococcus aureus* colonizationb in atopic dermatitis decreases disease severity. Pediatrics. 123 (5), e808–e814.

Kell, B., Hawkins, F., 2005. Collaboration in care: a case study. Paediatr. Nurs. 17 (4), 30–33.

Koning, S., van der Sande, R., Verhagen, A.P., et al., 2012. Interventions for impetigo. Cochrane. Database. Sys. Rev. 18, 1–CD003261. https://doi.org/10.1002/14651858.CD003261.pub3.

Kusari, A., Han, A.M., Virgen, C.A., et al., 2019. Evidence-based skin care in preterm infants. Pediatr. Dermatol. 36 (1), 16–23.

Lawton, S., 2014. Childhood atopic eczema: adherence to treatment. Nurse Prescribing. 12 (5), 226–231.

Lewis-Jones, S., Finlay, A., 1995. The Children's Dermatology Life Quality Index (CDLQI): initial validation and practical use. Br. J. Dermatol. 132 (6), 942–949.

Lynne, V., James, D., 2018. Meeting health educational needs of staff involved with children with epidermolysis bullosa in educational settings. Dermatol. Nur. 7 (4), 24–26.

Macartney, K., Mcintyre, P., 2008. Vaccines for post-exposure prophylaxis against varicella (chickenpox) in children and adults. Cochrane. Database. Sys. Rev. 3, CD001833. https://doi.org/10.1002/4651858.CD001833.pub2.

Martin, P.E., Eckert, J.K., et al., 2014. Which infants with eczema are at risk of food allergy? Result from a population-based cohort. Clin. Exp. Allergy. 45, 255–264.

Mazereeuw-Hautier, J., Vahlquist, A., Traupe, H., et al., 2019. Management of congenital ichthyoses: European guidelines of care, part one. Br. J. Dermatol. 180 (2), 272–281.

Mazereeuw-Hautier, J., Hernández-Martín, A., O'Toole, E.A., et al., 2019. Management of congenital ichthyoses: European guidelines of care, part two. Br. J. Dermatol. 180 (3), 484–495.

McAleer, M.A., Irvine, A.D., 2013. The multifunctional role of filaggrin in allergic skin disease. J. Allergy Clin. Immunol. 131 (2), 280–291.

Mooney, E., Rademaker, M., et al., 2015. Adverse Effects of Topical Corticosteroids in Paediatric Eczema: Australasian Consensus Statement. https://doi.org/10.1111/ajd.12313.

Moore, K., David, T.J., Murray, C.S., et al., 2006. Effect of childhood eczema and asthma on parental sleep and well-being: a prospective comparative study. Br. J. Dermatol. 154 (3), 514–518.

National Eczema Society, 2015. Fact Sheet: Complementary Therapies and Eczema.

National Eczema Society, 2016. All About Eczema: An information pack for schools.

National Institute for Health and Care Excellence (NICE), 2007. Atopic Eczema in Children: Management of Atopic Eczema in Children from Birth up to the Age of 12 Years. RCOG Press, London.

NICE, 2004. Tacrolimus and pimecrolimus for atopic eczema in children. Technology Appraisal Guidance (TA82).

Olsen, J.R., Gallacher, J., 2014. Epidemiology of molluscum contagiosum in children: a systematic review. Fam. Pract. 31 (2), 130–136.

Oranje, A.P., de Waard-van der spek, F.B., 2015. Recent developments in the management of common childhood skin infections. J. Infect. 71 (Suppl. 1), S76–S579.

Paller, A.S., Mercy, K., Kwasny, M.J., et al., 2013. Association of pediatric psoriasis severity with excess and central adiposity: an international cross-sectional study. JAMA. Dermatol. 149 (2), 166–176.

Patel, D., Levoska, M.L., Shwayder, T., 2018. Managing sleep disturbances in children with atopic dermatitis. Pediatr. Dermatol. 35, 428–433.

Penzer, R., 2010. Acne. In: Penzer, R., Ersser, S.J. (Eds.), Principles of Skin Care. Wiley-Blackwell, pp. 179–194.

Peters, J., 2001. Assessment of the dermatology patient. In: Hughes, E., Van Onselen, J. (Eds.), Dermatology Nursing: A Practical Guide. Churchill Livingstone, Edinburgh, pp. 19–39.

Public Health England, 2019. Health Protection in schools and other childcare facilities. Managing specific infectious diseases Chapter 9. http://www.gov.uk.

Rancé, F., 2008. Food allergy in children suffering from atopic eczema. Pediatirc. Allerg. Immunol. 19, 279–284.

Rajpopat, S., Moss, C., Mellerio, J., et al., 2011. Harlequin ichthyosis: a review of clinical and molecular findings in 45 cases. Arch. Dermatol. 147 (6), 681–686.

Reich, K., 2012. The concept of psoriasis as a systemic inflammation: implications for disease management. J. Eur. Acad. Dermatol. Venereol. 26 (Suppl. 2), 3–11.

Royal College of Nursing/ British Dermatological Nursing Group, 2008. Competencies for an Integrated Framework for Dermatological Nursing. Royal College of Nursing, London, pp. 48–49.

Royal College of Paediatrics and Child Health (RCPCH), 2011. Care pathway: eczema. Available from: www.rcpch.ac.uk/allergy.

Santer, M.S., Burgess, H., 2012. Experiences of carers managing childhood eczema and their views on treatment. Br. J. Gen. Pract. 62 (597), e261–e267. https://doi.org/10.3399/bjgp12X636083.

Santer, M.S., Burgess, H., 2013. Managing childhood eczema: qualitative study exploring carers' experiences of barriers and facilitators to treatment adherence. J. Adv. Nurs. 69 (11), 2493–2501.

Santer, M., Ridd, M.J., Francis, N.A., et al., 2018. Emollient bath additives for the treatment of childhood eczema (BATHE): multicentre pragmatic parallel group randomised controlled trial of clinical cost effectiveness. BMJ. 361, k1332. https://doi.org/10.11361/bmj.k1332.

Shah, K.N., Cortina, S., et al., 2015. Psoriasis in childhood: effective strategies to improve treatment adherence. Psoriasis. Targets. Ther. 5, 43–54.

Shallcross, L.J., Fragaszy, E., Johnson, A.M., et al., 2013. The role of the Panton-Valentine leucocidin toxin in staphylococcal disease: a systematic review and meta-analysis. Lancet. Infect. Dis. 13 (1), 43–54.

Shwayder, T., Akland, T., 2005. Neonatal skin barrier: structure, function and disorders. Dermatol. Ther. 18 (2), 87–103.

Stamatas, G., Nikolovski, J., et al., 2010. Infant skin microstructure assessed in vivo differs from adult skin in organization and at the cellular level. Pediatr. Dermatol. 27, 125–131.

Smith, S., Hong, E., Fearns, S., et al., 2010. Corticosteroid phobia and other confounders in the treatment of childhood atopic dermatitis explored using parent focus groups. Australas. J. Dermatol. 51 (3), 168–174.

Smith, S., Lee, A., Blaszcynski, A., et al., 2016. Pharmacists' knowledge about use of topical corticosteroids in atopic dermatitis: pre and post continuing professional development education. Australas. J. Dermatol. 57 (3), 299–204. https:www//doi.org/10.111/ajd.12339.

Sokolova, A., Smith, S., 2015. Factors contributing to poor treatment outcomes in childhood atopic dermatitis. Australas. J. Dermatol. 56 (4), 241–314.

Solman, L., Glover, M., Beattie, P.E., et al., 2018. Oral propranolol in the treatment of proliferating infantile haemangiomas: British Society for Paediatric Dermatology consensus guidelines. Br. J. Dermatol. 178 (5), 582–589. Available from: https://doi.org110.1111/bjd.16779S.

Strong, M., Johnstone, P.W., 2007. Interventions for treating scabies. Cochrane. Database. Sys. Rev. (3), CD00320. https://doi.1002/14541858.CD000320.pub2.

Takeichi, T., Akiyama, M., 2016. Inherited ichthyosis: non-syndromic forms. J. Dermatol. 43 (3), 242–251.

Tappel, A.C., Cresce, N., Zlotoff, B., 2018. What's the story? An analysis of children's books about atopic dermatitis. Pedriatr. Dermatol. 35 (5), 607–610. PLoS Med. 8 (2). www.plosmedicine.org/article/info%3Adoi2F10.1371%2Fjournal.pmed.1000395.

Tarr, A., Iheanacho, I., 2013. Should we use bath emollients for atopic eczema? BMJ. do1. 10.1136/b.

Tebrugge, M., Kuruvilla, M., et al., 2006. Does the use of calamine or antihistamine provide symptomatic relief from pruritis in children with varicella zoster infection? Arch. Dis. Child. 91, 1035–1036.

Thomas, K.S., Bradshaw, L.E., 2017. Silk garments plus standard care compared with standard care for treating eczema in children: a randomised controlled observational blind pragmatic trail (CLOTHES Trial). PLoS Med. https://doi.org/10.1371/journal.pmed.1002280.

Thomas, K.S., Dean, T., O'Leary, C., et al., 2011. A randomised controlled trial of ion-exchange water softeners for the treatment of eczema in children. PLoS Med. 8 (2), e1000395. Available from: www.plosmedicine.org/article/info%3Adoi2F10.1371%2Fjournal.pmed.1000395.

Tollefson, M.M., van Houten, V.K., Asante, D., et al., 2018. Association of psoriasis with comorbidity development in children with psoriasis. JAMA. Dermatol. 154 (3), 286–292.

van der Wouden, J.C., van der Sande, R., Kruithof, E.J., et al., 2017. Interventions for cutaneous molluscum contagiosum. Cochrane. Database. Sys. Rev. 17, 5–CD004767. https://doi.org/10.1002/14651858.CD004767.pub4.

Van Gysel, D., Lijnen, R.L., Moekti, S.S., et al., 2002. Collodion baby: a follow up study of 17 cases. J. Eur. Acad. Dermatol. Venereol. 16 (5), 472–475.

Voegeli, D., 2011. The vital role of emollients in the treatment of eczema. Br. J. Nur. 20 (2), 74–80.

Williams, H., Robertson, C., Stewart, A., et al., 1999. Worldwide variations in the prevalence of symptoms of atopic eczema in the international study of asthma and allergies in childhood. J. Allergy Clin. 103 (1 Pt1), 125–138.

Williams, H.C., Strachan, D.P., 1998. The natural history of childhood eczema: observations from the British 1958 birth cohort study. Br. J. Dermatol. 139 (5), 834–839.

Yang, E.J., Beck, K.M., Sekhon, S., et al., 2019. The impact of pediatric atopic dermatitis on families: a review. Pediatr. Dermatol. 36 (1), 66–71.

Yeoh, D.K., Bowen, A.C., Carapetis, J.R., 2016. Impetigo and scabies - disease burden and modern treatment strategies. J. Infect. 5 (Suppl. 72), S61–S67.

Negotiation of Care

24

Recognising and Responding to Child Maltreatment: The Role of the Children's Nurse

Rebecca Cooke, Annette Williamson, Julie Taylor

LEARNING OUTCOMES

- Define the major concepts associated with child protection.
- Assume professional responsibility in the recognition of and response to child maltreatment.
- Understand the consequences of child maltreatment.

- Recognise potential risk factors for and indicators of child maltreatment.
- Describe the changing landscape of child maltreatment.
- Access help and support for child protection practice.

INTRODUCTION

It is almost impossible to believe that parents, carers and other adults could inflict physical or sexual harm on a child, severely abuse them psychologically and emotionally, or neglect them to such an extent that their development is impaired. The truth is these kinds of acts (collectively known as *maltreatment*) happen every single day, with conservative estimates suggesting that in the UK alone about two children a week die at the hands of their parents/carers whilst thousands more endure cruel and intolerable circumstances that have long-term consequences (Munro et al., 2014). Although hopefully it will be infrequent, as a children's nurse there is no doubt that at some stage you are going to be confronted by children who have been maltreated, parents who conceal the truth about how their child has been injured, and families so chaotic or unable to cope that children are being negatively impacted. Much of this will not come to the immediate attention of health care staff, it will be suspected or inferred perhaps during routine care.

This chapter provides an introduction to child maltreatment, enabling you to understand the main issues about child abuse and neglect, how you might recognise it, and outline your responsibility to protect the child. The chapter will explore risk factors for maltreatment, interventions that help to protect children, the law surrounding child protection and professional accountability. Child maltreatment is an emotive subject and we acknowledge both the challenges and the need for emotional resilience. We use the term 'children' to mean children and young people under age 18. In England the word 'safeguarding' is used to denote measures to protect the health, well-being and human rights of vulnerable people (especially children). Although we mainly use the term child protection here, you may find local guidance and policy refer to safeguarding instead.

As a children's nurse it is important to recognise your professional responsibility in the management of child maltreatment. All nurses and midwives are expected to comply with national professional standards, which include safeguarding patients. In the UK the Nursing and Midwifery Council code identifies responsibility:

> … *for all nurses and midwives to raise concerns immediately if you believe a person is vulnerable or at risk and needs extra support and protection.*
> **Nursing and Midwifery Council, (2015: section 17)**

The scope of child maltreatment and its form has evolved in recent years in light of the digital age and reliance upon social media by children. This brings an array of new challenges to the forefront as perpetrators find novel ways to access children online.

A solid body of research demonstrates that child maltreatment is prevalent and impacts on the health and well-being of children in every society (Munro et al., 2014). Increasingly diverse populations due to globalisation and migration brings exposure to differing types of child maltreatment, for example, female genital mutilation, breast ironing and abuse linked to faith and belief.

🌐 WWW

Every year the NSPCC produces a summary report about the latest statistics for child abuse and neglect in the UK, known as 'How safe are our children'. Catch up with the latest report here: https://bit.ly/2u68Cdp.

There is significant evidence that the impact of child maltreatment can lead to poorer life chances due to the physical and psychological impact upon the child (Taylor and Lazenbatt, 2014). Negative childhood experiences increase the risk of future violence (both as victim or perpetrator), lifelong physical and mental health problems, and work or career opportunities. As such, early experiences are an important public health issue and may negatively impact work or career activities. Much of the foundational research in this area has been conducted by Felitti and colleagues on Adverse Childhood Experiences (ACEs) (Anda et al., 2006; Felitti et al., 1998), but interest in the issue is continuing still (Bellis et al., 2018).

The ACEs model demonstrates the longitudinal health and social burden of child maltreatment from a victim and societal perspective. The clear message from the ACEs programme is the need for early recognition and intervention to address social need before escalation to child maltreatment.

WWW

How ACEs influence health. Available from: https://bit.ly/2Msnl8l

Research and policy are constantly evolving surrounding child maltreatment. This chapter should therefore be read alongside your local and national child protection policies to gain further insight.

DEFINING CHILD MALTREATMENT AND THE INTERLINKING CATEGORIES OF ABUSE

The definition and consensus of what constitutes child maltreatment is internationally challenging (Alexander, 2017). Social, ecological and cultural differences influence behaviour, creating varied standards and expectations as to what are acceptable parental practices. For example, many would argue that corporal punishment of a child breaches human rights. Article 19 of the United Nations Convention on the Rights of the Child (UNCRC) (UN, 1989) requires States to protect children from 'all forms of physical and mental violence, injury or abuse' while in the care of parents, legal guardians and others caring for them. However, cultures differ, and for example, while in Sweden, Scotland and many other countries smacking has been banned for over 20 years, other countries (including England and United States) smacking a child is still legally and culturally acceptable as a way to enforce parental boundaries. However, there is a paradigm shift in attitudes to smacking in the UK, where there are campaigns to embrace alternative positive parenting techniques to implement boundaries for children. In Wales and Scotland particularly, there are moves to make smacking illegal (Astrup, 2018).

The UNCRC (UN, 1989) defines child maltreatment:

All forms of physical or mental violence, injury and abuse, neglect or negligent treatment, maltreatment or exploitation, including sexual abuse (Article 19).

Expanding on this, the World Health Organization (WHO) defines child maltreatment as:

All forms of physical and/or emotional ill-treatment, sexual abuse, neglect or negligent treatment or commercial or other exploitation, resulting in actual or potential harm to a child's health, survival, development or dignity in the context of a relationship of responsibility, trust or power.

WHO (2016)

There is general agreement that maltreatment definitions fall into four broad categories (HM Government, 2018a):

- Physical abuse: any physical harm to a child including shaking, hitting, poisoning, burning, suffocating, drowning.
- Neglect: persistent failure to meet a child's basic physical and psychological needs likely to result in severe impairment to a child's health or development.
- Sexual abuse: forcing or enticing a child to take part in contact or non-contact sexual activity.
- Emotional abuse: persistent emotional maltreatment likely to cause severe and persistent adverse effects on a child's development and self-esteem.

Table 24.1 provides further detail.

Fabricated or Induced Illness

As a children's nurse you should also be aware of the signs of fabricated or induced illness (FII). FII is a complex phenomenon and involves a parent or carer persistently presenting their child as ill to health professionals, when the child is in fact perfectly healthy. Examples of parental or carer behaviour include exaggeration or fabrication of their child's symptoms, or by deliberately inducing symptoms of illness – for example, by poisoning a child with unnecessary medication or other substances. FII may be considered following extensive clinical examinations and tests that conclude no explanation for the child's symptoms.

The potential warning signs of FII are:

- Symptoms only appear when the parent or carer is present.
- The only person noticing symptoms is the parent or carer.
- The affected child has an unusually poor response to medication or other treatment.
- The child's reported symptoms do not comply with the child's presentation.
- The parent or carer has a history of frequently visiting different hospitals or community medical centres for treatment.
- The parent or carer has good medical knowledge or a medical background.
- The child's daily activities may be restricted by parents or carers unnecessarily due to the potential fabricated illness, for example, non-attendance at school, non-participation in sport and leisure pursuits (NHS England, 2016).

Any concerns that may suggest FII should be reported to the designated child protection lead. FII is diagnosed by a senior, experienced paediatrician. Medical professionals who suspect FII should liaise with social services and the police, and follow local child protection procedures.

It is important to understand that categories of abuse are not stand-alone classifications, but are fluid and in many cases overlap. Taking a child-centred view, through their eyes we can

TABLE 24.1	**Main Categories of Abuse**		
Physical	**Emotional**	**Sexual**	**Neglect**
• Smacking/hitting (physical chastisement) • Burns/scolds • Human bites • Bruising • Shaking • Poisoning • Intracranial injury/eye trauma without history of trauma/medical condition • Drowning/suffocation • Fractures (e.g. ribs/legs/arms/skull in immobile babies) • Single/multiple fractures without history of trauma/medical condition • Female genital mutilation (FGM) • Fabricated or induced Illness • Honour based violence • Over/under feeding • Knife wounds • Terrorism/gang related injuries • Deliverance ceremonies for witchcraft exorcisms • Frequent accidents/attendance at emergency department • Breast ironing	• Negativity/hostility towards a child • Parental rejection • Blaming/scapegoat • Persistently critical • Exposure to distressing/frightening experiences (e.g. domestic abuse) • Verbal punishment (chastisement) • Deliberately humiliating/scaring/intimidating/isolating/ignoring a child • Conveying to the child they are worthless/unloved • Bullying/cyberbullying • Imposing age/developmentally inappropriate expectations • Making a child perform degrading acts • Threatening/shouting at a child • Never showing emotions in interactions with the child	• Sexual touching whether the child is dressed/undressed • Sex with a child under 13 years (rape) • Penetration of an object/body part inside child's mouth/vagina/anus • Forcing/encouraging participation in sexual activities • Grooming • Showing a child pornography • Child sexual exploitation for money/power/status • Making/viewing/distributing sexualised images/videos of a child • Sexting – sexual conversations via mobile phone • Sexually transmitted diseases • Unwanted pregnancy	On-going failure to meet a child's basic needs: **Physical** • Failing to provide food, clothes, shelter and supervision to keep them safe **Educational** • Failing to ensure child receives education **Emotional** • Failing to meet child's needs for nurture and stimulation **Health** • Failure to provide/access appropriate health and dental care • Ignoring medical advice/disguised compliance • Frequent injuries due to poor supervision • Poor dental hygiene/dental caries **Nutrition** • Obesity • Malnourishment

grasp the enormity of the immediate harm caused and long-term life impact. To illustrate, a case of physical abuse may cause an acute injury, for instance a burn. This can be managed with emergency treatment and pain relief, followed by repeated skin grafts as the child grows. The short-term emotional impact can display in excessive crying, feeling afraid, nightmares and bed wetting. In the longer term it can also lead to psychological trauma such as post-traumatic stress disorder and relationship trust issues. As they grow into adulthood, children carry the physical and emotional scars of abuse. Suicide, depression and self-harm is frequently associated with childhood physical and sexual abuse (Newbury and Arseneault, 2017).

> **ACTIVITY**
>
> The definition of child sexual exploitation (CSE) is as follows:
>
> *Child sexual exploitation is a form of child sexual abuse. It occurs where an individual or group takes advantage of an imbalance of power to coerce, manipulate, or deceive a child or young person under the age of 18 into sexual activity: (a) in exchange for something the victim needs or wants, and/or (b) for the financial advantage or increased status of the perpetrator or facilitator. The victim may have been sexually exploited even if the sexual activity appears consensual. Child sexual exploitation does not always involve physical contact; it can also occur through the use of technology (Department for Education, 2017).*

> **WWW**
>
> Watch the 2014 video 'Jasmin's Story'. Available from: https://bit.ly/2tRefL6.
>
> Think about child sexual exploitation (CSE) and discuss which categories this is described under when defining the abuse.

Understanding Risk Factors in Child Maltreatment

It is important that you have an understanding of the potential risk factors for child maltreatment that are often difficult to detect. Although there is no specific single risk factor that will definitively predict child maltreatment, 'multiples matter' (Spratt, 2012) and the more risk factors to which children are exposed, the greater the likelihood of harm. The framework for assessment (HM Government, 2018a) is core to developing a holistic understanding of the child's risk and protective factors (Fig. 24.1).

Decision-making in acute and community settings requires an evaluation of many complex factors and it can take a long time to gain sufficient experience to use practice wisdom in conjunction with the current situation and assessment. Effective care planning should reflect an assessment of the child's needs and parental capacity to fulfil the child's needs from a physical, social and emotional perspective.

Table 24.2 identifies potential risk factors that may increase vulnerability to child maltreatment. The presence of one or more risk factors will not necessarily result in child

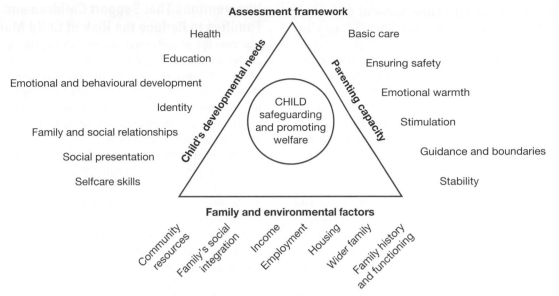

Fig. 24.1 Assessment framework. (https://bit.ly/2lTuIWb.)

TABLE 24.2 Risk Factors for Abuse[a]

Child Factors	Parent/Family Factors
<1 year of age – heightened risk of child maltreatment due to increased vulnerabilities as a non-mobile, non-verbal child. Statistically the greatest number of child deaths attributed to child maltreatment occur in the <1-year age group.	**Domestic abuse** – impacts emotionally and physically upon the child and is the key risk factor for abuse.
Disability or complex health needs – increases vulnerability due to potential immobility, speech and language needs, communication difficulties, learning needs.	**Substance misuse** – impacts upon parental capacity and child safety.
Adolescence – a time when needs may be overlooked or attributed to being a difficult teenager.	**Mental health needs** – parental capacity may be impaired and pose additional risk for the child.
Child is a young carer – looking after a parent can mean a child's needs are overlooked and unmet.	**Poor attachment between parent and child** can lead to internalising and externalising problems.
Mental health needs – increased risk if parental capacity is limited to support the child.	**Extreme poverty/debt** – impacts upon parental capacity and child safety.
Looked after children – A child may be in care due to abuse or neglect, and/or may be exposed to abuse or neglect whilst in the care system.	**Very young parents** – emotionally unprepared for parenthood, may be socially isolated and out of work.
Delayed physical/emotional/social development – environmental factors and parental capacity to meet the child's needs and provide appropriate stimulation through positive interaction with the child.	**Parents who have a history of abuse/neglect or have been in care** may not have learned how to be a parent themselves, or have very poor role models.
Preterm/low birthweight child – increased vulnerability due to additional needs and impact upon parental capacity.	**Family instability, dysfunction or chaos** – e.g. multiple partners, homelessness, criminality and prison.
Home-schooled children – may not have been seen outside of the home.	**Social isolation and lack of support e.g. extended family & friends** may include travelling families, being new to an area.
Friends with links to gangs – risk of child sexual exploitation.	**Significant stress,** e.g. divorce, bereavement, military families with deployment, injury, frequent moves.
Asylum seekers and refugees – linkages for both parents and children with prostitution, child sexual exploitation, drug smuggling, human trafficking, modern slavery, self-harm, unmet health needs and mental health issues.	

[a]These are not indicative of maltreatment, but the more risk factors there are, the more likely it may be that children might be vulnerable to abuse and neglect.

maltreatment, but the children's nurse needs to assess these risk factors alongside protective factors within the care planning process.

It is crucial to remember that risk factors are not indicators of abuse, but the more risk factors there are, the more vulnerable a child is to maltreatment, as the work on ACEs has so clearly demonstrated. A holistic assessment of the child's emotional, physical, psychological and environmental needs will help to determine what risk factors are present, but also what protective factors may also be present (such as the presence of a caring grandparent). Importantly a child aged under 1 year of age is at heightened risk of child maltreatment due to increased vulnerabilities, because they are non-mobile and non-verbal, and dependent on adults for every aspect of care. Statistically the greatest number of child deaths attributed to child maltreatment occur in this age group (Munro et al., 2014). As a children's nurse you need to constantly reflect the voice and journey of the child and although the under ones are largely non-verbal you should assess the child's overall demeanour in terms of child/parental relationship. The emotionally deprived child can demonstrate frozen watchfulness, lack normal babbling, or become quite rigid/tense upon handling (Evans et al., 2018). This is not intended as an exhaustive explanation, but a guide to potential indicators.

The children's nurse needs also to be aware of what physical or emotional or behavioural symptoms might be indicative of abuse in older children. Children who are ill or anxious or disabled may exhibit symptoms that can be mistakenly attributed to their illness or disability. However, it is important to be aware of signs that a child may be being abused or neglected. Potential indicators could be that the child:

- Is excessively watchful, anxious or withdrawn (internalising behaviour).
- Shows extreme behaviour (externalising).
- Acts in an inappropriately infantile or adult way.
- Has frequent injuries or bruising.
- Does not seem attached to caregiver.
- Shies away, flinches at touch or sudden movement.
- Is afraid to go home.
- Is always seeking food.
- Is inappropriately dressed for the weather.
- Has poor hygiene or filthy clothes.
- Has untreated illnesses or injuries.
- Is frequently unsupervised or plays in unsafe settings.
- Has difficulty walking or sitting.
- Displays sexualised behaviours with adults or other children.
- Has experienced a young pregnancy.
- Has a sexually transmitted disease.
- Runs away from home.
(Taylor and Bradbury-Jones, 2015)

🌐 **WWW**

The following WHO factsheet on child maltreatment is very useful. Available from: https://bit.ly/2FiYNww.

Interventions That Support Children and Their Families to Reduce the Risk of Child Maltreatment

The concept of early intervention with children and families can prove challenging for two reasons: first, the family's *perception* of 'need' may not be the same as yours; and second, there can be a subsequent resistance to change from the family. Acknowledgement and acceptance of early help is built upon effective communication between the children's nurse and the child and their family.

Early intervention to support the child and family can reduce the risk of potential maltreatment and improve outcomes for the child. For example, this might be negotiating appropriate housing for a child that has complex medical needs. It is important to be able to recognise such potential need at an early stage of the child's hospital admission as this may impact upon a safe discharge. The children's nurse should lead a coordinated response to ensure a positive transition from hospital to home, which will include discharge planning with all relevant agencies and family members involved in the child's care.

Other examples of early intervention include parenting support and you can play a key role in supporting families to develop positive parenting skills through teaching and supporting parents to care and play appropriately.

Some families and children will have needs that are beyond early intervention and require a further coordinated response from multiple agencies. This type of response is voluntary and therefore consent and positive engagement is required by the family to work with agencies. One example of this is the *Think Family* approach, which includes the allocation of an intensive family support worker for a short period of time. The family support worker will use evidence-based family-focused models to work with families to support change. The types of need that may require a *Think Family* support worker include children with health or behavioural problems or who have been involved in anti-social behaviour or criminal activity, poor school attendance, or who have parents with mental or physical health problems, or drug and alcohol dependence. Home life can be quite chaotic for some children and many families have been shown to benefit from the *Think Family* approach, as reductions in anti-social behaviour and risk of homelessness overall have declined (Ministry of Community, Housing and Health, 2018).

As a children's nurse you will be in a position to identify children or families that have needs that are so complex or significant that they need an immediate statutory social work assessment and intervention to prevent significant harm or serious risk to their health and well-being. Examples of the level of need that require a statutory response include: allegations of abuse or serious neglect or a suspicious injury in a child; domestic abuse; parents who are consistently unable to provide 'good enough' parenting that is adequate and safe; neglect of medical needs and basic care (e.g. food, warmth, stimulation); persistent non-compliance with and non-attendance to medical health needs and appointments, which impacts upon the child's well-being and potential prognosis; suspected sexual abuse.

In some instances, the level of need for the abused child requires removal from parental care due to the potential risk posed by parents. The child and their siblings are temporarily placed with foster carers via statutory or voluntary agreement with parents (this will be determined by the social worker based upon the assessed level of risk). A temporary placement in care may become long term and permanent. As a children's nurse you will meet children in care and therefore you need to consider their additional vulnerabilities. Children in care are four times more likely to experience mental health difficulty than their peers and those children leaving care are less likely to progress into education, employment and training. Children in care can be vulnerable to further abuse and neglect (Rahilly and Hendry, 2014).

As a children's nurse you need to be constantly aware of the risks of child maltreatment and should always escalate your concerns, even if you are not sure, to the nurse in charge or designated child protection lead and seek advice and support. **The safety and well-being of the child is always paramount.**

Serious Case Reviews

Child maltreatment is sometimes fatal. Internationally there is not a standardised process for the objective analysis of serious child maltreatment cases, that is, those where a child has died at the hands of their parents or carers, or where the abuse has been so severe it could have contributed to death. In England serious case reviews (SCRs) were until recently mandatory enquiries where abuse or neglect is known or suspected to be a factor in the child case, with similar processes in all the UK nations. In Scotland they are known as significant case reviews and in Northern Ireland, case management reviews. England and Wales have replaced SCRs with new regimes following calls to ensure improvements and improve the culture of learning from child protection cases. SCRs remain common terminology and continue to be published. Statutory guidance in England is known as *Working Together to Safeguard Children* (HM Government, 2018a) and defines serious child protection cases as those in which:

- abuse or neglect of a child is known or suspected; and
- the child has died or has been seriously harmed.

The purpose of SCRs and their counterparts has been to map out and reflect critically upon the journey leading up to a child's death/serious injury. They are not about blame, but about establishing the root cause of events and making recommendations to improve future interagency working, to protect children from harm. Many SCRs have changed the landscape of child protection (Table 24.3) and you might want to read about some of these cases. In 2013 the national case review repository provided a single place for publishing case reviews to initiate shared learning at a local, regional and national level (NSPCC, 2017).

 WWW

These reviews are available for all to read at: https://bit.ly/2nD8Mq1.

Change, however, is constant when striving to improve practices which protect and promote the welfare of children. The Wood Report (2016) called for a more flexible framework to ensure collective accountability and effective multi-agency actions in child protection. This was embraced by the government and propelled the launch of revisions to Working Together. England has entered a transitional period as reforms to child protection processes are implemented (Bray, 2018).

Local Safeguarding Children Boards (LSCBs) were phased out in 2019, replaced by local safeguarding partners, represented by police, health and local authorities. Safeguarding partners have new duties to make arrangements locally to protect children in their area. A National Panel has been established, tasked with managing complex cases and disseminating important lessons and recommendations.

Although in the throes of change, there are numerous key themes that can be drawn from SCRs to date (Brandon et al., 2010, 2016; Sidebotham et al., 2011):

- The 'voice of the child' is not obtained; instead the focus is on the parent/carer with the wishes and feelings of the child being omitted. For example, Victoria Climbié's primary language was French, but professionals did not get an interpreter to speak with Victoria (Laming, 2003). Victoria died from overwhelming abuse and neglect. Charlie and Charlotte experienced severe neglect, physical and sexual abuse by their mother, who had learning difficulties and their father, who had mental health issues. The voice of the children was not taken into account in decision making, risk assessment and planning (Hyde, 2018).
- Assuming someone else is managing the concern.
- Poor communication and documentation of the concern.
- Working in isolation from multi-agency professionals.
- Accepting information at face value instead of using professional curiosity to ask further questions and check the facts.
- Poor decision making and an inability to professionally challenge.
- Failure to interpret information gathered and take timely action.

Understanding barriers to embedding SCR lessons is the key to strengthening child protection practices and lessons need to be actively embedded in the organisational culture.

Professional Role and Accountability

As a children's nurse you are responsible for safeguarding those in your care and professionally you must respond to any child protection concerns. This includes:

- Protecting children from maltreatment.
- Preventing impairment of children's health or development.
- Ensuring that children grow up in circumstances consistent with the provision of safe and effective care.
- Taking action to enable all children to have the best outcomes (HM Government, 2018a).

Your roles and responsibilities will be outlined within your local policies and procedures underpinned by regional and national policy. As a children's nurse you should be

TABLE 24.3 **Serious Case Reviews Which Have Changed the Landscape of Child Protection**

Child's Name and Reference	Year	Child Protection Process Changes
Denis O'Neill	1948	Creation of the Parliamentary Care of Children Committee. *Children Act 1948*
Maria Colwell	1974	Area Child Protection Committees created. Encouraged integration of services.
Jessica Chapman and Holly Wells (Soham Murders) https://bit.ly/33MPbIA	2002	Safer recruitment of professionals in a position of trust. School staff must be trained in safeguarding. Database for all registered sex offenders. Introduction of a National Intelligence System.
Victoria Climbié https://bit.ly/3cfAK3B	2003	Minister for Children appointed. A national agency for children and families. Local committees and management boards to oversee children's services. Private fostering reviewed. Home education reviewed. A national child database. A 24-hour helpline for public to report concerns. Government Green Paper – Every Child Matters Initiated national child protection guidance (Working Together).
Peter Connelly https://bit.ly/2upxf4S	2009	Prompted a nationwide review of child protection processes. Creating greater transparency in child protection. Increased applications for care orders (Under section 31 of the *Children Act 1989*). Working Together (2010) guideline strengthened.
Kyra Ishaq https://bbc.in/2uembbC	2010	First SCR publicly published in full. New Police Public Protection Department Created.
Daniel Pelka https://bit.ly/3cc1nq9	2013	Fourteen lessons including: gain an interpreter to speak with the child, accurate record keeping, mandatory to report suspected abuse to local authority.
Ayeeshia-Jayne Smith https://bit.ly/33N1Nzo	2014	Highlights vulnerable adults, maternal mental health and domestic abuse. Minimising levels of violence. Professionals to speak with the vulnerable adult away from their partner.
Kayleigh Haywood https://bit.ly/3mMBTUX	2015	Grooming online – Internet safety training and heightened awareness.
Charlie and Charlotte https://bit.ly/2sLvbH3	2016	Initial child protection conference to be automatically convened when a parent becomes pregnant and there is history of care proceedings. Policy in place when children are not brought for health appointments. Children's wishes and feelings must be heard and understood.

competent in the identification and escalation of child maltreatment concerns. Professionally you are required to ensure that you are compliant with your employer's child protection training requirements. Your employer has a statutory responsibility for ensuring that all employees maintain their professional competence in child protection through training and supervision.

The core principles of child protection competence include:
- Knowledge of child maltreatment in its different forms and its impact on the child and family.
- Awareness of risk factors for abuse.
- Ability to effectively manage concerns about child maltreatment.
- Information governance and knowing the importance of sharing relevant information appropriately (including the consequences of failing to do so).
- Ability to seek appropriate advice and report concerns, feeling confident that they have been listened to and acted upon (Royal College of Paediatrics and Child Health, 2014).
- Awareness of the principles surrounding 'best interests' of children and young people.

The concept of best interests is complex. Parental refusal of treatment for their child, for example, needs to be carefully assessed and will include clinical indicators alongside the views of the child, family and health care professionals. Assessment of best interests and the impact of non-treatment upon the child may require referral and escalation (British Medical Association, 2018).

An important principle of effective child protection is the ability to escalate and where necessary challenge decisions and to be an advocate for the child. There may be instances when you feel that your concerns are not being taken seriously or you experience barriers to referring a child/family. Barriers to referral can occur internally within your organisation and externally from other services, but it is paramount that you ensure that child protection concerns are addressed and managed appropriately. You need to seek immediate advice from senior colleagues, your internal child protection specialist team and social services. Your employer will have a policy and process for escalation of child protection concerns. Professionally you are ultimately accountable for ensuring that your concerns have been addressed.

Legislation and Policy

Legislation and policies underpin and inform all decisions we make to keep children safe. A piece of legislation is a statutory law which has been developed by a governing body in order to regulate and authorise a sequence of events. A policy is a principle of action adopted by an organisation, which details how a sequence of events should be managed. Legislation and policies are important because not only do they hold individuals and organisations to account for their actions, but they also help determine the correct and most efficient way to manage a situation.

There are a number of key and primary pieces of legislation, which help to develop local and national policies for preventing and responding to child maltreatment. In the UK these are:

England: *Children Act 1989 (amended 2004)*.
Northern Ireland: *Children (Northern Ireland) Order 1995*.
Scotland: *Children (Scotland) Act 1995*.
Wales: *Social Services and Well-Being Act (Wales) 2014*.

These provide the key principles that all agencies must follow, including the paramountcy principle. The paramountcy principle means that the child's welfare should always be the prime focus and this means that as a children's nurse you should be child focused and advocate for the child when required.

Some policies are practised almost universally. The UNCRC (UN, 1989) is the most widely ratified treaty in the world, promoting 54 articles of equal rank that all children have either the right to, or freedom from.

There are four key general principles underpinning the UNCRC:

1. Non-discrimination (article 2)
2. Best interest of the child (article 3)
3. Right to life survival and development (article 6)
4. Right to be heard (article 12)

Consent to Share Information When You Suspect a Child Is Being Maltreated

Confidentiality and data protection are important from both legal and ethical perspectives. Information sharing is directed by legislation which guides safe sharing of information, that is, the EU General Data Protection Regulation (GDPR) introduced in May 2018 (EU General Data Protection Regulation, 2018). In England HM Government (2018b) identifies seven golden rules for information sharing, which include sharing information proportionately to need and where possible with consent. As a children's nurse there may be instances when you have a child protection concern, but the parents will not consent to a referral to children's social care. In this situation you must always act in the interest of the safety of the child and refer to children's social care. Seek support from your manager and your internal child protection or safeguarding team.

Consent to Treatment

People aged 16 years or over are entitled to consent to their own treatment, and this can only be overruled in exceptional circumstances. Like adults, young people (aged 16 or 17 years) are presumed to have sufficient capacity to decide on their own medical treatment, unless there is significant evidence to suggest otherwise.

Children under the age of 16 can consent to their own treatment if they are considered to have sufficient intelligence, competence and understanding to fully appreciate what is involved in their treatment. This is known as being Gillick competent, stemming from a 1982 case, which assessed whether doctors should be able to give contraceptive advice or treatment to those under age 16 without parental consent. The case has been superseded by the Fraser guidelines (Bainham, 2017) which are more widely used to help assess whether a child has the maturity to make their own decisions and to understand their implications. If the individual is deemed not to be Fraser competent then someone with parental responsibility should consent for them. Therefore you need to be clear in your assessment as to who has parental responsibility. A mother automatically has parental responsibility from birth. Fathers need to be married to the child's mother, be named on the birth certificate, or have applied for parental responsibility. In an emergency, where treatment is vital and waiting to obtain parental consent would place the child at risk, treatment can proceed without consent. Consent can be overruled (by the Court of Protection) if a young person refuses treatment, which may lead to their death or severe permanent injury.

Making a Good Quality Referral to Other Agencies

Children's needs are multi-layered; as they grow and develop they need a stable, loving environment which is safe from maltreatment. Parents/carers have responsibilities to ensure welfare and educational needs are met so children can achieve their full potential as they transition into adult life.

Each child and family is unique with their own life experiences based on social, ecological and cultural factors. Life circumstances are fluid and can change, leaving children sometimes vulnerable and at risk of significant harm. It is important to achieve a proportional response to any risks posed. If a child is believed to be suffering or likely to suffer significant harm it is imperative to take protective action and make a referral to Children Social Services.

A clear, legible and well-structured referral to Children's Social Services is the key to unlocking multi-agency targeted support and immediate statutory social service response to protect children from significant harm. To ensure the referral is processed smoothly through the front door of children social services, and achieve an optimal outcome for the child, it is important that content of the referral is clear and concise in terms of risk and protective factors and that medical terminology is explained in lay terms.

Student nurses will not be expected to make referrals until qualified, but in preparing for your role as a future nurse, you require a sound awareness of the process and how to articulate concerns. Prior to making the referral it is important to be clear of the desired outcome for the child; this will tailor the words and language used in the referral.

🌐 WWW

A good tool to assist in choosing the correct words can be found at: https://bit.ly/3mPPDyh.

Best practice is to promptly make a verbal referral when the concern presents, followed by a written referral, sent from and to a secure e-mail address (faxing is considered insecure) in line with the EU GDPR, 2018 (EU General Data Protection Regulation, 2018). Use the correct referral form for your place of work, matching the local authority (or relevant district if not in the UK) with the child's home address. It is always best to work with the family and gain consent for the referral unless this puts the child at risk of harm.

When writing the referral, it is important to consider who will be the recipient. A social worker will have the responsibility to screen the information, coordinate lateral checks (social, educational, health and police) then make recommendations to either:

- Take no further action – referral closed.
- Recommend for 'early help' intervention.
- Send the referral for a multi-agency professionals' discussion.
- Send the referral for a multi-agency strategy meeting.

Be mindful that important points can be missed in translation. The social worker will not have met the child and family or witnessed the concerns. They do not have a medical background so will require the presenting risks and impact for the child's health and well-being to be fully explained in simple terms. A balanced approach is required stating what is going well for the child, what are the risks and subsequent impact for the child.

Avoid using broad statements which can be open to interpretation, such as 'The child presented unkempt' or 'The mother appeared drunk'.

Instead document the facts as in the following examples:

1. The child was wearing dirt stained, threadbare clothes which had a stale odour to them. It was cold outside; the child was dressed in a t-shirt and he was shivering. The child's face and body were covered in dirt.
2. The mother was slurring her speech, pupils were dilated, she was unable to walk in a straight line and smelt of intoxicating liquor.

Box 24.1 lists the key points in making a good referral.

BOX 24.1   Key Points When Making a Quality Referral to Children Social Services

- ✓ Assess, be clear about your concern/category of abuse, take immediate action.
- ✓ The professional with the concern makes the immediate verbal and on-line secure referral.
- ✓ Consent obtained? If not, why (e.g. would put child in immediate risk of significant harm?).
- ✓ Keep language simple and concise, avoid medical jargon.
- ✓ Document child/family primary language and confirm interpreter has been used.
- ✓ Keep information factual – what did you see, hear, smell (e.g. substance misuse).
- ✓ Explain injury/illness/disabilities/child protection concern and the impact on child.
- ✓ Complete child and family tree details, permanent address and temporary if visiting.
- ✓ Be mindful of transferable risks to siblings – state where they are and who is caring for them.
- ✓ Child next of kin/legal guardian full details: name, date of birth and if they hold parental responsibility.
- ✓ Who is accompanying the child – any concerning behaviour?
- ✓ Child's journey – share relevant handover information from other professionals (e.g. police, ambulance, school).
- ✓ Capture child's voice – open questions: observe, listen and document.
- ✓ Parental capacity: consider risks (e.g. substance misuse, domestic abuse, learning difficulties, mental ill health).
- ✓ Protective factors: list those present and note their impact on the child.
- ✓ Document how the parent/carer interacts with the child.
- ✓ Risks of child sexual exploitation (CSE)? Use CSE screening tool and send with referral.
- ✓ Consider if the young person is a parent – where and who is caring for their child.
- ✓ Document multi-agency professionals involved with the child (e.g. GP, school, family support worker).
- ✓ Document the referrer's details: name, professional role, work address and contact number.
- ✓ Document what you think needs to happen to protect the child, make it clear if you want a statutory social care response.

Adults – Vulnerable Adults and Parental Capacity

While primarily focusing upon the needs of the child patient, the children's nurse also has a duty of care to the adult parents/carers of the child. Adult safeguarding means protecting an adult's right to live in safety, free from abuse and neglect. It is about people and organisations working together to prevent and stop the risks and experience of abuse or neglect, while at the same time making sure that the adult's well-being is promoted including, where appropriate, having regard to their views, wishes, feelings and beliefs in deciding on any action (Department of Health and Social Care, 2014).

All children are considered vulnerable by virtue of their age and immaturity, but which adults can be considered 'vulnerable'? This is sometimes fluid, as people may be vulnerable in different ways at different times of their lives. The following groups of people may be considered 'vulnerable adults':

- People with intellectual disabilities.
- People with a mental health condition such as dementia or personality disorder.
- People who are ill and need help to carry out normal daily functions.
- People with physical disabilities.
- People who have undergone a recent trauma – a bereavement, a divorce or loss of a job, for instance.
- People who, for whatever reason, are in abusive relationships.
- People who have no recourse to public funds or are homeless.

The children's nurse needs to consider the impact of the parent/carer's vulnerability upon their ability to care appropriately and protect their child. In some instances, it is important to consider the mental capacity of the vulnerable adult to advocate for their child, for example, learning disability, mental health needs. Assessment of mental capacity is underpinned by the *Mental Capacity Act, 2007* (England and Wales) and identifies whether a person is able to make their own decisions. This will be significant for the children's nurse when considering consent for treatment and capacity to care for the child at home.

You should always consider parental/carer mental capacity during the initial nursing assessment of the child and family's needs as this will potentially impact upon the longer term outcomes for the child's well-being. Additional advice and support should be sought from your internal safeguarding team and learning disabilities team where relevant. At the same time, you need to be careful to avoid generalisations or stereotypical thinking and be prepared to challenge instances where this may be happening.

Talking About Child Maltreatment Concerns and Child Protection Processes

In acute and community health care services professionals meet children and their families at a time when they are most vulnerable and distressed due to the presenting medical need. Bound by the Nursing Midwifery Council Code (2015) (Standards 7 and 17) nurses should not shy away from uncomfortable conversations. Using a non-judgmental, empathetic approach, professionals should openly share their child protection concerns and plan to refer to children social services. The only exception for non-transparency would be if this were to put the child at risk of immediate harm, for example, where fabricated or induced illness is suspected.

Self-awareness, interpersonal communication skills and emotional intelligence during the delivery of unfavourable information is a necessary part of nursing, but may take years to hone. Engaging in conversations about delicate and sensitive child protection issues and processes can trigger fear and a sense of feeling out of one's depth. However, a number

---

> ### BOX 24.2 Best Practice – How to Initiate a Child Protection Conversation
>
> - Determine if you are the best person to have the conversation. Understand your professional responsibilities and limitations.
> - Be self-aware and non-judgmental, prepare, breathe and calm yourself – address your thoughts and feelings as they could subconsciously show in your choice of words, tone and body language.
> - Be mindful of barriers to communication. Misinterpretation or lack of capacity to comprehend can arise from cultural/language barriers, mental health issues and intellectual difficulties.
> - Prior to the conversation be clear what and how much information you will share. Provide verbal and written information.
> - Think about the environment – is it conducive to achieving uninterrupted, confidential discussions?
> - Introduce yourself and your professional role. Conduct yourself in a polite and respectful manner.
> - A transitional statement is helpful to open discussions and prepare the family to receive unfavourable news. 'I understand the Consultant has explained they cannot find a medical cause for the fracture'; 'I am concerned you are taking risks with your safety and wish to work with you to change this'; 'I need to be direct and honest with you'.
> - Maintain open posture, good eye contact and professional boundaries.
> - Check that the information you have shared has been understood.
> - Avoid using medical jargon, keep it simple.
> - Explain the processes step by step with regular updates to help reduce anxiety of the unknown and reduce the risk of conflict.
> - Actively listen, gaining the wishes and feelings of the child and family.
> - Provide time for questions. If the answer is not known, endeavour to find out and feedback.
> - Expect a reaction, be prepared and keep safe.
> - Maintain accurate records of the conversation – this can be used as evidence in court.

---

of strategies can be built into everyday practice to improve confidence and competence when holding challenging conversations (Box 24.2).

Strategic Challenges to Safeguarding

Effective safeguarding is contingent upon strong multi-agency working. Therefore one of the key strategic challenges is the need for a cohesive response across many agencies. To achieve the best possible outcomes, children and families need to receive targeted services to meet their needs in a coordinated way.

Partnership working across agencies is often challenging due to geography, limited understanding of each other's roles and professionals working in isolation. Families may experience contact with multiple agencies, for example, health, education and social care, and there is a need for a joined up approach. Fragmented provision of services creates inefficiencies and risks disengagement by children and families. Local agencies are the front line when it comes to keeping children safe and it is vital that they work well together (HM Government, 2018a).

A shared understanding across agencies of the determinants of risk and child maltreatment are essential to creating effective partnership working. However, sometimes the interpretation of risk and child maltreatment can be contentious across agencies. A review of 38 serious case reviews of child maltreatment (Social Care Insitute for Excellence [SCIE], 2016) identified the challenges across agencies in working effectively together. These included disagreements about what early help means, or is needed, whether children's social care should be involved, confusion about medical terminology and not convening multi-agency strategy discussions in good time.

Political and economic factors can also create strategic challenges within child protection. Social inequalities and poverty can potentially increase the risk of child maltreatment. Childhood poverty can create additional stress for families and the potential for negative, harmful behaviour. There is interdependency between poverty and extended family support and the wider social and physical environment. Therefore the children's nurse should ensure that nursing care assessments of child and family needs includes an understanding of the family's social circumstances and their access to wider social support (Bywaters et al., 2016).

Emotional Challenges in Child Protection Work

Identifying and caring for children who have been maltreated is stressful and distressing and unless working specifically within a child protection role, it is not an everyday occurrence. Both human nature and juggling reactions to stress can pose a potential obstacle to effective practice. It is uncomfortable to disbelieve or think ill of, suspect or wrongly blame a parent or carer, and this can be coupled with fear of complaints, and fear for one's own safety or losing positive relations with families (NICE, 2013).

It is important to explore your own thoughts and feelings regarding child maltreatment and understand how you individually react to this stress. A lack of self-awareness can impact negatively on a person's abilities to recognise and respond to concerns or to cope in a crisis and these can impact on the wider team. A number of nurses, including student nurses, may have experienced maltreatment themselves in childhood. If this is the case, then child protection work may provoke unwelcome memories and emotions. It is important to confront these and where necessary, seek help. Robin, a survivor of child maltreatment, demonstrates courage in sharing inspiring words of wisdom (Box 24.3).

Acknowledging you may not have encountered child protection situations before, work with a peer you trust to reflect on the case study in Box 24.4 and work through the exercise at the end. Imagine you are the nurse and discuss the following questions:

- What feelings are emerging with this case for you as a person?

BOX 24.3   Robin's Advice to Nurses Who Were Maltreated in Childhood

As an adult survivor of child maltreatment, I have been faced with children who have been maltreated themselves during my employment at a school. They have been either introvert or troubled, displaying aggressive behaviour. My childhood experiences have given me a deeper insight and empathy towards these children. It has also hardened me because I wanted to live so my coping strategy is to survive. As a child I had no choice, I did not have the child protection services that are in place today, adults did not listen to a child. As an adult when you see the signs of maltreatment you think this child before me is suffering like I suffered but this hardened shell around you and inner resilience goes into automatic protective response to help them.

If a case reflects your own story this can trigger secondary trauma and flashbacks. It is important to be self-aware and know where to access help and support. Don't let this stop you from nursing, you are stronger than you know and can turn the negative into a positive. You will be in a unique position to help others with the skills to swiftly recognise maltreatment.

Robin, aged 67, with permission

- What are your concerns in relation to Isabel and her mother? How do you think this may impact on you emotionally, psychologically and physically?

Emotional Resilience

It is a misconception that repeated exposure to child maltreatment equates to professionals becoming used to the emotional impact that makes them in some way 'hardened' to the experience. Some people are more naturally attuned to coping with stress, but investing time to build a firm foundation of coping strategies protects our well-being. This becomes a foundation to developing emotional resilience. Building resilience is an important strategy in alleviating stress and reducing the risks of emotional burnout when encountering child protection cases (Delgado et al., 2017). Being resilient does not mean you are impervious to stress, but are able to bend and adapt to the challenges faced in a more calm and controlled manner. Resilience can be nurtured and continuously strengthened through experience, reflection and personal growth. Practising mindfulness may help to centre your focus on the here and now. It may assist students to develop self-awareness, see the bigger picture and enable greater empathy (Dean et al., 2017). Research into mindfulness exhibits benefits of lower levels of anxiety and depression with successful self-regulation and endurance of emotional stimuli (Egan et al., 2017). Emotionally resilient people can adapt positively to challenging situations, resolve problems with an optimistic attitude, and have a good support network. Emotional intelligence coupled with a strong self-belief and self-compassion are key characteristics (Delgado et al., 2017).

BOX 24.4 Isabel's Case Study

Isabel is 2 years old and has complex health care needs. Birth defects have resulted in abnormally narrow airways, so a tracheostomy is in place and she also has a gastrostomy for feeding. She lives in hospital, having been there since birth and has never been home. Isabel is having investigations for a potential genetic condition. She is developmentally delayed physically, but cognitively she is very bright and is learning basic sign language. There is a strong, positive bond between Isabel and her mother Marcia, a single parent. When Marcia goes home, Isabel refuses to eat her finger food and becomes withdrawn.

Marcia has a history of depression, anxiety and non-compliance with her prescribed anti-depressant medication. To be able to take Isabel home Marcia must be trained in tracheostomy care, gastrostomy management and basic life support – Isabel's life depends on Marcia being competent in all three skills.

Nurses have observed Marcia struggling to retain information, so staff have provided intense training over the past 8 months. Marcia is not following Isabel's care plan and nurses are constantly prompting her. Nurses have concerns Marcia may have an undiagnosed learning disability, but she clearly loves her daughter Isabel.

Children Social Services have now become involved due to concerns about parental capacity to meet Isabel's needs and have completed a parenting assessment on Marcia and found her unable to manage safely. Exhausting extended family support networks, there is nobody who can care for Isabel.

Marcia is informed by the social worker that Isabel will have to go into foster care and a pre-court proceedings meeting has been arranged.

Marcia tells the nurse if Isabel is taken into care she will choose not to see her again as she cannot cope with the pain and feels like taking her own life.

BOX 24.5 Noel and Steven's Case Study

Noel, aged 4 years 5 months and sibling Steven, aged 3 years have been brought to hospital by ambulance. Parents originate from Somalia and both speak English. Father is present and interacting well with the children. Noel appears protective of Steven and asks you for some food for his brother. Mother has been called, but is not attending the department as alleged to be at work.

Police share that they received a call from a member of the public at 7 am stating they had found Noel alone wondering the street wearing just a vest and underpants. It was cold outside and Noel was by the roadside. Police attended and Noel said he was looking for his brother, mummy and daddy. He had woken up at home and could not find them. Police took Noel back home and Noel showed them how he was able to open the apartment door and walk onto the street using the fire escape stairs. The apartment was damp and unclean, there was one mattress on the floor, no food in the cupboards and no toys. Father then returned home with Steven. The father keeps giving different accounts of what happened and denies that Noel was found in the street. Neighbours have reported they hear the children crying frequently and see the parents leaving the apartment without them. Police checks show father has a criminal history and a similar event occurred 1 month ago, currently being investigated by children social services.

Ambulance crew shared that Noel was very cold when they assessed him, slightly dehydrated and very calm, not upset he was alone. Noel said he does not go to nursery or school.

Using the Framework for Assessment (Fig. 24.2), imagine you are the nurse in the Emergency Department receiving the handover of care from the ambulance crew and police officer.

1. Explore your feelings, would you know what to do? Using the below anxiety scale, score how anxious you would be.
2. Under the subheadings **Risk Factors**, **Protective Factors** and **Unknown** pick out the relevant points and place them in the correct boxes. Practice identifying both vulnerabilities and any factors that would be protective for the children. Also think about any cultural factors and whether these would be important.

Resilience can be nurtured and continuously strengthened through experience, reflection and personal growth. Practising mindfulness may be beneficial to some people.

 WWW

A useful information sheet 'How to Manage Stress' can be obtained here: https://bit.ly/2GwnXZV.

Take time to explore the array of different ways people can positively address stress and reflect which work for you to create your own emotional resilience toolbox.

Supervision

Leadership in child protection is essential to drive best practice forward. The ability to raise concerns, take action and when required challenge decisions are skills professionals all require to protect children, young people and vulnerable adults from harm. Child protection work is often viewed as a specialism, despite recommendations from Laming (2003) and Munro (2011) which define safeguarding as 'everybody's business'.

Organisations are responsible to ensure their employees have child protection systems and processes in place and access to education and support to enable best practice (Royal College of Paediatrics and Child Health, 2014). Safeguarding supervision is a formal, accountable process where protected time facilitates reflection, decision making and providing a safe space to explore the emotional impact. Supervision endeavours to strengthen front line professional's skills in unearthing hidden harm, risk analysis, and child-centred, timely responses to child maltreatment. Take time to reflect on Noel and Steven's case study in Box 24.5. Using the framework for the assessment of children:

- What are the presenting risk, protective and unknown factors?
- Would this case cause you stress?
- What would be your proportional response in protecting the children?

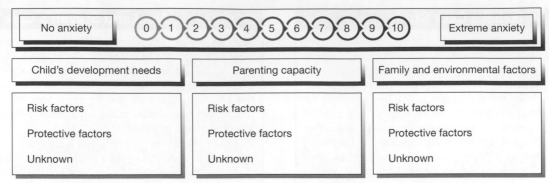

Fig. 24.2 Safeguarding supervision template: reflecting on the child, family and practitioner.

THE CHANGING LANDSCAPE OF CHILD PROTECTION

Target 16.2 of the 2030 agenda for Sustainable Development is to 'end abuse, exploitation, trafficking and all forms of violence against and torture of children' (WHO, 2018). However, the 21st century changing landscape brings globally diverse and multi-layered challenges to child protection. The digital age opens doors to easily accessible information and communication, creating both opportunities and risks. Computers, mobile telephones and newer technologies can be used by perpetrators of abuse to groom and control vulnerable children. In response to revelations of new and hidden child maltreatment, a plethora of laws and policies have been introduced and international efforts have designed a technical package INSPIRE: seven strategies for ending violence against children (WHO, 2018).

With freedom of movement and migration, health professionals need to be attuned to global forms of child maltreatment and the law, to be able to recognise and protect children at risk of significant harm (Phillimore et al., 2018). The following areas of maltreatment and useful websites/video links will provide a platform to broaden your knowledge on some of the global challenges faced and emphasise the importance of working together internationally to protect children.

Forced Labour, Modern Slavery and Human Trafficking

On 19 September 2017 during the 72nd meeting of the United Nations General Assembly, 37 Member States and Observer States endorsed 'A Call to Action to end forced labour, modern slavery and human trafficking'. These crimes include:

- Child sexual exploitation.
- Forced labour.
- Domestic servitude.
- Criminal exploitation – for example, organised theft, drug trafficking.
- Organ harvesting.

The United Nations define human trafficking as the recruitment, transfer, harbouring or receipt of persons by improper means (force, abduction, fraud, coercion) for an improper purpose (National Institute of Justice, 2018).

WWW

Further information can be obtained at: https://bit.ly/2vJX1CF and https://wb.md/2ECtGBO.
You might find the following BBC film helpful: https://bbc.in/2B9RavC.

Organ Trafficking

The trade of human organs to meet the transplantation shortage for financial gain is illegal in many jurisdictions. Victims may be recruited through deception and their consent may also be obtained through coercion or abuse of a position of vulnerability explains the United Nations Office on Drugs and Crime (UNODC, 2015). The WHO condemned the illegal organ trade in 1987 and has been instrumental in taking steps to stop organ trafficking.

WWW

More can be learned at: https://bit.ly/2KTrcvL.

War Zones, Torture, Rape and Terrorism

Krug et al. (2002) define collective violence as:

> *The instrumental use of violence by people who identify themselves as a member of a group – whether this group is transitory or has a more permanent identity – against another group or set of individuals, in order to achieve political, economic or social objectives.*

Violent conflicts and acts of terrorism between nations/groups have the following negative impact on civilians:

- Increased mortality and morbidity.
- Acute injuries and long-term disabilities.
- Psychological and behavioural issues, for example anxiety, suicidal tendencies, substance misuse, post-traumatic stress disorder.
- Increased risk of communicable diseases.
- Poor environment, lack of food/water/health care/shelter.

Female Genital Mutilation/Cutting

Female genital mutilation/cutting (FGM/C) is the partial or total removal of external female genitalia for non-medical reasons. It may also be known in some cultures as female circumcision, although this minimises the harm caused, likening it to male circumcision (only forms of FGM/C that remove only the clitoral hood are akin). Religious or cultural reasons may be given in mitigation of FGM/C, but FGM/C is nevertheless child abuse (NSPCC, 2018). FGM/C has been illegal in the UK since 1985. In 2003 it also became a criminal offence for UK nationals or permanent UK residents to take their children abroad for FGM/C. It is a mandatory reporting requirement to the police and children social services for any child under the age of 18 years at risk of/has had FGM/C (Home Office, 2016).

County Lines, Violence and Gangs

Thousands of vulnerable children and young people are being groomed and coerced by drug dealers and gangs to run drugs and money between urban and rural county lines in England and Wales. These children then recruit others via social media or in person. The National Crime Agency purports that gangs keep children in their service through drug dependency, threatening family, sexual exploitation, violence and intimidation (including knife and firearms). Emerging trends of violence-related crimes include ammonia and acid attacks (National Crime Agency, 2017).

Breast Ironing

Breast ironing is a hidden, painful female upon female gender-based violence, a physical mutilation against pubescent girls, resulting in lifelong consequences to their health and well-being. Originating from West Africa it is widespread mainly within certain regions of Cameroon but also reported in Guinea-Bissau, Chad, Togo and Benin and has spread across the globe (Tchoukou, 2014). Breast ironing practices continue in the UK due to population migration (Robinson, 2019).

Breast ironing is forced upon pubescent children in the belief that this tradition protects girls from sexual harassment and rape, and that it prevents early pregnancy and forced marriage (Pearsell, 2017). Typically performed by the mother but can be a female family relative, heated implements (i.e. grinding stones, spatulas, coconut shells) are used to pound, press or massage the naturally developing breast over a period of time to prevent or slow down breast growth to suppress womanhood. Other methods are binding girl's chests with an elastic belt/band to constrict natural breast growth (National FGM Centre, 2018; United Nations Women, 2013).
Health implications include:

- Severe pain/itching
- Fever/infection
- Dissymmetry/disappearance of breasts
- Tissue damage
- Discharge of milk
- Breast cancer
- Abscesses or cysts
- Trauma/psychological impact
- Social impact
  (National FGM Centre, 2017)

To download the breast ironing factsheet (2017) please see the link:

http://nationalfgmcentre.org.uk/wp-content/uploads/2018/04/About-Breast-Flattening-Leaflet-.pdf

To hear girls/women, share their own experiences of breast ironing please look at the following presentation and YouTube brief documentaries:
https://bit.ly/3kEmJ2o
https://bbc.in/3cogvAD
https://bit.ly/35ZubRz

Forced Marriage

A forced marriage is where one or both people do not (or in the case of people with learning disabilities, cannot) consent to the marriage and are pressured or abused to comply. It is important to distinguish this from an arranged marriage, where both parties have consented. Forced marriage is illegal in the UK where it is recognised as a form of violence against women and men, domestic/child abuse and a serious abuse of human rights (Foreign & Commonwealth Office, 2013). Forced marriage has been known to happen to girls as young as eight (British High Commission Islamabad, 2018).

The first UK successful forced marriage prosecution was in May 2018, where a mother was sentenced to 4.5 years imprisonment. The mother had tricked her daughter into going to Pakistan for an alleged family holiday, but the reality was to force her daughter to marry a relative 16 years her senior. Physical abuse and threats to burn the passport were made when the daughter protested to the arrangement.

 WWW

A useful video by the UK forced marriage unit: https://bit.ly/2w9D2ix.

'Honour' Based Violence

This is a violent crime or incident which may have been committed to protect or defend the honour of the family or community (Metropolitan Police, 2018). Usually linked to family members, it occurs when it is perceived that someone has shamed the family/community by behaving in a way which contradicts traditional beliefs/culture (e.g. not wearing traditional clothes, wanting to leave a marriage).

 WWW

A powerful documentary regarding the honour-based murder of Banaz Mahmod can be accessed by the following link: https://bit.ly/OkVYAI.

Key indicators for recognising modern slavery and other risks for refugees: https://bit.ly/2PckEvR.

CONCLUSION

This chapter cannot possibly cover every single aspect of child abuse and neglect that the children's nurse may encounter, but it has highlighted how you need to be vigilant at all times. Parents or carers who hurt children are unlikely to tell the entire truth, or can look to be complying with child protection plans when they are not. Some are just unable to cope, to a point where their child is negatively impacted. If you are

BOX 24.6   Signposts to Helpful Information

Organisation	Available	Telephone Number	Website
Black Association of Women Step Out (BAWSO) provide culturally sensitive and appropriate information and services to black and other minority ethnic groups		08007 318147	www.bawso.org.uk
Childline	24 hours	0800 1111	http://www.childline.org.uk/
Contact-A-Family (support for parents of children with disabilities)	9 am – 5 pm Monday to Friday	020 7222 2695	https://contact.org.uk/
Cry-sis (persistently crying and/or sleepless babies)	9 am – 10 pm Every day	08451 228669	http://www.cry-sis.org.uk/
Family Rights Group (support with child protection procedures)	9.30 am – 3 pm Monday to Friday	0808 801 0366	http://www.frg.org.uk/
Karma Nirvana Helpline Supports victims and survivors of forced marriage and honour based abuse		0800 599 9247	www.karmanirvana.org.uk
Kidscape (deals with bullying, stranger danger, threats of abuse)	10 am – 5 pm Monday and Tuesday	020 7730 3300 020 7823 5430 (Parent Advice Line) info@kidscape.org.uk (Email)	http://www.kidscape.org.uk/
Action for Children	9 am – 5 pm Monday to Friday	01923 361500 Ask.us@actionforchildren.org.uk (Email)	http://www.actionforchildren.org.uk
NSPCC Child Protection Adult Helpline (acts in cases of neglect and abuse of children)	24 hours	0808 800500 help@nspcc.org.uk (Email)	http://www.nspcc.org.uk/
National Association for People Abused in Childhood (NAPAC) (for adult survivors of abuse)	10 am – 9 pm Monday to Thursday 10 am – 6 pm Friday	0808 801 0331	http://www.napac.org.uk/
Refuge provider of specialist accommodation and services to women and children escaping domestic violence			www.refuge.org.uk
RESPOND (sexual abuse and people with learning disabilities)		020 7383 0700	http://www.respond.org.uk/
Women's Aid (emergency accommodation for abused women and children)	24 hours	0808 2000 247 helpline@womensaid.org.uk (Email)	http://www.womensaid.org.uk/

ever in doubt about a child or their family, do not hesitate to raise your concerns with your line manager or the lead child protection nurse or doctor. Most importantly, child abuse and neglect is emotive work and it is important to make sure you have support mechanisms and coping strategies in place.

REFERENCES

Children Act, 1989. c.41. Available from: http://www.legislation.gov.uk/ukpga/1989/41/contents (accessed July 4, 2018).

Department of Health & Social Care, 2014. Care Act Statutory Guidance. Available from: https://www.gov.uk/government/publications/care-act-statutory-guidance. [Accessed 4 July 2018].

EU General Data Protection Regulation 2018. Available from: https://gdpr-info.eu/.

Mental Capacity Act England and Wales, 2007. Available from: https://www.legislation.gov.uk/ukpga/2007/12/contents (accessed July 4, 2018)

Nursing & Midwifery Council, 2015. The Code: Professional Standards of Practice and Behaviour for Nurses and Midwives. NMC, London.

Alexander, R., 2017. Child Maltreatment Prevention. Definitions of Abuse and Prevention. STM Learning Inc., Florissant, MO.

Anda, R., Felitti, V., Brown, D., et al., 2006. Insights into intimate partner violence from the adverse childhood experiences (ACE) study. In: Salber, P., Taliaferro, E. (Eds.), The Physician's Guide to Intimate Partner Violence and Abuse. Volcano Press, Volcano, CA, pp. 77–78.

Astrup, J., 2018. The end of smacking? Community Pract 11 January 2018 Available: https://www.communitypractitioner.co.uk/features/2018/01/end-smacking#:~:text=As%20a%20campaign%20to%20help,'physical%20discipline'%20for%20children.

Bainham, A., 2017. Teenagers in care proceedings: welfare, rights and justice. Fam. Law 47, 505–512.

Bellis, M., Hughes, K., Ford, K., et al., 2018. Adverse childhood experiences and sources of childhood resilience: a retrospective study of their combined relationships with child health and educational attendance. BMC Publ. Health. https://doi.org/10.1186/s12889-018-5699-8.

Brandon, M., Bailey, S., Belderson, P., 2010. Building on the Learning From Serious Case Reviews. Department for Education, London. Available from: http://dera.ioe.ac.uk/852/1/DFE-RR040.pdf (accessed 4 July 2018).

Brandon, M., Bailey, S., Sorensen, P., et al., 2016. Pathways to Harm, Pathways to Protection: A Triennial Analysis of Serious Case Reviews 2011 to 2014 Final Report. Department for Education, London.

Bray, S., 2018. Working Together Proposed Changes. Stoke on Trent Safeguarding Children Board. Staffordshire County Council.

British High Commission Islamabad, 2018. UK conviction after mother forced daughter to marry in Pakistan. Available from: https://www.gov.uk/government/news/uk-conviction-after-mother-forced-daughter-to-marry-in-pakistan (accessed 4 July 2018).

British Medical Association, 2018. Children and Young People Ethics Toolkit. Available from: https://www.bma.org.uk/advice/employment/ethics/children-and-young-people/children-and-young-peoples-ethics-tool-kit (accessed 4 July 2018).

Bywaters, P., Bunting, L., Davidson, G., et al., 2016. The Relationship Between Poverty, Child Abuse and Neglect: An Evidence Review. Joseph Rowntree Foundation, York.

Children Act, 1989. c.41. Available from: http://www.legislation.gov.uk/ukpga/1989/41/contents (accessed 4 July 2018).

Dean, S.J., Foureur, M., Zaslawski, C., et al., 2017. The effects of a structured mindfulness program on the development of empathy in healthcare students. Nurs. Plus. Open. 3, 1–5.

Delgado, C., Upton, D., Ranse, K., et al., 2017. Nurses' resilience and the emotional labour of nursing work: an integrative review of empirical literature. Int. J. Nurs. Stud. 70, 71–88.

Department for Education, 2017. Child Sexual Exploitation: Definition and Guide for Practitioners. DfE, London.

Department of Health and Social Care, 2014. Care Act Statutory Guidance. Available from: https://www.gov.uk/government/publications/care-act-statutory-guidance (accessed 4 July 2018).

Egan, H., Mantzios, M., Jackson, C., 2017. Health practitioners and the directive towards compassionate healthcare in the UK: exploring the need to educate health practitioners on how to be self-compassionate and mindful alongside mandating compassion towards patients. Health Prof. Educ. 3 (2), 61–63.

EU General Data Protection Regulation, 2018. Available from: https://gdpr-info.eu/.

Evans, G., Cowley, L., Fox, S., et al., 2018. Every Psychologist's Responsibility: Safeguarding Children and Young People. British Psychological Association, London.

Felitti, V.J., Anda, R.F., Nordenberg, D., et al., 1998. Relationship of childhood abuse and household dysfunction to many of the leading causes of death in adults. The Adverse Childhood Experiences (ACE) Study. Am. J. of Preve. Med. 14 (4), 245–258.

Foreign & Commonwealth Office, 2013. What is Forced Marriage? Available from: www.gov.uk/forced-marriage (accessed 4 July 2018).

HM Government, 2018a. Working Together to Safeguard Children: A Guide to Inter-agency Working to Safeguard and Promote the Welfare of Children. DfE, London.

HM Government, 2018b. Information Sharing. DfE, London.

Home Office, 2016. Female Genital Mutilation. Home Office, London.

Hyde, C., 2018. Serious Case Review, Overview Report – Charlie and Charlotte. Local Safeguarding Children Board, Durham.

Krug, E., et al., 2002. World Report on Violence and Health. WHO, Geneva.

Laming, L., 2003. The Victoria Climbié Inquiry: Report of an Inquiry by Lord Laming. TSO, London. ISBN 0101573022, Cm 5730.

Mental Capacity Act England and Wales, 2007. Available from: https://www.legislation.gov.uk/ukpga/2007/12/contents (accessed 4 July 2018).

Ministry of Community, Housing and Health, 2018. Supporting Disadvantaged Families: Troubled Families Programme 2015–2020: Progress So Far. TSO, London.

Munro, E., 2011. Munro Review of Child Protection: Final Report – A Child-Centred System. Department for Education, London.

Munro, E., Taylor, J., Bradbury-Jones, C., 2014. Understanding the causal pathways to child maltreatment. Child. Abuse. Rev. 23, 61–74.

National Crime Agency, 2017. County Lines Violence, Exploitation and Drug Supply. National Briefing B Report. Accessed from: http://www.nationalcrimeagency.gov.uk/publications/832-county-lines-violence-exploitation-and-drug-supply-2017/file (accessed 4 July 2018).

National FGM Centre, 2018. Breast Flattening Factsheet. Available from: http://nationalfgmcentre.org.uk/wp-content/uploads/2018/04/About-Breast-Flattening-Leaflet-.pdf (accessed 12 May 2019).

National Institute for Health and Care Excellence (NICE), 2013. NICE Clinical Guideline 89: When to Suspect Child Maltreatment. NICE, London.

National Institute of Justice, 2018. Human Trafficking. Available from: https://www.nij.gov/topics/crime/human-trafficking/pages/welcome.aspx (accessed 4 July 2018).

Newbury, J., Arseneault, L., 2017. Measuring childhood maltreatment to predict early-adult psychopathology. J. Psychiatr. Res. 98, 57–64.

NHS England, 2016. Fabricated or Induced Illness. Available from: https://www.nhs.uk/conditions/fabricated-or-induced-illness/ (accessed 4 July 2018).

NSPCC, 2017. Child Protection in England. Serious Case Reviews. Available from: https://www.nspcc.org.uk/preventing-abuse/child-protection-system/england/serious-case-reviews/ (accessed 4 July 2018).

NSPCC, 2018. Female Genital Mutilation. Available from: https://www.nspcc.org.uk/preventing-abuse/child-abuse-and-neglect/female-genital-mutilation-fgm/ (accessed 4 July 2018).

Nursing & Midwifery Council, 2015. The Code: Professional Standards of Practice and Behaviour for Nurses and Midwives. NMC, London.

Pearsell, R., 2017. The harmful traditional practice of breast ironing in cameroon Africa. Bridges: An Undergraduate Journal of Contemporary Connections 2 (1).

Phillimore, J., Bradby, H., Knecht, M., et al., 2018. Bricolage as conceptual tool for understanding access to healthcare in superdiverse populations. Soc. Theor. Health. 17, 231–252. https://doi.org/10.1057/s41285-018-0075-4.

Police, M., 2018. Crimes of Honour Based Violence. Available from: https://safe.met.police.uk/crimes_of_honour/get_the_facts.html (accessed 4 July 2018).

Rahilly, T., Hendry, E. (Eds.), 2014. Promoting the Wellbeing of Children in Care: Messages from Research. NSPCC, London.

Robinson, F., 2019. Breast ironing. BMJ 365, l1790.

Royal College of Paediatrics and Child Health, 2014. Safeguarding Children and Young People: Roles and Competences for Healthcare Staff, third ed. RCPCH, London.

Sidebotham, P., Brandon, M., Bailey, S., et al., 2011. Serious and Fatal Child Maltreatment – Setting Serious Case Review Data in Context with Other Data on Violent and Maltreatment-Related Deaths in 2009–10. Department for Education, London.

Social Care Institute for Excellence (SCIE), 2016. Practice Issues from Serious Case Reviews – Learning into Practice. Available from: https://www.scie.org.uk/children/safeguarding/case-reviews/learning-from-case-reviews/ (accessed 4 July 2018).

Spratt, T., 2012. Why multiples matter: reconceptualising the population referred to child and family social workers. Br. J. Soc. Work 24 (8), 1574–1591.

Taylor, J., Bradbury-Jones, C., 2015. Child maltreatment: every nurse's business. Nurs. Stand. 29 (29), 53–58.

Taylor, J., Lazenbatt, A., 2014. Child Maltreatment and High Risk Families. Dunedin, London.

Tchoukou, J.A., 2014. Introducing the practice of breast ironing as a human rights issue in Cameroon. J. Civil Legal Sci. 3, 121. https://doi.org/10.4172/2169-0170.1000121.

United Nations, 1989. The United Nations Convention on the Rights of the Child. United Nations, Geneva.

United Nations Office on Drugs and Crime (UNODC), 2015. Vienna Expert Group Meeting on Trafficking in Organs. Available from: http://www.unodc.org/unodc/en/human-trafficking/2010/egm-vienna-organ-trafficking.html (accessed 4 July 2018).

Wood, A., 2016. Wood Report: Review of the Role and Functions of Local Safeguarding Children Boards. Department for Education, London.

World Health Organization, 2016. Child Maltreatment Factsheet. WHO, Geneva. Available from: http://www.who.int/news-room/fact-sheets/detail/child-maltreatment (accessed 4 July 2018).

World Health Organization (WHO), 2018. Violence Against Children Factsheet. Available from: http://www.who.int/media-centre/factsheets/violence-against-children/en/ (accessed 4 July 2018).

25

Cultural Aspects of Children's Nursing

Jim Richardson

LEARNING OUTCOMES

- Explore aspects of your own personal culture and the impact these might have on your professional interactions.
- Express what culture means as a term and appreciate the importance of taking culture into account in children's nursing work.

- Recognise what aspects of children's, and their families', responses are determined by their cultural background.
- Identify strategies for using ideas of culture in everyday children's nursing activity.
- Explore the dimensions of cultural safety.

WHAT IS CULTURE?

It seems difficult to pin down precisely what we mean by 'culture', although the term is in frequent use. The word contains shades of meaning that include 'race' or 'nationality'; we now talk of multi-cultural Britain and transcultural nursing. Equally, culture can be taken to mean the creative product of a society such as literature, music, etc.

An examination of what idea of culture this chapter is offering should help to clarify terms from the outset. The Nursing Council of New Zealand (2002, p 3) defines culture quite simply: 'culture refers to the beliefs and practices common to any particular group.'

Helman (2000, p 2) expands on this:

Culture is … a set of guidelines … which an individual inherits as a member of a particular society and which tells him/her how to view the world and learn how to behave in relation to other people. It also provides him/her with a way of transmitting these guidelines to the next generation.

Helman (2000) goes on to explain that culture can be seen as an acquired lens through which we see the world. This is a useful analogy because culture can be seen in this way as a sort of filter through which our experience of the world passes and which helps us to interpret it. From these definitions some characteristics of culture can be teased out:

- Culture is learned – therefore it is acquired. Children primarily learn their culture within the family and immediate community. Later, school life and peers contribute to the growing cultural sense of the child. In fact, it might be said that it is beliefs deriving from culture that dictate how we respond to children and our child-rearing practices.
- It is logical then that culture is passed from generation to generation. Some aspects of culture seem to change readily

between generations (we don't tend to think or behave exactly as our parents or grandparents do). On the other hand, once we have learned and internalised our cultural norms we might well be quite resistant to any change in these.

- Culture is dynamic – it changes while being passed between the generations (the generation gap). It might also change in response to the time, place and conditions within which a cultural group live.
- Culture helps us to identify the group to which we belong. By extension, it can help us to identify groups to which we do not belong. This can provide a potential source of a sense of solidarity within our group, but can also be the origin of friction between groups.
- Culture helps to identify core beliefs. This can include religious belief and spiritual responses. This aspect can be fundamentally important to people during periods of change, stress or crisis, for example, when a child is sick. This aspect of culture can also determine how people interpret health and ill-health, the causes of ill-health and which treatments should be used.
- Culture helps to define our core values. Culture influences us in how we judge what is 'right' and what is 'wrong' for example.
- Culture has a role to play in the development of our life habits and customs – the way we behave and dress, as well as the food that we eat, are determined by culture. How many of us, in times of stress or tiredness, prefer to eat familiar comforting food from our childhood?
- Culture gives us a pattern for living, it can give us a template for how to respond to crises and difficulties in everyday life.
- Culture is important to us because it dictates how we interpret and respond to the world around us. Without particularly reflecting on this, it can dictate our judgements on the views and actions of others. We tend to regard our own

way as correct and might view others as being wrong on the basis of this. For professional people like children's nurses this tendency might seriously affect the quality of our relationships with those we work with.

- Culture is thoroughly internalised. Having learned our culture in childhood, it is an integral part of ourselves and largely subconscious. When we encounter new situations we tend to see them through our cultural 'lens' and make rapid judgements, sometimes without much further thought.

These definitions can be seen to be broad. They indicate that culture is a feature of a wide variety of different groups (Wilkins, 1993). One of the bugbears of using cultural ideas in nursing in the past has been the tendency to see culture as being confined to ethnicity. Of course, ethnic groups can be seen as cultural groups, but so too can a range of other groups who share beliefs, values and customs. By extension, it is easy then to say that cultural issues concern us all. If we confine our inquiry about cultural aspects to other ethnic groups then we run the risk of not considering our own cultural responses.

If we continue in the vein of considering culture broadly, we create the opportunity of seeing a range of cultural groups that we might not otherwise see. It might even be argued that some of the perceived differences in beliefs and behaviours between men and women are based on cultural norms.

> ### 👤 ACTIVITY
>
> Suggest a range of cultural groups that might not necessarily be based on ethnicity.
>
> If we look at groups based on shared beliefs, values and customs on the list you compiled during the above activity we might find:
>
> - Groups based on age, for example, the elderly and youth might be seen as cultural or subcultural groups because although they largely share a world-view with society as a whole, they also have distinctive, slightly different perspectives from the majority.
> - Groups based on regional origin, for example, those originating from the north or the south of England, those from the Midlands and those from the southwest all carry with them distinct characteristics of groups from their home region. This is clearly illustrated when someone moves from their home region and is struck by the strange habits of the natives of their new home area.

> ### 👤 ACTIVITY
>
> - Stretch your imagination a little further and try to think of other areas that could be defined as cultural. An interesting perspective from the point of view of the children's nurse might be a suggestion that subcultures might be formed within the health care field.
> - Consider, with a view to the definitions of culture given earlier, to what extent children's nurses might form a subcultural group.

If we accept that nurses form a cultural group with a body of shared beliefs, values and customs, then by extension, children and their families do not belong to that group. It will often be observed that 'experienced' mothers – that is mothers whose child's health concerns have brought them into frequent contact with health care professionals – often seem to have learned the 'rules' of the culture of the health care world, including its language. One parent of a child in hospital observed to me that you could always tell 'experienced' mothers on a hospital ward; they are the ones who always have a packet of biscuits in their handbag!

It makes sense that parents unfamiliar with the health care context might find themselves bemused by the unspoken expectations and rules of the health care encounter. It is well documented that implementation of child and family care has been complicated by parents feeling uncertain about quite what is expected of them and not being clear about the unwritten 'rules' (Coyne, 1995; Darbyshire, 1994; Valentine, 1998).

> ### 👤 ACTIVITY
>
> - Think of a family you have cared for who is deemed by health care professionals to be 'difficult'.
> - To what extent do you think that cultural factors, for example, beliefs, values and customs common to a group, might have been implicated in this situation?

Examples like this illustrate how cultural misunderstandings or lack of insight can hamper collaborative work or even, in extreme cases, form the basis of conflict situations. From this it can be seen how important culture can be as a factor in the everyday work of children's nurses (Andrews, 1995).

Much of what you will read about cultural aspects of health care will appear to contradict this broad reading of what culture is. Many authorities will interpret culture as almost being synonymous with ethnicity. So when commentators describe Britain as being a multi-cultural society, they often mean a multi-ethnic society. It must be emphasised that the broad reading of what culture is does not negate in any sense the importance of ethnicity in health and social care. Ethnicity is a significant aspect of cultural care issues and caring for children from different ethnic groups often raises very clear cultural questions (Whiting, 1999).

> ### 🌐 WWW
>
> Find more material about ethnicity and health on the Department of Health website:
> - http://www.dh.gov.uk

One of the problems of considering cultural aspects of culture in children's nursing is that it can often seem very abstract, and this is often not helped by the complex, sometimes even obscure, language used to describe cultural concepts (Ahmann, 1994). Considering some of these ideas in more detail can be useful in illustrating how facets of cultural thinking can be useful in the everyday, practical world.

Ethnocentrism

Although this word appears fearsome it simply describes the situation where we consider our own personal cultural world view to be correct in all its detail. As we learn our culture from an early age – an important fact for children's nurses to bear in mind – it tends to be a deeply ingrained part of us. We do not usually consciously consider it when we are making judgements about our experiences. In this way our culture can be compared with Helman's lens, through which we filter everything that happens to us and colours our reaction to these experiences. Anyone who wears glasses will be aware of how quickly you become unaware of the glasses themselves when viewing the world around you.

 ACTIVITY

Think of a situation in which you have disapproved of something that someone else has said or done. Can you think of why you reacted in this way?

Because the cultural lens or yardstick against which you measure your experiences is often virtually subliminal, it can form the basis of the 'gut reaction'. Think of how you would feel if you went to eat at a friend's and were offered an unfamiliar or exotic food, such as snake, to eat. Your reaction would be based on your cultural concept of appropriate food to eat, which you learned in childhood. Of course, some of us are more daring and adventurous than others so you might enjoy the opportunity to sample some snake! This same kind of 'it's not my way' reaction can occur in any aspect of people's behaviour. A few years ago, I was involved in caring for the child in the scenario below. You can see that it is difficult sometimes to be clear as to quite why we react to situations in the way that we do – this is culture in action.

 SCENARIO

Five-year-old Rachel is being cared for following a traumatic fracture of her left femur. She is confined to bed on balanced traction. She is disorientated by what is happening and is often quite tearful. Her mother breastfeeds her in the morning and when she is settling to sleep in the evening. Many of the nurses on the ward are quite shocked by this.

 ACTIVITY

- Consider why the nurses might be feeling shocked in this situation.
- What might be the effect of their reacting in this way?

Ethnocentrism could be argued to be a part of all of us and will lead to us responding positively to those with whom we share a culture (Sprott, 1994). The other side of the coin is that we can respond negatively to people whose culture orientation leads them to behave or to value things that we do not. Clearly, we do not always demonstrate our reactions to others (nurses traditionally strive not to be judgemental) but it is all too easy for our reactions – positive or negative – to be communicated through channels such as body language. If we disapprove of someone's behaviour, which is based on their cultural orientation, and they become aware of our disapproval, then that could have a seriously negative effect on our working together if this occurs in a professional setting. Equally, we might be led to condone behaviours that are culturally acceptable to us, but that are not entirely constructive. Alcohol use among young people is widely acceptable within that age group within this community and is often talked of in a 'jokey' fashion.

Ethnocentrism is a natural part of us, but it is particularly important for children's nurses to reflect on how it leads us to respond and behave in our work with children and families. Children are especially vulnerable to cultural disapproval because they are learning their family's and community's culture (Chevannes, 1997). During this learning process their cultural self might be fragile and vulnerable to the disapproval or scorn of others. Cultural disrespect is potentially damaging. In this way, it can be seen how ethnocentrism can form the basis for prejudice, be it positive or negative. The process of reflecting on our cultural reactions based on ethnocentrism can help to improve our personal self-awareness and help avoid many harmful effects.

 WWW

A range of materials relating to cultural factors in children's nursing along with some exercises can be found on the Royal College of Nursing's website at:
- http://www.rcn.org/resources/transcultural

 SCENARIO

Three-month-old Matty, who was born at 34 weeks' gestation and had a very stormy start to his life, was recently discharged home into the care of his parents and big sister. He has come to outpatients with his mother and 6-year-old sister, Adele. Adele is bored and frustrated with the wait and has just been involved in a noisy disagreement with another child. Her mother reacts strongly and smacks her several times on the legs.

 ACTIVITY

- How do you feel about children being smacked by their parents?
- To what extent would you think that your views are culturally based?
- What kinds of messages do you give to those you disagree with on this question?

Any discussion about such matters is likely to generate a great deal of heat. It could be suggested that this is because such views are often determined by cultural values. The perspective we adopt in relation to such issues is ethnocentric; anyone agreeing with us is right and anyone disagreeing is wrong. Such automatically and unthinkingly assumed polar positions are unhelpful. It could be said that self-awareness is largely cultural self-awareness.

Stereotyping

Stereotyping is a close cousin of ethnocentrism. It can be defined as assuming cultural characteristics of a person (without asking them) based on our perception of the group that they belong to. An example of this might be when a nurse first meets the father of a child in their care. The father is wearing a turban. What does the nurse think? If the reaction is stereotypical it might run something like this: 'Oh, Mr S is a Sikh. I have nursed Sikh people before, they like to do A, B and C and they don't like D, E and F.'

Although these assumptions might be correct, they could equally well be quite wrong. People within cultural groups will naturally have individual and subgroup variations. Even within cohesive groups we do not share identical beliefs, values and customs. You need only listen to the sorts of debates that go on around the time of national elections to appreciate this. It is unhelpful to 'pigeonhole' people on the basis of assumed characteristics. The only way to know about people's culturally determined beliefs and habits is to ask them.

Culture Shock

Another feature of our cultural understandings being learnt early in life, deeply ingrained and often subconsciously acted on, is that we can rely on shared understandings and assumptions when we are within our cultural group. This is a comfortable, secure position to be in. However, if we move outside our group then we can no longer rely on these mutual interpretations. This can feel very disorientating. You might have noticed this when on holiday abroad; it is irritating when people do not do as you expect them to, for example, queue in an orderly fashion in a post office. A Southeast Asian refugee to the United States expressed his feeling of culture shock as feeling like a goat in a herd of cows. This is a vivid illustration of how culture shock can make you feel almost visibly different from those around you. Our shared understandings within our own cultural group

include many unwritten rules. Everyone in that environment understands and feels comfortable with these conventions; anyone new to the context is likely to feel discomfited.

It could be argued that the parents of a sick child experience a degree of culture shock when they come into contact with the hospital environment and health care professionals. Parents, and patients, often find it difficult to know what is expected of them and the rules that health care professionals expect them to abide by. This situation is not helped when children's nurses assume that parents have this knowledge and understanding. More open communication and clarity would go some way towards alleviating the discomfort and stress of culture shock.

Cultural Assessment

To be able to use all of these ideas in relation to culture it will be useful to examine a framework of cultural assessment. There are several of these (Giger and Davidhizar, 1995; Purnell and Paulanka, 1998; Tripp Reimer et al., 1984) and they generally do not vary greatly in terms of content. However, some are more practical than others in terms of clarity and ease of use in practice. Giger and Davidhizar (1995) offer a framework with six dimensions:

1. communication
2. space
3. social organisation
4. time
5. environmental control
6. biological variation

Giger and Davidhizar believe that each of these dimensions describes an area of human life that is universal and that is shared by all cultures, although there might be significant variation between cultural groups. Taken together, these universal dimensions illustrate the major culturally determined differences between people. Therefore if we use them as a system of assessment for cultural differences then we should identify and capture those issues in the care encounter that require culture sensitivity and understanding.

Communication

Communication is generally agreed to be a central part of the children's nurse's function. Communication is starkly illustrated as an issue when the nurse and patient/family speak different languages. However, it can be just as important when factors such as professional jargon or language that is too complex for the child to understand are used. Often, non-verbal communication is particularly challenging between people from different cultural backgrounds. Gestures carry different meanings in different groups and cultural norms, such as the use of eye contact, can vary a good deal. For some, avoiding eye contact, particularly with authority figures, is seen as simply polite; others would interpret this as shifty behaviour.

Space

We all have a sense of what is a comfortable distance between ourselves and others. This will vary with the degree to which the other is familiar to us. Too close feels vaguely threatening while too far away can feel rather cold. For us, as children's nurses,

---

👤 ACTIVITY

Consider your feelings when you first arrived in a clinical area that was quite different from anything you had experienced before, for example, the intensive care unit or operating theatre:

- What were your predominant feelings at that time?
- To what extent do you feel that these reactions were based on culture shock?

Return again to your reflection on the family you thought about in the earlier activity who were considered by health care professionals as difficult:

- Do you recognise any features of culture shock in that situation?

observing how people relate within their family and with strangers can give valuable clues as to their preferred style in this respect.

Wthin this category we can also consider social touching and what is and what is not tolerable for individuals and families. In some groups the handshake, before the Covid 19 pandemic, was socially important while for other groups a non-touch gesture of greeting and respect such as lightly touching your chest just over the heart was preferred.

Social Organisation

How we relate to each other as individuals and groups is strongly culture related. As they grow, children learn how to relate to their elders and parents. This can take the form of small children learning 'good manners', although what constitutes good manners changes over time and between cultural groups. That children should be 'seen and not heard' is not a value promoted in Western cultures today, but it is still a guiding principle for some groups. Similarly, some adults look askance on children behaving exuberantly in a public place, whereas for some groups it is to be positively encouraged. The respective roles adopted by men and women within communities and family groups are also determined largely by cultural norms.

Time

This dimension is important in children's nursing because it takes children a good deal of effort to understand this abstract notion. Small children can struggle with the idea of 'tomorrow' or 'at 2 o'clock'. Some groups value punctuality, whereas some are very much less concerned with this. Some cultures have a future orientation (e.g. 'Study hard for your exams and you'll get to university then you'll get a good job'.), and others are more past oriented (e.g. 'What do you want to go to university for? No one in our family ever has done so before'.). Others again might be present oriented and see the future as impossible to predict, whereas the past is gone and irrelevant. Each of those positions can influence how children and families react to misfortune or ill health.

Environmental Control

The variation between groups in terms of how they perceive their ability to affect events in their environment and lives is contained in this dimension. This will affect how they interpret the reason for events, for example, why a child becomes unwell, what causes this and what should be done about it. Therefore it will dictate what should be done, for example, if a child has a fever: perhaps nothing will be done – just wait and see; perhaps a drug (e.g. paracetamol) will be given; perhaps the child will be taken to a doctor or to consult a folk healer.

Biological Control

This is a very important dimension for nurses because it links to the variations seen under the environmental control category. Factors related to our place and group of origin are aspects of our cultural beliefs and customs in relation to life events. Rituals and required behaviours in the face of difficult challenges are affected by differences between cultures and these are often reflected in religious belief and practice. Dietary aspects also appear in this category – the foods we prefer and the effects we believe foods have on our bodies and health.

 ACTIVITY

Running through these categories, make a list of factors you and your family/community consider to be important in each dimension, for example, for the time dimension, do you consider punctuality to be important? Why?

Taking all of these factors together we can begin to get a picture of how complex, subtle and difficult to reveal and analyse cultural factors can be. However, it is not a hopeless picture. There are several approaches to working with cultural aspects in child health care. One is the promotion of cultural safety through self-awareness. This is an attractive idea because, as children's nurses, we seek to ensure the safety and well-being of the children and families in our care. In the past, culture was often not emphasised as a factor in nursing care and the potential for care to be culturally unsafe was considerable. This would occur when the beliefs, values and customs of children were ignored, or even worse scorned. Cultural safety is an orientation with an element of reaction to some previous attempts at developing transcultural nursing models. Some of these, although well-meaning, tended to emphasise differences between groups by examining what were sometimes exotically different groups (e.g. the weaning habits of Tibetan yak herders). These also ran the risk of stereotyping people (e.g. all Tibetan yak herders wean their babies at the same age and in the same way). Cultural safety does not concentrate on learning a shopping list of factors that identify a cultural group. Rather, within this framework the children's nurse works to achieve an understanding of their own cultural values. This reflection would also consider the nature of power within the nurse–child/family relationship. Obviously, if the nurse is basing professional and personal judgements on personal values, and also holds power in relation to the child and family, then the results could at best be non-constructive and at worst destructive.

Cultural safety consists of a set of ideas that have been evolving for some time in the social sciences and nursing. It is perhaps at its most developed in New Zealand. The context in New Zealand is particular: it is a post-colonial nation where the majority is descended from White European immigrants and the significant minority from the original inhabitants – the Maori. The last three decades of the 20th century saw a wide-ranging debate in New Zealand as to why outcomes for the Maori are worse on almost every dimension – and particularly in health – than for New Zealanders of European origin. The conclusion reached was that cultural oppression was a significant factor in this situation and solutions sought. The key features of cultural safety are described as follows:

The effective nursing or midwifery practice of a person or family from another culture, is determined by that person or family. Culture includes, but is not restricted to age or generation, gender, sexual orientation, occupation and socioeconomic status, ethnic origin or migrant experience, religious or spiritual belief and disability.

Nursing Council of New Zealand (2002 p 7)

The nurse or midwife delivering the nursing or midwifery service will have undertaken a process of reflection on their own cultural identity and will recognise the impact that their personal culture has on their professional practice. Unsafe cultural practice comprises any action which diminishes, demeans or disempowers the cultural identity and well-being of an individual.

Cultural safety in this system is based on each nurse gaining a knowledge and understanding of their own cultural values rather than trying to learn aspects of the culture of other groups (which runs the risk in any case of being stereotypical). Cultural safety can be said to be achieved when each child/family receives care that is based on all that makes them individual and unique. This can only be defined by those who are receiving that care.

It is not a major leap to appreciating that if this is achieved then the respect, trust and effective communication will be in place on which to base a constructive helping relationship. The Nursing Council New Zealand (2002) proposes a series of stages in learning to integrate culture into care:

- Cultural awareness: simply understanding that people differ on the basis of learnt beliefs and values.
- Cultural sensitivity: acknowledging that these differences are legitimate and gaining awareness of one's own cultural norms and how these might affect others.
- Cultural safety: the care delivered is culturally safe as defined by those receiving care.

Clearly, this represents a theoretical framework that could be further legitimated by testing through research. However, it does offer a number of very thought-provoking insights. It emphasises that culture will be an issue in most caring encounters and that skill in working with cultural aspects will be fundamental for all nurses.

🌐 WWW

Read more about the idea of cultural safety on the website of the Nursing Council of New Zealand:
- http://www.nursingcouncil.nz

Consideration of cultural safety practices in care delivery offers the opportunity to develop care skills which are culturally safe and satisfying within a context of child-centred care. The following skills will be required to achieve this:

- *Reflection* – this allows the children's nurse to consider themselves as players in care interactions, to learn from positive experiences and to use negative experiences to improve future performance.
- *Communication* – this is the key to achieving cultural safety. People who feel undervalued on the basis of their culture may well find it impossible to communicate with some they feel have more power and authority than they

do. All elements of communication used within interactions need to be taken into account, particularly the non-verbal. It will be important to create an environment and atmosphere conducive to open communication.

- *Use of fundamental values* – care interactions must be based on respect, dignity and kindness.
- *Empathy* – attempting to appreciate the nature of another person's viewpoint, and experience of a situation or interaction.
- *Motivation* – the desire and commitment to ensuring that care is culturally sensitive and safe.
- *Quality-driven* – the wish to ensure that, in every dimension, care is of the highest quality possible.
- *Leadership* – to define the significance and importance of culturally safe care and to identify a process to lead others through a process of implementing such practices (De and Richardson, 2008).

Unconscious Bias

One idea that has been developed of late, which supplements and adds detail to the concept of cultural safety, is that of **unconscious bias** (Bellack, 2015). Like cultural safety, unconscious bias is based on the assumption that we all have ideas about other groups of people, which we do not necessarily consider consciously, but which still drive our views on and reactions to people belonging to these groups. Such views might involve a wide range of groups that we perceive as different from ourselves based on factors such as age, class, ethnicity, sexual orientation and gender to name but a few (Teal, 2012).

An unconscious bias means that we might potentially respond negatively to others while not being aware of why we are reacting in that way (Duster, 2008). This makes such a reaction beyond our conscious control and can prove very damaging indeed in interpersonal interactions. Awareness of this flags up how important it is for professional children's nurses to address and control this phenomenon in order to ensure sensitive, insightful and satisfactory nursing interventions (Goldyne, 2007). Unconscious bias is becoming a focus in professional education and raising awareness of this factor in children's nurse education is aiming to enhance communication skills and ensure respectful and compassionate care tailored to each child and family (Haider, 2011, 2014).

👤 ACTIVITY

Access the Implicit Association Test inventory via your browser and undertake one of the unconscious bias scales. Reflect on the outcome of this and start to think about how you will use this information to direct your future professional learning.

SUMMARY

Culture can be argued to be a significant factor in nursing work and there have been several approaches for nurses to develop their knowledge and skills in this arena. Culture is defined widely as being a characteristic of the beliefs and practices of a wide range of groups, which might include:

- age or generation
- gender
- sexual orientation
- occupation and socioeconomic status
- ethnic origin or immigrant experience
- religious or spiritual belief
- disability

Taking cultural aspects into account is especially important for children's nurses because of the special and particular nature of children. Because culture is a learnt phenomenon that occurs during childhood, then children will be active learners of their own culture at the time of the care encounter. As a person's individual culture is incompletely learnt until later in childhood, then the child might be at risk of confusion and distress if disrespect is shown towards his or her culturally determined beliefs, values and customs. As active learners of culture, children might also be confused by encountering cultural norms that are at variance with those they are in the process of learning at home and within their community. Failure to take culture into account might result in a discriminatory, insensitive and inappropriate attempt at care, which is bound to fail.

REFERENCES

Ahmann, E., 1994. 'Chunky stew': appreciating cultural diversity while providing health care for children. Pediatr. Nurs. 29 (3), 320–324.

Andrews, M.M., 1995. Transcultural perspectives in the nursing care of children and adolescents. In: Andrews, M.M., Boyle, J.S. (Eds.), Transcultural Concepts in Nursing Care. Lippincott, Philadelphia JB.

Carter, B., McGoldrick, M., 1989. The Changing Family Lifecycle, second ed. Allyn & Bacon, London.

Chevannes, M., 1997. Nursing care for families – issues in a multicultural society. Br. J. Nurs. 6, 161–167.

Coyne, I., 1995. Parental participation in care: a critical review of the literature. J. Adv. Nurs. 21, 716–722.

Crain, W.C., 1988. Erikson and the eight stages of life. In: Crain, W.C. (Ed.), Theories of Development: Concepts and Applications. Prentice Hall, London.

Darbyshire, P., 1994. Living with a Sick Child in Hospital: The Experiences of Parents and Nurses. Chapman & Hall, London.

De, D., Richardson, J., 2008. Cultural safety: an introduction. Paediatr. Nurs. 20 (2), 39–43.

Duster, D., 2008. Introduction to unconscious racism debate. Soc. Psychol. Q. 71 (1), 6–11.

Epstein, N.B., Bishop, D.S., Levin, S., 1978. The McMaster model of family functioning. J. Marriage Fam. Counsel. 4, 19–31.

Erikson, E.H., 1963. Childhood and Society, second ed. Norton, New York.

Erikson, E.H., 1968. Identity: Youth and Crisis. Norton, New York.

Friedemann, M.L., 1989. The concept of family nursing. J. Adv. Nurs. 14, 211–216.

Friedman, M.M., 1998. Family Nursing: Theory and Practice, fourth ed. Appleton & Lange, Norwalk, CT.

Giger, J.N., Davidhazar, R.E., 1995. Transcultural Nursing, third ed. Mosby Year Book, St Louis.

Goldberg, S., 2000. Attachment and Development. Arnold, London.

Helman, C.G., 2000. Culture, Health and Illness, fourth ed. Butterworth Heinemann, Oxford.

Klein, M., 1940/1975. Mourning and its relation to manic-depressive states. In: Klein, M. (Ed.), The Writings of Melanie Klein, vol. 1. Hogarth, London.

Kroger, J., 1996. Adolescence as identity synthesis: Erikson's psychosocial approach. In: Kroger, J. (Ed.), Identity in Adolescence: Overview of Major Theorists, second revised ed. Routledge, London.

Levac, A.M., Leahey, M., 1997. Children and families: models for assessment and intervention. In: Fox, J. (Ed.), Primary Healthcare of Children. Mosby, Baltimore, MD.

Marcia, J.E., 1966. Development and validation of ego identity status. J. Pers. Soc. Psychol. 3, 551–558.

Marcia, J.E., 1979. Identity Status in Late Adolescence: Description and Some Clinical implications. Identity Development Symposium. Gronigen, the Netherlands.

Miller, P.H., 1993. Theories of Developmental Psychology, third ed. WH Freeman, New York.

Minuchin, S., 1974. Families and Family Therapy. Tavistock, London.

Nursing Council of New Zealand, 2002. Guidelines for Cultural Safety, the Treaty of Waitangi and Maori Health in Nursing and Midwifery Education and Practice. Nursing Council of New Zealand, Wellington.

Purnell, L.D., Paulanka, B.J., 1998. Transcultural Healthcare. FA Davis, Philadelphia.

Sprott, J.E., 1994. One person's 'spoiling' is another's freedom to become: overcoming ethnocentric views about parental control. Soc. Sci. Med. 38 (8), 1111–1124.

Stevens, R., 1983. The life cycle. In: Stevens, R. (Ed.), Erik Erikson: An Introduction. Open University Press, Buckingham.

Tripp-Reimer, T., Brink, P.J., Saunders, J.M., 1984. Cultural assessment: convert and process. Nurs. Outlook 32 (2), 78–82.

Valentine, F., 1998. Empowerment: family centred care. Paediatr. Nurs. 10 (1), 24–27.

Whyte, D., 1992. A family nursing approach to the care of a child with a chronic illness. J. Adv. Nurs. 17, 317–327.

Whyte, D., 1996. Expanding the boundaries of care. Paediatr. Nurs. 8 (4), 10–23.

Whyte, D., 1997. Explorations in Family Nursing. Routledge, London.

Wilkins, H., 1993. Transcultural nursing: a selective review of the literature 1985–1991. J. Adv. Nurs. 18 (4), 606–612.

Wong, D.L., 1995. Growth and development of children. In: Campbell, S., Glasper, E.A. (Eds.), Whaley and Wong's Nursing Care of Infants and Children, fifth ed. CV Mosby, St. Louis.

Whiting, L., 1999. Caring for children of differing cultures. J. Child. Health. Care 3 (4), 33–37.

Wright, L.M., Leahey, M., 1994. Nurses and Families: A Guide to Family Assessment and Intervention, second ed. FA Davis, Philadelphia.

FURTHER READING

Bellack, J.P., 2015. Unconscious bias: an obstacle to cultural competence. J. Nurs. Educ. 54 (9), S63–S64.

Bentovim, A., Bingley Miller, L., 2001. The Family Assessment: Assessment of Family Competence, Strengths and Difficulties. Pavilion Publishing, Brighton.

Duster, D., et al., 2008. Introduction to unconscious racism debate. Soc. Psychol. Q. 71 (1), 6–11.

Duvall, E., 1977. Marriage and Family Development. Lippincott, Philadelphia.

Goldyne, A.J., 2007. Minimising the influence of unconscious bias in evaluations: a practical guide. J. Am. Acad. Psychiatry Law. 35 (1), 60–66.

Haider, A.H., Schneider, E.B., Sriram, N., et al., 2014. Unconscious race and social class bias: its association with decision-making by trauma and acute care surgeons. J. Trauma Acute Care Surg. 77 (3), 409–416.

Haider, A.H., Sexton, J., Sriram, N., et al., 2011. Association of unconscious bias and social class biases with vignette-based clinical assessment by medical students. J. Am. Med. Assoc. 306 (9), 942–951.

Jones, E., 1993. Family Systems Therapy. John Wiley, Chichester.

Teal, C.R., Gill, A.L., Green, A.R., et al., 2012. Helping medical learners to recognise and manage unconscious bias towards certain patient groups. Med. Educ. 46 (1), 80–88.

Von Bertalanffy, L., 1968. General System Theory: Foundations, Development, Applications. Brazillier, New York.

26

Empowering Children and Young People and Families in Health Care

Sarah Reed, E. Alan Glasper

LEARNING OUTCOMES

- Understand the key drivers for empowering children and young people (CYP) and families in health care from United Kingdom (UK) perspectives.
- Explore the contexts, barriers and facilitators of CYP involvement in health care: in terms of their own health care, commissioning health care services and influencing the education of children's nurses. This will be considered

from CYP, parental/carer and health care professional's perspectives and examples explored.
- Consider the significance of empowering CYP in health care to support their self-care and transition to adult services.
- Consider the information provided to CYP and families when making health care decisions, during hospitalisations and the promotion of health literacy.

INTRODUCTION

This chapter explores principles and practices for the empowerment of CYP and families in health care contexts and the role of the children's nurse. It overviews the current directions of travel for empowering children to be involved in their own health care, drivers for this, barriers to this and the interventions to achieve this, alongside the importance of information and communication. The availability of information sources for empowering CYP in health is critically considered in terms of the opportunities, formats, and evidence base and health literacy. Empowerment is then explored in terms of the involvement of CYP and families in designing health care services that reflect their experiences and needs, including the mechanisms to support this from policy and practical perspectives. Finally, the contributions of CYP and parents/carers to pre-registration nursing education is explored, alongside the drivers and barriers to this.

EMPOWERMENT

The term 'empowerment' has become somewhat of a buzz word, yet it is often misunderstood. The term stems from the Latin word *potere*, meaning 'to be able' and is also linked to the word potent, meaning 'powerful, cogent, persuasive and having or exercising a great influence'.

However, the rhetoric of empowerment is somewhat different from the concreteness of strategies for empowerment that purport to enable people to make health-related decisions. Although the pursuit of empowerment strategies by nurses is a relatively recent phenomenon, it has become an integral component of advocacy. The term 'empowerment' is appealing perhaps because it conjures up images of power

and independence. The nursing profession has embraced advocacy as a method of promoting family-centred care but the methods of achieving its implementation have changed considerably over the years. From a position of interceding or pleading a case for families, children's nurses now act as guardians for their rights to autonomy and free choice. Indeed, current health promotion ideology accepts empowerment as enabling and supporting people to set their own health agendas and to take control of their health status through skills development and critical consciousness-raising.

Although there have been many innovations in advocacy, and empowerment is a real force within the field of child care, it must be stressed that CYP and families are sometimes passive bystanders in the process and this results in inequalities in the health care professional–family relationship. Through the provision of information to CYP and their families, these inequalities can begin to be addressed by empowering individuals to be more involved in their own health decisions. For the children's nurse there are many dimensions to empowerment, since each child or young person has a constantly evolving level of cognitive and social development that requires expert knowledge and flexibility in practice.

Policy Perspectives of Empowerment of CYP

The empowerment of service users, that is, individuals that use health and social care services, has been a key feature of the NHS modernisation agenda for more than a decade (Department of Health [DoH], 2000, 2003, 2004, 2006, 2008, 2010). Through involving service users, future health care services can be commissioned that respond to the needs of those using the services. The seminal policy document for children's nurses in this regard is the National Service Framework (NSF) for CYP and Maternity Services (DoH,

2004). This policy recognised that CYP are a distinct group to adults, requiring health care services that are developmentally responsive to their needs, for example, pre-school children require different approaches/services to those required by young people, and that CYP are best placed to inform these services. The NSF places a greater focus on delivering better information for children, young people and their parents on health and health services, and how to access them; and for monitoring and continual improvement of services. For a fuller discussion of child health policies see the relevant chapter of this book.

Children's Rights for Involvement in Their Health Care

Children and young people require health care which is developmentally responsive to their needs, since children pass through different stages of cognition and independence, which is different to the adult population (Coad and Evans, 2008). Empowering children to be involved in health care is a key role for children's nurses. The requirements to empower children and ensure their views individually and collectively are responded to come from international, national and legal conventions. Internationally, the driving force for empowering CYP in their health care comes from the United Nations Convention on the Rights of the Child (UNCRC) (UNCRC, 1989). The convention sets out 54 basic standards (Articles) for the care, treatment, protection and participation of children (under the age of 18) in society. It is an international, legal agreement signed and respected by governments. It was ratified by the UK government in 1991. Read about the UNCRC here: available from: https://www.unicef.org.uk/what-we-do/un-convention-child-rights/.

In the context of empowerment, there are articles of the convention that apply:

Article 12 – *Respect the views of the child in all matters affecting them and have their views considered and taken seriously.* For example, involving the young person in whether they would like their parents present for a personal procedure or asking about their understanding when consenting to a procedure.

Article 13 – *Freedom of expression of opinions.* For example, ensuring that the children with long-term conditions are actively encouraged to contribute during their medical consultations from an early age, in order to prepare them for transition to adult services. This is important for children's advocacy, as they will have different experiences/perspective to those of their parents.

Article 14 – *Freedom of thought.* The child has the right to think and believe what they choose. For example, the children's nurse should explore with the child what their understanding of their health care is and what their concerns are.

The Children's Commissioner for England is responsible for promoting and protecting the rights of children, as set out in the UNCRC (1989). The Children's Commissioner works independently of government and parliament, to stand up for the voices of CYP and ensure these are considered when decisions are being taken about them. This is achieved through directly engaging with CYP, gathering research evidence and making recommendations that prioritise and bring about sustained improvements for CYP (Children's Commissioner's Office, 2018).

SECTION ONE

Rationales for Empowering Children's Participation in Their Health Care

CYP are active citizens making decisions in their everyday lives which influence their personal circumstances. Therefore it is essential that professionals support them to do this in respect of their health care (Glasper and Evans, 2013). Developing life skills of citizenship, responsibility and personal independence are key to enabling CYP to achieve, promote and sustain their health, which impacts into adulthood. These life skills are taught as part of the school curriculum in the format of personal, social, health and economic education (PSHE) and children's nurses should actively promote opportunities for CYP to safely practise these. When children require input from health care services, whether electively, acutely or long-term, this can impact their developing independence skills. Empowering CYP to become involved from their initial health care contact provides them back some control of their situation. This issue is particularly significant when considered in the context of children with long-term conditions (LTC), who are expected to manage adaptations to enable their participation in daily life, for example, in the school environment where children are expected to negotiate their health care needs with school staff, in the absence of parents (Reed, 2015). Empowering CYP to participate in their health care requires approaches which take account of their individual desires for involvement and recognises their developing skills of independence.

Barriers Affecting CYP Empowerment in Their Own Health Care

When considering children's involvement in their health care, there are different types of barriers that include the attitudes of adults, the provision of appropriate information and health literacy provisions. Each of these barriers will be discussed in turn and the perspectives of CYP, parents/carers and health care professionals presented. The attitudes of parents/carers and health care professionals significantly influences the opportunities for CYP to be practically involved in their health care. Careful consideration is required of the potential control that adults exert over children in society that may restrict children's empowerment in health care. Davies and Randall (2015) recently undertook a literature review of the influences upon children's participation in health care, which identified that older children and those with greater health care experiences tended to be more involved in their health care. This finding was similarly identified by both children and by nurses, which Davies and Randall (2015) propose may reflect a societal bias that older children are more competent to be involved in health care. However, this makes assumptions about a child's age determining their capacity for involvement and does not recognise the capacity of young children to contribute to health care. The review identified significant influences of adult perspectives that impact CYP involvement, which included the health care professional's desires to maintain control and the weighting given to parental attitudes (when compared to CYP desires) (Davies and Randall, 2015). From the child's perspective, the review identified the lack of appropriate information available to CYP, which restricted their opportunities and abilities to become involved (discussed later). What emerges from this review is a key role of the children's nurse in managing the complex relationships between children, parents and professionals in health care experiences that prioritises children's rights for involvement. Furthermore, prioritising involvement needs to occur irrespective of the children's age and health care experiences, whilst recognising the appropriateness of information provision to enable this.

To overcome barriers and empower children's involvement requires children's nurses that champion inclusivity and health care organisations designed to support this. Children's nurses need to challenge their own assumptions about children's involvement, and at the same time actively seeking the individual CYP desire for involvement during each health care interaction. Consider the scenario where a young person with a long-term condition is hospitalised for an acute deterioration; they may choose for the nurse to undertake some of the therapies that they would usually self-manage at home or they may request additional support during this interaction. Through undertaking individualised approaches, involving actively finding out CYP desires and not presuming these, the nurse will be empowering and advocating for the CYP (Davies and Randall, 2015). Children's nurses require clear guidance and organisational policies that practically promote CYP involvement in their health care, in order that professional or parent/carer attitudes and fears about control do not preclude involvement. Challenging current practices and organisational cultures takes time, but this should not detract from promoting the rights of CYP in health care.

The articles from the UNCRC provide a framework to support children's nurses in their desire to put the child first and foremost in every health care interaction (UNCRC, 1989). Enabling understanding of the priorities for CYP in health care is best achieved by directly asking the CYP. The rationale for this is that their perspectives are likely to be different to that of an adult, since adults cannot return to the same frame of reference they had during childhood. Traditionally adults (parents) have spoken on behalf of children, as they are best placed to know their child, and this is particularly relevant with young children who are developmentally immature. However, this viewpoint does not consider children's potential to contribute to their health care. As discussed above, the realities of the extent of children's involvement in health care is significantly impacted by the attitudes placed upon this from parents and health care professionals (Davies and Randall, 2015). This reinforces the significance of the role of children's nurses in championing children's rights, but also the challenges for children's advocacy in practice, where the dynamic between CYP, families and professional partnership working is continually changing.

Advocating and respecting the rights of 'at-risk' children creates complex challenges for children's nurses in health care. Examples of 'at-risk' children include those who are acutely ill, have complex needs, for whom English is not their first language, or children cared for by social services. Advocating for these at-risk groups of CYP is particularly important, since they may not have the verbal abilities that adults traditionally respond to, limiting their opportunities to express their opinions. Without careful considerations, assumptions can be made about what is in the best interests of the child, which fails to take account of their developmental abilities. This requires creative approaches in practice from children's nurses to enable opportunities for empowering CYP, which may be facilitated initially through the parents/carers about how their child usually communicates verbally or non-verbally. Health professionals need to work with each child on an individual basis so that they can determine the level of involvement the child wants and feels comfortable with. For example, CYP with long-term conditions will have developed their own opinions of their health experiences and desires for involvement, based upon repeated contact with health care services. *The Children Act* (DoH, 1989) states that parents no longer have rights over their children; instead, parents have responsibilities towards their children and must have regard to their children's views when making any major decision affecting them. Practitioners should ensure that when working with children they listen to each child, provide appropriate information and take account of the child's wishes and feelings (DoH, 1989). To undertake these roles, children's nurses need educational preparation at pre- and post-registration levels, to develop skills when working to prioritise the rights of risk groups of CYP and families. What is clear is that children's nurses are in a unique position to influence each individual child's desires for involvement by positively empowering their voice in their health care, whilst recognising how professional and parental attitudes can restrict opportunities for involvement.

▶ REFLECT ON YOUR PAST

Consider children that you have cared for where it has been challenging to assess their views directly. What factors prohibited their engagement and what strategies did you employ to promote children's engagement? How do you think children's nurses can work differently in practice to uphold the rights of children? What can be done practically to overcome the barriers in health care from the child's perspective?

Empowering CYP to Undertake Self-Management and Transitioning to Adult Health Care Services

Empowerment is particularly significant when considered in the context of CYP learning to self-manage their long-term health conditions (LTC). Enabling CYP with LTC to develop skills they require to manage adaptations in their daily lives empowers them, providing control and lifelong skills to be able to manage their own health (Reed, 2015). This is an important part of child development, which promotes independence, self-efficacy in own abilities and reduces dependency upon parents/carers. Children and young people with LTC are required to self-manage in situations such as school or when playing at other children's houses, when their parents are absent. This is not to say that parents/carers do not play a significant role in the management of children with LTC, but that parents/carers need to be supportive and not fearful about developing CYP self-management abilities. To support the development of self-management skills, several interventions, for example, structured education, technical skills or behavioural support, have been established that have been shown to improve longer term health, self-efficacy (individuals confidence in abilities to manage their health needs), knowledge of their condition, problem solving skills, symptom management and health behaviours (de Silva, 2011). However, there is a lack of evidence relating to the effectiveness of self-care support interventions in children, when compared to the adults and health care professionals need to consider mechanisms to support children in the different contexts where they are required to self-care (Kirk et al., 2012a,b).

The transition of CYP from paediatric to adult health services represents a key time for promoting empowerment, where the young person with an LTC progresses to increasingly taking greater responsibilities in health care consultations. Transition from children's to adult health care services needs to be viewed as a gradual process rather than a one-off event, since it represents a step change in the way that health care consultations are conducted. In paediatric consultations, the parents/carers often lead the consultations and questions are often directed to/via them, whereas in adult consultations the young person will undertake this role in the absence of their parents. It is recommended that transition preparations begin from the age of 11 years, in order to coincide with when children are transitioning from primary to secondary school (Nagara et al., 2015). However, every CYP is an individual with a unique health and social experience, so this needs to be flexible. An evidence-based initiative that was trialled in the paediatric outpatient's department of Southampton Children's Hospital is the 'Ready Steady Go' transition preparation programme (Nagara et al., 2015). This evolved to work alongside young people (and their carers) to develop their skills and understanding of their condition, that is, the 'Ready, Steady' elements, leading on to empowering them to gradually prepare for the young person undertaking control of the clinic consultation with the lead health care professional, that is, the 'Go' elements. In practice, the young person would work through the series of 'Ready Steady Go' questionnaires (over a period of time) with the children's nurse to explore their understanding of the knowledge and skills they would require in order to be able to manage their health care confidently, in preparation for taking on greater involvement in clinic consultations. The programmes require commitment from health care professionals and health care organisations, to make the transitional care experiences truly focused upon the needs of CYP. Through these empowerment mechanisms, CYP can be better prepared and aware of opportunities for empowerment and take control of their health care.

Overcoming Barriers to CYP Involvement in Their Health Care: Information Provision and Communication

With the increasing growth and accessibility of the internet, CYP and their families have access to greater information sources than ever before in relation to health. The information available is vast, including promoting health for children/families, supporting particular health conditions and accessing NHS services and patient organisations/third sector services, both nationally and internationally. This information is available to CYP, their families and to health care professionals that support them. However, not all of the information available on the internet is evidence-based, reliable and the quality variable. It is therefore really important that children's nurses take time to review internet resources prior to recommending these and encourage CYP/families to exercise caution when researching internet sources that claim to provide information about health conditions/support.

Patient organisations and self-help groups have a rich history of providing information services for particular audiences. Importantly, they can provide a range of information in a variety of formats, languages and signposts to telephone and other forms of support. It should be noted that not all CYP and families will have internet access nor similar levels of health literacy; therefore it is important that a range of resources are available, for example, both paper and a range of electronic. A number of patient organisations provide access to a telephone support line, which provides a further mechanism for information but also direct support. The provision of digital/electronic information offers many advantages for CYP, since interactive App's, games and resources are available which appeal to CYP of different ages/stages of development. Patient organisations such as the Cystic Fibrosis (CF) Trust provide online forums for CYP that now enable them to communicate with one another, whereby historically CYP with CF were not allowed to mix, due to the risk of cross infection (CF Trust, 2018). In these respects, the internet has opened up empowerment opportunities for CYP through increasing access to information.

Through the internet, CYP and families have instant access to websites and App's covering a wealth of health information that includes health promotion, child development, healthy lifestyles, NHS and support services, parenting, and support for young people, as well as paediatric condition specific resources. Below are links to frequently accessed and useful websites that are pertinent for CYP and their families/carers:

- NHS Choices: https://www.nhs.uk (generic and paediatric specific conditions, medication and services).
- Great Ormond Street Children's Hospital (GOSH): https://www.gosh.nhs.uk/medical-information-0 (paediatric specific conditions, treatments, medications and support).

👤 **ACTIVITY**

Choose a specific condition and review the above three websites and critically analyse:

- How child focused (when compared to parent/carer) are the resources? Is there an area specifically for CYP to access?
- Have CYP been involved in the development and review of the websites? Are the resources subdivided for CYP of different ages?
- What key areas of information are addressed? What are the gaps?
- What is the quality of the evidence-base of the information provided?

- Healthier Together: https://www.what0-18.nhs.uk/ (resources aimed at CYP, parents and professionals).

In relation to the three websites, the Healthier Together website has a separate area specifically for CYP, whereas the others talk about issues/conditions that affect CYP. On the GOSH website, the resources aimed at CYP are delivered in the format of real stories from children's experiences, although the majority represent young people and parental perspectives. The NHS Choices website provides information pertinent to keeping children healthy and managing ill health in children, but this is largely from parent/carer perspectives. Within the CYP area of the Healthier Together website resource, support for CYP is provided under the following headings: staying healthy, growing up, sexual health, long-term conditions and mental health. Each of these topics are further subdivided with hyperlinks to address key issues pertinent from adolescent perspectives, for example, exam pressure, alcohol and drugs, anxiety, CAMHS, contraception and a dedicated section if support is needed immediately. A further advantage of the Healthier Together website resource is that it is devised to be used by health care professionals (who may not be paediatric trained) to act as a resource to ensure that children are given consistent information and high-quality care. This is a constantly evolving area and it is important for children's nurses to keep abreast of the quality and availability of resources that CYP/parents are accessing.

Providing Information About Hospital Experiences to CYP

The exchange of information takes place during any interaction between a health professional, the child and a member of the child's family. The children's nurse has a critical role in ensuring the child and his or her family has access to adequate, high-quality information. Children's nurses are among the best communicators in health care, ideally experienced to inform, educate and advise.

There are information points at each stage of the child's journey through the health care system. The nurse should be aware of these, and be in a position to provide additional information as required. Whereas some parents prefer not to have any information, the majority expect to have as much as can be made available. With the availability of information from the internet, it is important to assess the CYP and parental understanding of the hospital experience prior to providing information. The four main information points in the journey for the family with a hospitalised child are: preadmission, on admission, during the hospital stay and after discharge.

Preadmission to Hospital

Information provided before the child arrives in hospital should cover details about how to get to the hospital; travel issues, such as parking and cost of parking (often a significant concern to parents); how to get to the relevant department once inside the hospital; the ward routine, for example, doctors rounds, mealtimes, menu choices, facilities on the ward for CYP; accommodation and eating options for parents; how to raise concerns and details of key members of hospital staff. There should be a standard introductory leaflet to cover these issues, to accompany personalised information. The hospital's web address should be included. Some hospitals offer preadmission programmes and such provision features in standards set by the National Service Framework.

On Admission to Hospital

The nurse admitting the child is likely to be using a standardised admission sheet, which if set out well, will provide an ideal framework for exploring the immediate information needs of the family. It is particularly important here to explain the hospital's own signage system. For example, colour-coded directional signs and long place names such as 'paediatric rheumatology clinic' can be confusing.

During the Hospital Stay

Leaflets giving details of any investigations should be read through with the child and family. The nurse should explain any unfamiliar terms. The family should be given the opportunity to think about and write down any questions they may need answering. In addition to discussing these issues with appropriate staff, the family may require back-up with leaflets, or printed information from the hospital's own information systems or the internet (using websites such as those suggested above). A recent and useful repository of patient information leaflets for CYP and families has been collated into the Child Health Information Leaflet Directory (CHILD, 2017). This resource was created using information from regional and national NHS trust resources, charities, support groups and patient information sites. Information on this web resource is provided using hyperlinks within an alphabetically organised index. Importantly, users are able to download and print the resources, so that CYP and their families can have paper copies of information to review. This is important because internet access in hospitals can be challenging, and printing resources out for CYP/parents means they have a physical paper resource which they can refer to, whenever they feel they need to revisit information. This is available on the internet using this address: https://www.piernetwork.org/child.html.

ACTIVITY

- Select a condition leaflet to review from the CHILD resource and evaluate usability, range and quality of the resources available from the children's nurse and CYP perspectives.

After Discharge From Hospital

When a CYP is discharged from hospital, some nurses now provide business cards that give the telephone number on which the nurse can be reached. When 24-hour nursing advice service is not available, a telephone linked to voicemail is now standard practice to ensure calls can be followed-up. In addition, written information should be provided and the family should be aware of who to contact once the child is back at home. This is likely to include the relevant member of the multi-disciplinary team, but additional details of patient support groups and organisations should also be given. However, it is possible for families to 'drown in a sea of information' and not actually access the key facts they need to continue to care for their sick children.

The children's nurse is in an ideal position to ensure information is provided at a rate and volume appropriate to the needs of the family. Often, family members will ask when they need to know something but the nurse should get into the habit of checking that information needs are being met. It is also important to check that the family understands the information that is given; levels of illiteracy and low adult reading ages should not be underestimated. The child will not always ask for information and neither will the child's parents/carers.

Producing Local Patient Information Leaflets

Prewritten patient information leaflets are unlikely to satisfy all potential CYP/families and staff may wish to develop their own. Writing a family information leaflet may, on the surface, appear easy but the reality is more complex. Although they can be designed and produced using easily available desktop publishing software, the actual contents require careful consideration.

ACTIVITY

Reflect on your practice. You are keen to develop a leaflet for a child you are looking after:
- Where can you find out if such a leaflet already exists?
- Who should be involved with the development of the leaflet?
- Where and how could they meet together?
- What issues should they be made aware of in relation to national/local information policy?

Improving the Quality of Health Information Leaflets

When writing or reviewing patient information leaflets there are a number of considerations. These include whether the information and designs are:

- Comprehensible: does the reader understand the text?
- Usable/readable: can the reader apply the information?
- Accessible: can the reader find the information easily (or is it lost in a sea of ambiguous text)?

When applied to the contexts of nursing CYP, it is important to consider the age and developmental stage of the child or young person (or indeed family member) that it is aimed at. It is likely that a range of patient information leaflets will be required by CYP of different ages, for example, the information needs of a pre-school child compared with an adolescent. Therefore it is important to know the target audience. As highlighted in this chapter, the best informants of the content, readability and design of patient information leaflets are CYP and families themselves. Co-production of patient information leaflets, that is, shared collaboration and responsibilities between service users and health care professionals, provides a mechanism to enable information delivery and presentation that represents patient perspectives. A recent example that used co-production to inform a patient information leaflet involved the 'Safer Care Checklist project' undertaken by Cathy Pope at the University Hospital Southampton and NHS foundation trust (University of Southampton, 2017). Researchers worked collaboratively with young people in the hospital in order to design an inpatient leaflet which addressed the safety concerns of young people upon hospital admission, during their stay and when being discharged. Their concerns included topics such as: who can I ask if I have concerns, who can visit, where can I find the Wi-Fi code, what can I do and wear in hospital? These were different to the safety concerns of staff, which included ensuring children had wristbands with their name, date of birth and allergies detailed on them and that children understood the rationales for their medications. Co-production between the CYP and health care staff ensured that CYP perspectives were prioritised in the construction and phrasing of statements on the information leaflet and that the safety concerns of both parties were addressed.

Overcoming Barriers to Children's Involvement in Their Health Care: The Role of the School in Promoting Health Literacy

For CYP, their school/college plays an influential and significant role in the provision of health information. Within this learning environment, CYP are learning the skills which enable them to process information and make their own decisions in relation to their health. It is suggested by Hagell et al. (2015) that the capacity to process information and make decisions in relation to health are core elements for 'health literacy'. Health literacy can bring about positive changes on different levels including: changes for CYP, for example, better self-care; changes for schools, for example, enabling teachers to better support pupils with health conditions; and changes for local areas, for example, more appropriate use of health care services (Hagell et al., 2015). Health information is disseminated in the school curriculum through the

PSHE, although this is a non-statutory subject and schools, interpretations can vary. The national curriculum requires schools to make provisions for PSHE education, and importantly, from 2020 the Health and Relationship elements of PSHE will be compulsory in all schools (PSHE Association, 2018). Teaching staff are involved in delivering the PSHE elements to CYP, but they are supported by the school nursing workforce. To effectively promote health literacy for CYP, the teaching staff need to feel supported in delivering these health elements of the curriculum and this requires collaboration with school nurses. This is challenging with the current decline in school nurses and their responsibilities with delivering the Healthy Child Programme and the National Child Measurement Programme (DoH PHE, 2014; Munn, 2018). Initiatives such as the 'Monkey well-being' resources have been designed in collaboration with children's nurses and link to the health elements of the national curriculum, and support teachers to empower CYP health literacy (Greenop et al., 2012). What emerges is that schools have a key role in promoting health literacy and health empowerment for CYP.

SECTION 2

Empowering CYP Involvement in Commissioning Health Care Services

A different focus of empowerment relates to CYP being involved in planning and designing health care services specific to the needs of CYP. Patient and public involvement (PPI) or service-user involvement are terms that are used to capture the process of consulting with individuals, that is, users of health and social care services, to gain and use their views to influence health care services. This terminology (i.e. PPI) is also cited in the context of research, to ensure that health care research projects are undertaken, which represent the perspectives of service users. Patient and public involvement is part of wider step change in how health care professionals/organisations work with patients/clients, viewing them as equal partners in decisions and valuing the contribution that their experiences bring to health service designs. This is something that is now readily undertaken in adult health care services through PPI consultation events, but PPI events with CYP require a range of different/creative approaches, in order to capture the perspectives of CYP of different ages and abilities. As children have historically occupied a lower position in society relative to adults, traditionally their views have been sought by asking the parents about the child's experiences/needs (Punch, 2002). This represents a barrier to the involvement and representation of CYP voices in health care services designed for them. However, given appropriate opportunities and information, CYP can be empowered to provide contributions, based upon their experiences, which are different to the experiences provided by their parents. Therefore in order for service designs to be truly CYP focused, a range of developmentally-appropriate and flexible engagement

strategies need to be employed. Practical examples of these are discussed in the text below, for example, NHS Youth Forum and Children's version of the 'Friends and Family Test'.

Policies/Resources That Facilitate CYP Empowerment and Implementation of Their Perspectives in Health Care Service Designs

In 2011 the Department of Health (DoH, 2011) championed empowerment through publishing the 'You're Welcome – Quality criteria for young people friendly health services', which provided young people with a voice in commissioning health care services and set benchmark standards against which to monitor progress. In the same year, the Royal College of Paediatrics and Child Health (RCPCH, 2010) furthered empowerment through the publication of guidance for the participation of CYP in health services, which was aimed at paediatricians, senior children's nurses and leaders of health organisations. The RCPCH (2010) guidance justified the rationales for and evidence base around the participation of CYP, whilst providing principles for participation strategies and promoting a culture of participation. This guidance is designed by and aimed at practitioners, which although promotes CYP participation, it may not reflect the priorities CYP would identify if they had been involved in the design. These guidance documents set standards facilitating CYP involvement in health care service designs, but the enactment and translation into practice realities requires creativity, time and commitment to ensure empowerment is truly from CYP perspectives.

Further guidance which practically empowers contributions of CYP and their families/carers in health service design is provided through the NHS Institute for Innovation and Improvement toolkit (NHSI, 2013). The '15 steps challenge toolkit for children and young people's inpatient services' provides a series of questions and prompts to guide CYP, carers and professionals through their first impressions of a care setting, that is, within 15 steps of a ward setting they will have formed impressions about the quality of care provided (Glasper and Evans, 2013). The toolkit enables hospital services to understand the key priorities for high quality care from the perspectives of children and their families, based upon first impressions of a service for CYP (Glasper and Evans, 2013). Importantly, this toolkit was co-produced by children, families and professionals. The NHSI has produced 15 steps challenge toolkits for adults in primary and secondary care, but this toolkit was specific to CYP in inpatient services contexts.

A further mechanism to promote feedback from health care service users is the 'Friends and Family Test', which asks whether individuals would recommend the health services they received to their friends and families (Picker Institute, 2018). The results are published at monthly intervals on NHS England websites and apply across primary and secondary care. An adapted, child-friendly version of this test is available, which uses rating scales depicted both pictorially (as smiley faces similar to a pain assessment chart) and as words

(Picker Institute, 2018). These evidence-based toolkits were developed through focus groups with CYP, who advised on the toolkit content and wording, prior to piloting. This tool is specifically for children, but parents may elect to fill this out on their behalf if the children are younger or reluctant, so needs to be interpreted cautiously. These surveys facilitate and prioritise the perspectives and abilities of CYP as important users of health care, which addresses the earlier concerns noted in this chapter that information is not always available in child-friendly formats and is part of the gradual change in the culture of promoting the voice of children in health care.

NHS England Youth Forums

In England there are a number of good examples of PPI projects that have evolved, which champion CYP involvement in health care service development. National Health Service England (NHSE) has developed a Youth Forum, comprising 25 young people (aged 14–24 years), which works to enable young people to engage about their key health issues, from their perspectives and to be involved in decision making. The forum works in collaboration with NHSE, Public Health England and the Department of Health to contribute to local and national decisions. See website at: https://www.england.nhs.uk/participation/get-involved/how/forums/nhs-youth-forum/ for more information. A mixed-methods review of the experiences and impacts of the NHSE youth forum identified local, national and strategic impacts, as well as positive experiences for young people that included personal growth and sharing common desires to impart the voices of young people (Whiting et al., 2018). The review highlighted the investments, in terms of time and resources, required to facilitate young people's involvement in health service designs, and acknowledging limitations of this review, which included the low response rate (36%) (Whiting et al., 2018).

The NHSE youth forum produced guidance for patient participation groups with young people, to encourage involvement in a wide range of ways, including using social media, inviting young people to meetings or finding creative alternatives to meetings that would appeal such as community events at flexible times and listening/respecting the views of young people (NHSE, 2018). Importantly, the guidance recommends that feedback is provided to the young people in order for them to see the impact that their participation has upon health care services. Equally, this is important because young people may not recognise that their views are valued in society. This guidance has been designed for primary care services, but could equally apply to secondary/tertiary health care. Furthermore, it contains examples of practical applications and the impact they have made upon health service designs. Parallel guidance exists in child-health research, where young people advisory groups have been established to input their perspectives into research study designs; notably this has evolved in relation to reviewing research participant information sheets (Involve, 2018).

Barriers to CYP Involvement in Health Care Service Designs

Accessing CYP perspectives of health care services requires a range of different approaches when compared to those that are traditionally used with adult services users to find out their perspectives. This requires children's nurses to challenge the default position of asking the parents/carers, and prioritising how CYP can be given a voice in evaluating/designing their health care services. The aforementioned policies provide best practice standards for engaging the views of CYP in health care services, but these require commitment and time to translate them to reflect children's changing cognition levels. Projects to access CYP perspectives need to be designed in ways that appeal to CYP such as using technology or interactive group work, and arranged at times which fit around CYP busy lifestyles, for example, at weekends or during school holidays. Barriers in terms of gaining access to CYP are considered in the text below, in the contexts of their practical involvement in teaching children's nurses. Given appropriate information and opportunities, CYP are able to contribute to health care service designs and health care services need to be prepared to respond to their feedback. Furthermore, CYP can provide valuable insights into their experiences of consultation/feedback methods, to ensure these are truly CYP focused. Children's nurses need to keep abreast of current barriers and champion opportunities to promote CYP involvement.

SECTION 3

Empowering CYP and Families/Carers to Be Involved in the Education of Children's Nurses

Closely aligned with participation in commissioning health care services and research, are the rationales for involving CYP in the educational preparation of pre-registration children's nurses. Involving CYP in the education of children's nurses is key to ensuring that at the point of registration, children's nurses are educated to reflect the priorities from CYP and parents/carers perspectives. As children's nurses are advocates for CYP, it is imperative that their pre-registration education adequately prepares them for this role, but equally that the issues CYP perceive as important underpin this education.

In the United Kingdom, the Nursing and Midwifery Council (NMC) requires approved educational institutions to include the views of service users such as users of health and social care services, to contribute towards curriculum design of nursing programmes (NMC, 2018). The recently released NMC Educational Standards Framework requires that nursing programs are designed, developed, delivered, evaluated and co-produced with service users (NMC, 2018). The NMC encourages educational institutions to provide supportive evidence of this engagement and applies across all fields of nursing practice. This sets high standards for universities with regards prioritising, collaborating and continually engaging with service users. In University contexts, service user groups/forums provide mechanisms for CYP and parents to contribute to the design and assessment of nursing curriculums. There are potential disparities in terms of the ways in which universities choose to interpret these standards, but what is particularly pertinent for children's nursing education is how the views of CYP (across a range of ages and states of health) are sought and represented in the pre-registration curriculum. This represents a cultural change in academia, whereby service users are invited to share power/responsibilities with academics and this will take time to change. Providing meaningful involvement opportunities for CYP to contribute to nursing education requires creative approaches such as participatory research methods (see later) in order to meet the regulatory requirements that truly reflect and respect their perspectives.

Barriers and Facilitators to CYP Involvement in Children's Nursing Education

Inviting CYP to contribute to university education requires specific considerations, in terms of protecting, accessing and facilitating meaningful engagement that takes account of children's changing developmental status. Gaining access to CYP in order to engage their views is more challenging than with adults, because children are required to be in school/college during times when universities traditionally operate. This can be addressed by visiting CYP in pre-established groups such as at a local hospital, schools/college or scout groups, attending third sector patient groups, young carer groups or by hosting outreach events at university during and outside of school days. Even when CYP are in school, it can be challenging to release them to undertake engagement activities, since they have their own national curriculum requirements and rights to protected lunchtimes. Involving CYP requires careful planning, negotiation and respect for their commitments.

Making university engagement activities meaningful for CYP is important in order for them to feel valued, engaged and to create an environment conducive to gathering a range of perspectives (Carter and Brown, 2014). This can be achieved, for example, through engaging with children in the primary school setting using participatory research methods, such as arts-based activities or games, which appeal to children and also reflect primary school classroom practices (Carter and Ford, 2013). Furthermore, it is important for CYP to understand the value of their contributions and how these will be used to inform future nursing education. The children's nursing lecturer is an ideal facilitator who is experienced in working with children (and who have undertaken Disclosure & Barring Service [DBS] checks). Meaningful engagement can be enhanced when the outcomes are feedback to CYP, since this enables CYP to develop their skills of citizenship and understand the impacts of their contributions.

In order to meet the NMC Educational Standards, pre-registration children's nursing programs are required to be delivered and evaluated with CYP and their parents/carers (NMC, 2018). Directly involving CYP in teaching requires creative and sensitive approaches to ensure that the needs of both nursing students and young presenters are addressed. The feedback from paediatric nursing students highlights the unique insights gained when teaching is undertaken by CYP (Barnley, 2017; Carter and Brown, 2014). It can be daunting and stressful for CYP to speak about their health experiences to a lecture theatre or even to small groups of students, so this requires careful planning, preparation, and negotiation with carers and access to a group of well-supported contributors (Carter and Brown, 2014). In view of these challenges, alternative teaching approaches can include video or audio footage of CYP presenting their perspectives, including the use of podcasts and online blogs such as: www.healthtalk.org. However, restrictions and desires to protect CYP should not limit their opportunities for involvement in nursing education, as this is part of the professional role of children's nurses to promote children's advocacy and rights (NMC, 2018; UNCRC, 1989). Growing children's involvement in teaching pre-registration child field students requires commitment from universities to support the unique learning perspectives this brings to students' professional practice.

CONCLUSION

The empowerment of CYP in health care has gained momentum through increased opportunities and awareness that CYP want to be more involved in decisions about them. Through advances in the availability of health information, for example, via the internet and through the promotion of health literacy in schools, CYP are better informed and able to contribute to decisions about their health care. Policies and opportunities supporting the practical involvement of CYP in health care have progressed and include promoting self-care, commissioning of health services and influencing nursing education. However, these require time and commitment from adults, for example, children's nurses, other health care professionals and educators to facilitate, and ensure progression remains truly child centred, with the child first and foremost. Changing established health care practices and cultures will take time, but the benefits of empowerment will impact future generations of CYP and children's nursing practices.

REFERENCES

Barnley, R., 2017. Service user involvement in preregistration child nursing programs. Nurs. Child. Young People 29 (10), 38–40.

Brook, G., 2000. Children's competency to consent; a framework for practice paediatric. Nursing 12 (50), 31–35.

Carter, B., Ford, K., 2013. Researching children's health experience: the place for participatory, child centered, arts-based approaches. Res. Nurs. Health 36 (1), 95–107.

Carter, C., Brown, K., 2014. Service user input in pre-registration children's nursing education. Nurs. Child. Young People 24 (4), 28–31.

Child Health Information Leaflet Directory (CHILD), 2017. Available from: https://www.piernetwork.org/child.html (accessed 13 September 2018).

Children's Commissioner's Office, 2018. The Children's Commissioner for England. Available from: https://www.childrenscommissioner.gov.uk/about-us/the-childrens-commissioner-for-england/ (accessed 13 September 2018).

Coad, J.E., Evans, R., 2008. Is children's choice in health care rhetoric or reality? A scoping review. J. Adv. Nurs. 64 (4), 318–327.

Cystic Fibrosis (CF), 2018. Trust. Available from: https://www.cysticfibrosis.org.uk/news/introducing-the-new-forum (accessed 24 September 2018).

Davies, A., Randall, D., 2015. Perceptions of children's participation in their health care: a critical review. Issues Compr. Pediatr. Nurs. 38 (3), 202–221.

Department of Health (DoH), 1989. The Children's Act. Crown Copyright, London.

Department of Health (DoH), 2000. The NHS Plan: A Plan for Investment a Plan for Reform. Crown Copyright, London.

Department of Health (DoH), 2003. Building on the Best: Choice, Responsiveness and Equity in the NHS. Crown Copyright, London.

Department of Health (DoH), 2004. National Service Framework for Children and Young People and Maternity Services. Crown Copyright, London.

Department of Health (DoH), 2006. Our Health, Our Care Our Say. Crown Copyright, London.

Department of Health (DoH), 2008. High Quality Care for All. NHS Next Stage Review Final Report. Crown Copyright, London.

Department of Health (DoH), 2010. Equity and Excellence: Liberating the NHS. Crown Copyright, London.

Department of Health (DoH), 2011. Quality Criteria for Young People Friendly Health Services. Crown Copyright, London.

Department of Health Public Health England (DoH PHE), 2014. Maximising the School Nursing Team Contribution to the Public Health Aged Children. Crown Copyright, London.

De Silva, D., 2011. Helping People Help Themselves: A Review of the Evidence Considering Whether it is Worthwhile to Support Self-Management. The Health Foundation, London.

Glasper, E.A., Evans, K., 2013. Supporting children and young people: the 15 steps challenge. Br. J. Nurs. 22 (7), 292–293.

Greenop, D., Hughes, L., Avom, R., et al., 2012. Monkey's Guide to Healthy Living and NHS services. An Evaluation of the Implementation of Resources Designed to Support the Learning of Primary School Age Children in England. John Moores University, Liverpool.

Hagell, A., Rigby, E., Perrow, F., 2015. Promoting health literacy in secondary schools: a review. Br. J. School Nurs. 10 (2), 82–87.

Involve, 2018. The Young Person's Advisory Group. Available from: http://www.invo.org.uk/ypag-the-young-persons-advisory-group/ (accessed 9 August 2018).

Kirk, S., Beatty, S., Callery, P., et al., 2012a. Perceptions of effective self-care support for children and young people with long term conditions. J. Clin. Nurs. 21 (13–14), 1974–1987.

Kirk, S., Beatty, S., Callery, P., et al., 2012b. The effectiveness of self-care support interventions for children and young people with long term conditions: a systematic review. Child: Care Health Dev. 39 (3), 305–324.

Munn, F., 2018. Boost school nurse numbers to tackle obesity, says RCN. Nurs. Child. Young People 30 (4), 6.

Nagara, A., Mc Ginnity, P.M., Davis, N., et al., 2015. Implementing transition: ready steady go. Arch. Dis. Child. Educ. Pract. Ed. 100 (6), 313–320.

National Health Service England (NHSE), 2018. The NHS Youth Forums Top Tips to Involve Young People in Health Care Planning. NHSE, London.

National Health Service Innovation (NHSI), 2013. The 15 Steps Challenge for Children and Young People's Inpatient Services. NHSI, London.

Nursing and Midwifery Council (NMC), 2018. Part One: Standards Framework for Nursing and Midwifery Education. NMC, London.

Personal Social Health and Emotional Education (PHSE) Association, 2018. Curriculum Guidance. Available from: https://www.pshe-association.org.uk/curriculum-and-resources/curriculum (accessed 6 September 2018).

Picker Institute, 2018. The Children's and Young People's Friends and Families Test. Available from: http://www.picker.org/case-studies/recommending-friends-family-test-fft-children-young-people/ (accessed 9 August 2018).

Punch, S., 2002. Research with children: the same or different from research with adults? Childhood 9 (3), 321–341.

Royal College of Paediatrics and Child Health (RCPCH), 2010. Not Just a Phase: A Guide to the Participation of Children and Young People in Health Services. RCPCH, London.

Reed, S., 2015. What are the optimum research approaches to investigate the health care experiences of children with long term conditions within the infant school setting? A research proposal. Working Papers in the Health Sciences 1 (10), 1–4.

United Nations Convention on the Rights of the Child (UNCRC), 1989. Available from: https://www.unicef.org.uk/what-we-do/un-convention-child-rights/ (accessed 20 September 2018).

University of Southampton, 2017. Safer care checklists project – presentation at health foundation event. Available from: https://www.southampton.ac.uk/hws/news/2017/03/30-catherine-pope-health-foundation-event.page (accessed 20 September 2018).

Whiting, L., Roberts, S., Petty, J., et al., 2018. Work of the NHS England youth forum and its effect on health services. Nurs. Child. Young People 30 (4), 34–40.

27

Assessing, Planning, Evaluating and Recording Nursing Care for Children and Young People in Partnership

E. Alan Glasper

LEARNING OUTCOMES

- Appreciate the importance of undertaking and recording accurate and detailed observation and assessment of a child.
- Define the application of the nursing process and discuss its importance in delivering nursing care and conduct from range of nursing models an assessment of a child or young person.
- Discuss the application of the APIE and SOAPIE approaches to assessment.

- Use assessment data to make initial judgements about the child and family's need for general nursing care.
- Incorporate reassessment and evaluation of outcomes in developing a care plan.
- Recognise the complex nature of clinical reasoning and the roles of the child, family, nurse and multi-agency team in assessment, planning and evaluation of care.

INTRODUCTION

Assessment is the primary basis for planning and delivering nursing care to children, young people and families. Whether it is a comprehensive, holistic review of a child's health needs and problems, or a rapid, focused check on some aspect of their condition, assessment provides the information needed to agree with the child and family what needs to be done, when and by whom. To accomplish an assessment, clinical and other reasoning skills are required for the nurse to interpret assessment data and identify appropriate actions, using evidence where possible. Assessment and care planning should enable children, young people and their families to participate fully in the whole care process.

All aspects of care, from assessment to evaluation, are affected by the context in which the care takes place and in particular by the attitudes and values of the nurse and the care team. Working in partnership requires a specific focus for nursing assessment, planning and evaluation which is different to traditional disease focused models. This chapter gives a brief overview of how the nursing process can be used to assesses, plan and evaluate care for as sick child.

THE NATURE OF ASSESSMENT

In health care, the process of assessment attempts to answer the question 'What is (probably) going on here?' with some degree of certainty about what is happening, it is possible subsequent to a full assessment to formulate a plan of care that will address the child or young person's health problem.

However, there is much more to assessing and planning care than simply discovering the problem and deciding what to do. This chapter explores assessment and care planning in the context of child/family/nurse partnerships to provide insights into these complex interpersonal and clinical processes that are the cornerstones of clinical practice. Recording, communicating and evaluating planned care are also considered, with an emphasis on the clinical and information governance responsibilities of the nurse.

ASSESSMENT AND PLANNING IN CONTEXT

The Application of the Nursing Process to the Process of Assessment

When first learning about something as complex as nursing, it helps to use conceptual models that simplify the situation but demonstrate how things relate and where they fit in the real world of nursing practice.

Nursing theory is the applications of cognitive knowledge and understanding that can help nurses deliver the best possible care based on the best evidence. However, it is because children are fundamentally different from adults in a number of ways including being physiologically different, and they can become sicker much more quickly than adults that children's and young people's nurses need a cognitive toolkit to help them provide optimum care. To quote one of history's most famous 19th century children's hospital matrons, Catherine Jane Wood, 'sick children require special nursing and sick children's nurses require special training' (Wood, 1888).

Conceptual models and process models are used in nursing to clarify concepts important to the discipline and define relationships between them. The 'nursing process' was one such approach that was introduced from the United States to the United Kingdom in the late 1970s to help nurses focus on the assessment of each individual patient and their needs, rather than on the medical condition and 'what we always do for patients with such and such disease'. The whole purpose of using the nursing process is to help nurses assess, plan and deliver and evaluate their care to the child and family.

The nursing process is a simple but tried and tested model of assessing, planning and evaluating care that has held and stood test of time. Essentially the nursing process is made up of the following components known by the mnemonic APIE.

1. Assessment
2. Planning of care
3. Implementation of care
4. Evaluation of care

These components of the nursing process for assessing and planning care for sick children can be configured by using this mnemonic APIE. In using APIE this gives nurses a framework to follow throughout their working lives.

However, some nurses prefer to use the more detailed six step SOAPIE mnemonic model of the nursing process:

1. S = The identification of subjective data
2. O = The gathering of objective data
3. A = Assessment
4. P = Planning
5. I = Implementation
6. E = Evaluation

SOAPIE allows the nurse to also consider both subjective and objective criteria when assessing and planning care.

The ability to observe a child without even interacting with them is a skill that grows with experience and the subjective cues elicited during this period of observation may be invaluable in helping to identify actual or potential problems. Some nurses call this an across the room assessment, where objective observations such as the child's colour as in 'is cyanosis present' is noted, in addition to subjective criteria, for example, as in the child's general demeanour, or a sixth sense that something might be wrong but not always obvious. Parents are very much in tune with this subjective element. Subjective data can be considered before commencing the O or objective assessment of the child.

During this objective stage of the application of the nursing process the nurse will objectively assess a range of criteria including among others the child's pulse, respiratory rate, O_2 saturations, blood pressure, etc. In contemporary health care some children's hospitals use a range of electronic digital technology such as wearable communication devices, which enable nurses and other health care professionals to receive and read information about sick children such as bed position, personal data and importantly physiological status such as current early warning signs scores. In addition, some children's wards are using hand held digital devices which utilise mobile software information systems for monitoring the vital signs of children in hospital. (Glasper, 2019).

The whole of the assessment process can be guided and enhanced by the use of a nursing model and some nurses when applying either APIE or SOAPIE in their use of the nursing process to conduct an assessment of a child find it useful to use specific conceptual nursing models to guide them through the process.

Using Nursing Models to Undertake a Child Assessment

There are a number of conceptual models which have been designed by nursing theorists, but it is beyond the scope of this chapter to consider them all in detail. However, the two which are most frequently used in British health care environments such as hospitals are the activity of daily living models. These models can help a nurse assess a sick child by considering a range of pertinent activities. The Henderson and Roper Logan and Tierney activity of living models are very similar and are based around those activities that a human being would do for himself unaided if he had the necessary strength, will or knowledge (Henderson, 1978; Roper and Tierney, 2000).

The Activities of Daily Living (Henderson)

1. Breathe normally.
2. Eat and drink adequately.
3. Eliminate body waste.
4. Move and maintain desirable postures.
5. Sleep and rest.
6. Select suitable clothes, dress and undress.
7. Maintain body temperature within normal range by adjusting clothing and modifying the environment.
8. Keep the body clean and well-groomed and protect the integument.
9. Avoid changes in the environment and avoid injuring others.
10. Communicate with others expressing emotions, needs, fears or opinions.
11. Worship according to one's faith.
12. Work in such a way that there is a sense of accomplishment.
13. Play or participate in various forms of recreation.
14. Learn, discover or satisfy the curiosity that leads to normal development and health and use of the available health facilities.

The Activities of Daily Living (Roper, Logan and Tierney)

1. Maintaining a safe environment.
2. Breathing.
3. Communicating.
4. Mobilising.
5. Eating and drinking.
6. Eliminating.
7. Personal cleansing and dressing.
8. Maintaining body temperature
9. Working and playing.
10. Sleeping.
11. Expressing sexuality.
12. Dying.

It is important to stress that these activities of daily living are not just simple checklists, but each component needs to be considered in light of a number of factors, including:

- Biological
- Psychological
- Sociocultural
- Environmental
- Politicoeconomic
  (Timmins and O'Shea, 2004)

 ACTIVITY

> In your learning groups consider how these five factors might influence a nursing assessment of a child using an activity of daily living model of your choice.

Clearly very young children may not be developmentally able to perform their own activities of living or have a disability which prevents them from doing so and therefore rely on a parent or carer to do so. Although nursing models are useful in undertaking an assessment to then develop a care plan, increasingly nurses are relying on computer generated care plans or core care plans, which have standardised generic care prescriptions and which can be adjusted for individual children.

Similarly care pathways can be used to tailor care delivery to specific groups of patients. For example, a number of children's hospitals have been working with adult hospital colleagues to develop care pathways for young people in transition from child to adult services. The 'Ready Steady Go' care pathway, for example, developed by Nagra et al. (2015) has been designed to help professionals in children's and adults' services to work together to ensure a smooth and gradual transition for young people.

Such care pathways involve all the multi-disciplinary teams involved in the treatment and management of a child and provide a programme of care delivery involving all the professionals. For each clinical problem the essential steps involved in the care of the child are set out and planned with regard to that individual's expected progress. They provide a plan of desired patient outcomes, linked to an estimated time frame and the resources available. They can assist in the application of national evidence-based guidelines into local practice. Care pathways have the advantage of improving teamwork, reducing duplication of documentation and providing continuous records of care for a patient.

When using care pathways or predetermined core care plans it is important these should still be individualised. Some NHS Trusts have care planning software which allows nurses to produce a care plan for each child. When planning care the nurse must ensure that the goals of care are achievable.

ACTIVITY

> In your learning groups discuss other nursing models suitable for applying the nursing process to the care of sick children.

Three Pillars of Conducting an Assessment

The three pillars of assessment are:

1. Listening
2. Observing
3. Measuring

These are constant activities throughout the care process. Planned assessments such as hourly monitoring of pain level and ad hoc or opportunistic assessments, such as noticing a change in one child while attending to another, become the basis for changes to planned care, new assessments and new plans.

It can be helpful to distinguish between initial or generalised assessment of the kind that would be carried out at a first contact or admission in a non-emergency situation and focused assessment, where attention is directed at a specific state, behaviour, concern or situation.

The goals of an initial assessment are to identify:

1. Immediate and ongoing care needs related to the reason for the visit, contact or admission.
2. Other issues/areas of concern.
3. Health promotion needs and opportunities.

It is important to establish a baseline of assessment data that can be used to agree care aims, monitor progress and evaluate outcomes.

Using Specific Tools to Help Assess Sick Children

This is covered in depth in other chapters, but PEWs (paediatric early warning scores), sepsis bundles and the use of SBAR (situation, background, assessment, recommendation), which is a strategy used to facilitate prompt and appropriate communication about a sick child, are commonplace in the care of sick children. These techniques of assessment have been incorporated into the Royal College of Paediatrics and Child Health (RCPCH) suite of resources developed through the Situation Awareness for Everyone (SAFE) programme. Led by the RCPH, this was a 2-year project held in conjunction with 28 hospitals including Great Ormond Street Hospital for children. The resulting resource pack is primarily designed to offer children's units ways of enhancing their mechanisms to protect sick children from potential harms caused by unrecognised clinical deterioration, among others (Glasper, 2016).

Some nurses use the extended version of SBAR which is ISBARD, and is a technique to foster good communication when handing over the care of a sick child.

- Identify – yourself and the patient.
- Situation – what is the problem?
- Background – information to contextualise the problem.
- Assessment – your clinical assessment and prediction.
- Recommendation – what you think should happen.
- Decision.

Additionally, when a nurse has concerns about the management of a sick child in any context the RCPCH recommend the use of CUSS, the acronym for

- Concerns (about care or treatment delivery)
- Uncomfortable
- unSafe
- Stop

CUSS is a technique that uses a graded assertiveness approach to communicating when raising a concern regarding an instruction or process relating to a sick child. CUSS is a technique that helps nurses who are concerned about any aspect of a child's management to speak out. This advocacy role of the nurse is crucial in enhancing safe delivery of care.

Huddling is at the heart of the SAFE programme. Huddles are meetings to share and discuss important information safety information and the 'huddle' is the specific intervention that coordinates the primary aspects of the situation awareness. It is the vehicle that delivers the prime mission of ensuring that all information about a sick child is shared effectively, especially that which pertains to the identification of the sickest children, as well as those children who staff and parents are concerned about. Huddle membership should include all members of the multi-disciplinary team who might have insight into the particular needs of a sick child. The huddle can enable health care professionals to communicate effectively, and recognise and respond to the deteriorating child in a timely way.

👤 ACTIVITY

In your leaning groups go to the RCPCH website and download the SAFE toolkit. Practise the use of SBAR, ISBARD and CUSS with a range of scenarios from your practice.

Data that are collected by listening, observing, measuring and communicating with other professionals should be sifted and sorted to select what is relevant and then analysed to reach a conclusion on whether the situation is normal for this child, a problem, a risk and so on. If there are insufficient data to reach a conclusion, a further decision is required, that is, what more data do I need? To make good clinical judgements, the person doing the assessment draws on existing knowledge and past experience, and uses cognitive skills such as pattern recognition ('I've seen this kind of thing before') and ruling out by hypothesis testing ('It can't be infection because there's no fever'), to reach conclusions.

One of the benefits of reaching a firm conclusion is that this can be discussed openly. Many children's wards now have twice daily safety huddles where these kinds of individual patient concerns, which arise from the assessment process, can be discussed. However, your initial conclusion about what is making a child cry, for example, could lead you to take certain actions, which might be totally inappropriate unless you confirm your 'diagnosis' with the child or carer.

Knowledge from research and other evidence and personal experience of what works in these kinds of situations inform cognitive decision-making processes such as the narrowing of options and weighing-up pros and cons. Possible actions need to be balanced against available resources to arrive at an agreed plan of what is to be done, by whom and when.

Formulating a Care Plan

The primary goal of the assessment is to then initiate a care plan. When the assessment data has been collected the nurse may then commence the care planning process ideally with the child or young person and the carer where possible.

Some find it useful to use the acronym SMART when setting objectives of care.

S *Specific.* The objectives of care set by the nurse in consultation with the family must accurately specify what it is that will be measured as an indicator of achievement. Hence if the child is dehydrated and needs a certain volume of fluid intake then this can be specified by the hour or day.

M *Measurable.* The nurse should be in a position to accurately determine, for example, that the child has drunk the prescribed volume of fluid as specified in the nursing care plan or care pathway.

A *Achievable.* For example, was the specified volume of fluid prescribed for the child achievable in practice? Was the plan successful in achieving the objective set?

R *Realistic.* Were the targets set through the nursing plan objectives achievable given the resources available to the nursing staff, etc.?

T *Time.* Has a time-frame for achieving the specific child-focused nursing care plan objectives been set?

Developing a Care Plan

After subjectively and objectively assessing the child, the nurse is then in a position to list and prioritise the problems that require a nursing intervention. Each nursing problem or unfulfilled need as in the case of a developmentally immature child (or child with complex disabilities) will require an (SMART) objective of care. The actions needed to be undertaken by the nurse or carer to fulfil the objective and thus fulfil the unmet need or problem can be detailed on the care plan. To fulfil the evaluation stage of the APIE/SOAPIE nursing process formulae, it is necessary to include a review period on the action component of the care plan. This might be an hourly evaluation for a problem such as pyrexia.

Whether or not a formal care plan is written down, some level of planning takes place before any action is taken. Based on assessment findings (and on what they are hoping to achieve if goals have been set), the planners identify available options and make decisions about what needs to be done. The plan of care is a communication tool that should make it clear to all concerned who will be doing what, when and how. It can be as simple as a checklist or as complex as a step-by-step statement of a procedure with timed goals and expected outcomes: a plan in the child's home that will be used to inform a bank nurse providing respite care will need to be very detailed; a plan for a child seen in the emergency department with a fever may consist of a standard form with four actions to be ticked by whoever completes them (and space to write additional, individualised actions if required).

As computerised records and systems become more commonplace throughout the health service, 'e-pathways' will enable evidence-based standards to be better individualised and for individual differences to be analysed to provide improved evidence (de Luc and Todd, 2003).

Supporting Decision Making

A key role for the nurse working in partnership to plan care is to support decision making by the child/young person and family. The first step is to assess their decision-making preferences, not an easy task but one that acknowledges them as equals and establishes that their experiences and perspectives are valued and will be taken into account.

ACTIVITY

Think about your own most recent consultation with a doctor:
- How involved were you in the decision about what action to take?
- How involved would you have preferred to be?
- Having thought about this last question, choose your preference for that particular encounter from the list below:
  1. I would prefer to make the decision myself with information only.
  2. I would prefer to make the decision myself considering the doctor's view.
  3. I would prefer the doctor to make the decision, but considering my views.
  4. I would prefer the doctor to make the decision.

Having been involved in the decision about what to do, you are more likely to adhere to the course of action than if someone else has decided for you. As long ago as 1977, a doctor writing in the *Lancet* suggested that if doctors 'were willing to let go of the notion that they are responsible for controlling their patients', then patients who wanted to could 'make informed decisions on the basis of their own values' (Slack, 1977). Not all parents and children will want to participate in decision making, but the danger is in assuming that they do not wish to and ignoring their right to be heard.

The issue of consent and whether children are really given choices applies to all kinds of care decisions, from whether to proceed with a heart–lung transplant to what to have for breakfast. Alderson and Montgomery's (1996) seminal text addresses the challenges of health care decision making with children and parents. At the level of day-to-day practice, it is the values and attitudes of nurses and other team members that influence whether partnership in decision making is a reality. In addition, health care professionals need to have the confidence and be equipped with skills and tools with which to:
- assess preferences (which may change);
- assess competence (which will change);
- provide information without persuasion;
- 'teach' decision-making strategies;
- record and communicate decisions;
- support child and family when they have made their decision (even if you don't agree with it).

Benefits of Care Plans

1. Improved quality of care
2. Improved communication
3. Evidence-based practice
4. Reduced risk of litigation
5. Standardisation of care
6. Continuity of care
7. Child/family and staff satisfaction

A growing thread throughout health and social care in the UK is the concept of a single, shared multi-disciplinary patient record as a necessary requirement for ensuring continuity in an age when many different disciplines and services may be providing care for one child. A single record suggests a single assessment and one care plan for the child, something that many professionals believe would get rid of many of the communication failures and frustrations that parents and children experience. Although progress has been made towards a single electronic record it still has not come to fruition.

The Focus of Assessment

Even when single, shared patient records are a reality, nurses will still be responsible for the nursing elements of assessment and planning. But what are these, where do you start and how much do you cover? The obvious starting point is to identify those aspects of the health care of children and young people for which nurses are responsible. To some extent these are dictated by Health Service managers through role and job descriptions and can change over time and between settings. But the profession itself, in consultation with the public and other professional groups, defines the core focus of nursing work. The regulatory and professional bodies set standards for practice and education that specify what nurses are educated to do and how they will practise such as The Nursing and Midwifery Council 'Code' (NMC, 2015), for example.

Implementing Nursing Care

The implementation element of the care plan is crucial as this gives clear directions to the reader of the plan on how the care objectives are to be met. This might include specific instructions on the timing of infant feeds or how often specific physiotherapy is given to a child with cystic fibrosis.

Evaluating Care

All objectives of care and the nursing actions to implement them should be evaluated by the nurse responsible for the child. Amendments to the nursing care plan should be made in light of the evaluations. Once an objective has been achieved this can be deleted from the care plan. Conversely, if the recommended action failed to meet the objective then further changes to the care plan will be necessary.

Clinical Reasoning

One criticism of the nursing process is that it emphasises patient problems (it is sometimes referred to as a 'problem-solving process') and therefore is unsuited to health promotion and 'well person' elements of nursing roles. Although it clearly shows how a nurse could provide individualised, planned care, the process focuses on 'doing' steps, and thus hides the clinical reasoning that is required to sift through the available assessment data and to weigh up the evidence to make good clinical decisions.

Another way of looking at the same process is to consider the cognitive processes that underpin assessment, planning and evaluation, rather than the action steps. 'Clinical reasoning' is a general term covering the cognitive processes of diagnostic reasoning (also known as clinical judgement) and clinical decision making. Higgs (2000) provides an excellent overview of clinical reasoning in the health professions. Knowing about these clinical and cognitive processes can help direct your approach to care and will inform your practice in helping children, young people and families to carry out assessments themselves and make decisions about what actions to take in the light of their own findings.

 ACTIVITY

Imagine that you woke up this morning with a slight pain in your knee that has worsened during the day. List the things you might ask yourself or do to try to establish what the problem is. What knowledge have you drawn on to inform your 'diagnostic reasoning'?

Context for Care

Patient care and the clinical process do not take place in isolation. No matter how good the assessment is and how well planned the care, there are many other factors that influence whether the child's and family's expectations of care are achieved and their experience of nursing and health care is a positive one. The context of care, from the interpersonal relationships between family and staff to the prevailing political climate, heavily impact on the quality of the services and care provided. There are a multitude of factors that have an influence on the care process. At different times and in different situations the impact of the various factors will be different, but four of them are particularly important in nursing:

• Interpersonal: relationships and interactions between and among the child, the family and the clinical team.
• Financial: availability of and ease of access to specific services and resources, for example, equipment, staff and skill mix and time.
• Philosophical: the ethos of the team that pervades all aspects of care delivery.
• Ethical: recognition of rights, equity, etc.

REFLECT ON YOUR PRACTICE

Interpersonal Context

How could interpersonal relationships between members of a clinical team (an aspect of the interpersonal context) influence the quality of your nursing care? For example, what would happen if the nursing team does not feel able to question medical staff decisions? (Consider CUSS?)

Partnership Principles Applied to Assessing and Planning Care

Planning care should involve, where possible, the child and family to uphold the overarching family-centred care philosophy of children's and young person's nursing. Planning care involves reviewing all of the identified needs or patient problems and prioritising them.

Clearly, if a child has compromised respiratory efforts this must be prioritised before planning dietary intake, for example.

Care plans are frameworks through which nurses apply the nursing process in addressing the needs of their patients. A nursing care plan is a written statement of the patient's nursing problems and the measures that will be used to bring into effect a solution or mediate these problems.

Parental involvement in care can be visualised as moving along a continuum from nurse led to parent led care. Other conceptual models of nursing use similar constructs to help explain aspects of the relationship between nurses and patients, for example, Orem's view of the patient as totally dependent through to self-caring (Orem, 2001). These kinds of models and terms such as 'nurse led', 'patient-centred', 'child friendly' represent particular philosophies: ways of thinking and acting that directly influence the child's and families' experience of care. Even the language we use implies a particular way of thinking and acting. You might hear the term 'non-compliant' applied in a situation, for example, where a teenager with diabetes is admitted to hospital. 'Non-compliance' suggests that heavy-handed sanctions will be needed to get the patient to manage diet, exercise and insulin properly. If the teenager is described instead as 'making choices that can put her at risk' then the management approach is more likely to be one that reflects an understanding of adolescent needs.

Orem's Universal Self-Care Requisites

1. Air
2. Water
3. Food
4. Elimination
5. Activity and rest
6. Solitude and social interaction
7. Hazard prevention
8. Promotion of normality

REFLECT ON YOUR PRACTICE

Philosophical Context

Nurses often provide information to the child and family about the child's condition or treatment, reflecting a view of children and families as passive recipients of health care. What view would you be reflecting if instead of providing information you helped the child to find out where to get information for themselves?

The term 'partnership' is widely used in health and social care to represent the ideal or preferred relationship between agencies and between professionals and clients. In the nursing care of children and families it has come to mean a changing, negotiated, shared responsibility for care between child, family and nurse, with support and teaching provided (including teaching of nurses by the child and family). Family involvement in care may be a result of the negotiation of care responsibility, but this is not necessarily so. Conversely, nursing involvement in care may not be what the child and family want; respite care at home for the child with complex needs may be better provided by a social care assistant with specific training. A key principle of partnership working is that responsibility does not have to be shared equally; the extent to which the child, family member and nurse are ready for and able to contribute to the partnership dictates changes in responsibility, that is, for the child towards independent self-care and for some parents towards leading and delegating care. In some situations, the nursing team may only be able to offer limited services so the burden of care remains with the family.

Partnership complements other constructs valued by nurses caring for children and young people such as 'child-centred care' and respect for children's rights, particularly the right to be informed and to have a say in decision making. There is very little evidence of how children and parents view partnership working (as distinct from research into their views on involvement or participation in care), and little to indicate whether true partnerships are possible in a context where professionals have more power and there are limited resources. In Coyne's (1995) classic study, parents reported difficulties with lack of information, non-negotiation of roles, and feelings of anxiety and loneliness when caring for their child in hospital. However, by 2016 Coyne et al. were arguing that a conceptual move from family-centred care (FCC) to a child-centred care (CCC) approach was needed (Coyne et al., 2016).

Negotiated Roles

Kirk (2001) in a classic study investigated whether there was any negotiation of caring roles between professionals and parents of children with complex needs:

> From the parents' perspective, their initial assumption of responsibility for the care of their child was not subject to negotiation with professionals. Prior to discharge, feelings of obligation, their strong desire for their child to come home and the absence of alternatives to parental care in the community were key motivating factors in their acceptance of responsibility from professionals.

In this case professionals had concerns about whether parents were given a choice and the degree of choice they could exercise in the face of professional power. As parents gained experience in caring for their child, and as their relationships with professionals developed, role negotiation started to happen. Kirk concluded that professional expectations of parental involvement probably acted as a barrier to negotiation of roles and that parental choices were initially constrained by their feelings of obligation.

CHILD CONVERSATION

Kate Aged 11 Years With Asthma

Kate: Once I started doing it myself [the asthma diary] I could see much better how I was doing. I could tell the nurse how much Ventolin I'd needed and sometimes we could see what was making it worse. Once we decided for me to try taking Ventolin before going outdoors or for PE when it was cold outside.

Kate's mum: She was better at keeping the diary than me, at least at first. Now she only uses it when she's having problems and that helps her see what needs doing.

Applying a partnership approach to assessment alters the goals of care which now, in conjunction with the family, seek to identify:

- their immediate and ongoing care needs related to the reason for the visit, contact or admission;
- other issues/areas of concern;
- health promotion needs and opportunities;
- their experience and expectations of care and services;
- their readiness and preferences in relation to participation in care and decision making;
- to establish a baseline (as before).

Traditional, profession-centred models of care still exist where the carer, usually the mother, not the child or young person, is asked about the child's condition and progress. The clinician interprets the assessment information and informs the parent what needs to happen next. However, in most services it is accepted that the children and young people themselves are the best source of information and that seeking their views and involving them in decision making and self-care are beneficial not just in terms of outcome, but in making their whole experience of health care more positive.

Using the communication tools that are most familiar to children and young people, such as mobile phones and the internet, goes some way to improving the child friendliness of services. Although these approaches are still being evaluated, it is possible to envisage young people with diabetes, for example, managing their condition at home with internet-based decision support, e-mail advice and mobile phone text reminders for medication times. The 2019 NHS Long Term Plan's proposals for developing the use of digital technology to enhance patient care will fundamentally alter how children with long-term conditions are assessed and managed by health care professionals. New digital innovations such as Skype are a solution to this problem. Skype is one of a number of telecommunications application software products that allow users to see and hear through a video link between computers, tablets and mobile devices (Glasper, 2019).

But there is still a significant shift needed in the way professionals view the child and young person's world, particularly the child/young person with a chronic condition or disability. More locally delivered services and better use of technology will support moves from a world where the child/young person and the family must adapt their lives to fit around the condition and its management to a world where the condition and its management are adapted to their lifestyles. With more children's nurses as part of the primary care team supporting children and families at home there will hopefully be greater attention focused on assessment and intervention in relation to the safety and suitability of the child's environment, their access to community services and the appropriateness of those services. Simple solutions like having appointments outside of college hours seem obvious, but there are very few clinics that consider the needs and lifestyles of children and young people.

Traditional, disease-focused models of nursing assessment are very common and illustrate the need for improved understanding of the unique contribution of nursing. Reductions in medical staff numbers and advances in health technology mean that more and more nurses are taking on what were previously medical roles, from technical tasks to investigation, diagnosis and treatment of disorders. Evidence suggests that with appropriate education and training nurses can provide safe, high-quality clinical services. But the unique contribution that nursing care makes to improve the experiences and quality of life for children and families needs to be recognised, so that when nurses do take on new roles overall quality is not compromised.

It is impossible to totally separate the specific focus and contribution of nursing as nurses' work encompasses aspects of many other disciplines from play therapy to prescribing, and often substitutes for parental 'work', that is the continual care, protection, comfort, distraction and encouragement that parents provide to their children throughout their formative lives. However, a clear understanding of those situations that are the primary responsibility of nurses and those that are a collaborative responsibility helps to ensure that nurses meet the requirements of their professional role.

◎ EVIDENCE-BASED PRACTICE

Nursing or Medicine?

As long ago as 1997, Mason and Webb found that nursing records reflected children's medical/physical needs and care but that much practice was focused on psychosocial needs. When nurses were provided with a nursing framework for assessment, their clinical judgements were no longer described in terms of the primary medical diagnosis, but reflected the family-centred nursing model, including:
- continuity of usual care by parents;
- support for family members;
- impact of illness and hospitalisation;
- participation by parents in nursing and medical care.

As part of their collaborative role with medicine, nurses do include aspects of illness/injury management in their assessments such as:
- assessing any risks for complications of treatment;
- monitoring treatment progress;
- assessing the child/family ability to carry out treatment plans.

In collaboration with mental health and social care professionals working with children in need and their families, nurses may undertake diagnostic assessments related to development, behaviour, parenting capacity, family functioning and so on. As nursing specialist roles expand and more nurse-led services develop, assessments now incorporate tests and investigations relating to the child's medical condition. Combining nursing and medical or other discipline focused assessment is time consuming and complex, but marks the difference between the nurse with an expanded role and the nurse as 'doctor substitute'.

🔲 SCENARIO

A child is admitted to the day ward for minor surgery under general anaesthetic. As she had attended the clinic the week before, her height and weight are already noted. After greeting the child and mother and introducing herself, the nurse records the child's temperature, pulse and respirations, asks whether she has had a cough or cold in the previous few days and when she last had something to eat or drink. Having checked that the consent form is signed, the nurse asks whether the mother or child have any questions about the procedure.

This scenario is a good example of the clinical situation alone dictating the assessment. The nurse is using knowledge of what is important for ensuring a safe anaesthetic procedure, but is not using knowledge from nursing theory and research of what the child and the mother might be experiencing or other concerns and needs they may have. This is the crux of good nursing assessment:
- using knowledge from different sources (including from personal experience)
  ↓
- combining it with the results of holistic and focused assessment in order to
  ↓
- apply the knowledge appropriately to the individual child and family in order to
  ↓
- discover (and confirm with them) their care needs

🔲 PROFESSIONAL CONVERSATION

Theory Into Practice With Caution

Meena is a third-year children's nursing student.

We'd been studying psychological developmental stages and what they mean in terms of preparing children for surgery. So when I knew I'd be admitting a 4-year-old boy I thought carefully about what his understanding would be at that age about his body and the surgery and being in hospital. I was prepared with simple pictures of tubes going into the tummy and so on but he waved me away and seemed annoyed that I hadn't used the words gastrostomy, abdomen, etc. One of the staff nurses explained he'd been in and out of hospital since birth and had a better understanding of his condition than many of the nurses. It made me realise that, although applying theory in practice was important, I needed to use it to inform what I thought and did for each individual patient, not to make assumptions about what their actual needs were.

The following list summarises the scope of nursing assessment and also suggests a logical prioritisation of assessment topics:
1. Risk to life of child and risk of harm to child.
2. Communication – abilities, means, aids, language, etc. This is especially true of assessing children with autism or

a learning disability where special communication aides will need to be used.

3. Fears and anxieties – immediate concerns addressed.
4. Systematic and ongoing assessment – generalised, focused, changes, progress.
5. Preferences and needs related to participation in decision making and care.

The first priority must obviously be risks to life and risk of harm. Second, there must be a means of communicating and establishing a relationship with the child/young person and the parents/carer. When communication is possible, fears, anxieties and immediate concerns need to be identified and addressed. Appropriate, systematic assessment can then be carried out, including identification of other risks such as potential environmental threats or stress related to family disruption.

As stated earlier there are a number of frameworks or models which are available to help the nurse to decide what topics to cover in generalised assessment, such as the activities of living models.

REFLECT ON YOUR PRACTICE

Choose a clinical area that you have worked in and list the topics that you recall being the focus of nursing assessment. Would you add anything to your list?

Generalised assessment tools based on this kind of framework model give structure to assessments and reinforce the philosophy and values on which they are based. Whatever the clinical context, there will be a core set of items relevant to every child, young person and family such as their understanding of the situation and their special needs. As care needs emerge and a relationship is established, the child and family's preferences and readiness for participation in care and decision making and their information, learning and support needs can be identified.

Depending on the clinical context, specific assessment items will be prioritised, for example, respiration, hydration, skin integrity and pain level in intensive care; self-care, self-image, feeding regime and educational needs in the head injury rehabilitation unit. It would not be possible to publish all possible frameworks that might be appropriate for the many different health and nursing needs of children and young people. However, it is possible to list a set of principles for evaluation of those that are presently available, or to underpin the development of new ones. Most importantly, frameworks for comprehensive nursing assessment of children and young people must support the identification of health issues that require nursing intervention or referral to other team members. They should also:

- be child- and family-centred: consider the child's/young person's rights, responsibilities and relationships within the family and society;
- be holistic: covering physiological, physical, social, psychological and spiritual aspects of the developing child/young person;

- reflect partnership values: including consideration of child and family preferences related to care, and their involvement in care and decision making;
- be practical to use;
- be acceptable to children/young people and families;
- have a nursing focus: address the effects of the health issue and its management (not the diagnosis and treatment alone).

Although nursing assessment has a specific focus, as with all aspects of children's health care, team approaches to assessment should be considered. Many aspects of the child's care are managed by the whole team and joint or shared assessment approaches are becoming the norm.

Tools and Methods for Focused Assessment

Unlike generalised frameworks, most assessment tools measure just one aspect of the child's health status. Assessment tools can improve the quality and accuracy of assessments; their usefulness will depend on their purpose, content and practicality. The development and evaluation of assessment tools is complex and any measurement instrument needs to be reliable and valid. It should return consistent results when used repeatedly to measure the same thing and it should measure what it is supposed to be measuring. Signs and symptoms such as raised body temperature, weight loss and ulcerated lips are relatively easy to measure and quantify. However, most aspects of the child and family's responses to health problems and their management (i.e. nursing concerns) are subjective, variable and multi-faceted, making them difficult to recognise and even more difficult to 'measure'. Some paediatric and child health assessment instruments have been well researched, notably pain assessment scales.

As a general guide, any tool that is adapted from another setting or client group must first be validated for use with your client group in your clinical setting.

EVIDENCE-BASED PRACTICE
Transferability of Assessment Tools

Gharaibeh and Abu-Saad (2002) looked at the cultural validity, reliability and children's preferences of three pain assessment tools among Jordanian children. They found that the scales were valid and reliable but that there were gender differences in preference for particular scales, explained by the researchers as part of the socialisation process within the Arab culture.

PARENT CONVERSATION

Georgina is the mother of 17-month-old William.

Relying on Measurement Tools

The nurse in emergency department used an ear thermometer and said his temperature was normal. I knew he wasn't well. His temperature had been very high at home; he was pale, his head felt hot but his hands and feet were cold. She didn't seem to hear me saying to her that I thought his temperature was on the way up again (Mothers' sixth sense?).

Evaluation and Outcomes

Evaluation of the effectiveness of care for an individual child (and family) is an important part of nursing care. It needs to take place throughout the care process, with continual reassessment of their responses to interventions so that these can be changed or discontinued if they are ineffective or no longer needed. Initial assessment identifies health problems or issues that need addressing at the beginning of a care programme or episode; outcome evaluation identifies the extent of change in the health problem or achievement of goals related to the health issue.

A number of issues are related to the identification of what have been termed 'nursing sensitive patient outcomes' (those outcomes that are influenced by nursing care). The same difficulties that are faced when assessing less concrete aspects of the child's state, behaviour, feelings, etc., also apply in evaluation. The child and family's own reports of their experience and satisfaction with care are the most important evaluation evidence. However, nurses should supplement this evidence with outcome measures suited to the clinical setting, and where possible, derived from standards or benchmarks.

It may be difficult to differentiate the outcomes that are the result of nursing from those that result from interventions by others (including the child and family's own actions). However, it is important to consider 'nursing sensitive patient outcomes' for two main reasons: to monitor and improve effectiveness and to justify resources. Nurses do things for, with and to patients; they act on the results of assessments and decide what an appropriate course of action should be. If they don't evaluate the results of their actions (i.e. measure outcomes) they cannot know whether they made the right decision nor learn what works to provide evidence for future practice.

Much of the evidence we have about effectiveness and outcomes of care can be derived from intervention studies. For example, a study of the efficacy of tepid sponging to reduce fever in children (Sharber, 1997) used simple outcome measures of fever reduction and signs of discomfort (crying, shivering, goosebumps). Petryshen et al. (1998) used stability of physiological measures such as pulse and respirations as well as length of stay to evaluate the effectiveness of developmental care in very low birth weight babies.

Nursing interventions are directed at a number of child and family's responses to health problems and their management, from symptoms and behaviours through to their feelings and knowledge about their condition and how they cope with self-management at home and school.

Information Management and Keeping Accurate Records

As this chapter has shown, the clinical process of assessment involves a number of complex steps and all of these steps generate information about the child's and family's needs and preferences, care decisions that are made, things that are planned and done, and results or outcomes of what was done. Much of this information needs to be communicated and recorded and some of it will need to be used for other purposes such as audit and service planning. Recording, storing, communicating and using information is known as information management. The goal of information management is to ensure relevant information is in the hands of those who need it, at the time they need it, and in a format that they can understand and use. Patients, parents, staff and managers need information so they can make sense of the situation and make decisions about what to do. The child's health care record is the main tool for managing this information. Every professional who comes in contact with the patient needs to be able to make timely decisions about what care is needed and how best to deliver that care. If it is to be an effective information tool, the record should support this process of clinical decision making. All records must be legible, accurate, signed with designation stated, dated, timed, contemporaneous, be able to provide a chronology of events and use only agreed abbreviations. These 'patient-focused benchmarks' set standards for progress towards single, life-long, patient held records that are secure and support high-quality, evidence-based care. Care Quality Commission inspectors always review a sample of patient records for compliance to these benchmarks.

The purposes of the record dictate its format as well as its content. A key purpose of records is communication between disciplines, which suggests that moves towards a single record, used by all professionals and possibly held by the child or parent, will help to achieve 'fitness for purpose'. Another function is to serve as a secondary source of data: for audit, research and as evidence for legal or other enquiries.

Nurses are required to keep clear, intelligible and accurate (C I A) records and this is the gold standard toward which they should strive at all times (Glasper, 2011).

A good way to decide whether the content of your records and care plans are adequate is to ask the question: 'Can those coming after me find out from the record what they need to know to continue the care of this child?' This tests the fitness of the record for the purpose of communication to support continuity of care. A second question that tests the quality of the record for all other purposes is: 'Can those who need to know find out from the record what we found on assessment, what we did, and the results of our actions?' Working in partnership implies that the content of the record will reflect not just the nurse's view but the assessments, plans, actions and evaluations of the child/young person, parents and other members of the team.

Data to support audit, management and research can be obtained directly from these records or collected using specific data collection tools. One of the benefits of computerising patient records is that these will provide structured data that can be more easily aggregated and analysed.

Information Governance

An important part of information management is information governance, a quality framework that brings together legal requirements and professional guidance around record keeping, confidentiality, access to records, data quality, etc. The key principles of information governance are that information is:

H = held securely and confidentially

O = obtained fairly and efficiently

R = recorded accurately and reliably
U = used effectively and ethically
S = shared appropriately and lawfully

Good practice requires the nurse to ensure that children, young people and parents/carers are informed of what is recorded about them and who has access to that information so that they can choose whether to restrict access to the information in the record or withhold information they do not wish to be shared. This is even more important as electronic records are introduced in all health care settings making access easier.

CONCLUSION

There are several summary points to be made about assessment and care planning. First, admitting a patient is not the same as assessing a patient, and assessment is not just a tick box exercise. Second, there is no point doing a 'once only' generalised assessment as ongoing review is essential to monitor changes and the success of nursing interventions. Finally, without a nursing framework to guide the focus of assessment, care will focus solely on the medical/physical needs of patients and not the other aspects which are important. It is important to stress that the Care Quality Commission (the health care regulator for England) will examine individual child care plans when they inspect children's wards as part of an overall hospital inspection.

REFERENCES

Alderson, P., Montgomery, J., 1996. Health Care Choices: Making Decisions with Children. Institute of Public Policy Research, London.

Coyne, I.T., 1995. Partnership in care: parents' views of participation in their hospitalised child's care. J. Clin. Nurs. 4 (2), 71–79.

Coyne, I., Hallstrom, I., Soderback, M., 2016. Reframing the focus from a family-centred to a child-centred care approach for children's healthcare. J. Child. Health Care. 20 (4), 494–502.

de Luc, K., Todd, J., 2003. E-pathways: Computers and the Patient's Journey through Care. Radcliffe Medical, Oxford.

Gharaibeh, M., Abu-Saad, H., 2002. Cultural validation of pediatric pain assessment tools: Jordanian perspective. J. Transcult. Nurs. 13 (1), 12–18.

Glasper, A., 2011. Improving record keeping: important lessons for nurses. Br. J. Nurs. 20 (14), 886–887.

Glasper, A., 2016. Keeping sick children in hospital SAFE from harm. Br. J. Nurs. 25 (20), 1078–1079.

Glasper, A., 2019. A long-term plan for embracing digital health-care technology. Br. J. Nurs. 28 (3), 204–205.

Henderson, V., 1978. The concept of nursing. J. Adv. Nurs. 3 (2), 113–130.

Higgs, J., 2000. Clinical Reasoning in the Health Professions, second ed. Butterworth-Heinemann, Oxford.

Kirk, S., 2001. Negotiating lay and professional roles in the care of children with complex health care needs. J. Adv. Nurs. 34 (5), 593–602.

Nagra, A., McGinnity, M., Davis, N., et al., 2015. Implementing transition: Ready Steady Go. Arch. Dis. Child. Educ. Pract. Ed. 100 (6), 313–320.

Nursing and Midwifery Council, 2015. The Code: Professional Standards of Practice and Behaviour for Nurses and Midwives. NMC, London.

Orem, D., 2001. Nursing: Concepts of Practice. Mosby, St. Louis.

Petryshen, P., Stevens, B., Hawkins, J., et al., 1998. Comparing nursing costs for preterm infants receiving conventional vs developmental care. Neonatal Intensive Care 11 (2), 18–24.

Roper, N., Tierney, A., 2000. The Roper, Logan, Tierney Model of Nursing Based on Activities of Living. Churchill Livingstone, Edinburgh.

Sharber, J., 1997. The efficacy of tepid sponge bathing to reduce fever in young children. Am. J. Emerg. Med. 15 (2), 188–192.

Slack, W., 1977. The patient's right to decide. Lancet 296, 240.

Timmins, F., O'Shea, J., 2004. The Roper-Logan-Tierney (1996) model of nursing as a tool for professional development in education. Nurse Educ. Pract. 4 (3), 159–167.

Wood, C.J., 1888. The training of nurses for sick children. The Nursing Record. 6, 507–510.

28

The Management of Pain in Children and Young People

Alison Twycross, Jennifer Stinson, Rebecca Saul

LEARNING OUTCOMES

INTRODUCTION

The aim of this chapter is to outline current evidence-based practice in relation to the management of pain in children and young people primarily in hospital-based settings from the neonatal period onwards. The chapter starts by discussing why managing pain in children effectively is important. Following this, the anatomy and physiology of pain is outlined and current evidence in relation to managing pain in children and young people focusing on the management of procedural, acute and chronic pain is given. The information in this chapter prepares nurses to care for children across a range of inpatient settings, as well as providing guidance for managing pain outside of hospital.

WHY ASSESSING AND MANAGING PAIN IN CHILDREN AND YOUNG PEOPLE IS IMPORTANT

Managing pain effectively is an ethical imperative. The United Nations, in its Declaration on the Rights of the Child, states that:

Children should in all circumstances be among the first to receive protection and relief, and should be protected from all forms of neglect, cruelty and exploitation
United Nations, (1989)

Failing to provide children/young people with satisfactory pain relief can be considered a violation of their human rights. Indeed, the Declaration of Montreal identifies that access to pain management is a fundamental human right (IASP, 2015).

Unrelieved pain also has several undesirable physical and psychological consequences that affect the child/young person in the short and longer term (Table 28.1). There is also evidence that acute (postoperative) pain can result in chronic pain in a small but significant number of children/young people (Batoz et al., 2016; Rabbitts et al., 2017; Schug and Bruce, 2017). The consequences of unrelieved pain provide a clear rationale for why it is important to manage children/young people's pain effectively.

Given the consequences of not managing pain effectively it has been suggested mismanaged pain should be considered an *adverse event* (Chorney et al., 2010; Twycross et al., 2016). This is because even though the evidence to manage pain effectively is readily available in the form of clinical guidelines (Association of Paediatric Anaesthetists, 2012; Australian and New Zealand College of Anaesthetists and Faculty of Pain Medicine, 2015; Royal College of Nursing, 2009), children and young people still experience moderate to severe unrelieved pain while in hospital (Avian et al., 2016; Smeland et al., 2018; Walther-Larsen et al., 2017) and at home (Parker et al., 2018). Indeed, Chorney et al. (2010) argue that mismanaged pain is health care professionals' *dirty little secret* – a direct result of their management decisions (e.g. venepunctures, chest tubes and surgery). Without adequate treatment, the pain children and young people experience is often severe and above the threshold they or their parents find acceptable (Birnie et al., 2012).

When all the consequences of unrelieved pain are considered, managing children/young people's pain effectively can clearly be seen as an ethical imperative. Within this chapter we will be giving you the tools to manage acute, procedural and chronic pain in children and young people in hospital or other health care settings.

THE ANATOMY AND PHYSIOLOGY OF PAIN

To be able to manage a child/young person's pain effectively it is necessary to understand the anatomy and physiology involved. The processing of a pain signal involves physiological processes including transduction, transmission and modulation. These processes are explained pictorially in Fig. 28.1A–D.

Primary ascending nociceptors (pain nerves) transmit nerve impulses (action potentials) to the dorsal horn of spinal cord **(i)**. The structure of the axon influences the speed of nociceptor conduction. Small diameter, unmyelinated C-fibres have slow conduction speeds of as little as 1 metre per second (m/s) and transmit dull ache pain impulses, while large diameter, myelinated A-delta nociceptors conduct sharp stabbing

---

TABLE 28.1 Consequences of Unrelieved Pain

Physical Effects

Rapid, shallow, splinted breathing, which can lead to hypoxaemia and alkalosis

Inadequate expansion of lungs and poor cough, which can lead to secretion retention and atelectasis

Increased heart rate, blood pressure and myocardial oxygen requirements, which can lead to cardiac morbidity and ischaemia

Increased stress hormones (e.g. cortisol, adrenaline, catecholamines), which in turn increase the metabolic rate, impede healing and decrease immune function

Slowing or stasis of gut and urinary systems, which leads to nausea, vomiting, ileus and urinary retention

Muscle tension, spasm and fatigue, which leads to reluctance to move spontaneously and refusal to ambulate, further delaying recovery

Psychological Effects

Anxiety, fear, distress, feelings of helplessness or hopelessness

Avoidance of activity, avoidance of future medical procedures

Sleep disturbances

Loss of appetite

Other Effects

Prolonged hospital stays

Increased rates of re-admission to hospital

Increased outpatient visits

---

pain transmissions at up to 120 m/sec (Brodal, 2016a) **(ii)**. Second-order neurons carry action potentials along spinal pathways to the brain **(iii)**. Descending inhibition neurons release serotonin, noradrenaline and endorphins that inhibit the pain pathway **(iv)** (Lee et al., 2011).

Painful (noxious) sensations are conducted along nociceptors, towards the brain (where pain perception occurs), through the generation of action potentials. A-delta nociceptors are *unimodal*, responding to a specific high-threshold stimulus; either mechanical (e.g. needle-related procedures), or thermal (e.g. burning sensations). C-fibre nociceptors are *polymodal*, responding to multiple tissue-injury sensations, such as hot and cold (thermal), and mechanical and chemical stimuli. (Mason, 2017).

In response to tissue damage:

- Substance P is released by nociceptors **(A)**.
- Substance P triggers the release of bradykinin, serotonin and leukocytes and the release of histamine by mast cells **(B)**; it also plays a role in blood vessel permeability, resulting in oedema.
- This 'inflammatory soup' increases the sensitivity and activity of nociceptors (a process called *hyperalgesia*) **(C and D)**.
- Calcitonin gene-related peptide (CGRP) triggers vasodilation, causing the redness seen during tissue damage (Mason, 2017).
- Arachidonic acid is released from cell membrane phospholipids by the enzyme phospholipase **(E)**; it is converted to prostaglandin through the action of the enzyme cyclooxygenase (Simon and Hochberg, 2016). Prostaglandin is a key component of inflammatory soup and plays an important role in sensitising nociceptors (Mason, 2017).
- Cyclooxygenase (COX) exists in two forms: COX-1 acts as a 'housekeeping' enzyme, regulating the normal function

of the gastrointestinal tract, kidneys and platelet aggregation **(F)**. COX-2 is predominantly expressed in tissues during inflammation (Chan and Haroon, 2016) and prostaglandin produced via this route plays a role in pain, inflammation and fever.

An action potential is generated by nociceptors in response to a painful stimulus:

HANDY HINT: ANALGESIC DRUGS

Non-steroidal anti-inflammatories (NSAIDs) are non-selective and inhibit both COX-1 and COX-2 enzymes **(G)** (Sjøgren et al., 2015) accounting for their analgesic role, as well at their associated side-effects.

- Charged particles (ions) inside and outside the unstimulated nociceptor (pain nerve) are controlled by sodium–potassium ion pumps that maintain a high concentration of potassium (K^+) ions within the nociceptor, and sodium (Na^+) ions concentrated outside the cell.
- This maintains a *resting potential* across the nociceptor membrane of −70 millivolts (mV) **(a)**. In response to a pain stimulus **(b)**, Na^+ moves into the cell, changing the membrane potential to +55 mV as the inside of the cell becomes less negative *(depolarisation)* **(c)**.
- The membrane potential begins to return to normal as K^+ ions leave the cell *(repolarisation)* **(d)**.
- For a brief period the membrane potential is more negative than at resting state *(hyperpolarisation)*, the nociceptor is less excitable, causing a refractory state where no new action potential can be triggered **(e)**, preventing the action potential from spreading backwards **(f)**. Finally the sodium–potassium ion pump restores a resting potential **(g)**.

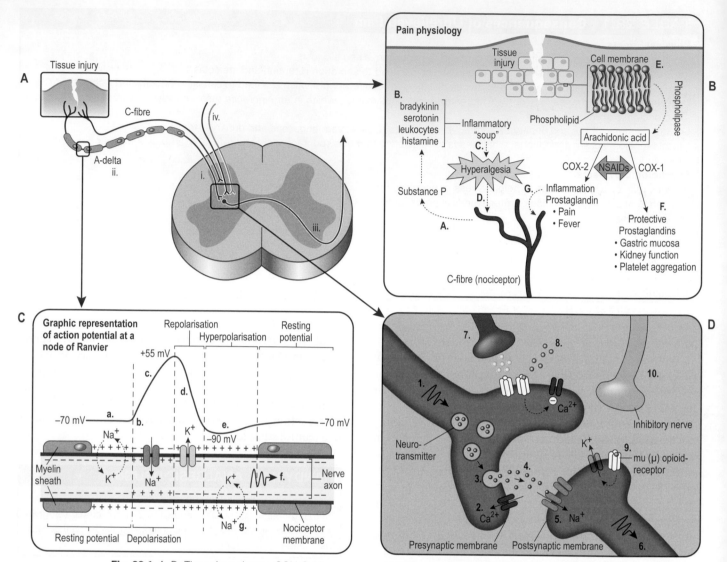

Fig. 28.1 A–D: The pain pathway. *COX*, Cyclooxygenase; *NSAID*, non-steroidal anti-inflammatory drugs.

• An action potential is completed within 1–3 ms and cycles of depolarisation and repolarisation at the axon membrane carry the nociceptive message in uninterrupted waves along C-fibres, or at unmyelinated sections of the axon (nodes of Ranvier) in A-delta fibres. (Brodal, 2016a).

HANDY HINT: ANALGESIC DRUGS

Local anaesthetics prevent the generation of action potentials by blocking Na^+ channels on the nerve cell membrane (Ramamurthi and Krane, 2007).

When an action potential arrives at the end of the primary nociceptor (**1**):

• Depolarisation of the presynaptic membrane opens calcium (Ca^{2+}) channels, (**2**) causing vesicles of neurotransmitter (e.g. glutamate) to fuse with the presynaptic membrane (**3**).

• Neurotransmitter is released into the space (synapse) between the primary and secondary nociceptor by exocytosis (**4**).

• Neurotransmitter attaches to receptors on the postsynaptic membrane opening sodium (Na^+) channels (**5**), causing depolarisation of the secondary pain neurone (Brodal, 2016b), allowing the nociceptive impulse to travel towards the brain (**6**).

• Pathways descending from the brain to the dorsal horn act as a control mechanism to amplify or reduce the pain signals. This process is called modulation (Briggs, 2010); for example, ß-endorphins act at endogenous opioid receptors, inhibiting pain neurotransmission (**7**).

HANDY HINT: ANALGESIC DRUGS

Exogenous opioids, such as morphine, tramadol fentanyl and oxycodone, mimic the effect of endorphins, attaching to mu (μ) opioid receptors on the presynaptic membrane to reduce Ca^{2+} influx (8) and on the postsynaptic membrane to enhance K^+ efflux (9); this combined effect decreases nociceptive transmission (Smith and Pappagallo, 2012).

- Descending modulation neurons from the brain release neurotransmitters serotonin and noradrenaline, which play a role in activating inhibitory neurons, reducing pain transmission (Steeds, 2013).

> **HANDY HINT: ANALGESIC DRUGS**
>
> Tramadol inhibits the reuptake of serotonin and noradrenaline enhancing this effect (10) (Smith and Pappagallo, 2012).

ASSESSING PAIN IN CHILDREN AND YOUNG PEOPLE

The stages of pain management are outlined in Fig. 28.2. Pain assessment is the crucial first step in ensuring children/young people's pain is managed effectively. If pain is not assessed, it is difficult to decide which interventions to implement or to evaluate the effectiveness of any pain-relieving strategies used and decide whether further action is needed. Current best practice guidelines indicate that we should do the following:

- Ask the child/young person about their pain using a developmentally appropriate self-report pain tool (if possible).
- Involve the parents/carers in decisions about their child/young person's pain management.
- Take the child/young person's behavioural cues into account.
- Note any physiological cues that may indicate the child/young person is in pain.
- Reassess pain following the implementation of pain-relieving interventions.
- Document pain assessments.

A systematic review of the evidence in relation to nurses' assessment of postoperative pain found that children/young people's behavioural cues are often considered more important than their self-report of pain and that a significant proportion of children/young people did not have pain scores recorded in the first 24 hours postoperatively (Twycross et al., 2015a). A recent study found that pain assessment tools were only used in 19% of children/young people; this fell to 9% for children/young people under the age of five years (Smeland et al., 2018). Further, simply recording a pain assessment does not necessarily impact on decision-making about which pain-relieving interventions are used (Twycross et al., 2013).

Self-Report of Pain

A child/young person's pain can be assessed using a self-report tool, behavioural indicators of pain and/or physiological cues. Self-report tools should normally be used with children/young people who are:

- old enough to understand and use a self-report scale
- not overtly distressed
- not cognitively impaired
  (Stinson et al., 2006)

Behavioural pain assessment tools should be used for older children/young people if they are overtly distressed.

Behavioural Indicators of Pain

Children/young people often exhibit behavioural cues indicating they are in pain (Table 28.2). These differ from child to child. Given this, a child/young person's normal behaviour needs to be ascertained – if possible, this is best done during the admission process as part of undertaking a nursing assessment. This is particularly important for children/young people with cognitive impairment; parents describe having an *embodied knowledge* of how their child expresses pain (Carter et al., 2017). It is important to remember for all children, that there is

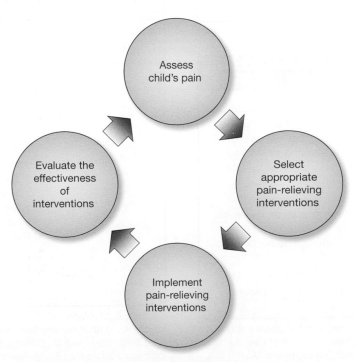

Fig. 28.2 The stages of pain management (Twycross and Williams, 2014).

evidence children/young people's self-reports of pain do not always correlate with their behaviour (Nilsson et al., 2008; Willis et al., 2003). So, behavioural cues only provide an *estimate* of how much pain a child/young person is experiencing.

Physiological Indicators of Pain

Physiological indicators can also be used to assess whether a child/young person is in pain. The evidence about how a child's physiological cues alter when they are in pain is summarised by Sweet and McGrath (1998) (Table 28.3). However, when used alone, physiological cues are not a valid clinical measure of pain as they can be affected by other factors. Given this, a pain assessment strategy that incorporates physiological and behavioural indicators as well as self-report is preferred (Arif-Rahu et al., 2012; von Baeyer and Spagrud, 2007).

Using Validated Pain Assessment Tools With Children/Young People of All Ages

It will often be necessary to have more than one pain assessment tool on a unit to cater for all patient groups. Whenever possible, pain assessment tools should use a *common metric* – e.g. all rate pain from 0 to 10. This means that a pain score of 5 will mean the same whichever pain assessment tool is

used. In this section the tools used most frequently in clinical practice are discussed.

WWW

Information about pain assessment tools that have been developed and validated for use with children of different ages and cognitive abilities are available (Australian and New Zealand College of Anaesthetists and Faculty of Pain Medicine, 2015; Royal College of Nursing, 2009).

The neonatal pain assessment tool that has been tested most often is the Premature Infant Pain Profile (PIPP) (Stevens et al., 1996) (Table 28.4) which has evidence of reliability, validity and ability to detect change (Stevens et al., 2010). The behavioural tools used most frequently for preverbal children are the FLACC (Face, Legs, Activity, Cry and Consolability) scale and the Children's Hospital of Eastern Ontario Pain Scale (CHEOPS). Commonly used pain assessment tools for cognitively impaired children/young people include the revised FLACC and the paediatric pain profile. For verbal children/ young people the use of a faces pain scale, a numerical rating scale or a visual analogue scale is recommended depending on their age and developmental level. Additional information about these pain scales can be found in Table 28.5.

TABLE 28.2	Behavioural Indicators of Pain	
Changed behaviour	Increased clinging
Irritability	Unusual quietness
Flat effect	Loss of appetite
Unusual posture	Restlessness
Screaming	Whimpering
Reluctance to move	Sobbing
Aggressiveness	Lying 'scared stiff'
Disturbed sleep pattern	Lethargic

TABLE 28.3	Physiological Indicators of Pain
Indicator	**Evidence**
Heart rate	Increases immediately following a pain stimulus and declines as pain diminishes, whereas in infants, an initial decrease is followed by a rise in heart rate.
Respiratory rate and pattern	There is conflicting evidence about whether this increases or decreases, but there is a significant shift from baseline. Breathing may become rapid and/or shallow.
Blood pressure	Increases when a child is in acute pain.
Oxygen saturation	Decreases when a child is in acute pain.

Sweet, S.D., McGrath, P.J., 1998. Physiological measures of pain. In: Finley, G.A., McGrath, P.J. (eds.), Measurement of Pain in Infants and Children, Progress in Pain Research Management. IASP Press, Seattle, vol. 10, pp. 59–81.

TABLE 28.4	The Premature Infant Pain Profile (PIPP)	
Indicators Used	**Considerations**
Postmenstrual age	• Preterm and term infants (e.g. 28–40 weeks gestation)
Behavioural state	
Heart rate	• Initially developed for procedural pain, requires further evaluation with very low birth weight neonates and with non-acute and postsurgical pain populations
Oxygen saturation	
Brow bulge	
Eye squeeze	
Nasolabial furrow	
	• Includes contextual indicators (e.g. postmenstrual age and behavioural state)
	• Indicators are scored on a four-point scale (0, 1, 2, 3) for a total score of 0–21 based on the gestational age of the infant
	• A score of 6 or less generally indicates minimal or no pain, while scores greater than 12 indicate moderate to severe pain
	• Pain assessments take 1 min
	• In the revised version (PIPP-R) postmenstrual age and behavioural state indicators are only applied if other variables indicate pain

Stevens, B., Johnston, C., Petryshen, P., et al., 1996. Premature Infant Pain Profile: development and initial validation. Clin. J. Pain 12, 13–22; Stevens, B.J., Gibbins, S., Yamada, J., et al., 2014. The Premature Infant Pain Profile-Revised (PIPP-R): initial validation and feasibility. Clin. J. Pain 30, 238–243.

TABLE 28.5 Pain Assessment Tools for Use With Preverbal Children, Children With Cognitive Impairment and Verbal Children

Tool	Description and Additional Information
Tools for Preverbal Children	
Children's Hospital of Eastern Ontario Pain Scale (CHEOPS) (McGrath et al., 1985) Available at: http://bit.ly/1SoSOZS	• Indicators: crying, facial expression, verbalisations, torso activity, whether and how child touches wound, leg position. • Intended for use in children aged 1–7 years but has been used in children 4 months to 17 years. • Validated for use with procedural and postoperative pain. • Indicators are scored on a four-point scale (0, 1, 2, 3) with a total score from 4 to 13. • Well-established evidence of reliability, validity and ability to detect change (von Baeyer and Spagrud, 2007). • Length of tool and confusing scoring system makes it complicated to use in clinical practice. • Cannot be used in intubated or paralysed patients.
FLACC (Merkel et al., 1997) See: http://prc.coh.org/PainNOA/ Flacc_Tool.pdf	• Indicators: facial expression, leg movement, activity, cry, consolability • Intended for use in children aged 2 months to 8 years but has been used in children aged 0–18 years. • Indicators are scored on a 0–2 scale, with a total score from 0 to 10 making it simple to use, score and interpret with high clinical utility (von Baeyer and Spagrud, 2007). • Validated for procedural pain in children aged 5–16 years (Nilsson et al., 2008). • Found to have clinical validity for postoperative, trauma related and cancer pain for children 0–2 years (Manworren and Hynan, 2003). • Validated for postoperative pain in children aged 1–5 years in one study (Hartrick and Kovan, 2002) and in children aged 4–18 years in another (von Baeyer and Spagrud, 2007). • Important to note that consolability requires (1) an attempt to console, and (2) a subjective rating of response to that intervention, which complicates the scoring. • Cannot be used in paralysed patients. Some preliminary data suggests it may be useful with ventilated patient (Voepel-Lewis et al., 2010), although one study found that the COMFORT-B scale was more reliable than the modified FLACC in paediatric intensive care (Johansson and Kokinsky, 2009). • Some evidence of reliability in the emergency department with children aged 6 months to 5 years (Kochman et al., 2017).
Tools for Children With Cognitive Impairment	
Revised FLACC (rFLACC) (Malviya et al., 2006) (Fig. 28.3)	• An amended version of the FLACC that allows an individual's pain behaviours to be incorporated within the tool. • Used in cognitively impaired children aged 4–19 years postoperatively (Malviya et al., 2006). • Also validated for procedural pain. • Indicators are scored on a 0–2 scale, with a total score from 0 to 10. • Simple to use, score and interpret (Voepel-Lewis et al., 2008; von Baeyer and Spagrud, 2007). • Nurses and parents considered the rFLACC a better tool for use in clinical practice compared to the (Chen-Lim et al., 2012). • Consider feasible for use in the acute care setting as relatively easy to use (Crosta et al., 2014). • Clinical utility has been rated higher than other tools for neurologically impaired children (Voepel-Lewis et al., 2008).
Paediatric Pain Profile (PPP) (Hunt et al., 2004, 2007) http://www.ppprofile.org.uk/	• Used to assess persistent daily pain in this group of children. • Includes the child's pain history, baseline and ongoing pain assessments as well as providing details about interventions and their effectiveness. • 20 items are rated on four-point Likert scale giving total scores of 0–60. (Scores greater than 14 usually indicate moderate to severe pain.) • Child is observed for 5 min before completing the pain assessment. • Use in the acute clinical setting limited by the length of time taken to complete the assessment and the teaching required prior to using it (Chen-Lim et al., 2012; Hunt and Franck, 2011). • Parents perceived the PPP as more accurate even though difficult to use in the clinical setting (Chen-Lim et al., 2012).

Continued

TABLE 28.5 **Pain Assessment Tools for Use With Preverbal Children, Children with Cognitive Impairment and Verbal Children—cont'd**

Tool	Description and Additional Information
Tools for Use With Verbal Children	
Faces Pain Scale-Revised (FPS-R) (Hicks et al., 2001) http://www.iasp-pain.org/Education/Content.aspx?ItemNumber=1519	• The Faces Pain Scale (FPS) (Bieri et al., 1990) was amended to ensure it was compatible in scoring with other self-rating and behavioural scales. • Six graphically depicted faces with neutral anchors. • Children told that the faces range from *no pain* to *as much pain as is possible*. • Scored 0–10. Intended for use in children 5–12 years old but has been used in children aged 4–18 years. • Demonstrates strong psychometric properties in children aged 4–17 years in with acute pain. Convergent validity may be questionable in children aged 4–7 years (Tsze et al., 2013). • Strongly recommended for use in acute pain. Limited evidence for postoperative and chronic pain (Birnie et al., 2019). • Quick and easy to use. • Translated into ≥35 languages. • Disadvantages: limited evidence regarding interpretability of scores and mixed evidence about the acceptability of the scale with children.
Wong-Baker FACES Pain Scale http://wongbakerfaces.org	• Six cartoon faces ranging from smiling to crying – faces graduate from smiling to tears. • Scored 0–5 or 0–10 (*but see note above about a common metric if using more than one pain assessment tool*). • Intended for use in children aged 3–18 years. • Quick and simple to use, requires minimal instruction. • Well-liked by children and health care professionals • Translated into more than 10 languages. • Readily available (free of charge) and easily reproduced by photocopying. • Wearable badges are available for purchase. • Disadvantages include: smiling *no pain* face results in higher reported pain scores compared to neutral face (Chambers et al., 2005), worst pain face has tears and not all children cry when in pain.
Numerical pain rating (NRS) scale	• Consists of a range of numbers (e.g. 0–10 or 0–00) that can be represented in verbal or graphical format. • Children told that the lowest number represents *no pain* and the highest number represents *the most pain possible*. • The child is instructed to circle, record or state the number that best represents their level of pain intensity. • Evidence that NRS is reliable and valid in children aged over 8 years and adolescents for acute pain (Bailey et al., 2010; Page et al., 2012; von Baeyer et al., 2009). • A verbal numerical rating scale was found to have strong convergent validity and reliability for children aged 6–17 years. Convergent validity was not as strong for children aged 4–5 years (Tsze et al., 2018). • NRS-11 (0–10 scale) strongly recommended for use in acute pain. Limited evidence for postoperative and chronic pain (Birnie et al., 2019).
Visual analogue scale (VAS)	• Requires the child to select a point on a vertical or horizontal 100 mm line where the ends of the line are defined as the extreme limits of pain intensity (no pain and the worst pain possible). • The child is asked to make a mark along the line to indicate the intensity of their pain. Recommended for children aged 8 years and older (Stinson et al., 2006). • Strongly recommended for use in acute pain. Limited evidence for postoperative and chronic pain (Birnie et al., 2019).

Adapted from Stinson, J., Reid, K., 2014. Chronic pain in children. In: Twycross, A., Dowden, S., Stinson, J. (eds.) Managing Pain in Children: A Clinical Guide, second ed. Oxford, Wiley Blackwell, p 179–211.

Name:	Hosp No:
DOB:	NHS no:

Revised FLACC scale

Great Ormond Street **NHS**
Hospital for Children
NHS Trust

	Scoring		
Categories	**0**	**1**	**2**
Face	No particular expression or smile	Occasional grimace or frown, withdrawn, disinterested; *appears sad or worried*	Frequent to constant frown, clenched jaw, quivering chin; *distressed looking face; expression of fright or panic*
Individual behaviours			
Legs	Normal position or relaxed; *usual tone and motion to limbs*	Uneasy, restless, tense; *occasional tremors*	Kicking, or legs drawn up; *marked increase in spasticity, constant tremors or jerking*
Individual behaviours			
Activity	Lying quietly, normal position, moves easily; *regular, rhythmic respirations*	Squirming, shifting back and forth, *tense or guarded movements; mildly agitated (e.g. head back and forth, aggression); shallow, splinting respirations, intermittent sighs*	Arched, rigid, or jerking; *severe agitation, head banging, shivering (not rigors); breath-holding, gasping or sharp intake of breaths; severe splinting*
Individual behaviours			
Cry	No cry/verbalisation (awake or asleep)	Moans or whimpers, occasional complaint; *occasional verbal outburst or grunt*	Crying steadily, screams or sobs, frequent complaints; *repeated outbursts, constant grunting*
Individual behaviours			
Consolability	Content, relaxed	Reassured by occasional touching, hugging, or being talked to, distractable	Difficult to console or comfort; *pushing away caregiver, resisting care or comfort measures*
Individual behaviours			

(Adapted from Malviya et al., 2006)

Revised FLACC – instructions for use
- **Individualise the tool:** The nurse should review the descriptors within each category with the child's parents or carers. Ask them if there are additional behaviours that are better indicators of pain in their child. Add these behaviors to the tool in the appropriate category.
- Each of the five categories: (F) Face; (L) Legs; (A) Activity; (C) Cry; (C) Consolability is scored from 0 to 2, which results in a total score between 0 and 10.
- **Patients who are awake:** Observe for at least 1–3 minutes. observe legs and body uncovered. Reposition patient or observe activity, assess body for tenseness and tone. Initiate consoling interventions if needed.
- **Patients who are asleep:** Observe for at least 5 minutes. Observe body and legs uncovered. If possible reposition the patient. Touch the body and assess for tenseness and tone.

Version no: 1.0	Version date: 15/04/2010	Document development lead: Jude Middleton	I:\Pain Control Service\Assessment\Revised FLACC\Revised FLACC Paperwork.doc

Fig. 28.3 Revised FLACC (Face, Legs, Activity, Cry and Consolability) scale.

⊚ EVIDENCE-BASED PRACTICE

A recent systematic review focusing on self-report tools for children/young people found that many studies were too poorly designed to be used to inform practice (Birnie et al., 2019). The key findings of this review are summarised below:
- Only eight pain assessment tools met the review's 'well-established assessment' criteria; the NRS-11, CAS, FPS-R/FPS, Pieces of Hurt (Poker Chip Tool), Oucher photographic and numerical scales, VAS and the faces scale.
- Based on available evidence, the NRS-11, FPS-R and CAS were strongly recommended for self-report of acute pain.
- Only weak recommendations could be made for self-report measures for postoperative and chronic pain.
- No measures were recommended for children less than 6 years old.

These results **do not mean** we should stop using pain assessment tools in practice. The results do indicate a need for further research and provides some guidance about the most effective tools to use.

When using a faces pain scale it is important to explain carefully how it is used to the child/young person. One way of doing this is to explain to the child/young person that each face is for someone who feels happy because there is no pain (hurt) or sad because there is some or a lot of pain:
- Face 0 is very happy because there is no hurt at all
- Face 1 hurts just a little bit
- Face 2 hurts a little more
- Face 3 hurts even more
- Face 4 hurts a whole lot more
- Face 5 hurts as much as you can imagine, although you do not have to be crying to feel this bad

Once you have explained this you can ask the child/young person to choose the face that best describes how they are feeling (Hockenberry et al., 2005).

Evidence indicates that children aged 3–4 years may not always be able to use the standard faces pain scales (von Baeyer et al., 2013). Unfortunately, there is no single test that can be used to screen children for their ability to use self-report pain scales (Besenki et al., 2007; von Baeyer et al., 2011). More recently it has been suggested that the validity and reliability of self-report tools with 3- to 4-year-old can be increased by having fewer response options or just asking about the presence of pain (Emmott et al., 2018; von Baeyer et al., 2017). This needs considering when deciding on the best strategy for assessing pain in children of this age.

The Importance of Documenting Pain Assessment Scores

Regular assessment and documentation of pain allows effective treatment and communication among members of the health care team as well as with the child/young person and their family. Despite this, it has been noted that some health care professionals do not always record pain assessments (Twycross et al., 2013; Smeland et al., 2018). Standardised forms and tools (e.g. admission assessment forms, observation charts) for the documentation of pain encourages initial assessment and ongoing reassessments.

MANAGING PROCEDURAL PAIN IN CHILDREN AND YOUNG PEOPLE

Painful procedures, such as venepuncture, cannulation and immunisations are routine parts of health care (APAGBI, 2012). However, whether planned or unscheduled, these procedures are associated with high pain intensity and are distressing to children and young people (Cohen et al., 2014). Examples of these procedures are given in Table 28.6.

Children/young people have reported that the pain from procedures is the worst thing that happens to them during a hospital stay (Friedrichsdorf et al., 2015). This is particularly the case for children/young people with cancer who often report experiencing more pain from procedures and cancer treatment than the disease itself (Twycross et al., 2015b). There is an increasing body of evidence suggesting children/young people's memories (past experiences) of pain affect how they react to future painful interventions (Noel et al., 2018). This means that children/young people's first experience with needle pain or other painful procedures sets the stage for future procedures. An evidence-based approach needs adopting right from the start to prevent unnecessary pain and suffering during future procedures. Two examples of campaigns that are helping to change practice in this area are highlighted later.

🌐 **WWW**
It doesn't have to hurt is a social media campaign working with parents to improve pain management for children: • http://itdoesnthavetohurt.ca/ (#itdoesn'thavetohurt).   The Children's Hospitals of Minnesota has adopted the *Comfort Promise* which is about *doing everything possible to prevent and treat pain*: • https://www.childrensmn.org/services/care-specialties-departments/pain-program/childrens-comfort-promise/.

TABLE 28.6 **Common Paediatric Painful Procedures**	
Immunisations	Dressing changes or wound care
Venepuncture	Insertion or removal of tubes (e.g.
Capillary sampling	urinary catheters, nasogastric
IV cannulation	tubes, drains)
Laceration repair	Subcutaneous reservoir access (e.g.
Fracture reduction	port-a-cath)
Diagnostic tests	Lumbar puncture (LP)
	Bone marrow aspiration (BMA)

Managing Procedural Pain in Children: Key Components

So how should we manage procedural pain in children/young people? Drawing on *#itdoesn'thavetohurt* and the *Comfort Promise* (Postier et al., 2018) alongside current research, six essential components to managing procedural pain in children emerge:

1. Preparing the child/young person.
2. Preparing and involving their parents.
3. Positioning the child/young person.
4. Using distraction or other psychological pain-relieving strategies.
5. Using topical anaesthesia.
6. Using sucrose or breastmilk for children aged 0–12 months.

Preparing the Child

Preparing the child/young person is an important part of undertaking a painful procedure. Procedural preparation has been identified as best practice in paediatric oncology (Flowers and Birnie, 2015) and shown to reduce children/young people's pain and anxiety during IV cannulation (Tunç-Tuna and Açikgoz, 2015). The preparation needs of children of different ages are described in Table 28.7. Table 28.8 provides some useful hints for health care professionals when communicating with children/young people. Play therapists can help prepare children/young people for procedures and support the health care team in setting the stage for a successful intervention (APAGBI, 2012).

Preparing and Involving Parents

A recent systematic review explored parents' experiences and information needs in relation to managing their child/young person's procedure related pain (Gates et al., 2018). Generally, parents want to be present during procedures and to be stoic for their child, but health care professionals do not always prepare them for their role in supporting their child/young person. Key to this preparation is explaining the language to use and not to use (Table 28.9).

Positioning the Child

In the past children/young people were often restrained so health care professionals could carry out painful procedures. It is now recognised that restraining a child for a painful procedure should be a last resort and only used in emergency

TABLE 28.7 Information Needs of Children

Age/Developmental Stage	Type of Information
Pre-schoolers and young children	• Include information about what they will see, hear, smell and feel during procedure, e.g. let them know it will feel cold when their skin is cleaned, that when the needle is inserted it 'will pinch for a little while, but this will go away'.
School-aged children	• Provide clear concrete explanations, e.g. 'It may tingle.' 'You might notice a cold feeling when the medicine goes in.' • Discuss why the procedure is necessary and how long it will take • Use analogies to explain things – e.g. describing a cannula as being 'like a plastic straw that is in your hand' • Explain function and operation of medical equipment in concrete terms • Allow medical play with equipment beforehand • Allow time before and after the procedure for questions and discussion
Adolescents	• Discuss why the procedure is necessary and how the results will be used • Explain long-term consequences of procedures including information about body systems working together • Discuss how the procedure may affect appearance (e.g. scar) and what can be done to minimise this • Emphasise any physical benefits of the procedure • Use models or computer images to aid understanding

Jaaniste, T., Hayes, B., von Baeyer, C.L., 2007. Providing children with information about forthcoming medical procedures: a review and synthesis. Clin. Psychol. Sci. Pract. 14, 124–143; Cohen, L., 2008. Behavioural approaches to anxiety and pain management for pediatric venous access. Pediatrics 122 (S3), S134–S139; Hockenberry, M.J., McCarthy, K., Taylor, O., et al., 2011. Managing painful procedures in children with cancer. J. Pediatr. Hematol. Oncol. 33 (2), 119–127.

TABLE 28.8 Helping Children Cope With Pain: What Health Professionals Can Do

• Give step-by-step information about what will happen during the procedure, including what the child will see, hear and feel, and why the procedure is necessary
• Children need truthful information to build trust in the health care professionals working with them
• Use age/developmentally appropriate language and avoid medical jargon
• Use medical play with young children – this allows them to use the equipment and adopt different roles, such as the nurse or doctor
• Avoid making promises that you cannot keep, e.g. 'It won't hurt' or 'It feels like a mosquito bite'
• Avoid high anxiety words such as *pain, hurt, cut* and *needle* or *shot*
• Use words such as *poking, freezing* and *squeezing* instead
• Do not suggest that the procedure will definitely hurt
• Be aware of possible misinterpretations of words and phrases such as *dye* or *put to sleep*
• Address children's concerns (e.g. *taking all my blood*)
• Consider using books or web-based resources describing the procedure for the child and/or parent
• Provide children with coping strategies they can use during the procedure such as distraction (Table 28.10)

Adapted from Young, K.D., 2005. Pediatric procedural pain. Ann. Emerg. Med. 45, 160–171; Jaaniste, T., Hayes, B., von Baeyer, C.L., 2007. Providing children with information about forthcoming medical procedures: a review and synthesis. Clin. Psychol. Sci. Pract. 14, 124–143; Kuttner, L., 2010. A Child in Pain: Health Professionalals Can Do to Help. Crown House Publishing, Bethel, United States.

situations. A decision to restrain a child/young person should be based on their best interests (Department of Health & Department for Education, 2017). A recent international study found that professional practices relating to holding vary considerably (Bray et al., 2018). This is clearly an area where there is a need to evaluate current practices and work with the child and parent to plan what strategies are going to be used. Often, having a younger child sitting on their parent's lap is effective while taking into account the impact of doing so on the parent.

Using Distraction and Other Psychological Pain-Relieving Interventions

Despite the evidence of its effectiveness, distraction is not used consistently by health care professionals (Cummings, 2015; Twycross et al., 2013). The evidence for the use of distraction and other psychological pain-relieving strategies can be seen in Table 28.10. There is increasing evidence that active methods of distraction appear to be more helpful than passive methods (Twycross and Stinson, 2014).

TABLE 28.9   Suggested Language to Use During Painful Procedures

Cohen (2008) suggests that the following language should be avoided during a panful procedure:	Instead he recommends using language such as:
• You will be OK; there is nothing to worry about (reassurance) • This is going to hurt/this won't hurt (vague, negative focus) • The nurse is going to take your blood (vague information) • You are acting like a baby (criticism) • It will feel like a bee sting (negative focus) • The procedure will last as long as …. (negative focus) • The medicine will burn (negative focus) • Tell me when you are ready (too much control) • I'm sorry (apologising) • Don't cry (negative focus) • It is over (negative focus)	• Tell me what you did in school today? (distraction) • It might feel like a pinch (sensory information) • First the nurse will clean your arm, you will feel the cold wipe, and next …. (sensory and procedural information) • Let's get your mind off it; tell me about the movie … (distraction) • Tell me how it feels (information) • The procedure will be shorter than [television programme or other familiar time for child] (procedural information, positive focus) • Some children say they feel a warm feeling (sensory information, positive focus) • When I count to three, blow the feeling away from your body (coaching to cope, distraction, limited control) • You are being very brave (praise, encouragement) • That was hard, I am proud of you (praise) • You did a great job doing the deep breathing, holding still …. (labelled praise)

Cohen, L., 2008. Behavioural approaches to anxiety and pain management for pediatric venous access. Pediatrics 122 (S3), S134–S139.

TABLE 28.10   Evidence to Support the Use of Distraction and Other Psychological Pain-Relieving Strategies

PSYCHOLOGICAL STRATEGIES		
Non-Pharmacological Strategy	**Physiology**	**Efficacy**
Distraction	Attention drawn towards an engaging task may disrupt neurocognitive pathways involved in pain perception (Sil et al., 2017).	Reduced pain and distress during immunisations (Chambers et al., 2009) and needle-related procedures (Birnie et al., 2014). Some evidence that verbal distraction, video distraction and music distraction along with breathing with a toy are useful strategies for managing the pain associated with immunisations in children and young people (Birnie et al., 2015). Promising evidence for the use of distraction for procedural pain in children with cancer (Bukola and Paula, 2017).
Hypnosis	Modulation of nociceptive input through downregulation of C and A-delta fibres and changes in pain-related activity in areas of the brain associated with pain activation (e.g. cortical pain matrix) (Liossi et al., 2014).	Pain and distress during needle-related procedures is reduced (Birnie et al., 2014; Birnie et al., 2018).
Interactive computer programs	Computer-generated distraction commands large parts of the conscious attention with fewer cognitive resources available to process nociceptive stimuli (Schmitt et al., 2011).	Immersive strategies (virtual reality) reduce pain during burns patients undergoing physiotherapy (Schmitt et al., 2011) and wound debridement (Hoffman et al., 2008).

Using Topical Anaesthesia

Topical anaesthetics are the mainstay of pharmacological interventions for managing needle-related pain in children/young people (Association of Paediatric Anaesthetists, 2012; Curtis et al., 2012). In addition to providing pain relief, the use of topical anaesthetics improves procedure success, decreases movement and increases accuracy. Health care professionals often debate which type of topical anaesthetic cream is best. However, *all* transdermal forms of topical local anaesthetic creams and patches (e.g. EMLA, amethocaine [tetracaine], liposomal lignocaine [lidocaine] 4% or 5%) are effective in reducing needle pain (2010 ENA Emergency Nurses Resources Development Committee, 2011). The important thing

TABLE 28.11	Evidence for the Use of Vapocoolant Spray and Cooling Vibration	
PHYSICAL STRATEGIES		
Non-Pharmacological Strategy	**Physiology**	**Efficacy**
Vapocoolant spray (ethyl chloride spray)	Biological and chemical processes imitated by tissue damage are slowed when skin temperature is reduced to 10°C. A-delta fibres (transmitting sharp pain) are more responsive to cooling than C-fibre nociceptors (Lane and Latman, 2009).	Limited evidence of efficacy (Schug et al., 2015).
Cooling vibration analgesia (e.g. Buzzy)	High frequency vibration stimulates Aβ mechanoreceptors and application of cold stimulates temperature receptors. Both share similar pathways with nociceptors at the dorsal horn. Stimulus of such pathways can compete with pain transmission (Moadad et al., 2016).	Lower levels of pain during cannulation (Moadad et al., 2016) and phlebotomy (Inal and Kelleci, 2012) in children over 4 years.

here is to be proactive and use whichever topical anaesthetic is available in your area of practice. More recently there has been discussion about the use of vapocoolant spray and Cooling Vibration Analgesia devices, such as Buzzy. The evidence for the use of these devices is summarised in Table 28.11.

Sucrose and Breastmilk for Children Aged 0–12 Months

Sucrose is a safe and effective method of reducing procedural pain from one-off events, such as heel lance, venepuncture and IM injection in pre-term and term infants (Stevens et al., 2016). The systematic review by Stevens et al. (2016) concluded that:
- Information about the optimum dose of sucrose remains inconclusive.
- Using sucrose in combination with other interventions, such as non-nutritive sucking, appears to be more effective than sucrose alone.

 WWW

The WHO Reproductive Health Library has published a review on sucrose for analgesia in newborn infants undergoing painful procedures:
- https://extranet.who.int/rhl/topics/newborn-health/care-newborn-infant/sucrose-analgesia-newborn-infants-undergoing-painful-procedures.

It is also worth noting that the results of another systematic review concluded that, if available, breastfeeding or breast milk should be used to relieve procedural pain in neonates undergoing a single procedure and that it was as effective as the administration of sucrose (Shah et al., 2012).

⊕ **WWW**

The WHO Reproductive Health Library has published a review on breastfeeding or breast milk for procedural pain in neonates:
- https://extranet.who.int/rhl/topics/newborn-health/care-newborn-infant/breastfeeding-or-breast-milk-procedural-pain-neonates.

Summary: Managing Procedural Pain in Children and Young People

Fig. 28.4 summarises which strategies should be used when preparing a child/young person for a needle procedure. While this figure relates to needle-related pain, the principles can also be applied to other types of procedural pain. The figure provides a useful summary of the steps we need to take when managing any type of procedural pain in children/young people and draws on current evidence in this area.

MANAGING ACUTE PAIN IN CHILDREN AND YOUNG PEOPLE

Within this section the pharmacological management of acute pain in children/young people is discussed. The physical and psychological strategies used to manage procedural pain can also be used to support children/young people in acute pain, although the evidence to support this remains limited.

Non-Steroidal Anti-Inflammatory Drugs

Non-steroidal anti-inflammatory drugs (NSAIDs) inhibit the cyclooxygenase (COX) enzyme non-selectively (both COX-1 and COX-2), thus blocking the synthesis of prostaglandins (Chan and Haroon, 2016), a key component of the 'inflammatory soup' involved in the sensitisation of peripheral nociceptors (see Fig. 28.1B). Many of the more common side-effects of NSAIDs are related to the regulatory role played by COX-1 (Dickman and Knaggs, 2008). However, when used in children/young people over 6 months of age, serious adverse events are rare (Schug et al., 2015):
- COX-1 is involved in the production of prostaglandins, which protect gastric mucosa, and their reduction can potentially lead to gastric or duodenal ulcers with symptoms including nausea, epigastric pain, diarrhoea or bleeding (Chan and Haroon, 2016).

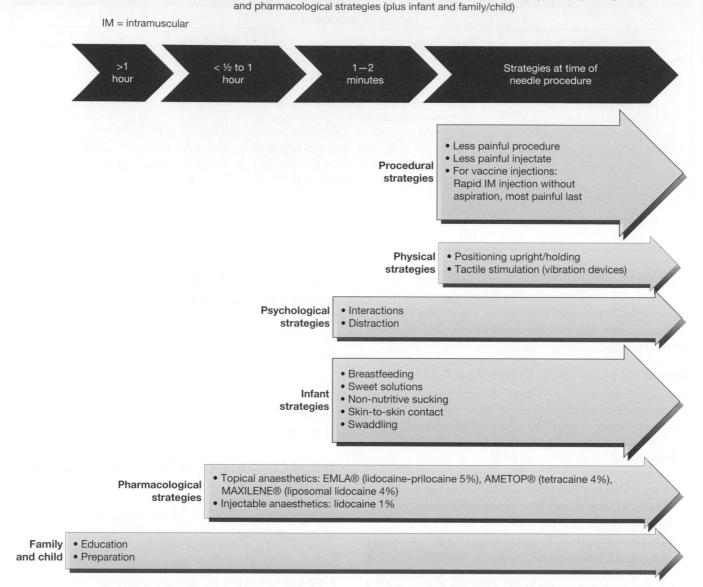

Fig. 28.4 Timeline for pain-relieving strategies prior to and during needle procedures: procedural, physical, psychological and pharmacological strategies (plus infant and family/child). [used with permission of Anna Taddio – citation awaited].

- Gastro-protective drugs are often co-prescribed with NSAIDs to reduce this risk (Smith et al., 2013); for example proton pump inhibitors, such as omeprazole or lansoprazole.
- COX-1 is involved in the synthesis of thromboxane in platelets and is required for platelet aggregation during coagulation.
- While NSAIDs do not appear to increase the risk of bleeding following tonsillectomy (Schug et al., 2015), they should be used cautiously in those at risk of platelet dysfunction; for example children/young people with cancer, because of the potential risk of bleeding (McCulloch and Collins, 2015).

- Prostaglandins play a role in renal vasodilation and glomerular filtration rate (GFR). In patients with decreased renal perfusion (renal disease, dehydration, etc.), inhibition of prostaglandin synthesis may cause acute renal failure by affecting this vasodilatory role of endogenous prostaglandins (Sjøgren et al., 2015).
- In patients with poor renal function inhibition of prostaglandins may also affect the nephrons regulation sodium and water balance, resulting in raised blood pressure or exacerbation of pre-existing hypertension (Sjøgren et al., 2015).
- NSAIDs appear to have an effect on osteoblasts involved in bone tissue healing (García-Martínez et al., 2015);

although, paediatric studies suggest that short-term use of NSAIDs following fractures or orthopaedic surgery does not clinically significantly affect bone growth or healing (Schug et al., 2015), with ibuprofen having the least adverse effect (García-Martínez et al., 2015).

- Although NSAIDs are used in neonates for closure of ductus arteriosus (Paediatric Formulary Committee [PFC], 2018), they are not prescribed for analgesia before 3 months of age, due to the risk of pulmonary hypertension or changes to cerebral or renal blood flow (Howard, 2013). Beyond this age, NSAIDs are effective in treating moderately severe pain and reduce opioid requirements following major surgical procedures (Schug et al., 2015).

Ibuprofen

Ibuprofen is the most commonly used NSAID (Smith et al., 2013). It is associated with fewest side-effects and has most supporting evidence for its safe use in children/young people (APAGBI, 2012). It is recommended as a take-home analgesic substitute for codeine (now contraindicated in children under 12 years), providing equal analgesic efficacy to oral morphine in the management of uncomplicated fractures (Poonai et al., 2014). Ibuprofen is available over the counter, although one in eight parents need help interpreting the dosing instructions regarding optimal therapy (Gill et al., 2013).

Diclofenac

Diclofenac differs from other NSAIDs in that, as well as inhibiting cyclooxygenase, it may also stimulate uptake and inhibit release of arachidonic acid (Smith et al., 2013). It provides effective perioperative analgesia, and the incidence of serious adverse events, such as gastric bleeding or allergic reactions, is rare (3 in 1000 children) (Standing et al., 2009) as is the incidence of bronchospasm (Short et al., 2000). High-dose diclofenac has been found to have similar cardiovascular risks to selective-COX-2 inhibitors, leading to its contraindication in large numbers of adult patients at risk of thrombotic cardiovascular events (Medicines and Healthcare products Regulatory Agency [MHRA] 2014). Consequently, some pharmaceutical preparations of diclofenac have become difficult to source (e.g. dispersible tablets), making accurate paediatric dosing challenging. The rectal bioavailability of diclofenac is high; thus suppositories can be a useful alternative (Schug et al., 2015) and diclofenac is also available in intravenous formats, where venous access is available.

Naproxen

Naproxen has commonly been used in the management of juvenile rheumatoid arthritis in children (Välitalo et al., 2012). It is associated with a smaller cardiovascular risk than other high-dose NSAIDs, which may explain its increased popularity. Naproxen has a longer elimination half-life than other NSAIDs (12–14 hours) making it useful following paediatric

day-case surgery (Korpela et al., 2007) although infants may have impaired clearance of naproxen (Välitalo et al., 2012).

Selective-COX-2 Inhibitors

Selective-COX-2 inhibitors 'coxibs' have been developed. However, they are associated with thrombotic cardiovascular events in adults (myocardial infarction, cerebrovascular accident) and evidence for use in the paediatric population is very limited (Schug et al., 2015).

Paracetamol

Paracetamol is one of the most frequently prescribed analgesic drugs for managing acute (McNicol et al., 2016) mild to moderate pain in children/young people (APAGBI, 2012). Like NSAIDs it has antipyretic and analgesic effects, but no anti-inflammatory properties and its mechanism of action is unclear (Anderson, 2014).

Paracetamol:

- Reduces pain scores following paediatric scoliosis and ophthalmic surgery (Schug et al., 2015); it has some efficacy in the management of short-term acute otitis media pain (Sjoukes et al., 2016).
- A single IV dose may provide effective analgesia for up to 4 hours in patients with acute postoperative pain (McNicol et al., 2016).
- Used in combination with ibuprofen may provide superior analgesia to either drug alone (Ong et al., 2010).
- Has a morphine-sparing effect perioperatively (Wong et al., 2013) and following major surgery in newborns (Ohlsson and Shah, 2015) and a fentanyl-sparing effect in young children postoperatively (Hong et al., 2010).

Although paracetamol affects prostaglandin production in a number of body organs, such as the brain, spleen, lung and kidney, it does not appear to affect platelets or the stomach mucosa (Botting, 2000) in the same way as do NSAIDs. A large-scale international retrospective study suggested that paracetamol administered during infancy and early childhood may be associated with an increased risk of asthma at 6–7 years of age (Beasley et al., 2008). However children/young people with mild asthma, using as-needed or short-term paracetamol, do not demonstrate increased incidence of asthma symptoms compared with children/young people taking as-needed ibuprofen (Lesko and Mitchell, 1999) and more research is required before changes to clinical practice are made (Lourido-Cebreiro et al., 2017).

It has also been suggested that paracetamol (or ibuprofen) administered prophylactically at the time of some infant vaccinations may interfere with the immune response (Prymula et al., 2009; Wysocki et al., 2016), although other studies challenge these findings (Sil et al., 2017). The advice to parents in the UK is to avoid prophylactic paracetamol, unless specifically advised to administer it (e.g. following MenB vaccine). However, paracetamol may be administered for post-vaccination pain, discomfort or fever (NHS Choices, 2009; NHS Scotland, 2018). Paracetamol should be avoided in neutropenic patients because of its potential to mask pyrexia (Bryant, 2003), a key indicator of potentially life-threatening infection (Barton et al., 2015), yet it may be used once broad-spectrum antibiotic therapy is initiated (Johnson, 2013).

Paracetamol has a long-standing safety record if used within recommended doses (Lavonas et al., 2010). However, up to 20% of general practitioners' oral paracetamol prescriptions included non-recommended dosages, such that younger children may have been at risk of over-dosage and older children under-dosing (Kazouini et al., 2011). *Weight-based guidelines* for the administration of oral paracetamol are, therefore, recommended for use by health care professionals, but are likely to be difficult for parents to interpret (Eyers et al., 2012b). *Age-related dose-banding* of liquid preparations of oral paracetamol in children aged 3 months to 12 years were introduced to increase administration safety and efficacy in the home (MHRA, 2011) but do not account for variation in body size within each age category (Eyers et al., 2012a) and clinical judgement should be used when administering paracetamol to children/young people who are overweight (Wiese et al., 2012). Because paracetamol clearance is lower and gastric absorption is delayed in premature neonates (Walker and Howard, 2002) specific dose regimes should be observed, based on the infant's gestational age (PFC, 2018). Intravenous (IV) paracetamol reaches therapeutic levels more quickly than oral or rectal administration (Uysal et al., 2011), although administration errors have been relatively common in children/young people, where incidents of 10 times the recommended dose have been reported (Beringer et al., 2011).

Opioids

Endogenous opioids (e.g. enkephalins, β-endorphins) are produced within the body and bind to opioid receptors causing an inhibitory effect (Steeds, 2013). Exogenous opioids are chemical compounds with similar structures to naturally occurring opioids (Spina, 2008). Most opioids have their analgesic effect through 'mu' (μ) opioid receptors, found on the terminals of peripheral primary afferent nociceptors: C and A-delta fibres, and on central secondary neurons. When opioid receptors are activated pre-synaptically, they decrease calcium influx, inhibiting neurotransmitter release. Post-synaptically opioid receptor activation increases potassium conductance, causing hyperpolarisation, which decreases the excitability of the neurone (Stannard et al., 2013) (see Fig. 28.1D).

Opioid medications have a number of side effects, therefore doses should be closely tailored to patients' individual needs in order to minimise their risk of occurring.

- Respiratory centres in the central nervous system (CNS) influence respiratory rate, tidal volume and respiratory responses to changes in arterial pCO_2 levels.
- Opioid action on these centres may cause sedation initially and can result in respiratory depression (Stannard et al., 2016); making sedation monitoring a useful early indicator (Strassels, 2014).
- Opioid action on peripheral opioid receptors on nerves supplying the gut may cause a reduction in gut motility,

resulting in constipation; they may also cause gastric-stasis which plays a role in opioid-related nausea and vomiting.
- Opioid-induced nausea and vomiting may also be caused by a central effect on the vomiting centre and chemoreceptor trigger zone in the CNS, and anti-emetics may be required.
- Multiple mechanisms may be involved in opioid-related pruritus (itching), including peripheral histamine release (Stannard et al., 2016) and central serotonin receptor (5-HT$_3$) involvement (Strassels, 2014). Treatment involves the cautious use of antihistamines, which can add to opioid-induced sedation, and 5-HT$_3$-receptor agonists, such as ondansetron (Stannard et al., 2016).

Codeine

Codeine analgesia is achieved through its metabolism in the liver by the cytochrome P450 enzyme, CYP2D6, to form morphine (see Fig. 28.5). Following a series of fatalities involving the ultra-rapid metabolism of codeine in children with obstructive sleep apnoea following adenotonsillectomy (Kelly et al., 2012) the MHRA (2013) recommended that it no longer be used for pain relief in children younger than 12 years and it should be avoided in all patients under 18 years old with sleep apnoea undergoing tonsillectomy or adenoidectomy.

Tramadol

Tramadol is a mixture of mirror-image molecules '(+) and (−) enantiomers', a so-called racemic mixture, both of which are involved in neurotransmission. The (+) enantiomer binds to mu (μ)-opioid receptors, but also inhibit serotonin (5-HT3)-reuptake and have a serotonin-releasing action. The (−) enantiomer inhibits the reuptake of noradrenaline (Bozkurt, 2005), enhancing descending inhibitory pain pathways modulated by the neurotransmitters serotonin and noradrenaline (Holdcroft and Jaggar, 2005) (see Fig. 28.1D). Tramadol is metabolised in the liver by the cytochrome P450 enzyme, CYP2D6, to form a potent active metabolite and opioid-receptor-agonist, O-desmethyltramadol (M1) (see Fig. 28.5). Because of its dual action, tramadol is described as an 'atypical centrally acting analgesic' (Schug et al., 2015).

While tramadol is metabolised along similar metabolic pathway to codeine, it is not clear if variations in *CYP2D6* allele expression affect its metabolism, analgesic effect or side-effect profile in the same way (Schug et al., 2015). The efficacy of tramadol may also be reduced when administered to a child/young person also receiving a 5-HT3 (serotonin) antagonist, such as ondansetron (Bozkurt, 2005). It has been suggested that tramadol may have the potential to be metabolised in an ultra-rapid manner, leading to its contraindication for treating pain in children younger than 12 years of age in the united States and New Zealand (Food and Drug Administration 2017, MEDSAFE 2020).

Tramadol is effective in managing mild, moderate (APAGBI, 2012) and severe acute pain (Marzuillo et al., 2014). It may provide appropriate analgesia in comparison to a placebo for postoperative pain, although further research is required (Schnabel et al., 2015). Tramadol has been also used in trauma settings and less frequently in management of pain in children/young people with sickle cell disease (Rodieux et al., 2018). Tramadol is a partial-agonist and has a significantly reduced incidence of respiratory depression (Stannard et al., 2016) and in comparison to other opioids has a reduced incidence of sedation, constipation, and nausea and vomiting (Bozkurt, 2005), its most common side-effects (Marzuillo et al., 2014).

Morphine

Morphine is the most commonly used intravenous opioid in children/young people (Chau and Koren, 2013) with an extensive history of use in the management of acute paediatric pain (Schug et al., 2015). Because of the long clinical experience of using morphine and its low cost it is usually the opioid of first choice (Strassels, 2014) and is safe and effective in children/young people of all ages when given using standard dosing schedules. Morphine is metabolised to morphine-6-glucuronide, which has analgesic activity, and morphine-3-glucuronide (Strassels, 2014), which may be linked to myoclonus in young children (see Fig. 28.5). The neonatal central nervous system is more sensitive to morphine, and morphine's half-life in neonates is more than double that of older children because of neonatal hepatic immaturity; therefore, lower doses are required initially, which can be titrated depending on the response of the individual neonate (Chau and Koren, 2013). Similarly, morphine's metabolites may accumulate in patients with reduced renal function (Strassels, 2014) as the active metabolite is excreted in urine (Stannard et al, 2016).

Oxycodone

Oxycodone is a semi-synthetic opioid analgesic which is being used more frequently in acute paediatric pain management. In comparison to morphine is has a higher oral bioavailability, swifter onset of action and a longer duration of action. It has a lower incidence of adverse effects (Schug et al., 2015) being less sedating than morphine and does not cause histamine release (therefore less pruritus) and may cause less nausea and vomiting (Kokki et al., 2004). It has been used for the management of moderate to severe pain in children/young people with cancer (Constance et al., 2017) and because of its relative lack of active metabolites, it may be used in children/young people with reduced renal function (Strassels, 2014).

MANAGING CHRONIC PAIN IN CHILDREN AND YOUNG PEOPLE

What Is Chronic Pain?

Chronic pain is a term used to describe persistent or recurrent pain lasting longer than three months (American Pain Society, 2012). New ICD-11 classification of chronic pain further differentiates the most common clinically relevant disorders including: (1) chronic primary pain, (2) chronic cancer pain, (3) chronic posttraumatic and postsurgical pain, (4) chronic neuropathic pain, (5) chronic headache and orofacial pain, (6) chronic visceral pain and (7) chronic musculoskeletal (MSK) pain (Treede et al., 2015).

The Pediatric Chronic Pain Task Force, which is part of the American Pain Society (APS), has provided a description of chronic pain in children:

> *Chronic pain in children is the result of a dynamic integration of biological processes, psychological factors, and socio-cultural context, considered within a developmental trajectory. This category of pain includes persistent (ongoing) and recurrent (episodic) pain in children with chronic health conditions (e.g. arthritis or sickle cell disease) and pain that is a disorder itself (e.g. migraines, functional abdominal pain, complex regional pain syndrome).*
>
> *http://www.ampainsoc.org/advocacy/downloads/ aps12-pcp.pdf*

Chronic pain in children/young people is a serious health problem because of its complex nature and can result in significant disability (Huguet and Miro, 2008; Zernikow et al., 2012a) and cost to families and the health care system (Groenewald et al., 2017) (e.g. cost for those with moderate to severe pain has been estimated to be $19.5 billion annually in the United States and high use of the emergency department, but not mental health care) (Groenewald et al., 2014; Tumin et al., 2018).

How Common Is Chronic Pain in Children and Young People?

There is growing evidence about the epidemiology of chronic pain in children/young people (King et al., 2011). However, there are inconsistent findings about prevalence with rates varying considerably across studies. King et al. (2011) systematically reviewed the nature and aggregated prevalence of chronic pain in children/young people from 41 studies carried out between 1999 and 2009. Prevalence estimates (median) range from 11% to 38%. De la Vega et al. (2018) conducted a secondary analysis of cross-sectional nationally representative data from the National Longitudinal Study of Adolescent to Adult Health to determine the prevalence rates and associated factors in young people with and without physical disabilities. They found that young people with physical disabilities experience chronic pain at a significantly higher rate than able-bodied peers, but the comorbidity of physical disability and chronic pain was not related to depression, anxiety or insomnia. These findings indicate that chronic pain is common in children and young people. Further, untreated chronic pain in children/young people incurs a high risk for the subsequent development of pain and psychological disorders in adulthood (Hassett et al., 2013).

The most common pain conditions are headaches, abdominal pain, back pain and musculoskeletal pain. Children/young people often report pain in multiple locations, with headache reported as the most disabling (van Gessel et al., 2011). It is estimated that 5%–8% of children/young people with recurrent and persistent pain will develop significant pain-related disability that increases with age (Huguet and Miró 2008) and about 3% will require intensive rehabilitation (Hechler et al., 2010). Pain prevalence rates tend to increase with age with the exception of abdominal pain (which is more prevalent in younger children) and girls generally report more pain than boys (Zernikow et al., 2012). Psychosocial variables impacting pain prevalence include anxiety, depression, low self-esteem, other chronic health conditions and low socio-economic status (King et al., 2011). Pain disorders associated with psychological factors are known as *somatoform disorders* with the most common in children/young people being conversion disorders (Cottencin, 2014).

Causes of Chronic Pain

Chronic pain may be part of an ongoing/long-term medical condition (e.g. sickle cell anaemia, juvenile idiopathic arthritis, haemophilia, cancer), develop following surgery (e.g. chronic postsurgical pain, phantom limb pain) Kozlowski et al., 2014, illness (post-viral) or injury (complex regional pain syndrome), or have no obvious cause (idiopathic; e.g. chronic widespread pain, recurrent abdominal pain and headaches). Chronic pain conditions can be nociceptive, neuropathic or mixed (combination of nociceptive and neuropathic) in nature and/or associated with psychological factors (Stinson and Reid, 2014).

Factors Triggering and Maintaining Chronic Pain

There are many factors that influence a child/young person's perception of and ways they behave when in pain. Many studies have provided evidence (primarily using cross-sectional studies) that a few isolated biological, physical, psychological (Randall et al., 2017; Simons and Kaczynski, 2012), family (Chow et al., 2016), and social factors (La Buissonnière-Ariza et al., 2018; Forgeron et al., 2018) play an important role in chronic pain in children/young people (Fig. 28.6). However, little is known about which factors or combination of factors predispose children/young people to chronic pain and disability.

Management of Chronic Pain in Children and Young People

The management of chronic pain involves the use of a range of psychological (mind–body techniques), physical and pharmacological interventions (Friedrichsdorf et al., 2016; Landry et al., 2015) that focuses on helping the child or young person to return to previous activities (Fig. 28.7). Key points in management of chronic pain in children are as follows:

- Many children and young people with chronic pain can be managed effectively by their family doctor.
- Referral to a multi-disciplinary paediatric pain programme should be considered for children with complex or ongoing chronic pain (Miró et al., 2017).
- The main goal of treatment is to return the child/young person to a functional state that will enable them to participate in daily activities, sports and return to school, rather than focusing solely on reducing or controlling the pain (Friedrichsdorf et al., 2016).
- A multi-disciplinary, multi-modal approach that incorporates the three Ps (physical, psychological and pharmacological interventions) is likely to be most effective.
- Decisions regarding the most appropriate treatments should be individualised and based on the assessment of the child/young person.
- Interventions should be aimed at treating any trigger factors, as well as the underlying cause(s) of the pain wherever possible.
- Treatment should also address pain-related disability with the goal of maximising functioning and improving quality of life. This approach includes specific treatment targeting possible underlying pain mechanisms, as well as symptom-focused management addressing pain, sleep disturbance, anxiety, or depressive feelings.
- Treatment must also include pain neuroscience education (Robins et al., 2016) and support of the parents' reactions to their child/young person's pain and how they can best support their child/young person (Friedrichsdorf et al., 2016).
- Parents of children/young people seen in a paediatric pain clinic want information about the causes of their child's pain and information on the various treatment options, as well as effective strategies to help their child cope with the pain (Friedrichsdorf et al., 2016).

Physical and Psychological Methods of Pain Relief

Using physical and psychological strategies in combination with pharmacological strategies optimises pain relief and improves functional outcomes.

Physical pain-relieving interventions. Chronic pain often leads children/young people to avoid physical activities because of fear of re-injury or because it exacerbates the pain (fear of movement is called kinesiophobia). Lack of muscle use leads to loss of muscle strength, flexibility, endurance and overall de-conditioning. Physiotherapy (physical therapy) is, therefore, an integral component and in certain instances (e.g. with CRPS), it is the cornerstone of treatment for children/young people with chronic pain (Booth et al., 2017; Landry et al., 2015). Despite the recognised importance of exercise and physiotherapy in treating children/young people with chronic pain, little research has been conducted to document the treatment effects or evaluate different therapeutic techniques (Campos et al., 2011; Kichline and Cushing, 2019).

Physiotherapy is usually administered on an outpatient basis with the ultimate goal of teaching the child/young person to continue the programme at home. Many patients with chronic pain will respond to lower exercise dosage than recommended for healthy aged peers; therefore it is important that exercise be started in a graded and paced manner and focus on active rather than passive modalities (e.g. massage). Regular exercise (e.g. with the goal of working up to 30–60 minutes three times per week) can also help improve sleep, mood, self-esteem and energy levels (Booth et al., 2017;

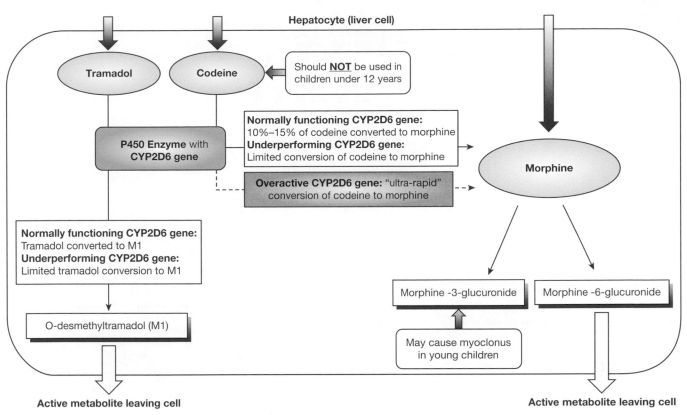

Fig. 28.5 Opioid metabolism.

Landry et al., 2015). Exercise programmes should be individually designed, enjoyable and tailored to the goals of the patient (e.g. return to a sport or age appropriate play activity). However, for any benefit to be realised, a minimum of two sessions per week on non-consecutive days with a minimum duration of 20 minutes (broken up into two 10-minute sessions over the day for deconditioned patients) should be done (Campos et al., 2011).

Psychological therapies. Many psychological therapies are used to manage chronic pain in children/young people. Often these therapies are integrated into a comprehensive cognitive behavioural therapy (CBT) programme that is directed at identifying and eliminating and/or reducing triggering factors that affect the child/young person's pain and disability. Such programmes usually include:

- education about the pain;
- learning cognitive behavioural pain coping skills (e.g. imagery, distraction and relaxation);
- stress management (for example, identifying and coping with stressful situations, using thought stopping, cognitive restructuring, assertiveness and problem solving);
- relapse prevention (Fisher et al., 2014).

A systematic review documented the effectiveness of CBT at reducing pain symptoms for children and young people with chronic pain (headaches, abdominal pain and MSK pain) immediately after treatment as well as reducing disability and depressive symptoms for some pain conditions (abdominal and MSK pain) (Fisher et al., 2014). However, there was

insufficient evidence about its impact on sleep and anxiety. CBT has been found to be effective in treating juvenile fibromyalgia (Kashikar-Zuck et al., 2012). CBT is also useful in reducing the emotional component of pain in children/young people with sickle cell disease (Anie and Green, 2012). There are also skills based psychological interventions targeting youth and their parents (Comfort Ability Pain Management Program) (Coakley et al., 2018).

There is growing evidence that CBT can be self-administered without a psychologist or nurse being physically present using the internet (Palermo et al., 2016). A systematic review of computer-based psychological pain treatment programmes for children and young people with chronic pain (including four randomised controlled trials) found that self-administered treatments delivered over the internet reduce pain intensity (Velleman et al., 2010). Recently there has been a rapid development in the use of smartphones (Lalloo et al., 2015; Minen et al., 2016) to provide pain self-management strategies. For example, Jibb et al. (2017) found significant reductions in pain intensity and pain interference and improvements in quality of life in children/young people using the Pain Squad+ app to manage cancer pain over 28 days. However, more research on the impact on clinical outcomes is required.

More recently, acceptance and commitment therapy (ACT) (Kemani et al., 2018) is being adopted as a treatment approach in chronic pain programmes (Pielech et al., 2017). This emphasises the acceptance of, or willingness to

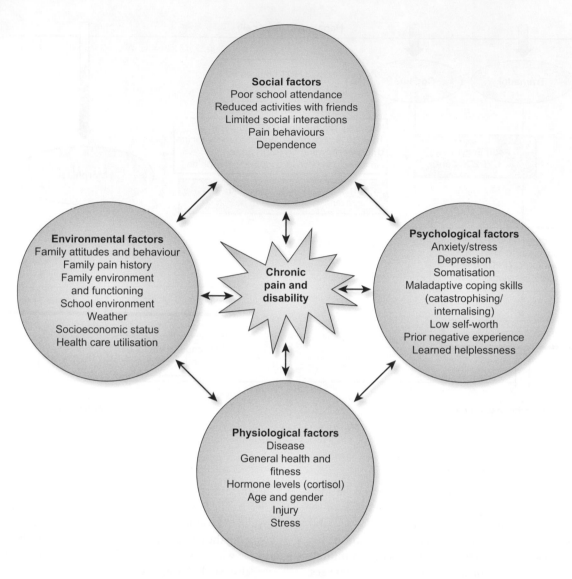

Fig. 28.6 Factors associated with children's chronic pain.

experience, pain and other interfering experiences (fear of pain with activities) rather than trying to control or reduce symptoms. The goal is to achieve functionality even in the presence of interfering pain and distress. There is emerging evidence of the effectiveness of this approach in children/young people with chronic pain (Kanstrup et al., 2016; Masuad et al., 2011; Wicksell et al., 2011) and as multi-family group therapy (Huestis et al., 2017; Kemani et al., 2018)

Sleep hygiene. Sleep disturbances are common in children/young people with chronic pain (Evans et al., 2017). Young people with chronic pain report poorer sleep quality, which is associated with increased pain intensity and pain interference and anxiety and depressive symptoms (Pavlova et al., 2017). Pain can interfere with the quality and quantity of sleep and insufficient sleep can cause daytime sequelae (behavioural and emotional changes) that undermine the coping skills necessary for effective pain management. Efforts should, therefore, be directed towards improving the sleep

hygiene (good sleep habits) of children/young people with chronic pain and address mental health issues.

 WWW

For specific strategies to improve sleep hygiene see the National Sleep Foundation at:
- http://www.sleepfoundation.org

Complementary health approaches (CAH) and integrative medicine. The National Centre for Complementary and Integrative Health in the United States defines complementary health approaches as practices (mind–body practices) and products (natural products, such as herbs and probiotics) that are not mainstream approaches (National Center for Complementary and Integrative Health, 2017). A recent study of CAM use by children/young people with pain in the United States using the National Health Survey data found that of

1. Evaluate child with chronic pain

- Complete medical and pain history
- Assess pain location, onset, duration, quality, variability, exacerbating and alleviating factors
- Assess associated disability including impact of pain daily life such as sleep, school, eating, social and physical activities
- Physical and neurological exam including appearance, posture, gait, growth parameters and vital signs
- Complete appropriate diagnostic tests

2. Diagnose the primary and secondary causes

- Current nociceptive and neuropathic components
- Attenuating physical symptoms
- Contributing psychological factors, social factors and biological processes

3. Select appropriate therapies to improve overall functioning and quality of life

Pharmacological	Physical	Psychological
• Analgesics • Adjunct analgesics • Anaesthetics	• Graded exercise program • Regular daily activity (e.g. walking, swimming, stretching) • Pacing	• Relaxation strategies • CBT • School reintegration • Sleep hygiene • Teach parents adaptive responses to child's pain

4. Implement pain management plan

- Provide pain diagnosis, feedback on causes and contributing factors
- Provide rationale for integrated treatment program
- Develop mutually agreed upon treatment goals
- Measure child's pain and functional improvement regularly
- Evaluate effectiveness of treatment plan
- Revise plan as necessary

Fig. 28.7 Treatment algorithm for children with chronic pain. *CBT,* Cognitive behavioural therapy.

the 26.6% of children/young people who reported chronic pain in the past year, 21.3% used CAM in contrast to 8.1% of children/young people without pain. The most commonly used CAM therapies were biologically based therapies (special diets and herbal supplements) (Groenewald et al., 2017) and manipulative or body-based therapies (chiropractic and massage). There are few high-quality empirical investigations that permit definitive conclusions to be drawn regarding the efficacy of CHA interventions for paediatric pain. For more information on CHA in chronic pain see the Centre for Complementary and Alternative Medicine at the National Institutes of Health (NIH) at: http://nccam.nih.gov/health/pain/chronic.htm.

Pharmacological Interventions

Pharmacological interventions are of benefit for some types of chronic pain, although research involving children/young people is lacking (Boulkedid et al., 2018). A recent systematic review of randomised controlled trials evaluating pain management interventions in children and young people with chronic pain found five trials evaluating analgesics or co-analgesics. Few of the medications prescribed are licensed for use in children (Grégoire and Finley, 2007) with the clinical indications and use extrapolated from research and clinical practice in adults with chronic pain. There is limited research supporting their use in children (WHO, 2012). Opioids are not indicated for primary pain disorders and are likely to cause more harm than benefit. Other medications, with few exceptions (i.e. anticonvulsants for neuropathic pain), are typically not first-line therapy (Friedrichsdorf et al., 2016).

Invasive Therapies

Non-invasive therapies are the mainstay of treatment of paediatric chronic pain conditions. A recent review of regional anaesthetics in treatment of complex regional pain syndrome in children/young people found only case series reports and no randomised controlled trials with weak evidence of their effectiveness (Rodriguez et al., 2015). More research is needed to determine their effectiveness using rigorous trials and determining which children/young people would benefit most from these invasive therapies given their risks. Invasive management should only be considered when standard conservative management has failed.

Multi-disciplinary Approach

The key to the success of chronic pain management in children/young people is adopting a multi-disciplinary, multi-modal rehabilitation approach (Odell and Logan, 2013). Because of the complexity of chronic pain, no single discipline has the expertise to assess and manage it independently. While not all children/young people require a multi-disciplinary approach, the services provided by multi-disciplinary pain treatment programmes (chronic pain clinics) are considered the optimal therapeutic model for the management of chronic pain (Friedrichsdorf et al., 2016; Landry et al., 2015). Specialised interdisciplinary chronic pain teams are the standard of care for children/young people with complex chronic pain conditions (Miró et al., 2017).

Summary: Managing Chronic Pain in Children and Young People

Chronic pain in children/young people is the result of a dynamic integration of biological processes, psychological factors and socio-cultural context, considered within a developmental trajectory. Chronic pain can occur as a result of a chronic medical condition, can develop following surgery, illness or injury, or have no obvious cause. Persistent and recurrent pains in childhood are common. Chronic pain can negatively impact all aspects of life and lead to pain-related disability. Children/young people's chronic pain can impact family functioning and result in significant economic costs. Those children/young people at risk of pain-related disability should be referred to a multi-disciplinary, multi-modal rehabilitative programme. Most chronic pain conditions can be treated using a combination of pharmacological, physical and psychological therapies.

SUMMARY

Within this chapter we have discussed why it is imperative to manage children/young people's pain effectively. We have provided information about the anatomy and physiology of pain as well as the pharmacology of analgesic drugs and some of the physical and psychological pain-relieving interventions available. Evidence-based practice in relation to pain assessment for all ages of children and young people has been outlined. The strategies for managing acute, procedural and chronic pain have also been discussed drawing on current evidence. Together the information provided in this chapter should prepare you for your role in managing the pain of children and young people in clinical practice.

REFERENCES

2010 ENA Emergency Nurses Resources Development Committee, 2011. Emergency nurses resource: needle-related procedural pain in pediatric patients in the emergency department. J. Emerg. Nurs. 37 (3), 246–251.

American Pain Society, 2012. Assessment and Management of Children With Chronic Pain: A Position Statement from the American Pain Society. Available from: http://americanpain-society.org/uploads/get-involved/pediatric-chronic-pain-statement.pdf (accessed 3 April 2019).

Anand, K.J.S., McIntosh, N., Lagercrantz, H., et al., 1999. Analgesia and sedation in preterm neonates who require ventilatory support: results from the NOPAIN trial. Arch. Pediatr. Adolesc. Med. 153 (4), 331–338.

Anderson, 2014. The non-steroidal anti-inflammatory drugs and acetaminophen. In: McGrath P.J., Stevens B.J., Walker S.M., Zempsky, W.T. (eds.), Oxford Textbook of Paediatric Pain. Oxford University Press, Oxford, pp. 560–568.

Anie, K.A., Green, J., 2012. Psychological therapies for sickle cell disease and pain. Cochrane Database Syst. Rev. (2), CD001916.

Arif-Rahu, M., Fisher, D., Matsuda, Y., 2012. Biobehavioral measures for pain in the pediatric patient. Pain Manag. Nurs. 13 (3), 157–168.

Association of Paediatric Anaesthetists of Great Britain & Ireland (APAGBI), 2012. Good Practice in Postoperative and Procedural Pain Management, second ed. Paediatr. Anaesth. 22 (Suppl. 1), 1–79.

Australian and New Zealand College of Anaesthetists and Faculty of Pain Medicine, 2015. Acute Pain Management: Scientific Evidence, fourth ed. Australian and New Zealand College of Anaesthetists, Melbourne.

Avian, A., Messerer, B., Wunsch, G., et al., 2016. Postoperative paediatric pain prevalence: a retrospective analysis in a university teaching hospital. Int. J. Nurs. Stud. 62, 36–43.

The Coxib and traditional NSAID Trialists' (CNT) Collaboration, Bhala, N., Emberson, J., et al., 2013. Vascular and upper gastrointestinal effects of non-steroidal anti-inflammatory drugs: meta-analyses of individual participant data from randomised trials. Lancet 382 (9894), 769–779.

Bailey, B., Daoust, R., Doyon-Trottier, E., et al., 2010. Validation and properties of the verbal numeric scale in children with acute pain. Pain 149, 216–221.

Barton, C.D., Waugh, L.K., Nielsen, M.J., et al., 2015. Febrile neutropenia in children treated for malignancy. J. Infect. 71 (Suppl. 1), S27–S35.

Batoz, H., Semjen, F., Bordes-Demolis, M., et al., 2016. Chronic postsurgical pain in children: prevalence and risk factors. A prospective observational study. Br. J. Anaesth. 117, 489–496. https://doi.org/10.1093/bja/aew260.

Beasley, R., Clayton, T., Crane, J., et al., 2008. Association between paracetamol use in infancy and childhood, and risk of asthma, rhinoconjunctivitis, and eczema in children aged 6–7 years: analysis from Phase Three of the ISAAC programme. Lancet 20 (9643), 1039–1048 372.

Beringer, R.M., Thompson, J.P., Parry, S., et al., 2011. Intravenous paracetamol overdose: two case reports and a change to national treatment guidelines. Arch. Dis. Child. 96 (3), 307–308.

Besenki, L.J., Forsyth, S.J., von Baeyer, C.L., 2007. Screening young children for their ability to use self-report pain scales. Pediatric. Pain Letter 9, 1–8.

Bieri, D., Reeve, R., Champion, G., et al., 1990. The faces pain scale for the self assessment of pain experienced by children: development, initial validation and preliminary investigation for ration scale properties. Pain 41, 139–150.

Birnie, K.A., Chambers, C.T., McGrath, P.J., 2012. When does pain matter? Acknowledging the subjectivity of clinical significance. Pain 153, 2311–2314.

Birnie, K.A., Chambers, C.T., Taddio, A., et al., 2015. Psychological interventions for vaccine injections in children and adolescents: systematic review of randomized and quasi-randomized controlled trials. Clin. J. Pain 31, S72–S89.

Birnie, K.A., Hundert, A., Chitra Lalloo, C., et al., 2019. Recommendations for selection of self-report pain intensity measures in children and adolescents: a systematic review and quality assessment of measurement properties. Pain 160 (1), 5–18.

Birnie, K.A., Noel, M., Chambers, C.T., et al., 2018. Systematic review and meta-analysis of distraction and hypnosis for needle-related pain and distress in children and adolescents. Cochrane. Database. Syst. Rev. 10, CD005179. https://doi.org/10.1002/14651858.CD005179.pub4.

Birnie, K.A., Noel, M., Parker, J.A., et al., 2014. Systematic review and meta-analysis of distraction and hypnosis for needle-related pain and distress in children and adolescents. J. Pediatr. Psychol. 39 (8), 783–808.

Booth, J., Moseley, G.L., Schiltenwolf, M., et al., 2017. Exercise for chronic musculoskeletal pain: a biopsychosocial approach. Muscoskel. Care 15 (4), 413–421.

Botting, R.M., 2000. Mechanism of action of acetaminophen: is there a cyclooxygenase 3? Clin. Infect. Dis. 31 (S5), S202–S210.

Boulkedid, R., Abdou, A.Y., Desselas, E., et al., 2018. The research gap in chronic paediatric pain: a systematic review of randomised controlled trials. Eur. J. Pain 22 (2), 261–271.

Bozkurt, P., 2005. Review article: use of tramadol in children. Pediatric Anesthesia 15, 1041–1047.

Bray, L., Carter, B., Ford, K., et al., 2018. Holding children for procedures: an international survey of health professionals. J. Child Health Care 22 (2), 205–215.

Briggs, E., 2010. Understanding the experience and physiology of pain. Nurs. Stand. 25 (3), 35–39.

Brodal, P., 2016a. Neuronal excitability. In: Brodal, P. (Ed.), The Central Nervous System, fifth ed. Oxford University Press, New York, pp. 32–43.

Brodal, P., 2016b. Synaptic Function. In: Brodal, P. (Ed.), The Central Nervous System, fifth ed. Oxford University Press, New York, pp. 45–55.

Bryant, R., 2003. Managing side effects of childhood cancer treatment. J. Pediatr. Nurs. 18 (2), 113–125.

Bukola, I.M., Paula, D., 2017. The effectiveness of distraction as procedural pain management technique in pediatric oncology patients: a meta-analysis and systematic review. J. Pain Symptom Manage. 54, 589–600.

Campos, A.A., Amaria, K., Campbell, F., et al., 2011. Clinical impact and evidence base for physiotherapy in treating childhood chronic pain. Physiotherapy Canada 63 (1), 21–33.

Carr, D.B., Goudas, L.C., 1999. Acute pain. Lancet 2051–2058.

Carter, B., Arnott, J., Simons, J., et al., 2017. Developing a sense of knowing and acquiring the skills to manage pain in children with profound cognitive impairment: mothers' perspectives. Pain Res. Manag. 2017, 2514920.

Chambers, C.T., Hardial, J., Craig, K.D., et al., 2005. Faces scales for the measurement of postoperative pain intensity in children following minor surgery. Clin. J. Pain 21, 277–285.

Chambers, C.T., Taddio, A., Uman, L.S., McMurtry, C.M., HELPinKIDS Team, 2009. Psychological interventions

for reducing pain and distress during routine childhood immunizations: a systematic review. Clin. Ther. 31 (Suppl. 2), S77–S103.

Chan, J., Haroon, N., 2016. Treatment: NSAIDs. In: Inman, R.D., Sieper, J. (Eds.), Oxford Textbook of Axial Spondyloarthritis. Oxford University Press, Oxford, pp. 189–198.

Chau, K., Koren, G., 2013. Principles of pain pharmacology in paediatrics. In: McGrath, P.J., Stevens, B.J., Walker, S.M., Zempsky, W.T. (Eds.), Oxford Textbook of Paediatric Pain. Oxford University Press, Oxford, pp. 429–435.

Chen-Lim, M.L., Zarnowsky, C., Green, R., et al., 2012. Optimizing the assessment of pain in children who are cognitively impaired through the quality improvement process. J. Pediatr. Nurs. 27, 750–759.

Chorney, J.M., McGrath, P.J., Finley, G.A., 2010. Pain as the neglected adverse event. Can. Med. Assoc. J. 182, 732.

Chow, E.T., Otis, J.D., Simons, L.E., 2016. The longitudinal impact of parent distress and behavior on functional outcomes among youth with chronic pain. J. Pain 17 (6), 729–738.

Coakley, R., Wihak, T., Kossowsky, J., et al., 2018. The comfort ability pain management workshop: a preliminary, nonrandomized investigation of a brief, cognitive, biobehavioral, and parent training intervention for pediatric chronic pain. J. Pediatr. Psychol. 43 (3), 252–265.

Cohen, L., 2008. Behavioural approaches to anxiety and pain management for pediatric venous access. Pediatrics 122 (S3), S134–S139.

Cohen, L.L., Cousins, L.A., Martin, S.R., 2014. Procedural pain distraction. In: McGrath, P.J., Stevens, B.J., Walker, S.M., Zempsky, W.T. (Eds.), Oxford Textbook of Paediatric Pain. Oxford University Press, Oxford, pp. 553–559.

Constance, J.E., Campbell, S.C., Somani, A.A., et al., 2017. Pharmacokinetics, pharmacodynamics and pharmacogenetics associated with nonsteroidal anti-inflammatory drugs and opioids in pediatric cancer patients. Expet. Opin. Drug. Metabol. Toxicol. 13 (7), 715–724.

Cottencin, O., 2014. Conversion disorders: psychiatric and psychotherapeutic aspects. Neurophysiol. Clin. 44 (4), 405–410.

Crosta, Q.R., Ward, T.M., Walker, A.J., et al., 2014. A review of pain measures for hospitalized children with cognitive impairment. J. Spec. Pediatr. Nurs. (JSPN) 19 (2), 109–118.

Cummings, J.A.F., 2015. Pediatric procedural pain – how far have we come? An ethnographic account. Pain Manag. Nurs. 16, 233–241.

Curtis, S., Wingert, A., Ali, S., 2012. The Cochrane Library and procedural pain in children: an overview of the reviews. Evidence-Based Child Health. 7, 1363–1399.

De la Vega, R., Groenewald, C., Bromberg, M.H., et al., 2018. Chronic pain prevalence and associated factors in adolescents with and without physical disabilities. Dev. Med. Child. Neurol. 60 (6), 596–601.

Dickman, A., Knaggs, R., 2008. Paracetamol and non-steroidal anti-inflammatory drugs. In: Dickman, A., Simpson, K.H. (Eds.), Chronic Pain (Oxford Pain Management Library). Oxford University Press, Oxford, pp. 15–24.

Emmott, A.S., West, N., Zhou, G., et al., 2018. Validity of simplified versus standard self-report measures of pain intensity in preschool-aged children undergoing venipuncture. J. Pain 18 564–557.

Evans, S., Djilas, V., Seidman, L.C., et al., 2017. Sleep quality, affect, pain, and disability in children with chronic pain: is affect a mediator or moderator? J. Pain 18 (9), 1087–1095.

Eyers, S., Fingleton, J., Eastwood, A., et al., 2012a. British national formulary for children: the risk of inappropriate paracetamol prescribing. Arch. Dis. Child. 97 (3), 279–282.

Eyers, S., Fingleton, J., Perrin, K., et al., 2012b. Proposed MHRA changes to UK children's paracetamol dosing recommendations: modelling study. J. R. Soc. Med. 105 (6), 263–269.

Fisher, E., Heathcote, L., Palermo, T.M., et al., 2014. Systematic review and meta-analysis of psychological therapies for children with chronic pain. J. Pediatr. Psychol. 39 (8), 763–782.

Flowers, S.R., Birnie, K.A., 2015. Procedural preparation and support as a standard of care in pediatric oncology. Pediatr. Blood. Canc. 62, S694–S723.

Food and Drug Administration (FDA), 2017. FDA Drug Safety Communication: FDA restricts use of prescription codeine pain and cough medicines and tramadol pain medicines in children; recommends against use in breastfeeding women. Available from: https://www.fda.gov/Drugs/DrugSafety/ucm549679.htm (Accessed 25 May 2018).

Forgeron, P.A., Chambers, C.T., Cohen, J., et al., 2018. Dyadic differences in friendships of adolescents with chronic pain compared with pain-free peers. Pain 159 (6), 1103–1111.

Friedrichsdorf, S.J., Giordano, J., Desai Dakoji, K., et al., 2016. Chronic pain in children and adolescents: diagnosis and treatment of primary pain disorders in head, abdomen, muscles and joints. Children 3 (4), 42.

Friedrichsdorf, S.J., Postier, A., Eull, D., et al., 2015. Pain outcomes in a US children's hospital: a prospective cross-sectional survey. Hosp. Pediatr. 5, 18–26.

García-Martínez, O., De Luna-Bertos, E., Ramos-Torrecillas, J., et al., 2015. Repercussions of NSAIDS drugs on bone tissue: the osteoblast. Life Sci. 15 (123), 72–77.

Gates, A., Shave, K., Featherstone, R., et al., 2018. Procedural pain: systematic review of parent experiences and information needs. Clin. Pediatr. 57, 672–688.

Gill, A., Davey, C., Kettle, N., et al., 2013. Parental understanding of dosing. Arch. Dis. Child. 98, e1.

Grégoire, M.C., Finley, G.A., 2007. Why were we abandoned? Orphan drugs in pediatric pain. Paediatr. Child. Health 12, 95–96.

Groenewald, C.B., Beals-Erickson, S.E., Ralston-Wilson, J., et al., 2017. Complementary and alternative medicine use by children with pain in the United States. Acad. Pediatr. 17 (7), 785–793.

Groenewald, C.B., Essner, B.S., Wright, D., et al., 2014. The economic costs of chronic pain among a cohort of treatment-seeking adolescents in the United States. J. Pain 15 (9), 925–933.

Hartrick, C.T., Kovan, J.P., 2002. Pain assessment following general anesthesia using the toddler preschooler pain scale: a comparative study. J. Clin. Anesthesia 14, 411–415.

Hassett, A.L., Hilliard, P.E., Goesling, J., et al., 2013. Reports of chronic pain in childhood and adolescence among patients at a tertiary care pain clinic. J. Pain 14 (11), 1390–1397.

Hechler, T., Dobe, M., Zernikow, B., 2010. Commentary: a worldwide call for multimodal inpatient treatment for children and adolescents suffering from chronic pain and pain-related disability. J. Pediatr. Psychol. 35 (2), 138–140.

Hicks, C.L., von Baeyer, C.L., Spafford, P.A., et al., 2001. The faces pain scale – revised: toward a common metric in pediatric pain measurement. Pain 93, 173–183.

Hockenberry, M.J., McCarthy, K., Taylor, O., et al., 2011. Managing painful procedures in children with cancer. Pediatr. Hematol. Oncol. J 33 (2), 119–127.

Hockenberry, M.J., Wilson, D., Winkelstein, M.L., 2005. Wong's Essentials of Pediatric Nursing, seventh ed. Mosby, St. Louis.

Hoffman, H.G., Patterson, D.R., Seibel, E., et al., 2008. Virtual reality pain control during burn wound debridement in the hydrotank. Clin. J. Pain 24 (4), 299–304.

Holdcroft, A., Jaggar, S., 2005. Core Topics in Pain. Cambridge University Press, Cambridge.

Hong, J.Y., Kim, W.O., Koo, B.N., et al., 2010. Fentanyl-sparing effect of acetaminophen as a mixture of fentanyl in intravenous parent-/nurse-controlled analgesia after pediatric ureteroneocystostomy. Anesthesiology 113 (3), 672–677.

Howard, R.H., 2013. Postoperative pain management. In: McGrath, P.J., Stevens, B.J., Walker, S.M., Zempsky, W.T. (Eds.), Oxford Textbook of Paediatric Pain. Oxford University Press, Oxford, pp. 269–279.

Huestis, S.E., Kao, G., Dunn, A., et al., 2017. Multi-family pediatric pain group therapy: capturing acceptance and cultivating change. Children 4 (12), 106.

Huguet, A., Miró, J., 2008. The severity of chronic pediatric pain: an epidemiological study. J. Pain 9, 226–236.

Hunt, A., Goldman, A., Seers, K., et al., 2004. Clinical validation of the paediatric pain profile. Dev. Med. Child. Neurol. 46 (1), 9–18.

Hunt, A., Wisbeach, A., Seers, K., et al., 2007. Development of the paediatric pain profile: role of video analysis and saliva cortisol in validating a tool to assess pain in children with severe neurological disability. J. Pain Symptom Manage. 33, 276–289.

Hunt, K.A., Franck, L., 2011. Special needs require special attention: a pilot project implementing this paediatric pain profile for children with profound neurological impairment in an in-patient setting following surgery. J. Child Health Care 15, 210–220.

Inal, S., Kelleci, M., 2012. Relief of pain during blood specimen collection in pediatric patients. MCN. Am. J. Matern. Child. Nurs. 37 (5), 339–345.

International Association for the Study of Pain, 2015. Declaration of montreal – declaration that access to pain management is a fundamental human right. Available from: https://www.iasp-pain.org/DeclarationofMontreal?navItemNumber=582 (accessed 26 July 2018).

International Association for the Study of Pain, 2017. IASP terminology. Available from: http://www.iasp-pain.org/Education/Content.aspx?ItemNumber=1698#backtotop (accessed 30 June 2018).

Jaaniste, T., Hayes, B., von Baeyer, C.L., 2007. Providing children with information about forthcoming medical procedures: a review and synthesis. Clin. Psychol. Sci. Pract. 14, 124–143.

Jibb, L.A., Stevens, B.J., Nathan, P.C., et al., 2017. Implementation and preliminary effectiveness of a real–time pain management smartphone app for adolescents with cancer: a multicenter pilot clinical study. Pediatr. Blood. Canc. 64 (10).

Johansson, M., Kokinsky, E., 2009. The COMFORT behavioural scale and the modified FLACC in paediatric intensive care. Nurs. Crit. Care 14, 122–130.

Johnson, P., 2013. Fever and neutropenia in the pediatric oncology patient. J. Pediatr. Health Care 27 (1), 66–70.

Kanstrup, M., Wicksell, R.K., Kemani, M., et al., 2016. A clinical pilot study of individual and group treatment for adolescents with chronic pain and their parents: effects of acceptance and commitment therapy on functioning. Children 3 (4), 30.

Kashikar-Zuck, S., Ting, T.V., Arnold, L.M., et al., 2012. Cognitive-behavioral therapy for the treatment of juvenile fibromyalgia: a multisite, single-blind, randomized, controlled clinical trial. Arthritis. Rheum. 64 (1), 297–305.

Kazouini, A., Mohammed, B.S., Simpson, C.R., et al., 2011. Paracetamol prescribing in primary care: too little and too much? Br. J. Clin. Pharmacol. 72 (3), 500–504.

Kehlet, H., Jensen, T.S., Woolf, C.J., 2006. Persistent postsurgical pain: risk factors and prevention. Lancet 367, 1618–1625.

Kelly, L.E., Rieder, M., van den Anker, J., et al., 2012. More codeine fatalities after tonsillectomy in North American children. Pediatrics 129 (5), e1343–e1347.

Kemani, M.K., Kanstrup, M., Jordan, A., et al., 2018. Evaluation of an intensive interdisciplinary pain treatment based on acceptance and commitment therapy for adolescents with chronic pain and their parents: a nonrandomized clinical trial. J. Pediatr. Psychol. 1–14.

Kichline, T., Cushing, C., 2019. A systematic review and quantitative analysis on the impact of aerobic exercise on pain intensity in children with chronic pain. Child. Health Care 48 (2), 244–261.

King, S., Chambers, C.T., Huguet, A., et al., 2011. The epidemiology of chronic pain in children and adolescents revisited: a systematic review. Pain 152, 2729–2738.

Kochman, A., Howell, J., Sheridan, M., et al., 2017. Reliability of the faces, legs, activity, cry, and consolability scale in assessing acute pain in the pediatric emergency department. Pediatr. Emerg. Care 33 (1), 14–17.

Kokki, H., Rasanen, I., Reinikainen, M., et al., 2004. Pharmacokinetics of oxycodone after intravenous, buccal, intramuscular and gastric administration in children. Clin. Pharmacokinet. 43 (9), 613–622.

Korpela, R., Silova, J., Laakso, E., et al., 2007. Oral naproxen but not oral paracetamol reduces the need for rescue analgesic after adenoidectomy in children. Acta. Anaesthesiol. Scand. 51, 726–730.

Kozlowski, L.J., Kost-Byerley, S., Colantuoni, E., et al., 2014. Pain prevalence, intensity, assessment and management in a hospitalized pediatric population. Pain Manag. Nurs. 15, 22–35.

Kristensen, A.D., Ahlburg, P., Lauridsen, M.C., et al., 2012. Chronic pain after inguinal hernia repair in children. Br. J. Anaesth. 109 (4), 603–608.

Kuttner, L., 2010. A Child in Pain: What Health Professionals Can Do to Help. Crown House Publishing, Bethel, United States.

La Buissonnière-Ariza, V., Hart, D., Schneider, S.C., et al., 2018. Quality and correlates of peer relationships in youths with chronic pain. Child. Psychiatr. Hum. Dev. 1–10.

Lalloo, C., Jibb, L.A., Rivera, J., et al., 2015. 'There's a pain app for that': review of patient-targeted smartphone applications for pain management. Clin. J. Pain 31 (6), 557–563.

Landry, B.W., Fischer, P.R., Driscoll, S.W., et al., 2015. Managing chronic pain in children and adolescents: a clinical review. PM&R 7 (11), S295–S315.

Lane, E., Latham, T., 2009. Managing pain using heat and cold therapy, 2014. Chronic pain in children after cardiac surgery via sternotomy. Cardiol. Young 24 (5), 893–899.

Lavonas, E.J., Reynolds, K.M., Dart, R.C., 2010. Therapeutic acetaminophen is not associated with liver injury in children: a systematic review. Pediatrics 126, e1430–e1444.

Lee, Y.C., Nassikas, N.J., Clauw, D.J., 2011. The role of the central nervous system in the generation and maintenance of chronic pain in rheumatoid arthritis, osteoarthritis and fibromyalgia. Arthritis Res. Ther. 13, 211–221.

Lesko, S.M., Mitchell, A.A., 1999. The safety of acetaminophen and ibuprofen among children younger than two years old. Pediatrics 104 (4), e39.

Liossi, C., Kuttner, L., Wood, C., Zeltzer, L.K., 2014. Hypnosis and relaxation. In: McGrath, P.J., Stevens, B.J., Walker, S.M., Zempsky, W.T. (Eds.), Oxford Textbook of Paediatric Pain. Oxford University Press, Oxford, pp. 560–568.

Lourido-Cebreiro, T., Salgado, F.-J., Valdes, L., et al., 2017. The association between paracetamol and asthma is still under debate. J. Asthma 54 (1), 32–38.

Malviya, S., Voepel-Lewis, T., Burke, C., et al., 2006. The revised FLACC observational pain tool: improved reliability and validity for pain assessment in children with cognitive impairment. Pediatr. Anesth. 16, 258–265.

Mann, E., Carr, E., 2006. Pain Management (Essential Skills for Nurses). Oxford, Blackwell.

Manworren, R.C.B., Hynan, L.S., 2003. Clinical validation of FLACC: preverbal patient pain scale. Pediatr. Nurs. 29, 140–146.

Marzuillo, P., Calligaris, L., Barbi, E., 2014. Tramadol can selectively manage moderate pain in children following European advice limiting codeine use. Acta. Paediatr. 103 (11), 1110–1116.

Mason, P., 2017. Somatosensation: from movement to pain. In: Mason, P. (Ed.), Medical Neurobiology, second ed. Oxford University Press, New York, pp. 309–328.

Masuad, A., Cohen, L.L., Wicksell, R.K., et al., 2011. A case study: acceptance and commitment therapy for pediatric sickle cell disease. J. Pediatr. Psychol. 36, 398–408.

McCulloch, R., Collins, J., 2015. Paediatric pain control. In: Cherny, N., Fallon, M., Kaasa, S., Portenoy, R.K., Currow, D.C. (Eds.), Oxford Textbook of Palliative Medicine, fifth ed. Oxford University Press, Oxford, pp. 632–648.

McGrath, P.J., Johnson, G.I., Goodman, J.T., et al., 1985. CHEOPS: a behavioral scale for rating postoperative pain in children. In: Fields, H.L. (Ed.), Advances in Pain Research. Raven Press, New York.

McNicol, E.D., Ferguson, M.C., Haroutounian, S., et al., 2016. Single dose intravenous paracetamol or intravenous propacetamol for postoperative pain. Cochrane Database Syst. Rev. 5, CD007126.

Medicines and Health Products Regulatory Agency (MHRA), 2011. More Exact Paracetamol Dosing for Children to Be Introduced. Medicines and Health Products Regulatory Agency, London.

Medicines and Healthcare products Regulatory Agency (MHRA), 2013. Codeine for analgesia: restricted use in children because of reports of morphine toxicity. Available from: https://www.gov.uk/drug-safety-update/codeine-for-analgesia-restricted-use-in-children-because-of-reports-of-morphine-toxicity (accessed 30 June 2018).

Medicines and Healthcare products Regulatory Agency (MHRA), 2014. Diclofenac: new contraindications and warnings. Available from: https://www.gov.uk/drug-safety-update/diclofenac-new-contraindications-and-warnings (accessed 30 June 2018).

Medication Safety Expert Advisory Group, Health Quality & Safety Commission, 2012. Paracetamol use in children--highlighting the risks. Nurs. N. Z. 18 (7), 25.

in the united States and New Zealand (Food and Drug Administration 2017, MEDSAFE 2020). Merkel, S.I., Shayevitz, J.R., Voepel-Lewis, T., et al., 1997. The FLACC: a behavioral scale for scoring postoperative pain in young children. Pediatr. Nurs. 23, 293–297.

Minen, M.T., Torous, J., Raynowska, J., et al., 2016. Electronic behavioral interventions for headache: a systematic review. J. Headache Pain 17 (1), 51.

Miró, J., McGrath, P.J., Finley, G.A., et al., 2017. Pediatric chronic pain programs: current and ideal practice. Pain Reports 2 (5), e613.

Moadad, N., Kozman, K., Shahine, R., et al., 2016. Distraction using the Buzzy for children during an IV insertion. J. Pediatr. Nurs. 31 (1), 64–72.

NHS Choices, 2009. Paracetamol affects childhood jabs. Available from: https://www.nhs.uk/news/pregnancy-and-child/paracetamol-affects-childhood-jabs/. (accessed 6 May 2018).

NHS Scotland, 2018. A Guide to Childhood Immunisations up to 5 Years of Age. NHS Health Scotland, Edinburgh. Available from: www.immunisationscotland.org.uk. (accessed 30 June 2018).

National Center for Complementary and Integrative Health, 2017. Complementary, alternative, or integrative health: what's in a name? Available from: https://nccih.nih.gov/health/integrative-health. (accessed 18 June 2018).

Nilsson, S., Finnstrom, B., Kokinsky, E., 2008. The FLACC behavioral scale for procedural pain assessment in children aged 5–16 years. Pediatr. Anesth. 18, 767–774.

Noel, M., McMurtry, C.M., Pavlova, M., et al., 2018. Brief clinical report: a systematic review and meta-analysis of pain memory-reframing interventions for children's needle procedures. Pain Pract. 18, 123–129.

Odell, S., Logan, D.E., 2013. Pediatric pain management: the multidisciplinary approach. J. Pain Res. 6 (1), 785–790.

Ohlsson, A., Shah, P.S., 2015. Paracetamol (acetaminophen) for prevention or treatment of pain in newborns. Cochrane Database Syst. Rev. 7 (10), CD011219.

Olkkola, K.T., Kontinen, V.K., Saari, T.I., et al., 2013. Does the pharmacology of oxycodone justify its increasing use as an analgesic? Trends Pharmacol. Sci. 34 (4), 206–214.

Ong, C.K., Seymour, R.A., Lirk, P., et al., 2010. Combining paracetamol (acetaminophen) with nonsteroidal antiinflammatory drugs: a qualitative systematic review of analgesic efficacy for acute postoperative pain. Anesth. Analg. 110 (4), 1170–1179.

Ozalevli, M., Unlügenç, H., Tuncer, U., et al., 2005. Comparison of morphine and tramadol by patient-controlled analgesia for postoperative analgesia after tonsillectomy in children. Pediatr. Anesth. 15 (11), 979–984.

Paediatric Formulary Committee, 2018. British National Formulary for Children. BMJ Group, Pharmaceutical Press, and RCPCH Publications 2016, London.

Page, M.G., Katz, J., Stinson, J., et al., 2012. Validation of the numerical rating scale for pain intensity and unpleasantness in pediatric acute postoperative pain: sensitivity to change over time. J. Pain 13, 359–369.

Palermo, T.M., Law, E.F., Fales, J., et al., 2016. Internet-delivered cognitive-behavioral treatment for adolescents with chronic pain and their parents: a randomized controlled multicenter trial. Pain 157 (1), 174.

Parker, R., McKeever, S., Wiseman, T., et al., 2018. An integrative review of interventions to support parents when managing their child's pain at home. Pain Manag. Nurs. 19, 139–156.

Pavlova, M., Ference, J., Hancock, M., et al., 2017. Disentangling the sleep-pain relationship in pediatric chronic pain: the mediating role of internalizing mental health symptoms. Pain Res. Manage 1–9.

Pielech, M., Vowles, K.E., Wicksell, R., 2017. Acceptance and commitment therapy for pediatric chronic pain: theory and application. Children 4 (2), 10.

Poonai, N., Bhullar, G., Lin, K., et al., 2014. Oral administration of morphine versus ibuprofen to manage postfracture pain in children: a randomized trial. Can. Med. Assoc. J. 186(18), 1358–1363.

Postier, A.C., Eull, D., Schulz, C., et al., 2018. Pain experience in a US children's hospital: a point prevalence survey undertaken after the implementation of a system-wide protocol to eliminate or decrease pain caused by needles. Hosp. Pediatr. Epub head of print.

Prymula, R., Siegrist, C.A., Chlibek, R., et al., 2009. Effect of prophylactic paracetamol administration at time of vaccination on febrile reactions and antibody responses in children: two open-label, randomised controlled trials. Lancet 374 (9698), 1339–1350.

Rabbitts, J.A., Fisher, E., Rosenbloom, B.N., et al., 2017. Prevalence and predictors of chronic postsurgical pain in children: a systematic review and meta-analysis. J. Pain 18, 605–614. https://doi.org/10.1016/j.jpain.2017.03.007.

Ramamurthi, R.J., Krane, E.J., 2007. Local anesthetic pharmacology in pediatric anesthesia. Tech. Reg. Anesth. Pain Manag. 11, 229–234.

Randall, E.T., Smith, K.R., Kronman, C.A., et al., 2017. Feeling the pressure to be perfect: impact on pain-related distress and dysfunction in youth with chronic pain. J. Pain 19 (4), 418–429.

Robins, H., Perron, V., Heathcote, L.C., et al., 2016. Pain neuroscience education: state of the art and application in pediatrics. Children 3 (4), 43.

Rodieux, F., Vutskits, L., Posfay-Barbe, K.M., et al., 2018. When the safe alternative is not that safe: tramadol prescribing in children. Front. Pharmacol. 9 (148), 1–13.

Rodriguez, M.J., Fernandez-Baena, M., Barroso, A., et al., 2015. Invasive management for pediatric complex regional pain syndrome: literature review of evidence. Pain Physician. 18 (6), 621–630.

Royal College of Nursing, 2009. The Recognition and Assessment of Acute Pain in Children – Recommendations: Revised. RCN Publishing, London.

Schmitt, Y.S., Hoffman, H.G., Blough, D.K., et al., 2011. A randomized, controlled trial of immersive virtual reality analgesia, during physical therapy for pediatric burns. Burns 37 (1), 61–68.

Schnabel, A., Reichl, S.U., Meyer-Frießem, C., et al., 2015. Tramadol for postoperative pain treatment in children. Cochrane Database Syst. Rev. 3, CD009574.

Schug, S.A., Bruce, J., 2017. Risk stratification for the development of chronic postsurgical pain. Pain Reports 2, e627. https://doi.org/10.1097/pr9.0000000000000627.

Shah, P.S., Aliwalas, L.L., Shah, V.S., 2012. Breastfeeding or breast milk for procedural pain in neonates. Cochrane Database Syst. Rev. Issue 12.

Short, J.A., Barr, C.A., Palmer, C.D., et al., 2000. Use of diclofenac in children with asthma. Anaesthesia 55, 334–337.

Sil, A., Ravi, M.D., Patnaik, B.N., et al., 2017. Effect of prophylactic or therapeutic administration of paracetamol on immune response to DTwP-HepB-Hib combination vaccine in Indian infants. Vaccine 35 (22), 2999–3006.

Simon, L.C., Hochberg, M.C., 2016. Non-steroidal anti-inflammatory drugs. In: Doherty, M., Hunter, D.J., Bijlsma, H., Arden, N., Dalbeth, N. (Eds.), Oxford Textbook of Osteoarthritis and Crystal Arthropathy, third ed. Oxford University Press, Oxford, pp. 297–304.

Simons, L.E., Kaczynski, K.J., 2012. The Fear Avoidance model of chronic pain: examination for pediatric application. J. Pain 13 (9), 827–835.

Sjøgren, P., Elsner, F., Kaasa, S., 2015. Non-opioid analgesics. In: Cherny, N., Fallon, M., Kaasa, S., Portenoy, R.K., Currow, D.C. (Eds.), Oxford Textbook of Palliative Medicine, fifth ed. Oxford University Press, Oxford, pp. 567–576.

Sjoukes, A., Venekamp, R.P., van de Pol, A.C., et al., 2016. Paracetamol (acetaminophen) or non-steroidal anti-inflammatory drugs, alone or combined, for pain relief in acute otitis media in children. Cochrane Database Syst. Rev. 12, CD011534.

Smeland, A.H., Twycross, A., Lundeberg, S., et al., 2018. Nurses' knowledge, attitudes and clinical practice in pediatric post-operative pain management. pain manag. Nurs. Times 19 (6), 585–598.

Smith, H.S., Apkarian, K., Argoff, C.E., 2013. NSAIDs and adjunctive pain medications. In: Brummett, C.M., Cohen, S.P. (Eds.), Managing Pain: Essentials of Diagnosis and Treatment. Oxford University Press, New York, pp. 35–65.

Smith, HS, Pappagallo M (2012) Essential Pain Pharmacology: The Prescriber's Guide 1st Edition. Cambridge Medicine.

Society for Paediatric Anaesthesia in New Zealand and Australia, 2017a. SPANZA advisory on tramadol – recommendations following FDA warnings about tramadol use in children. Available from: https://www.anaesthesiasociety.org.nz/wp-content/uploads/2015/11/17_05_SPANZA_Advisory_on_Tramadol_31_May_2017.pdf (accessed 3 May 2018).

Spina, D., 2008. Flesh and Bones of Medical Pharmacology. Mosby Elsevier, Philadelphia.

Standing, J.F., Savage, I., Pritchard, D., et al., 2009. Diclofenac for acute pain in children. Cochrane Database Syst. Rev. Issue 4.

Stannard, C., Coupe, M., Pickering, A., 2013. Opioid pharmacology. In: Tannard, C., Coupe, M., Pickering, A. (Eds.), Opioids in Non-cancer Pain (Oxford Pain Management Library), second ed. Oxford University Press, Oxford, pp. 5–20.

Steeds, C.E., 2013. The anatomy and physiology of pain. Surgery 31 (2), 49–53.

Stevens, B., Johnston, C., Petryshen, P., et al., 1996. Premature infant pain profile: development and initial validation. Clin. J. Pain 12, 13–22.

Stevens, B., Johnston, C., Taddio, A., et al., 2010. The premature infant pain profile: evaluation 13 years after development. Clin. J. Pain 26, 813–830.

Stevens, B.J., Gibbins, S., Yamada, J., et al., 2014. The premature infant pain profile-revised (PIPP-R): initial validation and feasibility. Clin. J. Pain 30, 238–243.

Stevens, B.J., Harrison, D., Rashotte, J., et al., 2012. Pain assessment and intensity in hospitalized children in Canada. J. Pain 13, 857–865.

Stevens, B., Yamada, J., Ohlsson, A., et al., 2016. Sucrose for analgesia in newborn infants undergoing painful procedures. Cochrane Database Syst. Rev. 16.

Stinson, J., Reid, K., 2014. Chronic pain in children. In: Twycross, A., Dowden, S., Stinson, J. (Eds.), Managing Pain in Children: A Clinical Guide, second ed. Wiley Blackwell, Oxford, pp. 179–211.

Stinson, J., Yamada, J., Kavanagh, T., et al., 2006. Systematic review of the psychometric properties and feasibility of self-report pain measures for use in clinical trials in children and adolescents. Pain 125 (1–2), 143–157.

Strassels, S.A., 2014. Opioids in clinical practice. In: McGrath, P.J., Stevens, B.J., Walker, S.M., Zempsky, W.T. (Eds.), Oxford Textbook of Paediatric Pain. Oxford University Press, Oxford, pp. 457–473.

Sweet, S.D., McGrath, P.J., 1998. Physiological measures of pain. In: Finley, G.A., McGrath, P.J. (Eds.), Measurement of Pain in Infants and Children, Progress in Pain Research Management, vol. 10. IASP Press, Seattle, pp. 59–81.

Taddio, A., Katz, J., 2005. The effects of early pain experience in neonates on pain responses in infancy and childhood. Pediatr. Drugs 7, 245–257.

Treede, R.D., Rief, W., Barke, A., et al., 2015. A classification of chronic pain for ICD-11. Pain 156 (6), 1003.

Tsze, D.S., von Baeyer, C.L., Bulloch, B., et al., 2013. Validation of self-report pain scales in children. Pediatrics 132, e971–e979.

Tsze, D.S., von Baeyer, C.L., Pahalyants, V., et al., 2018. Validity and reliability of the verbal numerical rating scale for children aged 4 to 17 years with acute pain. Ann. Emerg. Med. 71, 691–702.

Tumin, D., Drees, D., Miller, R., et al., 2018. Health care utilization and costs associated with pediatric chronic pain. J. Pain (in press).

Tunç-Tuna, P., Açikgoz, A., 2015. The effect of preintervention preparation on pain and anxiety related to peripheral cannulation procedures in children. Pain Manag. Nurs. 16, 846–854.

Twycross, A., Collis, S., 2013. How well is acute pain in children managed? A snapshot in one English hospital. Pain Manag. Nurs. 14, e204–e215.

Twycross, A., Finley, G.A., 2013. Children's and parents' perceptions of postoperative pain management: a mixed methods study. J. Clin. Nurs. 22, 3095–3108.

Twycross, A., Finley, G.A., Latimer, M., 2013. Pediatric nurses' postoperative pain management practices: an observational study. J. Spec. Pediatr. Nurs. (JSPN) 18, 189–201.

Twycross, A., Forgeron, P., Chorney, J., et al., 2016. Pain as the neglected patient safety concern: five years on. J. Child Health Care 25 (17–18), 2619–2628.

Twycross, A., Forgeron, P., Williams, A., 2015a. Paediatric nurses' post-operative pain management practices in hospital settings: a narrative review. Int. J. Nurs. Stud. 52, 836–863.

Twycross, A., Parker, R., Williams, A., et al., 2015b. Cancer-related pain and pain management: sources, prevalence and the experiences of children and parents. J. Paediatr. Oncol. Nurs. 32, 369–384.

Twycross, A., Stinson, J., 2014. Physical and psychological methods of pain-relief. In: Twycross, A., Dowden, S.J., Stinson, J. (Eds.), Pain Management in Children: A Clinical Guide for Nurses and Healthcare Professionals. Wiley-Blackwell, Oxford. pp. 67–84 and 86–111.

United Nations, 1989. Convention on the Rights of the Child. United Nations, New York.

Uysal, H.Y., Takmaz, S.A., Yaman, F., et al., 2011. The efficacy of intravenous paracetamol versus tramadol for postoperative analgesia after adenotonsillectomy in children. J. Clin. Anesth. 23 (1), 53–57.

Välitalo, P., Kumpulainen, E., Manner, M., et al., 2012. Plasma and cerebrospinal fluid pharmacokinetics of naproxen in children. J. Clin. Pharmacol. 52, 1516–1526.

van Gessel, H., Gabmann, J., Kröner-Herwig, B., 2011. Children in pain: recurrent back pain, abdominal pain, and headache in children and adolescents in a four-year period. J. Pediatr. 158 (6), 977–983.

Velleman, S., Stallard, P., Richardson, T., 2010. A review and meta-analysis of computerized cognitive behaviour therapy for the treatment of pain in children and adolescents. Child. Care Health. Dev. 36 (4), 465–472.

Voepel-Lewis, T., Malviya, S., Tait, A.R., et al., 2008. A comparison of the clinical utility of pain assessment tools for children with cognitive impairment. Pediatric Anesthesiology 106, 72–78.

Voepel-Lewis, T., Zanotti, J., Dammeyer, J.A., et al., 2010. Reliability and validity of the face, legs, activity, cry, consolability behavioral tool in assessing acute pain in critically ill patients. Am. J. Crit. Care 19, 55–61.

von Baeyer, C.L., Chambers, C.T., Forsyth, S.J., et al., 2013. Developmental data supporting simplification of self-report pain scales for pre-school children. J. Pain Symptom Manage. 14, 1116–1121.

von Baeyer, C.L., Jaaniste, T., Vo, H.L.T., et al., 2017. Systematic review of self-report measures of pain intensity in 3- and 4-year-old children: bridging a period of rapid cognitive development. J. Pain 18, 1017–1026.

von Baeyer, C.L., Spagrud, L.J., 2007. Systematic review of observational (behavioral) measures of pain for children and adolescents aged 3 to 18 years. Pain 127, 140–150.

von Baeyer, C.L., Spagrud, L.J., McCormick, J.C., et al., 2009. Three new datasets supporting the use of the numerical rating scale (NRS-11) for children's self-reports of pain intensity. Pain 143, 223–227.

von Baeyer, C.L., Uman, L.S., Chambers, C.T., et al., 2011. Can we screen young children for their ability to provide accurate self-reports of pain? Pain 152, 1327–1333.

Walker, S.M., Howard, R.F., 2002. Neonatal pain. Pain Rev. 9, 69–79.

Walther-Larsen, S., Pedersen, M.T., Friis, S.M., et al., 2017. Pain prevalence in hospitalized children: a prospective cross-sectional survey in four Danish university hospitals. Acta. Anaesthesiol. Scand. 61, 328–337.

Wicksell Olsson, G., Hayes, S., 2011. Mediators of change in acceptance and commitment therapy for pediatric chronic pain. Pain 152, 2792–2801.

Wiese, M.D., Sluggett, J.K., Wilson, C.J., et al., 2012. Perceived and actual paracetamol dosing in overweight and obese children. Eur. J. Hospital Pharm. 19, 438–442.

Willis, M.H., Merkel, S.I., Voepel-Lewis, T., et al., 2003. FLACC behavioral pain assessment scale: a comparison with the child's self-report. Pediatr. Nurs. 29, 195–198.

Williams, D.G., Patel, A., Howard, R.F., 2002. Pharmacogenetics of codeine metabolism in an urban population of children and its implications for analgesic reliability. Br. J. Anaesth. 89 (6), 839–845.

Wong, I., St John-Green, C., Walker, S.M., 2013. Opioid-sparing effects of perioperative paracetamol and nonsteroidal anti-inflammatory drugs (NSAIDs) in children. Paediatr. Anaesth. 23 (6), 475–495.

World Health Organization, 2012. WHO Guidelines on the Pharmacological Treatment of Persisting Pain in Children with Medical Illnesses. World Health Organization, Geneva.

Wysocki, J., Center, K.J., Brzostek, J., et al., 2016. A randomized study of fever prophylaxis and the immunogenicity of routine pediatric vaccinations. Vaccine 35 (15), 1926–1935.

Young, K.D., 2005. Pediatric procedural pain. Ann. Emerg. Med. 45, 160–171.

Zernikow, B., Wager, J., Hechler, T., et al., 2012. Characteristics of highly impaired children with severe chronic pain: a 5-year retrospective study on 2249 pediatric pain patients. BMC. Pediatr. 12 (1), 54–66.

29

Transition to Young Adulthood – A Particular Challenge for Developing Young People With Long-Term or Life-Limiting Conditions and Disabilities

Nick Medforth

LEARNING OUTCOMES

- Understand and apply the concept of 'transition' to planning and support arrangements for young people who are moving between children's and adult health and care services.
- Appreciate the evidence-based challenges in getting transition support right from the perspective of young people, families and professionals, particularly those

young people living with long-term or life-limiting conditions and disabilities.
- Outline the principles of best practice and explore examples of transition planning tools and pathways designed to assist professionals in enabling effective transition from children's to adult services.

INTRODUCTION

The life course perspective or life course theories that emerged in developmental psychology during the latter half of the 20th century inform our understanding of the development of the individual throughout their life course. Developmental psychologists were trying to explain the processes we humans share in our journey through our lives. They were also interested in those aspects that are unique to us as individuals. They focused on people's journey through childhood to adulthood from a biological perspective, looking at universal patterns and individual differences in biological growth and maturation. They also explored the connections between people and their shared experiences. The life course approach is not a theory in itself but an approach that draws on several disciplines. It includes a focus on the social environment and historical context within which the individual lives and factors that impact on well-being and healthy development. The role played by the individual in their own development is also important. Often understanding development throughout the life course has involved formulating ideas and concepts and making predictions based on evidence, which can then be applied to the 'real world'.

Different theorists have chosen to focus on specific aspects of development: physical, cognitive (thinking and learning), behavioural, social, emotional, language and cultural elements. Some see development as a series of distinct stages between which the individual makes significant leaps, while others see it as a steadier, more gradual process. Some theorists, like Jean Piaget and Sigmund Freud, have focused specifically on childhood, while others, such as Erik Erikson, have argued the need to recognise that development continues

throughout the life course, with significant stages experienced even in late adulthood. Erikson (1950), for example, suggested that the life course could be divided into eight distinct stages, each with a particular 'challenge' to be resolved. Somewhat controversially, he characterised adolescence as a period of role confusion involving a search for identity as the young person struggles to find out who they are, and the roles they will occupy as an adult. Above all, the life course approach involves an interest in the process of change as the individual grows, develops and progresses throughout their lifetime.

⊘ ACTIVITY 1

As a starting point, find a large piece of paper. Draw out a 'timeline' representing your own life course, from birth to your current age.

Think about your journey so far. On your timeline mark 'footprints' (with notes or drawings) to represent the most important developmental changes and life events or milestones you have experienced up to now. You might, for example, include those that relate to growing and developing; those that relate to learning, education and work; those that relate to family, social relationships or friendships, or those that relate to where you live and the world around you.

Consider the following:
- What have been your aspirations at different points?
- What kinds of opportunities have you had?
- Have you overcome any particular challenges and hurdles?
- What kinds of circumstances might have had a significant impact?
- Who might have helped you along the way … and how?

KEY CONCEPTS: TRANSITION AND TRAJECTORY

The American developmental psychologist Glen H. Elder was a key theorist who studied the long-term of effects of historical change on coping, adaptation and family relationships. He emphasised the impact of change over time and the interconnection of different roles, events and processes. Elder et al. (2003) make the distinction between the following concepts:

1. Trajectory – the long-term path of one's life experiences in a specific domain, such as health, education, career or family life.
2. Transition – a component within the trajectory marked by the beginning or close of an event, role or relationship.

 THINKING POINT

> How might these concepts be different from, but complimentary to the process of transferring from child to adult health and care services?

If you completed Activity 1 you will probably already have considered a number of different transitions and trajectories in your own life course so far. Examples in the education trajectory, for example, might have included joining a play-group or nursery, starting primary school, moving to secondary school, passing exams and progressing to college or university and working towards qualifications for a future career. You will probably also have considered other trajectories, such as friendships and relationships, and aspects of development, such as puberty where biological maturation plays a particular part. You might also have thought about your own developing identity: who you are and how you understand your place in your community and the wider world.

WHY IS TRANSITION TO ADULTHOOD AN IMPORTANT ISSUE FOR CHILDREN, YOUNG PEOPLE, FAMILIES AND PRACTITIONERS?

Progression from childhood to adulthood is a key transition too. Whilst childhood is defined legally, few teenagers will actually go to bed at 17 and wake up as an adult on their 18th birthday. Often a wide range of factors might define the process of becoming an adult and may mean many different things depending on your own life experiences, aspirations and expectations. You might, for example, have thought about it in terms of the things you are able to do or levels of independence and responsibility you have to take, or the kinds of opportunities, services and activities that become accessible to you.

 ACTIVITY 2

> Make a list of all the things you think:
> 1. Define childhood?
> 2. Determine when someone has become adult.
>   How would you describe the key differences?
>   When do you think adulthood begins? Is it the same for everybody?

Transitions do not necessarily occur at the same rate along each strand, and young people may negotiate transitions in several parallel trajectories at the same time. A young person might progress from school to college or university while at the same time leaving home, living independently of family for the first time, managing a budget and making new friendships and relationships. These examples may not reflect your own experiences, or those of young people you know, however transitions in whatever form are 'critical moments' in young people's life stories (Coles, 1995; Jones and Wallace, 1992). They also contribute to processes of social inclusion and exclusion. Young people recognise that these critical moments impact on their choices, chances and opportunities. Individual experiences may be shaped by family, well-being and illness, education, rites of passage, trouble, leisure and consumption, moving and relationships (Thompson et al., 2002).

Transition from childhood to adulthood is seldom straightforward; it does not necessarily follow a single path. Instead, it is shaped by individual life circumstances, opportunities and experiences. A range of factors and circumstances make adulthood more or less accessible. Furlong and Cartmel (2006) Jones, 2002). These include personal situations and social and geographical locations. Young people may be independent in some spheres of their lives, but dependent in others (Griffin, 1993; Jones and Bell, 2000). Transition to adulthood can bring additional challenges to young people who have long-term or life-limiting health conditions or disabilities, face mental health challenges themselves or have experienced other adverse childhood experiences, such as caring for a family member with a long-term condition, disability or mental health issue or exposure to violence, abuse or neglect. Transition for young people with mental health problems, for example, is particularly problematic. It is estimated that more than 25,000 young people in the UK transition from child and adolescent mental health services to adult mental health services each year. Many do not have a positive experience of transition. As a result, they may disengage from services and put their health and well-being at risk, with some reported cases of suicide shortly after transfer to adult services (Healthcare Safety Investigation Branch, 2019).

TRANSITION IN THE HEALTH AND SOCIAL CARE CONTEXT

How Can All Health and Care Services Aimed at Young People Be Friendly, Welcoming and Responsive to Their Needs?

The majority of documents and policy guidance referred to in this chapter reflects the United Kingdom context. However, much of the learning and many of the principles of best practice in transition support will be adaptable or transferable to practice in other countries. It must be acknowledged that there are gross inequalities in health status among childhood populations both within and outside the UK. The publication *Youth Matters* (Department for Education, 2005) and report *Bridging the Gaps: Health Care for Adolescents* (Royal College of Paediatrics and Child Health, 2003) raised awareness of the inadequacy of health services in responding to the needs of young people. Only 8% of health authorities contained adolescent provider units in their hospitals, and many young people did not access primary health care because of concerns about confidentiality, consent and privacy and the insufficient education of health professionals. In contrast to all other age groups, mortality among young people in the UK did not fall significantly in the second half of the 20th century and the early years of the 21st century (Royal College of Paediatrics and Child Health, 2003).

In 2005, the Department of Health published *You're Welcome – Quality criteria for young people friendly health services*, later refreshed and updated in 2011 (Department of Health, 2011, Public Health England 2017). The objective was to help commissioners and providers of health services to improve all National Health Service (NHS) and non-NHS health services, including hospital and community-based services, by making them more friendly, welcoming and responsive to young people. The Department of Health hoped that these criteria would, if implemented by 2020, greatly improve the care experiences of young people in the health service, leading to better health outcomes. *You're Welcome* asserts the principle that all young people are entitled to receive appropriate health care wherever they access it.

You're Welcome criteria had been designed to allow health services to determine how young person friendly they were by using a self-assessment tool that covered 10 themes. Theme 8 was specifically entitled 'Health issues and transition for young people'. This had seven components ranging from the identification of the health needs of young people as they emerged from transition into adult services through to the promotion of healthy lifestyles and the care and support of young people with complex health needs. The prime message of *You're Welcome* was that all young people should be entitled to receive appropriate health care wherever and whenever they access it and the Department of Health expects health providers to use these standards and benchmarks for reviewing and measuring their own compliance. However, although some clinical commissioning groups insisted that their provider services demonstrate that they fulfil *You're Welcome*, so far, many have not. This means that although many services will be welcoming, friendly and responsive to the needs of young people and young adult service users, it is still not possible to claim that this is a universal experience in the United Kingdom.

The Department of Health, Public Health England and NHS England sought to refresh the standards and accreditation process. They were aware of the continuing need to improve the quality of services for the 11.7 million young people aged 10–24 years in the UK who form 19% of the population. Several evidence-based reasons include a focus on both improving the public health and well-being of young people and responding to the fact that many long-term conditions and mental health problems emerge during childhood or adolescence. The British Youth Council, the Association for Young People's Health and Youth Focus North West are currently leading the work on the updated standards. The 2017 version of the *You're Welcome* standards have seven themes, each with eight specific criteria. The themes are: involving young people in their care and in the design, delivery and review of services; explaining confidentiality and consent; making young people welcome; providing high-quality health services; improving staff skills and training; linking with other services and supporting young people's changing needs.

Theme 7 (supporting young people's changing needs) specifically focuses on defining and assuring high-quality transition planning, preparation and support. It includes the following criteria:

- The service provides health care based on a young person's needs and abilities, not dictated by age alone.
- Referral systems foster a positive approach to healthy transitions with established systems of communication between all relevant health professionals, departments and services.
- There is clarity around the differing rules regarding different age ranges and consent. The information is shared with young people, parents and carers, and other relevant professionals.
- The service has a clear procedure to prepare young people for the transition from health services designed for children and young people to adult health services, consistent with current NICE guidance. Specific attention is given to the needs of young people with long-term health needs.
- Staff members are trained to help young people, and their parents or carers, with the transition to adult services from the age of 12 onwards. All young people with ongoing needs have an individual transition plan including a named key worker for each young person who will provide continuity during the transition process.
- The service provides publicity material specifically outlining the transition to adult services. The material is young people friendly and uses age appropriate language and images.
- In order for parents/carers to discuss health issues with young people, they are provided with relevant information and support in ways that are sensitive to different cultures and religions.

Theme 7 is just one example of the *You're Welcome* quality criteria. Together, they set out principles that will help health services to 'get it right for young people', whether in community, primary, secondary or tertiary care settings.

Policy Recommendations and Quality Standards Focusing Specifically on Transition and Transfer

Despite the complexities, transition is a familiar concept to health professionals, teachers, youth workers and others who are involved in direct work with children and young people. The number of polices published pertinent to young people's transition to adult services, and the ensuing debate about the process, has been growing over the past 30 years. This has led to attempts to define best practice in transition support within a legal framework, policy guidance and quality standards.

According to the *Care Act 2014* if a child or young person is likely to have needs when they turn 18 the local authority must assess them if it considers there is 'significant benefit' to the individual in doing so. This includes young people with long-term conditions, disabilities, mental health difficulties and young carers. There are two key issues in transition: becoming an adult and achieving independence and changes in the actual services used (Social Care Institute for Excellence, 2014).

The National Institute for Health and Care Excellence (NICE) published Quality Standard Q140 *Transition from children's to adult's services* in 2016 (NICE, 2016b). This quality standard covers the period before, during and after a young person moves from child to adult services. It can be applied in all settings where transitions from child to adult health or social care services take place. It covers all young people (aged up to 25) using child health and social care services who are due to make the transition to adult services. This includes young people with mental health problems, disabilities, and long-term, life-limiting or complex needs, and those in secure settings or under the care of local authorities. It describes high-quality care in priority areas for improvement. The aim is to help service providers identify best practice in supporting transition from child to adult services. This in turn will enable services to ensure that young people using health or social care services and their carers have a better experience of transition. The standards encourage services to focus on enhancing the way transition is planned and carried out before, during and after a young person transfers from child to adult services. The standards and guidance highlight overarching principles and the infrastructure required and focus on planning transition and providing support before and after transfer to adult services in all settings, including health or social care services. The overarching best practice principles include the following:

- **Involving young people and their carers** in service design, delivery and evaluation related to transition by co-producing transition policies and strategies with them; planning, co-producing and piloting materials and tools; asking them if the services helped them achieve agreed outcomes and feeding back to them about the effect their involvement has had.
- **Providing developmentally appropriate transition support**, taking into account the person's maturity, cognitive abilities, psychological status, needs in respect of long-term conditions, social and personal circumstances, caring responsibilities and communication needs.
- **Ensuring transition support is strengths-based**, focusing on what is positive and possible for the young person

rather than on a pre-determined set of transition options, and identifying the support available to the young person, which includes, but is not limited to, their family or carers.

- **Using a person-centred approach** to ensure that transition support treats the young person as an equal partner in the process and takes full account of their views and needs. This involves the young person and their family or carers, primary care practitioners and colleagues in education.
- **Supporting the young person to make decisions and build their confidence** to direct their own care and support over time, fully involving the young person in terms of the way transition is planned, implemented and reviewed.
- **Addressing all relevant outcomes**, including those related to education and employment; community inclusion; health, well-being, and emotional health; independent living and housing options.
- **Agreeing goals** and the transition plan with the young person at least annually, or more often as needs change.

The standards and guidance highlight that health and social care service managers in child and adult services should work together to ensure a smooth and gradual transition for young people. Suggestions of how this can happen in an integrated way include developing a joint mission statement or vision for transition and jointly agreed and shared transition protocols, and information-sharing protocols and approaches to practice. Service managers in adult and child services across health, social care and education sectors, should proactively identify and plan for young people in their locality with transition support needs. To be successful, every service involved in supporting a young person is required to take responsibility for sharing safeguarding information with other organisations. This needs to be in line with local information-sharing and confidentiality policies and involves ensuring that the young person is registered with a named GP (NICE, 2016b).

NICE (2016) recommends that the process and review should start from the age of 13 or 14, but not be based on a rigid age threshold. Transition planning should take place at a time of relative stability for the young person and consider their needs, capabilities and hopes for the future. The developing transition plan should be reviewed at least annually. Review involves all practitioners providing support to the young person and their family or carers, including the GP. The young person should be helped to identify a single practitioner or named worker to coordinate their transition care and support. This could, for example, be a nurse, youth worker or another health, social care or education practitioner, an allied health professional, the named GP or an existing key worker, transition worker or personal adviser. The role is to oversee, coordinate or deliver transition support, by working in partnership with the family and young person.

Throughout the process the key worker should promote independence in the young person. This could include assuring appropriate support in relation to health and well-being, including emotional health; social education and employment; community inclusion; and independent living and housing. The named worker should support the young person for the time defined in relevant legislation, or a minimum of 6 months before and after transfer, as negotiated with the young person. If they are based in child services, they will hand over their responsibilities as named worker to someone in adult services. For disabled young people in education, the named worker should liaise with education practitioners to ensure comprehensive young person-focused transition planning is delivered. This should involve peer advocacy and friends and mentors as active participants. Support after transfer to adults' services may be necessary if a young person does not attend meetings or appointments or engage with services. The NICE guidance provides further detailed suggestions on how this can be implemented.

NICE (2016) also highlights an organisational responsibility to develop an appropriate infrastructure to ensure that organisations are developing, championing and evaluating effective transition planning and related policies at a strategic level.

NHS England (2018) and the Royal College of Nursing (2018) have provided a range of transition-focused guidance documents and has appointed a National Clinical Director for Children, Young People and Transition to Adulthood. Cornish, J. (2015). They have provided specific guidance for service commissioners and service providers to help local services develop transition processes for young people with special education needs and disability, including specific guidance regarding personal health budgets and Integrated Personal Commissioning. NHS England highlights that there is an urgent need to improve the health and well-being outcomes of children and young people with the most complex health and care needs. Personal health budgets and Integrated Personal Commissioning are highlighted as a way of improving outcomes for young people who have one or more long-term conditions, mental health needs, a learning disability and/or autism, or a life-limiting condition. They are way of giving young people and families more choice and control over the care that they receive and how their health needs are met. This can promote independence and lead to improved quality of life and experience of care (NHS England, 2017).

The Care Quality Commission (2014) highlights that young people face numerous challenges when preparing for adult life, but without effective transition planning and support for young people with any form of disability, long-term or life-limiting condition or significant mental health problem, transition to adulthood can often bring even more difficulties. For the 40,000 children and young people with complex physical health needs, there are many additional hurdles. The transition from children's services to adults' services can be problematic and, for many, scary, particularly as young people may think, function and communicate very

differently from mature adults. Whilst their own care needs are changing, they will encounter significant differences in the expectation and culture of the services they move between. In many cases, they will be letting go of the same people who have looked after them for as long as they can remember, and as they transfer to an adult environment, they may need to consult several different health teams, therapy teams and adult social care services. Services focused on the needs of young adults rather than the general adult population would ensure that young people receive optimal care and management that they need to help reach full adulthood without mishaps.

☝ ACTIVITY 3

Imagine that you are a young person who has particularly challenging life circumstances because of one or more of the following:

- You were born with a learning disability.
- You struggle with anxiety and depression.
- You have a progressive visual or hearing impairment.
- You are living with a long-term medical condition.
- You have caring responsibilities for a close family member.
- You 'looked after' by your local authority rather than your biological family.

How might having one or more of these life circumstances have influenced your own development and life course transitions so far?

Are there any particular challenges as you move towards adulthood – what are they and why are they of concern?

How might you develop the skills and resilience to deal with them? Which might you find particularly difficult, in what way and why?

Are there any particular resources and sources of support that you think might help?

Caton and Kagan (2007) compared the transition experiences of young people with moderate learning disabilities with other vulnerable young people and their non-disabled counterparts and found that in many cases young people who are vulnerable or disabled may experience 'rushed' transitions, which are more stressful and difficult and may also lead to social exclusion. At the same time, out of necessity, they will often have to grow up much more quickly than do their non-disabled counterparts. A key pressure is negotiating uncoordinated and unresponsive services in which they have little involvement. Young people who have had other adverse childhood challenges describe similar experiences.

In the case of young people with learning disabilities, for example, transition is often very challenging, and at a period of their lives when they are also undergoing other profound physiological and psychological changes. Similarly, young people with mental health disorders, such as those with attention deficit hyperactivity disorder (ADHD), are particularly vulnerable during the transition period, and disruption of care during transition can adversely affect the health, well-being and potential of this vulnerable group (Young et al., 2016). Young et al. (2016) highlight that transition is often poorly experienced, and adherence to clear recommendations is necessary to ensure effective transition and prevent dropout from services. They conclude that transitions need to be planned through joint meetings involving referring and receiving services, patients and their families. Negotiation may be required to balance parental desire for continued involvement in their child's care, and the child's growing autonomy, recognising that transition is a process, not an event, and flexibility is important to accommodate individual needs.

Leonard et al. (2016) explored family experiences of transition involving young people who had intellectual disabilities, including Down syndrome, in Queensland, Australia, finding that there were similar difficulties. Parents were concerned about the capacity of their young adult to adapt and change to life in adulthood, their difficulty in navigating services, issues and challenges around the young person, building connectedness, strain on family well-being and finances and worry about the longer term future. They concluded that challenges and difficulties can, however, be overcome with provision of adequate information about financial assistance, the school transition programme and the building of informal community-based support.

Transition has been a key issue for the Council for Disabled Children (2011). Their Aiming High for Disabled Children Transition Support Programme report focused on learning from success and identifying key principles and actions supporting positive change for children, young people and families. They highlight nine areas to focus on in developing and improving services.

1. Participation of young people and families in the shaping of services.
2. Better information for families.
3. Simplifying access to services and planning with families.
4. Supporting families through the system: key workers and lead professionals.
5. National programmes as a catalyst for change.
6. Better data.
7. Workforce development and training.
8. Leadership.
9. Multi-agency engagement: strategic planning and the management of change.

The report highlights that multi-agency working across organisational boundaries is essential in providing the additional support that many children and young people who have special educational needs and disabilities require. If we are to continue to improve, this approach must be sustained. Incorporating the views of young people and families as service users in service developments is essential in developing credible, responsive and effective provision.

Why Are Some Young People Still Getting Lost in the Transition Process?

The report *Lost in Transition: Moving Young People between Child and Adult Health Services* (Royal College of Nursing,

2013) defines transition as the purposeful, planned movement of adolescents and young adults with chronic physical and medical conditions from child-centred to adult-orientated health care systems. The guidance document builds on previous versions, which illuminated some of the challenges and problems experienced by young people whose needs were overlooked or only partially met as they transitioned from child to adult services.

The current document draws on contemporary and systematically reviewed research evidence (Crowley et al., 2011) as well as good practice guidance (Children and Young People's Health Outcomes Forum, 2012; Department for Education and Skills, Department of Health, 2006; National Network of Parent Carer Forums, 2020; Royal College of Paediatrics and Child Health, 2013; 2019). It highlights how children and young people experience many significant transition points between health care services, as well as those between schools, university and other educational settings. All these transitional phases can have an impact on the young person's cooperation with treatment and continued engagement with supportive health care services.

The publication aims to provide health professionals who work with children and young people with information on the principles of good practice in arranging transitions: key-workers' roles in supporting effective transitions; young people's involvement; processes and protocols. It includes a list of recommendations for both service providing organisations and individual practitioners to make the transition for children and young people to adult services smoother. Standards focus on providing services that are seamless, flexible and based on the needs of the young person, rather than focused on the needs of the service. They also recognise that young people's needs are paramount, and key workers with appropriate specialist skills and knowledge and who are able to listen to and respond to the needs of young people need to be involved.

Successful transition is particularly important for the increasing number of young people with serious illnesses and disabilities who are surviving into adulthood. *Lost in Transition: Moving Young People Between Child and Adult Health Services* highlights a number of aspects of service provision that require careful consideration if we are to provide the best support possible. These include the following:

- Commissioning.
- Transition planning.
- Funding and budgets.
- Involvement and choice.
- Supporting carers.
- Working across different settings and professional boundaries.
- Training for professionals.
- Transfer between services.
- Learning from best practice to provide holistic integrated care.

Nurses, alongside other professionals and service providers, can play a key role in getting it right (Royal College of Nursing, 2013).

Despite practice guidance, examples of good practice and effective models, the experience of transition to adult services is by no means a universally positive experience. In his foreword to the Care Quality Commission (CQC, 2014) as well) report *From the Pond into the Sea* the Chief Inspector of General Practice, Professor Steve Field, expresses his frustration. He acknowledges that vast majority of practitioners and professionals are competent and deeply caring but 'we have a health and social care system that is not working, that is letting down many desperately ill youngsters at a critical time in their lives … the system is fragmented, confusing, sometimes frightening and desperately difficult to navigate. Too often instead of helping young people and their parents it adds to their despair.'

Professor Field reminds us that the CQC found a significant shortfall between policy and practice in good transition planning and commissioning of care. Through inspections, it has been transparent that this leads to confusion and frustration for young people, their families and the staff caring for them. Even more worryingly, young people can find themselves without essential care or equipment because of the different ways services are designed and provided, or while funding arrangements are resolved. Professor Field reminds us that it need not be like this.

The CQC is taking an increased interest in transition arrangements for young people when they inspect children's and young people's services in NHS trusts. *From the Pond into the Sea* indicates that greater emphasis is to be given to transition arrangements and providers will be encouraged to improve their services and, importantly, be challenged when inadequate care is revealed that fails to meet the needs of this vulnerable group. During inspections, CQC inspectors and their specialist advisers will seek evidence that children's and young people's services have the following:

1. Good planning for transition.
2. A good transition plan in place.
3. Health Passports for young people.
4. A lead professional to support young people and their families through transition.
5. Health care settings and services that are responsive to the needs of young people and their families when transferring to adult services.
6. Systems in place where the needs of parents as carers are assessed and addressed.
7. Processes in place that agree responsibility for funding at an early stage in the process of transition.

When Transition Goes Wrong: Tommy's Story

Tommy is a bright, articulate 18-year-old young man who lives with his mum, Paula, and dad, Joe. Tommy was born with epilepsy, which means that he is prone to tonic-clonic seizures. These are relatively well managed with medication under the careful supervision of a consultant neurologist, with the support of the epilepsy nurse specialist at his local children's hospital. These appointments continued until Tommy was 16. Up to that point Tommy and his parents were involved in all aspects of care and decisions regarding treatment.

Tommy attended a mainstream primary and secondary school with support from a teaching assistant. While at school Tommy had an integrated Health, Education and Social Care support plan, but this has not been in place since Tommy moved on to his local sixth form college to follow a course in Computing and Graphic Design. Fortunately, Tommy has a good circle of supportive friends both inside and outside of college. Tommy's course tutor knows that he has epilepsy and is worried that she is not confident in knowing what to do if he has a seizure in college. She thinks this should not be her problem – it is a job for health services. She has decided it is better not to tell Tommy's fellow students about his epilepsy, as she is worried that he will become stigmatised.

Paula and Joe understand that 'transition' means moving from child services to adult services as children mature. Paula recalls that the nurse specialist at the epilepsy clinic in the children's hospital did mention transition to her and Tommy when he was about 16 but she does not remember the detail. The nurse specialist told them that Tommy would soon be ready to transfer to the adult hospital. Paula, Joe and Tommy cannot remember any specific planning document being used and no written information was provided. Paula and Tommy remember the nurse saying that they would have a chat about the transfer to the adult hospital at a clinic appointment clinic nearer the time as they were currently working with the epilepsy team at the adult hospital hoping to set up a joint young people's clinic. Both Paula and Tommy were worried about having to get to know new people when he transferred to adult services as they felt that they trusted the staff they already knew at the children's hospital.

Tommy had always regularly attended his frequent appointments at outpatient clinics. When his latest appointment at the children's hospital was due Tommy needed to re-arrange that date and time and his subsequent appointment because of GCSE exams and a school trip. Paula telephoned the hospital to rearrange, confirmed the request in writing and was assured that new appointments would be sent out to them. When they failed to arrive, Paula contacted the hospital. The clinic receptionist told her that a decision had been made to discharge Tommy from the hospital because he did not attend the scheduled appointments and that this was a waste of valuable NHS resources. She advised Paula she would need to follow this up with Tommy's GP. This meant that Tommy no longer had access to the consultant who oversaw the management of his epilepsy. Tommy and his parents were most worried about the fact that they now were running short of Tommy's epilepsy medication and were unsure how his epilepsy would continue to be safely managed now and in the future. Paula contacted Tommy's GP who'd had no recent communication from the hospital.

Paula and Joe reflect saying that this was a crucial time for the family and yet a vital link was lost and no formal plan was in place to inform Tommy of what was to happen in the future. They had no opportunity to be involved in any of the planning, choices or decision making for the proposed transfer of

Tommy's care to adult services. They felt abandoned during the process, and had to learn to navigate the transfer to adult epilepsy services themselves, with some signposting from their GP. They say they are 'battle-weary' after spending several days making telephone calls to make sure that Tommy was not lost in the system, and found it difficult to arrange appointments at the adult hospital with consultants who did not already know Tommy. This involved repeated, lengthy and frustrating explanations about both the current situation and Tommy's medical history. It was not until they raised a complaint and sought the help of the hospital Patient Advice and Liaison team that they were able to resolve the situation.

Paula says that when Tommy is working at his computer his epilepsy is invisible, so the college has not really taken the time to really listen to and understand his needs.

Paula, Joe and Tommy think that an integrated transition plan, which incorporates Tommy's health, education and social care needs, is essential to ensure effective support for people like him in the future. To ensure that plans are implemented effectively there needs to be a named professional to take lead responsibility for coordinating arrangements and communication between adult services and the professional involved. Arrangements should not be left to chance as this means families falling through the net. An understanding of young people's lives outside of health services, including aspirations and educational priorities, needs to be acknowledged by health and social care practitioners, while schools and colleges should understand young people's health and care needs. To minimise disruption and maintain safe and effective care arrangements, families require a clear idea of who to contact for support when arrangements are not working.

What can research tell us to help us to get transition planning and support right for other young people like Tommy?

LONG-TERM CONDITIONS

Crowley et al. (2011) recognised that the transition and transfer between paediatric (child) and adult care services for young people with long-term conditions and disabilities is often poorly managed, with adverse consequences for health. They highlighted that although many agree that services need to be improved, there is limited empirical data to provide an evidence base for policy development. Crowley et al. (2011) aimed to address this gap by systematically reviewing the evidence of effectiveness of transitional care programmes in young people aged 11–25 with chronic illness (physical or mental) or disability. They hoped this would help to identify the successful components of transitional care and support.

They found that many of the studies were descriptive in nature and the majority focused on evaluating transitional care for young people who have diabetes mellitus. These programmes were targeted at improving patient education, staff continuity or service delivery. They concluded that existing evidence supports the use of educational programmes, joint paediatric/adult clinics and specific young adult clinics. A limitation they highlighted was that it might not be possible to transfer this approach to the transition support to young people with other conditions and disabilities. They caution that it is difficult to extrapolate from research focusing on young people who have diabetes to those requiring more complex service provision. For example, in ADHD, a major challenge comes from adult services being comparatively poorly developed, and managing transition for those with complex neurodisability requires comprehensive interagency coordination. They also identified some questions for possible future research priorities:

- How sustainable are improvements to disease management and health behaviours that have been established during the transition process?
- How do we determine the age-range at which transfer to adult services should take place, or if it should be a flexible process adapted to individual needs?
- Could new tools be used to assess transition readiness (as measured by self-management and advocacy skills)?
- Is it possible to identify which young people are most in need of, or likely to benefit from enhanced transition support?

The systematic review concluded that there remains much that can be done to improve the evaluation of existing transition programmes (and those in development) across the spectrum of long-term conditions and disability. It argued that demonstrating effectiveness of services is especially important during the current economic climate when cost-savings are demanded throughout the health service.

Campbell et al. (2016) recognised that the process of transition from paediatric services to adult health services is often associated with deterioration in the health of adolescents with chronic conditions. They conducted a systematic review to assist them in evaluating what works well and what factors act as barriers and facilitators of effective interventions. They uncovered a very small evidence base (four small studies) covering a limited range of interventions. These were developed to facilitate transition in a limited number of conditions such as spina bifida and diabetes. Interventions included 2-day transition workshops, technology-based and nurse-led interventions, with only 4–12 months follow-up. The authors concluded that these follow-up periods might not be long enough for any changes to become evident as a result as transition may be a much longer process. There was, however, some evidence of improvement in young people's knowledge of their condition and improvements in confidence and self-efficacy. The researchers concluded that for firm conclusions to be drawn, further rigorous evaluation of the longer-term outcomes of transition support is required.

MENTAL HEALTH TRANSITIONS – A GLOBAL CONCERN?

Nguyen et al. (2017) conducted another systematic review, this time focusing on models that aimed to prevent young people falling through the cracks between child and adolescent mental health services (CAMHS) and adult mental health services (AMHS). They highlight previous research that suggests inconsistencies in service delivery and practice standards for maintaining continuity of care as young people transition between CAMHS and AMHS. They found that research evidence from Australia, Canada, the United Kingdom and the United States have identified difficulties in obtaining access to care and providing coordinated and integrated services for young people transitioning to adult services. However, their systematic review enabled them to identify three models of care designed to optimise the transition experience.

What these three models have in common is that they all move the focus beyond health to incorporate a broader range of services, which working together can most effectively meet the transition support needs of young people facing mental health difficulties. Nguyen et al. (2017) concluded that there is limited available academic literature highlighting effective models of care that support continuity of care for young people receiving mental health services. The three models they did identify highlight some important considerations in achieving holistic and integrated care during this important stage of development:

- Complex and multi-faceted challenges exist when it comes to ensuring that transition-aged young people have appropriate continuity of care in mental health service delivery.
- Young people and families require support from multiple systems of care to address their diverse needs that extend beyond health services.
- Collectively, the identified models offer new insights into how services can be organised to better meet the needs of vulnerable young people. They highlight important gaps that must be considered when planning the delivery of services; for example, issues of sexuality, culture, finance and environment.
- These models of care reveal current silos (thinking and practice that is disconnected between organisations) in service design and delivery that can be overcome through enhanced collaboration.
- The three identified models of care suggest working together through an integrated and collaborative approach is essential for supporting continuity of care and facilitating successful transitions from CAMHS to AMHS.

The review concludes that in order to facilitate continuity of care and successful transitions to adult care, greater effort needs to be directed towards ensuring that services are client- and family-centred. They recommend using the knowledge and strategies found during the review to inform policy and to design effective client- and family-centred transition services.

PRIORITIES FOR FAMILIES

In the article *Still Lost in Transition* Medforth and Huntingdon (2017) report interview-based qualitative case studies, which included the perspectives of families who had recently undergone transition from child to adult services. Key messages from the families included the following points:

- To recognise the level of anxiety raised because young people may not be ready to act as adults in their new settings.
- Services need to appreciate that young people may still need their parents to advocate on their behalf.

- When transition is on the agenda the focus changes, forcing parents to make a significant adjustment and think about their child's future in terms of gifts, aspirations and what they are good at. This can be a 'huge switch' for parents.
- To recognise that families are expected to adapt to the needs and culture of services, rather than receiving responsive services that focus on the unique needs of young service users. This means that many young people with specific and complex needs are still 'lost in transition'.
- Prioritise the involvement of the young person throughout – they need to feel secure that they will receive a service that is at least as effective in meeting their needs as the service they are used to.
- A key worker or lead professional should manage the transition process and ensure integrated commissioning and services, taking the pressure of already exhausted and battle-weary parents and carers.
- Young people's worries include having to get to know new people, fears around safety and competence, and still needing parents there to explain and reassure.
- Advocacy services would be helpful, particularly for young people with severe learning disabilities.
- Having a young people's group and special clinics can help to make them feel less alone, unsure, anxious, unsafe or disempowered.
- Parents will have different feelings, and it can be scary seeing your child go out into the adult world (but it is like that for all parents).
- Transition plans should be in place for everyone so no one gets lost, particularly more vulnerable families who may not have the confidence to fight for services.
- Transition planning should start early (well before the point of transfer) and is best staggered at a manageable pace.
- Have a properly documented transition plan – you need the right tools; right time; right person to be effective so that no young people are left behind or without services. Practitioners should keep parents informed of outcomes of assessments, development of plans, what is happening and when actions have been completed.

The families asked practitioners not to promise the earth and then provide nothing – if you make promises, you should follow them through. To do this, the transition teams need to be multi-disciplinary and stay together. When it works well, they feel transition and transfer could be a very positive experience as many parents have lost sight of their child in all of the daily challenges they have to face. Hearing people saying positive things about the young person's future for the first time can be the hardest thing to hear but when you do 'it makes your heart sing'.

Professional Perspectives: Conversation With Julia, Transition Co-Ordinator at Broad Oak Children's NHS Trust

How would you describe your role as Transition Coordinator?

I work in a large NHS trust, which includes community services and children's hospital that is one of the busiest in the country and provides secondary and specialist tertiary care to children, young people and their families. The trust provides a range of services at the main Broad Oak Hospital site, including the full range of general and specialist medical and surgical services. The trust also offers inpatient and community child and adolescent mental health services. We treat everything from common illnesses to highly complex and specialist conditions from our main hospital site and across community sites and clinics throughout the region.

What are the main challenges from your perspective?

For young people who have a long-term condition like Asthma, Epilepsy and Diabetes, there are "like for like" adult services so transition planning and transfer to these adult services is relatively straightforward. It is much more challenging to co-ordinate care and support for families whose young people have more complex health conditions as the pathway for transfer to adult services is frequently not established. They are used to coming to the hospital and clinics, as they will have known us for the past ten or more years. They have learned to trust the staff they have come to know well over that time. The teams who provide their care, whether within the hospital or community services, work with the whole family, including parents and carers, brothers, sisters and grandparents. Often there is a different approach in adult services. Because of this, professionals will need to be able to adapt to working in a family centred way, understand specific communication needs and provide developmentally appropriate services.

It can be hard for young people to be suddenly expected to take complete responsibility for their care when they move over to adult services and it can be particularly hard for parents who find themselves excluded from decision-making. For professionals who are supporting young people to transfer to adult services a real problem is often finding like for like services who are appropriately experienced in meeting the needs of young people who have complex needs. Often adult services are geared up to meet the needs of older people. Because of this, some young people are still attending the children's hospital for clinic appointments and as inpatients because there is no suitable alternative. This was recognised to be a particular issue in a recent CQC Inspection at Broad Oak hospital.

My role is to support staff across the hospital in getting transition planning and support right for all young people and their families; for young people in general and in particular those who have complex health problems or disabilities. I could not do it on my own. We need to work together strategically across the trust. Together we develop policies, transition plans and pathways. We implement them to try to make sure that young people's transitions are well planned, well supported, appropriate and well informed. This means working in multi-disciplinary teams within particular specialist areas and across children's and adult services. It can involve consultants, G.P.s, key workers and service managers; specialist nurses, social services and allied health professionals. Often schools and colleges, youth and community organisations (and sometimes housing) are also involved.

What works well within your Trust?

Our staff have the best interests of children and young people at heart. It is in our DNA. We are good at working in partnership with families and involving children and young people in decisions about their care. We are experienced in getting transition planning and support right, with careful planning, where young people have only one common long-term condition such as Asthma, Diabetes or Epilepsy and we have good relationships with equivalent adult services. We can get it right even in specialist, but well-established services like Cystic Fibrosis, Haemophilia and Dialysis where we already have good partnerships with adult services. Where there is an identified lead in adult services to work with, and we have established good three-way communication between ourselves, the young people and their families and our adult colleagues it works particularly well. Well documented Transition Plans and Pathways that are clearly understood by everyone are essential. We have co-produced these with families and our adult colleagues after consulting with our children and young people's service-user group. We start the transition planning when the young person is at the age of eleven if they are ready and able. Transition planning becomes a real priority if we discover that a young person has slipped through the net somehow and is already near to the point of transfer to adult services but does not have a key worker or plan in place. My role also involves co-ordinating multi-disciplinary meetings to review the effectiveness and update transition planning processes on an annual basis and young people and parent's representatives, as well as partners from adult services contribute to these meetings. In the meetings we look at how we can develop the infrastructure locally to make sure we are meeting all of the relevant policy requirements and that our strategies ensure that we prevent young people falling through the gaps when it comes to transition and transfer.

What do you feel that you still need to improve?

We need to continue to work on developing effective Transition Plans and Pathways that work for young people who have complex health problems and those with long-term conditions, for example if the young person has a complex neuro-disability combined with other problems, where the future is uncertain, or where they are technologically dependant because they are on long-term ventilation. Working across geographical and regional boundaries, where models of service provision differ is also a challenge. Developing Plans and Pathways on their own is not enough. We need to work with adult service providers and community, education and social services to develop solutions where holistic and appropriate adult services do not exist. We need to keep the young people and their families at the centre and make sure that when we work across organisational boundaries we are able to keep teams together and maintain effective communication throughout. We also need to train and educate the people we work with to make sure that they understand what best practice in transition looks like. Research and audit helps us to understand what we do well and where we need to continue to improve. Listening to what our families and young people tell us is key. We need to take the time to ensure we provide a consistent, well-planned transition and transfer experience, whatever the young person's condition so that they build confidence and independence and can have the best possible start to their young adult life. Sometimes we might also need the support of an advocate for the young person if they struggle to communicate their wishes, aspirations, needs, ideas and feelings.

What are the best bits about your job?

The best things about my job are the wide range of committed and passionate people I work in partnership with and the sense of satisfaction we get when we know we have overcome hurdles and barriers together to get transition support right. We know we have done this when young people and their families are confident and happy to leave and tell us that they are satisfied with the arrangements we have put in place. Hearing our staff feedback that they are becoming more confident in supporting young people to move on is very encouraging too. My job is always challenging, sometimes frustrating but knowing that we can make a real difference to improving the transition experience of young people and their families is what gets me up in the morning.

EXAMPLES OF TOOLS TO SUPPORT THE TRANSITION PROCESS

Health Passports: Giving Young People a Say

Northumbria Healthcare NHS Foundation Trust, with the support of NICE, has worked in collaboration with Newcastle University on a 5-year Transition Research Programme to explore how health services can contribute most effectively to the successful transition of young people with complex health needs from childhood to adulthood (Newcastle University, 2017). As part of the project, the team worked with Up (their young people's working group) to co-design a Health Passport, along with a facilitator toolkit to enable others to facilitate similar co-production activities.

The team define a Health Passport as a booklet that you can carry with you when attending hospitals or other providers of health and disability services. A Health Passport contains information about how you want people to communicate with you and support you. The purpose of the project was to find out what young people thought about their Health Passports and, alongside professionals, explore what must be in a Health Passport, what could be in a Health Passport and what should not be in a Health Passport. The elements considered included:

- Hobbies and interests
- My home life
- My hopes and goals for the future
- A list of people who see the Education, Health and Care plan
- Where I live
- What I find difficult to do in school
- A plan setting out all of the support I am going to get
- How I learn
- What my parents want me to achieve
- What teachers want me to achieve
- How I want people to communicate with me
- What things I need to keep safe
- What my behaviour is like
- How I communicate
- What I want to achieve
- What support I need in school
- What I find hard
- Social care support I receive outside of school/college
- Things that scare me
- Teachers, doctors and support staff I like
- Who is important to me
- What I want to do when I am an adult
- If I have a boyfriend/girlfriend
- How I like to be supported
- My medical history
- What personal care I need help with
- My grades in school/college
- Things that annoy me
- Details about how I pay for support
- Date of birth
- My contact details
- NHS number
- Emergency contact details
- Details of medical conditions
- Medication
- Medical equipment I use
- My name
- Medical treatment plan
- Daily routine
- People who help me with decisions
- My doctor's name

The project team suggest that skilled and knowledgeable staff should facilitate similar activities in an appropriate setting, so that young people feel comfortable discussing their experiences and feelings and be actively involved in co-creating Health Passports that reflect their needs and aspirations. Facilitators will need to know the young people well, and be confident in supporting them to discuss and process their experiences as well as provide emotional support if difficult experiences or reactions emerge.

'Ready, Steady, Go' – Resources to Support a Whole Trust Approach

NICE (2017) highlights the *Ready, Steady, Go* programme as an example of good practice, which was successfully introduced at University Hospital Southampton NHS Trust. *Ready, Steady, Go* is a suite of resources designed to deliver high-quality transition for young people across all sub-specialities (Nagra et al., 2015). *Ready, Steady, Go* involves a 'traffic light' based system, which was developed in light of the NICE guidance on transition standards. It provides a tool that enables delivery on all the overarching principles in the NICE guidance. The resources include a six-minute video aimed at young people and their families in which young people experiencing transition share their stories and explain how the *Ready, Steady, Go* programme worked for them. They are freely available online at: https://www.uhs.nhs.uk/OurServices/Childhealth/TransitiontoadultcareReadySteadyGo/Transitiontoadultcare.aspx.

The resources also include information on:

- moving into adult care
- a transition plan template
- a parent questionnaire
- *Ready, Steady and Go* questionnaires for young people to complete at each stage of the transition process

The *Ready, Steady and Go* questionnaires for young people focus, for example, on the young person's developing knowledge about their condition and it is management; their developing self-advocacy skills; health, lifestyle and daily living; school, career and future; leisure; managing emotions; and understanding and information needs relating to transfer to adult care.

Ready, Steady, Go has a follow-on programme *(Hello to adult services)*, which provides a tool for health and social care service managers in child and adult services to work together in an integrated way to ensure a smooth and gradual transition for young people with education, health and care plans.

The team involved at Southampton explain how they implemented the project and evaluated its impact in a large NHS teaching hospital and with secondary and tertiary paediatric services, where it has now become a routine part of care. Within the hospital the programme is promoted through staff briefings and workshops and the use of posters in clinic. Uniquely, 4 weeks a year '11-plus clinic weeks' are held. All clinics during these weeks are intended for young people aged 11 years and over. The team ensure the physical environment is made young-person friendly. During these weeks, the young people start taking the first steps towards independence as they watch other young people like themselves go through the same process. The Southampton team says that seeing other young people and carers go through the programme also helps carers understand that letting the young people become more responsible for their care is expected and to be encouraged. During the Transition Clinic weeks health professionals are encouraged to adopt Ready, Steady, Go as part of their regular clinical practice. At Southampton this means that effective transition becomes part of their routine throughout the year.

The strengths of the programme, recognised by NICE (NICE and University Hospital Southampton NHS Foundation Trust, 2017), include that the full range of issues for good transition are addressed. The *Ready, Steady, Go* model is considered young-person friendly because it is easy to understand. This means it can be used to generate deeper discussion between the young person, carer and health care professional. The strengths of the tool and approach have led to wide and enthusiastic adoption and a consequent cultural change in health care practice. NICE recognises that *Ready, Steady, Go* empowers young people to manage their health care confidently and successfully in both paediatric and adult services. This leads to improved clinical practice, outcomes and patient satisfaction. The consequent benefits to the NHS need more evidence to confirm, but reduced costs, better disease control and fewer disease-related hospital admissions are suggested.

The Southampton team have found that *Ready, Steady, Go* provides a structured framework to ensure all issues are addressed so practitioners and their teams can start the programme themselves (Nagra et al., 2015). For anyone who is interested in implementing a similar programme they make the following suggestions.

Ideally set up a transition steering group involving an enthusiastic group of people and develop it to include members of the multi-disciplinary team, parents, young people, executive leads from the trust board, adult physicians, and administrators. They say that waiting for perfection leads to delay, so it is better to keep it simple and not over-complicate it. You can do it with or without an official transition, team or clinic; however Transition Champions are needed to convey the following:

- All members of the multi-disciplinary team are involved in transition, not just transition nurses.
- You do not need to identify an adult team prior to starting transition.
- Do not ask if the young person or carer wants to start on the programme, as the expectation is that everyone will.
- Start the programme early and go slowly. Remember small bite-sized pieces.
- Check progress and knowledge retention.
- There are many models for running a successful transition programme. See what works for you.
- Introduce *Ready, Steady, Go* sensitively to young people who have learning disabilities as some topics are especially difficult, for example sex, pregnancy and the future.
- Parents are encouraged to work through the programme as the young person's advocate.
- Start *Ready, Steady, Go* early, particularly in complex cases. Address the issues you can and signpost or seek help/advice early for those that are outside of your area of expertise (Nagra et al., 2015).

10 Steps to Improving Transition to Adult Services – An Evidence-Based Transition Pathway

Rogers et al. (2017) describe the development and implementation of an evidence-based transition pathway at Alder Hey Children's NHS Trust in Liverpool. The team at Alder Hey explain that they recognised the need for a unified approach to transition across the hospital and the wider network of health care providers, from both adult and child services. They set out to develop a simple, generic transition pathway, based on best practice evidence, flexible enough to be able to support highly complex patients, but simple and clear enough to be equally applicable for more straightforward transitions. The 10 Steps Transition Pathway was developed by combining evidence from a detailed literature review together with findings from a series of consultations – including interviews with GPs, focus groups and an online survey. The pathway was validated through a 1-day workshop, which included professionals, young people and parents. It outlines the important steps for a young person, their parents, and professionals, as the young person moves from child to adult services.

Step 1	Identify young people needing transition
Step 2	Empower young person and support parents
Step 3	Start transition plan
Step 4	Review multi-disciplinary team
Step 5	Refer on to lead adult services
Step 6	Joint reviews led by children's services
Step 7	Plan route into urgent care
Step 8	Young person confident to move into adult services
Step 9	Joint reviews adult services leading
Step 10	Young person settled in to adult services

Rogers et al. (2017) describe how the 10 Steps Pathway includes a number of innovative features not found in other transition resources:

- Reviewing the multi-disciplinary team and identifying a lead speciality to ensure that transition is coordinated.
- Use of the Special Transition Register to manage young people for whom timely transition is not possible or appropriate.
- Planning the young person's route into urgent (emergency) care.
- Support for young people with long-term conditions diagnosed in transition age.
- Scope to incorporate established transition preparation tools, such as *Ready Steady Go,* where appropriate.

The team at Alder Hey Children's NHS Foundation Trust is implementing and auditing the 10 Steps Transition Pathway across the hospital, speciality by speciality. They are supporting the implementation of the pathway buy providing a Transition Toolkit that includes the following:

- What good looks like: The young person-friendly guide for what to expect.
- Empowering the young person and supporting parents.
- Role of the lead consultant, key worker and GP.
- Transition map – speciality-by-speciality transition pathways.

- Special Transition Register – to actively support and monitor young people who remain under child services beyond normal transition age.
- 10 Steps Transition Policy for child and adult services with auditable standards.
- Competencies for multi-disciplinary transition training at universal, core and specialist levels.

The team argues that the growing toolkit of resources help make transition smooth, supported and empowered, and that the 10 Steps Transition Pathway is flexible enough to support transition of young people with the most complex health and social care needs.

Young Person-Friendly Guide for those who are transitioning with a life-limiting or life-threatening condition

Together for Short Lives is the leading UK charity for all children with life-threatening and life-limiting conditions and all those who support, love and care for them – families, professionals and services, including children's hospices. Their work helps to ensure that children can get the best possible care, wherever and whenever they need it. They produced *Stepping Up* in 2015, a guide to explore the process of transition and, in particular, how it can be improved to ensure that there are good outcomes for young people with complex and life-limiting health conditions. Together for Short Lives are not just concerned with the palliative care experience these young people and families. They recognise that complex, unpredictable and deteriorating health needs are often the element of a care package that makes it so difficult for young adults to achieve their goals. They argue that health care must underpin the provision of all other services so that young people and their families feel confident that their medical and nursing needs are met effectively, whatever setting the young people and family receive care in.

The authors of *Stepping Up* describe the difference between palliative care services for children and adults. Child services take an active and total approach to care from the point of diagnosis or recognition. They focus on enhancing the quality of life for the child or young person and family. Together for Short Lives highlight that one of the historical reasons for transition being so difficult for young people with life-limiting conditions is because of the differences between the services provided by adult hospice and palliative care services and those in the children's hospice and palliative care sector. They explain that put very simplistically, the adult palliative care sector has previously, by necessity of numbers, been more focused on those expected to die within the coming months or year, especially the elderly and those with cancer.

In *Stepping Up,* the aim is to encompass the concerns of young people, parents and carers and siblings. The transition journey is divided into three stages: preparing for adulthood, preparing to move on, and settling into adult services. At each stage the young-person focus is maintained and specific standards and service goals are outlined. Further detail on how these might be achieved is summarised in the table below by highlighting areas for service providers to focus on:

Preparing for Adulthood

Young Person

At the centre
Developmentally appropriate
Information
Supported to make decisions
Parents involved as young
person wishes
Key worker
Friendships
Relationships
School
Key worker supporting all
aspects of the move to
adult services

Service Goals

1. Young people are at the
centre of planning, using
person-centred planning
approaches.
2. Parallel planning takes
place.
3. Initial conversations about
transition take place with
the young person and their
family at a time and in a
place that suits them.
4. A follow-up meeting with
the young person and
family takes place.
5. The first multi-agency/
multi-disciplinary team
meeting takes place.

Standard 1

Every young person from
age 14 should be support-
ed to be at the centre of
preparing for approaching
adulthood and for the
move to adult services.
Their families should be
supported to prepare for
their changing role.

Preparing to Move On

Young Person

At the centre
Friendships
Relationships
Sexuality
Developmentally appropriate
Information
Advocacy
Self-advocacy
Self-management of condition
Short breaks
Able to talk about wishes for future

Service Goals

Young people and their parents are helped with the transition from family-centred to young
person-centred care.

Every young person has a key worker to facilitate continuity of care and prepare the way into
adult services.

Every young person is supported to consider future plans, supported by ongoing multi-agency
assessment.

Every young person is supported to identify adult services that can meet their needs.

Key worker supporting all aspects of the move to adult services.

Standard 2

Every young person is supported to plan proactively for their future. They are involved in ongoing assessments and developing a comprehensive holistic plan that reflects their wishes
for the future.

Service Goals

Transition planning continues to take place even during times of uncertainty.

Every young person has a documented end-of-life plan running alongside their plan for future life.

The young person's pain and other symptoms are dealt with effectively. Every effort is made to
ensure that the young person's death takes place according to their wishes and in their place of
choice wherever possible, with the young person's emotional, cultural and spiritual needs met.

Family members and other carers are supported, informed and involved.

The young person has the best quality of life and care to the end.

Parents should retain their parenting role after the death of the young person.

Standard 3

Every young person has an end-of-life plan that is developed in parallel with planning for ongoing care and support in adult services.

This standard applies to all stages of the transition journey.

Service Goals

Siblings should be supported and included in all decisions.

All professionals/agencies should be informed of the death with the parents' consent.

All family members should be supported according to their individual needs for as long as
they need it.

Child and adult services within health work together so that there is an overlap of care planning and care provision.

Services within all agencies should be engaged in planning for the specific needs of the
young person.

Ongoing reviews (at least annually) with the young person take place.

Settling in to Adult Services

Young Person

Friendships
Relationships
Sexuality
Self-management of condition
Meaningful occupation (leisure, education,
work)
Short breaks and holidays
Technology and adaptations
Independent living
Support in using personal budgets and man-
aging personal assistants

Service Goals

A key working function is provided for every
young person so that all the agencies providing care and support are coordinated.

All agencies ensure that age and developmentally appropriate services are available
that address the full range of a young
person's needs.

Palliative care services provide a single clinical overview for the young person and link
with other specialists involved in their care.

There is frequent review and communication
across services about care plans and end-
of-life decisions.

Primary health care services, including GPs,
develop a relationship with the young person and their families/carers.

Adult services in secondary care ensure there
is an appropriate lead clinician to take responsibility for young adults in their clinics
and admissions processes.

Short break or respite needs of young people
and their parents/carers are considered and
provided in the most appropriate setting.

Parents are included as appropriate.

Standard 5

Every young person is supported in adult
services with a multi-agency team fully engaged in facilitating care and support. The
young person and their family are equipped
with realistic expectations and knowledge
to ensure confidence in their care and support needs being met in the future.

The guidance provides exemplar case studies to illustrate their achievement in practice. It also highlights some issues for service providers to consider:

- Professionals in the children's sector need to 'let go' and really support young people to embrace transition to adulthood as a positive step.
- Professionals working in adult services need to reach out to young people to get to know them and to help them to feel comfortable and settled in new and unfamiliar adult services.
- Those in child and adult services will need to develop their skills and knowledge of communicating with young people. It is difficult both for staff trained to support younger children as well as for those used to working with older people.
- Professionals working in adult services in particular may need to develop skills and knowledge about the range of complex health conditions affecting this population of young people and the implications of these health conditions for their daily living.
- It is important that staff are familiar with the *Mental Capacity Act* and *Deprivation of Liberties Safeguards* and the implications of these when supporting young people as they move towards person-centred rather than child and family-centred care.
- It is important to also recognise that many young adults still need and want support from their families in some decision-making processes (Together for Short Lives, 2015).

End-of-life planning is a specific element of Stepping Up. Key goals in relation to this aspect of care planning include ensuring that transition planning continues to take place even during times of uncertainty and that every young person has a documented end-of-life plan running alongside their plan for future life. At the time of death, the young person's pain and other symptoms are dealt with effectively and every effort is made to ensure that the young person's death takes place according to their wishes and in their place of choice wherever possible, with the young person's emotional, cultural and spiritual needs met. During this time, family members and other carers are supported, informed and involved, and the young person has the best quality of life and care to the end. After death, parents are enabled to retain their parenting role and siblings are supported and included in all decision making. All relevant professionals and agencies should be informed of the death with the parents' consent and all family members should be supported according to their individual needs for as long as they need it.

Working Together to Get It Right: Lena's Story

Lena is a 20-year-old woman. She lives with her parents, Natalia and Anna, and brother, Ewan (17 years old). Lena has a neurodisability, which means that she has multiple complex needs, including limited mobility and epilepsy. Lena is also severely visually impaired. Lena is dependent on others to meet her day-to-day care needs. She uses a wheelchair and needs support to get ready in the morning and throughout her day, including with bathing and feeding, and with turns overnight.

Lena has communication difficulties, but is able to respond to questions and indicate her thoughts, ideas, needs, wishes and feelings when people take the time to listen. Her family are her main carers and advocates, skilled in supporting her communication and ensuring that her rights are maintained. This is summarised in the information documented in her Health Passport and Education, Health and Care Plan. While Natalia and Anna provide most of her care, they both have their own developing health problems, and require support that is funded jointly by health and social care commissioners. Personal budgeting arrangements mean they are able to make their own choices to buy in support through a local agency to help them meet Lena's day-to-day care needs.

Lena's parents have always been firm in their view that Lena deserved more than just following the path that was expected. They battle to ensure that decisions made on Lena's behalf are always in her best interest. Following her attendance at a special school during her primary years Lena attended both the special school and the local comprehensive. Maintaining attendance at the special school meant that Lena could continue to access essential speech and language support, physiotherapy and hydrotherapy and maintain her friendship with her best friend, while attending the high school 2 days a week enabled Lena to make new friends in her local community. Lena was also able to benefit from an adapted curriculum, unconstrained by pre-conceptions of her disability and tailored to her own needs, developing interests and aspirations. This enabled Lena to pursue her interests in fashion, creative arts and literature, with the support of a designated teaching assistant and carer who worked closely together.

Lena and her family understand the term 'transition' to mean the movement from child to adult education, health and social care services and that recent special educational needs and disability reforms mean that the transition period begins after the young person has started secondary school until they reach the age of 25. Natalia and Anna approached the school to discuss Lena's transition plan when she was in year 9. The special school initially led the transition planning process, with the support of professionals from health and social care, including her school nurse, speech and language therapist and physiotherapist.

Lena's health service transitions were staggered in order to make them more manageable. Lena's consultant neurologist and nurse specialist at the children's hospital played a coordinating role in ensuring a relatively smooth process, for example, enabling her to have an orthopaedic operation as an inpatient at the children's hospital at 18, before later transferring to adult services. Lena's epilepsy was initially managed through specialist services at the children's hospital, but she has now transferred to a specialist adult neurological centre. Natalia and Anna identify this as a positive aspect of the transition experience because the consultant neurologist at the adult centre met Lena twice in a special clinic for young people arranged in partnership with the neurology team at the children's hospital. This meant that Lena's new lead consultant was able to take time to get to know her and gain Lena's trust and confidence before she attended the adult service. The neurology team at the adult centre have also developed a young people's service-user group, which meets every month. Lena was invited to participate in the group. Here she met other young people who were facing similar challenges as they went through the transition process. Lena's dental care is now overseen by the local dental hospital and her transition to that service was smooth and well organised because the dental team at the children's hospital arranged joint clinics and family visits with the adult dentists.

Lena's transition plan and progress was shared with her GP (Dr Jones) and community matron (Sharon), who make sure that there is connectivity between the health, education and social care aspects of Lena's transition plan. Sharon works closely with Abbas, the manager of a Transitions Team established through social care services. The Transitions Team is based within a Community Hub, a facility shared with NHS, Education, and Youth Services. Dr Jones and Sharon are co-located within the Community Hub so communication with the Transition Team is easy to maintain. Through inter-agency working, they were able to ensure that Lena and her needs were always at the centre of the transition planning process.

Regular (monthly) transition planning meetings take place. These are hosted by the Transition Team with representatives from up to 20 partner agencies including the Children's Continuing Health Care team and community matrons, representatives from schools and colleges, commissioning and finance, Career Connect, housing and advocacy organisations and adult social care. These meetings enable the tracking and monitoring of transition plans for all young people with long-term conditions and disabilities, coordinating multi-agency support, bringing together community health services, social care and education to plan for what is going to happen when the young person turns 18. Ideally, the planning process will have commenced from 11 to 14 years (depending on the readiness of the young person) so Abbas's team are able to work with other agencies to assess needs and develop integrated Education, Health and Care Plans. Abbas explains that these are required in light of the *Children and Families Act 2014*. Abbas also considers Transition Guides produced by the Council for Disabled Children Transition Information Network useful planning tools (Council for Disabled Children Transition Information Network, 2019).

Abbas met Lena when she was 14, during a transition planning meeting at her special school, which the Children's Disability Team organised in partnership with the school nurse and Lena's teacher. Abbas was aware that Lena had supportive, well-informed parents, who were prepared to challenge the local authority to make sure that decisions taken were in Lena's best interests. Abbas also wanted to know how Lena herself felt about her future Transition Plan. Abbas was interested to know more about Lena's ideas about where she will live in the future, her continuing health and social care support needs, her aspirations for her continuing education and what she hoped for when her education was finished.

Ewan (Lena's brother) volunteered to act as an advocate for Lena when she found it difficult to express her ideas and thoughts. Abbas took time to listen to her views and understand her wishes and feelings. Lena said that she would like the opportunity to do more of the things she enjoys (including creative arts, fashion and literature). She also wanted the chance to make more friends of her own age and connect with other people who lived in her community.

The Transitions Team were able to continue to work with the family to explore options available locally to meet Lena's specific needs and interests. When Lena was 16 Abbas took Lena and Ewan to visit a local day centre and the further education college for a look round. Lena and Ewan told their parents the day centre and further education college had many activities that Lena would enjoy and they particularly liked the friendly and welcoming atmosphere at the day centre and the 'buzz' at the college. Lena could also continue to access physiotherapy and speech and language therapy at the day centre.

Abbas and the Transition Team helped the family to put arrangements in place so that Lena could continue her learning and development by attending the day centre 2 days a week and the FE college for 3 days. As Lena has additional 24-hour-care needs, transition planning involved working with commissioners of health and social care services to continue to fund her Personal Budget and ensure that appropriate support needed for Lena at home, as well as when she attends college and the day centre, was provided. Sharon made sure that this was in place and met with Lena's college tutors, carers and transport providers to make sure that Lena's support needs were fully understood and that they are confident in how to meet them. She maintains contact to help with any unexpected issues as they arise.

Lena is now continuing to pursue her interests and is learning some independent living skills. She has new friends at the college, and is getting involved in a cafe, fashion show and gardening project at the day centre. Anna and Natalia's longer-term aspirations are to support Lena to channel her enjoyment of fashion and creative arts to contribute to a community-based micro-enterprise involving production, decoration and selling of jewellery, scarves and T-shirts. Career Connect are helping to organise a placement for Lena at the community organisation that established the micro-enterprise. Ewan helps at the community garden when he can (planting under Lena's instruction!). Abbas has also enabled Ewan to get involved in a local voluntary sector organisation service for young adult carers to ensure that his support needs are not overlooked.

Anna and Natalia have recognised that other families may not be as confident as they are in advocating for young people. They understand how hard it is for parents to let go so that their young people can fulfil their potential, so they have worked with a local charity to develop and deliver a course to help. The course builds confidence and enables families to understand transition. This helps them to work with professionals to achieve the best outcome for the young person involved.

NHS England and NHS Improvement recognise that there is still much work to be done if we are to get transition planning, support and transfer to adult services right for all young people. NHS England, Leading Change, Adding Value Team (2018) At the time of writing, they are working with NHS trusts, clinical commissioning groups and other partners to drive continuing and rapid improvements and shared learning through an NHSi Transition Collaborative (NHS England, 2018).

👤 ACTIVITY 4

Reflect on your learning from reading the chapter.

1. Imagine you had to explain the concept of 'transition' to a young person accessing health services and their parents. How might you define it in terms they could understand?
2. Can you generate your own checklist of best practice principles to ensure effective transition planning and support for young people with long-term conditions and disabilities who are moving between child and adult services?
3. Consider who you might collaborate with to put these principles into practice.
4. Imagine you are working in an NHS Hospital Trust and you have been asked to develop a transition planning tool that can be used by professionals across the trust to develop transition plans for young people aged 11 and upwards. What might it look like and how could you ensure that young people and families are actively engaged in the process … who else might you need to work in partnership with?

REFERENCES

Campbell, F., Biggs, K., Aldiss, S.K., et al., 2016. Transition of care for adolescents from paediatric services to adult health services. Cochrane Database Syst. Rev. 29 (4), CD009794. https://doi.org/10.1002/14651858.CD009794.pub2 (accessed 5 July 2019).

Care Quality Commission, 2014. From the Pond into the Sea: Children's Transition to Adult Health Services. Care Quality Commission, Newcastle. Available from: https://www.cqc.org.uk/sites/default/files/CQC_Transition%20Report_Summary_lores.pdf (accessed 5 July 2019).

Caton, S., Kagan, C., 2007. Comparing transition expectations of young people with moderate learning disabilities with other vulnerable youth and with their non–disabled counterparts. Disabil. Soc. 22 (5), 473–488. https://doi.org/10.1080/09687590701427586 (accessed 5 July 2019).

Coles, B., 1995. Youth and Social Policy. UCL, London.

Cornish, J., 2015. Improving Transition for Children and Young People. NHS England, London. Available from: https://www.england.nhs.uk/blog/jacqueline-cornish-4/ (accessed 5 July 2019).

Council for Disabled 2011. Information and Learning from the Aiming High for Disabled Children Transition Support Programme: A Summary. London, England. Available from: http://www.councilfordisabledchildren.org.uk/media/136250/information_and_learning_from_ the_ahdc_tsp_report_summary.pdf (accessed 5 July 2019).

Council for Disabled Children, 2011. Learning from the Aiming High for Disabled Children Programme. Available from: https://councilfordisabledchildren.org.uk/sites/default/files/field/attachemnt/learning_from_the_ahdc_programme.pdf (accessed 5 July 2019).

Council for Disabled Children Transition Information Network, 2019. Transition Guides Council for Disabled Children. Available from: https://councilfordisabledchildren.org.uk/transition-information-network/information-and-support/transition-guides (accessed 5 July 2019).

Crowley, R., Wolfe, I., Lock, K., McKee, M., 2011. Improving the transition between paediatric and adult healthcare: a systematic review. Arch. Dis. Child. (6), 548–553. https://doi.org/10.1136/adc.2010.202473 (accessed 5 July 2019).

Department of Health, 2006. Transition: getting it right for young people : improving the transition of young people with long term conditions from children's to adult services. Available from dera.ioe.ac.uk. (Accessed 13 November 2020).

Department of Health, 2011. You're Welcome – Quality Criteria for Young People Friendly Health Services. Department of Health, London. Available from: https://assets.publishing.service.gov.uk/government/uploads/system/uploads/attachment_data/file/216350/dh_127632.pdf (accessed 5 July 2019).

Department for Education, 2005. Youth Matters Department for Education (Archived, 2013). Available from: https://webarchive.nationalarchives.gov.uk/20130320215804/https://www.education.gov.uk/publications/standard/publicationDetail/Page1/YGPSUM (accessed 5 July 2019).

Elder, G.H., Johnstone, M.K., Crosnoe, R., 2003. Chapter 1: The Emergence and Development of Life Course Theory in Handbook of the Life Course. Springer, Boston, pp. 3–19.

Erikson, E.H., 1950. Childhood and Society. Norton, New York.

Furlong, A., Cartmel, F., 2006. Young People and Social Change: New Perspectives, second ed. McGraw-Hill Education, Maidenhead, Berkshire, England.

Griffin, C., 1993. Representations of Youth: The Study of Youth and Adolescence in Britain and America. Polity Press, Cambridge.

Healthcare Safety Investigation Branch, 2019. Transition from Child and Adolescent Mental Health Services to Adult Mental Health Services. Available from: https://www.hsib.org.uk/investigations-cases/transition-from-child-and-adolescent-mental-health-services-to-adult-mental-health-services/ (accessed 5 July 2019).

Jones, G., Bell, R., 2000. Balancing Acts: Youth, Parenting and Public Policy. YPS for the Joseph Rowntree Foundation, York.

Jones, G., 2002. The Youth Divide: Diverging Paths into Adulthood. An Exploration of the Inequalities Existing between Different Groups of Young People As They Move into Independent Adulthood. Joseph Rowntree Foundation. Available from: https://www.jrf.org.uk/report/youth-divide-diverging-paths-adulthood (accessed 5 July 2019).

Jones, G., Wallace, C., 1992. Youth, Family and Citizenship, Buckingham (England). Open University Press, Philadelphia.

Leonard, H., Foley, K.R., Pikora, T., et al., 2016. Transition to adulthood for young people with intellectual disability: the experiences of their families. Eur. Child Adolesc. Psychiatry. 25 (12), 1369–1381. https://doi.org/10.1007/s00787-016-0853-2 (accessed 5 July 2019).

Medforth, N., Huntingdon, E., 2017. Still lost in transition? Compr. Child Adolesc. Nurs. 41 (2), 128–142. https://doi.org/10.1080/24694193.2017.1330370 (accessed 5 July 2019).

National Network of Parent Carer Forums, 2020. Thinking About Tomorrow: Preparing for Adult Life. Available at contact org.uk/advice-and-support/preparing-for-adult-life/. (Accessed 13 November 2020).

Nagra, A., et al., 2015. Ready Steady Go University Hospital Southampton NHS Trust. Available from: https://www.uhs.nhs.uk/OurServices/Childhealth/TransitiontoadultcareReadySteadyGo/Transitiontoadultcare.aspx (accessed 5 July 2019).

National Institute for Health and Care Excellence (NICE), 2016a. Transition From Children's to Adult's Services. Quality Standard [QS140]. Available from: https://www.nice.org.uk/guidance/qs140 (accessed 5 July 2019).

National Institute for Health and Care Excellence (NICE), 2016b. Transition from Children's to Adult's Services for Young People Using Health or Social Care Services. NICE Guideline [ng43]. Available from: https://www.nice.org.uk/guidance/ng43 (accessed 5 July 2019).

National Institute for Health and Care Excellence (NICE), 2017. Building Independence Through Planning for Transition Guide. A Quick Guide for Practitioners Supporting Young People. NICE. Available from: https://councilfordisabledchildren.org.uk/sites/default/files/field/attachemnt/NICE%20-%20Building%20independence%20through%20planning%20for%20transition.pdf (accessed 5 July 2019).

National Institute for Health and Care Excellence (NICE) 2017. Implementing Transition Care Locally and Nationally Using the "Ready, Steady, Go" Programme. NICE Shared Learning Database. Available from: https://www.nice.org.uk/sharedlearning/implementing-transition-care-locally-and-nationally-using-the-ready-steady-go-programme (accessed 5 July 2019).

Newcastle University and Northumbria Healthcare NHS Trust, 2017. Health Passports Workshop Facilitator Notes: A Practical Guide to Facilitate Focus Group Sessions Newcastle. Newcastle University. Available from: https://councilfordisabledchildren.org.uk/sites/default/files/field/attachemnt/Health%20Passports%20Facilitator%20Guide_0.pdf (accessed 5 July 2019).

Nguyen, T., Embrett, M., Barr, N.G., et al., 2017. Preventing youth from falling through the cracks between child/adolescent and adult mental health services: a systematic review of models of care. Community Ment. Health J. 53 (4), 375–382. https://doi.org/10.1007/s10597-017-0098-7 (accessed 5 July 2019).

NHS England, 2017. Personal Health Budgets and Integrated Personal Commissioning Quick Guide: Children and Young People. NHS England, London. Available from: https://www.england.nhs.uk/wp-content/uploads/2017/06/516_IPC-QG-Children-and-young-people_S7.pdf (accessed 5 July 2019).

NHS England, 2018. Commissioning for Transition to Adult Services for Young People with Special Educational Needs and Disability (SEND). NHS England, London. Available from: https://www.england.nhs.uk/wp-content/uploads/2018/07/send-quick-guide-commissioning-transition-adult-services.pdf (accessed 5 July 2019).

NHS England Leading ChangeAdding Value Team, 2018. Atlas of Shared Learning: Supporting Young People through Transition into Adult Care Services. NHS England, London. Available from: https://www.england.nhs.uk/atlas_case_study/supporting-young-people-through-transition-into-adult-care-services/ (accessed 5 July 2019).

NHS England. Board Report 27 September 2018. Agenda item 10. 36. Available from: https://improvement.nhs.uk/documents/3252/BM1864_Improvement_report.pdf. (Accessed July 5, 2019).

NHS Foundation Trust, 2017. Implementing Transition Care Locally and Nationally Using the 'Ready, Steady, Go' Programme. NICE Shared Learning Database. Available from: https://www.nice.org.uk/sharedlearning/implementing-transition-care-locally-and-nationally-using-the-ready-steady-go-programme (accessed 5 July 2019).

Public Health England, NHS England, Department of Health, British Youth Council, Association of Young People's Health, Youth Focus North West, 2017. You're Welcome Pilot 2017 Refreshed Standards for Piloting. London. Available from: http://www.youngpeopleshealth.org.uk/yourewelcome/wp-content/uploads/2017/02/YoureWelcome_RefreshedsStandards.pdf (accessed 5 July 2019).

Rogers, J., Brook, L., Aizelwood, L., et al., 2017. The 10 steps transition pathway: improving transition for children in hospital settings. Int. J. Nurs. 5 (2), 1–11. https://doi.org/10.15640/ijn.v5n2a1.

Royal College of Nursing, 2013. Lost in Transition: Moving Young People between Child and Adult Health Service. Royal College of Nursing, London. [Archived].

Royal College of Nursing, 2018. Children and Young People: Transition to Adult Services (Subject Guide). Royal College of Nursing, London. Available from: https://www.swswchd.co.uk/image/Clinical%20information/Transition/Lost%20in%20Transition%202013.pdf (accessed 5 July 2019).

Royal College of Paediatrics and Child Health, 2019. Transition to Adult Services; Best Practice, Resources, Young People's Experiences. Available at rcpch.ac.uk/resources/transition-adult-services. (Accessed 13 November 2020).

Social Care Institute for Excellence, 2014. The Care Act: Transition from Childhood to Adulthood. Available from: https://www.scie.org.uk/care-act-2014/transition-from-childhood-to-adulthood/ (accessed 5 July 2019).

Thompson, R., Bell, R., Holland, J., et al., 2002. Critical moments: choice, chance and opportunity in young people's narratives of transition. Sociology. 36 (2), 335–354. https://doi.org/10.1177/0038038502036002006 (accessed 5 July 2019).

Together For Short Lives, 2015. Stepping Up. A Guide to Enabling a Good Transition to Adulthood for Young People with Life-Limiting and Life-Threatening Conditions. Bristol, Together for Short Lives. Available from: https://www.togetherforshortlives.org.uk/wp-content/uploads/2018/02/ProRes-Stepping-Up-Transition-Care-Pathway.pdf (accessed 5 July 2019).

Young, S., Adamou, M., Asherson, P., et al., 2016. Recommendations for the transition of patients with ADHD from child to adult healthcare services: a consensus statement from the UK adult ADHD network. BMC Psychiatry BMC series – open, inclusive and trusted 16,301. Available from: https://doi.org/10.1186/s12888-016-1013-4 (accessed 5 July 2019).

30

Play for Children and Young People in Hospital and Healthcare Settings

Susan Fairclough,   Edited by Virginia Bennett

LEARNING OUTCOMES

- Understand the importance and benefits of play activities for children and young people
- Explore different types of play and interaction that health professionals and families can engage with to assist the child or young person.
- Understand the roles of Health Play Specialists and Play Leaders and how they are integral within the healthcare team.
- Recognise the value of play for children and young people the in all healthcare settings.

- Recognise the importance of play as a means of communication and interaction with children and young people and their families.
- Identify the benefits of developmental, therapeutic and specialised play for children and young people in healthcare settings.
- Identify how psychological preparation, distraction, diversional and participation therapies can help children and young people's ability to understand about what is happening to them.

THE ROLE OF PLAY FOR CHILDREN AND YOUNG PEOPLE

Play is the language of children and a vital part of every child's life. It is essential for normal growth and development, enabling a child or young person to develop physically, intellectually, emotionally, socially and verbally (Bee & Boyd, 2014). Through play, children acquire knowledge and learn new skills that prepare them to cope with the world around them (Whitebread, 2012). Play is therefore a crucial component of the care and support for children and young people helping them to adapt and deal with illness and injury. Children's nurses are instrumental in the promotion of all aspects of children and young people health and wellbeing and play forms a critical part of implementing public health agendas and accident prevention programmes, influencing children's understanding and behaviour (Warwick et al., 2009). Communicating healthy messages and engaging children and young people in fun and enjoyable educational activities to promote healthy messages and behaviours as well as facilitating recovery from illness and injury.

Play can mitigate against stressful interventions (Weaver et al 2007) for example where children and young people have faced traumatic, distressing or unpleasant procedures or situations. Play becomes particularly important when children and young people experience illness, injury or when a planned procedure or treatment is required. As children's nurses our duty is to ensure the children and young people's need are met holistically, and even when faced with the most critically ill and injured children and young people, the provision of play must feature. However, in busy health care environments such as children's wards and accident and emergency departments opportunities to provide play can be missed especially when the children and young people's condition is serious and much of the focus is on the resolving clinical symptoms. Moreover, in adult centric environments where staff are not equipped with the knowledge and skills required to care for children, play can often be overlooked. Such tensions form part of contemporary nursing practice where advancements in technology, the dominance of medical models of practice, and crises in skill mix and staffing can sometimes overshadow the most fundamental of children and young people needs. In this context, the importance of the role of children's nurses to advocate for the provision of play cannot be understated.

This chapter will introduce an overview of the emergence of play in children and young people care in hospital settings. The multiple functions of play for children and young people are outlined in Box 30.1. And further to this the chapter offers some insight into the role of play for children and young people with disability, and in preparing and minimising the effects of illness and hospitalisation on the children and young people. Children's nurses play a pivotal role in the care, support and promotion of health and wellbeing of children across a variety of settings. However, child focused contemporary healthcare relies on multidisciplinary teams working together with the child and family central to all aspects of care and support. The vital, innovative role of health play specialists and play leaders in facilitating and leading play across children's services is restated across the chapter. At key points in the chapter there are reflective activities aimed at developing critical thought and reflective learning.

with sick and vulnerable children in modern healthcare settings. Axline developed eight basic principles of non-directive play therapy that can be adapted and applied to the relationships that children's nurses and Health Play Specialists are required to develop with children (www.playtherapy.org.uk).

The children's nurse or health play specialist must:
- Develop a warm and friendly relationship with the child
- Accept the child as she or he is
- Establish a relationship with the child so that the child feels free to express their feelings
- Is alert to recognise the feelings expressed by the child and reflects this back for the child to gain insight to their own behaviour
- Maintains genuine respect, provide choice and opportunity for the children to solve their own problems or identify needs- all responsibility is with the child
- Does not attempt to direct the child's actions or conversations in any manner. Child leads, professional follows
- Does not hurry play therapy
- Establish limitations where necessary to ensure play is related to the world of reality and alert the child to their responsibility in the relationship.

THE DEVELOPMENT OF PLAY IN THE HEALTHCARE ENVIRONMENT

The need for all children to play remains constant wherever they may be receiving care, no matter what stage in their health or illness trajectory. The children and young people's right to play is enshrined in Article 31, of the UN Convention on the Rights of the Child (UNCRC 1989). In this context, all parties are required to promote *the provision of appropriate and equal opportunities for cultural, artistic, recreational and leisure activity* (p. 10).

Recognition of the influence that healthcare settings and organisations have in creating the conditions for the provision of play was initially acknowledged in The Platt Report (Ministry of Health, 1959). Leading on from this the formation of the National Association for the Welfare of Children in Hospital now named Action for Sick Children was formed and in 1975 the provision of play featured through the establishment of The National Association of Hospital Play Staff, today known as the National Association of Health Play Specialists. During this period there was an increasing recognition of

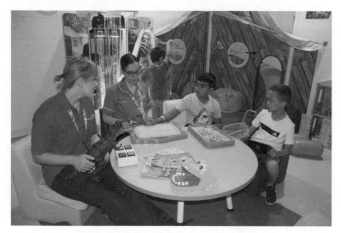

Fig. 30.1 Play Session in Playroom.

PRINCIPLES OF PLAY THERAPY

Whilst play is an essential activity for all children through which they learn and develop, children who are sick and vulnerable are likely to require therapeutic play. Play is termed therapeutic when there is an intended outcome beneficial for the child because of play haven taken place (Kool and Lawver, 2010).

There are two popular approaches to the promotion of play; directive therapeutic play and non-directive therapeutic play (Axline ,1974) although it is likely that a combination of these two approaches are observed in practice. Virginia Axline was psychologist whose research on children's play underpins approaches to modern play therapy

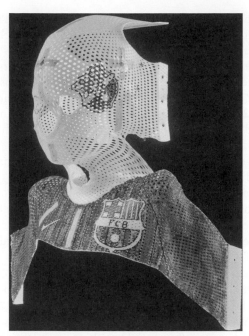

Fig. 30.2 Radiotherapy Masks Developed in The Christie Hospital, Manchester.

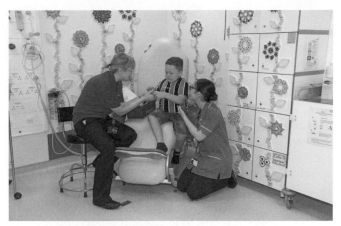

Fig 30.3 Distraction Therapy with Patients.

children's rights and that they should not be treated as small adults. Across the UK healthcare settings where children were in receipt of care, children's nurses and leaders in children's play services paved the way to advocate for more child friendly environments with play as the cornerstone. A gradual change in culture and attitude to the need for play provision in children and young people health services was championed by the emerging profession of health play specialists as part of children and young people healthcare teams in children's hospitals across the UK. This movement continues to emerge to date with experts in play blending imagination and reality to promote play provision in specialist emerging areas such as children and young people radiotherapy (Fig. 30.2). The importance of play children's lives continues to feature across contemporary child health policy to date (Royal College of Paediatrics and Child Health, 2018) with commissioning of children's play services an important established and growing area. Crucial to this continued growth are environments that foster attitudes and cultures where play is a normal, expected part of children and young people care and is encouraged and supported.

THE ROLE OF THE HEALTH PLAY SPECIALIST

With play as the central function of their role, health play specialists and play leaders are integral members of the multidisciplinary healthcare team for children and young people and enhancing the quality of care provided (Walker, 2006). They are involved in the design and delivery of play services and undertake a range of play methods, activities and interventions that ensure play forms part of every child's healthcare experience. Working closely with the multidisciplinary team,

health play specialists work with children's nurses to minimise the effects of what may be lengthy and uncomfortable treatments (Figure 30.3).

Although Health Play Specialists engage in many developmental therapeutic and patient experience activities, their focus is to alleviate any worries or misconceptions and to help the children and young people to cope with their changing health needs. Depending on the speciality, some health play specialists will be involved more in preparation i.e. preparing the child for operating theatre. In more specialist roles their expertise may be called on for long term one to one play interventions to help desensitise children and young people who have phobias and fears where a trusting therapeutic relationship is deepened through play (Kool & Lawver, 2010). Clearly health play specialists are an important resource and their expert play input is required across the children and young people healthcare journey. Prospectively, their skills may be called upon to ensure play features in the design and development of children and young people services for example the design of multi-sensory rooms, teenage facilities and outside play areas. In the tertiary hospital setting health play specialists may be members of an on-call rota to assist in complex care cases that requires specialist play interventions out of hours.

The key role of health play specialists and play leaders has been outlined. They are active members of the multi-disciplinary team influencing the quality of experience for the children and young people and their family during the healthcare journey.

> **ACTIVITY**
>
> Arrange some time with the health play specialists, observe, discuss and participate in play provision.

PROFESSIONAL BOUNDARIES AND PLAY

The unique language of play is a valuable form of communication when children and young people may be vulnerable and experiencing challenges physically and psychologically.

A rapport can be developed through play, particularly when a therapeutic approach is enacted, and very close, unique professional bonds may emerge with children and young people and their families. In this context promoting play sensitively with the children and young people, whilst carefully observing behaviour, expressions, emotions or memories is important in assessing and meeting their needs. In complex cases for example where the children and young people is receiving palliative care, it is appropriate to seek the help of a professional who has expertise and skills to meet such specific needs (Boucher et al., 2014). Axline (1974) suggests that children reveal their inner self through play and learn to understand themselves and others around them. In such close and personal exchanges, it is crucial to carefully observe professional boundaries in relation to disclosure of information that may raise safeguarding concerns and the emotional and mental health needs of the children and young people (Children Act, 2004; NMC, 2015).

THE ROLE OF PLAY IN CHILDREN'S NURSING PRACTICE

Given that play can reduce the psychological trauma of hospitalisation and is the vehicle through which children express and interact (Jolley, 2007), it is vital that play is an integral component of high-quality health care. As such it is critical that children's nurses have the knowledge, skills and attitudes to promote play as part of their nursing practice. Childhood injuries, illness and disability may compromise children and young people's ability to play, potentially causing a disruption to the continuum of their development and general wellbeing. To prevent these negative consequences, children's nurses must develop the knowledge and skills to promote play as part of all care, in all situations and settings, no matter the age or stage of the child's illness or injury. For the children and young people, play has many functions, and all are important for health and wellbeing (Box 30.1). The regulatory function of play enables children to deal with frightening and stressful situations, communicate emotions, fears, thoughts and experiences. This is particularly important for children and young people with illness or injury. Observing a child or young person engaged in a play activity can often look as if they are purely passing time, however from a child's perspective play does not have a purpose other than being fun and to express what happens to be occupying the child's mind at the time. Through play whether alone, one to one or in a group setting, children and

young people use play to learn to cope and live with illness, to adapt to their altered health status and for most children to move to recovery.

Observing a child play provides the children's nurse with a unique view of a child's holistic wellbeing and forms a vital component informing the holistic assessment of their needs (RCN, 2017). Knowledge about the types of play underpin all good holistic assessment and care delivery. The children's nurse will draw on knowledge about:

1. The expected developmental stage and attainment for child's age
2. The developmental attainment of the child prior to illness or hospitalisation (obtained by history taking usually from parents/ carers)
3. The effects of the illness upon the child manifested in the child's current willingness or ability to play

The key skills of good of nursing assessment involves the application of child development theory to nursing observation of the children and young people (Glasper et al., 2010).

Lev Vygotsky (1896 – 1934) reported 5 broad types of play that he claimed to influence children's learning and their psychological and physiological developmental function (Box 30.3).

PLAY AND THE CHILDREN AND YOUNG PEOPLE WITH DISABILITY AND COMPLEX HEALTHCARE NEEDS (CHCN)

Play is an integral part of every child's/young person's life. children and young people with learning disabilities and complex healthcare needs benefit from the use of play, interaction and therapeutic play during their hospital stay and as a means of coping with ongoing challenges of their condition. Therefore, it is essential that play is tailored to the children and young people's specific needs.

To meet the needs of the children and young people with a disability or CHCN, the social model of disability requires all health care professionals adapt their communication and skills to effectively meet the physical, social, emotional and cognitive needs of the children and young people. All health professionals have a duty to make reasonable adjustments as part of their practice to meet the needs of the children and young people with disability

---

BOX 30.3   Types of play

- Physical play
- Play with objects,
- Symbolic play,
- Pretence/ socio-dramatic play (role play)
- Games with rules

TABLE 30.1 Popular Types of Play Promoted in Healthcare Settings

Types of play	Description of play activity	Example of the situation where this play will be useful for recovery & wellbeing
Physical play	Physical play is an activity that requires movement. It involves either large motor skills such as running, jumping, throwing and hopping activities. The use of fine motor skills such as art and crafts, building, jigsaws, threading and musical instruments. Activities and games are interactive and fun (Fig. 30.4).	Often used in treatment assisting physiotherapists, occupational therapists, speech and language therapists and dieticians. Physical play encourages the child/young person to move and keep active and is also used to help assess the patient A team of professionals are likely to be involved to promote recovery and function i.e. A physiotherapist supporting a child who has a fractured femur who is immobilised in a Thomas Splint and balanced traction.
Imaginative Play- includes role play	Provides children and young people opportunity to use their naturally inquisitive minds to explore different scenarios. It can prompt conversation and is often a good opportunity to express themselves and discuss any fears or worries. These can often be acted out possibly even unknowingly through role play can help expression in a fun way. Provide an outlet of emotions and allow children/young people to express their feelings and opens communication. Assists the health, wellbeing and recovery process.	Play is guided by the child. Imaginative play and role play could include dressing up in staff costumes, hospital toy sets, hospital doctor's sets, dolls, houses and figurines such as play mobil ™. Widely used in preparation for hospital or a procedure such as pre-admission programmes (Fig. 30.5).
Outdoor play	Access to fresh air, and the outdoors The aim is to offer patients this as it is beneficial to their emotional and physical well-being. It also takes them out of the clinical area if they are well enough Promotes exercise and physical activity. May provide access to socialise with other children at play.	**Patient story:** As part of a daily routine, a young patient could go to the outside play area with the health play specialist, a nurse and parent. He was a patient on the High Dependency Unit (area of intensive care). He enjoyed the fresh air away from the clinical environment and sounds of all the intensive care monitors and equipment. He was able to engage in some physical activity although he had many restrictions. He enjoyed the outdoor environment and looked forward to his daily visits (Fig. 30.6).
Sensory play	Involve the child touching, smelling, hearing, tasting and using vision All ages can participate Especially beneficial to children or young people with additional needs and sensory impairment. children and young people with hypersensitivity or who are on the autism spectrum may like or dislike aspects of sensory play and, therefore reasonable adjustments must be considered. Multi-sensory play can be both calming and stimulating depending on the patient's needs	Include messy play such as sand, water, play dough or splashing paint. Use of music, multi-sensory environments, fibre optic lights, bubble tubes, interactive floor projector or wall projectors, tactile toys and equipment, ceiling mobiles, stories, water play, hand held activities and toys. Multi-sensory rooms are an excellent resource as they can offer stimulation or relaxation away from the busy clinical environment. The rooms are usually equipped with fibre optic lights, wall interactive panels, bubble tubes, sensory toys, floor and wall projectors plus interactive floors. Mobile multi-sensory equipment can be used on wards next to beds and in cubicles. Many hospitals have mobile multi-sensory units and projectors as well as those in situ in the multi-sensory rooms (Fig. 30.7). The wall and floor projectors can also be used in hospital entrances and ward entrances as they project images on the floor and walls for visual effects and can be interactive. Multi-sensory equipment is often used on the Intensive Care and High Dependency Units. Parents and staff have commented that when the sensory equipment is used with relaxing music the ward atmosphere is changed into a calming space and their perception of the bleeping monitors is not as prominent (Fig. 30.8).

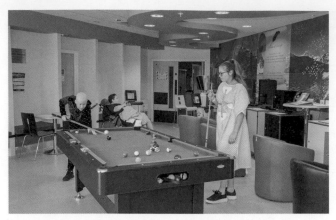

Fig. 30.4 Child/Young Person 11 Plus in the Teen Zone.

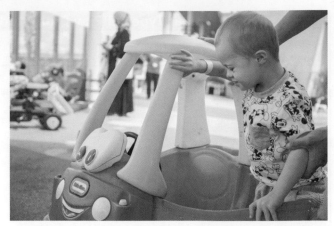

Fig. 30.6 Child in Outdoor Play and Sensory Garden.

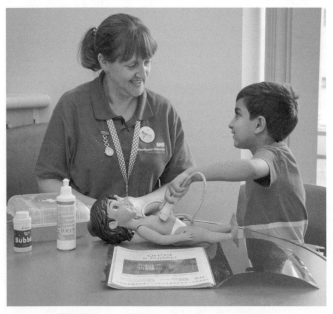

Fig. 30.5 Child/Children Engaged in Role Play).

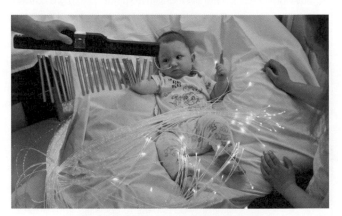

Fig. 30.7 Child in Multi-Sensory Room.

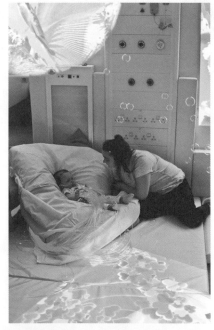

Fig. 30.8 Child with Projector/Wall and Floor.

(Disability Discrimination Act, 1995) and this should form part of the care plan. Accessing training in the use of alternative communication skills and aids, such as Makaton and Picture Exchange Communication Systems (PECS), has helped student nurses to communicate with children who have learning difficulties (Vinales, 2012). Play provides the essential means to achieve this, tailoring the environment to meet the needs of the children and young people. This may involve removing stressful and frightening stimuli and replacing these with calming, familiar play and activities that promote the children and young people's health and wellbeing.

The provision of a supportive environment e.g. without distractions for either staff or children and young people can reduce anxiety in people with learning disabilities or autism. Autistic people may be sensitive to aspects of the environment such as ambient noise, crowds and bright lights (NICE, 2018). Children and young people with Autism Spectrum Disorder can react to hospital admission in different ways and having access to a staff member with appropriate training and experience can reduce distress and improve the patient and staff experience (Pratt et al., 2011).

It is therefore key that children and young people with disability and CHCN are assessed for their individual holistic needs. Best practice involves person centred communication with the children and young people and their parents or carers (McCormack and McCance, 2016), whilst utilising the skills of specialist health play members of the team (Box 30.4. Blair (2013) has promoted the use of 'flagging' the needs of children and young people with disabilities and CHCN on the medical records and the hospital passports to make these more visible to the healthcare professional team. This creates good communication, promotes the retrieval of relevant information and enables a personalised plan of care that includes play and is tailored to the children and young people's individual needs.

 ACTIVITY

Write a short reflection about a children and young people's health condition or disability and how it affected their ability to play.

 REFLECT ON YOUR PAST

If you were the children's nurse caring for the child, how would you help support the child to play?

BOX 30.4   proposed Mandatory Training to Include Play as Part of a Reasonable Adaption for Children and Young People with Autism.

- Some children and young people have additional needs, learning disabilities, communication difficulties or are on the autistic spectrum and require bespoke interventions and care.
- Emeritus Professor Alan Glasper from the University of Southampton in 2019 promoted Oliver's Campaign spearheaded by Paula McGowan, following the death of her 18-year-old son Oliver in hospital. This campaign has lobbied the government to give additional training to all healthcare and social care staff in England about caring for people with learning disability or autism.
- The proposal for introducing mandatory training seeks to develop the practical skills of the workforce to ensure they can make reasonable adjustments in practice to improve the way people with a learning disability plus autistic people of all ages are supported.
- Play forms an important part of the adjustment for support for children and young people with autism and learning disabilities.
- The proposed mandatory training requires staff to have a basic understanding of the principles of the following legislation:
  - Mental Health Act (1983)
  - Children and Families Act (2014)
  - Autism Act (2009)

REDUCING THE EFFECTS OF HOSPITALISATION THROUGH PLAY

The negative effects of hospitalisation, illness or injury on the children and young people can be mitigated through the promotion of play. In this context play is a normalising activity that can help to transform a stressful situation and environment. The use of play in the design, organisation and delivery of care for children and young people protects them from psychological stresses and helps them and their family cope.

Contemporary children's healthcare philosophy is underpinned by the longstanding recognition that hospital admission needs to be as brief as possible and unless essential, avoided and care delivered in the home (Ministry of Health,1959; Department of Health England, 2004). Driven by this philosophy and a need to deliver prudent healthcare, a plethora of children's services, investigatory, medical and surgical procedures are carried out in outpatient and day service settings, with the average stay in hospital being dramatically reduced.

This change is in children and young people's best interest however it requires impeccable holistic preparation and a mix of psychological and practical support. The principles of play outlined in the following sections are invaluable for nursing practice as most children undergo some form of intervention when they are in hospital settings and have needs that requires healthcare professionals' intervention.

PRE AND POST PROCEDURAL PLAY

Firstly, not all children/young people are prepared for treatment procedures and blood tests etc. They may come into hospital as an emergency, medical emergency or accident. It is, therefore, important to know the techniques used can be beneficial for those not prepared as well as those who have had the opportunity to be prepared. Pain may be experienced during a procedure and this is often the primary fear for many children able to make this association. McCaffery and Beebe (1989) stated that distraction is a valuable asset of pain management and should be used in combination with prescribed evidence based pharmacological protocols.

THE ROLE OF PLAY IN DISTRACTION AND DIVERSIONAL THERAPY

The primary aim of distraction and diversional therapies is to take the children and young people's focus and attention away from the procedure itself (Box 30.6). A variety of techniques, methods and tools are used to do this. When distraction is successful, it can help to form a temporary barrier between the child's/young person's fearful mind and the physical experience of the procedure. This, in turn, can reduce any anxieties or perceptions of pain and take the child's/young person's thoughts away from the emotional turmoil they may be feeling inside.

Parents and carers need to support at this time also as they also may have anxiety and fears, and these may be conveyed to the children and young people. Some children and young people choose to participate and want to watch what is happening and may ask questions. It is important to find out whether they want to be distracted or watch the procedure and to provide choice for them to change their mind during the procedure. Many children and young people like to take part and be given a responsibility during the procedure like holding a plastic blood bottle or holding the stickers to give to everyone once the procedure is completed. Box 30.5 provides comprehensive guidance for the use of play and distraction during a procedure.

BOX 30.5 Guidance for the Use of Play and Distraction During a Procedure.

Preparation for the Procedure
- A calm child friendly environment is essential. The room where the procedure is to take place should afford privacy and all equipment required must be prepared before the child enters.
- Before any procedure takes place, it is useful to find out whether the child/young person wants to be distracted or participate and find out how they want or can communicate.
- Give the children and young people choice about options like positioning or if they want to sit on a parent's knee or on a chair. The positioning will depend on the procedure but the more choices the children and young people is offered the more they feel included and considered.
- Most procedures require the children and young people to remain still. This can be particularly difficult for very young children distraction and techniques may aid this. The techniques must relate to the child/young person's age and developmental ability as well as their choice. This can vary from many items in distraction boxes including:
  - pop-up toys
  - blowing bubbles
  - musical toys
  - interactive games
  - puppets
  - technology
  - conversation
  - storytelling
  - basic guided imagery (Fig. 30.9)
- Make sure everyone knows their role during the procedure, including parents, to ensure the distraction or participation therapy is effective, safe and successful. This avoids confusion and over stimulation that could threaten the success of the procedure.

During the Procedure
- Good timing and communication is essential and everyone should be aware of the plan.
- Children/young people get bored or lose interest or their clinical condition can quickly change so it is necessary to assess the children and young people and the situation and constantly and adapt the distraction methods accordingly.
- If distraction is commenced too early, the child/young person's focus may have been lost before the procedure has even begun.
- The child/young person should be allowed to cry if he/she wishes as it allows some release and be reassured and praised for keeping still while the procedure is being done.
- The person undertaking the procedure is the one to say when the procedure is finished.

Post procedure
- Positive reinforcement should be offered. All efforts of the child/young person should be praised whether the procedure was successful or not.
- Rewards given to the children and young people should be developmentally appropriate i.e. stickers, certificates of participation in a fun activity such as blowing bubbles.
- Invite the children and young people to reward the nursing and medical staff who undertook the procedure as this reinforces empowerment for the children and young people.
- Evaluate the procedure from the child and parent's perspective. Their feedback should be adopted into the care plan should future procedures be required.
- Provide the opportunity for the children and young people to undertake a play activity (post procedural play) or to do something that is normal for them. This facilitates expression of feelings in a safe way and encourages communication.
- Record the key observations and outcomes of the procedure
- (RCN, 2017)

BOX 30.6 Principles for Preparing a Child for a Procedure

There are some important things to remember when preparing a child or young person:
- Be honest.
- Use appropriate and child friendly language.
- Find out how the child communicates and what he or she would like to know.
- Use the correct terms for equipment to avoid confusion. Use the real names then explain what they do.
- Stay calm and relaxed to instil confidence and reassure the child and family.
- Be aware that the child may not necessarily be fearful of the procedure itself but may be worried about the implications.

With an intimate invasive procedure, the child may be embarrassed during the procedure or worried about the results.
- Consider timing when undertaking preparations. For some children/young people doing this too early can exacerbate fears because they have limited concept and understanding of time and so struggle to manage their fears in relation to this but, if done too late, when a child/young person is already distressed, it may not be successful because stress impairs the ability to absorb information.
- Always be vigilant and look for non-verbal clues to detect whether the child is paying attention.
- Spend time with siblings including them whenever possible.

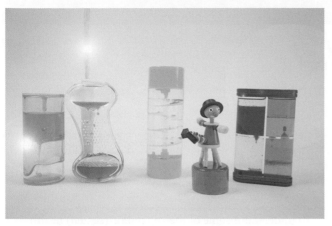

Fig. 30.9 Distraction Toys and Equipment.

DESENSITISATION THROUGH PLAY

Developing a fear or phobia is not unusual and desensitising children and young people occurs through play. This can be a lengthy process in which a child is subjected to controlled exposure of an object or situation that creates fear. The technique involves detailed planning and constant monitoring and must always be carried out under trained professional supervision. Health play specialists offer basic desensitisation however for more complex cases will be referred to a children and young people Psychology team. Box 30.6 provides an outline of the professional principals of desensitisation through play.

▎SUMMARY

And so, we end this chapter having provided a brief overview and examples of play as an integral part of the assessment, preparation and care that all children and young people have the right to receive when they are ill, injured or hospitalised. We have illustrated just a few of the innovations and developments in the promotion of play and have offered practical advice about the preparation and the use of distraction that can be readily adapted into children's nursing practice. We close the chapter with an exhortation to children's nurses to remember that when children are sick and admitted to hospital, they are at their most vulnerable. Play provides a link to normality for the children and young people, and for us as professionals, provides a window to their feelings and needs. Play can make a difference.

REFERENCES

Autism Act (2009) Available at https://www.legislation.gov.uk/ukpga/2009/15

Axline, V.M., 1974. Play Therapy. Ballantine Books, New York, USA.

Bee, H.L., Boyd, D.G., 2014. The Developing Child, 13th Edition. Pearson, New International, Harlow.

Blair, J., 2013. Everybody's life has worth: getting it right in hospital for people with an intellectual disability and reducing clinical risks. Clin. Risk 19, 58–63.

Boucher, S., Downing, J., Shemilt, R., 2014. The Role of Play in Children's Palliative Care. Children (1), 302–317.

Children Act (2004) available at: https://www.legislation.gov.uk/ukpga/2004/31

Children and Families Act (2014) available at http://www.legislation.gov.uk/ukpga/2014/6/contents/enacted

Department of Health (England), 2004. National Service Framework of Children, Young People and Maternity Services – Children and Young People Who Are Ill: Change for Children. Available at: https://www.gov.uk/government/publications/national-service-framework-children-young-people-and-maternity-services.

Disability Discrimination Act (1995) Available at http://www.legislation.gov.uk/ukpga/1995/50

Glasper, A., Aylott, M., Battrick, C., 2010. Developing Practical Skills for Nursing Children & Young People – Hodder Arnold. Publishers) Ltd.

Jolley, J., 2007. Separation and psychological trauma: a paradox examined. Pediat. Nurs 19, 22–25.

Kool, R., Lawver, T., 2010. Play Therapy: considerations and applications for the practitioner. Psychiatry (Edgmont) 7 (10), 19–24.

McCaffery, Beebe, 1989. Needle Phobia an Anaesthesiologist Perspective. J. Paediatr 122, 9–13.

McCormack, B., McCance, T., 2016. Person-Centred Practice in Nursing and Health Care: Theory and. Practice. John Wiley & Sons, Oxford.

Mental Health Act (1983) Available at: https://www.legislation.gov.uk/ukpga/1983/20/contents

Ministry of Health, 1959. The Welfare of Children in Hospital, Platt Report. Her Majesty's Stationery Office, London.

National Institute for Health and Care Excellence (NICE), 2018. Learning disabilities and behaviour that challenges: service design and delivery: NICE guideline [NG93]. available at: https://www.nice.org.uk/guidance/ng93.

Nursing and Midwifery Council, 2015. The Code. available at https://www.nmc.org.uk/globalassets/sitedocuments/nmc-publications/nmc-code.pdf.

www.playtherapy.org.uk (accessed on 19th June 2019) available at :https://playtherapy.org.uk/ChildrensEmotionalWellBeing/AboutPlayTherapy/MainPrinciples/AxlinePrinciples)

Piajet, J., 1963. The Origins of Intelligence in Children. Norton, New York.

Pratt, K., Baird, G., Gringras, P., 2011. In: Ensuring Successful Admission to Hospital for Young People with Learning Difficulties, Autism and Challenging Behaviour; A Continuous Quality Improvement and Change Management Programme. 38. Childcare, Health and Development, pp. 789–797.

Royal college of Nursing, 2017. Standards for Assessing and Monitoring Vital Signs in Infants, Children and Young People. RCN, London.

Royal College of Paediatrics and Child Health (2019) Facing the Future: Standards for Children in Emergency Care Settings. Available at https://www.rcpch.ac.uk/sites/default/files/2018-06/ftf_emergency_standards_digital_-_website_version.pdf

United Nations (UN), 1989. The United Nations Convention on the Rights of the Child. UN, Geneva.

Vinales, J., 2012. Evaluation of Makaton in Practice by Children's Nursing Students – Nursing Children and Young People. 25, pp. 14–17 3.

Walker, J., 2006. Play for Health: Delivering and Auditing Quality in Hospital Play Services. National Association of Hospital Play Specialists, London.

Weaver, K., Battrick, C., Glasper, E.A., 2007. Developing a Hospital Play Guideline and Protocol for Sick Children with Debilitating Fears. Child. Young. People's. Nur 1 (3), 143–149.

Whitebread, D., 2012. The Importance of Play. University of Cambridge.

World Health Organisation, 1996. Play in Hospital, 1st Ed. WHO, Geneva.

31

Sexual Health in Childhood and Young Adulthood

Debbie Fallon, Elizabeth Podesta

LEARNING OUTCOMES

- To understand the process of sexual development in utero and develop insight into disorders of sexual development (DSD).
- To have an awareness of healthy sexual development in children and young people.
- To explore the health and well-being experiences of LGBT young people.

- To understand some of the key public (sexual) health issues for children and young people, including unintended pregnancy and sexually transmitted infection.
- To gain insight into key policy issues including those related to sex and relationships education.
- To understand current child protection strategies that focus on sexual health.

INTRODUCTION

The sexual health care of children and young people is a complex topic that has evolved in the context of medical advancement and immense social change. These changes have been driven by a broadening understanding of gender, a greater appreciation of what constitutes adolescent sexuality and heightened awareness of childhood sexual exploitation (CSE) through high profile media coverage of CSE cases. These are challenging times for nurses in sexual health settings and specialist child protection settings, and also in the context of primary care, including schools.

Much of the visible work around children and young people's sexual health takes place under the umbrella of public health, focusing on health outcomes, such as the reduction of sexually transmitted infection (STI) or unintended pregnancy rates. Such work is informed by research, debate and global comparisons in search of 'what works best'. However, it can be challenging to provide effective youth-friendly sexual health services and sex and relationships education in the context of polarised public opinion about what is 'appropriate'. Health-care providers must rise to these challenges if they are to adequately meet the needs for children and young people, including marginalised groups, such as young people with disabilities, care experienced young people, or lesbian, gay, bisexual or transgender (LGBT) young people.

Importantly, and as the World Health Organization (WHO, 2006) definition shown later illustrates, we need to acknowledge that sexuality is part of sexual health, which means that sexual health is not just an issue for young people who are sexually active – it is an issue for all. In light of this, the chapter also explores contemporary understandings of sexual behaviour in young children.

In addition, this chapter considers some of the issues that arise when there are problems with the physical sexual development of the fetus in utero leading to a DSD. This is important because the care of these families is undergoing a significant philosophical shift as those infants who underwent surgery to 'normalise' their genitalia are now adults who are sharing the impact this has had on their lives.

SEXUAL HEALTH

The World Health Organization defines sexual health as:

> *… a state of physical, emotional, mental and social well-being in relation to sexuality; it is not merely the absence of disease, dysfunction or infirmity. Sexual health requires a positive and respectful approach to sexuality and sexual relationships, as well as the possibility of having pleasurable and safe sexual experiences, free of coercion, discrimination and violence. For sexual health to be attained and maintained, the sexual rights of all persons must be respected, protected and fulfilled.*
>
> *WHO (2006)*

 ACTIVITY

What human rights violations in relation to sexual health are you aware of that take place either in the UK or internationally? How many of these affect children or young people?

This definition of sexual health reflects the WHO definition of 'health' that was coined some 60 years earlier in 1946. Where it differs is in the addition of a reference to sexuality and an acknowledgement that sexual health cannot be achieved without respect for, or the protection of, certain human rights. Other definitions of sexual health (e.g. Public Health England, 2018) extend the description to emphasise that access to advice and services around contraception, sexually transmitted infections, HIV and termination of pregnancy are among these rights.

Although the WHO (2006) definition refers to *all persons*, discussions about sexual health can be complex for children's nurses because in contemporary society, issues related to sexual health and sexuality are generally discussed in terms of adult sexual activity. However, sexuality is a much broader concept than 'sex' since it has emotional, social, cultural and physical dimensions. Sexual development in childhood is part of sexuality, and it begins much earlier in life than puberty.

ACTIVITY

Could the WHO (2006) definition of sexual health be rewritten to more effectively reflect the experience and needs of children and young people in today's society? What would you include?

AGE-APPROPRIATE SEXUAL BEHAVIOUR

The topic of sexuality in children and young people can provoke uncomfortable feelings for some adults. This is because it is not a topic that is generally openly discussed, and because the many and varied cultural, ethical and religious views about appropriate sexual behaviour that an individual experiences through their own upbringing can influence what they consider to be either 'normal' or acceptable sexual behaviour.

ACTIVITY

What are the socially determined norms of acceptable sexual behaviour in your own community? Do any of these norms conflict with the WHO definition of sexual health?

Sexual behaviour is described as 'appropriate' when it is consistent with the child or young person's age and developmental status. In young children this behaviour generally reflects harmless curiosity that they can be distracted from with relative ease. Importantly though, age-appropriate sexual behaviour in children and young people only involves consensual activity with equals in terms of age and developmental status where no individual comes to either physical or emotional harm (National Society for the Prevention of Cruelty to Children [NSPCC], 2019a).

CONSENT IN THE LAW

Sexual activity involving children under 16 is unlawful in the UK *(Sexual Offences Act 2003)* this 'age of consent' reflects societal concerns about the vulnerability of children below 16 to exploitation or abuse. However, it is acknowledged that a minority of young people are sexually active below this age, and Crown Prosecution Service (CPS) guidance suggests that if these young people involved are of a similar age, and if the activity was mutually agreed and non-exploitative, then they should not be prosecuted. Children aged below 13 years, though, are considered to be particularly vulnerable and so any sexual activity with a child of this age is subject to the maximum penalties in law – whatever the age of the perpetrator (Department for Education, 2018).

Although professionals should have a good understanding of healthy sexual development in children and young people it can still be difficult for them to determine whether the sexual behaviours they may witness are appropriate or not. Equally, parents are not always aware of what to expect as a child develops sexually and so may struggle to identify or respond to what is adrift of appropriate behaviour and they may turn to health professionals for advice. Importantly, such an assessment may be the key to recognising whether the behaviour is simply healthy sexual development or whether the child or young person is exhibiting harmful behaviour that may indicate a need for further scrutiny. This means that understanding healthy childhood sexual development and issues of consent are central to the prevention of childhood sexual abuse.

Children learn from a very young age about what is acceptable to others through the process of primary socialisation, and so the way that a professional, parent or other trusted adult responds to a child or young person's sexuality is important as it can shape future behaviour. This can be something as simple as a toddler learning about when it is acceptable to take off their clothes and when it is not, or a more complex issue such as young people seeking sexual health advice or treatment. Adults that respond either verbally or non-verbally in a way that shows lack of understanding, or that indicates embarrassment or disapproval, are unlikely to be seen as trusted sources of support or information for children and young people, which may lead them to seek their answers from other potentially less reliable places.

There are a number of tools and guidelines designed to help both professionals and parents distinguish between healthy and harmful sexual behaviour. The young people's sexual health charity Brook, for example, has developed a Traffic Light Sexual Behaviours tool to categorise the sexual behaviours of young people as green (safe and healthy behaviour), amber (potentially outside of safe and healthy behaviour) or red (outside of safe and healthy behaviour) in order to provide professionals with a standardised criteria to aid decision making (Brook, 2012). The tool identifies age-appropriate behaviours in those aged 0–5 years, 5–9 years, 9–13 years, and 13–17 years, and is used in conjunction with a set of guidelines. The NSPCC (2019a) also provides a guide to stages of age-appropriate sexual behaviour using similar age bandings. This guide outlines how sexual behaviour emerges in infancy and moves through childhood to young adulthood, beginning for example with kissing and hugging, through to developing curiosity and discussion of private body parts using age-appropriate language in early childhood, and moving to increased curiosity about sex and sexual behaviour in pre-adolescence (aged 10–12 years). From 13 to 16 years, with the onset of puberty, the guide suggests that sexual behaviour may involve taking more interest in body parts, relationships and sexuality, using sexual language, talking about sex with friends, masturbating in private or experimenting sexually with the same age group through dating or longer lasting relationships.

Both guides emphasise that learning about sex and sexual behaviour is a normal part of childhood development but stress that children and young people do not all reach puberty or mature emotionally at the same chronological age. Health care professionals should be mindful of this, together with an awareness that children with cognitive impairments or developmental delay may not 'fit' neatly into these guides either. If a young person does exhibit harmful sexual behaviour either to a member of their family or to members of the public then health and social care professionals are directed to the National Institute for Clinical Excellence guideline *Harmful sexual behaviour among children and young people* (NICE, 2016).

ADOLESCENCE AND SEXUALITY

Puberty (focusing on physical development) and adolescence (focusing on psychosocial development) are essential concepts that underpin young people's sexual health. However, since these issues are discussed comprehensively in Chapters 2 and 12 they will be referred to rather than outlined in depth here.

Although sexuality develops across the lifespan, it is adolescence that is most commonly thought of as the time of 'emerging' sexuality because it is generally perceived as synonymous with puberty (Russell, 2005). As a period of noticeable physiological change that often coincides with both increased desire and increased opportunities for intimate relationships, adolescence and puberty create the conditions in which a young person's sexual self-perceptions begin to form (Horne and Zimmer-Gembeck, 2006). However, this combination of events means that adolescent sexuality can create concern and fear among some adults because they associate it with harmful or impulsive sexual behaviours and negative sexual health outcomes, such as unintended pregnancy or sexually transmitted infections. To date, a great deal of research resources have focused on addressing these concerns, for example exploring behaviours related to 'risky' sexuality, such as early sex, first sex and negative peer influences.

 ACTIVITY

Why do you think adolescent sexuality is a concern for adults? Are these fears supported by empirical evidence?

More recently, though, connections between adolescence and risky sexual behaviours have been tempered as research moves us towards a greater understanding of more positive aspects of adolescent sexuality (Tolman and McLelland, 2011) acknowledging that romantic relationships can be potentially protective for young people.

ACTIVITY

What are the potentially positive and protective features of adolescent romantic relationships?

In part, this shift reflects increased understanding and acknowledgement that young people can be effective decision makers when it comes to sexual activity. Research highlights that young people engage in sexual activities other than vaginal sex – and that they consider these activities to be less physically risky in terms of unintended pregnancy or sexually transmitted infection, and emotionally less likely to produce feelings of guilt or exploitation (Tolman and McLelland, 2011). Importantly for health professionals, this means that greater clarity is required regarding the use of the term 'sex' when consulting with young people. It is also important to ensure that our discussions of adolescent sexuality are not exclusively focused on heterosexual young people.

Sexual Orientation

Statistics for 2015 suggest that 1.7% of the total UK population identified themselves as lesbian, gay or bisexual but that this rose to 3.3% in those aged 16–24 (Hagell et al., 2017). In 2017 an estimated 4.2% of people aged 16–24 years identified as lesbian, gay or bisexual, which is a higher proportion than for other older age groups (Office for National Statistics, 2017). There is also a minority of young people who identify in a more diverse way, at times adopting a gay, lesbian, bisexual, or no specific sexual identity, or who may be actively questioning their identity, or who may engage in same-sex sexual activities, and/or may report same-sex attractions (Russell et al., 2009) and who may not be represented in official statistics. This demonstrates some of the limitations of such statistics, indeed data on gender identity as a whole in those below 16 years of age in the UK is very limited, and data on the proportion of individuals who identify themselves as transgender is also sparse.

We can gain some insight through small studies, such as the 2017 Stonewall School Report (Bradlow, et al., 2017), which analysed an online questionnaire completed by 3713 LGBT young people aged 11–19 years in the UK. In this study 16% of respondents identified as transgender and a further 8% said they were unsure of whether they were transgender or were questioning their gender identity.

Identifying as LGBTI can be a difficult experience for many young people, and seeking adult support can be challenging. Nearly half the LGBT young people who participated in the Stonewall 2017 study (Bradlow et al., 2017) experienced homophobic bullying at school, and this percentage rose to 64% for young transgender people with 9% of this group receiving death threats at school. Almost half of those bullied did not disclose this to anyone, but many (40%) truanted from school because of it. More than half of LGBT pupils stated that there is not an adult at school they can talk to about being LGBT and only 40% reported having an adult at home they could talk to about this. Worryingly, only 29% of the participants reported that teachers would intervene if they witnessed this bullying, and 68% reported that staff 'never' or only 'sometimes' challenged homophobic, biphobic and transphobic language used.

 ACTIVITY

What homophobic, biphobic or transphobic terms have you heard? Where did you hear them? Were they challenged? What do you understand by the term 'casual homophobia'? What do you think the impact of such language might have on a young person who is not yet 'out'? How could you safely challenge the use of such language?

 WWW

Stonewall provides an up to date and easy to understand glossary of terms at:
- https://www.stonewall.org.uk/help-advice/glossary-terms#t

In the absence of knowledgeable or trusted adults, nearly all of the young people in the Stonewall 2017 study (Bradlow et al., 2017) had used the Internet to help them understand more about their sexual orientation and/or gender identity. However, most of them had also seen homophobic, biphobic and transphobic content online with 40% experiencing online abuse. The report reveals stark consequences associated with a lack of emotional support, with 61% of lesbian, gay and bi young people in this study engaging in self-harm. This percentage rose to 84% for young trans people. Of the lesbian, gay and bi young people who participated in the study 22% also reported attempts to take their own life with this figure rising to 45% for the young trans people.

 ACTIVITY

What do you think the school nurse does to support young LGBTI pupils?

TRENDS IN YOUNG PEOPLE'S SEXUAL ACTIVITY

The extent of young people's sexual activity can sometimes be over-estimated by parents, the media and by young people themselves, so it is important to have robust evidence of trends to support sexual health interventions. One of the most important sources of information about sexual behaviour in the United Kingdom is the National Survey of Sexual Attitudes and Lifestyle (Natsal) which has been carried out every 10 years since 1990 and the latest data (Natsal-3) was conducted in 2013. However, this data relates to adults aged 16–74 years with the youngest age group in the data set being 16–24 year olds. A key source of data for those *under* 16 years of age is the Health Behaviour in School Aged Children (HBSC) survey which began in 1982 and is now a cross national survey of school pupils that takes place in 49 countries every 4 years

as part of a World Health Organization international alliance of researchers. The HBSC collects data on sexual behaviour but also a wider range of health and well-being issues, such as body image, mental health, relationships, tobacco and alcohol use, diet, and physical activity levels for 11-, 13- and 15-year-old boys and girls. In the UK, data for this survey is collected in England, Wales and Scotland. The Association of Young People's Health considers these surveys, as well as many other sources of evidence, as part of their *Key Data on Young People* publication to provide a useful comprehensive snapshot of young people's health, including sexual health.

First Heterosexual Intercourse

The majority (two-thirds) of both males and females in Natsal-3 reported that they did not have sex until after 16 years (Geary et al., 2016) which corresponds with the reported age of first heterosexual intercourse in the UK for several years now. The 2014 HBSC survey data, which looks at a younger age group, also reflects this, maintaining that by age 16 approximately one-third of young people reported that they have had sexual intercourse (Brooks et al., 2015). The average number of partners reported by the 16–25 year olds is under six (Hagell, 2014).

Use of Contraception

There is a wide range of freely available contraceptive methods in the UK, including condoms (through the C-Card scheme), oral hormonal contraception (the pill), emergency hormonal contraception, and long acting reversible contraception (LARC), such as intrauterine devices, injectable contraceptives and implants, which can be accessed from a variety of sources, including GPs, community clinics and sexual health services. Despite this, young people have higher unplanned pregnancy and abortion rates than older adults, pointing to less effective use of contraception, despite its availability. Recognised barriers to young people's access to contraception include service locations, opening times and appointment systems, confidentiality concerns, perceptions of service provider judgement, or simply lack of knowledge of services (Fallon, 2013).

There are some limitations to data about contraception use because survey questions need to aid recall and so ask (for example) about behaviour *over the last year* or *at last intercourse* and so cannot always capture the whole picture. According to the Natsal-3 survey, of the 75% of young people aged 16–24 who were heterosexually active, 86% reported that they had obtained contraceptives in the last year (Geary et al., 2016). The HBSC data on contraceptive use by those aged 15 suggests that the majority (85%) of those who had engaged in sexual intercourse reported using some kind of contraception at last intercourse. The most common method of contraception was condom use, reported by 61% of the boys and 57% of the girls, with the contraceptive pill reported as the second most common method, followed by the morning after pill or another method (Brooks et al., 2015). Those aged 16–24 who had engaged in vaginal sex in the last year reported that they were most likely to obtain contraceptives from general practice (young women), and retail outlets (young men), but both genders use a range of sources (Geary et al., 2016).

 ACTIVITY

The data tell us that the majority of young people use contraception during heterosexual sexual intercourse. What does this data NOT tell us about use of contraception?

Emergency contraception is a post-coital method of contraception that generally indicates either contraceptive non-use or concerns about contraceptive failure. Although the widening availability of emergency contraception initially created disquiet in some quarters (Fallon, 2013) current use is actually low in young women, used by under 3% for all ages up to 24 with the highest levels reported by 16–19 years olds where the rate is 23 per 1000 young women (Hagell, 2014). However, younger girls aged 13–15 in the most deprived areas of the UK were provided with emergency contraception at a rate three times higher when compared to girls of this age in the least deprived decile illustrating clear health inequalities (Hagell, 2014).

To date, much of the available empirical research about young people's sexual behaviour has focused on heterosexual activity and particularly on the circumstances or timing of first sexual (vaginal) intercourse or the use of contraception. However, the sexual practices of young people are changing – showing an upward trend towards oral and anal sex (Lewis et al., 2017) with young adults more likely to report oral sex than vaginal sex in the last year, and anal sex reported by nearly one fifth of 16–25 year olds in the last year. Noting trends is an important means of identifying gaps in our knowledge and allows associations between new patterns of sexual behaviour and sexual health to be discovered (Lewis et al., 2017) which can then inform public health efforts. Improved knowledge of these trends may also open up space to allow a conceptualisation of young people's sexual activity as a normative developmental process rather than a societal 'problem', which then has potential to improve the emotional well-being of young people.

 ACTIVITY

What kind of issues can arise when collecting research data about sexual health or sexual activity with young people? What are the threats to the reliability of this data?

THE CONSEQUENCES OF POOR SEXUAL HEALTH

The Framework for Sexual Health Improvement in England (Department of Health [DoH], 2013) is a public health policy that has a stated ambition to ensure that the sexual health needs of all young people are met – whatever their sexuality.

This policy outlines a range of policy goals to help young people up to the age of 16 years, which includes building their knowledge and resilience, improving the availability of good-quality sex and relationship education and improving their ability to seek and access effective confidential advice and support about well-being, relationships and sexual health. This is the policy that informs much of the sexual health work that children's nurses currently undertake.

The framework outlined the following factors that influence relationships and safer sex:
- personal attitudes and beliefs
- social norms
- peer influence
- religious beliefs
- culture
- confidence and self esteem
- misuse of drugs or alcohol
- coercion and abuse

According to Wilkinson et al. (2003) other factors influencing sexual health outcomes for young people are known as 'social determinants' or:

… the conditions in which people are born, grow, live, work and age. These circumstances are shaped by the distribution of money, power and resources at global, national and local levels. The social determinants of health are mostly responsible for health inequities – the unfair and avoidable differences in health status seen within and between countries.

The social determinants of health are factors that young people cannot control, such as poverty and deprivation, but not all young people who grow up in deprived circumstances experience poor sexual health outcomes. The Framework for Sexual Health Improvement in England (DoH, 2013) acknowledged this, suggesting that such young people are 'resilient' and highlighting the importance of identifying the assets that contribute to this resilience in order to help young people capitalise on them and survive life's challenges. These assets are very much focused on effective education so that children and young people understand issues around consent and sexual consent, and can recognise and take steps to avoid or seek help about abusive relationships. The framework (DoH, 2013) aims to equip young people with knowledge and awareness of the risks of unprotected sex and the benefits of delaying sex. In terms of emotional well-being the framework also aims to furnish young people with confidence and resilience and an awareness of the benefits of loving, healthy relationships.

Many concerns about poor sexual health relate to protection from, or diagnosis and treatment of, physical conditions associated with sexual activity. However, as the WHO definition of sexual health highlights, there is also a large social and emotional component to be accounted for in sexual health care. In many cases, emotional support is required because of the social stigma that accompanies some of these conditions when individuals are perceived to deviate from socially determined norms. Individuals may also require help to cope with the psychological impact of sexual coercion, exploitation or abuse.

Young people aged 16–24 years have significantly higher rates of poor sexual health, including STIs and abortions, than older people (Geary et al., 2016). These conditions most often manifest in adulthood or young adulthood, including unintended pregnancy or sexually transmitted infections, such as genital herpes, chlamydia, human immunodeficiency virus (HIV) or pelvic inflammatory disease, which may lead to ectopic pregnancies and infertility and are often the focus of public health interventions.

 ACTIVITY

> Make a list of the possible causes of poor sexual health. What public health interventions are you aware of that address these issues?

PUBLIC SEXUAL HEALTH ISSUES

Public health issues related to sexual health for children and young people are many and varied. Some, such as sexually transmitted infections, are particular risks for sexually active young people, but children's nurses may also care for babies who have contracted disease through mother-to-child transmission. A significant aspect of the nurse's role relates to education – not only in terms of safe sex and screening as a way of avoiding transmission, but also (as in the case of gonorrhoea) raising awareness of the potential problems with antimicrobial resistance where antibiotics are the key method of treatment.

Sexually Transmitted Infections

In terms of sexually transmitted infections, those under 25 years have diagnosis rates that are twice as high in men and seven times higher in women when compared to people aged 25–59 (Public Health England [PHE], 2017a) and perhaps unsurprisingly, they account for a significant proportion of new diagnoses. STI diagnoses among gay and bisexual men aged 15–24 are also significant, with 34% of cases genital warts, 24% gonorrhoea, 22% genital herpes and chlamydia and 13% syphilis among this age group in 2011 (DoH, 2013). These figures illustrate why addressing STIs is a public health priority. A number of STIs that relate particularly to children and young people are discussed below.

Chlamydia

Chlamydia is a bacterial infection and the most prevalent STI in England, but it is generally asymptomatic, which means that young people are often unaware that they have it. In 2017 there were over 126,000 chlamydia diagnoses made among 15–24 year olds (PHE, 2018a). Untreated, chlamydia can cause serious health problems, including infertility, but there is a now a national chlamydia screening programme that aims to control chlamydia through early detection and treatment. Routine tests via a urine sample or swab are recommended for all sexually active under-25s annually, or with each change of partner, and are available in a variety of locations including pharmacies and sexual health clinics. However, such services are dependent on availability of funds, and concerns have been expressed about a 13% decline in chlamydia testing of young people since 2015 (PHE, 2020). The Family Planning Association (2015) have previously reported the significant impact that lack of testing may have on young people including delayed diagnosis, undiagnosed infections and increased transmission.

Human Papillomavirus

The human papillomavirus (HPV) infects squamous epithelia including the skin and mucosae of the upper respiratory and anogenital tracts and genital infection by HPV is associated with genital warts and anogenital cancers in both men and women (PHE, 2014). There are around 100 types of HPV, but some are low risk and some are high risk. It is the low risk HPV types, responsible for genital warts, which are the most commonly diagnosed viral STI in the UK. However, persistent infection with high-risk HPV types is connected to cervical cancer (PHE, 2014). Approximately 40 of the 100 HPV types affect the genital tract and are transmitted through sexual contact or sexual intercourse with an infected individual. As with other STIs, the risk of contracting HPV is related to the number of sexual partners, the introduction of a new sexual partner, and the sexual history of any partner. Although the use of condoms reduces the risk of transmission, it does not eliminate it entirely, and as with HIV, HPV can be transmitted from mother to newborn baby. However, there are highly effective vaccines available to combat HPV, and in 2008 the national HPV immunisation programme was launched in England with the HPV vaccine made available to all girls in school year 8 (aged 12–13 years) with a 'catch-up' campaign for girls aged from 14 years to less than 18 years (PHE, 2014).

 EVIDENCE-BASED PRACTICE

> The Green Book (PHE, 2014) is a useful resource outlining vaccinations and vaccination procedures for health professionals.

Human Immunodeficiency Virus

HIV damages the cells of the immune system, thus reducing the ability of an individual to fight infection and disease. If the immune system is severely damaged by the HIV virus then the individual becomes susceptible to a number of potentially life-threatening infections and illnesses and this is described as acquired immune deficiency syndrome (AIDS).

In 2015 it was estimated that 101,200 people were living with HIV in the UK with approximately 13% of these unaware that they had it, which meant that they were not accessing effective treatment and potentially infecting others unknowingly (PHE, 2016). There is currently no cure for HIV but with early diagnosis and treatment most individuals will not develop AIDS-related illnesses and can live a near normal lifespan (PHE, 2016) which means that screening is vital. Screening is both free and universally available in the UK. Gay, bisexual and other men who have sex with men are advised to test for HIV and other STIs at least annually, and every 3 months if they are engaging in unprotected sex (PHE, 2017a), but late diagnosis remains a challenge in the UK with 42% of diagnoses occurring during the late stage of infection.

The virus is found in bodily fluids such as semen, vaginal and anal fluids, or the blood of in infected person, so is commonly transmitted through unprotected anal or vaginal sex or through sharing injecting equipment. HIV tends to be found mostly among men who have sex with men (MSM) and black African men and women. However, in 2016, 41 children were newly diagnosed with HIV, of these, 36 were born abroad and arrived in the UK at an older age (PHE, 2017b).

HIV can also be transmitted from a pregnant woman to her unborn child during pregnancy or childbirth or to the newborn via breastmilk if the mother has HIV. The overall prevalence of HIV among pregnant women in England was 2.2 per 1000, and 23 per 1000 in sub-Saharan African-born women (Townsend et al., 2014). Perinatal HIV transmission is now almost entirely preventable because of universal antenatal HIV screening, careful management of pregnancy, including appropriate antiretroviral therapy (ART), and mode of delivery (which may include a scheduled caesarean section), avoidance of breastfeeding and prophylactic use of antiretroviral medication for the newborn (Townsend et al., 2014). These improvements in diagnosis and treatment mean that the risk of mother-to-child transmission of HIV in the UK is now extremely low (below 0.5% between 2013 and 2015) (PHE, 2016).

Unintended Teenage Pregnancy

Unintended teenage pregnancy was acknowledged as a significant public health priority following the publication of the Teenage Pregnancy Strategy for England and Wales in 1999 (Social Exclusion Unit, 1999). This 10-year strategy identified teenage pregnancy as both a cause and a consequence of socio-economic inequality and called for radical changes in service provision in order to reduce the rates of unintended teenage pregnancy by half. Building upon a review of international evidence regarding the question 'what works?' the strategy called for better sex and relationships education, improved access to contraception and improved support for young parents. At the same time there were pharmacological advances and major political changes taking place that would expand the then very limited access to emergency contraception. The strategy showed disappointing results at the mid-point, but successes were built upon and more intensive guidance and tools were published to facilitate further progress. There were also further investments in contraception provision, and particularly in improving access to LARC. By 2011 there was a clear reduction in maternity and abortion rates, even in areas of socio-economic deprivation, and in England, under-18 conception rates fell by 51% between 1998 and 2014 to their lowest levels since records began in 1969 (Hadley et al., 2016). However, they remain among the highest in Western Europe (22.9 conceptions per 1000 women aged 15–17 in England and Wales in 2014) and abortion rates remain at 33 per 1000, for women aged 20, indicating the need for continued work to promote effective contraception to prevent unwanted pregnancy.

 WWW

A useful source of information about teenage pregnancy is the Teenage Pregnancy Knowledge Exchange:
• https://www.beds.ac.uk/tpke.

Female Genital Mutilation

Female genital mutilation (FGM) is a significant threat to the sexual health and well-being of many girls and young women in the UK. FGM describes any procedure that involves the partial or total removal of the external female genitalia, or any other injury to the female genital organs for non-medical reasons. There is no medical justification for FGM and it is recognised internationally as a serious violation of the human rights of girls and women (World Health Organization, 2012). Since it is nearly always carried out on minors without consent it is also a serious violation of the rights of children. This is a cultural practice that mainly occurs in countries across Africa, the Middle East and Asia and is undertaken by traditional circumcisers often using makeshift, unclean bladed instruments. However, in some settings health care providers perform FGM in the mistaken belief that the procedure is safer when medicalised, which is entirely contrary to the advice of both the WHO and the UN. There are currently more than 200 million girls and women alive today from all regions of the world that have experienced FGM (WHO, 2012). There are numerous immediate risks associated with FGM, such as haemorrhage, pain and infection, as well as later risks associated with sexual functioning such as decreased sexual desire, satisfaction or arousal. There are also obstetric risks including difficulties with labour, still birth or neonatal death, and there are undoubted mental health complications including anxiety, depression and post-traumatic stress disorder (WHO, 2016). The World Health Organization has produced guidelines to manage these (WHO, 2016).

 ACTIVITY

What are the physical and emotional harms that result from FGM? Why do you think this practice is carried out?

FGM has been illegal in the UK since 1985. The number of girls or women affected by FGM in the UK is currently unknown, but it is estimated to be around 137,000 (Macfarlane and Dorkenoo, 2015). Undoubtedly, FGM has been carried out in secret locations in the UK, but many girls are also taken out of the country to have the procedure. However, since 2003 any UK national or permanent resident who takes their child abroad to have FGM faces a maximum penalty of 14 years in prison (NSPCC, 2019b). School nurses and children's nurses working within local communities are ideally placed to identify if a girl or young woman is at risk (Royal College of Nursing [RCN], 2019). They may also be trusted by young women, their friends or siblings to the extent that they feel comfortable to disclose issues to them that raise safeguarding concerns. They may also witness behavioural changes that indicate a risk of harm, or that harm has already occurred, such as prolonged visits to the toilet that may indicate difficulties with urination following FGM (RCN, 2019).

It is mandatory for health and social care professionals and teachers in England and Wales to report known cases of FGM in those under 18 to the police (Home Office, 2016). While individual practitioners are not responsible for undertaking investigations in suspected cases of FGM, they should be aware of FGM as a consideration in any general assessment they undertake and know how to refer concerns (RCN, 2016). The RCN (2016) provides a helpful resource for professionals, and the Department of Health (DoH, 2015a) outlines the risk assessment, safeguarding and legislative procedures that professionals should follow.

👤 SCENARIO

A 7-year-old Somalian girl returns to primary school after an extended summer holiday visiting grandparents in Somalia. She appears withdrawn to her previous teachers and becomes agitated and upset when she has to go to the toilet. Her teacher speaks to her privately and the child discloses she had been 'cut' in a ceremony along with her cousins and other children in her grandparents' village in Somalia. She states this was a rite of passage and a normal part of growing up in her culture, but she has been experiencing a lot of pain when passing urine since. The teacher informs the school nurse who in turn reported the FGM to the police, social services and the child's GP as per their mandatory reporting policies.

Practice Reflection

The school nurse took appropriate steps to safeguard the child and ensure she was supported from a medical and psychological perspective following the FGM. It was established that the daughter was the eldest of three children, another of whom was female, and appropriate protective measures were put in place to prevent her being subject to FGM in future. The police and social services worked together to ensure the children were kept safe and protected from future risk of harm, and to ensure the parents were aware of the legal ramifications of allowing FGM to be performed on a child. Appropriate referral from the GP to a paediatric consultant allowed appropriate medical review and follow-up after the illegal procedure. The school ensured all staff had training on identifying risk factors for FGM and updated their website to include both local and national guidelines around FGM, the law and mandatory reporting.

DISORDERS OF SEXUAL DEVELOPMENT

For some families, it is an anomaly in a young child's physical sexual development that brings them in to contact with health services. The development of an individual in terms of their sex (male or female) is influenced by two complex physiological processes that take place in utero. The first of these processes is *sex determination*. This relates to an individual's chromosomal make-up which is established at the time the

egg and sperm fuse during reproduction. It is the sex chromosomes (allosomes) that determine whether an offspring is biologically male or female, with genetic males inheriting the sex chromosomes X and Y from their parents (XY) and genetic females inheriting the sex chromosomes X and X (XX).

The second process is *sex differentiation*, and this relates to hormonal action that takes place after fertilisation – affecting the embryonic tissues during growth in the womb. This is because every embryo, irrespective of its chromosomal make-up (XX or XY) possesses a pair of Wolffian ducts, which are the precursor structures for the male genital tract, *and* a pair of Mullerian ducts, which are the structures necessary for the development of female reproductive organs. This means that there is still the potential for *any* embryo to develop either male or female sex genitalia. It is during the first trimester of a pregnancy when the permanent development of the external sex organs (genitalia) and the formation of either testes or ovaries are established, and this occurs as the result of hormonal action on the embryonic tissues.

The hormones that impact upon this process are testosterone and anti-Mullerian (or Mullerian-inhibiting) hormone, and both are produced by the embryonic testes in a genetically male (XY) fetus. Testosterone works to stimulate the Wolffian ducts to develop into male sexual organs, and anti-Mullerian hormone causes the Mullerian ducts to shrink. In the genetically female (XX) fetus, these hormones are *not* secreted, and the *lack* of testosterone causes the Wolffian duct system to diminish while the lack of anti-Mullerian hormone allows the Mullerian ducts to develop into female sex organs. This process of sexual differentiation is completed at puberty.

Disorders of sexual development (DSD) arise when this complex process is disrupted, impacting on anatomical development (Davies and Cheetham, 2017). Babies may be born with 'atypical genitalia', which is where the outward appearance of the genitals is markedly different from that usually found in males and females, but there is still a reasonable degree of medical certainty about the sex of the child (Davies and Cheetham, 2017). This is sometimes established via pelvic ultrasound examination which suggests whether or not the newborn has a uterus. A rarer condition is 'ambiguous genitalia' where the appearance of the genitalia is so anomalous that clinical examination fails to establish either a typically or exclusively male or female sex in the newborn (Davies and Cheetham, 2017). Both of these conditions are part of the DSD group of conditions. The term DSD has been used since 2006, but the term 'intersex' is also commonly used, and historically, these conditions were often described as hermaphroditism. Disorders of sexual development occur for a variety of reasons, including hormonal imbalances or exposure to environmental pollutants. There are approximately 30 recognised DSDs, but the two examples discussed here are congenital adrenal hyperplasia and androgen insensitivity syndrome.

Congenital adrenal hyperplasia (CAH) is a family of autosomal recessive disorders characterised by a disordered enzyme pathway that causes a disruption to cortisol synthesis. Females with CAH who produce an excess of the hormone cortisol (which is similar to testosterone) will develop genitalia that is masculinised to some degree. They may develop an enlarged clitoris that is similar to a penis, or they may have partially fused labia, similar to a scrotum. The recessive genes responsible for CAH can also be found in males, but they do not have a significant impact on male sex differentiation. Females with this condition will go on to develop typical female external genitalia if they receive early hormonal treatment (Trapp et al., 2018; Speiser and White, 2003).

In androgen insensitivity syndrome (AIS) the body's receptors to male hormones (androgens) are faulty, which impacts on masculinisation. The extent of androgen insensitivity varies across individuals (it can be complete or partial) but in the most extreme cases individuals with male genetic composition (XY) will develop external genitalia that resemble the genitalia of a female (Hughes et al., 2012) but will not develop internal female reproductive organs and cannot menstruate or conceive a child. These individuals, though genetically male, may be typically raised as females and have a female gender identity (Hughes et al., 2012).

Although many intersex children do not have serious medical side effects or problems with normal bodily functions as a result of the DSD, it is a condition that has been 'shrouded in secrecy and shame' which means that parents may decide to conceal the details of their child's condition from others (Council of Europe, 2017; Sanders et al., 2008). Furthermore, surgery may be offered to 'normalise' the appearance of the genitalia thus avoiding an ambiguous gender identity. However, as awareness of intersex conditions grows, these aesthetic 'corrective' surgeries have become a source of controversy with several organisations condemning them as human rights violations and calling for an end to the practice (United Nations Human Rights Office of the High Commissioner, 2012). Much of the controversy relates to the lack of an infant's capacity to consent to treatment and the parental right to consent to treatment if it is in their child's *best interests*. Clearly these procedures are invasive and irreversible, and there can be no 'one size fits all' solution to such an individual experience, which means that it is not possible to determine whether the long-term impact on the individual will be of benefit or harm. In many respects the parents cannot really know whether such surgery will be in the best interests of their child at the time they are making such a serious decision. Parents rely on medical advice to guide them at this time of uncertainty and, motivated by a desire to do what they perceive as 'right' for their child, they may consider genital surgery to be a necessity (Sanders et al., 2008).

> ### 👤 ACTIVITY
>
> One cosmetic surgical procedure that intersex infants may be offered is a clitoral reduction of a clitoris that is subjectively considered to be too large. Given the discussion of FGM earlier, what are your thoughts about this?

As many of these infants reach adulthood we learn more about their experiences and the potential unintended psychosocial and physical consequences of normalising surgery,

such as pain, scarring, loss of sexual sensitivity, and a very real possibility that a child is assigned a gender in infancy that they struggle with as they grow and develop. Given that some intersex conditions may involve changes during or after puberty it is clear that surgical interventions carried out in infancy will also deprive some individuals of the opportunity to live in a gender they may choose at a later date. Indeed, individuals may choose an intersex identity rather than the accepted binary gender identity of female or male (Dreger, 2006).

The therapeutic management of intersex has also involved a tendency to advise families to conceal a child's intersex status (sometimes from the child themselves), which also has serious psychosocial consequences for both the child and their family, such as feelings of isolation, a loss of confidence in medicine, and potential to undermine the parent–child relationship (Sanders et al., 2008; Dreger, 2006). The UK does not currently legislate about specific 'normalising' surgeries, but the UN Human Rights Office of the High Commissioner (2012) has called for an end to such practices, and there is UN support for repeals to the laws that allow such treatments (Mendez, 2013). There are calls instead to offer such options to individuals when they are old enough to understand and give their own consent (Council of Europe, 2017).

> ### 👤 ACTIVITY
>
> Student activity: Binary gender identity. Think about how the use of the pronouns 'male' and 'female' (for example in public toilets) serve to discriminate against intersex individuals. What can be done to ameliorate this?

THE NURSE'S ROLE

So far, this chapter has highlighted some of the many and varied issues around children and young people's sexual health in the UK. The following section explores some of the roles that the children's nurse might play in addressing these issues.

Sex and Relationships Education

There is clear evidence to suggest that many young people lack basic knowledge about issues associated with puberty, with many girls, for example, experiencing menstruation before they have been taught anything about it (Sex Education Forum, 2016). It is also clear that young people on the cusp of sexual activity would benefit from knowledge of and access to effective contraception and an understanding of factors to reduce the risk of acquiring STIs in advance of this. These issues are key components of timely and effective relationships and sex education (RSE) but the provision of RSE has been the source of debate for many years in the UK, with progress hampered by repeated attempts and objections to providing comprehensive formal RSE in schools. Such objections are most often raised by individuals or organisations who are concerned that sex education may lead to sexual experimentation.

In 2008, the Department for Children, Schools and Families reviewed the provision of RSE in England and concluded that it was not taught well nor given sufficient classroom time to facilitate pupils' skills or the building of confidence in matters of sexual health. It was also found to lack relevance for many young people and failed to address lesbian, gay, bisexual and transgender young people's RSE needs or the needs of those with learning disabilities.

▶ REFLECT ON YOUR PAST

What are your own experiences of RSE both in and outside of school?

Children and young people want, and have a right to (UN, 1989), timely and accurate information about sex and relationships and their preferred sources of this information are school, parents and health professionals. Sex education in school provides a crucial opportunity to discuss sexual consent issues, providing young people with the skills to avoid and report abuse or exploitation, and a safe space to learn how to deal effectively with pressure to engage in unwanted or unprotected sex. Research indicates that young people who receive good-quality sex and relationships education at school are more likely to use contraception when they first have sex and are therefore less likely to have an unplanned pregnancy (Wellings et al., 2013).

The determination to provide high quality RSE is shared by the Department for Education (DfE) as highlighted in the DfE (2000) statutory guidance, the DfE (2019) draft guidance and by the Department of Health (2013) via the Sexual Health Improvement Framework. However, RSE provision in schools is ultimately bound by decisions made by head teachers and governing bodies around what, when and how the content is delivered, which means the uptake of DfE (2000) guidance is patchy. Private schools, for example, can opt out of teaching sex education, and all parents currently have the right to request that their child is withdrawn from sex education lessons. This means that some young people may leave the current education system having received no information at all about sex or relationships.

Current provision clearly does not meet the needs of LGBT young people either. The Stonewall 2017 study of LGBT school pupils (Bradlow et al., 2017) highlighted how they felt assumptions were often made that everyone in the class was heterosexual. Only 13% of the pupils surveyed were taught in school about healthy same-sex sexual relationships, and while 87% of the participants learnt about contraception and safe sex at school, only 20% learnt about this in relation to same-sex relationships. Similar disparities arose in terms of consent, where only 20% were taught about consent in relation to same-sex relationships with even fewer (17%) learning about violence or abuse in relation to same-sex relationships. For both of these issues the

statistics were even lower for LGBT pupils who attended a faith school. In the same way that heterosexual young people benefit from good sex education, the report highlights that LGBT pupils in schools that teach about LGBT issues are less likely to experience homophobic, biphobic and transphobic bullying when compared to schools that do not, which indicates that these important messages are reaching the whole school, and as a consequence, these young people report feeling safer and happier at school.

Another group who fare poorly in terms of RSE are children and young people with learning disabilities. This group is particularly at risk of sexual exploitation (Franklin et al., 2015) but are often denied age-appropriate advice, or are given ineffective advice from poorly trained professionals who lack experience with learning disability issues. The Department for Education (2017) explained that childhood sexual exploitation (CSE) is a form of child sexual abuse. It occurs where an individual or group takes advantage of an imbalance of power to coerce, manipulate or deceive a child or young person under the age of 18 into sexual activity (1) in exchange for something the victim needs or wants, and/or (2) for the financial advantage or increased status of the perpetrator or facilitator. The victim may have been sexually exploited even if the sexual activity appears consensual. Child sexual exploitation does not always involve physical contact; it can also occur through the use of technology.

Nurses are ideally placed to identify the warning signs and indicators associated with sexual exploitation, such as mental health problems, repeated alcohol and drug misuse, repeated pregnancies or repeated attendances at the emergency department (Gadda and Taylor, 2016; Littler, 2014). However, part of the solution is about education and Franklin et al. (2015) call for improved RSE for young people with learning disabilities, particularly around issues of consent, in order to reduce the risk of being groomed. The Department for Education (2017) also highlighted cases of CSE involving younger children, especially in the online sphere, and warned that if we fail to educate children and young people about CSE or other forms of sexual abuse in good time then they are left unprotected. They suggested that schools should consider how to provide effective, sensitive and age-appropriate education about these issues as part of a planned programme of study across key stages.

In 2019, following a long consultation, a proposal to update the DfE (2000) RSE guidance was made to address some of these issues and to account for the changing society within which children and young people are growing up, resulting in a new and updated draft guidance (DfE [2019]). A broader range of topics was proposed to include respecting that some people are LGBT and that these relationships are recognised and protected in law. Other topics for inclusion are puberty, safeguarding issues – such as sexual assault and FGM – forced marriage, pornography and sexting. The changes met with some opposition – particularly about the notion of teaching RSE in primary schools. Therefore schools retained some flexibility over what it is taught and when, based on the age, development and religious backgrounds of their pupils. Schools were also advised that parents should also be involved in these decisions in a timely manner. The government responded to the consultation in 2019 suggesting that relationships education should be taught in primary schools, that relationship and sex education should be taught at secondary schools and that health education should be taught at all state funded schools. Parents will still be able to withdraw their child from the sex education element of RSE, but only up to and until three terms before the child turns 16, and this is the same for parents of children with special educational needs. The changes are due to come into effect in September 2020.

Providing Timely and Effective Advice and Treatment

One of the key roles of the health-care professional is to provide confidential, timely and accurate sexual health information, treatment and advice in a non-judgemental way to young people in order to help develop the foundations of good sexual health. The capacity for health professionals to provide such advice and treatment to those aged 16 or under (including emergency contraception and abortion) was clarified following a change in the law in 1986 – Victoria Gillick v West Norfolk and Wisbech Health Authority and Department of Health and Social Security (1986).

This same law also established the health professional's duty to assess a young person's competence to discuss issues around consent, and to encourage them to talk to their parents.

 ACTIVITY

What sort of factors do you think should be considered when assessing young person's competence with regards to their sexual health and well-being?

Contraception is freely available in the UK and accessible via a wide range of services in primary care, via charitable and independent sector services, such as Brook, and in pharmacies and hospitals. However, young people often feel stigmatised when attending sexual health services and have expressed a desire for acknowledgement that their help-seeking is a responsible action (Fallon, 2013). It is important to foster confidence in young people so that they will attend sexual health services for timely treatment or advice to prevent pregnancy and STIs. This should account for diversity in terms of gender and sexuality, culture and ethnicity, disability and age to enable young people to make informed choices (DoH, 2011).

The Family Planning Association (FPA) is a UK-based sexual health charity that has developed a useful policy related to young people's sexuality (see below). Their policy points to the importance of professionals being equipped to deliver accessible, confidential, appropriate and welcoming sexual health services to young people in a non-judgemental way so that young people are able to safely develop the knowledge and skills required for safe and enjoyable sexual behaviour.

 EVIDENCE-BASED PRACTICE

1. The Family Planning Association (FPA) believes that young people need to be equipped with the knowledge and skills to develop sexual behaviour that is safe and enjoyable for them and their sexual partners.
2. FPA believes that young people's sexual development is often perceived in a negative way and should instead be viewed positively.
3. FPA believes that all sexual health service providers, including general practice, contraception and genitourinary medicine (GUM) clinics, young people's services and support services, must ensure that they are accessible, appropriate and welcoming to young people and should offer high-quality, confidential services.
4. FPA believes that the sexual health needs of young people are best served by multi-agency and multi-disciplinary approaches, and that young people should be fully consulted in the development of services.
5. FPA believes that protecting confidentiality is key in protecting young people's welfare. FPA is committed to the principle that under-16s – including those under 13 – should be able to get confidential sexual health advice and treatment, and we believe that professionals working with young people must protect their right to confidentiality in all but the most exceptional cases.
6. FPA supports young people's right to decide whether to continue or end a pregnancy. Young people who decide to become parents deserve to get the best support available and are damaged by negative stereotypes of teenage parents.

Family Planning Association, 2017. Young People and Sexuality Policy. Available from: https://www.fpa.org.uk/sites/default/files/young-people-policy-statement.pdf.

 EVIDENCE-BASED PRACTICE

Access to services in the community setting has had considerable attention but there is little discussion about the nurse's role in engaging with young people about their sexual health concerns in acute settings. Sanders et al. (2011) and Bray et al. (2013) suggest that some health professionals experience discomfort when discussing issues related to sexual health with young people and that though there is limited literature on acute service providers roles here, it seems we are particularly poorly equipped to hold opportunistic discussions in a hospital setting – despite a significant number of CYP accessing these services. Though young people tend not to seek advice this way, it seems they want to know that they could do so if they needed (Sanders et al., 2011; Bray et al., 2013).

EVIDENCE-BASED PRACTICE

There are a number of barriers to discussing sexual health with young people that health-care providers have identified, including:

1. embarrassment
2. lack of knowledge
3. fear of causing offence
4. conservative views
5. lack of time
6. lack of confidence broaching the subject
7. not seen as a priority

Bates (2011). Bates J (2011) Broaching sexual health issues with patients. Nursing Times [online]; 107: 48, 20–22.

 ACTIVITY

What can be done by (a) organisations and (b) individuals do to address the barriers identified by Bates (2011)?

Bailey et al. (2015) identified how both time and financial constraints can stifle opportunistic discussion with young people about sexual health, and therefore contribute to the failure to meet their needs in both primary and secondary care settings. However, nurses who work in non-sexual health settings, such as emergency departments or ward settings, should also be able to provide confidential sexual health advice as part of a holistic assessment or if they are approached. One approach to improving young people's health and well-being is for professionals to engage with 'Making Every Contact Count' (MECC) (PHE, 2016), which is an innovation that aims to capitalise on the many interactions that take place between health workers and the general public with a view to encouraging health behaviour change. Although much of the information for MECC focuses on improving health by addressing risk factors, such as alcohol, diet, physical activity, smoking and mental well-being, there are many opportunities in hospitals, schools and youth services where sexual health and relationship issues can also be discussed opportunistically, or where signposting young people to accessible youth friendly sexual health services can take place.

Two simple questions that children's nurses might consider are:

1. Is this the right time – has the young person prompted (however subtly) the conversation?
2. Have you demonstrated your openness to having a conversation or to listening?

In order to promote good sexual and reproductive health, professionals require an understanding of the needs of individuals, communities and populations related to sexual health, reproductive health and HIV and to be able to signpost them to the resources and services available. Health professionals should also have an understanding of specific activities or interventions that can prevent poor sexual and reproductive health and HIV (PHE, 2018b).

 ACTIVITY

Make a list of some common myths and misconceptions that children and young people have about sexual and reproductive health issues. Which local resources would you be able to point them to?

 ACTIVITY

Create a personal development plan related to children and young people's sexual health. Consider whether you have enough knowledge?. If you are female and a young male asks you questions about male anatomy and physiology or sexuality – are you equipped to deal with that question? Similarly, if you are male, do you have the knowledge to answer questions about female sexual health?

Sexual Health – The Nurse's Role in Safeguarding

There are many ways in which safeguarding and young people's sexual health are connected, and a central role for nurses working with young people is the recognition of, and response to, childhood sexual abuse and childhood sexual exploitation (CSE). There are a number of guidelines that all children's nurses and sexual health service providers must be aware of regarding child protection and safeguarding issues, including *Working Together to Safeguard Children* (DfE, 2018) and *What to Do If You're Worried a Child Is Being Abused* (HM Government, 2015). A key message across many documents and, indeed, a message that has threaded through this chapter, is that children's nurses should always seriously consider the possibility of abuse, FGM or CSE and to remember that children's nurses are often ideally placed to recognise warning signs. Given the potential physical and mental health consequences of sexual abuse for children and young people it is essential that nurses and other health professionals remain 'inquisitive' about abuse (Gadda and Taylor, 2015) when interacting with children and young people, working to improve their skills to identify the early signs of abuse, and to be confident to refer and collaborate with other professionals. The role of the children's nurse in safeguarding is outlined in more detail in Chapter 19.

REFERENCES

Bailey J, Mann S, Wayal S, et al. Sexual health promotion for young people delivered via digital media: a scoping review. Southampton (UK): NIHR Journals Library; 2015 Nov. (Public Health Research, No. 3.13.) Chapter 1, Introduction. Available from: https://www.ncbi.nlm.nih.gov/books/NBK326982/.

Bates, J., 2011. Broaching sexual health issues with patients. Nursing Times; 107: 48, 20–22.

Bradlow, J., Bartram, F., Guasp, A., Jadva, V., 2017. Stonewall (2017) School Report: The Experiences of Lesbian, Gay, Bi and Trans Pupils in Britain's Schools. Centre for Family Research, University of Cambridge.

Bray, L., Sanders, C., McKenna, J., 2013. Discussing sexual and relationship health with young people in a children's hospital: evaluation of a computer based resource. J. Clin. Nurs. 22 (23–24), 3447–3455.

Brook, 2012. Sexual Behaviours Traffic Light Tool. Available from: https://www.brook.org.uk/our-work/the-sexual-behaviours-traffic-light-tool.

Brooks, F., Magnusson, J., Klemera, E., et al., 2015. HBSC England National Report: Health Behaviour in School-aged Children (HBSC): World Health Organization Collaborative Cross National Study. University of Hertfordshire. Available from: https://assets.publishing.service.gov.uk/government/uploads/system/uploads/attachment_data/file/175496/DFE-00133-2011.pdf.

Council of Europe, 2017. Human Rights and Intersex People. Available from: https://rm.coe.int/16806da5d4.

Davies, J.H., Cheetham, T., 2017. Recognition and assessment of atypical and ambiguous genitalia in the newborn. Arch. Dis. Child. 102, 968–974.

Department for Children, Schools and Families, 2008. Review of Sex and Relationship Education (SRE) in Schools. A Report by the External Steering Group. Available from: https://webarchive.nationalarchives.gov.uk/20130323073713/https://www.education.gov.uk/publications/eOrderingDownload/SRE-Review-2008.pdf.

Department for Education (DfE), 2000. Sex and Relationship Education Guidance. Crown Copyright. https://www.pshe-association.org.uk/system/files/Sex%20and%20Relationship%20Education%20Guidance%202000.pdf.

Department for Education (DfE), 2010. Positive for Youth: A New Approach to Cross-Government Policy for Young People Aged 13 to 19. Crown Copyright. Available from: https://assets.publishing.service.gov.uk/government/uploads/system/uploads/attachment_data/file/175496/DFE-00133-2011.pdf.

Department for Education (DfE), 2017. Childhood Sexual Exploitation: Definition and a Guide for Practitioners, Local Leaders and Decision Makers Working to Protect Children From Child Sexual Exploitation. Crown Copyright. Available from: https://assets.publishing.service.gov.uk/government/uploads/system/uploads/attachment_data/file/591903/CSE_Guidance_Core_Document_13.02.2017.pdf.

Department for Education (DfE), 2018. Working Together to Safeguard Children. A Guide to Inter-agency Working to Safeguard and Promote the Welfare of Children. Crown Copyright. Available from: https://assets.publishing.service.gov.uk/government/uploads/system/uploads/attachment_data/file/779401/Working_Together_to_Safeguard-Children.pdf.

Department for Education (DfE), 2019. Relationships Education, Relationships and Sex Education (RSE) and Health Education Draft Statutory Guidance for Governing Bodies, Proprietors, Head Teachers, Principals, Senior Leadership Teams, Teachers. Crown Copyright. Available from: https://assets.publishing.service.gov.uk/government/uploads/system/uploads/attachment_data/file/781150/Draft_guidance_Relationships_Education__Relationships_and_Sex_Education__RSE__and_Health_Education2.pdf.

Department of Health (DoH), 2011. You're Welcome Quality Criteria. Available from: https://www.gov.uk/government/publications/quality-criteria-for-young-people-friendly-health-services.

Department of Health (DoH), 2013. A Framework for Sexual Health Improvement in England. Available from: https://www.gov.uk/government/uploads/system/uploads/attachment_data/file/142592/9287-2900714-TSO-SexualHealthPolicyNW_ACCESSIBLE.pdf.

Department of Health (DoH), 2015a. Female Genital Mutilation Risk and Safeguarding Guidance for Professionals. Available from: https://assets.publishing.service.gov.uk/government/uploads/system/uploads/attachment_data/file/525390/FGM_safeguarding_report_A.pdf.

Dreger, A.D., 2006. Cutting to the core: exploring the ethics of contested surgeries. New Eng. J. Med. 355 (15), 1626–1626.

Family Planning Association (FPA), 2015. Unprotected Nation: An Update on the Financial and Economic Impacts of Restricted Contraceptive and Sexual Health Services. Family Planning Association. Available from: https://www.fpa.org.uk/sites/default/files/unprotected-nation-2015-full-report.pdf.

Family Planning Association (FPA), 2017. Young People and Sexuality Policy. Available from: https://www.fpa.org.uk/sites/default/files/young-people-policy-statement.pdf.

Franklin, A., Raws, P., Smeaton, E., 2015. Unprotected Overprotected: Meeting the Needs of Young People with Learning Disabilities Who Experience, or Are at Risk of, Sexual Exploitation. Barnardo's, Essex. Available from: http://www.barnardos.org.uk/cse_learning_and_disability_report_2015a.pdf.

Gadda, A., Taylor, J., 2016. Child sexual exploitation: where are the nurses? J. Adv. Nurs. 72, 721–722.

Geary, R.S., Tomes, C., Jones, K.G., 2016. Actual and preferred contraceptive sources among young people: findings from the British National Survey of Sexual Attitudes and Lifestyles. BMJ Open 6, e011966. https://doi.org/10.1136/bmjopen-2016-011966.

Hadley, A., Ingham, R., Chandra-Mouli, V., 2016. Implementing the United Kingdom's ten-year teenage pregnancy strategy for England (1999–2010): how was this done and what did it achieve? Reprod. Health 13, 139.

Hagell, A., 2014. Sexual Health and Under 18 Conceptions. AYPH Research Update May 2014. Available from: https://www.youngpeopleshealth.org.uk/wp-content/uploads/2015/07/Sexual-health.pdf.

https://www.brook.org.uk/our-work/the-sexual-behaviours-traffic-light-tool.

Hagell, A., Shah, R., Coleman, J., 2017. Key Data on Young People 2017. Association for Young People's Health, London.

HM Government, 2015. What to Do If You're Worried a Child Is Being Abused: Advice for Practitioners. Crown Copyright. Available from: https://assets.publishing.service.gov.uk/government/uploads/system/uploads/attachment_data/file/419604/What_to_do_if_you_re_worried_a_child_is_being_abused.pdf.

Home Office, 2016. Mandatory Reporting of Female Genital Mutilation – Procedural Information. Home Office, London.

Horne, S., Zimmer-Gembeck, M., 2006. The female sexual subjectivity inventory: development and validation of a multi-dimensional inventory for late adolescents and emerging adults. Psychol. Women Q. 30 (2), 125–238.

Hughes, I.A., Davies, J.D., Bunch, T.I., et al., 2012. Androgen insensitivity syndrome. Lancet 380 (9851), 1419–1428.

Lewis, R., Tanton, C., Mercer, C., et al., 2017. Heterosexual practices among young people in Britain: evidence from three national surveys of sexual attitudes and lifestyles. J. Adolesc. Health 61 (6), 694–702.

Littler, N., 2014. School nurses' role in tackling child sexual exploitation. Br. J. School Nurs. 9 (10), 514–515.

Macfarlane, A., Dorkenoo, E., 2015. Prevalence of Female Genital Mutilation in England and Wales: National and Local Estimates. City University, London. Available from: https://www.city.ac.uk/__data/assets/pdf_file/0004/282388/FGM-statistics-final-report-21-07-15-released-text.pdf.

Mendez, J.E., 2013. Report of the Special Rapporteur on Torture and Other Cruel, Inhuman or Degrading Treatment or Punishment. https://www.ohchr.org/Documents/HRBodies/HRCouncil/RegularSession/Session22/A.HRC.22.53_English.pdf.

National Institute for Health and Care Excellence (NICE), 2016. Harmful Sexual Behaviour. Available from: https://www.nice.org.uk/guidance/ng55.

National Society for the Prevention of Cruelty to Children (NSPCC), 2019a. Healthy Sexual Behaviour. Available from: https://www.nspcc.org.uk/preventing-abuse/keeping-children-safe/healthy-sexual-behaviour-children-young-people/.

National Society for the Prevention of Cruelty to Children (NSPCC), 2019b. What Is FGM? https://www.nspcc.org.uk/preventing-abuse/child-abuse-and-neglect/female-genital-mutilation-fgm/.

Office for National Statistics, 2017. Sexual Orientation. UK: 2017. Available from: https://www.ons.gov.uk/peoplepopulationandcommunity/culturalidentity/sexuality/bulletins/sexualidentityuk/2017.

Public Health England (PHE), 2014. The Green Book. Available from: https://www.gov.uk/government/collections/immunisation-against-infectious-disease-the-green-book#the-green-book.

Public Health England (PHE), 2016. HIV in the UK 2016 Report. Available from: https://assets.publishing.service.gov.uk/government/uploads/system/uploads/attachment_data/file/602942/HIV_in_the_UK_report.pdf.

Public Health England (PHE), 2017a. Guidance HIV: Testing. Available from: https://www.gov.uk/guidance/hiv-testing.

Public Health England (PHE), 2017b. Towards Elimination of HIV Transmission, AIDS and HIV-Related Deaths in the UK. Available from: https://assets.publishing.service.gov.uk/government/uploads/system/uploads/attachment_data/file/675809/Towards_elimination_of_HIV_transmission_AIDS_and_HIV_related_deaths_in_the_UK.pdf.

Public Health England (PHE), 2018a. Sexually transmitted infections and screening for chlamydia in England, 2017. Health Protection Report 12 (20), 2018. Available from: https://assets.publishing.service.gov.uk/government/uploads/system/uploads/attachment_data/file/713962/hpr2018_AA-STIs_v5.pdf.

Public Health England (PHE), 2018b. Sexual and Reproductive Health and HIV: Applying All Our Health. Crown Copyright. Available from https://www.gov.uk/government/publications/sexual-and-reproductive-health-and-hiv-applying-all-our-health/sexual-and-reproductive-health-and-hiv-applying-all-our-health.

Public Health England (PHE), 2020. Sexually Transmitted Infections and Screening for Chlamydia in England, 2019. Crown Copyright.

Royal College of Nursing (RCN), 2016. Female Genital Mutilation: An RCN Resource for Nursing and Midwifery Practice, third ed. file://nask.man.ac.uk/home$/Downloads/005447.pdf.

Royal College of Nursing (RCN), 2019. Female Genital Mutilation. Available from: https://www.rcn.org.uk/clinical-topics/female-genital-mutilation.

Russell, S.T., 2005. Conceptualizing positive adolescent sexuality development. Sexual Research Society Polska 2 (3), 4–12. Berkeley.

Russell, S.T., Clarke, T.J., Clary, J., 2009. Are teens 'post-gay'? Contemporary adolescents' sexual identity labels. J. Youth Adolesc. 38 (7), 884–890.

Sanders, C., Carter, B., Goodacre, L., 2008. Parents' narratives about their experiences of their child's reconstructive genital surgeries for ambiguous genitalia. J. Clin. Nurs. 17 (23), 3187–3195.

Sanders, C., Pritchard, E., Bray, L., et al., 2011. Exploring young people's expectations and experience of discussing sexual and relationship health with professionals in a children's hospital. J. Clin. Nurs. 20 (11–12), 1705–1712.

Sex Education Forum, 2016. Heads or Tails? What Young People Are Telling Us About SRE. http://www.sexeducationforum.org.uk/sites/default/files/field/attachment/Head%20or%20tails%20-%20SRE%20-%202016.pdf.

Social Exclusion Unit, 1999. Teenage Pregnancy. London: SEU, Cmnd 4342. p. 139. http://webarchive.nationalarchives.gov.uk/20070402090838/http://dfes.gov.uk/teenagepregnancy/dsp_content.cfm?pageID=87.

Speiser, P., White, P., 2003. Congenital adrenal hyperplasia. New Engl. J. Med. 349, 776–788.

Stonewall Glossary. https://www.stonewall.org.uk/help-advice/glossary-terms#.

Tolman, D.L., McLelland, S.I., 2011. Normative sexuality development in adolescence: a decade in review, 2000–2009. J. Res. Adolescence 21 (1), 242–255.

Townsend, C.L., Byrne, L., Cortina-Borja, M., et al., 2014. Earlier initiation of ART and further decline in mother-to-child HIV transmission rates, 2000–2011. AIDS 28 (7), 1049–1057.

Trapp, C.M., Levine, L.S., Oberfield, S.E., 2018. Congenital adrenal hyperplasia. In: Radovick, S., Misra, M. (Eds.), Pediatric Endocrinology. Springer, Cham.

United Nations, 1989. Convention on the Rights of the Child. https://downloads.unicef.org.uk/wp-content/uploads/2010/05/UNCRC_united_nations_convention_on_the_rights_of_the_child.pdf?_ga=2.14010484.2104903152.1555422058-1324167575.1555422058.

United Nations Human Rights Office of the High Commissioner, 2012. Born Free and Equal. Sexual Orientation and Gender Identity in International Human Rights Law. https://www.ohchr.org/Documents/Publications/BornFreeAndEqualLowRes.pdf.

Wellings, K., Jones, K.G., Mercer, C.H., et al., 2013. The prevalence of unplanned pregnancy and associated factors in Britain: findings from the third National Survey of Sexual Attitudes and Lifestyles (Natsal-3). Lancet 382 (9907), 1807–1816.

Wilkinson, R., Marmot, M., World Health Organization, Centre for Urban Health, 2003. The solid facts: social determinants of health. In: Wilkinson, R., Marmot, M., Centre for Urban Health. World Health Organization, Copenhagen.

World Health Organization, 2006. Definition of Sexual Health. https://www.who.int/reproductivehealth/topics/sexual_health/sh_definitions/en/.

World Health Organization, 2012. Understanding and Addressing Violence Against Women: Female Genital Mutilation [Information Sheet]. WHO, Geneva. Available at www.who.int.

World Health Organization, 2016. WHO Guidelines on the Management of Health Complications from Female Genital Mutilation. https://apps.who.int/iris/bitstream/handle/10665/206437/9789241549646_eng.pdf;jsessionid=F797C9B903F21FA65BA2C7B0CE92C27?sequence=1.

Organisation of Children's Nursing

32

Health Problems of the Neonate

Kaye Spence

LEARNING OUTCOMES

- Using assessment strategies to be able to recognise a potentially vulnerable or sick neonate.
- Using evidence to understand the rationale for interventions.

- Apply knowledge of potential problems to minimise distress to the neonate and their parents.
- Evaluate and assess the care provided for a vulnerable or sick neonate in terms of outcomes.

GLOSSARY

Extremely low birth weight (ELBW) An infant with a birth weight below 1 kg.

Intrauterine growth retarded (IUGR) An infant with a symmetrical low birth weight below the 10th percentile.

Low birth weight (LBW) An infant with a birth weight below 2.5 kg.

Nasogastric feeding The practice of feeding an infant via a tube which is inserted through the nose and advanced to the stomach and normally left indwelling for up to a week.

Neonate Describes an infant from birth to 28 days.

NICU Neonatal Intensive care Unit.

Orogastric As with nasogastric but sited via the mouth.

Post-term An infant born after 42 weeks' gestation.

Preterm An infant born before 37 weeks' gestation.

Small for gestational age (SGA) An infant with an asymmetrical birth weight below the 10th percentile.

SCBU Special care baby unit.

Very low birth weight (VLBW) An infant with a birth weight below 1.5 kg.

INTRODUCTION

The history of neonatology began with French midwives and obstetricians. Even after specialised neonatal care began to develop in the USA in the 1950s and 1960s, the approach to care was primarily from an obstetric and anaesthetic viewpoint. Specialist neonatologists and neonatal nurses have emerged to care for the most vulnerable neonates as a specialty area of practice (NAO, 2007).

Specialised neonatal units, often located in large university hospitals, have evolved over the last 60 years to offer highly technological support to care for vulnerable and sick neonates. Preterm infants as young as 23 weeks' gestation, and weighing <500 g, to term neonates with respiratory, surgical or cardiac problems are cared for on these neonatal units. Environmental adaptation is necessary for survival (Lizarondo, 2016). Recently, the focus of care has been the relationship between neonatal nursing practice and long-term developmental outcomes (Burke, 2018; NICE, 2017). Studies have shown that the infant's

development is influenced by the care given, the presence of the parents and the environment (National Institute for Health and Care Excellence [NICE], 2017; Lizarondo, 2016). This has implications for nursing practice. In addition, nurses working in these challenging environments need to look after themselves as they are faced with many issues that can contribute to moral distress and burnout (Warren, 2017).

ACTIVITY

Read National Service Framework documents at:
- https://www.england.nhs.uk/wp-content/uploads/2016/02/national-maternity-review-report.pdf
- https://www.england.nhs.uk/commissioning/spec-services/npc-crg/group-e/e08/
- https://www.longtermplan.nhs.uk/publication/nhs-long-term-plan/

THE DEVELOPING BRAIN

Neurogenesis is the term used for the growth and development of the brain and neurons. The peak period of brain development in utero is around 3–4 months' gestation. Most neurons needed for the lifespan are created by 20 weeks; however, half may be later eliminated during development. The germinal matrix of the ventricles, the source of neurons and glial cells, has a rich supply of blood passing through delicate blood vessels, most active between 8 and 28 weeks' gestation. Haemodynamic changes can result in changes to the blood received by the brain, which can result in a bleed into the ventricles in the brain; this is known as an intraventricular haemorrhage (Stiles and Jernigan, 2010).

Neuroplasticity refers to the changes to the neural pathways and synapses due to changes in behaviour, environment, neural processes, thinking and emotion. Experience can change both the brain's physical structure and its function. Thus when caring for a premature infant it is important to keep this in mind as simple caregiving activities such as a nappy change can result in increasing the blood to the brain and a subsequent bleed. In addition, an environment of many stressors, such as bright lights, noise, activity, pain and stress can impact the developing brain.

The Synactive Theory of onatal Newborn Behavioural Organisation and Development (Als, 1986) provides a framework for health care professionals to have an understanding of the neonate's capabilities and interaction between five sub-systems of autonomic, motor, state, attention and interaction. Each infant is unique, and at a given moment has the ability to modulate and organise its own behaviour. The caregiver is often required to support the infant through coregulation to ensure the stress of the noxious environment of intensive care is kept to a minimum. Using the Newborn Individualized Developmental Care and Assessment Program (NIDCAP) approach, which is a complex, comprehensive, staff intensive, relationship-based intervention, the neonate and their family are supported (Als, 2009). Minimising stress is a primary goal and although many stressors cannot be avoided completely, most can be reduced or even eliminated. By recognising and monitoring infant stress, working with the parents, neonatal intensive care unit (NICU) staff can implement effective interventions that help these fragile neonates recover and thrive (Newnham et al., 2009). Evidence shows that repeated stress, especially that occurring during the critical early period of infant development, has profound and long-lasting effects on several physiological systems, including brain development (Brummelte et al., 2012).

PARENTS

Having a baby in the intensive care nursery is a stressful time for parents who may feel a sense of loss for the interrupted pregnancy or an unexpected outcome. They may feel a sense of isolation from others and each other. The inability to produce a healthy infant, coupled with the inability to protect an ill neonate from invasive and sometimes painful procedures, leaves the parents feeling inadequate. The birth of an ill or premature neonate has an overwhelming destabilising effect on parents, and many go through identifiable behaviours similar to a grief response. With empathetic care, parents can learn to cope and adapt as they are taught how to care for and become increasingly involved in their infant's life (Davila and Segre, 2018). Fathers have been shown to be particularly vulnerable and at risk of depression (Cyr-Alves et al., 2018) and will require support from the staff to enable them to also support their families. Psychosocial meetings are valuable and provide a forum to discuss current and anticipated problems that may arise during provision of neonatal care. Health care professionals endeavour to promote attachment between the infant and family in a supportive and nurturing environment. The Bliss Baby Charter has written six principles to help parents and health professionals provide best practice for preterm and sick neonates in hospital (https://www.bliss.org.uk/health-professionals/bliss-baby-charter/best-practice-bank).

Attachment

Currently, most neonatal units encourage parents to be with their infant/infants whenever they choose. A model of partnership between parents and staff can help alleviate some of the stressors faced through having their baby in hospital. With developmental care now being practised in most neonatal units, we are moving from a task-orientated model to one built on relationships. Filippa et al. (2017) found maternal voice, had beneficial effects on the preterm infant's physiological and behavioural stability. Having the mother present and getting her to talk, sing or read to her baby can help with the stressors of some care-giving activities as well as support the infant in their efforts to transition to sleep.

Neonatal units are busy, noisy, bustling places, caring for a range of infants, some of whom are very ill and require constant, highly technical care. Parents move through phases of fear, watching and touching, and research has shown that positive touch is essential to good developmental outcomes. It is therefore imperative that neonatal nurses are proactive in ensuring that contact and interaction are initiated as soon as possible after admission and are sustained until discharge, considering each parent's pace and ability to be confident in their care-giving (Raines and Brustad, 2012).

For nurses working with parents in the neonatal unit, caring for their baby should be seen as a privilege. There are ways that staff can minimise some of the stressors facing the families and Janvier et al. (2016) make the following recommendations:

- Be aware that parents experience both negative and positive impacts after an NICU experience. Communications with parents should be balanced.
- Remain humble. Avoid sentences such as: 'Parents don't understand' or 'If I were in their situation, I would not …' Too often, it is providers who do not understand.

- Remind parents often that their infant is lucky to have parents who love them.
- Let parents know that positive transformations are possible.
- Temper discussions about risks with words about something good happening, such as resilience, love, and the chances of healing.
- Help parents prioritise their energy and how to recognise what they can and cannot control.
- Inform parents that life will not always be like this, that the roller coaster will become a train with a known destination. That one day, it will be better.
- We can be there for parents at tough moments or avoid them. Be there.

Being welcoming and making as much time for parents as they want or need seems very simple, but it is important because it allows parents to relax and spend time getting to know their new infant. One of the most important aspects of this care is to include parents in plans and decisions about the care of their infant, by ensuring that they are fully informed and that their views are sought. As much written information as possible should also be given, as verbal information is soon forgotten in stressful situations.

Recognition of the mother by the infant is said to occur after eye contact over a 72-hour period. In infants without health problems, mothers spend many hours cuddling and gazing at their infant. This recognition is established within a few days but is delayed when an infant is ill. Therefore the neonatal nurse should encourage cuddling and gazing whenever possible to establish early recognition.

Kangaroo mother care (KMC) is defined as a combination of skin-to-skin contact, frequent and exclusive breastfeeding, and early discharge from hospital, with adequate follow-up (Jayasekara, 2016). It has been largely recommended for stable low birth weight (LBW) infants; however, all hospitalised infants will benefit. A recommended minimum of 1 hour a day can help infants grow as well as reduce stress levels in parents and increase attachment. Nurses need to be available to support the parents when KMC is initiated. However, to promote KMC requires staff to actively facilitate strategies, such as ensuring there is flexibility for parents' attendance with a focus on enabling mothers to drive the KMC initiative, with the support of midwives and nurses.

👤 ACTIVITY

- https://s3.eu-west-2.amazonaws.com/files.bliss.org.uk/documents/Health-professionals/Bliss-Baby-Charter/Bliss_Baby_Charter_Booklet.pdf?mtime=20180404152638.

  Using the link to the audit tool of the Bliss Baby Charter, review each principle and see how your practice matches the desired outcomes. Consider the improvements required by using the traffic light system described at the beginning.

COMMON NEONATAL DISEASES AND CONDITIONS

Caring for neonates in the NICU or Special Care Baby Unit (SCBU) requires nurses to have an understanding of some of the more common diseases and conditions encountered. This is not an exhaustive list, and the conditions included are those that can have a life-threatening risk to neonates.

NEONATAL HYPOTHERMIA

Hypothermia is a significant cause of morbidity and mortality in the neonate. Humans attempt to maintain their body temperature within a certain range to maintain metabolic functions. The normal temperature range for term neonates is 36.5°C–37.5°C per axilla, 35.6°C–37.3°C in preterm neonates and 36.7°C–37.3°C for low birth weight infants (Hodson, 2018).

Hypothermia occurs when the body's core temperature falls below 35°C. Neonates are at risk of hypothermia primarily because of their size because, although small, they have a large surface area in proportion to body weight, a large head size (through which heat is lost) in relation to the rest of the body, minimal fat reserves and poor insulation, as well as an immature hypothalamus, resulting in poor vasomotor control. Those neonates primarily at risk of cold stress are:

- preterm infants (born at less than 36 weeks' gestation);
- infants who are small for gestational age or with intrauterine growth restriction;
- infants with respiratory distress;
- infants who are transferred between hospitals or hospital departments for investigation, such as MRI.

Some neonates who have suffered an insult to the brain maybe be deliberately cooled to preserve the brain and reduce further ischaemic brain damage. These infants will be nursed in an intensive care unit, although the treatment may be commenced in the delivery room and other environments, but the neonate will require swift transfer to the NICU.

Temperature Regulation

Temperature regulation is a complex process. The hypothalamus, which is located at the base of the brain, is responsible for temperature regulation. Receptors in the skin, abdomen, spinal cord and internal organs provide the hypothalamus with information to maintain temperature balance. The hypothalamus produces hormones in response to temperature imbalance and, together with the autonomic and sympathetic nervous systems, regulates temperature (Knobel, 2014). For example, if the neonate is subject to reduction in body temperature, cold stress stimulates thermoreceptors to send impulses to the heat-promoting control centre in the hypothalamus, which in turn triggers responses to retain body heat. Vasoconstriction reduces heat loss through the skin. The adrenal medulla releases hormones that increase cellular metabolism and the thyroid gland releases thyroid hormone, which increases metabolic rate. Significantly, this requires an intact central nervous system. Furthermore, temperature regulation requires oxygen because it is an aerobic process. Glucose is also needed to carry out this aerobic process for heat production (Hodson, 2018).

Non-shivering thermogenesis is a significant and unique form of heat production in the neonate. Neonates generate most of their heat from the breakdown of brown fat. 'Brown fat' refers to the deeply red, highly vascularised areas surrounding an infant's scapular, clavicular and sternal areas. It is rich in fats and glycogen (Hodson, 2018). The full-term infant has sufficient storage of brown fat to maintain temperature for up to 4 days. Heat is generated by hydrolysis of triglycerides in brown fat utilising oxygen in the process. The responses to cold of neonates in a hypoxic state will be jeopardised. Non-shivering thermogenesis is inhibited by drugs, intracranial haemorrhage and hypoglycaemic states (Knobel, 2014).

Heat Loss

There are four main routes of heat loss: evaporation, convection, conduction and radiation (Hodson, 2018). Evaporative heat loss occurs when water is converted to water vapour during perspiration or respiration. Neonates, wet from amniotic fluid and delivered into a cool labour ward, can lose heat at a rate of 0.25°C/min. It is therefore important to dry the neonate thoroughly with warmed towels and dress them promptly. Convective heat loss is when the infant's heat is lost to surrounding cooler air, which is why it is important to dress infants and to keep them out of draughts.

Conductive heat loss occurs when the infant comes into direct contact with a cool surface. One way to prevent this would be to prewarm anything in contact with the neonate's skin, including weighing scales and caregivers hands. Finally, radiative heat losses occur when the infant radiates heat to a cold exposed surface such as a window. In this case the neonate should be nursed away from windows and a constant environmental temperature maintained (Chitty and Wyllie, 2013).

Effects of Cold Stress

The effect of cold stress is well documented (Pearlman and Kjaer, 2016). Constriction of skin blood vessels occurs in response to cold in neonates. The effect of peripheral vasoconstriction is to increase the core skin temperature gradient. Increased metabolic rate leads to increased oxygen consumption, lactic acid production, hypoglycaemia and, in very low birthweight infants, decreased surfactant synthesis and secretion. Blood coagulopathies also occur leading to increased capillary permeability and haemorrhage.

🌐 **WWW**

Up-to-date reviews of management of newborn thermal environments are available at:
- https://www.cochranelibrary.com/cdsr/doi/10.1002/4651858. CD004210.pub5/full

Neutral Thermal Environment

The neutral thermal environment (NTE) is the provision of an environmental temperature that minimises oxygen consumption and maintains normal metabolism. The neutral thermal environment varies according to the maturity of the neonate and whether the infant is nursed in an incubator or a radiant heater and is dressed or not. Infants less than 25 weeks' gestation will require an ambient temperature similar to what they had in utero, 35°C–37°C (Hodson, 2018; Freer and Lyon, 2011). Optimal weight gain and normal physical development occur when a neonate is cared for in a neutral thermal environment appropriate to their age and weight.

Nursing Management

Initially, a thorough assessment of the neonate and history are required. Does the neonate look pale? How does the infant feel? Is the infant cool to touch? Is there a difference between central and peripheral temperatures? A hypothermic infant may appear pale and is cool to touch. This is primarily due to vasoconstriction. Is there associated acrocyanosis, a blueish discoloration around the mouth, hands or feet? Is the infant tachypnoeic or in respiratory distress? A hypothermic infant may develop respiratory distress secondary to the body's attempt to maintain a normal temperature, consuming oxygen in the process. How does the infant handle? Is the infant irritable or lethargic? Behavioural changes may occur as cold stress continues.

A history should be taken to assist with assessment. Maternal history is important because infants of diabetic mothers are at higher risk of hypothermia due to rapid depletion of glycogen stores. Drugs that mother has received during labour may affect the infant after birth. Side effects of sedatives include hypothermia, hypoglycaemia, lethargy and respiratory depression. Check for external sources of heat loss, such as drafts from open doors, cold and wet surfaces – often these maybe the caregivers' hands.

An unstable temperature may indicate infection. If infection is present, a full blood count with differential will reveal elevated white cells and a positive result on blood culture analysis. Neurological sequelae, such as absent or poor temperature control and fitting may be significant, and a head scan may reveal an intraventricular haemorrhage (Kuzniewicz et al., 2017).

Neonates requiring specialist care should be initially nursed in a prewarmed incubator (38°C). Incubators prevent heat loss through radiation and convection. The very preterm infant requires high humidity to manage hydration, fluid balance and temperatures (Pearlman and Kjaer, 2016). Radiant warmers similarly prevent heat loss and allow easier access. Care to prevent overheating is vital, as hyperthermia can lead to dehydration, hypernatraemia, hyperbilirubinaemia and increased metabolic demands (Oatley et al., 2016: Lahana et al., 2018).

Preventative measures are initiated to maintain a normothermic state from delivery onwards. Neonates are initially dried with a warm towel and placed on the mother's abdomen, or dried and dressed (Chitty and Wyllie, 2013). However, vulnerable or sick neonates of less than 28 weeks' gestation maybe placed immediately after birth in a plastic bag to reduce heat loss. A caution is to ensure the infant is dried before placing in the bag (McCall et al., 2014). A hat is applied prior to transfer to a neonatal unit in an incubator. Minimal handling of an ill hypothermic neonate is important to minimise cold stress.

Rewarming

Slow rewarming of a mildly hypothermic neonate is advocated at about 1°C/h. However, in neonates with extreme hypothermia, defined as a core temperature less than 35°C, a more rapid warming may be used with caution to avoid the deleterious effects of metabolic acidosis and prolonged asymptomatic hypoglycaemia. During rewarming, vigilance is required of the infant's vital signs of heart rate, blood pressure and oxygenation (Morassutti et al., 2015).

Temperature Measurement

Although rectal temperature recording has been described as the gold standard for core temperature assessment, there are potential problems with this method, for example, bowel perforation and cross-infection. Their use is not currently recommended; however they may be used in neonates undergoing therapeutic cooling (Pearlman and Kjaer, 2016). Intermittent axillary measurement is the most commonly and frequently used method in neonatal care. Accuracy depends on consistent and universal measurement for a duration of 3 minutes at the same site. Continuous skin and core temperature measurements are recorded in critically sick neonates. A temperature gradient is significant, determining tissue perfusion (Bellini and Beaulieu, 2017).

 ACTIVITY

In the NICU or SCBU, describe measures taken to:
- prevent heat loss;
- warm-up a cold infant.

 WWW

Read the following standards developed by the European Foundation for the Care of Newborn Infants (ECFNI) on ways to involve parents in measuring their baby's temperature in the NICU/SCBU:
- https://newborn-health-standards.org/temperature-man-agement-infants/

NEONATAL HYPOGLYCAEMIA

Hypoglycaemia in the neonate is one of the most common clinical care issues facing nurses caring for neonates. Increasing evidence suggests that neonatal hypoglycaemia may have long-term neurological effects (Bellini and Beaulieu, 2017). Care is complicated by inconsistent definitive laboratory values of hypoglycaemia and by variable clinical signs and symptoms in term and preterm neonates.

Definition of Hypoglycaemia

Clinical hypoglycaemia is defined as a blood sugar level (BSL) low enough to cause symptoms and/or signs of impaired brain function. This is generally accepted as a BSL <2.6 mmol/L (Harris et al., 2014; van Kempen et al., 2020). Significant hypoglycaemia depends on the infant's age, weight and clinical status. Neonates are at risk of hypoglycaemia because of a lack of glycogen and fat stores (Sharma et al., 2017).

Gluconeogenesis

In response to adaptation to extrauterine life, the healthy neonate creates fuel from glycogen and fat. While postnatal hormones mediate this response, certain conditions predispose the neonate to hypoglycaemia. There are two main reasons for hypoglycaemia in neonates, the increased utilisation of glucose and the decreased production of glucose stores.

Glucose is obtained from two sources: glycogenolysis and gluconeogenesis. Initially, hepatic and muscle glycogen stores are broken down to form glucose and are rapidly utilised in the first 24 hours. The process of converting glycogen back into glucose is known as glycogenolysis (Bellini and Beaulieu, 2017).

In gluconeogenesis, glucose is formed from the breakdown of fats and proteins. Glucocorticoid hormones of the adrenal cortex mobilise proteins, and thyroid hormones mobilise proteins and fats, thus making glycerol available (Bellini and Beaulieu, 2017). Gluconeogenesis is regulated by changes in insulin and glucose ratios, catecholamine release, fatty acid oxidation and activation of liver enzyme production. Prior to stabilisation at an average blood glucose level of 3.6 mmol/L, neonatal blood glucose levels fall to their lowest level between 2 and 6 hours old (British Association of Perinatal Medicine, 2017).

Neonates at Risk of Hypoglycaemia

- Small for gestational age (intrauterine growth retarded)
- Preterm infants
- Hypoxic infants
- Infected infants
- Infants of diabetic mothers
- Hypothermic infants
- Infants with congenital heart disease

Infants primarily at risk of hypoglycaemia are small for gestational age (SGA) neonates. Reduced glycogen stores combined with increased glucose utilisation account for hypoglycaemic states. Preterm infants are also at risk of hypoglycaemia. In the low birthweight infant, reduced enteral or parenteral intake may explain low plasma glucose levels. Immature hepatocytes, impaired gluconeogenesis and glucogenolytic enzyme activity suggest that preterm neonates are dependent on continuous exogenous nutrition. Hypoxic neonates utilise glucose at an increased rate and are therefore at risk of hypoglycaemia (Sharma et al., 2017). The main problem is the reduced rate at which glucose is formed during anaerobic glycolysis. The problem is compounded by the fact that the neonate is unable to feed in the regular way due to hypoxic state (Bellini and Beaulieu, 2017).

Hypothermic infants are also at risk of hypoglycaemia. In an attempt to maintain temperature with normal levels the neonate utilises glycogen, and plasma glucose levels fall. Therefore early recognition of the effects of cold stress should involve consideration for administration of glucose intravenous infusion. Infants of diabetic mothers are one of the most common groups of neonates to experience hypoglycaemia. This is due to impaired glucose production and excessive insulin levels from prolonged intrauterine exposure to elevated blood sugar levels.

Infected infants frequently present with hypoglycaemia. Although this could be associated with inadequate calorie intake, it is mainly as a result of sepsis-induced increased metabolic rate. Inborn errors of metabolism may give rise to a defective gluconeogenesis.

Clinical Signs and Symptoms of Hypoglycaemia

- Abnormal cry
- Apnoea
- Cardiac arrest
- Coma
- Convulsions
- Cyanosis
- Hypothermia
- Hypotonia
- Jitteriness
- Lethargy
- Tachypnoea
- Tremors

Sequelae of Hypoglycaemia

A significant feature of neonatal hypoglycaemia is that an infant can have extremely low blood sugars without any signs or symptom. Although short-term neonatal hypoglycaemia will not cause central nervous system (CNS) damage, prolonged neonatal hypoglycaemia has serious consequences. Neuroglycopenia, the CNS depletion of glucose, can develop with apnoea leading to depression of consciousness and/or convulsions. In the long term, severe hypoglycaemia can lead to severe developmental abnormalities (Bellini and Beaulieu, 2017).

Nursing Management of the Hypoglycaemic Infant

Nursing management is dependent on a thorough assessment of the potentially hypoglycaemic neonate. Knowledge of the causes of hypoglycaemia (hypothermia, poor feeding history), a thorough history to include maternal risk factors (infant of a diabetic) and difficulties during or after delivery (prolonged labour, birth asphyxia), signs (intrauterine growth retarded infant) and symptoms, and a plasma glucose level are important. Care centres on the prevention of hypoglycaemia and the avoidance of risk factors is essential. The greatest risk factors are cold stress and poor feeding. Therefore, it is important to nurse an infant in a neutral thermal environment.

Unless contraindicated due to respiratory illness or birth asphyxia, early feeding is advocated.

Infants at risk of hypoglycaemia should be closely observed and have blood glucose levels monitored 4- to 6-hourly. If a blood sugar reading is less than 3.0 mmol/L, or BSL of below 2.6, a plasma glucose sample is obtained for analysis. If this result is lower than 2.6 mmol/L, the neonate is fed smaller amounts of milk more frequently by bolus intermittently or continuously via a nasogastric or orogastric tube. Fluid volumes are increased accordingly, usually calculated a day ahead of requirements. A hypoglycaemic neonate should be nursed in a warmed incubator or on a radiant warmer. Hypoglycaemic neonates with an apparently normal temperature may be working excessively to maintain their temperature within normal limits, thereby utilising glucose stores. Therefore it is important to monitor the infant's temperature closely. The neonate is monitored for symptomatic hypoglycaemia and for signs of respiratory distress. A repeat blood sugar level within an hour will indicate the need for further treatment. If the readings are consistently low, intravenous therapy is commenced.

Oral 40% dextrose gel is the first-line treatment for infants with neonatal hypoglycaemia and can be used from birth (Weston et al., 2016). The gel is applied to the inside of the cheek for initial care of infants with low blood glucose levels. The advantage of this treatment is that the baby can stay with the mother on the postnatal ward.

 ACTIVITY

Read the following article, and in particular the algorithm on page 80, for neonates at risk of hypoglycaemia whose mothers are breastfeeding. Consider how your practice is consistent with this evidence.
- Csont, L. G., Groth, S., Hopkins, P., et al., 2014. An evidence-based approach to breastfeeding neonates at risk for hypoglycemia. JOGNN, 43, 71–81. https://www.jognn.org/article/S0884-2175(15)31506-9/pdf.

NEONATAL NUTRITION

Meeting the nutritional needs of a sick and/or premature neonate is vital for their recovery, growth and brain development to enable optimal neurodevelopmental outcomes (Belfort and Ehrenkhrez, 2017). Breastfeeding is the desired outcome; however, depending on the age and severity of illness of the neonate, parenteral and enteral routes may be commenced first. An essential component of nutritional management is to individualise the nutritional requirements to ensure optimal growth.

Growth and Development

Physically, growth of the intestine and maturation of intestinal absorption continue to develop. At birth, the intestine is approximately 250 cm long and the stomach has a capacity of 90 mL. In terms of intestinal absorption, pancreatic function is immature, hence there are limited enzymes for fat and carbohydrate breakdown. Therefore, neonates are at risk of malabsorption characterised by intolerance to feeds. Inadequate liver enzymes can lead to physiological jaundice, a common treatable illness of infanthood. Intestinal mucosal immunoglobulin levels are low and neonates are at increased risk of infection; Glycogen stores are depleted in periods of extreme stress of hypoglycaemia and hypothermia. In neonates, gluconeogenesis is impaired thereby limiting compensatory responses to adverse conditions of illness. This highlights the importance of adequate nutritional support. In addition to intestinal growth and maturation, the motility function of the gut continues to develop. A measure of gastrointestinal motility is the passage of stools in the first 24 hours of life. However, the more premature the infant the greater the delay in defaecation. Enteral feeding and early trophic feeds promote gastric emptying and the release of hormones that can stimulate peristalsis in term and preterm infants. In neonates, however, the rate of gastric emptying is prolonged.

The importance of growth as an indicator of adequate nutrition needs to be closely monitored in hospitalised neonates (Cooke, 2016). Regular measurements of weight, length and head circumference in a consistent way and an audit of the fluid and nutritional requirements is an important part of the nurse's role.

Neonates are weighed on admission and twice weekly thereafter, depending on clinical stability, diagnosis and need. Weights and head circumferences are plotted on graphs called percentile charts. For example, infants on the 10th percentile or graph line means that 10% of the population of infants are smaller and 90% are bigger. Typically, neonates lose 5% to 10% of their bodyweight in the first week of life. Preterm infants have a higher body water content so may appear to lose more. Infants should have regained their birth weight by 2 weeks of age. Accurate measurements are vital, and infants should be weighed on the same scales at the same time of day, and head circumferences measured weekly on the same day. All weights and head circumference measures are checked by two persons to ensure accuracy.

Nutritional Requirements

Ideally, the healthy preterm neonate should gain 15 g/kg/day in weight, 1 cm in length per week and 1 cm in head circumference per week, whereas the term neonate is expected to gain approximately 20–30 g/day. Accurate calculation of feeds is essential to ensure the correct volume fluid, on average 150 mL/kg/day, and calorific intake, on average 115 mL/kg/day (Cooke, 2016). Insensible losses, which mostly occurs through the permeable skin barrier, may be high in some neonates, are taken into account.

Breastfeeding is recommended nutritionally because human milk provides easily digestible protein, fat, carbohydrate and water for normal growth in the term infant. In terms of anti-infection, breast milk provides immunoglobulins (IgA), leucocytes, complement, lactoferrin and lysosome, which protect the infant from neonatal infections and reduce the incidence of necrotising enterocolitis, a complication of ischaemic bowel disease. Breast milk also contains growth

hormones, minerals and trace elements necessary for organ maturation and growth. Apart from the nutritional benefits of breastfeeding, the physical and emotional benefits have been well documented, especially for sick or preterm infants (American Academy of Pediatrics [AAP], 2012). Breast milk given to very low birthweight infants may need to be supplemented as these infants require a higher protein and calorific intake. These infants are also at risk of hyponatraemia and therefore may need sodium supplements. Calcium and phosphorus supplements reduce the risk of bone growth disorders of prematurity, such as metabolic bone disease. Iron stores of infants born at 32–34 weeks' gestation or less are deficient and therefore supplemental iron is given with feeds. Folic acid and vitamins are given also (AAP, 2012).

Although breast milk is the preferred source of neonatal nutrition, it should be noted that infections such as cytomegalovirus, herpes, hepatitis B and HIV can be transmitted through breast milk. Furthermore, certain drugs are excreted in breast milk, and women taking these drugs should therefore not express milk. Neonates in some countries may be more at risk from bottle feeding so caution is required as recommended by the World Health Organisation. (WHO 2020)

Standard infant formulae have been modified to imitate breast milk. Special preterm formulae have been developed to meet high protein and mineral requirements of low birthweight infants. Accurate calculation of fluid requirements is essential to promote infant well-being. In terms of the need for iron and vitamins, new formula feeds compensate for this, so these may be needed, but not necessarily.

Parenteral Nutrition

Total parenteral nutrition is the administration of total nutritional requirements prescribed intravenously to the infant unable to have enteral feed. It is characterised by the gradual increase in fluid, proteins, fats and glucose concentrations to promote normal growth. Electrolytes are monitored on a daily basis and adjusted accordingly. Light-sensitive vitamins and trace elements are also added to the intravenous solution and caution during administration is required by covering the bag and tubing with an opaque cover. Total parenteral nutrition can be given via a peripheral venous line. However, because of the vein sclerosing nature of highly concentrated solutions, central venous lines are the preferred method of administration. The trend is to reduce the duration of parental nutrition due to complication of cholestasis. Often both parental and enteral feeds are used, gradually decreasing parenteral and increasing enteral feeds as tolerated.

When parenteral nutrition is used in the NICU, nurses need to be vigilant to ensure the complications associated with its use are avoided. Infants should be monitored regularly for their fluid intake and output, their tolerance of dextrose by measuring both blood and urine glucose, and their tolerance of lipids by monitoring plasma turbidity, either by observing a sample of settled blood or spinning a sample of blood. Preterm infants have poor tolerance of both glucose and fat when infused above physiological levels; therefore nurses need to ensure that the infusion rate remains constant and avoid the temptation to 'catch up' with volumes when the infusion has been disrupted (Uthaya and Modi, 2014).

Enteral Nutrition

Infants who have difficulties with sucking, or who are unable to suck, can be fed into the stomach orogastrically, nasogastrically or transpylorically into the small intestine. Caution is required to ensure the tube is correctly placed and secured to ensure safety from movement or accidental dislodgement. Gastric feeding may be continuous via syringe pump or intermittent by hourly to 4-hourly bolus feeds. Assessment for complications is essential. Feeds should be reassessed:

- if gastric aspirate every 3–4 hours is greater than the volume of feed;
- if there are signs of intestinal obstruction, for example, abdominal distension, the presence of bile-stained aspirates or vomitus and failure to pass faeces, or passage of blood-stained stools;
- if feeding triggers apnoeic attacks;
- if the infant is suspected of necrotising enterocolitis.

 ACTIVITY

Read the following resource from the NHS regarding the safety requirements for placing gastric tubes. Neonates are particularly susceptible to errors and it remains the nurse's responsibility to ensure safe practice.

- https://improvement.nhs.uk/documents/193/Resource_set_-_Initial_placement_checks_for_NG_tubes_1.pdf

Neonates tolerate small amounts of milk and feed frequently. There is a well-coordinated suck and swallow reflex which develops from 34 weeks' gestation onwards. This has implications for feeding preterm infants.

The way in which adequate nutritional intake is achieved depends primarily on neonatal well-being and level of maturity. In a well neonate, suck feeds – by breast or bottle – is initiated as soon as possible after delivery and infants are fed on demand. Healthy preterm infants require a nasogastric tube and 2nd- to 3rd-hourly feeds commenced, as they gradually transition to suck feeds as they mature. Very immature or sick neonates will require nutrition provided by parental nutrition and then enteral feeds are slowly introduced (Harding et al., 2018).

Non-nutritive sucking is the practice of giving the neonate a pacifier during tube feeding to help the infant associate sucking with the feeling of having a full stomach and improves the sucking reflex. NNS enables the neonate to develop taste and smell to assist in the transition to suck feeds. (Lipchock et al., 2011)

Mothers are encouraged to express breast milk for their infants when they cannot initially have milk feeds. Expression of breast milk will initiate and maintain lactation. Successful breast expression depends on thoughtful patience and guidance. Breast pumps (electrical or hand) and a breastfeeding room are widely available on neonatal units. Initially, mothers are encouraged to express every 3 hours to stimulate milk

production. Breast milk can be frozen for up to 3 months. Once defrosted, it should be used within 4 hours. Breastmilk is also used for mouth care when neonates cannot take suck feeds. It is placed on a pacifier and given to the infant in small drops that are not swallowed.

The transition from tube to suck feeds can be problematic if there is no consistency in support from the health care team. The transition can be traumatic for both the infant and the family if the introduction of suck feeding and the transition process is not approached carefully (Jones, 2012). The transition from tube to suck feeding can take 10 to 14 days for healthy preterm infants (Griffith et al., 2018). However, variation in practices may delay the identification of infant readiness leading to the delay of the introduction of suck feeding and increasing hospital length of stay.

 WWW

Read about the Department of Health (DoH) infant feeding report at:

- https://www.gov.uk/government/publications/infant-feeding-commissioning-services

Suck Feeds

Sucking feeds are a great enjoyment for an infant and should be seen as a pleasurable experience. The first suck feed should ideally be a breastfeed; if this cannot occur, then the parent should be the first person to offer the feed to their baby. Using the principles of developmental care, the neonatal nurse assesses each infant's individual behavioural cues during care-giving and adapts the environment and their interactions accordingly to enhance the infant's strengths and self-regulation capacities (White-Traut et al., 2017). Feeding readiness cues and maturational competence for preterm neonates provide more useful information in guiding the neonatal nurse as to when to initiate suck feeds (Crowe et al., 2016). Suck feeds are infant-driven in that the infant will provide cues to their readiness (Lubbe, 2017). These include:

Early Cues – I'm hungry

　Stirring

　Mouth open

　Turning head

　Rooting

Mid Cues – I'm really hungry

　Stretching

　Increased physical movement

　Hand to mouth

Late Cues

　Crying

　Agitated

　Colour turning red

There may be disruptions to establishing suck feeds. For instance, prolonged ventilation with an orally placed endo-tracheal tube (ETT) can interfere with the normal function of the mouth and swallowing (Hardy et al., 2018). Oral disorders can interfere with feeding where the normal negative pressure of feeding is impaired in infants with unilateral and bilateral cleft lip and palate; a prosthetic palate will alleviate feeding difficulties. Pierre–Robin syndrome is characterised by poor muscular development and retromicrognathia. Feeding is problematic, but this can be overcome with the use of soft, elongated teats.

👤 ACTIVITY

Reflect on Your Practice

What feeding-related advice would you give to a first-time mother of a severely ill neonate?

INFECTION IN THE NEONATE

Neonatal sepsis is an important cause of mortality and morbidity among infants, above all in very low birth weight (VLBW) and preterm infants. Neonates are susceptible to infection due to an immature immune system. Infections are classified according to the time and mode of infection – early onset sepsis (EOS) is caused by maternal intrapartum transmission during the first 7 days following birth or during the first 72 hours for VLBW infants. Late-onset sepsis (LOS) is when there is a positive culture after 7 days from birth. Late onset is mostly caused by a nosocomial organism acquired in the hospital (Cortese et al., 2016)

Immunity

Initially, the neonate is protected by maternal immunoglobulins that cross the placenta in utero. Immunoglobulin G (IgG), which is present at birth, carries specific antigens to diseases that the mother has encountered, and therefore the infant can produce antibodies in response. IgG potentially offers protection against tetanus, diphtheria, measles, rubella and mumps, as well as common strains of streptococci (Verklan and Walden, 2015). IgM produced by the fetus offers protection from Gram-negative bacteria such as *Escherichia coli*. IgA is present in breast milk and protects the infant from gut infection.

There are two types of lymphocyte-mediated immunity in the neonate:

- Cellular immunity, produced by B cell and T cell lymphocytes, enables the infant to produce some antigens in response to infections.
- Humoral immunity, produced by immunoglobulins, offers protection from viruses and bacteria (Hong and Lewis, 2016).

Nursing Care

Nursing care centres on prevention of infection and assessment and early diagnosis of sepsis. Ways to prevent infection are adherence to strict hand washing techniques and wearing gloves by all staff and parents (Verklan and Walden, 2015). Infected infants should be nursed in isolation to protect other infants. Equipment should be cleaned regularly. Mothers should be encouraged to provide breast milk for their infant, and parental education on the importance of prevention of infection is advocated.

Frequent assessment of the neonate is vital to identify early signs of infection. Signs of infection in the neonate are often subtle. Is the infant quiet? How does the infant look: pale, mottled, jaundiced, presence of a rash? How does the infant handle: irritable, lethargic? How does the infant feel: hot, cool? How is the infant's breathing: fast, slow, using accessory muscles of respiration, nasal flaring? How does the infant feed: slowly, disinterested, vomiting, large aspirates? A septic infant's condition can deteriorate rapidly due to limited compensatory mechanisms.

PAIN IN THE NEONATE

For nurses, one of the most challenging situations is managing pain in the patient who cannot speak. It is well established that the neonate can feel pain; however, how pain is assessed remains a challenge (Anand, 2017; Bellini and Beaulieu, 2017). Compared with older children, neonates are more sensitive to pain and vulnerable to its long-term effects (Schwaller and Fitzgerald, 2014).

Physiology of Pain

Nociception, that is pain perception, is transmitted via pathways in the peripheral and central nervous systems and is fully established by 37 weeks. Research has shown that pain inhibitory pathways are immature at birth, suggesting a developmental hypersensitivity to pain (Verriotis et al., 2016). This means that preterm infants may be at greater risk of pain than the term infant.

Behavioural and physiological responses to pain are observed to determine levels of pain in the neonate. Facially, an infant in pain has a furrowed brow, eyes that are closed tightly, nostrils flared, a mouth that is unnaturally opened and a grey pallor to face. In terms of movement, an infant in pain will initially display sharp, tense movements and will withdraw the affected limb. As pain intensifies, or is prolonged, the infant will lie still with clenched fists, altered breathing and little eye movement. Fingers and toes will be held tightly curled and the infant will cry almost all of the time. The nature of the cry is important. A prolonged, intense, high-pitched cry indicates severe pain. The severity of pain may compromise the infant's respiratory status. A mewing pitiful cry together with apnoea indicates a pre-respiratory failure state. Physiologically, there is increased heart rate, blood pressure is also raised, oxygen saturations fall and there is evidence of palmar sweating. There are differences in the behavioural response between term and preterm neonates and vigilance is required during observations to ensure the cause and context of the painful stimuli are identified (Bellieni et al., 2014).

👤 ACTIVITY

During your placement on the neonatal unit, make a list of the painful procedures that you have observed. Note the infant's response and how the pain was controlled. What measures are used to alleviate the infant's pain?

Nursing Care

The aim of nursing care is to prevent pain and to minimise discomfort in neonates. Therefore infants should be assessed using an appropriate stressor scale (Newnham et al., 2009) and/or neonatal pain scale (Bellieni et al., 2014; Harrison et al., 2015). Non-pharmaceutical methods are incorporated into the nursing care plan to minimise environment-induced distress. For example, the care of neonates should be consolidated to avoid continuous disturbance. Infants should be handled gently with pre-warmed hands and equipment, and offered gentle reassurance. Minimal handling of ill infants is advocated. Quiet periods during the day should be observed to promote rest. A daytime/night-time pattern should be established. Infants should be shielded from bright lights. Noise levels should be kept to a minimum and alarms attended to promptly. Infants should be contained within soft boundaries to promote a sense of security. Thoughtful use of electrodes and tape is important. Physical pain during blood sampling or intravenous cannulation can be minimised with the administration of oral sucrose via a pacifier (Harrison et al., 2015). Also, breastfeeding effectively reduces pain in term neonates undergoing minor invasive procedures (Harrison et al., 2015). In terms of pharmaceutical management of pain, effective pain relief is essential if indicated. Opioids may be administered frequently; paracetamol is also administered. Regular administration of analgesia is important in pain management; however, caution is required and the doses should be monitored with regular pain assessment (Carbajal et al., 2015).

⊕ WWW

For further reading on pain prevention strategies, see:
- http://pediatrics.aappublications.org/content/pediatrics/early/2012/10/02/peds.2011-3848.full.pdf

  For guidelines for recognition and assessment of pain in neonates, see:
- https://link.springer.com/article/10.1007%2Fs40138-016-0089-y

  For prevention and management of pain stress in the neonate, see:
- https://www.cps.ca/en/documents/position/prevention-management-pain-neonate

---

NEONATAL RESPIRATORY PROBLEMS

The most common reason for admission to a neonatal unit is for respiratory difficulties. Respiratory difficulties can be present at delivery, requiring prompt resuscitation and admission to the neonatal unit for further treatment, but they can also occur during the postnatal period. The commonest causes of respiratory distress in preterm infants is respiratory distress syndrome and transient tachypnoea of the newborn, whereas in term infants it is likely to be meconium aspiration (Jackson, 2018).

Clinical Signs of Respiratory Dysfunction

- Cyanosis: the infant becomes 'blue' due to lack of circulating oxygen.
- Tachypnoea: the breathing rate is in excess of 60 breaths/min.
- Sternal and intercostal recession: this becomes evident as the work of breathing becomes harder. It is more pronounced in preterm infants who have a more pliable rib cage.
- Grunting: infants expel air explosively over a partially closed glottis to attempt to retain some function residual volume so as to maintain alveolar distension (Rubarth and Quinn, 2015).

 ACTIVITY

Discover how neonatal staff monitor infants for these signs of respiratory difficulties.

Respiratory Distress Syndrome

The most common respiratory difficulty in preterm infants is respiratory distress syndrome, also known as hyaline membrane disease, which is a disease of prematurity and is due to a lack of surfactant and structural immaturity (Reuter et al., 2014). In the very preterm infant, the disease is usually present at delivery and needs immediate treatment. In infants of greater gestational age, the disease can be seen to worsen gradually over a period of several hours. All of the clinical signs of respiratory distress are seen.

Respiratory distress syndrome is a disease directly resulting from the fact that the lungs are underdeveloped and the normal system of gaseous exchange is disturbed. One of the main problems is that the squamous epithelial type 2 cells producing surfactant are too immature and so insufficient amounts of surfactant are produced. Surfactant is necessary to reduce the surface tension of the alveoli, allowing continuous partial distension, and thus maintenance of functional residual capacity (Reuter et al., 2014).

Diagnosis is usually assumed when an x-ray, performed when the infant is at least 4 hours of age, shows a typical 'ground glass' appearance. Duration of this disease is usually 5–7 days.

Treatment

- The severity of the disease can be reduced significantly by the use of antenatal steroids.
- Artificial surfactant is given to any infant with respiratory distress syndrome.
- Inspired oxygen is given to maintain oxygen saturations between 85% and 93%.
- Continuous positive airways pressure (CPAP) or intermittent positive pressure ventilation (IPPV) can be used to maintain functional residual volume and to ensure that adequate gaseous exchange is maintained (NICE, 2019).

> ### ACTIVITY
>
> Discover how continuous positive airways pressure works and how it is administered. What are some of the specific nursing care that are required?

Transient Tachypnoea of the Newborn

The most common condition causing respiratory difficulties in the term infant is transient tachypnoea of the newborn (TTN). This condition is most often seen in infants who are delivered by caesarean section. The infant absorbs pulmonary alveolar fluid during labour and delivery. This loss of physiological function with caesarean section is thought to be very significant because the presumed aetiology of tachypnoea of the newborn is transient pulmonary oedema (Jackson, 2018). Clinical signs of respiratory distress may be seen, depending on the severity of the condition.

The chest radiograph may show increased perihilar interstitial markings and increased pleural fluid, especially in the minor fissure. The duration of the condition is usually 1–3 days.

Treatment

- Inspired oxygen to maintain oxygen saturations above 95%.
- Continuous positive airways pressure or intermittent positive pressure ventilation if maximal inspired oxygen fails to maintain adequate gaseous exchange.

Neonatal Pneumonia

Pneumonias may occur at any gestational age. They may be congenital, that is onset from birth to 48 hours of age, or nosocomial, that is onset after 48 hours of age. They are usually caused by bacteria or a virus. The poorly developed immune system of the neonate makes them more prone first to contracting pneumonia and second to a rapid acceleration of the condition. Pneumonias are even more likely to occur in ventilated neonates and those infants who weigh less than 1000 g (Jackson, 2018). In preterm infants, the pneumonia is often difficult to distinguish from other causes of respiratory distress.

The chest radiograph may show consolidation, interstitial infiltration or, particularly in group B streptococcus pneumonia, a 'ground glass' appearance, which often makes the diagnosis difficult to separate from other causes of respiratory distress. The diagnosis of pneumonia is also made by blood cultures, white blood cell count and C-reactive protein count. The duration of the disease is likely to be 5–7 days but may occasionally be prolonged – up to 3 weeks.

Treatment

Administration of antibiotics is started immediately, and the choice will be determined by the most common organism. Currently antibiotics of choice are ampicillin and gentamicin (Jackson, 2018).

- Specific antibiotic treatment once the organism/sensitivity is known.
- Inspired oxygen to maintain oxygen saturations appropriately.

- Continuous positive airways pressure or intermittent positive pressure ventilation may be used if maximal oxygen fails to maintain adequate gaseous exchange.

> ### ACTIVITY
>
> - Name two bacteria and two viruses that cause neonatal pneumonia.
> - What is a normal white cell count from birth to 1 week of age?

Principles of Nursing Management for Infants With Respiratory Distress

- Ensure continuous positive airways pressure or ventilation endotracheal tubes are in the correct position to promote effective ventilation. Secure tubes to minimise trauma to the infant's face and accidental dislodgement.
- Observe for signs of deterioration in condition and report to medical team promptly.
- Maintain oxygen saturations between 90% and 93% in preterm infants and greater than 95% in term neonates with particular attention to alarm settings (Sola et al., 2014).
- Administer analgesia as prescribed; observe for signs of stress and/or pain.
- Reposition the infant 6-hourly or as condition permits.
- Ensure minimal handling of infants observing for signs of stress.
- Support parents to assist to care for their infant while on respiratory support.

Persistent Pulmonary Hypertension of the Newborn (PPHN)

This condition occurs when there is a high resistance in the pulmonary vessels resulting in shunting of blood across the open fetal channels of the foramen ovale (in the heart) and/or the patient ductus arteriosis. This results in pulmonary vasoconstriction, pulmonary hypoplasia or pulmonary hypertension. It is more commonly found in term or late preterm infants who have had some asphyxia at birth (Parker and Kinsella, 2018).

Management

The goal is to correct hypoxia and acidosis (major contributing factors), increasing and maintaining systemic blood pressure while decreasing pulmonary vascular resistance, maintaining oxygenation and reducing any iatrogenic effects of the ventilator support (Fraser, 2015; Cabral and Belik, 2013).

Inotropic support with dopamine, dobutamine and milrinone to ensure there is an adequate cardiac output to maintain systematic blood pressure. These drugs require diligent care to ensure the administration of consistent doses and the infant closely observed for fluctuations in their autonomic responses to handling (Cabral and Belik, 2013).

Inhaled nitric oxide maybe used as a pulmonary dilator, which may reduce the need for extracorporeal membrane oxygenation (ECMO) in the majority of infants. This is often used in conjunction with high frequency ventilation (Bendapudi and Barr, 2014).

The principles of caring for a neonate with respiratory distress apply.

Meconium Aspiration Syndrome

Meconium passed at or before delivery and inhaled in the presence of hypoxia is known as meconium aspiration syndrome (MAS). MAS is a disease of term or post-term infants and is rarely seen in infants born at less than 36 weeks of gestation (Parker and Kinsella, 2018).

When asphyxia occurs with chronic hypoxia these neonates are at risk of PPHN (Fraser, 2015). They often present with respiratory distress with signs of tachypnoea, nasal flaring and retractions, which may be mild or prolonged and is often accompanied by cyanosis. Nail beds may be stained a yellow-green from the meconium in the amniotic fluid and the skin is often dry, cracked and stained.

A chest x-ray can show a barrel-like shape with over-inflation of the lungs, which is secondary to the obstruction of the small airways. A right to left shunt of blood through the ductus arteriosus can result in hypoxaemia and hypercapnia (Martin et al., 2015; Fraser, 2015).

Management

- If infant has no respiratory effort at delivery the infant will require intubation, ventilation and sedation to enable oxygenation and prevent hypoxia.
- Inotropic support may be required to sustain blood pressure in the presence of increased pulmonary pressures and shunting through the ductus arteriosus.
- Arterial blood gas (ABG) ABGs to determine degree of respiratory compromise and type of therapy needed.
- Assisted ventilation, initially conventional but may need high frequency ventilation or inhaled nitric oxide if PPHN develops.
- Surfactant replacement therapy has been shown to reduce the risk of air leaks, lessen the need for ECMO, and improve gas exchange but has not had an impact on mortality (Martin et al., 2015; Fraser, 2015).

Jaundice

Physiological Jaundice

Hyperbilirubinemia occurs when the level of bilirubin exceeds the normal range, and jaundice refers to the yellow discoloration of the skin. Jaundice is one of the most common conditions in newborn babies; approximately 60% of term (gestational age of 37 weeks or more) and 80% of preterm babies develop jaundice in the first week of life (NICE, 2014). It occurs as the life of the red blood cells ends and they are broken down. When red blood cells are destroyed in the liver and the spleen via the reticuloendothelial system, the globin is preserved for reuse and the haem is further broken down. This process produces bilirubin in a fat-soluble/water-insoluble form called unconjugated bilirubin. It cannot be excreted in bile or urine and must be further converted in the liver so that a conjugated, water-soluble bilirubin is produced that can be excreted by the body (Bellini and Beaulieu, 2017).

The bilirubin is carried to the liver for conjugation in the circulating blood. Binding sites are located on the albumin carried in the plasma and the bilirubin binds to these sites until it is passed into the liver cells (the hepatocytes). Once in the hepatocyte, uridine diphosphate-glucoronal transferase joins the bilirubin with a water-soluble glucuronide to create bilirubin monoglucuronide. This is called conjugated bilirubin; this structure is water soluble. It is transferred into the bile for excretion in the stool. In the neonate, several factors combine to overload this normal function (Martin et al., 2015).

In utero the foetus has a high haemoglobin level of 18–22 mg/dL as a result of the high number of circulating red blood cells. This allows sufficient transport of oxygen from maternal to fetal cells. At birth these cells are no longer required and must be destroyed. This is helped by fetal red blood cells having a lifespan of 80–100 days. The increased number of red blood cells being broken down means that there are increased amounts of unconjugated bilirubin (Bellini and Beaulieu, 2017).

The mechanisms for the transfer and breakdown of bilirubin, ex utero, can take several days to become fully activated. The more preterm the infant, the longer this process can be delayed. This adds to the amount of unconjugated bilirubin.

Once bilirubin has been conjugated and transferred to the intestine, it can be broken down by bilirubin gluconidase, an enzyme found in the small intestine. In the neonate, the passage of stool is slow for the first few days of life and this allows more breakdown by the enzyme. Normal gut flora inhibits this process but it is several days before normal gut flora is present. Also, in breastfed infants there is a continued lack of normal gut flora, which also allows more breakdown. This often causes what is known as 'breast milk jaundice'.

These combined factors result in more unconjugated bilirubin than there are binding sites. Some of this bilirubin can be stored in the skin, which is what gives the infant their yellow colour. There is a limit to how much can be stored in the skin and the excess is carried in the circulating blood with nothing to bind to. This is called 'free' bilirubin. Free bilirubin passes easily through the blood–brain barrier, where it is transferred into the brain cells. This can result in 'kernicterus', which causes brain damage. It is for this reason that it is necessary to provide treatment to restrict the amount of free bilirubin in the circulating blood (Martin et al., 2015).

👤 ACTIVITY

- Find out which method of treatment for jaundice is used in your local neonatal unit.
- What are the thresholds for commencing phototherapy?

Any infant who appears jaundiced will have a blood test to measure the serum bilirubin level. If the level is high, treatment will be given. The serum bilirubin level will be tested regularly. Once it falls to low levels, treatment will be discontinued. Assessing whether the levels are high enough for treatment can be done by plotting the level against a universal chart.

Non-Physiological Jaundice

The most common cause of non-physiological jaundice is incompatibility of blood groups. Rhesus blood proteins are highly antigenic, causing severe jaundice This problem used to be more common than it is now because the introduction of anti-D for any antenatal event and post-delivery for women whose partner has a different blood group has reduced the incidence of this condition significantly.

ABO incompatibility is probably more common than Rhesus incompatibility but is usually mild and does not require treatment other than phototherapy. However, in some instances the condition is very severe and requires prompt and efficacious management.

The best treatment commences antenatally with all pregnant women being screened for blood group and for antibodies. Sometimes there is no indication of problems until hydrops is seen on scan. It is possible for some foetuses to have in utero transfusions to maintain the pregnancy until viability. Fetuses are affected to varying degrees. In the most severe cases, there is fetal anaemia, cardiac failure, oedema and hydrops. The prognosis is poor and only immediate exchange transfusions provide any hope of survival.

In less severe cases, the infant may appear normal at birth, but signs of clinical jaundice become apparent within hours of delivery. Jaundice is never a normal finding before 24 hours of age, and if there is any doubt, a serum bilirubin level must be measured. If there is any indication of problems, blood for a Coombs test should be taken at delivery.

Treatment with phototherapy is invariably successful. This is the use of a specific wavelength of light onto the skin. This light wavelength causes a chemical reaction in the bilirubin stored in the skin. This reaction changes the stored unconjugated bilirubin into conjugated bilirubin, which can be excreted. One of the side effects of phototherapy treatment is that it accelerates the digestive process, resulting in diarrhoea. This actually enhances the reduction of bilirubin because it allows less time for bilirubin gluconidase to break down the conjugated bilirubin. The light can be delivered by a light-box placed over the cot or incubator. This means that the infant must be naked for the light to fall on the skin. Infants may need to be transferred to an incubator if they are unable to maintain their core temperature when naked. Phototherapy can also be given via a 'biliblanket': a fibreoptic light source is used to provide the appropriate wavelength of light into a specially developed small rectangular 'blanket', which can be wrapped around the infant's torso and used underneath the clothes. This causes less disruption to the infant and is more acceptable to parents. Treatment usually lasts for 3–7 days.

Phototherapy is the first choice for the treatment of jaundice. There are two modes, conventional and intensive. Conventional phototherapy is where three to four globes or a biliblanket are used so the bilirubin level will decrease by 25% to 50% in the first 24–48 hours of therapy in the absence of underlying haemolysis. The infant is nursed naked to allow for maximum exposure. Intensive phototherapy involves irradiance in the blue-green spectrum (430–490 nm) and is delivered to as much of the infant's body surface area as possible. If total bilirubin does not fall or continues to rise despite intensive phototherapy, then the likelihood of ongoing haemolysis is high and an exchange transfusion will be required (NICE, 2014).

An exchange transfusion aims to remove the affected blood and replace it with blood that has normal erythrocytes and a normal bilirubin level. Thus it will relieve anaemia and help to prevent kernicterus. Assessing whether an exchange transfusion is required can be done by plotting the serum bilirubin level against a universal chart. If the serum bilirubin level is above this number then an exchange transfusion should be given. In severe cases, several exchange transfusions may be required before the infant's condition becomes stabilised.

WWW

For current British neonatal practice for jaundice, see:
- https://www.nice.org.uk/guidance/cg98/evidence/full-guideline-245411821

ACTIVITY

- Describe what a Coombs test is and why it is helpful.
- How may a sample bilirubin level be measured
- What are the principles of undertaking an exchange transfusion?

Nursing Care

- The infant's eyes are covered during phototherapy with a firmly placed eye shield. There is a risk of airway obstruction so these infants must always have a cardio-respiratory monitor attached.
- By undressing infants, they are exposed to the risk of hypothermia and it may be best to nurse them in an incubator or open heating source.
- The use of the phototherapy lamp can increase the ambient temperature surrounding the infant. The set incubator temp should be reduced by 1°C for all infants already being nursed in an incubator.
- Care should be taken to change infants regularly to avoid skin problems.
- Nappies should be used to ensure gonads are protected at all times.
- Feeding and interaction with parents should be actively encouraged. Up to 4 hours in 24 hours out from under the phototherapy lamp does not affect treatment levels as treatment is rate-limited.

- Attention to good nutrition and adequate fluids is essential to avoid dehydration and/or weight loss.
- Constant reassurance of family members is usually required.
- Consider the other neonates in the nursery and staff in ensuring the light is deflected.

Surgical Conditions

Many neonates are born with a congenital abnormality that requires surgery in the neonatal period. It is beyond the scope of this chapter to cover all such conditions and these infants are cared for in specialist neonatal units with access to surgeons, specialist nurses and facilities.

The following resources are available for those wanting more information.

Meeker, T. (Ed.), 2018. The surgical neonate. Adv. Neonatal Care. 18 (1), 1–2. https://doi.org/10.1097/ANC.0000000000000463.

Jain, L., 2012. The surgical neonate. Clinics in Perinatology 39 (2), xiii–xiv.

Spence, K., 2013. Chapter 25: surgical considerations in the newborn and infant. In: Kenner, C., Lott, J.W., 2013. Comprehensive Neonatal Nursing Care (5th ed), Springer https://connect.springerpub.com/content/book/978-0-8261-0976-7/part/part04/chapter/ch25.

Discharge

Preterm and sick infants and their families experience an unfamiliar and often overwhelming journey through the neonatal intensive care unit (NICU). When the time comes to plan their discharge, parents may seem unsure about their ability to care for their baby at home. Supporting and involving parents in the discharge process helps to ensure their confidence in caring for their infant once they are back home (Fong, 2017).

In preparation for discharge, parents should be assessed on their ability to provide safe care. Simple care-giving, such as bathing, positioning on the back to sleep, handling and feeding as well as cardiopulmonary resuscitation are demonstrated and discussed. The home environment preparation for supplies and required equipment and community resources are discussed by the discharge nurse/s. Guidance on car seat use and transporting their baby home is also given. Follow-up appointments are made and many NICUs have a developmental follow-up programme that enables an assessment to be done to ensure the milestones are being achieved.

Some units have an early discharge programme with a coordinator to support these vulnerable infants and their families when they go home. Often reassurance and initial follow-up is appreciated. There are many support groups available and health care professionals need to be aware of their local resources.

 ACTIVITY

Check the information for both parents and health care professionals on the Bliss website. This will help you become aware of the resources available and ways to support parents when they take their baby home.
- https://www.bliss.org.uk/

SUMMARY

Neonatal nursing is as challenging as it is rewarding. As neonatal care continues to evolve, it is important for nurses to develop evidence-based practice and to keep abreast of changes. Individualised developmentally supportive care is a framework for ensuring protection of the developing brain.

Parents are the important mainstay for infants in neonatal units and all health care professionals should strive to keep families informed and involved in the care of their baby in the NICU/SCBU. A neonate's outcome rests in nurses' hands.

REFERENCES

Als, H., 1986. A synactive model of neonatal behavioural organization: framework for the assessment of neurobehavioural development in the premature infant and for support of infants and parents in the neonatal intensive care environment. In: Sweeny, J.K. (Ed.), 1986. The High-Risk Neonate Developmental Theory Perspectives. Physical and Occupational Therapy in Pediatrics, vol. 6, pp. 3–55.

Als, H., 2009. NIDCAP: testing the effectiveness of a relationship-based comprehensive. Pediatrics 124, 1208–1210.

American Academy of Pediatrics (AAP), 2012. Policy statement. Breastfeeding and the use of human milk. Pediatrics 129 (3), e827–e841.

Anand, K.J.S., 2017. Defining pain in newborns: need for a uniform taxonomy? Acta Pediatrics 106, 1438–1444.

Bellieni, C., Tei, M., Buonocore, G., 2014. Should we assess pain in newborn infants using a scoring system or just a detection method? Acta Pediatrics, 1–4.

Bellini, S., Beaulieu, M., 2017. Neonatal Advanced Practice Nursing: A Cue Based Approach. Springer Publishing Company, New York.

Belfort, M.B., Ehrenkhrez, E., 2017. Neurodevelopmental outcomes and nutritional strategies in very low birth weight infants. Semin. Fetal Neonatal Med. 22, 42–48.

Bendapudi, P., Barr, S., 2014. Diagnosis and management of pulmonary hypertension in the newborn. J. Paediatr. Child Health 24 (1), 12–16.

British Association of Perinatal Medicine, 2017. Identification and Management of Neonatal Hypoglycaemia in the Full Term Infant – Framework for Practice.

Brummelte, S., Grunau, R.E., Chau, V., et al., 2012. Procedural pain and brain development in premature newborns. Ann. Neurol. 71 (3), 385–396.

Burke, S., 2018. Systematic review of developmental care interventions in the neonatal intensive care unit since 2006. J. Child Health Care, 1–18.

Cabral, J., Belik, J., 2013. Persistent pulmonary hypertension of the newborn: recent advances in pathophysiology and treatment. deJ. Pediatric 89 (3), 226–242.

Carbajal, R., Eriksson, M., Courtois, E., et al., 2015. Sedation and Analgesia Practices in Neonatal Intensive Care Units (EUROPAIN): Results from a Prospective Cohort Study. Available from: www.thelancet.com/respiratory.

Chitty, H., Wyllie, J., 2013. Importance of maintaining the newly born temperature in normal range from delivery to admission. Semin. Fetal Neonatal Med. 18 (6), 362–368.

Cooke, R.J., 2016. Improving growth in preterm infants during initial hospital stay: principles into practice. Arch. Dis. Child. Fetal Neonatal Ed. 101 (4), F366–F370.

Cortese, F., Scicchitano, P., Gesualdo, M., 2016. Early and late infections in the newborn: where do we stand? A review. Pediatr. Neonatol. 57, 265–273.

Crowe, L., Chang, A., Wallace, K., 2016. Instruments for assessing readiness to commence suck feeds in preterm infants: effects on time to establish full oral feeding and duration of hospitalisation. Cochrane Database Syst. Rev. (8), CD005586. https://doi.org/10.1002/14651858.CD005586.pub3.

Csont, L.G., Groth, S., Hopkins, P., Guillet, R., 2014. An evidence-based approach to breastfeeding neonates at risk for hypoglycemia. J. Obstet. Gynecol. Neonatal Nurs. 43, 71–81. Available from: https://www.jognn.org/article/S0884-2175(15)31506-9/pdf.

Cyr-Alves, H., Macken, L., Hyrkas, K., 2018. Stress and Symptoms of Depression in Fathers of Infants Admitted to the NICU. J. Obstet. Gynecol. Neonatal. Nurs. 47 (2), 146–157. https://doi.org/10.1016/j.jogn.2017.12.006.

Davila, R.C., Segre, S.C., 2018. A nurse-based model of psychosocial support for emotionally distressed mothers of infants in the NICU. J. Obstet. Gynecol. Neonatal Nurs. 47 (1), 114–121.

Fraser, D., 2015. Respiratory disorders. In: Verklan, T.M., Waldren, M. (Eds.), Core Curriculum of Neonatal Intensive Care Nursing, fifth ed. Saunders, Imprint of Elsevier. St. Louis, Miss.

Filippa, M., Panza, C., Ferrari, F., et al., 2017. Systematic review of maternal voice interventions demonstrates increased stability in preterm infants. Acta Pediatrics 106, 1220–1229.

Fong, E., 2017. Evidence Summary. Discharge of Pre-term Infants: Facilitating Family's Readiness for Discharge, vol. 2017. The Joanna Briggs Institute EBP Database, JBI@Ovid, p. JBI12959.

Freer, Y., Lyon, A., 2011. Temperature monitoring and control in the newborn baby. J. Paediatr. Child Health 22 (4), 127–130.

Griffith, T.T., Bell, A.F., White-Traut, R., et al., 2018. Relationship between duration of tube feeding and success of oral feeding in preterm infants. J. Obstet. Gynecol. Neonatal Nurs. 47 (5), 620–631.

Harding, C., Mynard, A., Hills, E., 2018. Identification of premature infant states in relation to introducing oral feeding. J. Neonatal Nurs. 24, 104–110.

Hardy, C., Senese, J., Fucile, S., 2018. Rehabilitation of infant oral feeding difficulties: a survey of occupational therapists practice approaches. Occup. Ther. Health Care 32 (1), 14–27.

Harris, D.L., Weston, P.J., Battin, M.R., et al., 2014. A survey of the management of hypoglycaemia within the Australian and New Zealand neonatal network. J. Paediatr. Child Health 50 (10), E55–E62.

Harrison, D., Bueno, M., Reszel, J., 2015. Prevention and management of pain and stress in the neonate. Res. Rep. Neonatol. Dovepress 5, 9–16.

Hodson, W.A., 2018. Temperature regulation. In: Gleason, C.A., Juul, S.E., (Eds.), 2018. Avery's Diseases of the Newborn, tenth ed. Elsevier, Philadelphia.

Hong, D.K., Lewis, D.B., 2016. Chapter 4: developmental immunology and role of host defenses in fetal and neonatal susceptibility to infection. In: Remington and Klien, 2016. Infectious Diseases of the Fetus and Newborn, eighth ed. Saunders (Elsevier), Philadelphia.

Jackson, C.J., 2018. Respiratory disorders in the preterm infant. In: Gleason, C.A., Juul, S.E. (Eds.), Avery's Diseases of the Newborn, tenth ed. Elsevier, Philadelphia.

Janvier, A., Lantos, J., Aschner, J., et al., 2016. Stronger and more vulnerable: a balanced view of the impacts of the NICU experience on parents. Pediatrics 138 (3), e2/0160655.

Jayasekara, R., 2016. Evidence Summary. Kangaroo Mother Care: Low Birth Weight Infants. The Joanna Briggs Institute EBP Database, JBI@Ovid, p. JBI6046.

Jones, L.R., 2012. Oral feeding readiness in the neonatal intensive care unit. Neonatal Netw. 31 (3), 148–155.

Knobel, R.B., 2014. Fetal and neonatal thermal physiology. Newborn Infant Nurs. Rev. 14 (2), 45–49.

Kuzniewicz, M.W., Puopolo, K.M., Fischer, A., et al., 2017. A quantitative risk approach to the management of neonatal early onset sepsis. JAMA Pediatrics 171 (4), 356–371.

Lipchock, S., Reed, D., Mennella, J., 2011. The Gustatory and Olfactory Systems during Infancy: Implications for Development of Feeding Behaviors in the High-risk Neonate. Clin. Perinatol. 38, 627–641. https://doi.org/10.1016/j.clp.2011.08.008.

Lahana, A., Delanaud, S., Erbani, R., Glusko-Charlet, A., Durand, E., Haraux, E., Ghyselen, L., Libert, J., Tourneux, P., 2018. Warming the premature infant in the delivery room: Quantification of the risk of hyperthermia. Med. Eng. Phys. 59, 70–74. https://doi.org/10.1016/j.medengphy.2018.06.002.

Lizarondo, L., 2016. Evidence Summary. Development Care: Preterm or Ill Neonates. The Joanna Briggs Institute EBP Database, JBI@Ovid, p. JBI16368.

Lubbe, W., 2017. Clinician's guide for cue-based transition to oral feeding in preterm infants: an easy-to-use clinical guide. J. Eval. Clin. Pract. 24 (1), 80–88.

McCall, E., Alderdice, F., Halliday, H., et al., 2014. Challenges of minimizing heat loss at birth: a narrative review of evidenced-based thermal care interventions. Newborn Infant Nurs. Rev. 14 (2), 56–63.

Martin, R.J., Fanaroff, A.A., Walsh, M.C., 2015. Fanaroff and Martin's Neonatal-Perinatal Medicine: Diseases of the Fetus and Infant. Elsevier/Saunders, Philadelphia.

Morassutti, R.F., Cavalin, F., Zaramella, P., et al., 2015. Association of rewarming rate on neonatal outcomes in ELBW infants with hypothermia. J. Pediatr. 167, 557–561.

Newnham, C.A., Inder, T.E., Milgrom, J., 2009. Measuring preterm cumulative stressors within the NICU: the neonatal infant stressor scale. Early Hum. Dev. 85 (9), 549–555.

National Audit Office, 2007. Caring for Vulnerable Babies: the Reorganisation of Neonatal Services in England. Available at: https://www.nao.org.uk/report/caring-for-vulnerable-babies-the-reorganisation-of-neonatal-services-in-england/.

National Institute for Health and Care Excellence (NICE), 2014. Jaundice in Newborn Babies under 28 Days. Quality standard [QS57]. Available from: http://nice.org.uk/guidance/qs57.

National Institute for Health and Care Excellence (NICE), 2017. Developmental Follow-Up of Children and Young People Born Preterm. NICE Guideline [NG72]. Available from: http://nice.org.uk/guidance/ng72.

National Institute for Health and Care Excellence (NICE), 2019. Specialist Neonatal Respiratory Care for Babies Born Preterm. NICE Guideline [NG124]. Available from: http://nice.org.uk/guidance/ng124.

Oatley, H., Blencowe, H., Lawn, J., 2016. The effect of coverings, including plastic bags and wraps, on mortality and morbidity in preterm and full-term neonates. J. Perinatol. 36, S83–S89. https://doi.org/10.1038/jp.2016.35.

Parker, T.A., Kinsella, J.P., 2018. Respiratory disorders in the term infant. In: Gleason, C.A., Juul, S.E. (Eds.), Avery's Diseases of the Newborn, tenth ed. Elsevier, Philadelphia.

Pearlman, J., Kjaer, K., 2016. Neonatal and maternal temperature regulation during and after delivery. Anesth. Analg. 123 (1), 168–172.

Raines, D.A., Brustad, J., 2012. Parent's confidence as a caregiver. Adv. Neonatal Care 12 (3), 183–188.

Reuter, S., Moser, C., Baack, M., 2014. Respiratory distress in the newborn. Pediatr. Rev. 35 (10), 417–429.

Rubarth, L.B., Quinn, J., 2015. Respiratory development and respiratory distress syndrome. Neonatal Netw. 34 (4), 231.

Schwaller, F., Fitzgerald, M., 2014. The consequences of pain in early life: injury-induced plasticity in developing pain pathways. Eur. J. Neurosci. 39 (3), 344–352.

Sharma, A., Davis, A., Shekhawar, P.S., 2017. Hypoglycaemia in the preterm neonate: etiopathogenesis, diagnosis, management and long-term outcomes. Transl. Pediatr. 6 (4), 335–348.

Sola, A., Golombek, S.G., Montes Bueno, M.T., et al., 2014. Safe oxygen saturation targeting and monitoring in preterm infants: can we avoid hypoxia and hyperoxia? Acta Paediatrics 103 (10), 1009–1018.

Stiles, J., Jernigan, T.L., 2010. The basics of brain development. Neuropsychol. Rev. 20 (4), 327–348. https://doi.org/10.1007/s11065-010-9148-4.

Uthaya, S., Modi, N., 2014. Practical preterm parenteral nutrition: systematic literature review and recommendations for practice. Early Hum. Dev. 90, 747–753.

van Kempen, A., Eskes, P., Nuytemans, D., et al., 2020. Lower versus traditional treatment threshold for neonatal hypoglycemia. N. Engl. J. Med. 382 (6), 534–544. https://doi.org/10.1056/NEJMoa1905593.

Verklan, T.M., Walden, M. (Eds.), 2015. Core Curriculum of Neonatal Intensive Care Nursing, fifth ed. Saunders, imprint of Elsevier. St Louis, Miss.

Verriotis, M., Chang, P., Fitzgerald, M., et al., 2016. The development of the nociceptive brain. Neuroscience 338, 207–219.

Warren, I., 2017. Creating a holding environment for caregivers. J. Perinat. Neonatal Nurs. 31 (1), 51–57.

Weston, P.J., Harris, D.L., Battin, M., et al., 2016. Oral dextrose gel for the treatment of hypoglycaemia in newborn infants. Cochrane Database Syst. Rev. (5), CD011027. https://doi.org/10.1002/14651858.CD011027.pub2.

White-Traut, R., Liu, L., Norr, K., et al., 2017. Do orally-directed behaviors mediate the relationship between behavioral state and nutritive sucking in preterm infants? Early Hum. Dev. 109, 26–31. https://www.who.int/news-room/fact-sheets/detail/infant-and-young-child-feeding.

33

The Role of the Community Children's Nurse (CCN): Managing Care at 'Home'

Sarah Adrienne Hughes

LEARNING OUTCOMES

- Consider the benefits of supporting sick children in their own home.
- Discuss the effects of nursing in the 'home' setting on relationships between nurses, children and their carers.
- Understand the importance of managing risk: accurate and effective assessment of the potentially deteriorating child by nurses, parents and carers.

- Explore the concept of care at home: supporting the independence and development of the child as an expert in their own self-care.
- Consider how community children's services could be evaluated and developed to meet children's care needs in 21st-century childhoods.

GLOSSARY

Carer(s) While most children will experience a conventional family setting with at least one parent, many live in alternative families, so this term is used to denote the main person(s) who provide help and support with a child's day-to-day living.

Childhood Term used to denote the experience of children in their own lives when undertaking their everyday routines and tasks.

Community children's nurse (CCN) A nurse who has undergone specialist post-graduate training. The term is also used in this chapter to denote children's nurses working in the 'community' setting.

Community/home Environments where a child normally lives or inhabits and their care takes place (e.g. schools, playgroup).

PART 1: THE DEVELOPMENT OF THE ROLE OF THE CCN

Community nursing schemes were set up as early as the 1950s as an alternative to acute hospital care, and by the mid-1990s, there were over 120 teams across England (Cain et al., 1995), with almost 200 teams identified by Whiting et al., in 2009. A long history of government reports (Platt, CHSC, 1959; Department of Health and Social Security [DHSS], 1976; House of Commons Select Committee, 1997; Department of Health [DoH], 2009; DoH, 2011) supported the idea that children were at an advantage if nursed at home. In considering the 21st-century world, the notion that 'children should only be nursed in an acute setting if needed' (Platt, 1959, Para 18) has enabled services to expand and shift care to the 'community' setting (Carter and Coad, 2009). Care of the 'acute, but stable' child and those who were technologically dependent, has also been increasingly delivered in educational settings with specialist support and training (RCN, 2018), important to ensure the best possible 'childhoods' (Randall, 2016). It is now difficult to estimate how many CCN teams there are in current service provision, but in a report written for 'WellChild'

(Whiting, 2017), it was estimated that approximately 6800 CCNs would be needed for the current 0–18 population.

As can be seen in Fig. 33.1, care of children in the community can be commissioned or provided by a number of stakeholders, in both the NHS as well as the private and voluntary sectors. Fig. 33.1 depicts a variety of settings with the child and family at the centre. CCN teams can be located or managed within a wide range of services and work between teams to provide a network to support children and home and to develop best practice. Teams led by qualified specialist practitioners (CCNs) continue to assess, care for, evaluate and support families and children to manage health needs at home and at school.

Community Children's Nurse Competencies and Skills

The Queen's Nursing Institute (QNI) (2018, p 2) identified the role of the community children's nurse as 'enabling children and young people to remain safely in the community and their transition to adult services in due course'. They published 'Voluntary Standards for Community Children's Nursing Education and Practice', which contained four

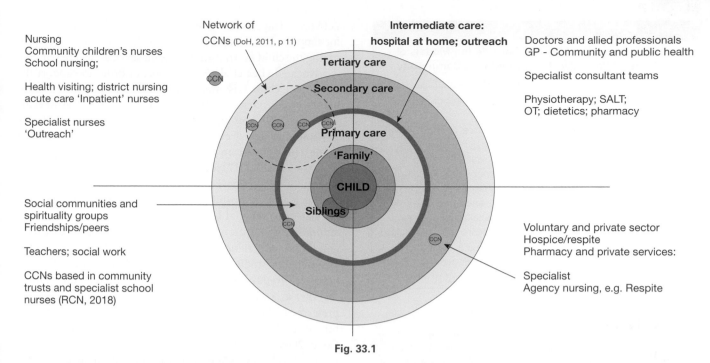

Fig. 33.1

domains. Nineteen key elements within the Clinical Care Domain (QNI, 2018, pp 3–4) were identified, which included: 'clinical expertise ... in a variety of community settings', including promotion of good mental health and well-being; accurate and evidence-based assessment and reassessment skills; 'co-production' of care intervention plans and partnership with young people and their carers within therapeutic relationships; supervision and appropriate accountability of the delivery of care. Risk management and the implementation of strategies to manage risk were also considered key in protecting Children and young people, carers, health care practitioners and the public.

You may wish to read the voluntary standards if you are considering a career in the community setting. However, you do not need to undertake the formal CCN training to work within a community team. Teams are made up of a variety of members, each with an appropriate range of skills relating to the Children and young people that they are supporting. For example, there are specialist teams who provide information and support for particular conditions, which include carers, health care assistants, nursing associates and junior children's nurses, as well as team leaders with further expertise. Alternatively, teams might work primarily with a particular community or area, providing much more generalised care, working closely with a health visiting, district nursing or social services team (Bee et al., 2018; DoH, 2011; Parker et al., 2011).

Videos of CCNs from QNI Scotland are available at: https://www.qnis.org.uk/what-is-community-nursing/standards/community-childrens-nursing-standards/.

The Work of the CCN

Initially, modern CCN teams were developed for specific conditions and interventions, providing a limited weekday service, but they now coordinate a range of care packages and nursing interventions across the week and out of hours.

However, Carter and Coad (2009) identified that this was not universal across the UK. Services might involve the supervision, support and training of outside agencies, of support workers to provide respite in the home, and liaison with private-sector hospice services for those with life-limiting conditions. Bee et al. (2018) highlighted the need for children's services to be equitable and an effective use of NHS resources. However, they did not find a statistically significant reduction in admissions in their meta-review. As research identifies the increasing effect of poor childhood health and lifestyle on the long-term health of adults, minimising the effects of ill-health in childhood and improving health outcomes for children and young people are increasingly being considered more important. New research in genomics has identified that this can affect our genetic blueprints (somatic mutations) (Genomics England, 2018).

The work of the CCN will depend on the health needs of their caseload and the communities in which they serve (DoH, 2011) and can be highly complex (Carter and Coad, 2009). This could be direct assessment and co-produced care planning and delivery by a variety of people, as well as reassessment and maintenance activities, such as venepuncture and psychological support at home. It may be acute administration of intravenous medication, or longer-term prescribing for those with long-term care needs (subject to appropriate training and competence). Collaboration with an ever-increasing range of other services and agencies is also an important part of the team's function in meeting mental and physical health needs. Effective discharge planning and dynamic communication (Noyes et al., 2013, p 975) are also vital.

Transitional care is considered elsewhere in this textbook; however, historically, CCNs have also empowered patients to find the 'right' support once transfer to adult services has been initiated (Table 33.1). For example, patients with cystic fibrosis now live far longer and require local specialist services.

TABLE 33.1

'Four Areas of Need' (DoH, 2011, p 4)	Considering Models of Children's Community Nursing
• Children with acute and short-term conditions • Children with long-term conditions • Children with disabilities and complex conditions, including neonates and those requiring continuing care • Children with life-limiting and life-threatening illness, including those requiring palliative and end-of-life care	• Hospital at home • Palliative or end-of life care • Outreach vs in-reach services, e.g. managing the needs of technology-dependent children • Specialist versus generalist care, e.g. managing the needs of a specific illness or symptom, such as an eating disorder

👤 ACTIVITY

Explore different models of care of the sick child at home.
- Spend about an hour searching online for examples of local community services for sick children: remember to also consider mental health and child and adolescent mental health (CAMHs) services.
- Where are they based and what areas do they cover? Create a diagram or map of your area. What is meant by the term 'community' in the examples that you have found?
- Considering the type of young patient that you have observed being nursed at home, where would resources be best placed in your area? What do we mean by the term 'patient'? What would be a better term?

PART 2: PUTTING THE CHILD AT THE CENTRE: THE IMPORTANCE OF CHILDHOOD AND 'HOME'

Family centred care is discussed elsewhere in this book; however, there are many reasons why putting the child at the centre of what we do is important. O'Dell and Leverett (2010) identified a number of ways to understand factors affecting the child and their development. The child will always be 'socially' located within a 'family' unit that in itself is subject to financial, social and physical factors that can affect health. The child is shaped by that environment, as well as the values and routines of their family (Super and Harkness, 1998) and it is the security of these routines and support networks for both child and family that is interrupted by constant or long-term admission to hospital (Randall, 2016). Added to this, Eshenbeck et al. (2018) reviewed trends regarding the differing needs of the growing child for developing and maintaining resilience in the modern world, vital for coping with long-term conditions or sudden acute illness. They explored six coping strategies developed through middle-childhood through to adolescence: social support seeking; problem solving; avoidance strategies; emotion regulation; anger management and using media. As the child develops, strategies start to include peers and other

networks. The education service is also used as a mechanism for support. This is important to consider, especially when preparing the child for transition to adult services, where self-care is advocated (Bee et al., 2018). Thus, in order to support the developing child, it is important to maintain a caring environment that considers the 'child's view of the world' (Castor et al., 2017, p 2788). 'You know that a child thrives in their home environment and if everything is as ordinary as possible, at home.' (Response from participant: Castor et al., 2017, p 2788.)

Castor et al. (2017) identified several benefits of caring for sick children at home. For the child, who could become bored and/or fearful in hospital, they identified how worries were alleviated by being at home, where children could feel more autonomous, be more easily distracted and able to access childhood experiences (Randall, 2016). They highlighted a number of studies that outlined the importance of maintaining everyday life and how parents try to keep their family together as a way of 'feeling in control'. Home care was often preferred by families, and this was replicated in a report commissioned by the House of Commons in 2009 (Carter and Coad, 2009). The financial burden of having a sick child was reported to be less while being cared for at home, but Castor et al. (2017) cautioned that this must be in the best interest of the child.

Access to a Childhood

In Chapter 2, Randall (2016) identified the importance of childhood for the developing young person. CCNs consider the child first, while identifying the need for carers to feel in control of what will be required at home in order to feel safe and supported. Pragmatic children's nursing focuses on the importance of 'living a childhood' (Randall, 2016, p 36) and a new way of perceiving the needs of a child in the context of time and space. It identifies the role of the children's nurse to also act to inform the child's building knowledge about themselves. This perspective changes the care dynamic to the child (and their legal best interests) leading the care negotiations separate or ahead of the main carer and/or nurse, becoming more important as the child returns to their home and routines and as they mature. The change in ability to self-care can thus be nurtured from a young age, rather than starting to consider it at adolescence when the effects of an interrupted childhood may start to emerge (Randall, 2016).

Child as 'Developing Expert' and Their Relationship With CCNs

It is becoming increasingly important in both health care and social sciences that children are seen as 'competent interpreters of their everyday life' (Mason and Danby, 2011, p 186; O'Reilly et al., 2016). Historically, parents were not allowed to see their children in hospital and could only visit at set times (Platt, 1959). The importance of 'parents as experts' cannot be denied when supporting the care of sick children, especially neonates and young children (Denman, 2014). In the 21st century, children are seen to have a greater voice, and Randall (2012) identified that they also want to be more involved with their own care and to be nursed by people who engage with them appropriately. Mason and Danby (2011) also suggested that by understanding how children 'constructed their own worlds', new opportunities for enabling those working with them would arise. Joint planning, or coproduction of care involves input from the child or young person, the parent and the nurse in order to identify appropriate, justified and reasonable care goals to be developed.

CCNs work predominantly outside the acute care setting, in what could be considered the realm of the child and the family (Mason and Danby, 2011). While children and young people are in a clinical hospital setting, they perceive the 'rules' to be regulated by the hospital staff (Randall, 2016), but at home or in school, their family or 'peer' rules are more applicable. Kirk et al. (2012) identified the need to engage children and young people in promoting self-care. However, once in the community setting, there are many factors that can affect a sense of community, confidence, independence and empowerment. For example, a young person with type diabetes may go to a fast food outlet and eat with friends, not wanting to appear different by examining the calories, or going to a public toilet to mask the administering of insulin. The nurse might then decide to talk to the young person about the use of insulin pump technology, based on the *young person's desire* to have more flexibility. A key finding in a recent research paper that asked adolescents about their experiences of living with asthma highlighted that they 'wanted their asthma to be acknowledged but not to the point that they were defined by their asthma' (Jonsson et al., 2017, p 23).

👤 ACTIVITY

Discuss the role of the children's nurse with a young person. Locate and read the following article:

Randall, D., 2012. Children's regard for nurses and nursing: a mosaic of children's views on community nursing, 91–104. https://doi.org/10.1177/1367493511426279.

What questions might you ask a child or young person when first meeting them? List five questions and discuss them with a child or young person, their mentor or parent (with permission from the child or young person). *This need not be a sick child*, but it would be interesting to compare Randall's findings with your own.

How does the age of the child affect the questions that you might ask? Use the questions to find out what young people most expect from the people caring for them.

PART 3: MANAGING RISK: NEGOTIATING ROLES AND CARE RESPONSIBILITIES OF THE NURSE, CHILD, AND/OR CARER

Defining Risk

The main issues in managing care in a clinical setting versus a 'social space' designed for living, are the expertise, appropriate equipment and space, and the necessary skills and knowledge of the main carer, which are often assumed to be vastly different.

- A ventilated patient needs piped oxygen, an 'expert' carer and back up equipment (Naupane et al., 2015).

- A child with asthma, who has fast onset of respiratory symptoms, will need emergency access to equipment and medication, such as nebulised salbutamol (Isik et al., 2019).
- A young adult with mental health needs may resist attempts by health-care professionals to assess their need for safety (O'Reilly et al., 2016).
- A school aged child who is has a severe peanut allergy will need the expertise of those who supervise him at school to be able to administer adrenaline (RCN, 2018).

When considering risk in health care, the World Health Organization (n.d.) considers the following four steps:

1. Identification of the risk.
2. Assessment of the likelihood, or frequency, of the risk.
3. Reduction or elimination of the risk.
4. 'Cost' or the potential outcome of the risk occurring.

If a circumstance is highly likely to happen, but with low potential harm associated with it, then reducing the risk by being prepared, may be acceptable. However, even with a small likelihood of the high potential of 'severe harm occurring' may be deemed 'substantial' or 'intolerable' (HSE Risk Matrix, n.d.). The CCN also needs to consider risk to herself and the carer (NMC, 2018).

The greatest risk for any child is the potential for their health to deteriorate rapidly, or actions that would put them in danger. Risk assessment is important for the child and family to consider when agreeing to take on care at home. They need to know what to do in an emergency, within the context of their understanding and skills of assessment. Teaching about signs and symptoms of deterioration, such as within an Asthma Plan (NICE, 2018), as well as what to do and who to contact, is vital. This may mean calling emergency services, which is important to consider when living rurally or going on holiday away from their usual community. Babies with apnoea, or those on oxygen, may need immediate resuscitation to have the best possible chance of survival, and require their parents and/or carers to receive training on what to do if they stop breathing (Murray and Joseph, 2016).

Parents may have a different perceived risk for children who are taking on more self-care, especially when supporting young people with mental health needs. Young adults with diabetes will need to know how to manage their blood glucose level, or to use modern insulin pumps within school (RCN, 2018), and those who experience suicidal thoughts will need to be risk assessed in relation to seeking appropriate help when required. Managing risk could be considered resilient behaviour as the child takes on more responsibility, or it could provide the potential for young people to rebel. The high risk of mental health consequences for those with complex care needs or learning disabilities is also key, considering both the child and carers (Foundation for People with Learning Disability, 2014).

As well as the immediate risks to the child, there may also be risks associated with the equipment that is required to care for a sick child at home. There will be limitations in terms of the living space in most homes and close negotiation with other services will be required to enable children with complex needs to live a childhood at home. This may be as simple as working with the local community pharmacist to deliver or install home oxygen delivery systems, while highlighting the risk of having oxygen at home and in the car, for example, friction toys creating sparks, which can exacerbate the risks.

More complex care negotiation of risks, including the use of technology and disposable equipment, will require much more planning, for example: safe electric connections; good telephone signal; respite and parental support; and appropriate space for moving and handling. As young people grow, their moving and handling needs will change and lifting equipment may not fit within the home, or the household budget. Safety can be a factor when considering financial, access and housing issues.

Negotiating Self-Care

Bee et al. (2018) highlighted the lack of research regarding the negotiation of care with and for children and young people. Most studies consider specific medical conditions rather than the overall nursing requirements of a range of complex care needs and the interventions that they need.

In negotiating and facilitating self-care, a number of other resources and agencies are required. For example, the safety of the child and young person must come first in line with safeguarding legislation and policy, as well as the extra needs of 'looked after children' (DfES, 2015).

Technical equipment, such as apnoea alarms, saturation finger probes and 'hospital' beds, are often required and will need to be supplied and maintained. Increasingly, these are now contracted through private suppliers or charitable donation, but this is not mirrored throughout the UK. CCNs are often instrumental in negotiating or sourcing the equipment, as well as teaching children and their carers how to use it, for which they are accountable. Anecdotally, in some instances, patients and carers are becoming more expert in the maintenance of their technical equipment than their nurses.

Disposable equipment is prescribed through primary care, and processes for re-ordering and delivery can minimise disruption to family life and thus, childhood. For more complex needs, such as dialysis or nutrition via a percutaneous device, some private companies will take on the re-ordering and delivery if you prescribe their products, providing equipment such as fridges if required.

Finally, documentation of agreed care and what has been done must be completed, and this will need to be negotiated with the young person and their carers. It may take the form of hand-held nursing notes, but increasingly 'passports' and other documents are used in relation to coordinated care: for example, advice re-positioning and enabling the intake of nutrition. The child should not need to keep revisiting what their needs are: collaboration, communication and cooperation are vital in reducing the impact on living. This is also vital in moving between agencies such as school and home, as well as between services, for instance, visits to tertiary services for ongoing orthopaedic revision.

> ### 👤 ACTIVITY
>
> Explore how a young person with a long-term condition, such as cystic fibrosis, might be included in a much-anticipated school trip.
>
> The young person's mainstream school is planning a three-day trip to London relating to a science GCSE project. They will visit the Science Museum and one of the London universities and take a boat trip on the Thames.
>
> Imagine you are the young person with the long-term condition: what would be your main concerns and what do you think you would miss out on by not attending the trip? What effect might this have on you?
>
> Imagine you are the parent of a 15-year-old managing cystic fibrosis, who requires interventions, medication and frequent intravenous antibiotics. What would be your concerns about the risks associated with the trip?
>
> What support and guidance can you find to help the young person, their carer and the school to help mitigate any risks?

PART 4: EVALUATING CARE WITH THE CHILD AND FAMILY

A key part of any care plan is the evaluation and reassessment of need (Reeve et al., 2015, p 93) identified the importance of considering: 'structure', 'process', and 'outcome' when evaluating plans, as well as 'sustainability', 'quality of care', and other determinants of health. As a child develops and starts to grow and take on more self-care – or not – it is important to consider these when supporting them in the community. If the child has a physical disability, they may require a lot of therapy and other interventions throughout their life. The CCN can help by talking things through with both child and carer, providing a sounding board for decision making, scaffolding future decision-making for the young person. They can also help to minimise visits away from home, by working with others to bring appointments together if possible. Frequent visits to hospital can severely disrupt childhood, but can also serve as support to carers, and respite may also be required. This enables the young person to access other experiences outside parental control, and the carers to get a rest. It can be a chance for the young person or their siblings to access other services, such as talking therapy or an equipment review: 'E loves staying away from home and it is like an adventure for her' (Helen House, 2019). Children with complex care needs may have limited childhood opportunities if independence is difficult.

However, acute care needs, or regular monitoring, may better served at home by teaching self-care or by the nurse negotiating to undertake this at home, outside school hours, to improve access to schooling and childhood (Randall, 2016). Thus, evaluation must also include other agencies, such as the acute ward area (Neupane et al., 2015), teachers and other therapists. Access to funding and equipment will also change as the young person reaches adulthood.

The QNI (2018) identified a number of ways in which CCNs can be expected to work with children and young people, while collaborating with a range of other stakeholders.

The other three domains of their document considered: 'Management and Leadership'; 'Facilitation of Learning for Other Healthcare Professionals'; and 'Evidence, Research and Development'. The final section will identify current evaluation of experiences.

Developing Services for Future Health Care for Children at Home

Callery et al. (2011) interviewed children, parents and professionals in considering what was important about providing care to children and young people in the community: reduction in hospital admission; the feeling of empowerment by parents undertaking care; access to a community nursing service and sufficient advice and education about the health care need. Parker et al. (2011) also identified CCN services that were 'closer to home'. Randall (2012) found that the child's regard for nursing was not dependent on the nurse nor their actions. From the point of view of professionals, Castor et al. (2017) identified concerns of nurses about care for children at home being centred on feeling inadequate and challenged, despite identifying the importance of 'adapting to child's care'. They also identified increased competence and satisfaction when undertaking that care, as well as the requirement for time to care, good teamwork, collaboration with acute services, early referral and cooperation. In their review of services, Hill and Coyne (2012, p 279), identified four key areas for consideration in developing CCN services for the 21st-century child: 'Inclusiveness; Partnership; Comprehensiveness; and Flexibility'. Carter and Coad (2009, p 27) identified the need further develop and provide 'responsive systems and resources'.

This chapter considered the role of the community children's nurse, competences required, and relationships and partnerships with and for children requiring care at home. It identified the importance of risk management and collaboration with a wide range of stakeholders in their aim to keep children safely at home.

REFERENCES

Bee, P., Pedley, R., Rithalia, A., et al., 2018. Self-care support for children and adolescents with long-term conditions: the REfOCUS evidence synthesis. Health Serv. Deliv. Res. 6 (3). https://doi.org/10.3310/hsdr06030.

Cain, P., Hyde, V., Howkins, E., 1995. Community Nursing: Dimensions and Dilemmas. Arnold, London.

Callery, P., Kyle, R.G., Banks, M., et al., 2011. Moving Care Closer to Home: An Evaluation of the Costs and Effects of Different Models of Caring for Acutely Ill Children at Home. Final Report, Commissioned Report, Manchester University.

Carter, B., Coad, J., 2009. Community Children's Nursing in England. Available from: https://assets.publishing.service.gov.uk/government/uploads/system/uploads/attachment_data/file/215710/dh_124901.pdf.

Castor, C., Hallstrom, I., Hannson, H., Landgren, K., 2017. Home care services for sick children: healthcare professionals' conceptions of challenges and facilitators. J. Clin. Nurs. 26 (16–18), 2784–2793. https://doi.org/10.1111/jocn.13821.

Denman, S.J., 2014. Parents as experts on children with disabilities: being prepared for the long-haul. Int. J. Disabil. Dev. Educ. 61 (4), 434–440. https://doi.org/10.1080/1034912X.2014.956003.

Department of Education (DfES), Department of Health (DoH), 2015. Promoting the Health and Well-Being of Looked-After Children. Available from: https://assets.publishing.service.gov.uk/government/uploads/system/uploads/attachment_data/file/413368/Promoting_the_health_and_well-being_of_looked-after_children.pdf.

Department of Health and Social Security (DHSS), 1976. Fit for the Future: The Report of the Committee on Child Health Services (The Court Report). HMSO, London.

Department of Health (DoH), 1997. Government Response to the Reports of the Health Committee on Health Services for Children and Young People, Session 1996–97. The Stationery Office, London.

Department of Health (DoH), 2008. Better Care: Better Lives. Available from: https://www.nsf.no/Content/662656/Bedre%20Behandling,%20bedre%20liv%20ENGLAND.pdf.

Department of Health (DoH), 2009. Healthy Lives, Brighter Futures: the Strategy for Children and Young People's Health. Available from: https://webarchive.nationalarchives.gov.uk/20130104164640/http://www.dh.gov.uk/en/Publicationsandstatistics/Publications/PublicationsPolicyAndGuidance/DH_094400.

Department of Health (DoH), 2011. NHS at Home: Community Children's Nursing Services. Available from: https://assets.publishing.service.gov.uk/government/uploads/system/uploads/attachment_data/file/215708/dh_124900.pdf.

Eschenbeck, H., Schmid, S., Schröder, I., Wasserfall, N., Kohlmann, C., 2018. Development of coping strategies from childhood to adolescence. Euro. J. Psycho. 25 (1), 18–30. https://doi.org/10.1027/2512-8442/a000005.

Foundation for People with Learning Disability, 2014. Feeling Down: Improving the Mental Health of People Living With Learning Difficulties. Available from: www.mentalhealth.org.uk/sites/default/files/feeling-down-report-2014.pdf.

Genomics England, 2018. Cancer Genomics. Available from www.genomicsengland.co.uk/understanding-genomics/cancer-genomics/.

Health and Safety Executive (HSE), (no date). Risk Matrices. Available from: http://www.hse.gov.uk/risk/index.htm.

Helen, Douglas House, 2019. Max's Story. Available from: www.helenanddouglas.org.uk/family-stories/max-story/.

Hill, K., Coyne, I., 2012. Palliative care nursing for children in the UK and Ireland. Br. J. Nurs. 21 (5), 276–282.

Isik, E., Fredland, N.M., Freysteinson, W.M., 2019. School and community-based nurse-led asthma interventions for school-aged children and their parents: a systematic literature review. J. Pediatr. Nurs. 44, 107–114. https://doi.org/10.1016/j.pedn.2018.11.007.

Jonsson, M., Schuster, M., Protudjer, J.L.P., Egmar, A.-C., Kull, I., 2017. Experiences of daily life among adolescents with asthma – a struggle with ambivalence. J. Pediatr. Nurs. 35, 23–29.

Kirk, S., Beatty, S., Callery, P., Milnes, L., Pryjmachuk, S., 2012. Perceptions of effective self-care support for children and young people with long-term conditions. J. Clin. Nurs. 21 (13–14), 1974–1987. https://doi.org/10.1111/j.1365-2702.2011.04027.x.

Mason, J., Danby, S., 2011. Children as experts in their lives. Child Indicators Res. 4, 185–189. https://doi.org/10.1007/s12187-011-9108-4.

Ministry of Health, 1959. The Welfare of Children in Hospital (Report of the Committee – Chairman Sir H. Platt). HMSO, London.

Murray, C.H., Joseph, R.A., 2016. Transition from NICU to home: are the parents ready to manage any emergency? An evidence-based project. Neonatal Network 35 (3), 151–155. https://doi.org/10.1891/0730-0832.35.3.151.

Naupane, B., McFeeters, M., Johnson, E., Hickey, H., Pandya, H., 2015. Transitioning children requiring long-term ventilation from hospital to home: a practical guide. Paediatr. Child Health 25 (4), 187–191. https://doi.org/10.1016/j.paed.2015.01.007.

NICE, 2013 updated 2018. Asthma. Quality Statement 2: Written Personalised Action Plan. Available from: www.nice.org.uk/guidance/qs25/chapter/Quality-statement-2-Written-personalised-action-plan.

Noyes, J., Brenner, M., Fox, P., Guerin, A., 2013. Reconceptualizing children's complex discharge with health systems theory: novel integrative review with embedded expert consultation and theory development. J. Adv. Nurs. 70 (5), 975–96. https://doi.org/10.1111/jan.12278.

O'Dell, L., Leverett, S., 2010. Working with Children and Young People: Co-constructing Practice. Palgrave Macmillan, Basingstoke.

O'Reilly, M., Nina, J., Muskett, T., 2016. Children's claims to knowledge regarding their mental health experiences and practitioners' negotiation of the problem. Patient Educ. Counsel. 99 (6), 905–910. https://doi.org/10.1016/j.pec.2015.10.005.

Parker, G., Spiers, G., Cusworth, L., Birks, Y., Gridley, K., Mukherjee, S., 2011. Care closer to home for children and young people who are ill: developing and testing a model of service delivery and organization. J. Adv. Nurs. 68 (9). https://doi.org/10.1111/j.1365-2648.2011.05893.x.

Queens Nursing Institute (QNI), 2018. The QNI/QUIS Voluntary Standards for Community Children's Nurse Education and Practice. Available from: www.qni.org.uk/wp-content/uploads/2018/09/QNI-and-QNIS-voluntary-standards-for-CCN.pdf.

Randall, D., 2012. Children's regard for nurses and nursing: a mosaic of children's views on community nursing. J. Child Health Care 16 (1), 91–104. https://doi.org/10.1177/1367493511426279.

Randall, D., 2016. Pragmatic Children's Nursing: A Theory for Children and Their Childhoods. Routledge, Abingdon.

RCN, 2018. Meeting Health Needs in Educational and Other Community Settings: A Guide for Nurses Caring for Children and Young People. RCN.

Reeve, C., Humphreys, J., Wakerman, J., 2015. A comprehensive health service evaluation and monitoring framework. Eval. Progr. Plann. 53, 91–98. https://doi.org/10.1016/j.evalprogplan.2015.08.006.

Super, C.M., Harkness, S., 1998. The development of affect in infancy and early childhood. In: Woodhead, M., Faulkner, D., Littleton, K. (Eds.), Cultural Worlds of Early Childhood. Routledge, Abingdon.

Whiting, M., 2017. Caring for Children '24-7'. Available from: www.wellchild.org.uk/wp-content/uploads/2017/01/Caring_for_children_24-7.pdf.

World Health Organization. Topic 6: Understanding and Managing Clinical Risk. Available from: www.who.int/patientsafety/education/curriculum/PSP_mpc_topic-06.pdf.

34

Leading Innovation and Improvements in Children's and Young People's Nursing Through Best Evidence

Jane Coad, Joseph C. Manning

LEARNING OBJCTIVES

- Describe evidence-based practice in the context of nursing children, young people and their families.
- Understand the role of professional experience and expertise to evidence-based practice.
- Describe the process for developing a research question, identifying the best available evidence and appraising the evidence.

- Appreciate the need for children's nurses to meaningfully and authentically seek the views, values and preferences of children, young people and their families to integrate into their practice, including a variety of ways in which this can be done.

◎ EVIDENCE-BASED PRACTICE

Evidence-Based Practice in the Context of Nursing Children and Young People

In the last 20 years, nursing children and young people has undergone significant transformation. This is in response to the changing health needs of children and young people, rising numbers of children with complex and long-term conditions, advances in medicines and technologies to support care, and changes to the way care is organised and delivered. This has had profound implications for the children's nurse as it has resulted in changes to the expectation and scope of their professional practice. Subsequently, it is essential that nurses support their practice by integrating: (1) their clinical expertise, (2) the best available evidence and (3) patient preferences in order to deliver safe and effective care.

These three components form what is defined as 'evidence-based practice' or EBP (Sackett et al., 1997) which has been adapted to the setting of children and young people's care (Fig. 34.1). However, being an effective evidence-based practitioner brings a number of challenges. The sheer volume of information and research can be overwhelming. Even a simple search on a topic will generate volumes of conflicting evidence. The appraisal and evaluation of this evidence requires a specific skillset and can be daunting. Furthermore, seeking the views

of children, young people and their families and meaningfully integrated these to inform nursing care can be challenging.

Drawing on the evidence, this chapter will provide a systematic and structured approach to addressing these challenges. We have introduced in the following pages that using the best external evidence requires a number of steps:

1. Clearly identify the child or young person's problem and needs based on accurate assessment and current professional knowledge and practice.
2. Research the literature for relevant research to develop your question.
3. Evaluate the research evidence using established criteria regarding scientific merit. Choose interventions and justify those with the most valid evidence.
4. Utilise prior experience and patient preferences in order to deliver safe and effective care.

However, whilst this seems fairly straightforward, it can sometimes feel unclear where to start or overwhelming due to the volume of information available. Let us consider these elements further in the next section which is based on practical reflections of both authors.

PRACTICAL REFLECTIONS

Formulating Research Questions

The first step to accessing the best available evidence to improve care is to develop and define a research question. Whilst this is sometimes very hard to do, it is worth the effort as the more clearly focused the question, the more likely it is to locate the most appropriate evidence to answer

the question. Arguably, questions can simply be broad, but to enhance their focus many professionals use frameworks to formulate their question. The most widely used include the 'PICO' framework for quantitative research questions (Sackett et al., 1997), or the 'SPIDER' framework for qualitative research questions (Cooke et al., 2012). These frameworks are described in Fig. 34.2. The advantages of using these frameworks are that they help to narrow the question

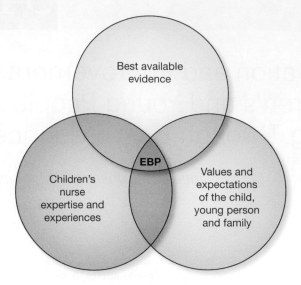

Fig. 34.1 Evidence-based practice *(EBP)* triad in the context of children's nursing.

P	Patient	Who is the treatment being delivered to? Consider their ages, disease or condition.
I	Intervention	What treatment is being delivered?
C	Comparison (optional)	Do you want to compare the intervention with another treatment or standard care?
O	Outcome	How is the effect being measured? What impact are you interested in?
S	Sample	What children, young people and families are you focusing on? Consider their ages, disease or condition.
PI	Phenomenon of Interest	What phenomena are you interested in exploring and understanding?
D	Design	What study designs or approaches are used to understand the phenomena? This could include interviews, observations, focus groups.
E	Evaluation	How is the phenomena being evaluated? This could include through the experiences, perceptions, descriptions, views of children, young people and families.
R	Research type	What type of research are you wanting to identify? Qualitative, quantitative or mixed methods research?

Fig. 34.2 Description of PICO and SPIDER frameworks.

down to a realistic, manageable focus. Conversely, the limitations of the evidence base in the field of children and young people may mean this can be very challenging in identifying any relevant information.

Two Scenarios

Two different scenarios as worked examples have been drawn using published papers relevant to children's nursing. They demonstrate the application of each framework in developing a comprehensive question.

1. Carter et al. (2015) study aims to determine the effectiveness of exercise intervention on depressive symptoms of young people with depression. Using the PICO framework, the following elements can be extracted:

   Population = young people aged 14–17 years with depression

   Intervention = exercise intervention + standard treatment

   Comparison = standard treatment

   Outcomes = depression severity (measured using the Children's Depression Inventory 2 (Kovacs, 2014))

   Using these components, it is then easier to compose a structured research question:

   What is the effectiveness of an exercise intervention plus standard treatment when compared with standard treatment alone on the depressive symptoms of young people (aged 14–17 years) with depression?

2. A qualitative study by Manning et al. (2017) aimed to explore childhood critical care survivors' experiences of long-term psychosocial well-being. Using the SPIDER tool, the following elements could be extracted:

   Sample = children and young people aged 6–18 years that had survived an emergency admission to the Paediatric Intensive Care Unit.

   Phenomenon of **I**nterest = long-term psychosocial well-being

   Design = narrative, interviews

   Evaluation = perceptions, experiences

   Research type = qualitative

   Using these elements, it should then be easier to compose a structured research question as below:

   What are the qualitative perceptions and experiences of long-term psychosocial well-being of children and young people (aged 6–18 years) who have survived an admission to the paediatric intensive care unit?

👤 ACTIVITY 1

Now think about your clinical practice and identify a problem that you need evidence to solve. Make a list and then decide on one issue only. Decide whether this problem needs quantitative or qualitative research to answer it. Listed in Table 34.1 are some points to help you make this decision. Now select the PICO or SPIDER framework to develop your question. Try and be as specific as possible, as this will help when going to the next stage in identifying the evidence.

Accessing the Evidence

Once the question has been identified from Activity 1, the next task is to find the best available evidence to help answer it. Many will tell you that you can just embark on a broad search, but to really answer that question we would recommend that you use a systematic approach. This is to not only answer the question, but will also help to ensure that you do not miss anything; this also means that another person could come along and repeat the process. This structured and transparent approach is recognised as a quality standard.

TABLE 34.1 Features of Quantitative and Qualitative Research Approaches

Quantitative	Qualitative
Aims to test a hypothesis or address a specific research question	Aims to discover, explore or build understanding of a particular practice/topic
Approach will include measurement and testing	Approach involves observing and interpretation
Sample includes large numbers which are often selected using probability sampling approaches (such as random selection)	Small samples selected using non-probability methods (such as convenience sampling)
Data is collected using precise measurements using validated and structured instruments	Data is collected using semi-structured or unstructured interviews, field notes, participant observations and reflections
Data analysed to identify statistically significant relationships/differences	Data analysed to identify patterns, themes and features

The first stage in this process is to identify where you want to search for evidence. There are numerous places you can search that include search engines, online databases and libraries. However, access may be limited depending on whether you are affiliated with a university or health care organisation that subscribes. The most common and convenient place for searching is by using online databases. These index a whole range of evidence that can be searched and accessed electronically. The most common online databases are listed in Table 34.2 and should be selected based on the focus or topic of your question. An example from the child health literature is from a review conducted by Coad et al. (2017). The purpose of the review was to establish from previously published evidence whether a blended diet was a safe and realistic option for children with tube feeding needs. Five electronic databases (PubMed, MEDLINE, CINAHL, PsychINFO and Google Scholar) were selected due to their relevance to the topic/phenomena being explored that included: nutrition, health care, children, families, experiences and outcomes.

Once you have identified where you will search for the evidence you need to develop a search strategy. A search strategy is defined as an organised structure of key words

TABLE 34.2 List of Databases Used to Identify Evidence in Health Care

Database	Description
British Standards (BS) Online	The full text of British Standards, covering: specifications for products, dimensions, and performance; methods; codes of practice; guides and glossaries. Also find British Standards equivalents to International Organization for Standardization (ISO) and European (EN) standards. Updated daily.
CAB Abstracts Online	Covers human health, food and nutrition, agriculture, environmental issues, genetics, plant and animal science. CAB Abstracts includes information about research articles, books, conference proceedings and reports. Coverage from 1973 onwards.
CINAHL	Covers nursing and allied health. Search for journal articles, books, dissertations and conference proceedings. Coverage from 1960 onwards.
Cochrane Library	Cochrane reviews represent the highest level of evidence on which to base clinical treatment decisions. Search these and other reliable sources, including other systematic review abstracts, technology assessments, economic evaluations and individual clinical trials. Coverage from 2005 onwards.
EMBASE	Search for journal articles in biomedicine and pharmacology. The database is updated weekly and can be searched back to 1980. A current awareness service provides alerts for newly added content. Compared to Medline, EMBASE has a more European bias, and only about one-third of the journals are covered in both databases.
Hinari: research in health	One of the world's largest collections of biomedical and health literature. HINARI Access to Research in Health Programme covers up to 14,000 journals (in 30 different languages), up to 33,000 e-books, up to 70 other information resources. No access to subscription content.
HMIC database	This database brings together the bibliographic databases of two UK health and social care management organisations: Department of Health (DH-Data) and King's Fund. HMIC enables you to search for journal articles, books, Department of Health policy documents and unpublished material in the area of UK and international health and social care management and policy. The two HMIC databases are updated six times a year and records go back to 1983. A free current awareness service provides e-mail alerts to newly added content.
Index to Theses	Covering all subjects this database is the most comprehensive available record of doctoral theses from the United Kingdom and Ireland. The collection offers listing of theses, with abstracts accepted for higher degrees by universities in the United Kingdom and Ireland, since 1716.
Maternity and Infant Care	The Maternity and Infant Care database has over 100,000 references relating to midwifery, pregnancy and childbirth, from 1971 onwards. Each reference includes full bibliographic information, an author abstract or summary, and is subject indexed with key words to enable easy searching of the database. The database also includes pre-prepared 'standard' searches.

Continued

TABLE 34.2   List of Databases Used to Identify Evidence in Health Care—cont'd

Database	Description
Medline	Search for journal articles and other reference types in medicine, dentistry and nursing, including biomedicine, medicine, nursing, dentistry, allied health, pre-clinical sciences. This includes material from across the biological and environmental sciences, psychology, and chemistry. The database is updated frequently and can be searched back to 1950. A current awareness service provides alerts for newly added content.
Ovid databases	More than 100 core and niche databases to support a variety of research needs in a wide range of disciplines including clinical medicine, pharmacology and more. The powerful combination of Ovid's rich database implementation with Ovid's advanced search features, natural language processing, sophisticated linking technology, and customisable display options, offer a unique, integrated database solution ideal for all users.
ProQuest Dissertations and Theses	This database lists details of more than two million doctoral dissertations and master's theses from 1861 in all disciplines. Divides into: Dissertation abstracts A: The humanities and social sciences, and B: The sciences and engineering. Coverage is international. Dissertations published from 1980 onwards include 350-word abstracts written by the author. Master's theses published from 1988 onwards include 150-word abstracts. Titles available as PDF formats include free 24-page previews. The full text of most documents can be purchased online.
PsycINFO	Contains journal articles, books, dissertations and theses in core psychology disciplines, behavioural sciences and mental health. It covers 1881 to the present day. A current awareness service provides alerts for newly added content. Updated weekly.
PubMed	A service of the US National Library of Medicine that includes over 16 million citations from the journals in the Medline database as well as biomedical articles from further life-science journals. This version of Medline also includes PreMedline, references to articles that have been published but not yet included in the full version of Medline. The search interface is less easy to use than our normal Medline service, and many of the records in PreMedline don't have abstracts, but this is one of the most up to date biomedical databases available. Also includes some links from references to full text journals. A current awareness service provides links for newly added content.
Scopus	Scopus is a large abstract and citation database of peer-reviewed literature from more than 18,500 journals and quality web sources, with smart tools to track, analyse and visualise research. Coverage starts from 1823.
Social Care Online	Free database provided by the Social Care Institute for Excellence (SCIE). Updated daily resources include legislation, government documents, practice and guidance, systematic reviews, research briefings, reports, journal articles and websites. Every resource listed includes an abstract. Links to full text are also included where available. Social Care Online is a particularly useful resource for staff, students and researchers working in social work and social care.
Web of Science	Search for journal articles using three databases; Science Citation Index, Social Science Citation Index and Arts and Humanities Citation Index.

Adapted from https://library.leeds.ac.uk/subjects/1161/healthcare.

used to search a database. This involves using the PICO or SPIDER framework to identify what search terms you will use. Again, using the Coad et al. (2017) review paper as an example, they used a modified version of the PICO (omitting the 'C') to develop their search strategy and set this out in a simple table (shown in Table 34.3). It is important to include a range of terms/words that are used to describe the same thing. For example, Coad et al. (2017) used the terms 'child', 'teenage', 'adolescent', 'young adult', 'young person' to search for literature relating to children and young people. The researchers were able to apply these terms to searching all of the identified databases, which ensured a consistent, transparent and replicable approach.

Listed below are some terms and tips that will assist in your database searching:

- Boolean operators – connect your search terms together to either narrow or broaden your set of results. The three basic Boolean operators are: AND, OR and NOT. For example: art(s) based or arts-based methods (title) AND Coad (author) AND 2019 (year).

include various term endings and spellings. This is achieved by putting a truncation symbol [*, ? or #], which is determined by the database, at the end of the word. For example: child* = child, childs, children, childrens, childhood.

- Wildcards – are used to substitute a symbol for one letter of words which are spelled in different ways but have the same meaning. For example: colo?r = color, colour.

ACTIVITY 2

Using your research question developed in Activity 1, identify three online databases where you will search for your evidence. Remember to consider what types of evidence you want to identify and the topic of your question. Then develop a search strategy from your research question. Identify the key terms that you will use to search the databases. Once you have undertaken the above, log on and have a go at your searching.

TABLE 34.3 Search Strategy Developed by Coad et al. (2017)

Child	AND	Blended Diet	AND	Gastrostomy
OR young people		OR Blend*		OR enteral
OR teenage		OR homemade		OR tube*
OR Young adult*		OR pureed food		
OR adolescen*				
OR adult				

Coad, J., Toft, A., Lapwood, S., et al. 2017. Blended foods for tube-fed children: a safe and realistic option? A rapid review of the evidence. Arch. Dis. Child. 102, 274–278.

Selecting and Appraising the Evidence

Undertaking Activity 2 might have highlighted to you that selecting the best evidence to inform your practice is not a simple task. It will be determined in part by your inclusion and exclusion criteria as suggested in the list below:

Inclusion criteria

- Studies need to be published in the language of preference (such as English).
- Studies within a time constraint of the review. This might be a few years to much longer, depending on the parameters set.
- Studies set internationally or in one country only, such as the UK.
- Studies specific to the group – such as age, development, condition.
- Studies that specifically explore your topic.
- Specific additional criteria, for example, studies that examined the topic in adults but can be easily transferable to children and young people. Decide on this at an early stage.

Exclusion criteria

- Studies which did not focus on original research (e.g. literature reviews).
- Study criteria not fitting the inclusion list above.

SEMINAR DISCUSION TOPIC

We now recommend you consider one case study which you use in a seminar discussion. Look at the inclusion and exclusion of Coad et al. (2017) to understand what types of papers they wanted to include in their review.

Inclusion and exclusion criteria will vary according to defining features, such as what type of evidence it is (e.g. opinion, systematic review, observational study), how it was conducted (e.g. study design) and how convinced you are to any conclusions drawn. As such, evidence is ranked on study types based on the rigour (strength and precision) of their research methods. The hierarchy of evidence (characterised by a pyramid shape) is the most widely accepted, albeit contested, schema and is presented below (adapted from Muir Gray, 1997):

I. Strong evidence from at least one systematic review of multiple, well designed, randomised controlled trials.
II. Strong evidence from at least one robustly designed randomised, controlled trial of appropriate size.
III. Strong evidence from well-designed trials without randomisation, single group, cohort, time series or matched case-control studies.
IV. Evidence from well-designed, non-experimental studies from more than one centre or research group.
V. Opinions of respected authorities based on clinical evidence, descriptive studies or reports of expert committees.

The convention is that the higher up in the hierarchy the study design is positioned, the more rigorous the methodology and hence the more likely it is that the study design can minimise the effect of bias on study results (Hoffmann et al., 2013).

In addition to understanding where the evidence you have identified is situated in the hierarchy of evidence, it is also fundamental that the quality of the evidence is appraised. Critical appraisal aims to identify methodological flaws in research and allow the reader/user of the evidence an opportunity to make informed decisions about the quality of it. However, critical appraisal can be a daunting task as it may be unclear where to start and focus your critique. Furthermore, the focus will be different according to different types of evidence and their methodology. Therefore there are a number of different tools available that help to support the appraisal of the quality of evidence. The following links provide access to these tools/checklists:

CASP Appraisal Checklists. A set of eight critical appraisal tools for systematic reviews, randomised controlled trials, cohort studies, case control studies, economic evaluations, diagnostic studies, qualitative studies and clinical prediction rule: https://casp-uk.net/casp-tools-checklists/.

Critical Appraisal Tools, Centre for Evidence-Based Medicine, University of Oxford. Critical Appraisal worksheets for systematic reviews, diagnostic and prognostic studies, randomised controlled trials, and qualitative studies: https://www.cebm.net/2014/06/critical-appraisal/.

Critical Appraisal Tools, Joanna Briggs Institute, The University of Adelaide. Checklists available for case control studies, case reports, case series, cohort studies, diagnostic test accuracy studies, economic evaluations, prevalence studies, quasi-experimental studies, randomised control trials, systematic reviews, text and opinion, analytical cross sectional studies and qualitative research: https://joannabriggs.org/critical-appraisal-tools

To help put this seminar discussion into practice please complete Activity 3.

👤 ACTIVITY 3

Find research paper(s) that explores a problem relevant to your nursing practice:

- Write down a short list of what type of evidence has been used to study the problem.
- What other types of design could be used to study this problem?

Utilising Prior Experience and Patient Preference

The one aspect not covered so far in the chapter is how prior experience and knowledge inform the research question, and how evidence is drawn upon to improve and innovate. This is a vital issue in the UK, as we are all very aware that the National Health Service (NHS) faces the challenge of improving quality of care while coping with significant pressures of funding and staffing. These challenges are substantial, and in some parts of the UK, quality is reported on as needing much improvement (Alderwick et al., 2017). Consequently, prior experiences of health care practitioners and patients is crucial.

Utilising Prior Experience in EBP

Working in the context of children and young people, one aspect that quickly becomes clear is that diversity of specialties, conditions, care and needs is vast. EBP is an essential part of improving practice; however, providing a well-rounded EBP approach requires nurses to draw on all of their life and health care experiences. It involves health care professionals taking action in their own contexts and realities, developing experience, questioning, problem solving and decision making. Many of the traits listed are thus elements of leadership.

This brings with it some challenges. Many health professionals may have little expertise including time to access and appraise the research evidence. Making a clinical or nursing decision is different than an EBP decision, and whilst experience is normally a key component of the EBP process, as described earlier in this chapter, in reality this may be harder to enact. Working together in teams can facilitate all stages of the EBP process and a combination of experiences can be a powerful tool for change. We have provided Activity 4 to bring your experience and learning from this section into practice.

👤 ACTIVITY 4

Using your problem and evidence from Activities 1–3, print out the evidence you have collated and appraised.

You could ask the ward manager and then leave it at the 'nurses' desk' or in the break room with your name on it.

Now find a time to discuss this with one colleague (mentor etc.), or your team of colleagues.

Keep in your mind this is important as it will help the care of your patients and their families.

Capturing and Involving the Views of Children, Young People and Families in EBP

Support for obtaining the views of children and young people on services comes not only from philosophical and legal standpoints, but also from the EBP paradigm. According to the seminal paper from Sackett et al. (1996), EBP requires health professionals to use clinical expertise to integrate systematic research evidence appropriately into their interventions, with due regard for patient preferences. In short, better understanding of children and young people's perspectives as patients enables us to ensure care meets any individual's context and/or needs.

Ideally, this in turn should lead to improved patient engagement and thus to improved outcomes for patients (Horne et al., 2013).

Children and young people are increasingly becoming involved in research as a part of the research team – including acting as interviewers – partly following the trend towards user involvement in research and partly to reduce the power imbalance that exists between an adult interviewer and a child. Traditionally, in adult qualitative research, attempts are made to match interviewer and interviewee for age, social position, gender and ethnicity (Mahon et al., 1996), to avoid any power imbalance between researcher and subject. More recently, even in the adult research methods literature, it has been recognised that this is not always possible. Instead, honesty about the nature of the differences has been advocated (Mallory, 2001). This provides a possible approach with children – to discuss with them the differences between themselves as researchers and/or as research participants and the coercive effect such power imbalances may have.

However, this can be complicated by tensions between children and young people's and parent/carers' perspectives and interests. Each may have different understandings of health problems and different goals for care so any research questions need to respect those wishes and concerns.

Increasingly participatory research methods are being used with children which engage children in the research process (Coyne and Carter, 2018b). Children from middle childhood upwards have participated in projects as researchers (Alderson and Morrow, 2011; Coad and Evans, 2008; Coyne and Carter, 2018a). Coad and Evans (2008) describe five levels of children's participation in research from simple participation as research respondents to child/young person-led research teams with adults facilitating the process.

This chapter has so far presented the EBP approach in four sections. Underpinning any EBN approach is the need to consider all the issues and how to overcome any challenges. The following sections outline issues relating to ethics and project complexity of researching with children and young people.

Ethics and Governance in Children and Young Peoples Research

The protective approach to children and young people has meant that traditionally they were often left out from being involved in research. However, for the last 20 years there has been enlightened change to such ideas, and indeed to not conduct research with children and young people would now be viewed as unethical (Darbyshire, 2000; McIntosh et al., 2000).

It is therefore important to conduct research with and for children and young people, but to do so in such a way as to ensure their voluntary participation. Children and young people need to be able to make an uncoerced and informed decision before consenting to their participation in research. Even when children are not 'Gillick competent', that is, of sufficient understanding and intelligence to fully understand what is proposed, opportunities need to be provided with sufficient amounts of appropriately formatted information to enable children to assent or dissent to their involvement (see Box 34.1 for definitions of consent, assent and dissent).

BOX 34.1   A List of Terms and Their Definitions Used in Research With Children and Young People

- Informed consent: an interactive process between subject and researcher involving disclosure, discussion and a complete understanding of a proposed research activity, and which culminates in the individual freely expressing a desire to participate.
- Parental consent: all of the components of informed consent and should include consideration of the implications of research involvement for the child.
- Assent: an interactive process between a child and researcher involving disclosure, discussion and a limited understanding of a proposed research activity, wherein the child freely expresses a preference for participation but has insufficient maturity to make a fully informed and autonomous decision.
- Dissent: an interactive process between a child and researcher involving disclosure, discussion and a limited understanding of the proposed research activity, wherein the child freely expresses an objection to the participation but has insufficient maturity to make a fully informed and autonomous decision.

Whenever children are involved as researchers, ethical problems must be addressed around the child protection issues mentioned previously. Nuffield Council on Bioethics (2015) guidelines for research with children and young people are very clear about the need to protect the child from unnecessary physical harm. The guidelines state that the decision concerning whether the research is allowed to take place should be based on an assessment of the balance of potential benefit against potential harm. In research involving physical procedures, the degree of 'harm' involved is relatively predictable. The psychological impact on the child is less predictable, but it is well recognised that it may occur at the time of the research or at a later date (Mahon et al., 1996; Nuffield Council on Bioethics, 2015). Research projects involving children and young people should include strategies for the emotional support of children immediately after data collection and the provision of information about sources of help for the future. Throughout the research process, researchers need to monitor the child's non-verbal signs for any indication of unwillingness to take part or to continue with the research (Alderson and Morrow, 2011)

Children and young people need to feel emotionally safe with any individual to be able to talk about their views or experiences or to submit to physical investigations (Latif et al., 2017). Appraisers of research should consider how children and young people were put at ease, for example, using ice-breaking techniques (Borland et al., 1998). Children's understanding of what is involved in a project is affected by the way information is presented in terms of the content and the pace of information giving (Oulton et al., 2016).

Activity 5 gives you the opportunity to explore the ethics and governance of conducting research with children through published studies from the literature and to understand some of the approaches used to ensure children and young people are involved.

👤 ACTIVITY 5

Find a research study article in the literature involving children and identify
- Using a highlighter tool/pen identify the procedures used to obtain consent to participation in the research from children and young people.
- Make notes on the extent to which consent is discussed in the article.
- Make notes on how the process for seeking consent took place.

PROFESSIONAL CONVERSATIONS

Methodological Challenges in Children and Young People's Research

The final section of this chapter will focus on our reflections of using qualitative approaches with children and young people. Some children and young people will be content to talk, enabling the use of interviews for data collection; others might feel more comfortable drawing or taking pictures of relevant objects and places (Coad, 2007). Children and young people are then encouraged to talk about the resulting images, as shown in the study by Manning et al. (2017). Researchers, initially in the social science field (Matthews and Tucker, 2000), and now in the field of child health (Coad, 2007; Coad and Lewis, 2004), emphasise the importance of using methods which interest and therefore engage children and which are within the child's ability. A wide range of data collection methods have been used from drawings and photographs (referred to earlier) to poetry, drama, role play and video (Kirby, 1999). When children's and young people's interest in both the research process and the topic is engaged, the resulting data will be much richer, providing greater insights into the world of children and young people.

Furthermore, a range of designs including evaluation, exploratory, descriptive, case and mixed approaches, are available to researchers in order to answer their research question. However, the greater the difficulty in defining precisely what, exactly, are the questions being explored or tested and how they relate to each other, the greater the likelihood that you are dealing with a complex project.

The evidence for children's nursing practice can therefore be complex and require skilled interpretation. Knowledge of both quantitative and qualitative research methods is required to assess evidence, particularly about complex interventions. We suggest you undertake Activity 6 to work through some of these complex issues.

👤 ACTIVITY 6

- Identify one complex intervention from your area of practice. List the possible issues and challenges.
- If you were undertaking a project on that issue what might be your challenges? Make a list of those issues.

SUMMARY

This chapter has set out the approach to evidenced-based practice, which is rooted in research evidence with consideration of professionals and individual children, young people and families' preferences. Nurses who care for children, young people and their families need to be proficient at the EBP process, which takes time and development of skills and knowledge to ensure the process is systematic and robust. Activities included in this chapter have allowed the reader to develop fundamental evidence-based practice skills, such as developing a research question, identifying the best available evidence and appraising the evidence.

REFERENCES

Alderson, P., Morrow, V., 2011. The Ethics of Research with Children and Young People: A Practical Handbook. SAGE Publications Ltd, London.

Alderwick, H., Charles, A., Jones, B., et al., 2017. The Health Foundation. Making the Case for Quality Improvement: Lessons for NHS Boards and Leaders. The Kings Fund, London.

Borland, M., Laybourn, A., Hill, M., Brown, J., 1998. Middle Childhood. The Perspectives of Children and Parents. Jessica Kingsley Publishers, London.

Carter, T., Guo, B., Turner, D., et al., 2015. Preferred intensity exercise for adolescents receiving treatment for depression: a pragmatic randomised controlled trial. BMC Psychiatr. 15, 247.

Coad, J., 2007. Using art-based techniques in engaging children and young people in health care consultations and/or research. J. Res. Nurs. 12, 487–497.

Coad, J., Evans, R., 2008. Reflections on practical approaches to involving children and young people in the data analysis process. Child. Soc. 22, 41–52.

Coad, J., Lewis, A., 2004. Engaging Children and Young People in Research: Literature Review for the National Evaluation of the Children's Fund (NECF). NECF, London.

Coad, J., Toft, A., Lapwood, S., et al., 2017. Blended foods for tube-fed children: a safe and realistic option? A rapid review of the evidence. Arch. Dis. Child. 102 (3), 274–278.

Cooke, A., Smith, D., Booth, A., 2012. Beyond PICO: the spider tool for qualitative evidence synthesis. Qual. Health Res. 22 (10), 1435–1443.

Coyne, I., Carter, B., 2018a. Being Participatory: Researching with Children and Young People: Co-constructing Knowledge Using Creative Techniques. Switzerland: Springer.

Coyne, I., Carter, B., 2018b. Participatory Research in the Past, Present and Future. Being Participatory: Researching With Children and Young People. Switzerland: Springer.

Darbyshire, P., 2000. From research on children to research with children. Neonatal, paeditric and child health nursing 3 (1), 2–3.

Hoffmann, T., Bennett, S., Del Mar, C., 2013. Evidence-Based Practice across the Health Professions-E-Book. Australia: Elsevier Health Sciences.

Horne, R., Chapman, S.C.E., Parham, R., Freemantle, N., Forbes, Cooper, V., 2013. Understanding patients' adherence-related beliefs about medicines prescribed for long-term conditions: a meta-analytic review of the necessity-concerns framework. PLoS One 8 (12):e80633.

Kirby, P., 1999. Involving Young Researchers: How to Enable Young People to Design and Conduct Research. Joseph Rowntree Foundation, York.

Latif, A., Carter, T., Rychwalska-Brown, L., et al., 2017. Co-producing a digital educational programme for registered children's nurses to improve care of children and young people admitted with self-harm. J. Child Health Care 21, 191–200.

Mahon, A., Glendinning, C., Clarke, K., et al., 1996. Researching children: methods and ethics. Child. Soc. 10, 145–154.

Mallory, C., 2001. Examining the differences between researcher and participant: an intrinsic element of grounded theory. Schreiber, R.S. and Stern, P.N. (Eds) Using grounded theory in nursing Springer Publishing Company, Inc, New York: 85–95.

Manning, J.C., Hemingway, P., Redsell, S.A., 2017. Stories of survival: children's narratives of psychosocial well-being following paediatric critical illness or injury. J. Child Health Care 21, 236–252.

Matthews, H., Tucker, F., 2000. Consulting children. J. Geogr. High. Educ. 24 (2), 299–310.

McIntosh, N., Bates, P., Brykczynska, G., Dunstan, G., Goldman, A., Harvey, D., Larcher, V., McCrae, D., McKinnon, A., Patton, M., Saunders, J., 2000. Guidelines for the ethical conduct of medical research involving children. Royal College of Paediatrics and Child Health: Ethics Advisory Committee. Archives of Diseases in Childhood 82 (2), 177–182.

Muir Gray, J., 1997. Evidence-Based Healthcare. Churchill Livingston, London.

Nuffield Council on Bioethics, 2015. Children and Clinical Research: Ethical Issues. Nuffield Council on Bioethics, London.

Oulton, K., Gibson, F., Sell, D., et al., 2016. Assent for children's participation in research: why it matters and making it meaningful. Child Care Health Dev. 42, 588–597.

Sackett, D.L., Rosenberg, W.M.C., Gray, M.J.A., Haynes, B.R., Richardson, S.W., 1996. Evidence Based Medicine: what is it and what it isn't. Br. Med. J. 312, 71–72.

Sackett, D.L., Richardson, W.S., Rosenberg, W.M.C., Haynes, R.B., 1997. Evidence-Based Medicine - How to Practice and Teach EBM. Churchill Livingstone, New York.

35

Caring for Children With Critical Illness

Peter McNee, Philip Davey

LEARNING OUTCOMES

- Demonstrate an understanding of the key concepts of children's intensive care nursing.
- Explain the principles of respiratory and cardiovascular support within the intensive care setting.

- Consider the role of the children's nurse as part of the multi-professional team in helping to maintain respiratory support and haemodynamic control.
- Discuss the physical and psychological care of the child with critical illness and their family.

GLOSSARY

Afterload The load against which the left ventricle ejects after opening the aortic valve.

Cardiac contractility Contractile capability of the heart.

Cardiac output The volume of blood that the heart pumps in 1 minute.

Central venous pressure A measure of pressure in the right atrium.

Chronotropic Agent that acts to increase heart rate.

Compensated shock Blood flow is normal or increased and may be maldistributed; vital organ function is maintained.

Compliance The ease with which the lungs and thorax expand during pressure changes.

Endotracheal intubation Insertion of endotracheal tube into the trachea either through a patient's nose or mouth and directly through the larynx between the vocal cords into the trachea to open and maintain airway.

Fibrosis Replacement of lung epithelium and elastic fibres with fibroblast scar tissue.

Frank-Starling's law An increase in preload leads to an increase in stroke volume.

FRC Functional residual capacity is the pool of air left in the lungs at the end of total expiration.

Heart rate The number of cardiac contractions that occur in 1 minute.

Hypoxia An inadequate supply of oxygen.

Inotrope Agent that acts to improve myocardial contractility and enhance stroke volume.

Irreversible shock Inadequate perfusion of vital organs; irreparable damage; death cannot be prevented.

Minute volume Amount of gas inhaled and exhaled in 1 minute.

PEEP/CPAP Positive end expiratory pressure, or continuous positive airway pressure, is the baseline pressure and controls functional residual capacity in the patient's lung.

PIP Peak inspiratory pressure indicates the maximum pressure that has occurred during the last ventilatory cycle.

Preload The load on the ventricle before ejection.

Shock Circulatory system failure to supply oxygen and nutrients to meet cellular metabolic demands.

Stroke volume The amount of blood ejected by both ventricles with each contraction.

Systemic vascular resistance The resistance against which the left ventricle must eject to force out its content with each beat.

Tidal volume The amount of gas or air breathed in or out in one breath.

Uncompensated shock Microvascular perfusion is compromised; significant reductions in effective circulating volume.

INTRODUCTION

There are a range of terms which describe the clinical space where children's intensive care is delivered. These include Paediatric Intensive Care (PIC), Paediatric Critical Care Unit (PCCU) and Children's intensive care. For the purposes of this chapter, PIC will be used.

Paediatric critical or intensive care can be described as the delivery of care to children who are in need of closer monitoring, observation and interventions that are unable to be delivered in acute inpatient wards (Royal College of Paediatrics and Child Health [RCPCH], 2014).

Nurses are an important element of the team of staff that care for the critically ill child, and this is reflected by the high nurse-to-patient ratio – ideally 1:1 – that is characteristic of critical care. To understand what critical care is, we must focus on the social context in which it occurs. The role encompasses an independent as well as interdependent element. Although critical care nurses work one-to-one so that they can truly focus on each patient, they will contribute as part of a team when the need dictates. In addition, nursing and therapeutic intervention in PIC extends beyond the patient. It includes the interface with technology, for example the lines, monitors and the organ support machinery.

WHAT IS CRITICAL ILLNESS?

Across the UK and Ireland between 2015 and 2017 there were around 20,000 admissions each year to PIC (Paediatric Intensive Care Audit Network Report, 2018). There are, however, many differences in health care facilities available in PICs across the UK relating to the case mix of patients admitted and the intensive care resources available in particular units. For example, a hospital with a cardiac surgery programme will increase the number of patients that unit admits with that condition. Although a wide variety of diseases may lead to critical illness, the fundamental interventions required are limited. The common pathway of deterioration in critical illness occurs as a result of the progressive deterioration of respiratory and circulatory function with increasing respiratory failure or shock associated with the pathophysiological consequences of organ damage and dysfunction leading to cardiopulmonary failure (Advanced Life Support Group [ALSG], 2016).

ORGANISATION OF PIC SERVICES

Critical illness is characterised by the acute loss of physiologic reserve but in many cases the course of illness is prolonged and often the underlying cause may be difficult to discern. Moreover, despite a child having a recognised critical illness there is great interpatient variability. In the past children with critical illness were nursed in a range of settings, including general adult intensive care units, depending on geographical location. In the UK, paediatric intensive care developed in an ad hoc and fragmented way. Now, however, after 25 years of effort, care has moved to a more integrated service.

Concerns about paediatric intensive care were first raised by the British Paediatric Association (BPA) in the 1980s, and again in 1993 when it published its report on paediatric intensive care. The BPA report highlighted the fragmented configuration of paediatric intensive care provision, demonstrating that only 51% of children were cared for in paediatric intensive care units, 20% in adult intensive care units and 29% in children's wards (BPA, 1993). Furthermore, only 36% of paediatric intensive care units provided a retrieval service. Concerns were also expressed regarding the lack of physical facilities, lack of education and training of both medical and nursing staff and poor staffing levels available to care for these critically ill children.

In 1996, an inquiry into the death of a child named Nicholas Geldard, who died in a paediatric intensive care unit in 1995 after inappropriate transport for management following a spontaneous cerebral haemorrhage, was published

(Ashworth, 1996). In response to this, the Department of Health (DoH) requested an inquiry into paediatric intensive care services with a view to developing a policy framework for paediatric intensive care (NHS Executive [NHSE], 1996). The inquiry found that PIC had developed in an ad-hoc manner and was a low-volume high-cost service with very little in the way of national standards or an evidence base on which care was delivered. Ten of the 29 units in existence had three beds or fewer which led to scrutiny of their ability to provide critical care services to those children admitted to the units. In 1997 'Paediatric Intensive Care: a Framework for the Future' was published (NHSE, 1997a). This report alongside NHSE (1997b) 'Paediatric Intensive Care: a Bridge to the Future' set out a strategy for developing and integrating the service for critically ill children within a geographical area, and so centralise the skills and experience of medical and nursing staff. The central recommendations of the report were delivered with lead centres identified within each region. Lead centres had to be in hospitals which also delivered the full range of tertiary care for children, had skilled staff in all disciplines in order to both deliver care and act as training centres, and had to provide 24-hour retrieval services in their region. There are local and geographical differences in how services are delivered, for instance Wales has one PIC based in Cardiff which serves South Wales. Children requiring PIC in North Wales would be transferred to Alder Hey in Liverpool.

Today, children requiring intensive care are no longer cared for in general children's wards and centres that do not meet the standards as laid out by the NHSE framework document. Quality of paediatric intensive care is not only reliant on a centralised and standardised service, but also – importantly – the effectiveness and appropriateness of treatment within a child and family-orientated environment (Paediatric Intensive Care Society [PICS], 2015). To facilitate this, nurses working in PIC undertake a specifically designed, competency-based course to equip them with the knowledge, skills and understanding that underpins effective paediatric intensive care nursing practice.

 WWW

Read the NHS Executive Report, *Paediatric Intensive Care 'A Framework for the Future'* online:
- http://www.ihrdni.org/315-016-1.pdf
    Consider how PIC is organised and delivered in your country or region.

IDENTIFYING LEVELS OF PAEDIATRIC CRITICAL CARE

Clarke (2012) identifies that PIC can be recognised from other forms of care by the severity of illness that the child or young person presents with. They may present in the emergency department or children's assessment unit, then require admission to a ward with escalation of treatment in high dependency and ultimately they may be in a paediatric intensive care unit. Originally the (NHSE, 1997) identified levels of care as being level 1 equivalent to high dependency care, and levels 2 and 3 being PIC. The Paediatric Intensive Care Society (2015) has

TABLE 35.1   Paediatric Critical Care Units Levels of Care: Paediatric Intensive Care Society (2015) Quality Standards for the Care of Critically Ill Children

Paediatric critical care unit (PCCU)	A discrete area within a ward or hospital where paediatric critical care is delivered.
Level 1 PCCU	A discrete area or unit where Level 1 paediatric critical care is delivered. With Paediatric Critical Care Network agreement, CPAP for bronchiolitis may be initiated or continued in a number of Level 1 PCCUs.
Level 2 PCCU	A discrete area or unit where Level 1 and Level 2 paediatric critical care are delivered. Other than in specialist children's hospitals, Level 2 PCCUs should be able to provide, as a minimum, acute (and chronic) non-invasive ventilation (both CPAP and BiPAP support) and care for children with tracheostomies and children on long-term ventilation, but should not be expected to deliver specialist Level 2 interventions such as ICP monitoring or acute renal replacement therapy. Within specialist children's hospitals, Level 2 units may provide some or all of these additional specialist interventions.
Level 3 PCCU	A unit delivering Level 2 and Level 3 paediatric critical care (and Level 1 if required). This unit may also be called a paediatric intensive care unit (PICU).

BiPAP, Biphasic/bilevel positive airways pressure; *CPAP,* continuous positive airway pressure; *ICP,* Intracranial Pressure.
Paediatric Intensive Care Society (PICS), 2015. Quality Standards for the Care of Critically Ill Children, 5th ed. PICS, London. Available from: http://picsociety.uk/wp-content/uploads/2016/05/PICS_standards_2015.pdf.

refined the levels of care and associated descriptors over time, and provided further detail on the interventions that would be required at each level (Table 35.1).

 ACTIVITY

Analyse the categories of intensive care as defined by the PICS Quality Standards. Discuss in your learning group how these levels of care and facilities, including staff skills and expertise, compare with a general paediatric ward.

 SCENARIO

Introducing Daniel

The Badger Ward paediatrician and nursing staff were concerned about the condition of 15-month-old Daniel, who weighed 13 kg and was developing increased respiratory distress since admission 4 hours earlier. Daniel had been admitted to Badger Ward as a referral from his GP and was accompanied by his parents, Emma and Alan. Daniel had a 2-week history of an upper respiratory tract infection, which over the previous 2–3 days had worsened, with decreased appetite and fluid intake. Since admission to Badger Ward, Daniel's respiratory distress had markedly increased. Initial treatment was directed towards alleviating his respiratory distress and included 30% oxygen and intravenous antibiotics. Despite this therapy there had been no evidence of improvement. The paediatrician contacted the paediatric intensive care unit (PICU) intensivist to review Daniel on Badger Ward.

The paediatric intensivist and an experienced PIC nurse equipped with emergency bag and retrieval trolley responded immediately to this request. On assessment they found that Daniel was in obvious respiratory distress. He was irritable and reluctant to leave his mother's arms. His pulse rate was 180 beats/min, and was 65 breaths/min with grunting and sternal and intercostal chest recession. Inspiratory stridor and expiratory wheeze were readily audible and his tidal volume was decreased.

Daniel was transferred to PICU on the retrieval trolley on his mother's lap.

 ACTIVITY

Consider Daniel's situation and the PICS levels of care. What was the rationale for Daniel's admission to PICU?

Relating back to Chapter 27, consider why the critical care team who assessed Daniel decided to transfer him to PICU in his mother's lap, without further intervention on Badger Ward.

SCENARIO

On admission to PICU, additional vital signs were obtained:
- Daniel was awake and irritable and appeared exhausted
- respiratory rate had increased from 60 to 70 breaths/min
- his recession appeared pronounced
- oxygen saturation: 95% in 50%
- pulse rate had increased from 174 to 200 beats/min
- radial and dorsalis pulses were weak and thready
- his skin was cool, dry and pale
- capillary refill: 4 s
- blood pressure: 90/60 mmHg
- he was conscious and responding to his mother
- blood glucose: 1.7 mmol/L
- axilla temperature: 38.5°C
- no skin rash noted
- an arterial gas was obtained: pH 7.25, pCO_2 7.6, pO_2 22, base deficit −3

Rapid Cardiopulmonary Assessment

Recognition of potential respiratory failure, based on clinical evaluation of the child, is vital (ALSG, 2016). Intubation and ventilation of a child with potential respiratory failure will be considered if a child fails to improve after initial oxygen therapy or if further deterioration is observed. An individual must be able to support three specific functions:
- Protect the airway
- Adequately ventilate
- Adequately oxygenate

A failure to perform any one function will result in respiratory failure. Respiratory failure is the most common reason for admission to PIC (Davies and McDougall, 2019) and is defined as a major abnormality of gas exchange (Hazinski, 2013) and is an absolute indication for intubation and mechanical ventilation. However, not every patient who is intubated has a primary pulmonary pathology. Intubation and ventilation may serve to support the cardiovascular system. For example, for patients in cardiogenic shock, the demands of the respiratory system may precipitate cardiovascular collapse. Supporting the patient with mechanical ventilation can reduce the demands on the heart, allowing it to recover. Intubation can also serve to protect the airway for those who cannot do it themselves, for example patients in coma as a result of a head injury. Moreover, mechanical ventilation offers the option of hyperventilation for patients with intracranial hypertension with evidence suggesting that keeping the pCO_2 at the lower end of normal may provide some benefit (National Institute for Health and Care Excellence [NICE], 2014; Davies and McDougall, 2019).

ACTIVITY

Analyse the data collected during a rapid cardiopulmonary assessment of Daniel, and arterial blood gas, and list the factors that support the decision to intubate and ventilate.

Respiratory Support
Intubation

Intubation and ventilation are always performed with caution, as anaesthetic agents as well as positive pressure ventilation will exacerbate hypovolaemia. Assessment of Daniel's perfusion indicates a degree of hypovolaemia; therefore he was given 260 mL (20 mL/kg) of normal saline as an intravenous bolus with good effect observed by an improvement in his heart rate and perfusion. In addition, he was administered broad-spectrum intravenous antibiotics.

Intubation is a painful and unpleasant procedure and should never be performed on a conscious or semi-conscious patient. Unless the child has completely collapsed, the medical practitioner, usually an anaesthetist or intensivist, will perform what is called rapid sequence induction. This means inducing anaesthesia and giving muscle relaxants. Examples of common drugs used in this procedure are morphine (analgesic), midazolam (sedative) and rocuronium (muscle relaxant); it remains the responsibility of the practitioner carrying out the intubation to select appropriate combinations of drugs to ensure safe administration at the correct dose (see *BNF for Children* [BNFc 2020/2021]). When the drugs are being prepared for rapid sequence induction, equipment should be prepared and checked to be in good working order to ensure a safe procedure, as displayed in Fig. 35.1.

As the sedation and anaesthetic agent of choice is administered intravenously and the child starts to lose consciousness,

SCENARIO

Daniel was intubated with a size 4.5 mm endotracheal tube. Initial ventilation parameters were:
- respiratory rate: 30 breaths/min
- inspiratory time: 0.8 s
- tidal volume: 180 mL
- Positive end expiratory pressure (PEEP): 5 cm H_2O

Synchronised mandatory ventilation (SIMV) mode was selected; resultant peak inspiratory pressure (PIP) was 28 cm H_2O. Analgesia and sedation were maintained with continuous infusions of morphine and midazolam, respectively.

the child will be preoxygenated with 100% oxygen using a bag-valve-mask device for at least 1–2 minutes. This ensures that the child is in optimum condition prior to the procedure of intubation. Once the child is assessed to be unconscious and bag-valve mask-ventilation is established, the paralysing agent is administered intravenously. A nasogastric tube should be passed to empty gastric contents and left of free drainage, thus preventing aspiration. It is also useful for decompression of gas accumulated in the stomach during bag-valve-mask ventilation. During the intubation procedure the medical practitioner may ask an assistant to apply cricoid pressure. This is external compression of the trachea to decrease the probability of aspiration and inflation of the stomach, and also enhances visualisation of the glottis. Care must be taken to apply cricoid pressure symmetrically. Once the endotracheal tube is in place, observations are made to confirm that the tube is in the correct position. This is done by:
- observing for bilateral chest movement with ventilation;
- auscultation using a stethoscope to ensure breath sounds heard clearly over the anterior and posterior chest and in both axillae;
- confirming that there are no breath sounds over the stomach;
- confirming that O_2 saturations are improving;
- confirming that the heart rate is stable and within normal limits;
- the endotracheal tube is then secured in place and a chest x-ray ordered for formal confirmation of tube placement;
- measurement of expired CO_2 by capnography (ALSG, 2016).

Mechanical Ventilation: Physiological Principles and Effects

Mechanical ventilatory support is the major supportive treatment used in critical care. A mechanical ventilator is simply a machine used to replace or supplement the natural function of breathing. It is usually a temporary measure until the patient can breathe adequately without help. Ventilation is simply the movement of gas into and out of the lungs. To safely and effectively provide care for intubated infants and children who are receiving assisted ventilation, it is necessary to have an understanding of the fundamental

Action	Rationale
Suction apparatus with appropriate size suction catheter.	Relatively small amounts of mucus accumulation, oedema or airway obstruction can reduce airway patency or obscure view of the vocal cords for intubation.
Assemble appropriate sized and working bag valve mask device.	To ensure effective ventilation.
Positioning to achieve optimal airway patency is essential to bag valve mask. A shoulder roll may be used to help extend the neck and position the airway in a neutral position (nose perpendicular to the ceiling). An airway adjunct may also be used if head position is difficult to maintain	A child under the age of 2 years has a large, heavy head with prominent occiput, short chubby neck and a large tongue. Furthermore, sedation and CNS dysfunction will exacerbate these effects.
Assemble appropriate sized and working laryngoscope and blade. Check adequate illumination from bulb. 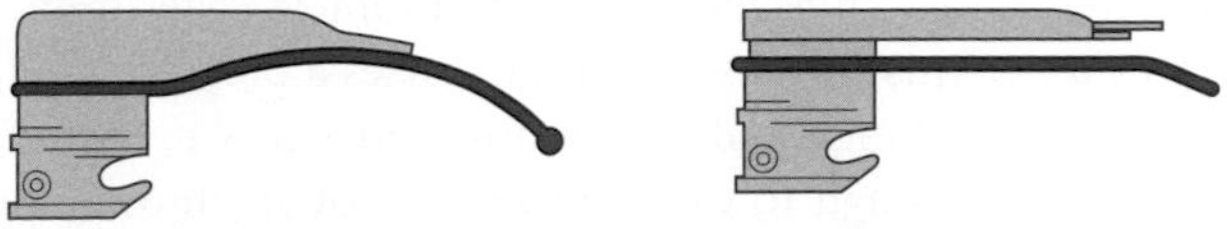	A straight laryngoscope blade is better in younger children as it is used to pick up the floppy epiglottis. A curved laryngoscope blade is better in older children who have a stiff epiglottis where the blade is placed in the vallecula.
Assemble the correct size endotracheal tube (ETT) plus one a size above and one size below. 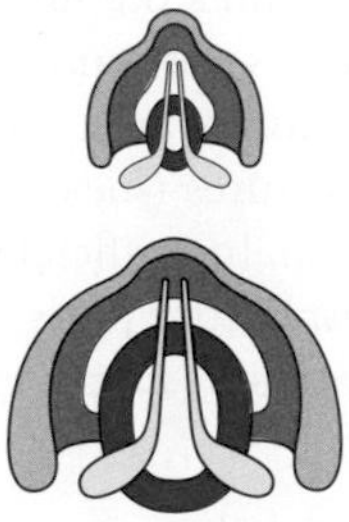	The narrowest part of the airway in a child under 8 years at the level of the cricoid cartilage which is cone-shaped. An ETT may pass through the vocal cords easily in the young child but be too large to pass through the cricoid cartilage. Select the correct size uncuffed tube carefully using a broselow tape, a recognised chart of the formulae: $$\frac{Age + 4}{4}$$ For the child under 2 years: Age　　　　kg　　　ETT Newborn　　3.5　　　3.5 3 months　　6.0　　　3.5 1 year　　　10　　　4.0 2 years　　　12　　　4.5
Assemble ETT with introducer if wanted. 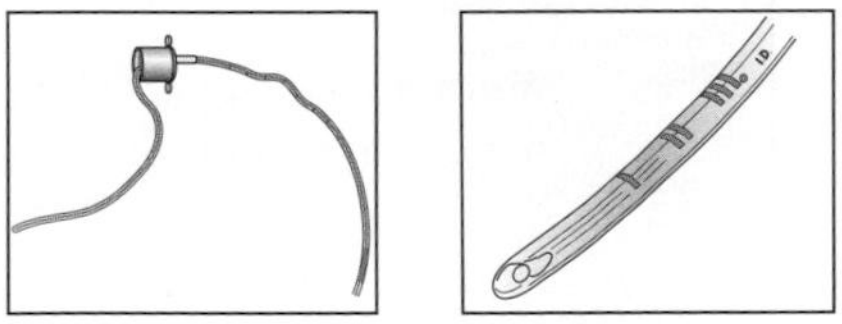	The practitioner intubating may request an introducer. This makes the tube more 'stiff' which makes intubating easier. When inserting the introducer take care to ensure that it does not protrude beyond the tip of the ETT itself as this may cause tissue trauma to the trachea. Many bend the top of the introducer over the connector after checking for profusion as a further safety mechanism.
Assemble tape ready cut to secure ETT in place.	This enables stability of the ETT in place. Various methods of securing an ETT exist. Find out how your PICU prefers to secure an ETT.
Stethoscope.	To confirm ETT placement prior to the formal confirmation of a chest X-ray.

Fig. 35.1 The action and rationale for preparation prior to intubation. *CNS,* Central nervous system; *PICU,* paediatric intensive care unit.

physiological principles of lung function and the physiological effects of assisted ventilation in terms of both gas exchange and pulmonary mechanics and have an appreciation of the particular disease process leading to the need for assisted ventilation.

Ventilation and Perfusion Relationship

The primary function of the lungs is to enable gas exchange between inspired air that reaches the alveoli and the blood of the pulmonary capillaries. Ventilation is the process of gas movement in and out of the lungs (Kline-Tilford et al., 2013).

This activity of gas exchange is crucial for homeostasis and is interdependent with the circulatory system's prime role of blood transport. Gas exchange is deemed to be adequate if oxygen tensions (PaO_2) and carbon dioxide tension ($PaCO_2$) are maintained within normal limits. To enable adequate gas exchange, it is crucial that oxygen and carbon dioxide move between air and blood by simple diffusion across the alveolar surface. More specifically, there is a balance between ventilation (V) and perfusion (Q). However, it is more complicated than this. V and Q are not evenly distributed throughout the lung. Fig. 35.2 illustrates how V increases from apex to the base of the lung and Q increases from apex to base relatively more than perfusion. During normal quiet breathing in an upright position the bases of the lung receive about 50% more ventilation than the apices. This is due to:

- gravity
- variations in airways size (remember Poiseuille's law, Chapter 4)
- variations in alveolar elastic properties (surfactant – to be discussed later)

If oxygen is not delivered to alveolar capillaries, or the alveolar surface is damaged, oxygen and/or carbon dioxide elimination may be impaired, V and Q are not balanced and respiratory failure ensues. In a single lung unit V and Q must be matched to allow gas exchange (Fig. 35.3).

Mechanical ventilation is an attempt to normalise the patient's ventilation–perfusion ratio. However, perfusion is determined by:

- the amount of oxygen in the blood
- the oxygen binding capacity of haemoglobin
- cardiac output

Therefore when a patient is being ventilated, therapeutic interventions must also be taken to optimise perfusion by ensuring there is a sufficient delivery of inspired oxygen, concentration of haemoglobin and cardiac output. We will look at cardiac output in more detail later.

The Mechanics of Breathing

Three factors affect the mechanics of breathing:

- Force (pressure)
- Displacement (volume)
- Rate of displacement (flow), which comprises compliance and resistance

These factors are all interrelated:

Pressure = Volume ÷ (Compliance + Resistance),

that is, Pressure = Volume ÷ Flow.

During normal inspiration the mechanical contraction of the inspiratory muscles causes the thoracic cage to enlarge in volume. This increased volume causes a pressure gradient between the lungs and the atmosphere. This pressure differential is enough to cause an in-rush of air into the lungs (Boyle's law). The work that the inspiratory muscles perform represents the negative pressure applied. Fig. 35.4a shows the changes in airway pressure in the mouth during spontaneous quiet breathing. Airway pressure during inspiration is negative, allowing air to enter the lungs, and is positive during expiration. Also, there is normally a brief pause, when airway pressure remains at atmospheric pressure. Fig. 35.4b shows the upper airway pressures (measured at the mouth) during mechanical ventilation. In artificial ventilation, the ventilator must provide the inspiratory pressure provided by the inspiratory muscles in normal respiration. This is done by creating

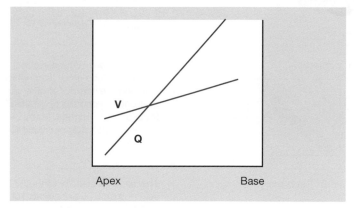

Fig. 35.2 The ventilation *(V)* and perfusion *(Q)* relationship.

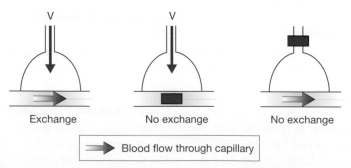

Fig. 35.3 A simple illustration of ventilation *(V)* and perfusion *(Q)* mismatch.

a positive intrapulmonary pressure whereby air is pushed out of the ventilator into the lungs of the patient, thus raising the pressure in the airways relative to atmospheric pressure. This resultant increase in intrapulmonary pressure forces the lungs to expand. It is important to remember that artificial ventilation fundamentally alters normal airway pressures. This fact accounts for most of its benefits and complications.

In the equation Pressure = Volume ÷ (Compliance + Resistance), compliance and resistance are assumed to remain constant and are illustrated by Fig. 35.5a. However, this is not the case in cardiopulmonary illness. With stiff lungs (reduced compliance) patients tend to take rapid, small breaths, to minimise elastic workload as in Fig. 35.5b. With high airway resistance, for example in asthma, patients take large slow breaths (Fig. 35.5c). As can be seen in Fig. 35.5, the inspiratory lung volume is low in both instances. Thus their combined effect is a greater load presented to the ventilator. Pressure, volume and flow change over time in illness,

therefore they are considered variable. From the equation of motion, the ventilator must control one of these variables. A mechanical ventilator will control airway pressure, inspired volume or inspired flow.

But there is more to compliance. Compliance refers to the effort required to stretch the lungs and chest wall. High compliance means that the chest all and lungs expand easily whereas low compliance means that they resist expansion. In the lungs, compliance is related to two main factors: surface tension and elasticity (Tortora and Derrickson, 2014). To achieve compliance, alveolar lung units have an important lung property – they are elastic. They can be expanded by small forces and return to their resting state. Two components are responsible for their elastic behaviour:

- elastic tissue consisting of elastic and collagen fibres embedded in alveoli walls and around bronchi;
- the surface tension reducing effect of surfactant increases compliance.

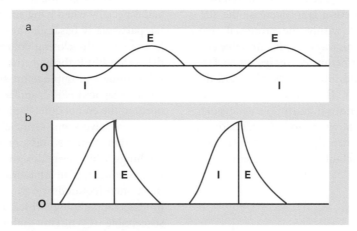

Fig. 35.4 Changes in airway pressure during *(a)* normal spontaneous breathing versus *(b)* artificial mechanical ventilation.

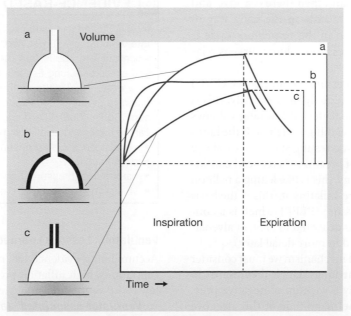

Fig. 35.5 The effects of compliance and airway resistance on lung volume. *(a)* The effect of normal compliance; *(b)* the effect of reduced compliance; *(c)* the effect of increased airways resistance.

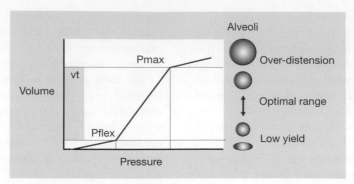

Fig. 35.6 Alveolar compliance and the pressure–volume curve.

Compliant lungs will inflate with very low pressures (Kline-Tilford et al., 2013). The lung contains a foamy phospholipid fluid commonly known as surfactant. Pulmonary surfactant is produced by types I and II alveolar pneumocytes. Surfactant is a complex mixture of both lipids and proteins which line the epithelial surface of the lung (Been and Zimmermann, 2007). Surfactants' primary function is to decrease the surface tension of the lining fluid within the bronchial tree. Without surfactant, pulmonary airways become unstable and have decreased compliance. Surfactant decreases the surface tension in the alveolar air–liquid interface alveoli to aid the diffusion of gases (Dixon, 2012). This mechanism stabilises the alveolus at the end of inspiration and prevents alveolar collapse at the end of the expiratory period. A reduction in production of surfactant will directly affect gas exchange. General causes of reduced surfactant production are:

- acidosis
- hypoxia
- hyperoxygenation
- pulmonary oedema
- atelectasis

To help understand this concept, think about blowing up a balloon. At first it is difficult, and then there is a 'give' and the balloon inflates easily. This occurs in the same way in the lungs. The greatest workload in the respiratory cycle is in early inspiration where the pressure–volume curve is relatively flat (Fig. 35.6).

Once the steep part of the pressure–volume curve (PVC) (the P_{flex}) is reached, the lung suddenly inflates easily; this is the inflection point. The PVC is flattest at low lung volumes and consequently the work of breathing is highest. If the lungs were left filled with air so that the resting state is at or above the inflection point, the work of breathing is reduced considerably. Going back to our analogy, this is like letting a balloon deflate incompletely and then re-inflating it. This is the basis for positive end expiratory pressure (PEEP), which is a continuous constant pressure of gas delivered to prevent alveolar collapse (PEEP will be discussed in more detail later).

Finally, the last physiological mechanism we must consider is closing volume. In health, the lungs dangle downwards in the pleural cavity, supported by a vacuum of negative pressure. As you would expect, the magnitude of this negative pressure is greater in the apices than in the bases. The effect of this is to splint the airways open at the end of the tidal volume (normal expiration) – the expiratory reserve volume (ERV) (McCance and Huether, 2002) (Fig. 35.7). Apical alveoli are more inflated at rest than basal. But during inspiration, because the latter are at a steep part of the pressure–volume curve, the gas turnover (see Fig. 35.6) is greater. However, in illness, further confounded by upper airway compromise, and especially when lying supine, there is a tendency for distal, particularly basal airways to collapse in expiration. This is known as the closing volume. If this is not addressed by delivering PEEP through the ventilator, eventually the closing volume will impinge on and begin to exceed functional residual capacity (FRC) and atelectasis (alveolar collapse) will occur at the end of quiet expiration.

As we have seen, artificial ventilation is unlike normal ventilation. Positive pressure ventilation can be injurious to the lungs, which were designed as a negative pressure circuit receiving oxygen at 21%. Moreover, artificial ventilation is most often required by patients with underlying lung or cardiovascular pathology which makes the lung tissue even more susceptible to ventilator-induced lung injury and cardiovascular complications.

⊚ EVIDENCE-BASED PRACTICE

Intubation and ventilation carry their own risks although both interventions are life saving. Evidence has been mounting since the late 1980s that mechanical ventilation can cause and exacerbate lung tissue injury (Dreyfus et al., 1985; Kolobow et al., 1987). Although most of this evidence has originated from animal studies, clinical reports support this concern (Bohn, 1998). There are a range of complications which can be experienced including:

- ventilator-associated pneumonia
- oxygen toxicity
- barotrauma (pressure)
- volutrauma (shearing forces)

Ventilation: Lessons Learned

Accumulating evidence has revealed that high oxygen concentrations, high inflation pressures, large tidal volumes and low PEEP ventilation strategies are damaging to the lungs:

Ventilator-associated (acquired) pneumonia. Ventilator-associated pneumonia (VAP) is a hospital-acquired infection in patients who are mechanically ventilated. The

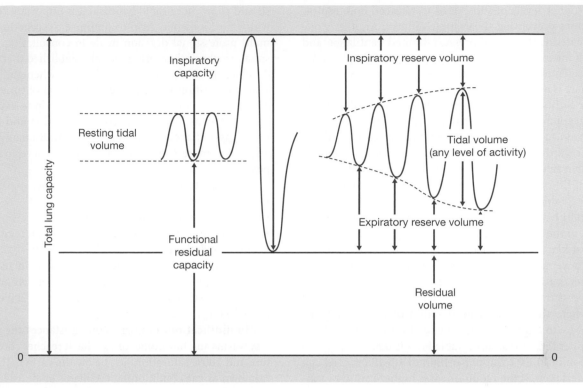

Fig. 35.7 Lung volumes.

infection is not present at the initiation of ventilation but develops more than 48 hours later (Wright and Romano, 2006). VAP contributes to increased mortality, morbidity and increased duration of stay (Melsen et al., 2009). Intubated patients are at risk of VAP due to the change in first-line host defences relating to intubation with an endotracheal tube being passed directly into the airway. Diagnosis can be difficult due to a range of definitions and surveillance protocols, but treatment is directed at the organisms which are most likely to have caused the pneumonia (Foglia et al., 2007).

Oxygen toxicity. Breathing high levels of inspired oxygen can cause oxidant injury within the lung parenchyma and airway; this is known as oxygen toxicity (Macintyre, 2005). Oxygen in supraphysiological concentrations is injurious to the lung, particularly in concentrations over a fraction of inspired oxygen (FiO_2) of 0.60 (Robb, 1997a). PEEP is frequently increased in order to allow a reduction of FiO_2 (Hazinski, 2013).

Barotrauma. Positive pressure ventilation is non-physiological and causes pulmonary injury. The higher the pressures used, the greater the potential for injury. This is referred to as barotrauma and is typically associated with excessive airway pressures leading to extra-alveolar air and also includes pneumothorax, pneumomediastinum, pneumoperitoneum and subcutaneous emphysema. What exactly qualifies as a dangerous pressure is not known (Bohn, 1998); however, ensuring that ventilation pressures are minimised is an essential component of lung protective strategies to minimise incidence and improve the clinical outcomes for ventilated children (Jauncey-Cooke et al., 2010).

Volutrauma is caused by excessive tidal volumes, which produce regional lung over-distension leading to lung injury. Mechanical ventilation with varied tidal volumes will lead to degrees of lung injury even when peak airway pressures are identical (Rotta and Steinhorn, 2007). Volutrauma results from the distension of the lungs caused by increased transpulmonary pressures rather than high airway pressures. Volutrauma is manifested by disruption of the alveolar capillary membrane and alterations in gas exchange. The propensity for volutrauma is related to the volume of lung available and to regional differences in compliance. In, for example, pneumonia, where lung volume is significantly diminished and compliance is reduced, the risk of volutrauma is increased (Kerr, 1997).

Shearing forces caused by repeated expansion of collapsed alveoli is injurious to the lung by causing the release of inflammatory mediators independent of over-distension or oxygen concentration (Bohn, 1998). The concept of 'shear' injury along with the increase in dead space to tidal volume ratio prevents the use of high rates to compensate for small tidal volumes/low pressures.

Strategies to reduce lung injury. In response to these findings, respiratory experts have espoused the use of lung protective ventilator strategies (Kerr, 1997). One strategy is to use sufficient PEEP to raise FRC above closing capacity without compromising cardiac output, and as a consequence, oxygen delivery. This strategy keeps alveolar units on the steep part of the compliance curve (see Fig. 35.6). Higher levels of PEEP help to maintain:

- alveolar recruitment (the 'open lung' approach)
- reduce V/Q mismatch and progressive hypoxaemia
- achieve lower tidal volumes (4–8 mL/kg)

Thus, higher levels of PEEP lead to reduced end inspiratory volumes preventing shear/stretch injury. Another strategy advocated is the use of pressure-limited ventilation and increasing mean airway pressures by permissive hypercapnia and hypoxaemia (Reynolds et al., 1993; Rotta and Steinhorn, 2007). There is no research evidence to dictate what acceptable oxygen or carbon dioxide levels are. The general philosophy is that an acceptable level is determined by what intensivists are willing to do to get there, considering the research findings available regarding the causation of lung injury. For example, if an oxygen saturation of 95% can only be achieved through using a PEEP of 12 cm H_2O and a FiO_2 of 1.0 (100%), this is not acceptable in the light of the best available evidence. Both high PEEP and high inspired-oxygen concentrations are injurious to the lung. However, if achieving a carbon dioxide level of 5.4 kPa results in a peak pressure of 30 cm H_2O, this might be acceptable as this carbon dioxide level is acceptable.

In general, Kline-Tilford et al. (2013) note:
- Peak pressures greater than 35 cm H_2O are not acceptable and where this occurs consideration of transferring the patient on to High Frequency Ventilation should be given.
- The upper limit for an acceptable FiO_2 is 0.60.
- Titration of PEEP to an upper limit of 10–12 cm H_2O can be undertaken. If the requirement is higher invasive monitoring cardiac output should be considered.

Ventilator parameters will be set by the intensivist who will consider the patient's current clinical status and objective data obtained from monitoring and blood gas results. The overall goal of mechanical ventilation is not to achieve a target blood gas value, but to maximise oxygen delivery while minimising pulmonary injury as gas exchange and lung function improve.

Inhaled nitric oxide (iNO) was originally thought to be the 'magic bullet' for improving V/Q mismatch in severe respiratory failure (Tibballs, 1998). NO is a powerful pulmonary dilator which has been shown to improve oxygenation in some patients.

Given its ability to vasodilate blood vessels, be delivered as a gas (act on blood vessels that perfuse ventilated alveoli: selective pulmonary vasodilatation) and its short half-life (no systemic hypotension), it was studied with great interest. NO can be used in patients who have reversible pulmonary hypertension or V/Q mismatch, for example, neonates with persistent pulmonary hypertension of the newborn or post-operative cardiac patients (Davies and McDougall, 2019). There have been a range of clinical trials using NO specifically in acute respiratory distress syndrome (ARDS). It was found that there was no clinically discernible benefit in mortality or the duration of ventilation in either adults or children (Adhikari et al., 2014).

Positioning. There are options, beyond adjusting the ventilator, which have implications for nursing. Body positioning affects ventilation/perfusion (V/Q) matching and therefore arterial oxygen levels. Accumulation of secretions and atelectasis can occur in the dependent regions of the lungs, therefore regular position changes will help to avoid problem areas developing. Position can also affect a child's FRC. A reduction in FRC will make a child more vulnerable to atelectasis and allow more rapid hypoxia. It is important to consider which positions may help to optimise oxygenation; this is a multi-professional decision made in consultation with a respiratory physiotherapist. It is well established that atelectasis develops in the dorsal areas of the lung when patients are in a supine position for any extended period of time (Ganong, 2001). 'Prone positioning' a patient can help re-expand these collapsed areas, improve alveolar ventilation and hence improve gas exchange (Ball et al., 2001). Additionally, the chest wall has a more favourable compliance curve in the prone position.

The benefits of prone positioning include:
- optimise the v/q mismatch
- more uniform alveolar ventilation
- reduce atelectasis particularly in the dorsal region
- improve drainage of secretions

Studies have shown some improvement in oxygenation with prone positioning; however, this is not demonstrated in survival and ventilator-free days (Curley et al., 2005; Mancebo et al., 2006).

Humidification. In normal circumstances the upper airway warms and humidifies air, so that it reaches core temperature and 100% saturation just below the carina. This process is known as gas conditioning (Williams et al., 1996). During gas conditioning inspired air is also cleaned and filtered of foreign particles by the mucociliary transport system, which extends from the nasopharynx towards the bronchioles (Tortora and Derrikson, 2014). Thus gas conditioning optimises gas exchange and protects delicate lung tissue. Intubation and mechanical ventilation bypass this defence mechanism and the gas exchange function of the lung. The placement of the endotracheal tube physically shifts the conditioning, and heat and moisture recovery functions further down the airway, which would not normally be required to give up heat and moisture.

Hence in the intubated patient, the mucociliary transport system is the sole remaining mechanical defence system. The mucociliary transport system's function depends on the:
- thickness of the mucus
- depth of the aqueous layer
- cilia beat frequency

If the temperature of inspired gas is less than core temperature, the beat frequency of the cilia will reduce and the gas will be heated to a suboptimal temperature causing the relative humidity of the gas to be reduced. Less than optimal humidification results in a compromised mucociliary transport and pooling of mucus in the lower airways, thus restricting gas exchange and being an ideal site for bacterial colonisation (Centers for Disease Control [CDC], 1994). Furthermore, the gel layer will lose moisture and become thicker. If suboptimal humidification is allowed to continue, cell damage might occur and the process of gas conditioning will move deeper into the lung. Increased thick mucus and reduced clearance of secretions from small airways results in reduced airway patency and lung compliance (Williams et al., 1996). Effective humidification will maximise lung defence by reducing exposure to contaminants invading the airways by increasing clearance of contaminants through suctioning. Humidification can be achieved either through passive heat and moisture exchangers or through active heated humidifiers. Both systems have advantages and disadvantages, but it has been found that in patients who have copious secretions, heat humidification is more beneficial (Siempos et al., 2007).

Cardiovascular Complications: Lessons Learned

Mechanical ventilation through its delivery of positive intrathoracic pressure has an adverse effect on the heart. Consequently, patients require close assessment and monitoring of their cardiovascular function. Increasing intrathoracic pressure which occurs with positive pressure ventilation decreases venous return to the right side of the heart and subsequent cardiac output (Dixon, 2012; Davies and McDougall, 2019). Therefore patients may need additional fluid volume to maintain cardiac output. The nurse must be mindful to observe cardiovascular parameters in relation to ventilator airway pressure. Decreased cardiac output due to positive pressure ventilation is often ameliorated by fluid administration. The degree of cardiac compromise may often limit the amount of PEEP that a child can tolerate and hence what the intensivist is willing to use.

Modes of ventilation. The goals of assisted ventilation are to achieve adequate gas exchange while at the same time minimising damage to the lungs or interference to the circulation. The review of the risks and side effects of positive pressure ventilation possibly goes some way towards explaining why there are so many modes of ventilation available today.

This chapter will now turn to a brief synopsis of the common approaches to ventilation based on physiological principles. It is by no means exhaustive or complete, and is not intended to be. For a more exhaustive discussion of management issues surrounding mechanical ventilation of the sick child, refer to one of the major intensive care texts, such as *Nursing Care of the Critically Ill Child* (Hazinski, 2013).

Ventilators (Fig. 35.8) deliver gas to the lungs using positive pressure at a certain rate. The amount of gas delivered can be limited by time, pressure or volume. The duration can be cycled by time, pressure or flow. The basic terms used with ventilators are the following:

- Peak inspiratory pressure (PIP): indicates the maximum pressure that has occurred during the last ventilatory cycle
- Positive end expiratory pressure (PEEP): pressure applied at the end of expiration in order to maintain functional residual capacity thereby maintaining alveolar volume resulting in increased arterial oxygenation
- Functional residual capacity (FRC) describes the volume of gas that remains in the lungs at the end of normal expiration
- Pressure above PEEP (PAP)
- Mean airway pressure (MAP) is the average airway pressure measured from one inspiration to the start of the next
- Inspiratory time (Ti): shown in seconds. Settings will reflect the normal for the child's age

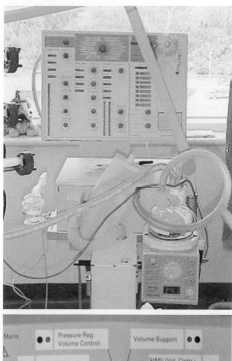

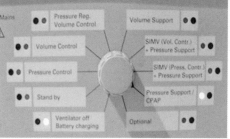

Fig. 35.8 A ventilator *(top)* and a close-up of the control panel *(bottom)*.

- Expiratory time (Te): shown in seconds again will reflect the normal for the child's age
- Tidal volume (TV): equates to the volume of gas inspired and expired in one single breath (6–8 mL/kg)
- Minute volume (MV): refers to amount of gas expired by the lungs in 1 minute. Minute volume = TV × Frequency

The common ventilation modes illustrated in Fig. 35.9 are the following:

- Assisted control mode (AC): the ventilator will guarantee that the patient receives a set tidal volume or peak airway pressure with every breath. The patient can breathe 'above' the set rate but will receive full support regardless of their effort.
- Intermittent mandatory ventilation (IMV): the ventilator supports breaths only at the set rate and interval. Breaths 'above' the set rate are not supported.
- Synchronised intermittent mandatory ventilation (SIMV): the ventilator synchronises an IMV 'breath' with the patient's effort. If, for example, the set rate is 10, then every 6 seconds the patient will receive a machine triggered breath. In between those 10 breaths, the patient is free to breathe but those breaths are not supported. These breaths can be supported if a 'pressure support mode' is added.
- Pressure support or pressure control mode (PS/PC): the ventilator supplies pressure support but no set rate. A patient needs to generate a certain amount of work to

trigger it. Additionally, a patient has to breathe through an endotracheal tube that is almost always narrower than their own airway and ventilate the increased dead space imposed by the ventilator circuit. A patient may not be able to generate adequate tidal volumes for these reasons. To compensate for this increase in the work of breathing, pressure support is given.

Irrespective of mode, whenever a breath is supported by the ventilator, the limit of the support is determined by a pre-set pressure or volume. Thus if volume is set, pressure varies, and conversely, if pressure is set, volume varies according to the patient's lung compliance.

In continuous positive airway pressure (CPAP), PEEP is elevated baseline airway pressure (Fig. 35.10). The two terms 'PEEP' and 'CPAP' are used interchangeably and can lead to confusion. The concept of PEEP is that a pressure is applied at the end of expiration to maintain alveolar recruitment, and can therefore improve oxygenation and ventilation. Airway pressure is kept positive and not allowed to return to atmospheric. PEEP is usually set at between 4 and 10 cm H_2O, which is usually enough to ensure that the patient receives sufficient tidal volume (Pearson, 2002). It can also stent open areas of trachea malacia (abnormal softening) and thereby improve ventilation and oxygenation even if these areas in of themselves do not participate in gas exchange. CPAP differs from PEEP. An advantage of this approach is that CPAP can be delivered non-invasively either by nasal prong or mask (Fig. 35.11). This approach is designed to reduce the work of breathing by actively assisting the inspiratory and expiratory phases of respiration (Davies and McDougall, 2019). CPAP restores FRC and allows for normal respiration with normal pressures.

As ventilator technology has advanced, newer modes have been developed, such as pressure-regulated volume control (PRVC), volume support, inverse ratio (IRV), airway-pressure release ventilation (APRV) and high-frequency oscillatory ventilation (HFOV). Some are variations of volume or pressure modes and some are completely unrelated to conventional mechanical ventilation. The approach to respiratory management and ventilation will be based on the patient's condition and their response to interventions.

Ventilator settings. The initial settings prescribed and set by the intensivist for both volume and pressure are similar. Except in volume control a tidal volume is set at usually 8–10 mL/kg and in pressure control the peak airway pressure is set. The starting peak airways pressure is set at what is needed to adequately inflate the patient's chest and

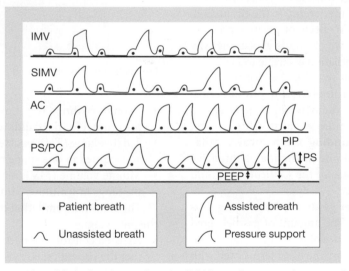

Fig. 35.9 Ventilator modes. *AC*, Assisted control mode; *IMV*, intermittent mandatory ventilation; *PEEP*, positive end expiratory pressure; *PIP*, peak inspiratory pressure; *PS/PC*, pressure support or pressure control mode; *SIMV*, synchronised intermittent mandatory ventilation.

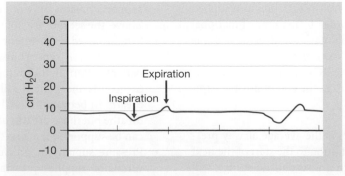

Fig. 35.10 Continuous positive airway pressure (CPAP) – pressure wave.

generate breath sounds and is usually 15–20 cm H_2O above PEEP. The starting breath rate is usually one that would be physiologically appropriate for the age of the patient. Immediately after intubation patients are usually placed on a FiO_2 of 1.0 and are weaned down as long as the oxygen saturations remain acceptable. PEEP is usually set at 5 cm H_2O and then increased as needed to achieve acceptable oxygen saturations with a FiO_2 less than 0.6 (Pearson, 2002) (Fig. 35.12).

Respiratory assessment and monitoring of the ventilated child. Clinical observation of the ventilated child is mandatory. Generally, it is the PIC nurse who observes, assesses, communicates, monitors, analyses and interprets data in

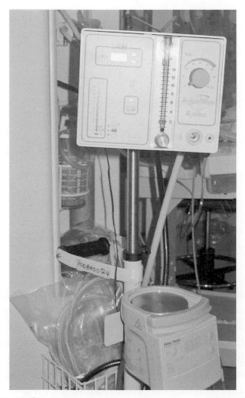

Fig. 35.11 Continuous positive airway pressure (CPAP) driver.

order to effectively care for the critically ill child 24 hours a day (Fig. 35.13). In addition to the usual respiratory and cardiovascular observations discussed in Chapter 4, the critical care team must observe adaptation of the child to the mode of ventilation. This will be based on clinical assessment and interpretation of laboratory results such as arterial blood gases.

👤 ACTIVITY

To ensure patency of the airways, the nurse must ensure that active humidification is set to administer inspired gas at 37°C and 100% relative humidity in the lungs to assist lung clearance of secretions from the endotracheal tube by suctioning using an evidence-based technique. Trauma, infection and cardiopulmonary compromise are well-documented adverse events associated with a poor suction technique:

• Read the review by Davies et al. (2015).

👤 ACTIVITY

Fig. 35.12 presents a simple paradigm to help explain how medical practitioners decide which ventilation parameter to alter based on the results of an arterial blood gas. Use the figure to determine what parameters might be altered by the intensivist in response to the arterial blood gas below taken 4 hours after Daniel was intubated and ventilated:

• pH 7.56, pCO_2 3.2, pO_2 20.0, base deficit –5.
• oxygen saturations were 100%.

Analyse your local PIC observation chart and note the breadth of data that are collected at least hourly.

Consider the similarities and differences to the data you would collect on a child receiving oxygen therapy on a children's medical ward.

This is achieved by: observing the child's work of breathing and spontaneous chest movement against ventilator-induced chest movement; regular 3- to 4-hourly blood gas analysis (as often as quarter-hourly if the child is unstable); constant cardiorespiratory observation; monitoring

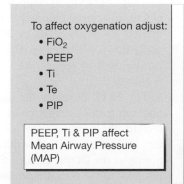

To affect oxygenation adjust:	To affect ventilation adjust:
• FiO_2 • PEEP • Ti • Te • PIP	• Rate • Vt
PEEP, Ti & PIP affect Mean Airway Pressure (MAP)	Alveolar ventilation is determined by the expired minute volume (VT x RR)

Fig. 35.12 Simple paradigm to explain likely ventilation setting changes. *FiO₂*, Fractional concentration of oxygen in inspired gas; *PEEP*, positive end expiratory pressure; *PIP*, peak inspiratory pressure; *RR*, respiratory rate; *Te*, expiratory time; *Ti*, inspiratory time; *TV*, tidal volume.

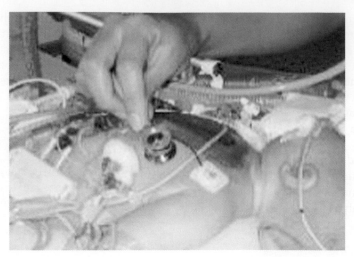

Fig. 35.13 Nursing assessment.

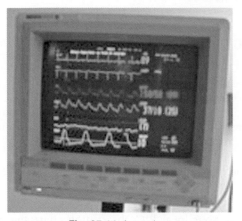

Fig. 35.14 A monitor.

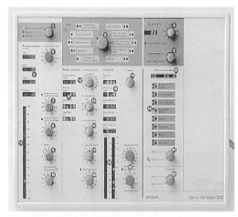

Fig. 35.15 Ventilator board.

and hourly recordings together with ventilator observations. 'Monitoring' is a term usually reserved for automatic visual display of patient data such as temperature, pulse, respiration and blood pressure (Fig. 35.14). A continuous monitoring system, with safety alarm limits set, providing a minute-by-minute accurate picture of the child, means that effective decision making is carried out in 'real time' and at the 'right time'. In the critical care environment, the capabilities and complexity of modern technology are used to their best advantage. Deciding what needs to be monitored is complex but fundamentally essential in the care of the critically ill patient.

In addition to the respiratory monitoring techniques covered in Chapter 4, the nurse observing the ventilated child will monitor end tidal carbon dioxide (ETCO$_2$) and record ventilation parameters, which are analysed in the light of the child's vital signs, pulse oximetry and arterial blood gas results in collaboration with the medical team (Fig. 35.15).

Capnography is the measurement of carbon dioxide (CO$_2$) in each breath of the respiratory cycle. The capnograph displays a waveform of CO$_2$ (measured in kPa or mmHg) and it displays the value of the CO$_2$ at the end of exhalation, which is known as the end tidal CO$_2$ (Fig. 35.16). The capnograph sensor is placed between the endotracheal tube and the breathing circuit.

ETCO$_2$ provides a non-invasive method of evaluating ventilation and is helpful in assessing placement of the endotracheal tube. CO$_2$ is exhaled through the trachea and not usually from the oesophagus and so the measurement of CO$_2$ in the expired air distinguishes tracheal from oesophageal intubation. Provided the patient has a stable cardiac status and stable body temperature, an ETCO$_2$ with a normal capnograph trace approximates to the partial pressure of CO$_2$ in arterial blood (PaCO$_2$) (normal PaCO$_2$ is approximately 4.6–6 kPa) (Dixon, 2012). The arterial PCO$_2$ is normally 0.3–0.7 kPa higher than the ETCO$_2$ reading and thus can be used to reduce the frequency of blood gas analysis required.

Fig. 35.17 illustrates the different components of the capnograph trace. The first phase occurs during inspiration. The second phase is the onset of expiration, which results in a rapid increase in CO$_2$. The third phase, the expiratory plateau, occurs as the CO$_2$ is exhaled from all the alveoli. The highest point (4) of the plateau is known as the ETCO$_2$ and marks the end of expiration. Phase four is the onset of inspiration. If the

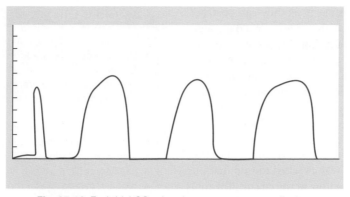

Fig. 35.16 End tidal CO_2 showing on a caprogram display.

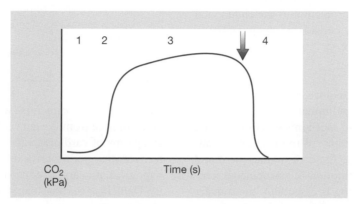

Fig. 35.17 The capnograph trace.

waveform does not return to the baseline during inspiration this indicates that re-breathing of exhaled gas is occurring and is accompanied by a rise in $ETCO_2$ reading. Sudden loss of the capnograph, that is a decrease to zero, should alert the clinician to a catastrophic event such as oesophageal intubation, total obstruction, or ventilator malfunction. An exponential decrease of $ETCO_2$ can be seen due to loss of pulmonary blood flow as in cardiac arrest or sudden hypotension for example. A gradual decrease in $ETCO_2$ indicates decreased production such as in hypothermia. Rising $ETCO_2$ can be seen either due to increased CO_2 production, such as in sepsis, malignant hyperthermia, or due to decreased CO_2 elimination when there is decreased alveolar ventilation (Bhende, 2001).

SCENARIO

One hour after intubation, the nurse noted that Daniel's heart rate was 145, blood pressure 130/92 mmHg, respiratory rate 30 breaths/min and oxygen saturation 100%. Ominously, the $ETCO_2$ that had been reading 5.6 kPa had increased to 9.7 kPa.

PROFESSIONAL CONVERSATION

Michael, a registered children's nurse new to PIC, summons his mentor for help and records this learning episode in his reflective diary.

Trouble-Shooting

If after intubation or at any time during ventilation therapy a child's condition deteriorates, the pneumonic 'DOPE' is a useful tool to help make a systematic patient assessment and perform appropriate interventions when waiting for the arrival of the intensivist who had been asked to attend Daniel. Is the deterioration as a result of:

- D = displaced tube?
- O = obstructed tube?
- P = pneumothorax?
- E = equipment?

Assess A: the airway first – is the tube still in? Is it in the right position? The endotracheal tube was still at 13 cm at the lips. Had the endotracheal tube not been in place it would have been removed and bag-valve-mask ventilation instituted.

Assess B: breathing next – is the chest rising? Had the chest not been seen to rise with ventilation, Daniel would have been disconnected from the ventilator and bag valve inflations given to eliminate the ventilator circuit as the problem. 'Bagging' by hand can also allow the facilitator to gauge compliance.

Are breath sounds present and equal? Changes in breath sounds? Endotracheal tubes can become obstructed with secretions or be dislodged especially if the patient moves (or is moved). Need for endotracheal tube suction? Mucous plugs can block lower airways as easily as they can obstruct the endotracheal tube. A suction catheter was placed through the endotracheal tube to be certain that it was patent and to rule out obstruction by mucous plug. It was patent and suction did not return any abnormal secretions. The chest rise appeared to be symmetrical bilaterally and breath sounds were unchanged on auscultation. We noted the increasing blood pressure and administered sedation. Despite these actions the problem persisted.

The entire ventilatory circuit from the level of the endotracheal tube back to the ventilator was checked to find that the tubing was kinked thus restricting flow in the circuit. The tubing was repositioned to relieve the obstruction and Daniel's $ETCO_2$ started to decrease immediately back to its previous level. If this had not revealed a problem and the child's vital signs were stable, we would have considered the potential of malfunction of the $ETCO_2$ device.

Extubation

As discussed earlier, children require respiratory support for many pulmonary and non-pulmonary problems. In the majority of cases, intubation and mechanical ventilation are necessary until the underlying cause of the respiratory failure is improved or resolved. The focus of management and care is thus facilitating the resumption of spontaneous ventilation that is 'weaning'. Weaning is essentially the transfer of demands from the ventilator to the child. It is important to assess the individual child's ability to handle the increased demands that extubation will place upon the child. In practice the critical care team is always weaning the child by progressively reducing ventilator support settings as the child's condition improves, thus minimising the adverse effects of ventilation. Progressive reduction of rate, FiO_2 and PEEP demands that the child does more, and is guided by arterial blood gas results. A child is usually ready to be extubated when they are:

- cardiovascularly stable;
- able to protect own airway;
- FiO_2 0.40 or less with appropriate oxygen saturations for the child's condition;
- PEEP 5 cm H_2O or less;
- breathing at a comfortable physiological rate;
- good cough and gag reflex;
- sedation discontinued or minimal;
- tolerates pressure support/CPAP ventilator modes as these compensate for the added work of breathing via a ventilator circuit and endotracheal tube (Pearson, 2002; Dixon, 2012; Hazinski, 2013).

As with any clinical procedure it is important to discuss weaning and extubation with the family and make clear that there is a possibility that the child may experience respiratory fatigue and need to return to some form of airway support, whether that be CPAP or ventilation.

Haemodynamic Control

In this scenario, Daniel is admitted to PICU and a rapid cardiopulmonary assessment was undertaken by the

> ### 👤 SCENARIO
>
> On admission to PICU, additional vital signs were obtained:
> - Daniel was awake and irritable and wanting to remain in Emma's lap
> - respiratory rate: 70 breaths/min
> - marked sternal and intercostals recession
> - oxygen saturation: 95%
> - heart rate: 200 beats/min
> - radial and dorsalis pulses: weak and thready
> - skin was cool, dry and pale
> - capillary refill: 4 s
> - blood pressure: 90/60 mmHg
> - he was conscious and responding to his mother Emma
> - he appeared exhausted
> - blood glucose: 1.7 mmol/L
> - axilla temperature: 37.5°C
> - no skin rash noted
> - an arterial gas was obtained: pH 7.25, pCO_2 7.6, pO_2 22, base deficit −3

admitting critical care nurse which was documented as above. You will note from the data collected that there are signs and symptoms of cardiovascular instability for example marked tachycardia, poor perfusion (capillary refill >2 seconds), hypoglycaemia and a reduced level of consciousness. In reality, Daniel's cardiovascular status would have been managed almost simultaneously with his respiratory failure by the critical care team, following a systematic ABCDE approach. However, for the purposes of this chapter, respiratory support and haemodynamic control have been artificially separated for ease of presentation and to facilitate learning in a step-by-step approach.

Haemodynamic Principles

The management of the critically ill child is based on knowledge of fundamental physiological variables. Through technological advancements, monitoring of the haemodynamic status has developed from non-invasive monitoring of a single parameter to more invasive monitoring of multiple parameters that we see in today's clinical practice. This allows a comprehensive analysis of haemodynamic status, enabling health care practitioners to not only provide effective treatment but importantly to anticipate deleterious events and intervene proactively in advance.

Haemodynamics refers to the forces, such as preload and afterload, that affect the circulation of blood throughout the body. Critical care nurses assess the stability of these factors when they take a blood pressure or palpate a pulse. Although the interaction of these forces is quite complicated, the concepts can be more easily understood by substituting the word 'stretch' for preload and 'resistance' for afterload. Preload and afterload are closely related. Put simply, they reflect the heart's effectiveness in managing blood flow out of its chambers, that is, cardiac output. This chapter will now turn to a more detailed explanation and discussion of the determinants of cardiac output introduced earlier.

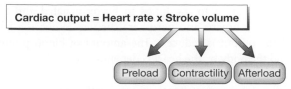

Fig. 35.18 Determinants of cardiac output.

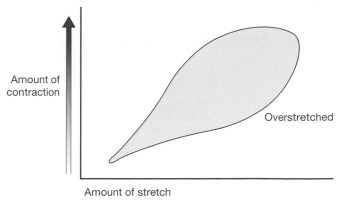

Fig. 35.19 The Frank–Starling mechanism.

Cardiac Output

Cardiac output (Fig. 35.18) is defined as the volume of blood pumped by the heart in 1 minute, and is represented by the equation:

Cardiac output (CO) = Stroke volume (SV) × Heart rate (HR).

Stroke volume (SV) is the amount of blood pumped by the heart in one contraction. Thus an increase in SV or HR causes an increase in cardiac output and conversely a decrease in SV or HR results in a decrease in cardiac output. An adequate cardiac output is essential to supply oxygen and nutrients to major organs and peripheral tissues. It is important to remember at this point, that in order for tissues and organs to perform their function, the cellular structure of each needs to be oxygenated, provided with nutrients and have metabolic by-products removed. This process is reliant on a stable haemodynamic state. For example, a reduction in cardiac output may diminish blood flow to the brain and result in an altered level of consciousness. An alteration in heart rate, contractility, preload and afterload can affect cardiac output and therefore tissue and organ function can be affected.

What is contractility? Contractility of the heart is its ability to shorten the cardiac muscle fibres and generate an ejection force during each contraction. The contractility of the heart can be influenced by what is known as the preload. Preload is the force that stretches the contractile muscle fibres, the myofibrils, of the resting heart. This 'stretch' is determined by the amount of blood present within the left ventricle prior to contraction. The greater the volume of blood in the left ventricle, the greater the stretch on the myofibrils the greater the contractile force and, therefore, the greater the preload. An adequately filled and stretched left ventricle should briskly contract to eject blood. However, there is a point where the stretch (fill) is insufficient and cardiac output is diminished. Likewise, there is a point where the stretch (fill) is too extreme that output is diminished. This relationship between preload (stretch) and contractile force is explained by the Frank-Starling mechanism (Fig. 35.19).

Starling's mechanism states that, up to a point, the more the myofibrils are stretched in diastole, the more forcefully the heart contracts in the next systole. A simple analogy is an elastic band. If we apply a moderate stretch to the elastic band it will 'ping' back with moderate force. Likewise, if we apply a strong stretch to the elastic band it will 'ping' back with greater force. However, if we repeatedly provide too great a force to the elastic band it will very quickly lose its elasticity and fail to do its task. It is much the same with the myofibrils in the heart: if over-burdened, they will eventually fail; this is represented in Fig. 35.19. It must be remembered, however, that children, particularly under the age of 8 years, have insufficient myocardial contractile proteins to significantly increase contractility and are therefore largely dependent on an increase in heart rate to maintain cardiac output.

Stroke volume is affected by preload, contractile force and afterload. As discussed, preload is the amount of blood delivered to the heart during diastole but this is in turn dependent on venous return. Venous return can be affected by variable venous capacitance known as afterload, which can increase or decrease blood return to the heart (preload).

Understanding Afterload

Afterload is the resistance against which the heart must pump. When the heart overcomes resistance, the blood can be ejected. Sources of resistance include blood pressure (BP), systemic vascular resistance (SVR), and the condition of the aortic valve. When there is arterial vasoconstriction, as in shock or aortic valve narrowing as in aortic stenosis, the ventricle has to create a greater amount of pressure to overcome that resistance – a useful analogy is that it is akin to opening a door against a strong wind.

What Is Shock?

As previously stated, the body's cells require a constant supply of oxygen and nutrients and elimination of carbon dioxide and waste products. These needs are fulfilled by the circulatory system in conjunction with the respiratory system, central nervous system and gastrointestinal system. The ultimate goal of this integrated control of the circulation is to maintain blood flow to the tissues to the optimum extent; this is known as tissue perfusion. Normally the body can compensate for some reduction in tissue perfusion through a variety of compensatory mechanisms. However, when compensation fails, shock develops. Shock has been defined as '... acute, life-threatening syndrome of circulatory dysfunction resulting in inadequate delivery of oxygen and other nutrients to meet metabolic demand' (ALSG, 2016, p 67). It is characterised by a loss of normal cellular function caused by anaerobic cell metabolism and acidosis leading to a loss of normal cell function and cell death. This will progress to organ dysfunction if it is not recognised and appropriately treated, and ultimately death of the child will follow (Fig. 35.20).

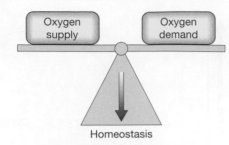

Fig. 35.20 Homeostasis.

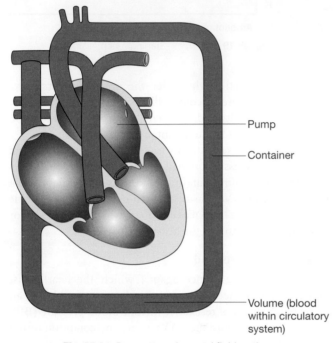

Fig. 35.21 Pump, container and fluid analogy.

Metabolism in normal conditions is aerobic (respiration with oxygen). In contrast, metabolism in poorly perfused tissues is anaerobic (respiration without oxygen). In aerobic respiration, glucose metabolism in the presence of oxygen is broken down into carbon dioxide, water and energy. If there is insufficient oxygen available to the cell then glucose metabolism without oxygen produces lactic acid and this accumulates along with other metabolic acids (Marieb, 2016). Over time, this build-up of the acidic metabolites creates an environment that is not conducive to normal cell function.

Using a well-known analogy (ALSG, 2016) (Fig. 35.21), the causes of shock involve one or more of the following dysfunctions of the body's:

- pump (cardiogenic)
- fluid volume (hypovolaemic)
- vessels (distributive)
- resistance to flow (obstructive)
- capacity for blood to release oxygen (dissociative)

Inadequate tissue perfusion can result in derangement of any of these components. The heart is the pump of the circulatory system. Put simply, it receives blood from the venous system, pumps it to the lungs to be oxygenated and then pumps it to organs and peripheral tissues. When the heart 'fails' the output is reduced. The amount of blood pumped around the body by the heart is dependent on:

- heart rate
- ability to empty the heart, which depends on:
  - contractility
  - resistance to flow and blood pressure
- ability to fill the heart, which depends on:
  - amount of blood returning for re-circulation
  - filling pressures versus compliance

Blood is the fluid of the cardiovascular system. Blood is a viscous fluid that is thicker, more adhesive and slower moving than water. As the cardiovascular system is essentially a closed system, an adequate volume of blood must be present to fill the system. Blood transports oxygen, carbon dioxide, nutrients, hormones, metabolic waste products and heat.

The blood vessels which include arteries, arterioles, capillaries, venules and veins serve as the container for the cardiovascular system. This container provides a continuous, closed, pressurised pipeline that moves blood under the control of the autonomic nervous system, which delivers haemoglobin saturated with oxygen to diffuse into cells at end organs. The vessels regulate blood flow to different areas of the body by adjusting their size and re-routing blood through the microcirculation. Contraction of venous circulation increases preload and stroke volume, but contraction of arterioles increases afterload and blood pressure. The microcirculation is responsive to local tissue needs. Capillary beds can adjust size by opening and closing pre- and post-capillary sphincters to supply undernourished tissue or bypass tissue with no immediate needs. Therefore blood flow is dependent on peripheral resistance, which in turn is dependent on internal diameter, length of the vessel and blood viscosity.

Signs of poor tissue perfusion include: temperature instability between core and peripheral temperatures; reduced capillary refill time and a capillary refill gap between central and peripheral perfusion; and a reduction of urine production. Tissue perfusion is dependent on the circulatory system, consisting of pump, container and fluid. But equally as important are conditions for optimal uptake, effective oxygenation and utilisation of oxygen in the body (Hazinski, 2013). The conditions are:

- adequate concentration of oxygen – ideally 97%–100% of haemoglobin is saturated with oxygen;
- oxygen diffuses across the alveolar–capillary membrane;
- adequate number of haemoglobin molecules attached to red blood cells to enable transport of oxygen;
- adequate and efficient off-loading of oxygen at the tissue–cellular level.

These conditions are often referred to as the 'Fick principle' where the efficiency of cell oxygenation is maximised by all these elements working in synergy to achieve homeostasis.

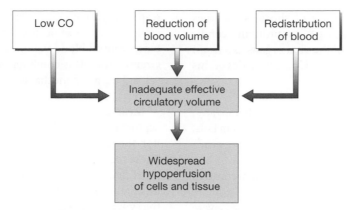

Fig. 35.22 Common pathway. *CO,* Cardiac output.

In summary, it can be seen that shock is a cellular state of imbalance resulting in inadequate tissue perfusion, and can be caused by either one or a combination of the following components (Fig. 35.22):

- An inadequate pump:
  - inadequate preload
  - inadequate contractile strength
  - inadequate heart rate
- An inadequate fluid volume:
  - insufficient fluid volume
- An inadequate container:
  - excessive dilation without increase in fluid volume
  - excessive SVR

Stages of Shock

Shock is progressive in nature and follows three recognised stages (ALSG, 2016). These are commonly identified as:

- compensated shock
- uncompensated shock
- irreversible shock

Compensated shock. In the initial stage, cardiac output and perfusion are decreased and the body uses compensatory mechanisms to perfuse and preserve major organs by way of a series of reflex mechanisms involving the central nervous system and neurohormonal systems. Increased production of angiotensin and vasopressin allow reflex compensatory mechanisms to occur in the micro-circulation and macro-circulation in the kidney. This enables the kidney to increase reabsorption of water and salt resulting in reduced urine output. For this reason, this stage is often referred to as 'compensated' shock. In compensated shock, systolic blood pressure will likely be within normal parameters, while the diastolic blood pressure may be raised. These subtle indicators make shock difficult to detect at this stage, especially in children who usually have healthy organs, and therefore efficient compensators.

Uncompensated shock. If left untreated, the compensatory mechanisms will become overwhelmed and shock will progress to 'uncompensated shock'. The reduced cardiac output results in the ineffective shunting of blood to vital tissues resulting in severe hypoperfusion. Poor perfusion of tissues results in anaerobic metabolism in the cells, a by-product of which is lactate. This combined with an increase in carbonic acid, due to the poor removal of carbon dioxide of the cells, results in acidosis. This in itself reduces the ability of cardiac fibres to contract and is compounded by a loss of autoregulation of the microcirculation and increased capillary permeability. These effects cause a reduced blood volume to the right side the heart. Reduced blood flow and reduced contractility are the two primary causes of reduced cardiac output in uncompensated shock. This in turn reduces blood pressure, which reduces coronary artery perfusion. Myocardial oxygen demand then exceeds myocardial oxygen supply. Imbalance of arterial blood supply to the myocardium causes arrhythmias, muscle ischaemia and a self-perpetuating cycle of reduced cardiac output and cardiac failure occurs.

In addition, prolonged depletion of cardiac output results in:

- reduction in cerebral blood flow;
- renal tubules to become ischaemic;
- prolonged vasoconstriction causes ulceration of the stomach wall allowing bacteria and toxins to cross into the bloodstream;
- bilirubin is not metabolised by the underperfused liver and waste products build up;
- cell death causes release of enzymes from the pancreas, which depress the myocardium;
- ischaemia of alveolar cells inhibits surfactant production in the lungs causing alveolar collapse, atelectasis, and reduced pulmonary compliance leads to acute respiratory distress syndrome (ARDS);
- increased pulmonary vascular permeability causes interstitial and intra-alveolar oedema.

In this stage of shock, due to the loss of homeostasis in the circulatory system, platelet adhesion can occur, triggering the coagulation systems to trigger and thus result in disseminated intravascular coagulation (DIC). With swift treatment and critical nursing care, this stage of shock has potential to be reversed.

Irreversible shock. The final stage of shock, sometimes also referred to as the 'refractory stage', is a profound condition where there is major failure of the vital organs as a result of being starved of oxygen for too long. Characteristics of this would be:

- hypotension is unresponsive to drugs and fluids;
- severe hypoxaemia is unresponsive to oxygen therapy;
- anuria and build-up of toxic waste as the renal system fails;
- liver causes hyperglycaemia and build-up of waste products and allows no metabolism of drugs;
- pancreatic dysfunction further affects myocardial contractility, haematologically;
- multiple emboli form, intravascular clotting and severe coagulopathy;
- neurologically, there is reduced response to stimuli and sympathetic stress response due to failure of the medulla causing circulatory failure and death eventually occurs.

Early Recognition of Shock

Shock is a common cause of morbidity and mortality in children and therefore early recognition is essential. The outcome for children once shock has progressed to being uncompensated is, in general, very poor (Hazinski, 2013). Early recognition of the child in compensated shock and prompt and appropriate intervention as a result has been shown to reduce mortality and secondary morbidity. As outlined in compensated shock, the early indicators of shock are subtle and difficult to detect. To recognise the initial body response to a loss of cardiac output, the nurse must be fully cognisant of the compensatory mechanisms used by the cardiovascular system. In addition, a thorough knowledge and understanding of the pathophysiology of different types of shock together with a high index of suspicion facilitates recognition of these subtle signs and symptoms. It is to a physiological description of the compensatory mechanisms of shock that this chapter now turns.

Shock: Compensatory Mechanisms

Young children are able to maintain a normal cardiac output and thus remain normotensive until vascular and cardiac de-compensation is imminent (Crain and Gershal, 2012). It is therefore essential that the nurse can recognise the initial signs of shock; a high index of suspicion can help to raise your awareness of the subtleties of compensation. Ask yourself if the child is at risk:

- Does the child have mild increases in heart rate, blood pressure, respiratory rate, capillary refill time and irritability?
- Does the child have a history of diarrhoea, vomiting and decreased oral intake?
- Has he or she had surgery recently?
- Has he or she got allergic symptoms and recent exposure to a known allergen?
- Has he or she got a congenital heart defect?

The cardiovascular system is regulated by many feedback control loops; as the body detects a reduction in blood pressure, there are a number of physiological reflex and hormone responses that attempt to restore normal blood pressure. This compensated raise occurs through increasing vascular resistance, central blood volume and cardiac output (Waugh and Grant, 2014). This combination of neural, hormonal, chemical and humoral mechanisms maintains tissue perfusion and protects cells.

Mean arterial blood pressure (MAP) is sensed by baroreceptors located in the aortic and carotid bodies which monitor the circulation closely for changes in blood pressure. These receptors control arterial pressure mainly by adjusting heart rate and arteriolar vessel radius. Baroreceptors respond to small changes in vascular tone and pressure and message the sympathetic nervous system (SNS) to decrease vagal tone which increases heart rate and decreases coronary artery resistance thus improving myocardial oxygen supply (Fig. 35.23). MAP is also the basis for autoregulation by the heart, lungs and brain.

Arterioles are the primary sites that contribute to systemic vascular resistance (SVR). If the oxygen and nutrient requirements of the tissues are greater than can be supplied, autoregulation of the tissue help regulate and enrich the blood flow. Autoregulation of the brain, heart and kidneys efficiently ensures maintenance of perfusion when the MAP is mildly diminished. This automatic adaptation of the radius of an arteriolar vessel in an organ to maintain constant blood when the mean pressures are fluctuating protects functioning of that organ (Marieb, 2016). In addition, in the microcirculation, adrenergic control of the arterioles is a major determinant of blood flow into the capillaries. In response, the adrenal gland will increase catecholamine release. Catecholamines consist of adrenaline and noradrenaline which are endogenous vasoconstrictors that cause added vasoconstriction in an added attempt to improve cardiac output (Martini et al., 2018). Catecholamines also enhance cardiac contractility and heart rate. Constriction of blood reservoirs such as the skin, skeletal muscle, liver and spleen disgorge blood to be shunted from the capillary beds to flow directly from arterioles into the venous system, thus increasing circulating blood volume (Figs 35.24 and 35.25). This arteriovenous shunting helps to redirect blood flow to vital organs. Arteriovenous shunting is one reason a child's blood pressure alone is not a sole indicator of peripheral tissue perfusion, and further assessment of peripheral temperature and capillary refill time is required.

Renin production is increased as a result of decreased renal perfusion, which leads to angiotensinogen production, eventually yielding angiotensin which is a potent vasoconstrictor. Antidiuretic hormone (ADH) is released from the posterior pituitary gland, and is another potent vasoconstrictor which prevents the elimination of water. The continued failure of the kidneys to eliminate and excrete hydrogen ions causes a metabolic acidosis and consequent decrease in blood pH, which in turn further impairs myocardial function and cardiac output. Aldosterone is released, stimulated by ADH, causing sodium reabsorption in the renal distal tubules; as water follows sodium, this helps to conserve both sodium and water. Retained sodium assists in the reabsorption of tissue

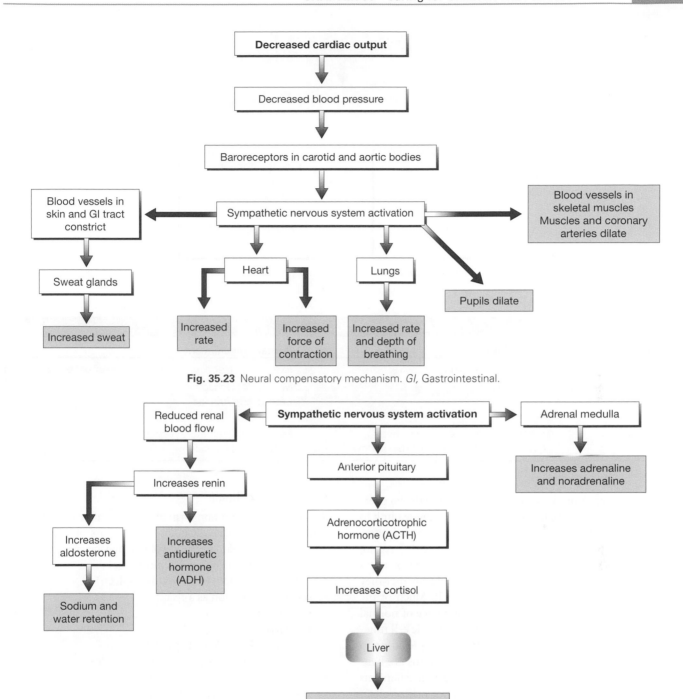

Fig. 35.23 Neural compensatory mechanism. *GI*, Gastrointestinal.

Fig. 35.24 Hormonal compensatory mechanism.

fluids (see Fig. 35.24). Decreased mean arterial pressure leads to arteriolar constriction, which together with decreased pressure in capillaries leads to decreased hydrostatic pressure that, due to reabsorbed sodium, is less than osmotic pressure; this assists an increased reabsorption of fluid from the tissues (Rhoades and Bell, 2009).

Chemoreceptors located locally in tissue beds sense the hypoxia due to the now-inadequate blood flow to the tissues as a result of systemic circulation constriction, and cause further vasoconstriction (Marieb, 2007). The cells become starved of oxygen. Tissue begins to metabolise anaerobically and the patient becomes acidotic. Respiratory

function during shock is very important in compensation. In response the body begins to hyperventilate in order to blow off excess carbon dioxide, resulting in respiratory alkalosis (see Fig. 35.25). This hyperventilation will also help to improve venous return (pump model). In summary, the mechanisms for restoring cardiovascular homeostasis are:

- redistribution of blood flow: attempt to preserve perfusion to vital organs
- augmentation of cardiac output:
  - increased heart rate
  - increased peripheral resistance
- restoration of intravascular volume: arteriovenous shunting

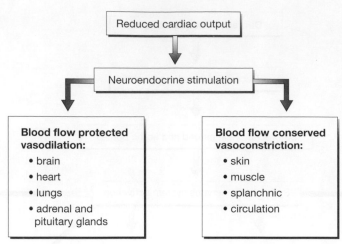

Fig. 35.25 Chemical compensatory mechanism.

TABLE 35.2	**Classification and Causes of Shock**	
Classification	**Clinical Causes**	**Primary Mechanism**
Hypovolaemic	Circulating fluid volume loss	Exogenous blood, plasma, fluid or electrolyte loss
Cardiogenic	Pump failure	Myocardial ischaemia Cardiac arrhythmias Cardiac failure
Distributive	Increased venous capacitance and extra-cardiac obstruction of blood flow	Massive inflammatory response, e.g. septic and anaphylactic shock

These compensatory mechanisms will eventually be overwhelmed and begin to fail, and circulatory failure leading to multi-organ failure will ensue if not recognised and if intervention is not aggressively initiated (Urden et al., 2016). Again, blood pressure is not the key to deciding whether or not a child is in shock, although it does help to decide whether they are in compensated or uncompensated shock. Much of the body's response revolves around the maintenance of normal aerobic metabolism and thus maintenance of viable cell function and measurement of the degree of tissue oxygenation in vital organs. The body's compensatory mechanisms are beneficial in the early stages but these homeostatic mechanisms soon become counterproductive. Nurses play a major role in recognising shock and play a direct role in influencing timely and appropriate intervention in conjunction with medical colleagues.

Types of Shock

Any reduction of blood volume by whatever means (pump, container, fluid) can cause shock. Shock is classified according to the causes to three classes (Table 35.2):
- Hypovolaemic
- Cardiogenic
- Distributive

It is important to be aware that more than one type of shock may be present at the same time.

Hypovolaemic Shock

This is the most common form of shock in infants and children (Fuhrman et al., 2017). It is caused by a loss of intravascular volume. The decrease in blood volume may be caused by:
- external blood loss (e.g. haemorrhage)
- internal blood loss (e.g. ruptured spleen)
- severe dehydration as a result of:
  - vomiting
  - diarrhoea
- excessive plasma loss (e.g. burn)
- excessive diuresis (e.g. diabetic ketoacidosis)
- third space loss (e.g. peritonitis)

A child's body can tolerate a loss of 20%–25% circulating volume prior to a drop in blood pressure and cardiac output. In hypovolaemic shock the body attempts to maintain circulation despite the deficit.

👤 ACTIVITY

Hypovolaemic shock is a volume problem:
- What signs and symptoms would you expect to see in a child in hypovolaemic shock?

Cardiogenic Shock

Cardiogenic shock occurs in acute heart disease and is caused by an inability of the heart to pump sufficient blood. Inadequate function of the heart may be caused by heart failure that is weak cardiac contraction, from any cause. Cardiac output falls despite normal or elevated blood volume and cardiac pressures.

Causes include:
- myocardial ischaemia
- arrhythmia
- congenital heart disease
- cardiomyopathy due to drug toxicity

 ACTIVITY

Cardiogenic shock is a pump problem:
- What signs and symptoms would you expect to see in an affected child?

Distributive Shock

Distributive shock is a container problem caused by abnormal and excessive vasodilatation. This leads to misdistribution of fluid from the circulatory system to the tissues causing loss of afterload and SVR. Examples are:
- neurogenic shock (rare)
- anaphylactic shock from an allergen, e.g. bee sting, peanuts and medications
- septic shock

Neurogenic Shock

Neurogenic shock occurs due to widespread and massive vasodilation due to imbalance of the parasympathetic (overstimulation) and sympathetic (understimulation) stimulation of vascular smooth muscle. Interruption of the sympathetic nervous system, which normally maintains muscle tone, results in persistent vasodilation. This overwhelming vasodilation results in pooling of the blood in the peripheries resulting in poor perfusion of the heart, brain and kidneys. It presents classically with hypotension, without tachycardia or vasoconstriction. Therefore the child will have warm, dry skin and a slow heart rate. Whilst this type of shock is rare in children, it can be caused by trauma resulting in spinal cord injury above T6 (Cameron, 2018).

Anaphylactic Shock

Anaphylactic shock is the widespread immune and inflammatory response with rapid respiratory and circulatory effects (ALSG, 2016). The pathological response is similar to that of neurogenic shock, that is: vasodilation, increased vascular permeability causing peripheral oedema causing relative hypovolaemia and smooth muscle constriction leading to bronchoconstriction and dyspnoea. Individuals present with an almost immediate response to the inciting antigen with any combination of the following: cutaneous manifestations such as urticaria, erythema, pruritis, angioedema; respiratory compromise with stridor, wheezing, bronchorrhoea, respiratory distress; and varying degrees of circulatory collapse with tachycardia, vasodilation, hypotension.

Septic Shock

Septic shock is classified as a distributive shock. However, it is a combination of problems with the pump, container and fluid and is characterised by a:
- loss of preload
- loss of afterload/SVR
- loss of contractility

Septic shock is the most common cause of death in PICU, with mortality rates shown in studies as high as 73% if fluid resuscitation of 20 ml/kg is not initiated in the first hour of treatment (Davies, 2019). A well-known cause of septic shock is meningococcal septicaemia; studies show a fatality rate of 49% if the patient is diagnosed with sepsis when they first receive medical help (Seymour and Wiersinga, 2018). A purpuric rash known as purpura fulminans is usually seen in meningococcal disease and constitutes a medical emergency.

 ACTIVITY

Use this link to this British Medical Association website and study the photographs of the non-blanching purpuric rash usually seen in meningococcal septicaemia:
- https://www.meningitis.org/meningitis/check-symptoms

The term sepsis is used to identify a clinical syndrome that occurs when a person reacts adversely to an infection. Whereby an uncontrolled body system response rapidly escalates to severe sepsis and septic shock, with the patient developing organ dysfunction as a result (Wiersinga and Seymour, 2018). Although bacterial infection is the most common cause, fungal, viral and protozoa infections may also cause septic shock (Long et al., 2018).

Whatever the initial cause of the infection, patients with sepsis and its accompanying systemic inflammatory response syndrome (SIRS) have overwhelming inflammation followed by a common pathway consisting of a systematic inflammatory cascade activated by inflammatory mediators and toxins (Gormley-Fleming and Peate, 2018). These mediators stimulate the release of cytokines, which act to amplify the inflammatory response and lead to systemic endothelial damage. Exposure of tissue and presence of cytokines stimulate the coagulation cascade. Coagulopathy leads to intravascular thrombus formation. In addition, diffuse endothelial injury leads to vasodilation and increased capillary permeability resulting in leakage of plasma in to the interstitial spaces (Porth, 2011). Therefore there is progressive vasodilation and maldistribution of blood flow, which ultimately causes organ hypoperfusion. A substance known as myocardial depressant factor (MDF) is secreted by the pancreas in response to hypoperfusion and ischaemia. MDF decreases myocardial contractility and results in ventricular dilatation, thus further compromising cardiac output (Cameron, 2018). To further complicate matters, in response to the pro-inflammatory

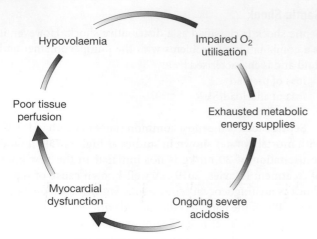

Hypovolaemia

Impaired O₂ utilisation

Poor tissue perfusion

Exhausted metabolic energy supplies

Myocardial dysfunction

Ongoing severe acidosis

Fig. 35.26 Pathophysiological cycle.

mediators, excessive anti-inflammatory mediators are also released which then cause immunosuppression.

The clinical features of septic shock depend on where the child is in the inflammatory response continuum. In the early phase of septic shock, cardiac output is well maintained or even increased. The vasodilation may result in warm skin, warm extremities and normal capillary refill; this is known as warm shock (Kalil, 2018). In this situation a child is normotensive but may have a widened pulse pressure as vasodilation decreases diastolic blood pressure (DBP) and increased cardiac output raises systolic blood pressure (SBP). A progression from warm to cold shock occurs as hypovolaemia and ventricular dysfunction occur.

This progression can be rapid in small children because of their limited ability to maintain the increased cardiac output (Gormley-Fleming and Peate, 2018). In response to a fall in cardiac output, catecholamines are released causing vasoconstriction. Increasing vasoconstriction compromises oxygen delivery and leads to anaerobic metabolism and lactic acid production. Acidosis in the capillary beds causes the arterioles to dilate and the venules to constrict causing pooling and stasis of blood. Hypotension develops as intravascular volume is further depleted from ongoing capillary leak, and progressive myocardial depression occurs (Fig. 35.26). If the cycle of depleted intravascular volume, poor tissue perfusion, impaired oxygen utilisation, exhausted metabolic energy supplies and myocardial dysfunction is not broken, the child will progress to vascular collapse, irreversible multiple system organ failure and death (Gormley-Fleming and Peate, 2018).

Haemodynamic Monitoring

Haemodynamics refers to the functional state of the heart and circulatory system as it relates to the perfusion of the body's tissues with oxygenated blood. A person's haemodynamic state can be measured invasively or non-invasively and can be used to support diagnosis, monitor response to interventions and titrate therapy. Haemodynamic instability occurs when there is inadequate perfusion to support normal organ function (Fuhrman et al., 2017). It is important, therefore, to monitor the physiological responses of patients, as this not only allows the assessment of physiological reserve but will also give a baseline against which the effectiveness of any applied treatment can be judged. Knowledge of the principles of haemodynamic monitoring and correct interpretation of data is important as a failure to do so can result in significant morbidity, or indeed, mortality of the patient. In the critically ill and haemodynamically unstable patient, tissue oxygenation is determined by measuring components of cardiac output such as heart rate, arterial blood pressure, central venous pressure, arterial oxygenation and haemoglobin. In complex situations such as septic shock, pulmonary artery pressure monitoring may also be used. We will now introduce the concepts of arterial blood pressure and central venous pressure monitoring.

? ACTIVITY

Septic shock is a pump, container and fluid problem:
- What signs and symptoms would you expect to see in a child in 'cold' shock?

Arterial blood pressure (ABP) is measured by a catheter commonly placed in the radial, brachial or tibial artery and which is kept patent using a continuous infusion of intravenous heparin saline, 1 unit per mL at between 0.5 and 2 mL/h depending on the size of the child. Arterial pressure is measured at its peak, which is the SBP, and at its trough, which is the DBP. The SBP is determined by the stroke volume, contractility, systemic arterial resistance and preload. The SBP is a clinical indicator of afterload. The DBP is affected by systemic arterial resistance and heart rate. Systemic mean arterial pressure (MAP) is defined as the mean perfusion pressure throughout the cycle:

Mean arterial pressure (MAP) = Systemic vascular resistance (SVR) × Cardiac output (CO)

Pulse pressure is the difference between systolic and diastolic pressure and is normally about 40 mmHg. An increased pulse pressure may be the result of increased SV or contractility and is common during fever and anaemia. An acute decrease in pulse pressure may indicate an increase in SVR, decreased SV or decreased intravascular volume (Klabunde, 2012). In summary, because of the multiplicity of factors that contribute to ABP, interpreting changes in arterial pressure and its components (SBP, DBP, MAP and pulse pressure) as indicative of any single factor may lead to an erroneous assessment of a patient's condition. Furthermore, however, numerically satisfactory ABP or MAP values are not necessarily related to adequate perfusion and organ system function. For optimal management of critically ill patients, ABP data must be integrated with information gained from clinical assessment of patient's status. This is particularly important in the management of the critically ill child. In children, blood pressure is not a reliable indicator of a failing cardiovascular system as they have effective compensatory mechanisms. Therefore once these have failed and the blood pressure begins to drop, this is a late sign of shock (Coyne et al., 2010).

Central venous pressure (CVP) is measured by a catheter that is placed in the right atrium and attached to a transducer which amplifies the energy signal and displays its wave form onto a monitor using a similar set-up to an arterial line as described earlier. Venous pressure is a term that represents the average blood pressure within the thoracic vena cava near to the right atrium. Thus determination of the CVP provides a direct measurement of the changes in the pressure of blood returning to the heart. CVP is a useful tool for assessing the volume status of a patient. Since veins dilate and collapse passively depending on how much blood (volume) they contain, the pressure of blood in large veins depends directly on the patient's 'volume status'. The more fluid in the venous system the higher the central venous pressure is. A normal CVP is 2 to 6 mmHg in the self-ventilating patient (Lippincott, 2009). CVP is influenced by a number of factors that affect venous return, circulating blood volume and cardiac performance, including:

- cardiac output
- respiratory activity
- contraction of skeletal muscles (particularly legs and abdomen)
- sympathetic vasoconstrictor tone
- gravity

A decrease in cardiac output either due to decreased heart rate or loss of heart contractility results in blood backing up into the venous circulation (increased venous volume) as less blood is pumped into the arterial circulation. The resultant increase in thoracic blood volume increases CVP. An increase in total blood volume as occurs in renal failure or with activation of the renin–angiotensin–aldosterone system will increase venous pressure. Venous constriction elicited by sympathetic activation of veins, or by circulating vasoconstrictor substances, for example, catecholamines, decrease venous compliance, thereby increasing venous pressure. It is important to remember that increased intrathoracic pressure associated with positive pressure ventilation causes a reduction in CVP.

Treatment of Shock: Always Starts With ABCs

Airway needs will vary depending on the aetiology of shock, from no intervention to aggressive intervention. In our scenario, Daniel was assessed to be in respiratory failure and was immediately intubated and ventilated. However, sometimes a patient can be in shock but be breathing adequately and oxygenating well. Given the knowledge that shock syndrome causes excessive oxygen demand, it is advised that these patients are always given 100% oxygen via a non-rebreathe bag regardless of good saturations (ALSG, 2016). Often, these patients ultimately need intubation and respiratory support to help them compensate for profound metabolic acidosis.

Daniel had progressed rapidly to respiratory failure accompanied by signs and symptoms of shock. He exhibited marked tachycardia, cold extremities with delayed capillary refill and poorly palpable peripheral pulses; these are suggestive of hypovolaemia. However, Daniel's history of upper respiratory tract symptoms and fever suggested an infectious aetiology. The rapid deterioration to a shock state from what earlier in the day appeared to be a seemingly benign prodrome in an otherwise healthy child made the critical care team suspicious that this might be sepsis. Therefore, unless an alternative diagnosis is very clear, a third-generation cephalosporin antibiotic is given as soon as a blood culture is taken (ALSG, 2001). As is often the case, the precise aetiology of Daniel's illness was not clear. Despite this, the clinical findings indicated the need for prompt intervention.

SCENARIO

On admission to PICU, Daniel's circulatory assessment found:
- heart rate: 200 beats/min
- radial and dorsalis pulses: weak and thready
- skin was cool, dry and pale
- capillary refill: 4 s
- blood pressure: 90/60 mmHg
- prior to intubation, 20 mL/kg normal saline was given rapidly

ACTIVITY

Refer to Chapter 22 in ALSG (2016), *Advanced Paediatric Life Support: A Practical Approach*, where techniques for achieving vascular access are described.

Antibiotic therapy, although essential in addressing the underlying cause, does not treat septic shock as severe sepsis involves a disturbance in the immune system response towards the original infection. Additionally, antibiotics do not directly improve tissue perfusion or the associated delivery of oxygen and nutrients. Furthermore, oxygen therapy is of limited benefit because the primary problem is not inadequate oxygenation but inadequate transport of oxygenated blood. Remember that in severe sepsis a patient has excess coagulation and inflammation and impaired fibrinolysis with disruption of the endothelial layer. The endothelial wall disruption includes markedly increased capillary permeability and vasodilation. The vasodilation that occurs causes a relative hypovolaemia. Therefore treatment of septic shock must be aimed at recovering function at the microcirculatory level so that dysfunctioning organs can begin to function again.

Circulation

Irrespective of aetiology, initial shock therapy is directed at restoring circulating blood volume and perfusion. Fluid resuscitation is the mainstay of initial haemodynamic management. Optimal cardiac output is dependent upon volume, heart rate and contractile fibres in the myocardium achieving the appropriate amount of stretch. Therefore replacing lost volume will support cardiac output by increasing preload, thus enhancing cardiac muscle stretch and subsequent contraction, the optimum effect of the Starling mechanism. Thus a simple fluid bolus helps to improve a patient's haemodynamic status.

If not already available, vascular access should be obtained as quickly as possible once a 'shock state' is recognised. The Advanced Life Support Group (2016) recommends that medical practitioners make peripheral intravenous attempts over a maximum of 60 seconds and progress to immediate placement of an intraosseous needle if unsuccessful. Replacement must be made using a fluid bolus of 20 mL/kg of isotonic fluids given within a 10- to 20-minute period. Normal saline is the solution of first choice because it is ubiquitously available and carries minimal risks. However, repeated administration of iso-oncotic crystalloid solution boluses can lead to extravasation of fluid from the intravascular to the interstitial space, especially in situations where there is increased capillary permeability, for example in septic shock. In these circumstances, colloids may be administered as they have an important effect on the intravascular space. When infused, the osmotic colloid pressure on the intravascular space increases. As a result, fluid is drawn from the interstitial space into the intravascular space. Therefore the blood is rehydrated by osmosis (Alderson et al., 2001).

 ACTIVITY

Read Docherty and McIntyre (2002), which includes a simplified interpretation of the arguments and discussion offered in the Cochrane Review (Alderson et al., 2001).

 ACTIVITY

Daniel is given 20 mL/kg normal saline over 10 minutes. His circulation should then be re-assessed:
• What will you assess, why and how?

 SCENARIO

Despite a transient improvement after an initial bolus of 20 mL/kg normal saline with a heart rate of 130 and capillary refill of 3–4 seconds, Daniel requires further fluid therapy. After 60 mL/kg (3 × 20 mL/kg boluses), Daniel remains pale with a heart rate 160 beats/min, SBP 70 mmHg, capillary refill of 5 seconds and pulse oximetry that is not picking up. A central line has been inserted and Daniel has a CVP reading of 4 mmHg. He is started on dopamine at 4.0 mcg/kg/min and dobutamine at 10 mcg/kg/min administered via the central venous line.

A 2 mL/kg bolus of 10% dextrose in addition to maintenance fluids commenced and has improved his blood glucose from 1.7 to 4.2 mmol/L.

 ACTIVITY

Refer to the *BNF for Children* (BMA et al., 2017–18) and review the actions, dosage and side effects and nursing implications for the administration of the following inotropic agents: adrenaline, noradrenaline, dopamine and dobutamine.

As severe sepsis worsens, the benefits of fluid therapy are reduced, mainly because fluid therapy alone cannot address the cellular problem of increased capillary permeability as seen in severe sepsis. The fluid bolus has little effect on CVP. The widespread endothelial damage, vasodilation and capillary permeability are so great that pressure cannot be developed in the system. Because myocardial depression and vasodilation may be features of the patient's septic shock, inotropic agents may be valuable in restoring adequate perfusion. An inotrope is an agent that improves myocardial contractility and enhances stroke volume.

In patients with no significant improvement after two or three fluid boluses, particularly if sepsis is expected, inotropic agents are used to maintain arterial pressure. The agents most commonly used are catecholamines. Dopamine and dobutamine are both catecholamines but have different profiles as they activate different specific receptors. Their main course of action is through adrenergic receptors:
• α: peripheral vasculature stimulation: vasoconstriction
• β1: myocardium stimulation: inotropy and chronotropy
• β2: lungs and peripheral vasculature stimulation: smooth muscle relaxation (vasodilation and bronchodilation)

Dopamine is the gold standard as the initial vasopressor support of septic shock because of its versatility and its activation of dopamine receptors, thus possibly protecting the kidneys and preventing acute renal failure due to tubular necrosis. Dopamine, a precursor of adrenaline (epinephrine), administered as a continuous infusion, affects preload by causing vascular constriction or dilation through its effect on the sympathetic nervous system. Dopamine acts on α, β and dopamine receptors. Low-dose dopamine, 2–4 mcg/kg/min, has peripheral vasodilating effects but causes little or no increase in force of myocardial contraction (positive inotropy). However, low-dose dopamine may help to maintain splanchnic circulation and promote renal perfusion via dopamine receptor action. Dopamine affects β receptors at 5–10 mcg/kg/min and α receptors at >10 mcg/kg/min. If unable to meet haemodynamic goals with dopamine, medical practitioners will have a low threshold for switching or adding other agents such as adrenaline, noradrenaline and dobutamine, which have been shown to be beneficial in the hemodynamic support of septic shock. Dobutamine, a synthetic catecholamine, is also administered as a continuous intravenous infusion and acts primarily on β1 receptors. Dobutamine increases myocardial contractility (inotropic effect) and heart rate (chronotropic effect), and therefore increases stroke volume. It also causes peripheral vasodilation decreasing afterload. Overall dobutamine improves cardiac output.

Monitoring the Child in Shock

 SEMINAR DISCUSSION TOPIC

Shock is an altered state of tissue perfusion severe enough to induce derangements in normal cellular function. Neuroendocrine, hemodynamic and metabolic changes work together to restore perfusion. Treatment of shock is primarily focused on restoring tissue perfusion and oxygen delivery while eliminating the cause. The general goal is to maximise oxygen delivery and minimise oxygen demand and thereby enhance perfusion: Haemodynamic goals:
• mean arterial pressure >60 mmHg
• heart rate within normal parameters

- central venous pressure > 8 but <15 mmHg
- capillary refill <2 seconds

Organ perfusion goals:
- CNS: improved sensorium
- skin: warm, well perfused
- renal: urine output >1 mL/kg/h

Oxygen delivery adequacy:
- arterial oxygen saturation >95%
- Hb concentration >10 g/dL
- lactate <2 mmol

ACTIVITY

Work with colleagues to determine the implications for nursing in working collaboratively to achieve these goals.

FAMILY-CENTRED CRITICAL CARE – EXPLORING THE EVIDENCE

The hospitalisation of a child with a life-threatening illness constitutes a major stress experience for both the child and parents, endangering the child's and the parent's biological, social and psychological integrity. Infants and children admitted to intensive care (Fig. 35.27) require immediate stabilisation and life support that is frightening, invasive and likely to alter the appearance of the infant or child with an uncertainty about outcome. Nurses must be knowledgeable of the impact this phenomenon has on children and their families and the factors influencing their adjustment to this stressful experience to assist children and their families in developing positive, adaptive coping mechanisms. NICE (2013) set out guidance that aims to ensure the provision of care meets the needs of patients, service users and carers ensuring their views are reflected in the planning of health and social care services and enhance quality of care.

Family-centred care moves beyond the rhetorical theoretical recognition of the centrality of the child and family in health care. A family-focused multi-professional critical care team views the child and family as a unit to be cared for and organises care delivery around them as a unit as opposed to the more traditional patient-centred model. Managing this complexity requires the interprofessional team to think wider than their own individual expertise and to take the broader perspective of the child, family and other experts involved in the delivery of care (Nichols and Shaffner, 2016). However, providing family-centred care in a critical care setting is not a simple endeavour and is often misconceived as a list of interventions, for example open visiting. Family-centred care is a philosophical approach to care that recognises the needs of the family as well as the important role that they play during a child's critical illness, therefore it should be more accurately referred to as family-centred critical care in this setting. Although providing family-centred critical care means that the critical care team recognise their responsibility to help the family, as well as the child, survive the crisis of an illness and have an obligation to endeavour to meet their fundamental needs, it is important to stress that meeting a child's needs should always be the priority for both the child's family and the critical care team.

Research has indicated the fundamental needs of the family of the critically ill child as the need for honest and open information, the need for reassurance and support and the need to be in partnership with health care professionals regarding their child's care. These needs must be ascertained from individual families and from individuals within a family, and interpreted accurately. Thus it is important that nurses receive clarification about what these needs are and what they entail whilst at the same time recognising their dynamic nature. Empowering child and family participation in experiences that enhance control and independence and build on their strengths in the critical care environment demands advanced effective communication skills of the nurse and multi-professional team and the establishment of therapeutic relationships under stressful conditions.

Much research has been carried out in an endeavour to understand parental experiences of intensive care and the needs of family members of the critically ill child. A critique of this literature reveals through positivistic studies, which attempt to quantify parental feelings and experiences, that paediatric intensive care units (PICUs), for patients and their families, are almost certainly one of the most stressful hospital environments because the outcome is often uncertain.

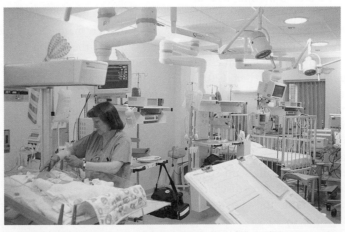

Fig. 35.27 Paediatric intensive care unit (PICU) environment.

Oxley (2015) studies the effects on children and their families with regards to their PICU experiences and post-traumatic stress (PTS). While children were not the primary focus of this study, it was noted that admission to a paediatric intensive care unit (PICU) can leave a child traumatised. The study reviewed the lived experience of parents through their child's admission to PICU; the key times of high emotion and stress started with the beginning of the journey and the child deterioration leading to PICU admission. The transfer to PICU was the greatest and most consistent anxiety-inducing element of the journey. It was also established that the emotional trauma of having a child in PICU does not end when the child is discharged but continues for the several months that follow. It was noted that removal of all stress from parents in this situation is unattainable, but care can be delivered in a way to make the experience less traumatic. Suggestions for improving care were linked to good communication and positive transfers to PICU, which could potentially reduce parental anxiety and make the experience less traumatic. Some parents also felt a loss of confidence in their parenting ability following a child's acute admission to a PICU, and co-production of care and involving family in care procedures will help them feel involved and grow their confidence. As parents may experience post-traumatic stress syndrome following an admission to PICU post discharge, support is also recommended.

Colville and Pierce (2012) conducted a longitudinal study of 66 child–parent pairs to establish the incidence of post-traumatic stress in a child or parent following a PICU admission. Using the Children's Revised Impact of Event Scale (CRIES-8), assessments were made at 3, 12 and 18 months following discharge. Forty-four per cent of child–parent pairs contained at least one member who were experiencing symptoms of post-traumatic stress 12 months after discharge. Those with symptoms increased over time, with the highest incidence for a child or parent to suffer symptoms being 3–12 months' post-discharge. It was noted that parents were more likely to suffer post-traumatic stress when their child was admitted to PICU non-electively. The finding that almost half of families were still experiencing significant post-traumatic stress symptoms 12 months after discharge and the fact that many experienced delayed reactions, after 3 months, indicate a need for long-term follow up and monitoring to ensure families have the support they need to minimise the impact of PICU admission on their future mental health.

One strategy to overcome long-term psychological effects of intensive care has been studied by Mikkelsen (2018). Mikkelsen explored children's and families' experiences of intensive care using diaries that were constructed by the child and family through their PICU journey. These were then used after discharge to facilitate discussion and reflection of their stay in a paediatric intensive care unit. The study collected data from five children and their families using semi-structured interviews between 4 and 6 months following discharge. Three significant themes emerged from the study. Firstly was the value of the diary to the entire family to seek meaning, explanation and coherence from the experience. The diaries also helped to create memories and importantly provide pictures to illustrate the family's journey. The findings suggested that a diary can serve as a catalyst for discussion and support the coping processes of the child and family. The study also finds that children who have been cared for in PICU have a sense of unreality about their experience, and the diary could help fill in some missing gaps in their journey to support the children in understanding their story. Recommendations for practice include:

1. Personalised diaries written by family members and the multi-interprofessional team, during a child's stay in the paediatric intensive care unit. It is recommended that entries should be age-appropriate and sufficiently detailed to describe the event being captured. When the event is being described, it is important to leave room for the child to insert their own interpretation and reaction to the event. The diary should also contain photographs and images of the child whilst a patient in the intensive care surroundings. If these diaries stimulate open discussion of the child's and family's experience of intensive care, there is further study needed to explore the impact of these diaries on post-traumatic stress disorder following an admission to PICU.

2. Family presence in invasive procedures and resuscitation is much debated in the literature and several researchers document the benefits of family presence during these (McAlvin and Carew-Lyons, 2014). The emerging themes in the evidence include knowing that everything possible was being done for their child; reducing anxiety and fear; feeling of being comforting and helpful to their child and the staff; sharing critical information about their child and the child's condition; maintaining the child–family relationship; closure on a life shared together; and facilitating the grieving process in the critical care environment and later at home.

👤 ACTIVITY

Analyse the evidence-based proposed advantages and disadvantages of family presence during resuscitation listed in Table 35.3. Consider the question:
- Do the advantages of allowing parents to be present during their child's resuscitation outweigh the potential disadvantages?

Although many family members and health care providers support the option of family presence, family members frequently are not given the option to remain with their child during invasive procedures and resuscitation efforts. This separation during treatment occurs for a variety of reasons. Health professionals express concern that: the event may be too traumatic for the family; clinical care might be impeded; family members might become too emotional or out of control; staff may experience increased stress with family present; unit rooms are too crowded; staff are focused on the child and may not be available to assist family members; there is a shortage of nurses and there is the risk of increased liability. Interestingly, parental presence at resuscitation has been fully supported by the UK Resuscitation Council since 1996,

TABLE 35.3 Advantages and Disadvantages of Family Presence During Invasive Procedures and Resuscitation

Advantages	Disadvantages
Holistic approach: acknowledges role of family	Family may disrupt procedure/resuscitation efforts
Child/family bond facilitated	Health care staff perceive that they may not be able to show
Family can observe efforts of health care team	emotion
Family see that all that can be done is done	Fear of litigation due to lack of understanding
Imagination is more fearsome than reality	Observer effect may inhibit staff performance
Reduce litigation because of openness	May cause psychological damage to family
Family can provide comfort	Long-term effects on family unit not known
Families perceive that they are participating in procedure/	Increases stress of staff involved
resuscitation	Child's privacy may be violated
Facilitates bereavement process	Resuscitation efforts may be unnecessarily prolonged
Facilitates relationship between family and staff	Interference of procedure/resuscitation
	Distraction of focus from child
	Family anger/violence towards staff

despite the controversy and in advance of much of this research. Every critically ill child is a member of a family system and family is usually the major source of support for the child during times of stress, crisis and decision making.

Research studies have shown that most families want the option to be present during invasive procedures, during their child's medical procedures and at the time of their child's death.

SUMMARY

Topics for this chapter were chosen because of their importance to children's morbidity and mortality and their prevalence as problems in intensive care. This chapter has considered the respiratory support, haemodynamic control and family-centred critical care required by a child with life-threatening illness on a paediatric intensive care unit. It demonstrates the principles of intensive care, which require that nurses apply specialist evidence-based knowledge and skills in the direct provision of care to manage a dynamic and rapidly evolving illness process in collaboration with medical and allied profession colleagues. The challenge is to provide this technologically sophisticated care in a compassionate environment and facilitate in-depth interaction between the critically sick child and their family.

REFERENCES

Adhikari, N., Dellinger, R., Lundind, S., et al., 2014. Inhaled nitric oxide does not reduce mortality in patients with acute respiratory distress syndrome regardless of severity: systematic review and meta analysis. Crit. Care Med. 42 (2), 404–412.

Advanced Life Support Group (ALSG), 2016. Advanced Paediatric Life Support: A Practical Approach To Emergencies, 6Th. John Wiley & Sons.

Alderson, P., Scherhout, G., Roberts, I., et al., 2001. Colloids versus Crystalloids for Fluid Resuscitation in the Critically Ill. The Cochrane Library, Oxford, p. 4.

Ashworth, W., 1996. Inquiry into the Care and Treatment of Nicholas Geldard. North West Regional Health Authority, Manchester.

Ball, C., Dams, J., Boyce, S., et al., 2001. Clinical guidelines for the use of the prone position in acute respiratory distress syndrome. Intens. Crit. Care Nur. 17, 94–104.

Been, J.V., Zimmermann, L.J., 2007. What's new in surfactant? Eur. J. Pediatr. 166 (9), 889–899.

Bhende, M.S., 2001. End-tidal carbon dioxide monitoring in pediatrics – clinical applications. J. Postgrad. Med. 47, 215–218.

British Medical Association and Royal Pharmaceutical Society of Great Britain 2020/2021 BNF For Children.

Bohn, D., 1998. New ventilation strategies. In: Duncan, A. (Ed.), Paediatric Intensive Care. BMJ Books, London, pp. 41–91.

British Paediatric Association (BPA), 1993. The Care of Critically Ill Children. Report of the Multidisciplinary Working Party on Paediatric Intensive Care. BPA, London.

Cameron, P., 2018. Textbook of Paediatric Emergency Medicine, third ed. Elsevier, London.

Centers for Disease Control (CDC), 1994. CDC guidelines. Resp. Care 39 (12), 1191–1236.

Clarke, D., 2012. Introduction to paediatric intensive care. In: Dixon, M., Crawford, D. (Eds.), Paediatric Intensive Care Nursing. Wiley-Blackwell, Oxford.

Colville, G., Pierce, C., 2012. Patterns of post-traumatic stress symptoms in families after paediatric intensive care. Intensive Care Med. 38 (9), 1523–1531.

Coyne, I., Timmins, F., Neill, F., 2010. Clinical Skills for Children's Nursing. Oxford University Press, Oxford.

Crain, E., Gershel, J., 2012. Clinical Manual of Emergency Pediatrics. Cambridge University Press, Cambridge.

Curley, M., Hibberd, P., Fineman, L., et al., 2005. Effect of prone positioning on clinical outcomes in children with acute lung injury. J. Am. Med. Assoc. 294 (2), 229–238.

Davies, J., McDougall, M., 2019. Children in Intensive Care: A Survival Guide. Elsevier, London.

Davies, K., Monterosso, L., Bulsara, M., et al., 2015. Clinical indicators for the initiation of endotracheal suction in children: an integrative review. Aust. Crit. Care 28 (1), 11–18.

Dixon, M., 2012. Care of an infant or child with a respiratory illness and/or need for respiratory support. In: Dixon, M., Crawford, D. (Eds.), Paediatric Intensive Care Nursing. Wiley-Blackwell, Oxford.

Docherty, B., McIntyre, L., 2002. Nursing considerations for fluid management in hypovolaemia. Prof. Nurse 17 (9), 545–549.

Dreyfus, D., Basset, G., Soler, P.S., Saumon, G., 1985. Intermittent positive pressure hyperventilation with high inflation pressures produces pulmonary microvascular injury in rats. American review of Respiratory Diseases 132 (4), 880–884.

Foglia, E., Meier, M., Elward, A., 2007. Ventilator-associated pneumonia in neonatal and pediatric intensive care unit patients. Clin. Microbiol. Rev. 20, 409–425.

Fuhrman, B., Zimmerman, J., Carcillo, J., et al., 2017. Fuhrman & Zimmerman's Pediatric Critical Care. Elsevier, Philadelphia.

Ganong, W.F., 2001. Review of Medical Physiology, twentieth ed. Lange Medical Books, New York.

Gormley-Fleming, E., Peate, I., 2018. Fundamentals of Children's Applied Pathophysiology. John Wiley and Sons, Chichester.

Hazinski, M.F., 2013. Nursing Care of the Critically Ill Child, third ed. Elsevier, New York.

Jauncey-Cooke, J., Bogossian, F., East, C., 2010. Lung protective ventilation strategies in paediatrics: a review. Aust. Crit. Care 23 (2), 81–88.

Kalil, A., 2018. Septic shock clinical presentation: history, physical examination, complications. [online] Emedicine.medscape.com. Available from: https://emedicine.medscape.com/article/168402-clinical.

Kerr, M., 1997. Paediatric ventilatory care. In: Morton, M.S. (Ed.), Paediatric Intensive Care. Oxford University Press, Oxford, pp. 109–151.

Klabunde, R., 2012. Cardiovascular Physiology Concepts. Wolters Kluwer Health/Lippincott Williams & Wilkins, Philadelphia.

Kline-Tilford, A.M., Sorce, L.R., Levin, D.L., et al., 2013. Pulmonary disorders. In: Hazinski, M.F. (Ed.), Nursing Care of the Critically Ill Child, third ed. Elsevier, New York.

Kolobow, T., Moretti, M.P., Fumagalli, R., et al., 1987. Severe impairment in lung function induced by high peak airway pressure during mechanical ventilation: an experimental study. Am. Rev. Respir. Dis. 135 (3), 312–315.

Lippincott's Nursing Procedures, 2009. Fifth ed. Lippincott Williams & Wilkins, Ambler.

Long, S., Prober, C., Fischer, M., 2018. Principles and Practice of Pediatric Infectious Diseases. Elsevier, Philadelphia.

Macintyre, N., 2005. In: Mason, R. (Ed.), Murray and Nadel's Textbook of Respiratory Medicine. Elsevier, Philadelphia.

Mancebo, J., Fernandez, R., Blanch, L., et al., 2006. A multicenter trial of prolonged prone ventilation in severe acute respiratory distress syndrome. Am. J. Respir. Crit. Care Med. 173 (11), 1233–1239.

Marieb, E., 2016. Human Anatomy and Physiology, tenth ed. Pearson, Harlow.

Martini, F., Nath, J., Bartholomew, E., 2018. Fundamentals of Anatomy & Physiology. Pearson Education Limited, Harlow.

McAlvin, S., Carew-Lyons, A., 2014. Family presence during resuscitation and invasive procedures in pediatric critical care: a systematic review. Am. J. Crit. Care 23 (6), 477–485.

McCance, K., Huether, S., 2002. Pathophysiology: The Biological Basis for Disease in Adults and Children. Mosby, London.

Melsen, W.G., Rovers, M.M., Bonten, M.J., 2009. Ventilator associated pneumonia and mortality: a systematic review of observational studies. Crit. Care Med. 37 (10), 2709–2718.

Mikkelsen, G., 2018. The meaning of personal diaries to children and families in the paediatric intensive care unit: a qualitative study. Intens. Crit. Care Nur. 45, 25–30.

National Institute for Health and Care Excellence (NICE), 2013. Patient and Public Involvement Policy. NICE, London.

National Institute for Health and Care Excellence (NICE), 2014. Head Injury Triage, Assessment, Investigation and Early Management of Head Injury in Children, Young People and Adults. CG 176 (Partial Update of NICE CG56): Methods, Evidence and Recommendations. NICE, London.

NHS Executive (NHSE), 1996. Paediatric Intensive Care. NHSE, Leeds.

NHS Executive (NHSE), 1997a. Paediatric Intensive Care: A Framework for the Future. Report of the National Co-ordinating Group on Intensive Care to the Chief Executive of the NHS Executive. NHSE, London.

NHS Executive (NHSE), 1997b. Paediatric Intensive Care: A Bridge to the Future. Report of the Chief Nursing Officer's Taskforce to the Chief Executive. NHSE, London.

Nichols, D.G., Shaffner, D.H., 2016. Roger's Textbook of Pediatric Intensive Care. Wolters Kluwer, Philadelphia.

Oxley, R., 2015. Parents' experiences of their child's admission to paediatric intensive care. Nurs. Child. Young People 27 (4), 16–21.

Paediatric Intensive Care Audit Network for the UK, 2018. PICANET Annual Report. University of Leeds and Leicester, Picanet.

Paediatric Intensive Care Society (PICS), 2015. Quality Standards for the Care of Critically Ill Children, fifth ed. PICS, London. Available from: http://picsociety.uk/wp-content/uploads/2016/05/PICS_standards_2015.pdf.

Partrick, D.A., Bensard, D.D., Janik, J.S., et al., 2002. Is hypotension a reliable indicator of blood loss from traumatic injury in children? Am. J. Surg. 184 (6), 555–559.

Pearson, G., 2002. Handbook of Paediatric Intensive Care. WB Saunders, London.

Porth, C., 2011. Essentials of Pathophysiology. Wolters Kluwer Health, Philadelphia.

Reynolds, E.M., Ryan, D., Doody, D., 1993. Permissive hypercapnia and pressure-controlled ventilation as a treatment of severe adult respiratory distress syndrome in a pediatric burn patient. Crit. Care Med. 21, 468–475.

Rhoades, R., Bell, D., 2009. Medical Physiology. Lippincott Williams & Wilkins, Philadelphia.

Robb, J., 1997. Physiological changes occurring with positive pressure ventilation: part one. Intens. Crit. Care Nur. 13, 293–307.

Rotta, A., Steinhorn, D., 2007. Conventional mechanical ventilation in pediatrics. J. Pediatr. 83 (Suppl. 2), S100–S108.

Royal College of Paediatrics and Child Health (RCPCH), 2014. High Dependency Care for Children: Time to Move On. RCPCH, London.

Siempos, I., Vardakis, K., Kopterides, P., et al., 2007. Impact of passive humidification on clinical outcomes of mechanically ventilated patients: a meta-analysis of randomized control trials. Crit. Care Med. 35 (12), 2843–2851.

Tibballs, J., 1998. Clinical aspects of nitric oxide therapy. In: Duncan, A. (Ed.), Paediatric Intensive Care. BMJ, London.

Tortora, G., Derrickson, B., 2014. Principles of Anatomy and Physiology, fourteenth ed. Wiley, New York USA.

Urden, L., Stacy, K., Lough, M., 2016. Priorities in Critical Care Nursing, seventh ed. Elsevier, Missouri.

Waugh, A., Grant, A., 2014. Ross & Wilson Anatomy & Physiology in Health and Illness, twelfth ed. Churchill Livingstone Elsevier, London.

Wiersinga, W.J., Seymour, C.W., 2018. Handbook of Sepsis. Springer International, New York.

Williams, R., Rankin, N., Smith, T., et al., 1996. Relationship between the humidity and temperature of inspired gas and the function of the airway mucosa. Crit. Care Med. 24 (11), 1920–1929.

Wright, M., Romano, M., 2006. Ventilator-associated pneumonia in children. Semin. Pediatr. Infect. Dis. 17 (2), 58–64.

36

Emergency Care, Out of Hospital Care, Emergency Department Assessment and Inpatient Care

Liz Gormley-Fleming

LEARNING OUTCOMES

- Demonstrate an understanding of pre-hospital care and emergency care services for children and young people in contemporary health services.
- Understand how the triage process is operationalised in the children's emergency departments.

- Appreciate positive attributes of the environment of care in emergency departments in the overall care of children.
- Consider how the philosophy of family-centred care is promoted in emergency departments.
- Appreciate the role of children and young person's nurse in the emergency department.

THE EVOLUTION OF EMERGENCY CARE FOR CHILDREN AND YOUNG PEOPLE

The concept of emergency care as a designated facility was first recommended following the Standing Medical Advisory Committee of Central Health Services investigation into NHS acute hospital arrangements for receiving and stabilisation of acutely ill and injured patients in 1961. The subsequent report that followed this inspection, and for the first time formally recognised this concept of 'casual attendees' within the casualty department.

Many subsequent reports, including the court report *Fit for the Future* (Department of Health and Social Security [DHSS], 1976), *Welfare of Children and Young People in Hospital* (Department of Health [DoH], 1991), *Children First, a Study of Hospital Services* (Audit Commission, 1993) and *The Patient's Charter – Services for Children and Young People* (DoH, 1996), all advocated and determined recommendations and standards for health services, with specific reference to A&E services for children.

During the 1990s most families would have contacted their general practitioners (GPs) when they had concerns about their child. However, changes in the GP contract and their working practices in 2004 has resulted in the need to create a multiplicity of emergency care settings. Subsequently many children and families now self-refer to urgent care services.

Since the original *Accident and Emergency Services for Children* was published in 1999 and updated in 2007, significant changes have continued to evolve in urgent care provision. Care for children is now delivered in urgent care centres, walk-in centres, minor injury units, pharmacies, emergency departments (EDs) and major trauma centres. The emergency care of children is regarded as a sub-specialty of emergency medicine.

The National Service Framework (NSF) for children, young people and maternity services (DoH, 2003) includes specific recommendations for accident and emergency departments. These include physical separation between children and adult areas within emergency departments, and environments that are accessible, safe and suitable for babies, children and families.

The 2018 *Standards for Children and Young People in Emergency Care* relate to all aspects of emergency care for children and young people (Royal College of Paediatrics and Child Health [RCPCH], 2018). This set of standards embraced the child's journey and has adopted a whole systems approach acknowledging the importance of self care and support in the community as prerequisites for reducing avoidable hospital admissions and reduced lengths of stay. The intent was also to reduce variation in services and to raise the profile of the care children and young people require when they become acutely unwell.

The emphasis is very much on improving safety and reducing preventably child death (Glasper, 2016). Audit is now a feature of everyday NHS practice so access to impact of these standards should enable enhancement of practice.

Significant changes in the delivery of pre-hospital care and emergency hospital care for children and young people has occurred, particularly in the last 10 years. This landscape continues to develop at pace, although emergency care for children and young people continues to be under great pressure. The changes to this provision have occurred as our understanding of the importance of pre-hospital care continues to improve. This is now recognised as essential in achieving positive outcomes for the child or young person.

In addition, there is a more informed understanding about why children and young people access these services Keeble & Kossarova (2017). New models of care delivery have been implemented as a result of this which are cost effective and efficient with an emphasis on keeping children out of hospital at all cost.

The Facts – Who Attends for Emergency Care?

Discussions rarely centre around the emergency admission of children to hospital. This is despite of the fact children and young people are the most frequent users of A&E. Children and young people account for nearly one-third of the total population in England (Office for National Statistics, 2018). This is approximately a total of 16.6 million children and young people.

During 2016 there were 425 A&E attendances for every 1000 children/young people compared to 345 A&E attendees for every adult aged over 25 years (per 1000) (NHS Digital, 2017).

In 2016, there were 23.57 million in attendance at A&E. Sixty-five per cent of these were at a major emergency department. This was a 5.2% increase over the previous year (Baker, 2017). A quarter of these were less than 19 years of age.

Annually there are 2,000,000 accidents in the home alone in the 0- to 15-year-old age group. Sixty-two children die as a result of accidents in the home and 25,000 children 0–4 years will attend A&E following accidental poisoning. There are 58,000 accidents per year that occur on the stairs and 67,000 that occur in the kitchen; 76,000 children 0–14 years will be admitted for treatment and 40% of these will be under 5 years of age; 13 children per day will attend A&E following a burn or scald. Around 500 children, mainly under-5s, are admitted to hospital, and a further 2000 attend A&E departments every year as a result of bath water scalds.

Ninety per cent of all children attending A&E do so between 8.00 a.m. and midnight; the remaining 10% attend between midnight and 8.00 a.m. The busiest period for children in A&E is between midday and 4.00 p.m., when over 55% children attend for unscheduled care; 80% of children with traumatic injury arrive between 4.00 p.m. and midnight.

Kmietowicz (2018) identified that attendance at the ED is growing twice as fast as the population. Attendances by young people with mental health disorders have seen a steep rise in the last 5 years (Young Minds, 2018). The incidences of intentional self-harm have increased from 18,291 in 2011 to 21,904 in 2018. The incidences of young people attending A&E with a diagnosed psychiatric condition has risen threefold. Data from 2011 shows that there were 9372 attendances and in 2018 this figure was 27,487. Infants experience more emergency admissions than any other age group. The 1- to 4-year-old age group has also seen an increase in the number of emergency admissions over the last 10 years (Keeble and Kossarova, 2017). The most common conditions diagnosed on emergency admissions in the 0- to 24-year-old age group are listed below in Fig. 36.1. The only age group that has seen a slight decrease in attendance is the 15- to 34-year-old age group (NHS, 2018).

1	Viral infection
2	Acute bronchitis
3	Upper respiratory tract infections
4	Abdominal pains
5	Gastro-intestinal infections
6	Acute and chronic tonsillitis
7	Poisonings
8	Epilepsy, convulsions
9	Asthma
10	Upper limb fractures

Fig. 36.1 Ten most common diagnosed conditions on emergency admissions. (NHS Digital, 2017. Hospital Accident and Emergency Activity 2016–17. Summary Report. NHS, Leeds.)

These findings are similar to those found by MacFaul and Werneke (2001). Fifty-six per cent of children presented with one of three problems: breathing difficulty (25%), fit (16%) or feverish illness (15%). Feeding problems and diarrhoea together accounted for a further 21%. Some of the conditions listed in Fig 36.1 are preventable admissions. With effective management and treatment in the community the need for emergency care could have been mitigated.

There has been a rise in infants being admitted with perinatal conditions and jaundice, in particular, and this has doubled in the last 10 years.

The NHS England Urgent and Emergency Care review (2013) Identified that the ED was the most appropriate health care setting for many people, but that 40% of patients who attended ED were 'avoidable' attenders. In other words, this group of patients could be managed more effectively and efficiently by other services.

TRANSFORMING URGENT AND EMERGENCY CARE

A comprehensive review of the NHS urgent and emergency care system in England, chaired by Professor Sir Bruce Keogh, NHS Medical Director, was commenced in 2013. This was one of the priorities of the clinical commissioning groups (CCGs) in their planning guidance: Everyone Counts: Planning for Patients 2013/14. Working with clinical experts, patients and delivery partners from both urgent and emergency care systems their remit was to develop an evidence base for change and identify principles that would underpin change. The implementation phase of this programme commenced in 2015. A range of interventions were rolled out to achieve the objectives set by urgent and emergency care (UEC) programmes with the expectation that these would positively impact on patient experience and behaviour. Twenty-three UEC networks were established with the goal of harnessing expertise within local health care systems.

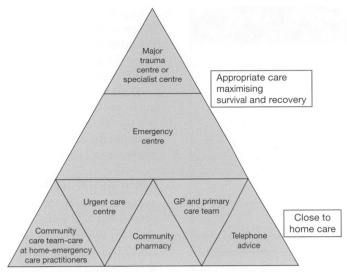

Fig. 36.2 Urgent and emergency care networks. *GP*, General practitioner.

The NHS Five Year Forward View (2014) set out a positive vision for the future based around new models of care. It sought to explain the need to redesign urgent and emergency care services in England for people of all age groups with physical and mental health problems and the new models of care required to meet these needs. A fundamental shift in the way UEC services were provided to all age groups was detailed in this plan NHS (2010). Improving out-of-hospital services to enable care to be delivered close to home and avoid hospital admission was a priority. A safe sustainable system that delivered high quality care consistently was decreed as the ultimate goal. This was outlined in the good practice guide: *Safer, Faster, Better: Good Practice in Delivering Urgent and Emergency Care* (2015). The development of the urgent care network provided a fundamental shift in the provision of emergency and urgent care. The ambition is to meet the patients urgent care needs as close to their home as possible (Fig. 36.2) and if hospital care is required then the patient should be taken to the most appropriate hospital to maximise survival and recovery from life-threatening conditions.

URGENT CARE SERVICES

A Network Approach to Urgent Care

In light of the *Five Year Forward View, The Right Time, The Right Place,* the Keogh *Urgent and Emergency Care Services Review* and the *National Unscheduled Care Essential Actions Improvement Programme*, work was commenced across the UK to address the required changes to urgent and emergency care services. At a time of transition into new models of care, it is particularly pertinent for providers and service planners to work together to meet standards to ensure locally delivered, safe and high quality urgent and emergency care for infants, children and young people.

Urgent care services for children and young people were required to be integrated and a whole systems approach taken. Multi-disciplinary training and attainment of specific competencies were advocated. Shared protocols, staff training, staff rotation and ongoing quality improvement and monitoring were

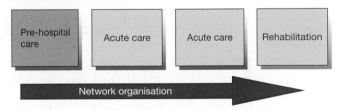

Fig. 36.3 Major trauma pathway.

established across regional networks. A key feature of the network approach to urgent care is the use of referral pathways and clinical guidelines. This is an attempt to improve consistency in care and unwarranted variations across the care provision in the networks. An example of a pathway is found in Fig. 36.3.

This requirement extended to telephone triage as this may be conducted by non-clinical staff who utilise clinical decision support software to triage via telephone.

The ambulance service is often the starting point of emergency care for the child and young person. Uniformity in the provision of equipment and medication was advised along with competency in caring for sick and injured children by all immediate care practitioners (RCPCH, 2012). Good trauma care involves getting the right treatment by the right people in the most expedient manner.

Currently the NHS offers a range of emergency care centres: minor injury units, walk-in centres, urgent care centres and urgent treatment centres. All provide unique services. The ambition of the NHS Long Term plan (2019) is to embed Urgent Treatment Centers consistently across the NHS regions in England to support the provision of consistent out of hospital urgent care. The urgent care model of care has been developed to provide urgent care to people in non–life-threatening situations. These are GP led and operate for a minimum of 12 hours per day. Referral may be made by your GP or NHS 111. Self-referral is also permissible. The ambition is that UTCs will treat common ailments, leaving EDs free to treat the seriously injured or ill patients. The types of injury/illness seen in an urgent care centre are outlined in Table 36.1.

TABLE 36.1 **Conditions Seen at an Urgent Care Centre**

Ear, nose and throat (ENT) infections
Minor scalds and burns
Minor lacerations
Suspected fractures
Minor head injuries
Bites and stings
Skin infections and rashes
Minor eye problems
Respiratory conditions
Abdominal pain
Diarrhoea and vomiting
Emergency contraception
Urinary tract infections
Feverish illnesses

The staffing model for an UCT should include children and young people (CYP) nurses who can assess and treat the child and support their families. One of the key principles of this model is that UTCs should be co-located alongside the Emergency Department (ED) in the acute setting where CYP nurses will be employed. UTCs are required to have protocols in place to manage the critically ill child who may arrive unexpectedly. Child protection information systems should be in use in a UTC to ensure that information is shared as necessary with NHS and social care colleagues (NHS, 2017a).

Pre-hospital Emergency Care

Pre-hospital care refers to the care given to the seriously ill or injured child or young person before they arrive into the emergency department. It will involve doctors, critical care paramedics and other emergency services.

The need for emergency care in the community for CYP is relatively rare as they only account 5%–10% of all cases who require an ambulance. Nonetheless, traumatic injuries are the leading cause of mortality and morbidity in the CYP age group. The small number of cases and the paucity of data on pre-hospital care outcomes for CYP is identified as a gap in the provision of quality care for CYP compared to the adult patient (Seid et al., 2012; International Federation of Emergency Medicine, 2014). The pre-hospital care team may have limited exposure to the seriously ill/injured CYP. Paediatric trauma accounts for only a very small percentage of paediatric intensive care unit (PICU) admissions – currently just 2.8%. This is one of the consistent anxieties of the pre-hospital team (Reavley, 2014). However, the development of theoretical knowledge and understanding together with the practice scenarios through simulation can enhance the team's skills. The relatively recent inclusion of recognition of the sick or injured child into curriculum for pre-hospital care providers will assist with improving the knowledge, skills and needs of the seriously ill/injured CYP.

Pre-hospital care for children and young people provides an unrivalled opportunity to significantly improve their outcomes in the presence of serious illness or trauma. The period of time that immediately follows the injury or onset of serious illness is often referred to as the 'golden-hour'. During this period of time, the emergency care team play an essential role in assessing stabilisation and transportation to a definitive care facility Ley et al., (2015).

Definitive care for the seriously injured or sick child cannot be provided outside of the secondary care setting. Prompt transport to a designated appropriate care setting must occur once the child has been stabilised and appropriate treatment interventions undertaken.

Pre-hospital Transfers

Transfer to the appropriate medical facility is undertaken by paramedics and other appropriately trained specialists. It is usual for the receiving hospital to be notified so they will be advised of the imminent arrival of the seriously injured or sick child and have mobilised their trauma team or paediatric resuscitation team.

However, parents and carers are often unaware of the severity of illness and injury that children suffer. Often because of their size, children are 'scooped up' and brought by people unaware of the risks they are taking by escorting children in critical conditions by private car, public transport or taxi. Only 6% of children attend emergency departments by ambulance.

Taking this figure into account, it is important that A&E staff are aware that seriously ill and injured children often arrive in the emergency department 'in arms', and should receive early triage for this very reason. Conveying to the public the message about appropriate use of ambulances in urgent and emergency situations has been ongoing for years. The nationally available NHS 111 telephone advice service is available for parents and carers who need advice for children over the age of 5 years who are unwell. The nurses can provide emergency advice about a child's health status and mobilise an ambulance if necessary.

Major trauma bypass tools (RCPCH, 2018) have been developed and include protocols for children to transfer them to major trauma centres, thus bypassing their local hospital's emergency departments. There are occasions when the child may be transferred to the nearest medical facility as in the event of ongoing resuscitation or when life or limb are compromised. Local hospitals must ensure they have skilled staff, trained in advanced paediatric life support skills, available at all times to safely resuscitate and stabilise the seriously ill child until they can be retrieved to a specialist centre.

The 'ASHICE' or 'ATMIST' format of pre-hospital communication (Table 36.2) is recommended as the communication tool between the emergency care team at the scene and the receiving emergency department (Advanced Life Support Group, 2017).

MAJOR TRAUMA, TRAUMA TEAM AND EMERGENCY CARE TEAMS

Major trauma remains the most frequent cause of death in the UK for children aged between 1 and 18 years of age

TABLE 36.2 ASHICE and ATMIST Tools for Handover Communication	
ASHICE	**ATMIST**
A – age	A – age
S – sex	T – time of injury
H – history	M – mechanism of injury
I – illness/injury	I – injury sustained
C – current condition	S – signs and symptoms
E – expected time and mode of arrival at the emergency department	T – treatment given so far

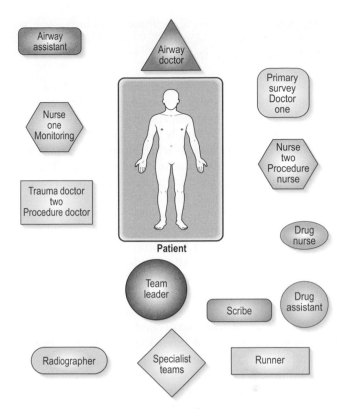

Fig. 36.4 Positions of the trauma team. (National Institute for Health and Care Excellence [NICE], 2016. Major Trauma: Service Delivery. Clinical Guideline [CG40]. NICE, London.)

and is a serious public health issue. Thirty-one percent of deaths in children aged 1–4 years, increasing to 48% of deaths in the 15- to 18-year age group, is attributed to trauma. Road traffic accidents resulting in high energy, blunt trauma is the most common mechanism of injury. The formation of trauma networks in the UK in 2012 saw the creation of designated major trauma centres. The driver for change to children's emergency care was based on evidence from adult patients where there were improved outcomes if treated in designated emergency care centres. This requires the use of a pre-hospital screening tool which considers the patient's condition and distance to emergency department.

There are 27 major trauma centres in the UK:
- 11 of these treat adults and children.
- 11 treat adults only.
- 5 treat children only.

Given that accidents are the foremost cause of death in children over 1 year of age, response to the care of the most seriously ill and injured children must be delivered speedily and following a professionally competent model, backed up by the right facilities. A team approach allows critically ill and traumatised patients optimal chances for survival.

As already identified, there has been a dramatic increase in the number of children attending hospital and particularly with head injuries in the last decade, and this accounts for up to one-third of the incidence of accidental death in childhood. While there has been a marked improvement in the long-term outcome for children with traumatic brain injuries, there is an associated health impact for the child and their families (Parslow et al., 2005). A systematic approach to the initial assessment and early management of head injuries is crucial to the long-term outcome (National Institute of Clinical Excellence [NICE], 2016).

Seriously injured children and young people are described as having major trauma and this is measured on a scale referred to as the Injury Severity Scale (ISS). It is an anatomical scoring system. This ranges from a score of 1–75 with the latter being the most severely injured. A score of greater than 15 is defined as major trauma, and 9–15 is classified as moderate severe trauma. The challenge

of determining an ISS for a child at the time of injury may not be possible as a full diagnostic assessment is required. A system of triage is employed to identify those who are most likely to have had a major trauma, and these patients are referred to as 'candidate' major trauma (NHS, 2013a). This category of patients is then transferred to a major trauma centre. On arrival to the resuscitation bay, the child's care is handed over to the team leader. The trauma team will be in position to continue treatment. Each member has a clearly defined location (Fig. 36.4).

Trauma Teams

The education requirements for trauma teams are now well established and competence in a range of advanced skills but also leadership and risk management are now considered essential. Training to deliver appropriate care for all health care professionals must include the following topics:
- Advanced life support: paediatric and neonatal.
- Team resource management in the trauma resuscitation room.
- Management of catastrophic haemorrhage.
- Airway management including the indication for rapid sequence induction anaesthesia and the role of the assistant.
- Recognition and management of key life-threatening interventions (e.g. pneumothorax, cardiac tamponade, management of chest drains, emergency thoracotomy).

- Intravenous access: central, peripheral and intraosseous.
- Management of head injuries.
- Pelvic and long bone fractures.
- Pain management.

Major trauma units (MTUs) will have approved protocols for telephoning and calling in consultants to aid with decision making and case management. In addition, there will be transfer protocol and protocols for accepting patients back from the MTU and referral to rehabilitation centres. Mercer et al., 2018 Best practice guidelines, for example, NICE will be used in the management of the care the patient requires. Table 36.3 outlines the roles and responsibilities of the trauma team. There may be slight variations to this, but generally the responsibilities of the roles remain unchanged.

Established timelines for the management of CYP who are admitted to MTUs do exist. After handover from the pre-hospital team, the team leader will lead and direct the care of the child until they are transferred to theatre, PICU or to another specialist centre (e.g. neurology, cardiac). This may include airway management, insertion of chest drains, focused assessment with sonography for trauma (FAST) scan, computed tomography (CT) scan, reduction of limb fractures, dressing of open wounds, fluid resuscitation, management of haemorrhage, administration of analgesia.

The time frame for treating the seriously ill child on arrival to resuscitation bay is essential if optimum outcomes are to be achieved (Mercer et al., 2018; NICE, 2016). Below is an outline of how this is operationalised:

Time −15 minutes: the team will assemble prior to the arrival of the child, and role will be allocated. This includes making introductions and sharing of known facts. If a 'code red' has been declared then the transfusion laboratory should be contacted and a transfusion pack ordered for delivery to the resuscitation bay.

Time T, on arrival into the resuscitation bay: the pre-hospital team will commence handover. This is referred to as a 'sterile' handover and the assembled trauma team will be silent. Questions may be asked once handover is complete. A communication tool is utilised to give structure to the handover and also ensures it is complete. Initial assessment is commenced.

Time 0 includes immediate actions. This will include a systematic assessment CABCD:

- Control of catastrophic haemorrhage,
- Airway,
- Breathing,
- Circulation,
- Disability.

Oxygen will be administered via non-rebreather mask. Intravenous access will be obtained. If it is not possible to obtain intravenous access, then intraosseous access will be attempted. Blood samples will be obtained at this point. A blood sample for a full blood count, urea and electrolytes, group and cross match/save and a venous blood gas will be required.

Time 5+: Five minutes after arrival, a review of CABCD is undertaken with each response from each team member directed to the team leader. Further treatment interventions are considered, e.g. chest x-ray, x-ray of pelvis. Additional intravenous access may be obtained. A FAST scan may be undertaken. A key intervention at this time is the administration of analgesia. The risk and benefits of this will need to be considered.

Time +15 minutes: a decision may be made to transfer the child to CT or Theatre if indicated. If a blood transfusion is required it is at this point that it will be administered. On the direction of the team leader, a secondary survey will now be undertaken if time critical interventions are not required. Preparation for transfer is commenced. This will involve securing intravenous lines, secure patient (vacuum mattress), wounds will need to be dressed and any splints applied will need to be reassessed at this point.

20–30 minutes after arrival: the child should be ready to transfer to either the operating theatre, CT, PICU/HDU or the ward. A 'Command Huddle' between the team leader and senior team member will discuss and identify the next steps of treatment for the child following completion of the initial assessment. The outcome of the huddle will be shared with the team by the team leader. All medication administered should be confirmed and records made. At this point the team leader and senior nurse will meet with the family and update them on their child's condition.

Once the initial assessment has been completed and immediate treatment delivered, the team leader will evaluate the child's response to treatment and direct the next stages of care Groenesteng-Kreb et al., (2014). A team huddle will take place with the senior team members and team leader deciding on the next stages of treatment. Communication with the family is essential at this time. Decisions about the ongoing care of the child will be made and arrangements for safe transfer to either theatre, CT, a definitive care area (PICU/HDU) or ward will commence. A team debrief should happen as soon as possible. This enables the team to reflect on their actions, learn for the future and evaluate their performance. Audit documentation should be completed as all major traumas are audited via the Trauma Audit and Research Network (TARN).

Standards for Emergency Care

The RCPCH (2018) standards aim to ensure that urgent and emergency care services are fully integrated with the child receiving the right care in the correct environment at the correct time. The *Standards for Children and Young People in Emergency Care* (RCPCH, 2018) relate to all aspects of emergency care for children and young people. The scope of this publication is to provide health care professionals and commissioners with a clear set of standards that are applicable to all urgent and emergency care settings. The aim is to improve the experience and outcomes for children and young people on their journey through urgent and emergency care service. The 2018 edition incorporated chapters on mental health and care pathways. It also identified the need for community nursing support for early discharge and follow-up care from emergency care settings.

TABLE 36.3 Role of the Trauma Team Members

Role	Responsibilities
Team leader – ED Consultant, Paediatrician	Be clearly identifiable, stands at end of bed and has sight of patient and team; a hands-off role. Responsible for prioritising care and making all critical decisions. All instructions and feedback are communicated through to the team leader. Assembles team prior to arrival of patient. Designates roles and responsibilities in pre-team briefing before patient arrives. Identifies skill set of the team. Confirms equipment is ready and that team are wearing appropriate PPE. Ensures CT/theatre are informed (if likely to be required). Orders blood to be brought to resuscitation area in the event of a code red.[a] Starts the clock when patient arrives in resuscitation bay. Receives handover from pre-hospital emergency team–quiet environment, hands off handover. Manages a thorough, safe assessment of the patient and ensure trauma team members are informed of the care priorities. Seeks specialist advice and performs a succinct handover to the team who will be providing definitive care for the patient. Is clear that the team leader role has been handed over to the definitive care team. Completes contemporaneous records and audit requirements. Debriefs team. Meets with family/carers.
Airway doctor: Anaesthesia/PICU Consultant/Registrar or Anaesthetic Registrar	Prepares airway equipment prior to arrival of patient. Communicates with drug nurse to prepare required emergency drugs. Sets up and checks ventilator. Key responsibility is to perform airway assessment and management of airway. Communicates findings to team leader. Intubates patient as required utilising intubation check list, and establishes patient on ventilator in discussion with team leader. Use of airway adjuncts as required and ensure patient is oxygenated. Ensure cervical spine immobilisation and manages 20-degree tilt to enable inspection of patient's back. Manages airway during any transfers (CT, theatre, PICU). If patient is alert then ascertains AMPLE history: A – allergies M – medication P – past medical history L – last meal/food E – everything else that might be relevant. May insert nasogastric tube. Provides assurance to patient if they are alert and updates them on what is happening. Completes contemporaneous record of assessment, care given and decision making.
Airway assistant	Prepares equipment. Removes clothing from patient. Assists with intubation. Accompanies airway doctor with transfers.
Trauma doctor 1 – ED Registrar but may be PICU Registrar. Primary survey	Completes 'WETFLAG' calculations prior to the arrival of the child based on an estimation of their weight. Ensures relevant equipment is ready: vac mat, splints, pelvic binder. Undertakes primary survey. Communicates findings to team leader. May take AMPLE history if possible. Orders relevant imaging following discussion with team leader. Undertakes secondary survey as appropriate. Keeps patient warm. Prescribes all medication and fluids and makes sure it is all signed for. Completes contemporaneous records, highlighting findings from primary and secondary surveys. Treatments required but not yet implemented must be included in records and highlighted.
Trauma doctor 2: ED Registrar/PICU Registrar/Junior Doctor	Prepares IV and IO access equipment and rapid infuser. Gains IV or IO access. Take blood samples, ensures they are sent and utilise track care paediatric order set. Informs team leader of results. Communicates with blood bank, ensures any blood required is prescribed, checked and signed for. Administration of tranexamic acid if required and not previously administered at scene of trauma. Applies pelvic binder if required and if not in situ already. Performs chest decompression and inserts chest drain. Performs CPR. Prescribes and administers analgesia. Assists with 20-degree tilt for secondary survey. If required and trained, performs FAST scan as instructed by team leader.

Continued

TABLE 36.3	**Role of the Trauma Team Members—cont'd**
Role	**Responsibilities**
Nurse 1 – Monitoring Nurse: ED Nurse/PICU Nurse	Prepares warming devices - Bair hugger.
	Prepares monitoring equipment.
	Warms IV fluids and primes giving sets.
	Prepares chest drain(s).
	Applies monitoring equipment: three-lead ECG, BP cuff, SpO_2 probe, defib pads.
	Sets monitors to required cycling time.
	Reports vital signs to team leader and scribe.
	Records patient's temperature by the most appropriate means.
	Have scissors ready and remove all of the patient's clothing and store securely.
	Cover patient with Bair hugger/sheets/blankets.
	Collects urine sample if required.
	Assists with procedures: line insertion, catheter insertion/drains.
	Prepares for safe transfer.
Nurse 2 – Procedures Nurse. ED Nurse/ENP/PICU Nurse	Remove all the patients clothing with nurse one.
	Assists with securing IV access.
	Prepares IO kit.
	Prepares and assists with advanced procedures: chest drain insertion, arterial lines, central lines, urinary catheters.
	Assists with 20-degree tilt
	Manages the administration of blood and blood product transfusion.
	Performs CPR.
	Prepares for transfer.
Drugs Nurse: Senior ED Nurse/ PICU Nurse	Clearly identifiable and delineated by wearing suitable coloured apron.
	Has no other task during resuscitation procedures other than drug and fluid preparation and administration.
	Prepares drug chart prior to arrival of patient.
	Prepares fluid boluses based on estimated weight of patient.
	Prepares drugs as requested: anaesthetic agents, antibiotics, analgesia, emergency drugs using resuscitation guidelines.
	Prepares intravenous fluids for infusions and additional fluid boluses.
	Checks all drugs and intravenous fluids with second staff member making sure they have been prescribed, signed for and are labelled clearly.
	Ensures all drugs and fluids administered are signed for by the clinician who administered them.
	Ensures controlled drug records are accurate, updated and signed.
	Prepares and organises any drugs required for the transfer of the patient to CT/theatres/definitive care location.
Radiographer	Ensures all team are wearing lead aprons as required.
	Performs imaging following primary survey and as ordered by team leader.
	Performs imaging following secondary survey as ordered by team leader.
	Discusses with CT radiographer availability of CT scanner.
Scribe – ED Nurse	Utilises ED trauma recordkeeping document pack.
	Records the names, grades, roles allocated, and specialties of all staff present and time of arrival.
	Notes time of arrival of patient into resuscitation bay. Ensures clock is started when patient arrives.
	Records all vital signs including GCS, completes PEWS scores. Communicates trends in physiological findings to team leader.
	Records all findings and procedures undertaken noting salient points from primary survey.
	Records drug doses, time given and route of administration.
	Documents time of transfer to CT/theatres.
	Compiles all documents and patients' belongings prior to transfer. Packs evidence bags as required.
	Applies wrist and allergy bands onto patient.
Family support: ED Nurse/ENP/ Junior Doctor/ Play Specialist/ Support Worker	Meets family on arrival and stays with them throughout resuscitation - this may be in the resuscitation bay or in the relative's room.
	Identifies personnel to the family and their roles.
	Provide updates for the family regarding their child's care.
	Contact other family members on behalf of the family.
	Contact other hospital support staff – Chaplin/Spiritual leader as required.
	Provide refreshments for the family as required.
	Sit with family during updates from medical staff.
	In the event of the death of their child, remain with the family at all times; when they are being informed and while they are in the ED.

TABLE 36.3	Role of the Trauma Team Members—cont'd
Role	**Responsibilities**
Runner – Health Care Support Worker	Informs and directs trauma/specialist teams to correct resus bay.
	Processes blood gas analysis and returns result to team leader.
	Collecting and ensuring blood samples are delivered to laboratory.
	Obtains O-negative blood from blood bank as directed by team leader
	Obtains blood products from blood bank as directed by team leader.
	Obtains any equipment required by team leader from PICU/theatres.
Specialist teams: E.G. burns, vascular, neurological, cardiac, orthopaedic teams	Assist with secondary survey.
	Performs advanced procedures as indicated by the team leader.
	Provides expert advice.

aMajor haemorrhage protocol.

CPR, Cardiopulmonary resuscitation; CT, computed tomography; ECG, electrocardiogram; ED, emergency department; ENP, emergency nurse practitioner; FAST, focused assessment with sonography for trauma; GCS, Glasgow Coma Scale; PEWS, Paediatric Early Warning Scores; PICU, paediatric intensive care unit; PPE, personal protective equipment.

There are a total of 70 standards for children's and young people's emergency care, including the following themes:

1. Service design: an integrated urgent care service
2. Environment in emergency care settings
3. Management of the sick or injured child
4. Staffing and training
5. Safeguarding in emergency care settings
6. Mental health, substance and alcohol misuse
7. Major incidents involving children and young people
8. Death of a child
9. Safe transfer
10. Information systems and data analysis
11. Research for paediatric emergency care

The Royal College of Paediatricians and Child Health (RCPCH, 2018) stipulates that a nominated consultant anaesthetist, suitably trained in paediatric anaesthesia, should be responsible for children's services. It is important to train the right team members, with the right skills and abilities; successful results in a trauma situation are determined by the training and abilities of the trauma team.

A paediatrician should be included in the emergency care team for seriously traumatised children. After initial resuscitation and stabilisation, children should be transferred to the care of paediatric surgeons in a specialist facility with paediatric intensive care back-up.

Any hospital receiving and caring for the severely injured child must have on-site support from paediatricians and paediatric anaesthetists.

CHILDREN'S NURSES IN EMERGENCY DEPARTMENTS

The development of A&E nursing has been at the forefront of role extension within the UK and the development of a faculty of emergency nursing within the Royal College of Nursing (RCN) has allowed nurses working within the domain to agree and establish levels of clinical competencies (RCN, 2010 and 2015). The RCPCH (2018) standards identify that there must be at least two registered children's nurse in the department per shift and they must possess recognisable post-registration trauma and emergency training. This requirement includes advanced life-support training. It is very helpful that this set of standards mandates training requirements. The Emergency Nurse Practitioner is now an established role in many children's ED departments throughout the UK.

Safety in Hospital

Improving safety in hospitals for children has been the quest of the RCPCH for a number of years. They decreed that robust systems are required to prevent necessary mortalities and morbid items for preventable sequelae (RCPCH, 2016).

Situational awareness considers the perspective of everyone involved in the care of the child, including the child and their families, as well as doctors, nurses, allied health professionals and support staff, with a view to enabling the correct clinical decisions to be made.

The primary aim of the Situation Awareness for Everyone (SAFE) programme was to reduce avoidable error and harm to sick children in hospital by building a safety-based culture Glasper, (2016).

In addition, the introduction of the SAFE programme sought to:

- Improve communication between all health care professionals involved in the care of the child.
- Reduce avoidable errors and harm in the acute care setting.
- Reduce the gap in health outcomes for children in the UK compared with other countries.

The SAFE resource consists of six separate elements, which when employed together form a safe approach. These are:

1. Quality improvement
2. Patient safety culture
3. Structure communication
4. Recognising deterioration
5. The 'huddle'
6. Evaluation and spread

Structured communication has been identified as a necessary strategy to reduce poor outcomes for children in hospital. The key to effective communication when providing care for the sick child is the health care team knowing the precise information about that child and family. Confidence to express ones view as part of the health care team is essential if there are to be no barriers in communication. The SAFE resource recommends the use of communication tools such as Situation, Background, Assessment, Recommendation (SBAR or CUSS (Concern, Uncomfortable, unSafe, Stop). The CUSS tool is most often initiated during a procedure or if instructed to perform a task. The SBAR tool is now widely applied to everyday communication. The use of structured communication is a key element in providing safe and effective care.

The use of early warning scores has helped to identify the deteriorating child and enable rapid treatment. Used across neonatal care and in the care of children and young people, the primary aim of the huddle is to ensure all the information about a patient is known to all who need to know it. It involves the multi-disciplinary team. This mechanism proactively shares all the required information to those that have a vested interest in knowing that information in order to make effective decisions about care.

The Environment in the Emergency Department

Often, the first point of contact or portal of entry to hospital is through the emergency department (ED). The ED can be a distressing place, full of unfamiliar sights and sounds and little opportunity to prepare children for this experience. Depending on their particular stage of cognitive development, children will interpret the situations into terms they can conceptualise. In turn, the child's perceptions and experiences in the A&E or emergency room will affect future attendances; the right staff and the right environment can have a dramatic impact (Dudley et al., 2015). The provision of services for children should be appropriate to their cognitive and developmental needs. Children are now mainly cared for in designated areas. Privacy is important and the provision of play facilities is now standard. They should be attended to by staff who have been suitably trained and educated to care for children and trained in emergency management and procedures.

Triage, Streaming and 'See and Treat' in Emergency Department

Children who arrive at the ED are unselected on arrival, even if referred by an urgent care centre or GP. Triage has been widely adopted and is generally considered an efficient way of 'sorting' those very urgent needs from those with less urgent needs, and in managing emergency departments. Triage, however, can only be truly effective if the process takes place on arrival. Triage also needs to be a continual process, so that deterioration in children with initially lower priority can be recategorised.

Triage is an integral part of the modern emergency department. The use of a recognised triage system has many advantages for the emergency department, including reference to a recognised decision-making structure and support in the form of a professionally accepted and validated system. Many units use the Manchester triage system, which is a method of identifying high-priority patients. The word 'triage' comes from the French 'to sort' and has its origins in the management of battlefield casualties. There are a number of definitions and Scoble (2004), for example, describes triage as a process of nurse assessment of a patient on arrival in an

---

BOX 36.1   Triage Categories

Triage Category 1
- People who need to have treatment immediately (in practice, within 2 minutes) are called immediately life-threatening patients.
- People in this group are critically ill and require immediate attention. Most would have arrived at the emergency department by ambulance. They would probably be suffering from something like a critical injury or cardiac arrest.

Triage Category 2
- People who need to have treatment within 10 minutes are called imminently life-threatening patients.
- People in this group would probably be suffering from something like a critical illness or very severe pain. People with serious chest pains, difficulty in breathing and severe fractures are included in this group.

Triage Category 3
- People who need to have treatment within 30 minutes are called potentially life-threatening patients.
- People in this group would probably be suffering from something like severe illnesses, major bleeding from cuts, major fractures or dehydration.

Triage Category 4
- People who need to have treatment within 1 hour are called potentially serious patients.
- People in this group would probably have less severe symptoms or injuries with something like a foreign body in the eye, sprained ankle, migraine or earache.

Triage Category 5
- People who need to have treatment within 2 hours are called less urgent patients.
- People in this group probably have minor illnesses or symptoms that may have been present for more than a week, like rashes or minor aches and pains.

Triage categories 1–5 were previously described as resuscitation, emergency, urgent, semi-urgent and non-urgent.

---

emergency department. All the definitions are consistent in that they describe triage as the categorising of sick or injured patients according to severity in order to coordinate care and ensure the most efficient use of emergency department staff and facilities (Box 36.1).

The Manchester triage system uses 52 flow charts, which allocate patients to one of the five national triage categories described above. Willis describes an enhancement to the Manchester triage system known as CWILTED (Willis, 2001):
- C = Condition: area of pain, problem, child protection.
- W = Witness: name, position and designation of person who actually saw the incident; if nobody saw the incident write 'none'.
- I = Incident: mechanism that caused the injury.
- L = location: home address, school, childminder (name and address), park or play area.
- T = Time: time accident occurred and date, time first aid given (including medication), time of last meal.

BOX 36.2 Methods of Relieving Childhood Pain in Emergency Departments

- Local anaesthesia infiltrated into the wound: simple and safe but potentially painful. This can be counteracted by using a small-bore needle or a warmed solution.
- Topical anaesthesia: EMLA (not for infants under a year) or Ametop (not for infants under 1 month). Good for preparing for cannulation or venipuncture but not for use in open wounds or mucous membranes which makes them unsuitable for use in the cleaning or suturing of wounds.
- Field block: local anaesthesia is injected around the perimeter of a wound or abscess a centimetre away from the edge. Takes longer to work but prevents the reduction of the desired anaesthetic effect, which occurs when local is infiltrated into infected areas, which have increased vascularity.
- Peripheral nerve block: this involves the injection of local into the area of a peripheral nerve to provide anaesthesia to the area of the body distal to the area being infiltrated. Commonly used to provide femoral (good for fractures of the shaft of femur before x-ray and application of traction) or digital nerve block (good for avulsed finger nails or draining of paronychia).
- Paracetamol: good for mild pain (can be given rectally).
- Non-steroidal anti-inflammatory drugs such as ibuprofen: not recommended for children younger than 1 year but useful for moderate pain, especially that caused by musculoskeletal trauma. Contraindicated in patients with a history of gastrointestinal bleeding or renal impairment. Can cause bronchospasm in asthmatic children.
- Nitrous oxide: in a mixture of 70% with 30% oxygen this gas is effective for venous cannulation. It is painless to administer and the children can control their own dispensation through a mouthpiece. In a 50:50 mixture, nitrous oxide has good analgesic effect.
- Opioids: codeine is a good drug for mild to moderate pain; its effect is enhanced when it is combined with paracetamol. Morphine is an excellent choice for severe pain such as that caused by burns or fractures; the intravenous route is preferred. Diamorphine administered intranasally has been shown to be effective in children with fractures of the long bones. Pethidine has a shorter duration than morphine with less sedative effects. However, pethidine can cause nausea and sometimes convulsions. Fentanyl is a synthetic opioid that can be administered intravenously or intranasally. It has a rapid onset and short duration but can cause respiratory depression. It should be used with caution in emergency departments. Ketamine has analgesic, anaesthetic and dissociative state properties but also has side effects and known complications. It should only ever be used by experienced clinicians in a controlled environment with access to full resuscitation equipment (Royal College of Emergency Medicine 2020). Paracetamol oral solution/suspension is available in 120 mg in 5 mL and 250 mg in 5 mL.
- 1% lidocaine is most commonly used for local anaesthetic infiltration prior to suturing children's wounds. This drug comes as 10 mg/mL and maximum dosages to achieve local anaesthesia are 3 mg/kg.

- E = Escort: it should not be automatically assumed that an accompanying adult is a parent. Does this person have parental responsibility? If they did not witness the accident, how do they know what happened?
- D = Disability: initially this was called 'description', but this tended to repeat 'condition' and triage staff have modified this to be disability caused by the incident or diagnosis, if known at the time. Willis (2001) notes that the staff in one emergency department reverted to 'description', that is, to mean what the appearance of the child, their behaviour and so forth, because 'disability' did not always appear appropriate when the child had a medical presentation.

Immediate and continued triage requires nursing staff to be constantly available and assigned to triage duties. This is often difficult with a less than optimal nursing establishment. The emergency situation that can be visualised is more likely to take precedence than the potential one waiting for triage. One needs to be reminded of the 'duty care' to all patients and the emergency department shift coordinator holds the ultimate responsibility for deployment of nursing and medical colleagues.

Streaming

Streaming is now used more commonly than triage. This is the process of allocating patients to specific areas or services so they will receive efficient and effective care. This objective is to ensure the patient is located in the correct area/service and the correct health care professional will manage their health needs. This may include locating a patient to a specialist service within a hospital. As an example, if the child has an eye injury, they could be sent to the Ophthalmology Department. Safety is paramount when streaming is used and the system must incorporate safeguards so continued assessment and observations of the child as clinically indicated will be undertaken. Streaming may be:

- Simple streaming: based on clinical assessment alone
- Complex streaming: involves an assessment of priority and acuity, correct service at the correct time

Streaming should be performed as soon as possible after arrival in the ED, ideally within 15 minutes (Royal College of Emergency Medicine [RCEM], 2017).

'See and Treat'

This system refers directly to seeing and treating patients who have presented with a minor illness or injury. This is often the type of patient that the Emergency Nurse Practitioner will see. The episode of care can be completed quickly, which is advantageous to the child and family. A streaming system may be in place directing the flow of 'See and Treat' patients. However, safeguards must be in place so the child that requires immediate attention receives it and is not left waiting,

Early Warning Scores

Early warning scores help detect alterations to the physiology of the child, which lead to a deteriorating health status. Paediatric Early Warning Scores (PEWS) have been developed to provide a common language in order to identify the seriously unwell and deteriorating child. By using a PEWS in the ED, a baseline is formed from which improvement or deterioration can be detected. PEWS should not be used in isolation for streaming (RCEM, 2017) as there is a risk of missing the child with a significant pathology that may not have fully manifested at the time of triage or streaming.

The use of early warning scoring systems is now usurping many traditional systems of assessing the child in the emergency department. The vital signs that must be recorded are heart rate, respiratory rate and blood pressure. Oxygen saturation and amount of oxygen being administered should also be recorded (Gormley-Fleming, 2017). There are many variations of early warning scores in use, which may require measurement of different physical signs. PEWS enable health care professionals to intervene early and prevent deterioration of the child's condition.

Recognition and Assessment of Pain

Integral to the process of triage, children have their pain assessed. Triage priority is often determined by severity of pain. This allows for the child's pain to be managed at the earliest opportunity. Once pain management is determined and the child made more comfortable, it may be possible to recategorise to a lower priority.

Pain assessment in the emergency department is often difficult, particularly with children. Having sustained an injury or illness causes the child anxiety. Children will be frightened of being in a strange environment and not knowing what is going to happen next, and often think that what happened is their fault and fear punishment. Children often imagine the worst outcome of their pain, or they will deny their pain entirely. Many health care professionals hold unfounded beliefs that because children are not crying, they cannot be in pain. By the same rule it is often said 'that children who make the loudest noise usually experience the least pain'.

Pain assessment tools should be used at the time of the initial assessment. The ideal pain assessment tool in the emergency department should be age appropriate, user friendly, and simple and quick to use. As part of the initial assessment, analgesia should be administered within 20 minutes of the arrival of the child (RCPCH, 2018).

Verbal descriptor scales when working with children are extremely helpful. Depending on their cognitive stage of development, children often are unable to express the intensity of their pain. By understanding the mechanism of injury and the effect the injury has on the child, it is not unreasonable to anticipate the level of pain when a child is unable to express the intensity.

ACTIVITY

- What methods of pain relief are available to emergency nurses to administer?
- Discuss the role of distraction and complementary therapies.

SCENARIO

Kate is a 10-year-old female. She lives with her parents and younger sibling Alice. Kate travels to school by school bus. She was anxious to get home and stepped out from the front of the school bus and was hit by a car travelling at approximately 30 miles per hour. She was flung up into the air and landed on her back onto the road. The emergency services were alerted, and first aid was commenced by the bus driver. Kate was maintaining her own airway and was making incomprehensible sounds. Her right leg was abnormally angulated and there was mid-thigh swelling. She had a laceration to her forehead, occiput and right ear. Her right forearm was also grossly angulated. The ambulance team arrived and performed an initial assessment and concluded that as this was a major trauma the assistance of the pre-hospital major trauma care team was required. The air ambulance was dispatched. Her level of consciousness deteriorated at the scene. Glasgow Coma Scale (GCS) was 12. She had decreased air entry on her right side. There was a poor peripheral pulse to her right foot. She had a grade 2 radial pulse in her right wrist. She was becoming agitated. Following systematic assessment Airway, Breathing, Circulation, Disability, Exposure, a decision was made to transfer to the MTU. She was intubated for the transfer as she was becoming increasingly agitated, immobilised to protect her cervical spine, her fractures were reduced and splinted, intravenous access was secured, and fluids were administered. She was placed in a position that allowed a 20- to 30-degree head tilt upwards position. By the time she arrived at the MTU her condition started to improve.

On arrival, Kate is taken into the paediatric resuscitation area, where the emergency team are waiting. Handover is given to the team and the team leader acknowledges that the Kate is now in their care. A primary survey is commenced – Airway, Breathing, Circulation, Disability – to determine if there is any immediate threat to life.

What are the priorities in the management of her injuries?

As the nurse responsible for communicating with the family, plan how you will describe her injuries and likely treatment to her parents.

Refer to the NICE guideline CG176 (2019): *Head Injury: Assessment and Early Management*. What would best evidence suggest for the management of Kate's head injury as she has presented – agitated, incomprehensible sounds, decreasing GCS and sluggish pupils.

FAMILY-CENTRED CARE IN THE EMERGENCY DEPARTMENT

Previously, families have not been allowed to participate in or be present at certain invasive procedures involving children in emergency departments. However, families are now viewed as partners in the delivery of care and the barriers that impede the implementation of family-friendly protocols and procedures have been removed. The admission of parents/guardians to areas of the hospital that have traditionally excluded them has been slow, and emergency departments have only recently acknowledged that the presence of parents during invasive procedures is actually helpful, not only for the practising nurse, but also for the child and family as a whole. Eppich and Arnold (2003) previously describe how family members can contribute to the overall care of the child during such procedures, and furthermore, can be present during cardiopulmonary resuscitation (CPR). A large body of evidence suggests that parental presence during hospital procedures is helpful to a child during a stressful procedure (Glasper and Powell, 2000). The improved understanding of the parental concerns adds an 'acceptable sensitivity' to the diagnosis. The value of the parental concern on admission to the ED must never be overlooked. However, the balance between a helpful presence at a time of emotional turmoil should be weighed up. In most cases, the parent will wish to be present and post-resuscitation care should be offered through normal support mechanisms.

ACTIVITY: A PROFESSIONAL CONVERSATION

Anisha is a third-year student who is in her final semester of her children's nursing programme. She is undertaking a clinical placement in an emergency department in a secondary care environment.

There are not always sufficient children's nurses on duty to ensure that all children are appropriately managed due to staff sickness. Anisha is working an early shift with her practice assessor Sally and they are reflecting on an event the previous day, when a mother was refused entry to the resuscitation room. The 18-month-old child was not successfully resuscitated, and the mother later complained that she regretted not being present during this last period of her child's life.

Discuss this scenario with a colleague/peer.

Paediatric Resuscitation

Although paediatric events that require resuscitation are rare, it is important that all nurses understand the principles of successful resuscitation. Castle (2002) suggests that most district general hospitals will have less than one paediatric cardiac arrest per week. It is the rarity of this event that makes it emotionally difficult for those in emergency departments. Parra et al. (2018) showed that relatives want to be present during their child's resuscitation. The parents all reported feeling nervous, but they trusted the emergency team were doing the best for their child. It is, however, important to recognise that there are both positive and negative aspects of family presence during this stressful event. Although family presence during a resuscitation procedure is becoming more usual in emergency departments, many members of the interprofessional team still have concerns and doubts about it. The nurses should take into account the views of relatives, although resuscitation procedures should never be compromised by the presence of family members. Evidence suggests

that it can improve the grieving process for families and be helpful to patients who survive (Bauchner, 2014).

Paediatric Intensive Care

The team approach allows critically ill or traumatised patients optimal chances for survival. The distribution of trauma deaths has been described as being 'trimodal'. Fifty percent of all trauma deaths occur before medical attention can be provided. The first peak in mortality occurs at the time of injury or shortly after. The second peak of the trimodal experience occurs within the first hours of injury. It is in this phase that the emergency care team response can make a difference in provision of care to prevent death as a result of 'airway, breathing and circulatory problems'. The term the 'golden hour' is often used to describe this second phase of the trimodal theory. Having survived the initial trauma, resuscitation and stabilisation patients who die in the third trimodal stage commonly die in intensive care from multi-system failure.

The paediatric intensive care report *Framework for the Future* (NHS Executive, 1997, p 7) describes three levels of care for the critically ill or injured child. Level one, often referred to as high-dependency care, is greater than that care provided on an acute paediatric ward or department. Children requiring level-one care require close observation, continuous heart monitoring, non-invasive blood pressure monitoring or single organ support not including respiratory support. Children who fall into level one may be experiencing severe breathing difficulties like croup, suspected intestinal obstruction or poisoning. Level two is defined as the level of care for children requiring assisted ventilation either due to respiratory absence or single system failure requiring respiratory support. Level three is defined as children with multi-system failure requiring advanced respiratory support.

Safeguarding

Children's nurses must be able to recognise potential problems in relation to children and their interaction with their immediate family or carers. All health care staff must be competent enough to recognise maltreatment and take appropriate actions to safeguard the child. The employer has a duty to ensure appropriate training is in place for all staff and this is an explicit part of all NHS employment contracts. Each organisation is responsible for determining and maintaining their own quality standards in regard to safeguarding. They need to ensure policies and processes are in place and that there is safeguarding culture embedded throughout the organisation. This will include recruitment policies, training and education, risk assessments and risk registers, mechanisms for reporting and evaluation critical incidents, review and audit of policies and processes and an appraisal system (RCPCH, 2013). It is also important that all staff have an appreciation of the role of external regulators such as Care Quality Commission (CQC). There should be two nominated leads for safeguarding; a consultant and a senior nurse.

Child protection issues are often identified when observing the dynamics between the child and family. While undertaking assessment of any child it is important to identify non-verbal information as much as the verbal information gathered. The non-verbal clues might indicate lack of eye contact, withdrawn body posture, facial expression and tone of voice. These are all factors that can encourage or discourage the flow of information between the nurse and the parents.

Nurses who use verbal cues such as open-ended questions, active listening and empathy, can demonstrate to the parents that what they are saying is important and is helping in the care of their ill child. This is a continual process and should be two-way between the parent and nurse to facilitate the development of trust and confidence in the nursing and medical staff. This can begin the development in care of a partnership with the parents.

Social interaction manifests in numerous forms of non-verbal communication; children's nurses use non-verbal cues to eliminate, amplify or expand on what is expressed in words. The use of eye contact during conversations is a process by which each individual demonstrates attention and involvement in the conversation by regularly looking into the eyes of the other; staring intently can indicate evasiveness. Facial expressions, gestures and body posture can convey what is really meant, even when nothing is actually said.

In the case of major trauma as a result of non-accidental injury care pathways should be utilised (Davies et al., 2017).

It is important that the ED nursing staff have access to training and ongoing safeguarding supervision appropriate to their role. Safeguarding advice should be accessible 24 hours a day from a paediatrician who had completed advanced training in safeguarding.

The Role of Play

The provision of therapeutic play facilities within emergency departments is of crucial importance in the management of children attending. A good hospital play therapist will be aware of a child's developmental needs and can often determine the toys and therapeutics that each child needs for distraction from painful procedures.

Emergency Paediatric Nurse Practitioners

The expansion of roles within the emergency departments was first described by Jones and Smith (1998), who articulate the challenge of assessing and treating children in the emergency department for independent practitioners. To date, there is no national recognised course for the training and development of registered children's nurses to become emergency nurse practitioners (ENPs). However, there has been an area of growth around clinical assessment of children, although again this has yet to gain national recognition. Yet little is known about the impact of the ENP in the children's ED Feetham et al (2015), Crouch & Brown (2018). However, some early evaluations show the advantage of such roles. Muller et al. (2018) identified that the presence of ENPs improved patient flow through the ED. One of the challenges of this role is that they have been developed in response to local demand and case mix resulting in inconsistencies in job descriptions, education requirements and scope of practice. The 2017 Health Education England framework has identified a cross-discipline focus with key principles. This should enable a consistent approach in developing the core capabilities and a credentialing process.

SUMMARY

The emergency care of children and young people has changed significantly in the last decade. First contact emergency care for children and young people is a growing area of nursing. A number of national initiatives highlight the pivotal role of emergency departments in the care of sick children and their families.

Children and young people nurses will continue to play a big role in ensuring that emergency care for their client group is commensurate with the age group, continuum of growth and development. Health promotion must be a feature of emergency care and has not been considered within the context of this chapter.

REFERENCES

Advanced Life Support Group, 2017. Pre-Hospital Paediatric Life Support. A Practical Approach to Emergencies, third ed. Wiley Blackwell, Oxford.

Audit Commission, 1993. Children First: A Study of Hospital Services. HMSO, London.

Baker, C., 2017. Accident and Emergency Statistics: Demand, Performance, and Pressure. Briefing paper 6964. House of Commons Library.

Bauchner, H., 2014. Parental presence during cardiopulmonary resuscitation: uncommon but yet necessary. J. Dis. Child. 99 (4).

Crouch, R., Brown, R., 2018. Advanced clinical practitioners in emergency care: past, present and future. Br. J. Hosp. Med. 79 (7).

Davies, F.C., Lecky, F.E., Fisher, R., et al., 2017. Major trauma from suspected child abuse: a profile of patient pathway. Emerg. Med. 34, 562–567.

Department of Health and Social Security (DHSS), 1976. Fit for the Future (the Court Report). The Report of the Committee on Child Health Services. HMSO, London.

Department of Health (DoH), 1991. Welfare of Children and Young People in Hospital. HMSO, London.

Department of Health (DoH), 1996. The Patient's Charter – Services for Children and Young People. HMSO, London.

Department of Health (DoH), 2000. The NHS Plan: A Plan for Investment, a Plan for Reform. The Stationery Office, London.

Department of Health (DoH), 2003. Online. Available from: https://assets.publishing.service.gov.uk/government/uploads/system/uploads/attachment_data/file/199953/Getting_the_right_start_-_National_Service_Framework_for_Children_Standard_for_Hospital_Services.pdf.

Department of Health (DoH), 2004. The National Service Framework for Children, Young People and Maternity Services. Online. Available from: http://www.dh.gov.uk.

Dudley, N., Ackerman, A., Brown, K., et al., 2015. Patient and family centred care of children in the emergency department. Pediatrics 135 (1), 255–272.

Feetham, J.E., Christian, W., Benger, J.R., et al., 2015. Paediatric ED reattendance rates: comparing nurse practitioners and other clinicians. Emerg. Med. 32, 379–382.

Glasper, E.A., 2016. Keeping sick children in hospital SAFE from harm. BJN 25 (20).

Glasper, E.A., Powell, C., 2000. First do no harm: parental exclusion from anaesthetic rooms. Paediatr. Nurs. 12 (4), 14–17.

Gormley-Fleming, E., 2017. Pews. In: Gormley-Fleming, E., Martin, D. (Eds.), Clinical Skills Children and Young Peoples Nursing. Clinical Skills at a Glance. Wiley Blackwell.

International Federation of Emergency Medicine, 2014. International Standards for Children in Emergency Departments. Victoria, Australia.

Kanani, A.N., Hartshorn, S., 2017. NICE clinical guideline NG39: major trauma: assessment and initial management. Arch. Dis. Child. Educ. Prac. Ed. 102, 20–23.

Keeble, E., Kossarova, L., 2017. Quality Watch. Focus on Emergency Hospital Care for Children and Young People. What Has Changed in the Past 10 Years? Nuffield Trust.

Keogh, B., 2018. Urgent Care and Emergency Review. NHS. Leeds Available from: https://www.nhs.uk/NHSEngland/keogh-review/Pages/about-the-review.aspx. (accessed 29 December 2018).

Kmietowicz, Z., 2018. A & E attendance in England are growing twice as fast as population. BMJ 362.

Ley, E., Webb, T., Chester, A., et al., 2015. Essex and Herts Air Ambulance: a focused case series for pre-hospital practice. Case 5: management of paediatric trauma. J. Paramedic Pract. 7 (9), 438–445.

MacFaul, R., Werneke, U., 2001. Recent trends in hospital use by children in England. Archive of Disease in Childhood 85, 203–207.

Maurice, S.C., O'Donnell, J.J., Beatie, T.F., 2002. Emergency analgesia in the paediatric population. Part II: pharmacological methods of pain relief. Emerg. Med. J. 19, 101–105.

Mercer, S.J., Kingston, E.V., Jones, C.P.L., 2018. The trauma call. BMJ 361 k2272.

Muller, K., Chee, Z., Quynh, D., 2018. Using nurse practitioners to optimize patient flow in a pediatric emergency department. Pediatr. Emerg. Care 34 (6) 396–388.

National Institute for Health and Care Excellence (NICE), 2019. Head Injury, Triage, Assessment Investigation and Early Management of Head Injuries in Infants, Children and Adults. Clinical Guideline [CG176], 4th ed. NICE, London.

National Institute for Health and Care Excellence (NICE), 2016. Major Trauma: Service Delivery. Clinical Guideline [CG40]. NICE, London.

NHS, 2013/14. Everyone Counts: Planning for Patients 2013/14. NHS, Leeds.

NHS, 2013a. National Standard Contract for Major Trauma of All Ages. NHS Commissioning Board, England.

NHS, 2015. Transforming Urgent and Emergency Care Services in England. Safer, Faster, Better: Good Practice in Delivering Urgent and Emergency Care. A Guide for Local Health and Social Care Communities. NHS, Leeds.

NHS, 2017a. Urgent Treatment Centres-Principles and Standards. NHS, England.

NHS, 2018. Summary Report 3. Hospital Accident and Emergency Activity 2017–18.

NHS Advisory Group, 2010. Regional Networks for Major Trauma. NHS, Leeds.

NHS Confederation, 2003 Getting the Right Start: Standard for Hospital Services. Briefing June N87.

NHS Digital, 2017. Hospital Accident and Emergency Activity 2015–16. NHS Digital (accessed March 4, 2019).

NHS Digital, 2017. Hospital Accident and Emergency Activity 2015/16. NHS Digital. Available from: www.content.digital.nhs.

uk/catalogue/PUB23070/acci-emer-atte-eng-2015-16-rep.pdf (accessed 3 January 2019).

NHS Digital, 2017. Hospital Accident and Emergency Activity 2016–17 Summary Report. NHS, Leeds.

NHS East of England, 2013. TEMPO Guidelines. NHS, East of England Trauma Network.

NHS England, 2014. Five Year Forward View. Available from: https://www.england.nhs.uk/wp-content/uploads/2014/10/5yfv-web.pdf.

NHS Executive, 1997. Paediatric Intensive Care: A Framework for the Future. Report of the National Co-Ordinating Group on Intensive Care to the Chief Executive of the NHS Executive. NHSE, London.

Office for National Statistics, 2018. Hospital Accident and Emergency Statistics Parliament UK. Available from: http//:researchbriefing.files.parliment.uk//research. (accessed 20 January 2019).

Parra, C., Mele, M., Alonso, I., et al., 2018. Parent experience in the resuscitation room: how do they feel? Eur. J. Pediatr. 177 (12), 1859–1862.

Parslow, R.C., Morris, K.P., Tasker, R.C., 2005. Epidemiology of traumatic brain injury in children receiving intensive care in the UK. Arch. Dis. Child. 90, 1182–1187.

Reavley, P., 2014. The challenges of pre-hospital paediatric trauma care. J. Paramedic Pract. 6 (10), 18–22.

Royal College of Emergency Medicine, 2017. Initial Assessment of Emergency Department Patients. Safe, Efficient, Effective Care. RCPCH, London.

Royal College of Nursing, 2010. Maximising Nursing Skills in Caring for Children in Emergency Departments. RCN, London.

Royal College of Nursing, 2015. National Curriculum and Competency Framework Emergency Nursing (Level 1). RCN, London.

Royal College of Paediatrics and Child Health (RCPCH), 2012. Standards for Children and Young People in Emergency Care Settings. RCPCH, London.

Royal College of Paediatrics and Child Health, 1999. Accident and Emergency Services for Children: Report of a Multidisciplinary Working Party. RCPCH, London.

Royal College of Paediatrics and Child Health (RCPCH), 2013. Safeguarding Children and Young People: Roles and Competencies for Health Care Staff. Intercollegiate Document, third ed. RCPCH, London.

Royal College of Paediatrics and Child Health (RCPCH), 2016. Introduction to the S.A.F.E Resource Pack. RCPCH. (accessed March 8, 2019). Available from: https://www.rcpch.ac.uk/resources/safe-system-framework-children-risk-deterioration#introduction.

Available from: Royal College of Paediatrics and Child Health (RCPCH), 2018. Facing the Future: Standards for Children and Young People in Emergency Care Settings. RCPCH, London.

Royal College of Emergency Medicine, 2020. Ketamine Procedural Sedation for Children in the Emergency Department. RCEM, London.

Seid, T., Ramaiah, R., Grabinsky, A., 2012. Pre-hospital care of pediatric patients with trauma. Int. J. Crit. Illn. Inj. Sci. 2 (3), 114–120.

Tiel Groenesteng-Kreb, D., van Maarseveen, O., Leenen, L., 2014. Trauma team. British Journal of Anaesthesia 113 (2), 258–265.

Willis, M.A., 2001. Cwilted. Emerg. Nurse 8 (9), 18–22.

Young, M., 2018. A&E Attendances by Young People with Psychiatric Conditions Almost Double in Five Years-New Figures. Press release. Available from: https://youngminds.org.uk/about-us/media-centre/press-releases/ae-attendances-by-young-people-with-psychiatric-conditions-almost-doubled-in-five-years-new-figures/.

37

Pharmacological Interventions, Calculations, Administration and Evaluation

Arija Parker

LEARNING OUTCOMES

- To be able to outline the roles and responsibilities of a children and young person's (CYP) nurse in relation to safe management of medicines.
- To self-assess numerical ability via a diagnostic assessment and review the process of calculating medications for children and young people.
- To have a baseline knowledge of the key pharmacological principles that underpin our practice and knowledge of how children and young people are different from

adults and so need special considerations during the prescribing, administering, monitoring and evaluation processes.

- To explore the issue of working in a concordant way with children, young people and their families so promoting adherence to medication regimes.
- To explore how children learn about numbers to aid the process of promoting independence and self-efficacy in relation to management of medicines.

INTRODUCTION

This chapter offers a brief, though comprehensive, introduction to the safe management of medicines when working in partnership with children, young people and their families/carers. The management of medicines is a significant part of our workload as children's nurses whether working in acute or community settings, where medicines will be prescribed, administered and taken by most children during the course of their childhood – even if this is only an occasional dose of paracetamol and vitamins – or administering the immunisation schedule. The chapter covers pharmacology and interventions that support the knowledge base a nurse needs to possess to work with other health care professionals and service users, a section on how to calculate safely and accurately, the principles of safe administration and how to evaluate the effectiveness of the process overall – has the medicine that has been administered had the therapeutic outcome that was desired?

The Nursing and Midwifery Council (NMC) (2018) nursing and midwifery education and training standards that guide practice in the UK are used to focus and structure the discussion, realising that this is an introduction to the key principles where further research will be needed to generate deeper knowledge in this key area of our practice. The first section on numeracy and medicine-related calculations serves to develop curiosity and interest and deeper reflection when thinking not only about our own attitudes and abilities when working with numbers, but also those of children, young people and the adults around them and how we work with them to gain numerical proficiency. The next section offers some guidance on how to ensure safe administration of medicines and this is followed by a review of the knowledge base needed in relation to the pharmacokinetics and pharmacodynamics as they relate

to the physiology of children and young people so children are not viewed as 'little adults' in relation to the prescribing and administration of medicines. The chapter concludes with a review of how we can work in partnership working with children and families to promote adherence in relation to medication regimens, as well as promote self-efficacy in medicines management with children and young people who have long-term conditions and are taking medicines on a daily basis.

At the heart of this chapter is the key aim, as taken from Platform 4, Part 3 of the NMC Standards of Proficiency (2018), providing and evaluating care requires that:

> *… registered nurses take the lead in providing evidence-based, compassionate and safe nursing interventions. They ensure that the care they provide and delegate is person-centred and of a consistently high standard. They support people of all ages in a range of care settings. They work in partnership with people, families and carers to evaluate whether care is effective and the goals of care have been met in line with their wishes, preferences and desired outcomes.*
>
> *NMC (2018, p 16)*

Within this proficiency are the central tenets of safe medication administration where the knowledge base is sound and robust and based on the best evidence base and human physiology, which is child focused.

CALCULATING TO PROMOTE SAFE ADMINISTRATION OF MEDICINES

The place of calculation skills as part of safe administration of medicines to children and young people.

The NMC Standards for Proficiency require that 'at point of registration the registered nurse will be able to demonstrate the numeracy, literacy, digital and technological skills required to meet the needs of people in their care to ensure safe and effective nursing practice' (Platform 1: Being an accountable practitioner). Furthermore, in Platform 4 and subsection 4.14 'understand the principles of safe and effective administration and optimisation of medicines in accordance with local and national policies and demonstrate proficiency and accuracy when calculating dosages of prescribed medicines' (NMC, 2018, p 18).

A poor numeracy ability continues to be a significant problem for the UK population as a whole, which includes nurses and the adults in the families they work in partnership with. Government statistics suggest that 17 million adults, that is 49% of the working-age population, have the numeracy level expected of primary school children. The total cost to the UK economy (to the Exchequer, employers and individuals) has been put at £20 billion a year. This has an impact on levels of income for individuals and also their health and well-being, in addition to their children's health and well-being. The impact on productivity in the workplace is also significant just when reflecting on the role of the CYP nurse and how emotions, particularly confidence, around working with numbers will impact on the care provided (National Numeracy, 2017).

This section considers what skills nurses need and offers some strategies on how to improve numeracy skills, where most of the 'how to?' of the basics with numbers – that is adding, subtracting, multiplying and dividing from first principles is included in the PowerPoint presentation supporting this chapter. It includes numeracy-related guidance to revise the basic numerical skills that underpin the calculations skills nurses need, practice examples and links to numeracy resources. There is a wealth of information and resources accessible online. Numeracy books, chiefly written by nurses, that cover all fields of nurses, identify the many different ways of navigating the nurse's way through the world of numbers to help gain proficiency (Parker, 2015). Even if numerical skills are excellent, learning may still progress and develop in the move from administering medicines to also prescribing medicines as part of the future role of the CYP nurse (NMC, 2018).

ACTIVITY

Access the PowerPoint presentation: review and practise basic numeracy skills so able to work from first principles.

Although the purpose of this chapter is not to focus on the negative aspects of medicine administration – we should always have a focus on safe medicine administration – it is worthwhile having a look at some of the errors that will aid our personal assessment of risk to gain proficiency. The National Patient Safety Agency (2007) found that the most serious errors were caused by errors in medicine administration (41%) and prescribing (32%). Medication errors with children were reported from all stages of the medication process, although the majority involved administration of the medicine itself (56%). The main causes are as follows:

Prescribing errors – where medicines prescribed as volume of liquid rather than actual dose and also calculation errors, that is, 5 mL instead of 250 mg.

Dispensing errors – due to labelling errors.

Administration – intravenous drug errors are most common, although other errors may be giving a drug such as paracetamol when a previous dose given was not recorded, a drug being given to the wrong patient or giving the wrong amount, that is, millilitres instead of milligrams.

Additionally, there is a whole list of errors including wrong dose, strength or frequency errors, weighing scale errors and weight in pounds not kilograms. Other factors relate to the environment and human resources such as poor lighting, poorly designed medical devices, confusing labelling, inadequate staffing and the systems of checking that support safe practice. Pentin et al. (2016) offer a comprehensive review of all the factors that contribute to errors in children's nursing practice where the final point made relates to challenging any uncertainties that are present in the overall process – if not sure it is vital to ask questions and check before proceeding with medicines administration.

ACTIVITY

Reflect on Your Numeracy Ability

Have a go at the diagnostic assessment included in the PowerPoint presentation, without using a calculator. Use this to reflect on your ability and identify areas in numeracy practice and calculation dosages which need development.

'To Use' or 'Not to Use' a Calculator

Many nurses are totally dependent on calculators, and numeracy assessments undertaken pre-registration and post-registration usually allow for use of a calculator. However, the use of calculators should not replace the underpinning mathematical knowledge and skill needed to calculate correct medicine dosages (NMC, 2007). Since writing this chapter the NMC guidance has changed and been superceded by other guidance though the quotation is still relevant.

From a numeracy perspective the following quotation is the Gold Standard in relation to nursing with numbers in this chapter and is as follows:

To be numerate means to be competent, confident and comfortable with one's own judgements on how to use mathematics in a particular situation and if so what mathematics to use, how to do it, what degree of accuracy is appropriate and what the answer means in relation to the context.

Coben (2000, p 35)

Relationship Between Numbers and Words – The Language of Numeracy

The fact that literacy and numeracy walk together hand-in-hand cannot be overemphasised, where how a nursing numeracy question is written and phrased has a major impact on how it is interpreted and understood. It can often be difficult to unpick the written language to actually comprehend what needs to be done with the numbers. Once this is done the numeracy problem is usually easy to solve. The prescription chart, if well designed and correctly completed, should help reduce any risk of misunderstanding in relation to numbers and words.

Interpreting the Prescription Chart

The following guidance is taken from the British National Formulary (BNFc, 2019).

- Prescriptions should be written legibly in ink, and in the case of children under 12 years of age, include the age of the child as well as the date of birth and weight of the child.
- Strength of liquid preparations should be clearly stated, e.g. 250 mg/5 mL.
- Unnecessary use of decimal points should be avoided, e.g. 2 mg not 2.0 mg.
- Quantities less than 1 gram should be written in milligrams, e.g. 500 mg not 0.5 g.
- When decimals are unavoidable a zero should appear in front of the decimal point, e.g. 0.5 mg not .5 mg.
- Micrograms and nanograms should not be abbreviated.
- Units should not be abbreviated.

Convention in the BNF is that millilitres should be abbreviated as mL, though ml is recognised as an SI abbreviation. Whether administering 1 mL or 5 mL, the abbreviation remains the same, but 's' should never be added, e.g. 5 mLs is incorrect.

Names of medicines should be written clearly and not abbreviated, using approved titles only. It is preferable to write directions in English without abbreviations, although it is recognised that some Latin abbreviations are used (BNF, 2019). These abbreviations are included in the table below.

Abbreviation	Latin Meaning	English Meaning
a.c.	ante cibum	before meals
ad lib	ad libitum	use as much as you desire; freely
alt. h.	alternis horis	every other hour
Amp		Ampoule
Aq	Aqua	Water
Bis	Bis	Twice
b.d./b.i.d.	bis in die	twice a day or 12 hourly
Cib	cibus	with food
dieb.alt.	diebus alternis	every other day
gtt(s)	guttae(s)	drop(s)
h, hr	hora	hour
Mane	mane	in the morning
m.d.u	more dicto utendus	to be used as directed
Neb	nebula	a spray
Noct	nocte	at night
Od	omne in die	every day/once daily

Abbreviation	Latin Meaning	English Meaning
Per	per	by or through
p.c.	post cibum	after meals
p.o.	per os	by mouth or orally
p.r.	per rectum	Rectally
Prn	pro re nata	as needed
q.d.s or q.i.d	quater die sumendus or quattuor in die	four times a day (or 6 hourly)
SL		sublingually or under the tongue
Stat	statim	Immediately
Sup	supositorium	Suppository
Susp		Suspension
Syr	syrupus	Syrup
Tab	tabella	Tablet
t.d.s.	ter die sumendum	three times a day (or 8 hourly)
t.i.d.	ter in die	three times a day

Math anxiety and lack of confidence in relation to working with numbers is prevalent in society. This is seen in relation to nurses as a professional group, where some nurses and many children and their parents/carers may have *dyscalculia*, the numeracy equivalent of dyslexia (the term used in relation to use of language and writing).

Dyscalculia is a 'condition that affects the ability to acquire arithmetical skills, where those affected have difficulty understanding simple number concepts, lack an intuitive grasp of numbers and have problems learning facts' (Dfes, 2001).

 WWW

Access the following online resources to find out more:
- Dyslexia, dyspraxia and dyscalculia – toolkit for nursing staff (RCN, 2010). Available from: https://www.rcn.org.uk/professional-development/publications/pub-003835.

Using Nursing Formulae

Within a numerical context a formula can be defined as a mathematical rule or relationship expressed in symbols or alternatively a set of symbols and numbers that expresses a fact or rule. For example, $A = \pi r^2$ is the formula for calculating the area of a circle or $E = mc^2$ is Einstein's famous formula relating energy and mass. A formula is a type of equation which shows the relationship between different variables where an equation defines the relationship between two things that are equal, that is, x + 2 = 5. The equals sign defines the relationship.

The children's nursing formula contains the variables of amount in mg and mL (or number of capsules, tablets, etc.), which can sometimes confuse nurses because we are not using the same units, that is, linking mL and mg where giving medicines in suspension form. Learning a formula can be useful, although it is important to recognise the derivation and understand the principles that underpin it so that the result you get is meaningful and real.

The most common way of calculating amounts of medicine required is by using the formula as follows, though more than one method can be used. It helps to recognise that a formula is a calculation based on fractions, ratios and proportions to be able to use the formula effectively as well as efficiently. It is useful to find a way that works and is understood from first principles.

Fig. 37.1 The Children's Nursing Formula

$$\frac{\text{What you want?}}{\text{What you have got?}} \times \frac{\text{What amount it is supplied in?}}{1} = ?$$

This is referred to in various ways in different nursing contexts as demonstrated in the text that follows. Identify the wording that makes more sense to you and use a consistent approach.

Fig. 37.2 Alternative Wording

$$\frac{\text{Strength required}}{\text{Stock strength}} \times \text{Volume of stock solution} = ?$$

OR The NHS formula $\frac{\text{Need}}{\text{Have}} \times \text{Stock} = ?$

The following is a worked example using a variety of ways to calculate the amount needed, including the formula.

Worked Example

Sam aged 2 years has developed an otitis media and has been prescribed a course of antibiotics, flucloxacillin 250 mg. It is available in a suspension consisting of 125 mg of medicine in 5 mL liquid.

How much will you administer?

Start by estimating what the final amount of suspension should be. The prescribed amount, 250 mg, is bigger than 125 mg (as supplied) so you will need more than 5 mL. The final number must be bigger than 5 mL.

The amount can be calculated in many different ways. What follows are some suggestions:

Method 1: Using mental arithmetic.

Some of you at estimations stage will have already identified the amount to be given. Look at the relationship between the numbers involved. How does 250 relate to 125? Can you see that 250 is two times bigger than 100? Therefore you will need twice the amount of liquid, that is, 10 mL.

Method 2: Using proportion.

Using proportion notations calculate as follows:

$5 : 125 :: ? : 250$ **SO** $5 / 125 :: ? 250$ **SO** $5 / 125 \times 250 = ?$

$$\frac{5}{125} \times \frac{250}{1} = 10 \text{ mL}$$

OR
We have 125 mg of the medicine in 5 mL solution, which as a ratio is 125:5.

We need 250 mg.

$$250 \div 125 = 2 \times 5 = 10 \text{ mL}$$

Method 3: Using the children's nursing formula.

$$\frac{\text{What you want}}{\text{What you have got}} \times \text{What volume it is supplied in} = \text{Amount required}$$

$$\frac{250}{125} \times 5 = 10 \text{ mL}$$

Method 4: Another way could be to work out how much of the suspension is equal to 1 mg.
i.e.

$$125\text{MG} = 5\text{ML} \text{ SO } 1\text{MG} = \frac{5}{125} = 0.04 \text{ ML}$$

We need 250mg so we need to multiply 0.04 by 250 = 10mL

The key message that has to be delivered at this stage is to find a method that works and then to practise, practise, practise so that using calculating skills becomes second nature. This can develop confidence and competence to enable safe and comfortable practice.

INTERVENTIONS TO PROMOTE THE SAFE ADMINISTRATION OF MEDICINES TO CHLDREN AND YOUNG PEOPLE

How medicines are administered will be dependent on the health care/social care organisation and the policies that have been developed. This will be influenced by the clinical or community setting and patient/client groups. These are based on the principles developed by the Royal Pharmaceutical Society (RPS) and Royal College of Nursing (RCN) in 2019. They specify that medicines are to be administered in accordance with a prescription, Patient Specific Direction, Patient Group Direction or as directed by Government regulations and legislation.

A useful tool for ensuring safe practice will guide personal practice and this exists in various formats from the Five Rights as the most common version of this tool, to as many as 10 Rights (Edwards and Axe, 2015).

The Rights of Medicine administration are one way of remembering what needs checking in relation to the prescription and the child/young person receiving the medicine – the patient. The key five are discussed first and are then followed by an additional five as suggested by Edwards and Axe (2015).

1. **Right patient** – check verbally by asking the child and/or parent/carer (name and date of birth) and visually (patient name band against prescription chart and by looking at the child). At the same time ensure that you communicate with the child and parent/carer by explaining what you are doing as well as why medication is being given to ensure you have informed consent to proceed.

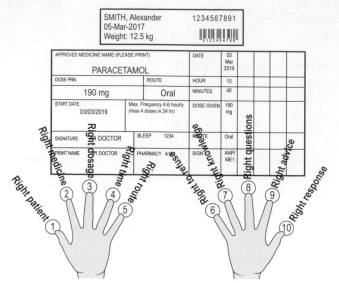

Fig. 37.3 Rights of medicine administration.

2. **Right medicine** – check that the medicine is prescribed by using generic or non-proprietary name (not the trade, patented or brand name), that is, salbutamol not Ventolin, paracetamol not Calpol. It is also important to check dosage strength, that is, paracetamol 120 mg in 5 mL or 250 mg in 5 mL, as one example.

3. **Right dose** – check the dose – the prescriber and the giver of the medication both have a legal responsibility to know what the correct dose is. In children's nursing, medicines are prescribed on the basis of weight so ensure that the child's age and weight is recorded on the prescription chart.

4. **Right time** – check when and how often the medicine should be given, as well as when it was last given, in addition to checking the expiry date.

5. **Right route** – check whether the medicine is to be given orally, parenterally or cutaneously (see abbreviations commonly used later, that is, p.o., IV, etc.).

6. **Right to refuse** – this applies to both the nurse and patient, where many factors will contribute to the nurses decision to give or not give a medicine, which starts with checking the documentation – check that the prescription chart is legible, check for allergies, check for any specific actions you may need to do before giving medication, that is, checking observations and ensure that you sign that you have given the medicine.

7. **Right knowledge** – an in-depth knowledge of how the pharmacokinetics and pharmacodynamics of the medicine as discussed later in this chapter.

8. **Right questions** – is the medicine the best medicine for the individual patient prescribed in a concordant manner by working in partnership with the patient to promote adherence. In relation to children this will relate to how the medicine is supplied, that is, an oral dose of a suspension rather than a tablet and certainly avoiding a route by injection wherever possible. Are

there other health care professionals to support and give advice and are resources such as drug formularies available? The BNF is readily accessible on a mobile device.

9. **Right advice** – the people who prescribe or administer the medicine should be able to give advice about its actions and side effects, as well as finding out about the patient's – child and parent's/carer's – preferences and health beliefs around the medication being administered. This will also ensure you have consent to give the medicine.

10. **Right response** – this includes the monitoring that needs to be done to ensure that the medicine is acting in the way it is meant to as well as identifying any potential harm that may need further reporting via the Yellow Card system (BNF, 2019).

> **⊳ REFLECTION POINT**
>
> Again, it is worth reflecting on and developing a personal approach to remembering the 'rights', or putting some order or structure to the checking process, where adding extra rights such as the right to refuse, right attitude and right expiry date might make the process more meaningful for you. See Fig. 37.3

PHARMACOLOGICAL KNOWLEDGE NEEDED TO SUPPORT SAFE ADMINISTRATION OF MEDICINES TO CYP

With respect to having the right knowledge to administer medicines in Platform 4 subsection 4.15 of the NMC (2018) Standards of Proficiency, nurses at the point of registration need to:

> … *demonstrate knowledge of pharmacology and the ability to recognise the effects of medicines, allergies, drug sensitivities, side effects, contraindications, incompatibilities, adverse reactions, prescribing errors and the impact of polypharmacy and over-the-counter medication usage.*
> **NMC (2018, p 18)**

What follows is a basic outline of some of the key physiological processes that need to underpin our knowledge base in relation to how medicines have an effect on children and young people. The key pharmacological processes where nurses need to have knowledge are pharmacokinetics and pharmacodynamics. The words 'drug' and 'medicine' are used interchangeably in many information sources, although the keyword 'medicine' is used mostly as the preferred term. The word 'drug' tends to have negative connotations whereas a medicine has a more therapeutic perspective on action.

Pharmacokinetics is 'what the body does to the drug' or the study of how a drug (or medicine) is absorbed, distributed, metabolised and excreted, thus ensuring that the principles that result can ensure safe and effective therapeutic

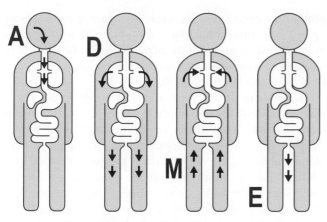

Fig. 37.4 ADME diagram.

TABLE 37.1 Routes of Administration

Route	Description	Example of Medicines
Oral	By mouth as liquids, capsules, tablets	Paracetamol, ibuprofen, antibiotics
Intravenous	Injected into a vein	Morphine
Intramuscular	Injected into a muscle	Immunisations
Subcutaneous	Injected under the skin	Insulin
Intrathecal	Injected into the subdural space	Chemotherapy, i.e. methotrexate
Sublingual	Under the tongue	Ondansetron
Buccal	Between gums and teeth	Midazolam
Rectal	Into the rectum usually in the form of a suppository	Paracetamol; diazepam
Vaginal	Into the vagina as a solution, tablet, cream or gel	Clotrimazole
Ocular	Into the eyes in the form of a liquid, gel or ointment	Chloramphenicol
Otic	Into the ear in the form of ear drop solutions or suspensions	Antibiotic and steroid based drops
Intranasal	Into the nasal passages usually in a spray form	Influenza immunisation for children
Inhalation	Into the airways using inhalers or nebulisers	Salbutamol
Topical	Applied to the skin	Emollients and steroid based creams and ointments
Intradermal	Into the dermis just below the epidermis	Vaccines
Transdermal	Applied to the skin using patches	Analgesics such as fentanyl, hormones and nicotine replacement therapy

administration of medicines to patients. What is vital is that the medicine is in the right place, at the right concentration for the right amount of time. The way children respond to

medicines, particularly neonates and infants under the age of 1, is very different from adults. Health care professionals caring for children need to be very aware of the special considerations we need to afford children when administering medications, including the physiological differences. This includes the impact the medicine has on the child, as well as developmental differences in relation to how the medicine will be given to and taken by the child.

Pharmacodynamics refers to 'what the medicine does to the body' and looks at the relationship between medicine concentration at the site of medicine action and the effect that results including the time course and intensity of therapeutic and adverse (side) effects.

Figure 37.4 outlines the key processes involved in the pharmacokinetics of what the body does to the drug and these processes will be considered in turn.

Absorption is how the medicine enters the body and is the process by which fluids and other substances such as nutrients and medicines are taken up by the body tissues, where the main site of absorption is the small intestine. The bioavailability of a medicine is the amount of a medicine, given orally, that reaches the systemic circulation of the child or young person. It is affected by the form and solubility of the medicine as well as the extent of drug metabolism before reaching the systemic circulation, as well as the amount of food in the gastrointestinal (GI) tract.

As already mentioned, the rate of absorption will be determined by route of administration, where it is given and the solubility of the medicine, that is, the medicine formulation. If it is in a liquid formulation, the medicine will be absorbed more rapidly. If the child is generally warm the uptake into the bloods stream will be improved. If an oral medication is administered the nurse will need to take account of gastric emptying times and gut motility, which may reduce the absorption of the medicine. Obviously the first challenge that CYP nurses will face is the taste, smell and texture of the medicine that will dictate whether a child will even take a medicine in the first place (Eidelmann and Abdel-Rahman, 2016). Children will favour sweeter formulations; however, medicine formulations are rarely palatable. This is important from a safety perspective both in terms of accidental ingestion as well as the potential damage that can be caused in the form of dental caries.

From birth to the age of 2–3 years the gastric mucosa is immature and gastric acid production is reduced. Medicines such as penicillins, which are partially broken down by gastric acids in an adult, will be absorbed in higher amounts in children. Reduced levels of gut flora will increase the bioavailability of medicines like digoxin, therefore will need to be used with care with children. These differences are restricted to the stomach where intestinal pH is similar to that of adults. Gastric emptying is also age related, and also of consideration is that medicines that require bile salts to facilitate absorption need to be administered in a more water soluble format in the first few months of life, for example fat soluble vitamins. Absorption will be affected by common childhood illnesses such as gastroenteritis, which will increase GI motility and so decrease absorption. The route of administration needs to be given some careful consideration (Kelly, 2001).

Other issues to think about in relation to children and their developmental stage and behaviour is the chosen route. A large surface area like the lungs will ensure that nebulised medication will be absorbed very efficiently. For a child receiving salbutamol via nebuliser, this can only happen if the child can cope with the mask, the noise of the nebuliser and the time it takes for the nebuliser to be completed. Clearly the problems we have in administering certain medicines to children will have an impact on how they are absorbed, that is, the need to use liquid formulations as opposed to tablets. We also have to be aware of the potential problems of high sugar content in some syrups (which improve the taste, so children will take them, but can cause dental caries), as well as use of tartrazine, which may cause hyperactivity in some children. In neonatal settings, medicines not available in suitable concentrations necessitate the use of complex dilutions thus increasing the risk of medicine errors. It is also vital that instructions are followed where medicines should not be crushed or broken unless clearly stated on the medicine itself and approved by the pharmacists dispensing the medicine (Pentin et al., 2016).

Other points to consider are that the use of the intramuscular route is unpopular for children for obvious reasons; however, physiologically it is not a reliable route for neonates due to poor muscle mass and reduced blood flow to the muscles that results from their immaturity. Medicines that rely on enzyme activity will demonstrate variable bioavailability in children, where adult levels are achieved at different ages. In relation to topical administration – children have thinner stratum corneum – absorption is increased in newborn and young infants. Medicines like corticosteroids will be absorbed excessively need to be used with care.

In relation to medicines administered orally they will go through what is called 'first pass' metabolism where the medicine is absorbed from the GI tract, will pass into the hepatic portal system to the liver, where some of the medicine will be inactivated the first time they pass through the liver. This explains why some medicines will be given via different routes. Medicines that undergo significant first pass metabolism include paracetamol and morphine, and explains why different doses are given when administering via different routes.

Distribution is the way in which the medicine is transported to the source tissues and is dependent on circulatory function; core organs have the best distribution and the skin the worst distribution. This will be affected by cardiac output, regional blood flow, how the medicine binds to plasma proteins, lipid solubility as well as the age of the patient. It is the free drug that has the effect. The key difference with children is that an infant's body weight has a higher percentage of water. At birth in an infant, 80% of total body weight is water, which drops to adult percentage of 60% by the end of the first year of life. Water-soluble medicines are diluted to a greater extent; therefore higher doses may be required to produce the required plasma concentration. Serum albumin and total protein concentrations are decreased during early infancy up to 1 year. Protein binding is also affected; therefore lower protein binding in newborn infants needs to be considered when prescribing medicines such as phenytoin and ampicillin (Batchelor and Marriott, 2013).

Metabolism is the first stage of medicine clearance whereby a medicine is chemically altered to aid elimination from the body. The primary site of medicine metabolism is the liver, along with other organs such as the lungs, kidneys, blood and intestines. With children, the key difference from adults is that as a result of metabolic immaturity, medicines will be cleared by the liver more slowly so the medicine therapy needs to be closely monitored. Medicines that are highly metabolised are given a lower milligram per kilogram dose for infants compared with older children due to differences in enzyme levels. Hepatic clearance can be higher in infants as liver blood flow is increased, which may increase the first pass effect (Batchelor and Marriott, 2013). Bacterial colonisation of the intestine, which varies with age, will have an effect on medicines that are metabolised in the intestines. This can reduce the bioavailability of medicines such as nifedipine, midazolam and verapamil.

Excretion involves excreting the metabolites of the medicine from the body via kidneys for the most part. The rate of excretion will depend on the type of medicine, where again the immaturity of the neonate and infant may necessitate the need for reduced doses of some medicines, which we need to be aware of. Infants' values of urinary pH are lower, which increases the reabsorption of weakly acidic medicines.

The glomerular filtration rate (GFR) is 2–4 mL per minute in a neonate, doubles by 1 week of age and reaches adult values by the end of the first year of life. Creatinine is used to measure GFR in children where a reduction in medicine dosage is needed if creatinine clearance is less than normal GRF (Batchelor and Marriott, 2013).

When prescribing medicines for children, health care professionals also need to consider any underlying disease processes for children with longer term conditions, where, for example, children with type 1 diabetes have slower gastric emptying times.

This creates an acronym ADME, which is a useful way of remembering the processes as well as remembering that responses to medicines are not always predictable and there are variations in individuals from child to child, adult to adult.

Pharmacodynamics is the impact the medicine has on an infant or child's body, where there will be a physiological and biological response. It is not always directly related to the pharmacokinetics. This requires end-point measurement that is validated in children, where children cannot be treated like small adults. The best way of doing this is based on age, body weight or body surface area or a combination of all of all of these (BNF, 2019).

An important concept to understand is the half-life of a medicine, which is the time taken for the activity of a medicine to reduce to half its original level. A steady state concentration is achieved when the amount of medicine eliminated over a specific time interval is equal to the amount of medicine entering the plasma at the same time interval. So, for example:

- Medicine plasma levels reach a therapeutic level after four to five half-lives from the time of initial dose.
- Dosages should be given with every passing half-life to achieve a steady state concentration.

In the previous example the repeat doses should be given four hourly. A 500 mg medicine with a half-life of 4 hours enters the blood stream at 10 am. At 2 pm it will have a plasma concentration of 250 mg. At 6 pm it will have a plasma concentration of 125 mg.

This covers the basic underpinnings of health care knowledge of how medicines work and why we need this knowledge.

 ACTIVITY

Access a pharmacology textbook for nurses to find out more about the detail of these processes.

THE PRESCRIPTION – WHY CYP ARE DIFFERENT AND NEED SPECIAL CONSIDERATION?

In Platform 4, subsection 4.16, of the NMC (2018) Standards, at point of registration a nurse is required to 'demonstrate knowledge of how prescriptions can be generated, the role of generic, unlicensed, and off-label prescribing and an understanding of the potential risks associated with these approaches to prescribing' (p 18).

This section will clearly and concisely cover the essential aspects in relation to how a prescription is generated and by whom. There are many people involved in this process of prescribing and administration: the prescriber (who can be a doctor, dentist, midwife or a nurse amongst many others), the pharmacist, the nurse (or person who gives the medicine), as well as the patient themselves who may be self-administering the medicine in addition to taking it.

The Multi-Professional Team

While the CYP nurse will be working with doctors and other allied health professionals it is important to emphasise the role of the hospital pharmacist. Hospital pharmacists are experts in the field of medicines. They work closely with medical and nursing staff to ensure patients receive the most appropriate treatment, and provide help and advice to patients in all aspects of their medicines. They advise on the selection of medicines, the dose, preparation and route of administration for individual patients. They provide information about potential side effects and ensure that new treatments are compatible with existing medication in terms of physical and clinical interactions. In addition, they monitor the effects of treatment to ensure that it is safe and effective. Pharmacists have a responsibility to follow their standards of conduct, ethics and performance as issued by the General Pharmaceutical Council (2017).

All pharmacy professionals contribute to delivering and improving the health, safety, and well-being of patients and the public. Professionalism and safe and effective practice are central to that role. As guided by the GPS (2017) Pharmacy professionals must:

1. Provide person-centred care
2. Work in partnership with others
3. Communicate effectively
4. Maintain, develop and use their professional knowledge and skills
5. Use professional judgement
6. Behave in a professional manner
7. Respect and maintain the person's confidentiality and privacy
8. Speak up when they have concerns or when things go wrong
9. Demonstrate leadership

Legal and Ethical Aspects of Prescribing and Administering Medicines for Children and Young People

For medicines to be marketed in the UK they need to have a product licence or what is now known as a marketing authorisation (MA), thus ensuring that the medicine is safe, effective and of suitable quality to use with people as guided by the Medicine and Healthcare Products Regulatory Agency. This authorisation is age related; as a result, many medicines prescribed to children are outside the terms of the MA, because of the lack of clinical trials providing the evidence to support safety for children. Beyond the consent issues in relation to participating in trials, there are also other ethical issues preventing drug trials being conducted with children and young people.

As a result, health care practitioners have to prescribe on the basis of best evidence, including BNF and UK medicines information centres, and this is referred to as 'off licence' or 'off label' use. The vast majority of medications that are used in newborn babies are licensed. However, there are instances when children are required to take medication that is either unlicensed or off-label. These are often needed when there is a lack of suitable licensed medication for use in children, and consequently, a lack of appropriate formulations that children can take in suitable volumes.

The Changing Role of the Nurse – Children and Young People's Nurse as Prescriber

Platform 4, subsection 4.17, requires that a registered nurse at point of registration be able to 'apply knowledge of pharmacology to the care of people', in this case infants children and young people and their parents and carers, demonstrating the ability to progress to a prescribing qualification following registration.

The term 'non medical prescriber' is used to support the developing roles of health care practitioners who now prescribe as part of their health care role, where there are differences in prescribing rights related to professional registration compared with doctors and dentists (Davies and Nuttall, 2016). The focus on the shift and changes in health care roles that now incorporate prescribing practice has been guided by patient safety, effective use of resources, skills and competences of various health professionals, changes in clinical practice and public expectations (Department of Health, 1999). This encompasses significant changes in relation to legal, ethical and professional practice, which for nurses does mean undertaking a course post-registration to ensure that they are competent in this field of practice. The aims for changes in the pre-registration curriculum in the UK indicate that student nurses need to be prepared to progress to achieve a prescribing qualification following registration.

Davies and Nuttall (2016) identify the specific skills that non medical prescribers who are prescribing for children will need, which include understanding the terminology, differences in the pharmacokinetics as they happen in children and that child specific formularies and evidence should be used to support CYP prescribing practice.

> ### 🔒 ACTIVITY
>
> List all the medicines which are used regularly in your day-to-day practice. Access the BNF and electronic medicines compendium (emc) to update your knowledge of mechanisms of action, side effects and interactions to add to your existing knowledge.
> - Available from: https://www.medicines.org.uk/emc.

WORKING IN PARTNERSHIP WITH CHILDREN AND FAMILIES – EVALUATING CARE AND PROMOTING ADHERENCE TO MEDICATION REGIMENS

Platform 4 in the NMC (2018) Standards requires that at point of registration nurses will be able to:

> … *demonstrate the knowledge and skills required to support people with commonly encountered physical health conditions, their medication usage and treatments, and act as a role model for others in providing high quality nursing interventions when meeting people's needs.*

Concordance is defined as the process of the consultation in which prescribing is based on a partnership (Horne et al., 2006). Factors that affect concordance will include age and stage of development, autonomy, lack of insight, gender, socio-economic status, the complexity of the treatment, influence of others, the setting where the discussions are taking place, fears and anxieties, as well as mental health and well-being in general, as well as experience of coercion (WHO, 2003).

Adherence is the extent to which a patient's behaviour matches an agreed action (Horne, 2016), where the emphasis on working in a partnership and child/family-centred manner to avoid the situation where we tell people what to do and expect them to do as they are told.

The National Institute for Health and Care Excellence (NICE) guidelines (2009), which focus on medicine adherence, identify four components to the working relationship: patient involvement in decisions about medicines, supporting adherence, reviewing medications and promoting communication between health care professionals. The issue of non-adherence in relation to managing medicines is an ongoing problem with a cost to the individual child and family, along with the NHS budget in terms of the cost of medication that is being wasted and not used appropriately. It is estimated that the cost of medicine waste to the NHS per year is £300 million, where one significant cause is non-adherence to medication regimes. The most common reasons for non-adherence included forgetfulness, stopping medicines because the child is no longer symptomatic, misunderstanding instructions and resistance/refusal by the child to take the medicines. The ideal dosage for children's medicines will involve the minimal dosage and frequency, will be easy to tolerate with minimal impact on day to day life and will be convenient and easy to administer and take (Chappell, 2015). This is not always possible, as already identified with the use of 'off label' or unlicensed use of medicines for children.

In trying to overcome the risk of non-adherence the CYP nurse develops considerable expertise in working within a triadic model of communication – with child and parent/carer. Callery and Milnes (2012) explored these communication processes in relation to asthma medication reviews to find that the dyads of nurse–parent, nurse–child and parent–child interacted to form the triadic relationship. This had features of what they described as therapeutic alliances where there was potential for cooperation and conflict within the dyads and triad. This illustrates the point that the communication that needs to take place to ensure adherence to medicines prescribed is complex, where the complexity of the dyad and triad needs to ensure that the information conveyed is clear and understanding is clear within the relationships.

What is also important, especially for children and young people with long-term conditions, is that they are enabled to develop the skills of self-care with the help of the adults that are around them. This involves monitoring symptoms, managing medicines, knowing when to ask for medication assistance and having the communication skills to interact with health care professionals (Buford, 2004).

Meah et al. (2009) examined the sense of responsibility in relation to medicine self-management, as it develops in children's lives in relation to 7–12 year olds, and their ability to recognise symptoms of asthma and know how and when to use inhalers. This was dependent on those in parental roles giving their children opportunities to take responsibility. This in spite of their fears of life-threatening consequences if they did not fully take parental responsibility and act as good, responsible parents. This will have an impact on nursing roles as they work and communicate within the triadic relationship.

The nursing role, when working with CYP and their families, is knowing the medicines, mechanism of action, interactions and side effects and sharing this information with child, young person and family whilst ensuring the message is received and understood.

REFLECT ON PRACTICE

How do you manage to use a triadic model of communication to gain the information you need while giving advice to promote adherence to the medicines being taken by children, where there might be some disagreement between either yourself and the parent or child, or between parent and child?

To enable the development of a sense of responsibility and promote self-care from a young age, it is helpful to understand how children learn about how to use numbers. (Parker, 2015). What follows is a brief overview of how children learn about numbers and use them in their day-to-day lives.

 ACTIVITY

How children learn about numbers? Have a look at the National Curriculum in England: Mathematics Programmes of Study (2013) at Gov.uk. This will guide nursing practice as part of the process of teaching and offering advice particularly in relation to managing medicines given to children with long-term conditions such as asthma and diabetes, where promoting independence and 'self-efficacy' has to be the aim of our practice even for very young children.

In general terms, by 30 months, children can understand, through observation, what the process of counting is. By the age of 3 years most children recognise that there are separate words to describe quantities of something. They may not always get them in the correct order. Four-year-old children are able to subitise and do finger counting and start looking at and defining quantities, for example, with two stacks of bricks identifying which is more or less. They will know that each word for a number occurs in a fixed sequence and each only applies to one object in a collection. They also know that the last number word is the total number of objects in that collection. They can count to five and some can count to 10 (Sousa, 2007).

Sousa (2007) continues to identify that children are able to understand the commutative rule that a + b = b + a, at around the age of 5 years. He argues that a significant change in thinking occurs at around the age of 5 years where children start developing skills learned in earlier years into a hierarchy. Six-year-old children have developed a mental number line where they have developed a central cognitive conceptual and structure for whole numbers. They can use counting skills in a broad range of new contexts, read hours on a clock and know which two identically sized monetary values is worth the most.

Sousa (2007) discussing estimation argues that this is an important skill to have and is an extension to the brain's natural ability to subitise. Children are very quick to notice if halves of a cake are not equal when asked to share, but within math teaching the emphasis on getting the answer right seems to account for poor estimation skills that persist into adulthood. As nurses, we are so focused on getting the correct answer we are unwilling to estimate to check that our answer

is correct. It is all about finding a balance between allowing children to find their own ways of completing numeracy tasks and so developing an understanding of how, what and why as opposed to rote learning using one method. Most children find addition easy to understand though multiplication is much more complex and these problems can persist into adulthood. There needs to be an understanding of four related concepts: quantity, problem situations requiring multiplication, equal group, and units relevant to multiplication.

In addition to advancing skills in relation to shape and measurement and handling data, 8-year-old children are able to manipulate two number lines and are able to work with two variables – they can understand place value and can use mental arithmetic to solve double digit addition problems. They can read hours and minutes on the clock and can solve monetary problems where you might be dealing with pounds and pence. Ten-year-old children can manage two number lines structure and include a third variable, are developing a deeper understanding of the whole number system and can compute three-digit numbers and understand the principles of borrowing and carrying. They are able to work out which time is longer when working in hours and minutes.

This is important to know when discussing health care needs with the child and family, which include some numerical component; for example, in management of asthma, when counting the number of 'puffs' of an inhaler might be needed, or how many clicks of insulin to give when using a pen for a 5-year-old child with type 1 diabetes mellitus. This developmental information will also aid the process of developing the skills to self-care where 10-year-old children want to be responsible for their own health care needs and require this skill as they move from primary school to secondary school settings.

Explaining the numbers is vital both for child and parent. Some of the issues of supplying medicines, particularly in liquid formulations, volumes administered may be so small that they are difficult to measure, necessitating supplying the medicine in a different concentration. This can cause confusion for child and parent, for example, the parent remembers the dosage volume but not the dosage units (Chappell, 2015). It is not only necessary to communicate how to give medicines to children, but it is also vital to reinforce this with written information, including the following resources that are accessible online.

 WWW

Useful resources for children and parents/carers can be found with Medicines for Children. Available from: <https://www.medicinesforchildren.org.uk/>.

To summarise, this chapter has considered the roles and responsibilities that a CYP nurse has in relation to the whole process from prescribing to administering medicines to CYP, and doing this in a concordant manner by working in partnership with children, young people and their families and carers. This has been achieved by self-evaluating issues around safety via an audit of numeracy skills as well as reviewing the knowledge needed to understand how medicines work and why children are different physiologically from adults. The content of the chapter is closely aligned to the proficiencies required to practise as a registered nurse, to allow for a personal review of how children's nursing skills match to knowledge and evidence base, so ensuring safe administration of medicines to children and young people. This ensures therapeutic outcomes for all involved in the process – particularly the infant, child and young person.

REFERENCES AND WEBSITES

Buford, T.A., 2004. Transfer of asthma management responsibility from parents to their school age children. J. Pediatr. Nurs. 19, 3–12.

Batchelor, H.K., Marriott, J.F., 2013. Paediatric pharmacokinetics: key considerations. Br. J. Clin. Pharmacol. 79 (3), 395–404.

British National Formulary (BNF), 2019. Available from: https://bnf.nice.org.uk/.

British National Formulary for Children (BNFC), 2019. Available from: https://bnfc.nice.org.uk/.

Callery, P., Milnes, L., 2012. Communication between nurses, children and their parents in asthma review consultations. J. Clin. Nurs. 21, 1642–1650.

Chappell, F., 2015. Medication adherence in children remains a challenge. Prescriber 31–34.

Coben, D., 2000. Numeracy, Mathematics and Adult Learning. .

Cowen, M. (2010) Dyslexia, dyspraxia, dyscalculia: A toolkit for nursing staff, RCN. Available from: https://www.distancelearningcentre.com/policies_and_procedures/Dyslexia_Dyspraxia_and_Dyscalculia_Toolkit.pdf

Department for Education and Schools (2001) The National Numeracy Strategy, DfES. Available from: https://content.ncetm.org.uk/itt/fe/SEN/nns_dyslexia051201.pdf

Department of Health, 2009. Allied Health Professions, Prescribing and Medicines Supply Mechanisms Scoping Project Report. The Stationary Office, London.

Edwards, S., Axe, S., 2015. The ten 'R's of safe multidisciplinary drug administration. NursePrescribing 13 (8), 352–360.

Eidelmann, C., Abdel-Rahman, S.M., 2016. Pharmacokinetic considerations when prescribing in children. Int. J. Pharmacokinet 1 (1), 69–80. Available from: https://www.future-science.com/doi/pdf/10.4155/ipk-2016-0001.

General Pharmaceutical Council, 2017. Standards for pharmacy professionals. GPS. Available from: https://www.pharmacyregulation.org/sites/default/filcs/standards_for_pharmacy_professionals_may_2017_0.pdf.

Horne, R., 2006. Compliance, adherence, and concordance implications for asthma treatment. Chest 130 (1), 65S–72S.

Kelly, J., 2001. Minimising potential side effects of medication at different ages. Professing Nurse 17 (4), 259–262.

Meah, A., Callery, P., Milnes, L., et al., 2009. Thinking 'taller': sharing responsibility in the everyday lives of children with asthma. J. Clin. Nurs. 19, 1952–1959.

National Numeracy, N., 2017. A New Approach to Making the UK More Numerate. Available from https://www.nationalnumeracy.org.uk/sites/default/files/nn124_essentials_numeracyreport_for_web.pdf.

National Numeracy link to resources to help families with under 13's. Available from: http://www.familymathstoolkit.org.uk/.

National Institute for Health and Care Excellence (NICE), 2009. Medicines adherence: involving patients in decisions about prescribed medicines and supporting adherence. CG76 Available from: https://www.nice.org.uk/guidance/cg76.

Nursing and Midwifery Council (NMC), 2018. Future Nurse: Standards of Proficiency for Registered Nurses. Available from: https://www.nmc.org.uk/globalassets/sitedocuments/education-standards/future-nurse-proficiencies.pdf.

Nursing and Midwifery Council (NMC), 2007. Future Nurse: Standards of Proficiency for Registered Nurses, NMC.

National Patient Safety Agency, 2007. Safety in Doses: medication safety incidents in the NHS. Available from: https://nationalpatientsafetysuite.vctms.co.uk/assets/content/35497/story_content/external_files/NRLS-0486-safety-in-doses-PSO-2007-v1.pdf.pdf.

Nuttall, D., Rutt-Howard, J., 2016. The Textbook of Non-medical Prescribing, second ed. Wiley- Blackwell, Chichester.

Parker, A., 2015. Numeracy in Children's Nursing. Wiley Blackwell, Chichester.

Pentin, J., Green, M., Smith, J., 2016. Undertaking safe medicine administration with children: part 1. Nurs. Child. Young. People 28 (6), 35–42.

Royal Pharmaceutical Society, 2019. Professional guidance on the administration of medicines in Healthcare settings. RPS Available from: https://www.rpharms.com/Portals/0/RPS%20document%20library/Open%20access/Professional%20standards/SSHM%20and%20Admin/Admin%20of%20Meds%20prof%20guidance.pdf?ver=2019-01-23-145026-567.

Sousa, D.A., 2007. How the Brain Learns Mathematics. Corwin Press, Thousand Oaks, CA.

World Health Organisation, 2003. Adherence to Long-Term Therapies: Evidence for Action. World Health Organisation, Geneva: World Health Organisation.

38

Children and Surgery

Hannah Liversedge

LEARNING OUTCOMES

- Gain an overview of the nature of paediatric surgery.
- Understand the role of parents and family-centred care in paediatric surgery.
- Gain an overview of some common paediatric procedures.
- Understand the principles of safer surgical care.

- Understand the importance of education for parents and children throughout any surgical experience.
- Understand the ethical and legal ramifications of surgery on children.
- Understand the flow through the operating theatres: preparation, admission, induction, procedure/surgery/anaesthetic, recovery, discharge and education.

WHY CHILDREN NEED SURGERY

Paediatric surgery was not considered a specialised area separate to adult surgery until the first half of the 20th century (Mooncy, 1997). It encompasses a wide range of surgical procedures and differing ages, from premature infants weighing as little as 500–600 g to adolescents. There are many reasons why children need surgery. These can range from congenital malformations to accidental and non-accidental injuries, or a variety of disease processes (Shields and Werder, 2002). A number of characteristic conditions and/or injuries for the varying age groups have been detailed in Table 38.1. These are representative of the general trends and are not indicative of all age groups or all types of surgery. Detailed descriptions of these procedures can be found at the end of the chapter. Surgery to repair or stabilise fractures is also common in childhood; this is discussed in more detail in the Orthopaedic chapter of this book.

Standards for Paediatric Surgery

The Royal College of Surgeons' (RCS) Children's Surgical Forum have produced guidelines for a variety of paediatric surgical situations, which have been endorsed by professional bodies including the Royal College of Nursing (RCN) and the British Association of Paediatric Surgeons (BAPS), among others. These guidelines cover topics ranging from safeguarding to emergency care, and can be found on the RCS and BAPS websites. The document providing standards for children's surgery contains recommendations that all children's nurses working in surgical environments will need to be familiar with (RCS, 2013). They recognise that children should be cared for by people trained to look after them, in services that have been designed with them in mind and can cater to their specific needs.

Particularly important to the children's nurse is the instruction that both children and families should be involved in the design of clinical services. Among the multi-disciplinary surgical team, nurses are well-placed to advocate for children and young people to be represented when services are being redesigned or implemented for the first time. General recommendations for involving children and parents in service design have been issued, adapted from experiences in neonatal care (Bedford Russell et al., 2014). This may be of interest to nurses wanting to involve children in the redesign of surgical services. The RCS (2013) standards also state that frequent communication with the family should occur throughout the hospital stay, and that parental access should be encouraged, for example, in the anaesthetic room and recovery areas. These topics are discussed in more detail later.

It is best practice for children undergoing surgery to be looked after by registered children's nurses throughout the care pathway, although this will not always be possible with emergency or highly specialist surgery. In these circumstances, there must be liaison with a named children's nurse. All children's nurses and support workers in surgical environments must be trained in pain assessment and management, which is also discussed in more detail later. The 'Governance and leadership' section of the standards further recognises the importance of children's nurses in leadership roles, identifying that children's surgical services should have a specific children's nurse lead.

The Role of the Family

In times past, parents (the child's natural parent, step-parent, legal guardian or carer) were excluded from the hospital during a child's admission (Glasper and Charles-Edwards, 2002; Jolley and Shields, 2008). Such attitudes are now not widespread and parents are encouraged, and often expected, to stay for the duration of the child's admission. However, parental presence in the operating room is a more contentious issue.

TABLE 38.1   A Sample of Paediatric Surgical Cases for Different Age Groups

Age	Type of Surgery	Figures
0–2 years	Hernia repair (most common – inguinal)	38.2
	Repair of tracheo-oesophageal fistula	
	Diaphragmatic hernia repair	
	Repair of gastroschisis and exomphalos	38.2–38.5
	Insertion of ventricular-peritoneal shunts for hydrocephalus	
	Circumcision (medical and cultural)	38.6
	Correction of congenital abnormalities (removal of extra digits, cleft palate repair, repair of imperforate anus)	
	Craniofacial surgery for congenital abnormalities such as fusion of cranial sutures	38.7
	Hypospadias repair	38.8, 38.9
	Eye surgery such as probing of tear ducts and examination under anaesthetic for tumours	
2–5 years	Common ENT (ear, nose and throat) procedures such as:	
	• insertion of grommets	
	• adenoidectomy	38.10
	• tonsillectomy	38.12
	Urological surgery such as cystoscopy and ureteric reimplantation	
	Lacerations, dog bites	
	Repair of fractured limbs	
	Dental restorations and extractions for multiple dental caries	
	Eye surgery for squint repair	
	Burns grafts for scald burns	
	Brain tumours	
5–10 years	ENT: adenoidectomy, tonsillectomy	38.10, 38.12
	Repair of fractured limbs	
	Accidental injuries	
	Appendicectomy	38.13
	Orthopaedic surgery for congenital skeletal deformities	
	Brain tumours	
10–15 years	Accidental injuries	
	Lacerations	
	Repair of fractured limbs	
	Torsion of testes	
	Laparoscopic appendicectomy	38.13
	Bone tumours	
	Burns, grafts for flame burns	

Fifty years ago, admission to hospital was portrayed as a positive, growth-promoting experience for children (Jessner et al., 1952; Oremland and Oremland, 1973) and the experience of overcoming the emotional trauma associated with surgery was extolled as character-forming (Blom, 1958); as late as 1992, Lansdown suggested that children could gain psychologically from a hospital admission. However, studies of the psychological trauma encountered by children and their parents before admission have highlighted the importance of adequate preparation of children for hospital admission and surgery (Strachan, 1993) (Box 38.1).

Children have needs different to adults (Price, 1994). The most important factor differentiating the needs of children from those of adults is their level of physical and psychological development.

A Child's Eye View of the Operating Room

Children are smaller and less developed physically and emotionally than adults, so have different visual and psychological perspectives to adults. Consequently, the environment of the operating room looks different to a child (Figs 38.14 and 38.15). Also, children lack the rationalisation skills that would allow them to integrate the environment perceptually, and so may become frightened.

The paediatric operating room environment must be planned with this in mind and should be as 'child-friendly' as possible, with pictures and cartoons on the walls, bright curtains and hangings and colourful mobiles. Children are small, so pictures on walls need to be at relevant heights, for example, the bottom of walls for children who walk into the operating room, and higher for children who arrive on a trolley. Toys, books and television are needed, as the children may not be pre-medicated and will play until taken into the theatre. If possible, and if the parent is adequately prepared, parents should stay with the child until the child is anaesthetised, either in an induction room or in the operating theatre itself. Operating room dress is often redundant for children and they can be admitted to the operating room in their own pyjamas or clothes, providing that these allow appropriate access for the surgery and for the surgical team to manage any perioperative emergencies (Fig. 38.16).

ETHICS AND THE LAW IN PAEDIATRIC PERIOPERATIVE SETTINGS

Informed Consent

Most hospitals have rigid, mandatory policies for obtaining consent for an operation from a parent before their child's surgery. It is imperative that the parents are fully informed as to the reason for the operation, what is going to happen to their child and the risks involved (Steven et al., 2008). By law in many countries, it is the duty of the surgeon to explain the procedure and accompanying risks (Perera, 2008), and the anaesthetist has responsibility for explaining the anaesthetic and its implications to the patient before the operation (Australian and New Zealand College of Anaesthetists (2020)). It is the nurses' responsibility to ensure that the child (if able) and the parents have been told and that they understand what has been said (Daly, 2009). This confirmation is done pre-operatively by nurses on the ward, and by the nurse who receives the patient in the operating suite. In some hospitals, it is the admitting nurse in the operating suite who must check that the consent form has been signed; in others, the child cannot leave the ward for the operating room until the consent form is signed. Except in the most extreme emergency situations, no operation can begin without a signed consent form.

In some hospitals, older children have the right to sign their own consent forms, although usually, by law, it must be countersigned by the parent. The child must understand what they are signing, must understand what the operative procedure is and what it is for, and must be informed of the risks involved. Teenage patients have reported that one of the worst aspects of undergoing major surgery is the associated loss of control, with some feeling that they have not been given the opportunity to make their own choices about the surgery (Rullander et al., 2013). Although adolescents still need parental support from both a legal and an emotional standpoint, every effort should be made to involve teenagers in making informed decisions about their own care (RCS, 2015). Any communication with a child has to be age appropriate; tools such as puppets and calico dolls are useful explanatory tools with younger children.

Parents and children need to know what to expect. Even for the most informed, intelligent and knowledgeable person of any age, operating theatres and procedures are frightening, anxiety-causing events. The role of the paediatric perioperative nurse is to alleviate as much anxiety as possible for both children and parents (Shields and Waterman, 2002).

Privacy

Children's privacy can be greatly compromised within the operating theatre. Some children are far more 'body-aware' and modest than many adults and to expose them unnecessarily is to affront their personal dignity, more so if they are anaesthetised. The anaesthetised child has no control over what is happening, their body may be exposed for the operation and there are numbers of people within the operating theatre at any one time. Theatre suites often have little provision for private conversations, and procedure boards with patients' names and details are often on view to anyone who enters the suite. Perioperative nurses must ensure that children's privacy is respected at all times. Keep the patient covered as much as possible, restrict visitors to the operating theatres and conduct conversations about private information away from heavy traffic areas. If a surgeon briefs the family on completion of a procedure,

this should be done in a separate room away from other people (Fallatt et al., 2007).

Patients' Rights

Every child, regardless of sex, race, religion or class, has the right to be cared for with dignity and respect. This is as true in the perioperative area as in any other part of a health care facility (Perera, 2008). Extraordinary procedures, an alien environment, odd smells and sounds, people in bizarre clothes and strange surroundings make up the milieu of the operating room suite. Many children and parents' perceptions of an operating theatre are gained from the media, and often these are unrealistic. Some are terrified at the thought of entering such a foreign place, while others may have had multiple surgeries throughout childhood and have negative associations with the operating theatre. Regardless, everyone undergoing surgery will require support. Nurses have the communication skills to make children and their families less frightened by touch, reassurance, talking and explaining what is happening.

Parents and children have the right to know that their safety and spiritual, emotional and physical well-being are assured while in the care of perioperative nurses (Ireland, 2006). Children often have operations for life-threatening illnesses, possibly for palliative care or to improve quality of life. Parents often accept the risks of a new procedure in the hope that their life will be improved. Nurses are most often those who recognise the fear and foreboding felt by the children and parents and are most able to support them effectively.

Children and parents from a culture different to the prevailing culture of the hospital have a right to have their religious and spiritual needs met. For example, Muslim parents will feel much more comfortable about their child having an operation for removal of a body part if they know they have the choice to decide if that body part will be given to them to dispose of according to their religious laws (Ebrahim, 1995). Similarly, if blood transfusions might be required during the operation, discussion of this should form part of the informed consent process. Nurses are best situated to find out the wishes of people and to afford them the opportunity of having their wishes respected.

Children and parents always have choice and it is an important part of operating room procedure to ensure these choices are open to the patient. If, at the last minute, a patient decides that they cannot go through with a procedure, then those wishes must be respected, although obviously in a life-threatening emergency the best interests of the child must be considered. Nurses require good counselling skills to talk with the family, help address any queries and issues, and allow them to discuss the issues with the appropriate person, be it the surgeon, the anaesthetist or both. The nurse assumes the role of patient advocate and coordinates communication for the child and family so their best interests are assured.

PRE-ADMISSION PROGRAMMES

Many paediatric hospitals or services use preadmission programmes as a means of educating children and caregivers about what to expect. This can be done in person, or via video if the family is unable to visit in person (SickKids, nd). Because this occurs before admission, it is generally in a more relaxed environment, which in turn is more conducive for child and parent education. The child may have a visit to the theatre admission area, and if possible, the recovery room, and receive an explanation as to what to expect during their own admission to theatre. If it is anticipated that the child will be admitted to intensive care following surgery, a visit to the intensive care unit to meet some of the staff may be helpful, although this should be carefully managed as it can be overwhelming for both children and parents. Pre-admission clinics save time on the day of surgery, particularly for day-surgery procedures, and are a means of obtaining an informed surgical consent in advance, gaining a familiarity in the theatre environment and allaying anxieties. Information sheets, particularly for day surgery, can be given to children and parents at this stage, or posted to those unable to attend the clinic. Structured pre-operative preparation can reduce post-operative analgesia consumption and emergence delirium (Kain et al., 2007).

Not all paediatric surgery is planned, and pre-admission programmes will therefore not be appropriate in all situations. Nonetheless, wherever possible, it is important to talk with children and their parents prior to surgery in order to explain what the process will be like. For example, it may be helpful to explain to children that they will wake up in a different environment, and that their parents will be called once they are awake.

Pre-Operative Assessment

For children undergoing planned surgery, the pre-operative assessment is likely to take place in the weeks preceding admission. This crucial aspect of surgical care will identify any individual/family history of surgical or anaesthetic complications, assess the risk associated with the surgery for the individual patient, and provide essential information to both the child and family, as well as the team carrying out the surgery. For example, environmental exposure to tobacco smoke increases the risk of anaesthetic complications, and should therefore be taken into consideration while planning the surgery (Chiswell and Akram, 2017). It is also important to have baseline observations taken pre-operatively, probably on the day of the operation, which will allow health care professionals to quickly identify any deterioration.

Some areas have trialled pre-operative nurse practitioner-led clinics or other interventions, with the view of combining or effectively coordinating different aspects of pre-operative care, such as educational aspects and health assessment, with some evidence of positive outcomes

(Hines et al., 2015). The seven main tasks associated with pre-operative nursing care are as follows: pre-operative screening and assessment; coordination; communication and collaboration; patient and family education; patient and family-centred care; pre-operative contact with a patient; and scheduling (Turunen et al., 2017). The location and timeline of these aspects of care will vary depending on type of surgery and local policy, but all are essential components of providing good pre-operative nursing care to children and their families.

PURPOSE AND ROLE OF THE WORLD HEALTH ORGANIZATION SURGICAL SAFETY CHECKLIST

The World Health Organization (WHO) launched the surgical safety checklist (SSC) in 2008, and it was mandated throughout the NHS in 2009. It is now in standard use worldwide. This functions as a series of steps that all staff members involved in surgery should follow when carrying out any surgery, with some specific responsibilities assigned to specific staff, such as nurses or anaesthetists (Fig. 38.1). The intention of the SSC is to reduce errors and adverse events, thereby reducing morbidity and mortality in surgical settings (Haynes et al., 2009). At the time of introduction, it was estimated that half of all surgical complications were avoidable (Gawande, 1999; Kable et al., 2002).

In the adult population, there is good evidence that effective introduction of the SSC reduces surgical complications and mortality, including in hospitals that already have a high standard of care (de Vries et al., 2010). The effects of implementing the SSC into paediatric settings are mixed (Lagoo et al., 2017), although improvements have been found in low-resource hospitals carrying out high-risk surgeries (Jenkins et al., 2014). The effectiveness of a paediatric SSC is likely to depend on local implementation efforts, as well as cultural and contextual factors that have yet to be fully explored (Lagoo et al., 2017).

The SSC is often adapted for individual areas and specialties. Some areas have implemented paediatric-specific SSCs that includes pictures and child-friendly language, in order to allow for greater participation of children and their families (Pires et al., 2012). Others have incorporated the SSC into surgical care pathways and paperwork, to promote greater consistency between ward, theatre, and recovery. Nurses working in a surgical environment should therefore familiarise themselves with local policies and guidance related to the use of the SSC.

One of the advantages of the SSC is that it promotes multi-disciplinary collaboration and cooperation in order to obtain good outcomes for patients. All stages of the checklist as originally conceived require input from both nurse and anaesthetist, with the third stage additionally requiring the involvement of the surgeon. A recent study suggests that the use of the SSC increases individual staff awareness

Surgical safety checklist

Before induction of anaesthesia	Before skin incision	Before patient leaves operating room
(with at least nurse and anaesthetist)	(with nurse, anaesthetist and surgeon)	(with nurse, anaesthetist and surgeon)

Before induction of anaesthesia
(with at least nurse and anaesthetist)

Has the patient confirmed his/her identity, site, procedure, and consent?
☐ Yes

Is the site marked?
☐ Yes
☐ Not applicable

Is the anaesthesia machine and medication check complete?
☐ Yes

Is the pulse oximeter on the patient and functioning?
☐ Yes

Does the patient have a:

Known allergy?
☐ No
☐ Yes

Difficult airway or aspiration risk?
☐ No
☐ Yes, and equipment/assistance available

Risk of >500 mL blood loss (7 mL/kg in children)?
☐ No
☐ Yes, and two IVs/central access and fluids planned

Before skin incision
(with nurse, anaesthetist and surgeon)

☐ Confirm all team members have introduced themselves by name and role.
☐ Confirm the patient's name, procedure, and where the incision will be made.

Has antibiotic prophylaxis been given within the last 60 minutes?
☐ Yes
☐ Not applicable

Anticipated critical events

To surgeon:
☐ What are the critical or non-routine steps?
☐ How long will the case take?
☐ What is the anticipated blood loss?

To anaesthetist:
☐ Are there any patient-specific concerns?

To nursing team:
☐ Has sterility (including indicator results) been confirmed?
☐ Are there equipment issues or any concerns?

Is essential imaging displayed?
☐ Yes
☐ Not applicable

Before patient leaves operating room
(with nurse, anaesthetist and surgeon)

Nurse verbally confirms:
☐ The name of the procedure
☐ Completion of instrument, sponge and needle counts
☐ Specimen labelling (read specimen labels aloud, including patient name)
☐ Whether there are any equipment problems to be addressed

To surgeon, anaesthetist and nurse:
☐ What are the key concerns for recovery and management of this patient?

This checklist is not intended to be comprehensive. Additions and modifications to fit local practice are encouraged.   Revised 1 / 2009   © WHO, 2009

Fig. 38.1 World Health Organization (WHO) surgical safety checklist. (Available from: https://apps.who.int/iris/bitstream/handle/10665/44186/9789241598590_eng_Checklist.pdf;jsessionid=D915D0BA43BE-651A5E17EA035562295A?sequence=2.)

of their responsibility for patient safety, as well as improving multi-disciplinary teamwork between nurses, surgeons, and anaesthetists (Ayabe et al., 2017).

For the ward-based children's surgical nurse, responsibilities related to the SSC are likely to include checking and recording that the child is wearing the correct nameband, that the child's allergy status has been confirmed, and that informed consent has been obtained prior to transfer to theatre. Ensuring that these steps have been completed will prevent any delay upon arrival in the induction room. For the theatre nurse, responsibilities will include completing accurate instrument, sponge, and needle counts, identifying any equipment problems that need addressing, and confirming that specimens are accurately labelled. All team members, including nurses throughout the surgical environment, should be prepared to speak up should any step of the checklist be skipped, as this will contribute towards improving surgical safety.

FLOW THROUGH THE OPERATING ROOMS

Admission: Theatre Reception

The first port of call in the operating rooms is the theatre reception area. Sometimes termed the 'holding bay', it is the

 WWW

Visit the Great Ormond Street Hospital YouTube channel and listen to Ryan's story about having surgery on his right leg. Available from:
- https://www.youtube.com/watch?time_continue=337&v=ye41tMv4TIM

 WWW

Visit the University Hospitals of Morecombe Bay NHS Foundation Trust YouTube channel to see one example of how a surgical team has incorporated the SSC into their practice. Available from:
- https://www.youtube.com/watch?v=w325Dy7MJcc

public face of theatre. Unlike adults having surgery, the children often walk in with their parents, as they may not have been pre-medicated. They may ride in on a toy vehicle, or babies may be carried in by their parents. If the child is experiencing heightened anxiety, the anaesthetist may have ordered a pre-medication. Clonidine has become one of the drugs of choice as a pre-medication to alleviate anxiety and provide post-operative analgesia (Bergendahl et al., 2006). The role of the nurse in this area is to check the incoming child to ensure the name band is labelled correctly with the correct spelling, date of birth, weight and possible allergies. The child's identification band must be checked with the accompanying notes and x-rays, scans or pathology results to ensure they match the patient. The consent is confirmed by checking both written and verbal consent and confirming the type and location of surgery that the child and family believe they are about to undergo.

A pre-operative checklist is completed to ensure that fasting times have been adhered to, that the presence of allergies and their reactions are documented, and that child and parent understand the procedure. During this admission, the nurse can ask the child and parent if they need to speak to the surgeon or anaesthetist once again before surgery. To alleviate anxieties, a relaxed, friendly, professional demeanour works best. This is the last stage for the child and their family before undergoing their anaesthetic, and can be a time of heightened emotions for both parties. Distraction works well at this time. Children's television and children's videos are often used as a distraction tool. Some operating rooms make use of volunteers, who help in play activities. Toys, books and ride-on cars and bikes can be effective. Some operating room staff encourage smaller children to ride a toy motor bike or car directly into the induction room, which keeps them distracted right up to anaesthetic induction. Of course, a quick assessment of the child's compliance needs to be done to ensure they can be coaxed off the bike or out of the car when it is time to do so. The aim is to minimise any pre-operative anxiety as it is associated with adverse post-operative outcomes such as emergence delirium and increased pain (Zeev and Kain, 2007).

 ACTIVITY

> Search the Cochrane Library for a copy of the review about the use of clonidine as a pre-medication for post-operative analgesia in children (Lambert et al., 2014).

Induction

Paediatric anaesthetic induction is the process where an anaesthetist administers an anaesthetic agent either as a gas via a mask or intravenously. The child is usually cannulated to provide intravenous access essential for the anaesthetic and for the administration of emergency drugs should the child suffer laryngospasm and require emergency intubation to maintain an airway. Both processes (gas or intravenous or a combination of the two) anaesthetise the child, who is then ventilated by means of an endotracheal tube, a laryngeal mask airway or a Guedel airway with a ventilator bag and mask. Physiological signs are monitored. Electrocardiograph

adhesive pads are placed on either side of the chest and one on the left flank. An oxygen saturation monitor is placed on the finger or toe so that the child can be safely monitored during surgery, and a blood pressure cuff is applied for further monitoring. The type of intubation and cannulation required depends on the type of surgery being performed. Once cannulated and intubated, the child is ready to be transferred onto the operating table and positioned appropriately for surgery.

The use of an induction room for paediatric anaesthesia is increasing. It provides a number of functions. Firstly, it means that the instrument nurse can set up for the case in the theatre separate to the induction room, and may facilitate case turnover. Additionally, based around the principles of family-centred care, it allows a parent or caregiver to accompany the child until they are anaesthetised. Assessment of the child's developmental needs would suggest that they might experience during traumatic events, including the induction of anaesthesia, and it has been proposed that parental presence at induction could alleviate this. However, to date, there is limited evidence that parental presence at anaesthesia induction makes a significant difference to the child's anxiety, although the presence of both parents during induction may significantly reduce parental anxiety (Manyande et al., 2015; Erhaze et al., 2016). The presence of parents during induction should therefore be assessed on an individual basis by the anaesthetist, who will take into consideration a number of factors. This should include discussion with children as well as their parents. Generally, for emergency anaesthetics when the standard fasting time is not possible, a rapid sequence induction is required and it is not common routine to have parents present.

Parental education is an effective means of reducing parental anxiety. The provision of information during the pre-operative admission process may reduce anxiety and improve understanding of the anaesthetic and surgical process (Bellew et al., 2002). It is important that the accompanying adult is forewarned as to what to expect when the child is anaesthetised, because once induced, the child does not look to be merely asleep but looks lifeless (Box 38.2). This can be extremely distressing for the parents and some will become upset and have to be escorted from the induction room. Obviously, this is not the positive scenario sought during parent-present inductions.

Studies have found that it can be counterproductive to bring an anxious parent into the operating room without adequate preparation (Chan and Molassiotis, 2002). Given sufficient education and reassurance before the day, and escorted immediately from the induction room once the child has received the anaesthetic agent, the process should successfully alleviate anxieties of the family by having the parent present until the child is unconscious, and the parent is comforted by remaining with their child instead of leaving them among strangers (see Fig. 38.17). However, it is important to remember that parental presence in the induction room alone is not sufficient to reduce child anxiety (Manyande et al., 2015), and to use additional methods such as play, distraction, and, if appropriate, pre-medication for reducing the child's anxiety.

The Operation

Once anaesthetised, the child is transferred from the induction room onto the operating table and is positioned as required. For example, the child may lie supine (which is the case for the majority of procedures) but could be placed prone or in a lateral position. Patient monitoring systems, such as oxygen saturation and an exhaled carbon dioxide monitor, are connected. These two non-invasive monitors provide the most valuable information to the anaesthetist regarding the child's condition during surgery (Binda and Mestad, 2000). Blood pressure is monitored at regular intervals. If the surgery is major, arterial lines and central venous lines are inserted and taped securely so as not to dislodge once the child is positioned, prepared and draped. Most importantly, the airway is taped and secured and the child is not repositioned until the anaesthetist has control over the airway.

It is the instrument nurse's responsibility to check the patient's identification band with the chart, and to check the consent form. Usually the scout nurse shows these to the instrument nurse, who is already 'scrubbed' and has set up for the case. The instrument nurse checks patient positioning and placement of the diathermy plate (Fig. 38.17). The presence of allergies is re-checked. The child is then 'prepped' (using an antiseptic skin preparation such as aqueous betadine or chlorhexidine) and draped. Mayo tables and instrument trolleys are moved into position, suction and diathermy are connected before the surgeon puts knife to skin. The surgeon generally checks with the instrument nurse and the anaesthetist if they are ready to begin.

The instrument nurse's legal responsibility is to maintain a correct count of any instruments or swabs that have been placed in or around the wound, and to ensure that all are removed from the wound before it is closed. There are a standard three counts completed by the instrument nurse and the scout nurse together: the first before the commencement of surgery, and after all accountable items have been taken onto the sterile field. The second is completed at the initial stages of wound closure and the third when the surgeon commences closing the skin. Dressings are applied, drapes and diathermy removed, and when the anaesthetist is satisfied that the child's condition is stable, the child is extubated (unless transferring directly to intensive care intubated) and transferred to the post-anaesthetic care unit (PACU).

Post-Anaesthetic Care Unit

When the child arrives in the PACU the immediate tasks of the registered nurse are to secure the intravenous line, check that the child is breathing, ensure the airway is clear, reposition the airway (e.g. by supporting the jaw) if necessary, apply the oxygen saturation monitor, and place an oxygen mask on or next to the child's face, depending on the level of alertness and tolerance of the mask. Airway obstructions can occur in paediatric patients, particularly in those arriving deeply anaesthetised without mechanical airway support such as jaw support or a Guedel airway (Holm-Knudsen and Rasmussen, 2009). Once these tasks have been done, the registered nurse checks the wound site for bleeding, assesses the pain level and documents vital signs. This process of checking, assessing and documenting is repeated at 5-minute intervals for the duration of the child's stay in PACU, or less frequently if the child's condition is stable and the stay in PACU is extended. This is at the discretion of the registered nurse caring for the child. Because children's metabolism is rapid, they wake from anaesthetic much more rapidly than adults and can become quite active. For this reason, the nurse to patient ratio for paediatric recovery units is routinely 1:1.

The child remains in the PACU until he or she is awake and responsive to stimuli (such as calling their name), maintaining their own airway, oxygen saturation is satisfactory on room air, pain is fully controlled and the wound dressing remains dry and intact. If any bleeding has occurred, the wound is reinforced and if significant, reassessed by the surgeon in case the child needs to return to theatre.

Pain Management

Approximately 75% of children will say that they have considerable pain on the first day after surgery (Binda and Mestad, 2000), and children's pain is less likely to be appropriately assessed and managed than that of adults (Vittinghoff et al., 2018). The European Society for Paediatric Anaesthesiology have recently released specific guidance on post-operative pain management for several common paediatric surgeries, including inguinal hernia repair, adenotonsillectomy and others (Vittinghoff et al., 2018).

Neonates are at risk of respiratory depression following the use of narcotics. For this reason, neonates require close monitoring if narcotics are required, preferably in an intensive care unit, and may need to remain intubated for their initial post-operative recovery. There is a greater risk of respiratory depression in any paediatric patient than in adults following narcotic use (Lundeberg and Lonnqvist, 2004). An emergency scenario in the PACU is more likely to involve a respiratory arrest than a cardiac arrest. Close monitoring by experienced paediatric anaesthetic nursing staff is required.

When the child has undergone a major or significantly painful procedure, narcotic analgesia is administered by means of a metered dose system, which releases the prescribed amount (Lundeberg and Lonnqvist, 2004). This can be patient-controlled analgesia (PCA) if the child is able to understand and use the device, or parent- or nurse-controlled analgesia (NCA) if the child is too young or not capable of administering a dose. Initially, these infusions may have a continuous background infusion and the parent, nurse or child can administer a bolus dose as prescribed according to a milligram per kilogram ratio. The pump is set with limits as to the number of bolus doses per hour. The child's level of pain and vital signs are closely monitored.

The role of the registered nurse in pain management is primarily one of acute assessment of the degree and severity of pain, and liaison with the anaesthetist to administer analgesics to bring the child's pain under control (Jonas and Worsley-Cox, 2000). Experienced paediatric nurses are essential for this assessment because children may withdraw from those around them in response to their pain. In inexperienced hands this could be interpreted as an absence of pain. It has also been suggested that adolescent patients may avoid requesting analgesia as they do not wish to burden busy staff (Rullander et al., 2013).

An increased understanding of the effectiveness of analgesia given as a pre-medication has markedly reduced the initial post-operative pain experienced by many children, particularly in the case of day-procedure surgery. In fact, pain is one of the factors inhibiting discharge following surgery and can significantly add to the health costs of day-case admissions if the child requires overnight stay for pain management. Prior to discharge of day cases, or indeed any children who have undergone surgery, it is important to provide specific education about analgesia to parents, as many have misconceptions about the safety of post-operative analgesia and may be reluctant to administer adequate pain relief to their child (Zisk Rony et al., 2010).

In children who have undergone major surgery, the assessment of pain and decisions about pain management can be complex. As noted above, it is essential to ensure that children's pain is managed effectively following surgery, both for their immediate well-being and in order to assist with their recovery. However, prolonged use of opiates and benzodiazepines in paediatric intensive care environments has been linked to increased disturbing hallucinations and delusional memories, which may increase a child's risk of developing post-traumatic stress disorder (PTSD) related to their admission (Colville et al., 2008). Close liaison with paediatric pain specialists may be required in order to ensure that children receive effective pain management with minimal negative side effects.

Codeine and co-codamol are not suitable for children who have undergone adenoidectomy, adenotonsillectomy, or tonsillectomy due to differences in the metabolism of this drug and the risk of adverse drug reactions (Prows et al., 2013).

Discharge From the Post-Anaesthetic Care Unit

Once the child has satisfied the PACU discharge requirements, including maintaining their own airway, satisfactory oxygen saturation on room air, controlled pain and a dry and intact wound dressing, they are ready to be transferred back to the wards. As with the admission of parents into the induction room, it is now becoming standard practice in many PACUs to admit the parents once their child is stable and awake. However, the same principles apply in terms of educating and preparing the parent prior to their admission to PACU and reassuring them when they see their child (Smith and Dearmun, 2006). If the parent is ill informed and not prepared for their visit to PACU they may become overcome with emotion. The role of the registered nurse is to support and explain procedural details and to outline the pain relief provided, and the location and type of dressings their child may have. Reassurance is the key word, and remaining calm, professional and friendly helps to comfort both the parent and child. The ward staff can be contacted to collect the child at the same time as the parents are invited into PACU. In this manner the parents and staff can benefit from the handover of the child's care.

Regular observations should continue once the child is transferred back to the ward. The frequency and nature of these will be determined by local policy, the type of operation the child has had and any peri-operative complications. For instance, paediatric eye surgery is associated with a high incidence of post-operative nausea and vomiting (Davies and Sale, 2017), and nurses should therefore be alert to the importance of checking a child's level of nausea while assessing their vital signs. The RCN *Standards for Assessing, Measuring and Monitoring Vital Signs in Infants, Children and Young People* suggest that as a basic guideline, heart rate, respiratory rate and blood pressure should be checked every 30 minutes for 2 hours, and then hourly for 4 hours. Vital signs must also be assessed prior to discharge (RCN, 2017). Some children may require more frequent observation depending on their degree of stability.

Any concerns or signs of deterioration should be escalated rapidly according to local policy. Use of an early warning system such as PEWS may be helpful in identifying deterioration (RCN, 2017), but this does not replace clinical judgement. Some operations are associated with a high incidence of particular post-operative emergencies, and both recovery and ward-based surgical nurses need to be aware of these. Post-tonsillectomy haemorrhage, for example, is a serious and potentially lethal emergency, and occurs in between 2.1% and 12% of patients (Spektor et al., 2016). Any sign of post-operative bleeding should therefore be escalated immediately to the ENT surgical team.

 ACTIVITY

Review the "Post-operative care" section of the RCN *Standards for Assessing, Measuring and Monitoring Vital Signs in Infants, Children and Young People* (starts on page 13). Available from:

- https://www.rcn.org.uk/professional-development/publications/pub-005942

 ACTIVITY

Review the European Society for Paediatric Anaesthesiology (ESPA) guidance on post-operative pain management in children, especially the ESPA Pain Management Ladder. Available from:

- https://onlinelibrary.wiley.com/doi/full/10.1111/pan.13373

PARENTS IN POST-OPERATIVE RECOVEMRY

Parent presence at the induction of anaesthesia is discussed earlier, and is likely to be appropriate in most circumstances (Fig. 38.19). Although research about parents present at induction (PPI) has been extensive, little research exists about the presence of parents in the PACU. It can be assumed that similar benefits to parental anxiety accrue, and it may be surmised that children will be reassured to see their parents soon upon coming around, although empirical evidence is lacking.

Standing Orders

Standing orders (Shields and Waterman, 2002), that is, orders written by a team within a unit (usually, in this case, comprised of the head anaesthetist, nurse in charge of the PACU, and if different, the nurse in charge of the operating room) are often used in situations such as PACU where the nurses work autonomously. They save time while providing safe practice guidelines for care while a child is in the unit. A sample of standing orders for the post-operative recovery of children who have had adenotonsillectomy are shown in Box 38.3 at the end of this chapter.

The PACU provides the first point of contact for the parents as to what to expect after their child's surgery and provides the initial education of care and discharge planning advice. This education needs to be reiterated by the ward staff, and the child's condition reassessed before discharge.

Issues Affecting Discharge Planning and Parental Anxiety During the Child's Discharge From the PACU/Recovery Unit

Discharge

Children of various ages require different strategies for discharge planning, and different surgeries will require different in-hospital recovery periods. It is important to ensure the parents are comfortable about taking the child home and that they are fully prepared to do so. Similarly, the child, if old enough, must feel secure about going home. Children of appropriate ages should be involved in all stages of planning for their care, as should their parents.

In practical terms, discharge can be routine: when the child is awake, there is no bleeding from the wound site, the child has eaten and drunk and there is no vomiting or fever. There will be specific considerations for individual surgeries. The parents must be educated about:

- the child's care;
- potential later complications;
- when to call the hospital if something is wrong;
- what the ward and accident and emergency (A&E) telephone numbers are;
- what drugs to give and when and how;
- when the child can return to a normal diet;
- when the child can return to school, preschool, kindergarten or childcare;
- how to identify infection;
- when it is safe for the child to resume normal activity;

- dressing and wound care;
- potential changes in the child's behaviour relating to the hospital admission, how to recognise them and what to do about them;
- appointment for the follow-up visit to the doctor or clinic.

COMMON PAEDIATRIC SURGERIES

Hernia Repair

Hernias are one of the most common congenital abnormalities found in infants (Fig. 38.2). There are several different types of hernia affecting both male and female children. The most frequently occurring hernias are indirect and direct inguinal hernias and hydroceles. Hernias occur when the processus vaginalis (a peritoneal diverticulum that extends through the inguinal ring) remains as a patent conduit with the peritoneal cavity instead of closing off and disappearing.

During male hernia repair, the hernial sac is dissected from the testicular structures; this dissection contains the risk of injury to the testicular blood flow (Palabiyik, 2009).

Circumcision

Circumcision was once routinely performed at birth in many countries, although this custom has now mostly disappeared. However, it remains a reasonably common procedure, although it is now performed for cultural/religious and medical reasons. There is some controversy surrounding male circumcision. In the UK about one-quarter of circumcisions are performed for religious reasons (Mukherjee, 2009). Medical

During fetal development, the processus vaginalis attaches itself to the testes and is pulled down into the scrotum as the testes descend. If the processus vaginalis remains patent it is a potential hernia. Twenty per cent of individuals have a patent processus but remain asymptomatic. If bowel or other contents from the abdomen enter the processus it becomes an actual hernia. If only peritoneal fluid enters the processus it becomes a communicating hydrocele (Weber and Tracy, 2000).

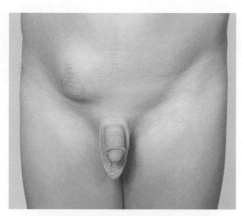

Fig. 38.2 Inguinal hernia in a child.

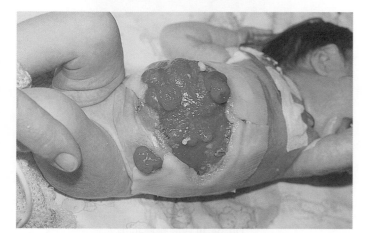

Fig. 38.3 Gastroschisis.

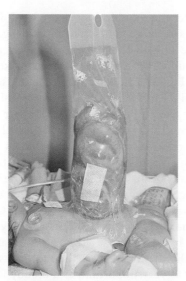

Fig. 38.4 Repair of gastroschisis.

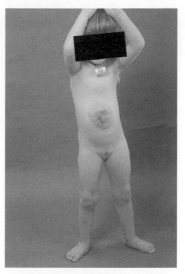

Fig. 38.5 Child with healed gastroschisis at age 3 years.

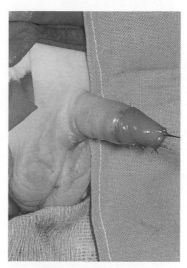

Fig. 38.6 Circumcision.

Circumcision is usually performed under general anaesthetic and a penile nerve block. The surgeon makes a blunt dissection between the glans and the foreskin, the collar of the foreskin that has been isolated is then excised usually using diathermy, and the shaft skin is then sutured to the subcoronal skin using interrupted absorbable sutures (Fig. 38.6).

Hypospadias and Repair

Hypospadias is one of the most common congenital anomalies. It occurs in 1:200 to 1:300 live births. The aetiology of hypospadias has been linked to environmental influences. There has been an increase over the past 30 years of male reproductive abnormalities occurring alongside the increased production and use of synthetic chemicals. Concerns have been raised that such environmental factors may play a role in the aetiology of hypospadias, undescended testes and lowered sperm count (Baskin and Ebbers, 2006). Hypospadias (Fig. 38.8) is a developmental abnormality in which the urethra opens onto the ventral surface of the penis. The opening can occur anywhere from glans to the scrotum (Winship

circumcisions are required for two main conditions: *phimosis*, which is an inability to retract the foreskin, indicated by a ballooning of the foreskin on urination (Raynor, 2000); and *paraphimosis*, which occurs when the foreskin which has retracted cannot be pulled back down, leaving it forming a stricture around the head of the penis.

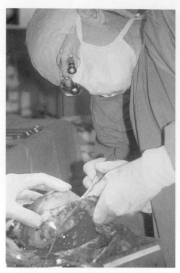

Fig. 38.7 Craniofacial surgery.

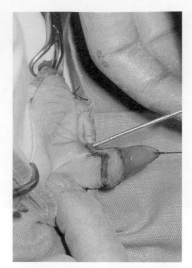

Fig. 38.9 Hypospadias repair.

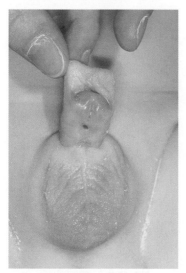

Fig. 38.8 Hypospadias.

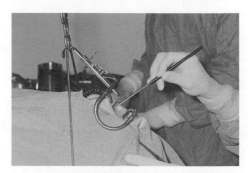

Fig. 38.10 Adenoidectomy.

et al., 2017) (Fig. 38.9). Surgical repair of hypospadias is often two-staged. The repair involves the formation of a flap using the meatus to create a neourethra that opens at the tip of the glans. An indwelling catheter is left in situ for 7–10 days post-operatively, or until the dressing is removed.

Adenoidectomy

Adenoidectomy is a common ear, nose and throat (ENT) procedure on children, particularly 2- to 5-year-olds. Some children in that age bracket have tonsils and adenoids so enlarged that they obstruct their breathing, particularly during sleep. Snoring is often an indicator. Paediatric sleep disorders such as obstructive sleep disorder are often associated with behavioural problems, poor school performance and decreased quality of life. Adenotonsillectomy resolves sleep disorder behaviours in 80% of children, and improves quality of life and behaviours (Mitchell, 2008). General anaesthetic is given and the child lies supine, with

a gel roll under the shoulders to tilt the head back (Herron et al., 2002). The surgeon inserts a mouth gag, which both depresses the tongue and holds the jaw open. Two rods are used to support the gag in place and to keep the head in position (Fig. 38.10). An adenotome is used to scrape the adenoidal tissue from the adenoidal bed. Diathermy is not routinely used for adenoidectomy, rather haemostasis is obtained by firmly packing a swab into the adenoidal bed. This is removed after about 5 minutes and may be replaced with a fresh swab if bleeding persists. Adenoidal bleeding usually occurs if the adenoidal tissue has not been sufficiently scraped away. In this instance the surgeon may re-curette the tissue with the adenotome. Occasionally, suction diathermy is needed to cauterise any vessels that continue to bleed. Because Raytec swabs are routinely packed into the adenoidal space for haemostasis, the scrub nurse's count is very important, as a bloody Raytec is difficult to see and may cause a serious airway obstruction if left undetected.

Recent studies have suggested that suction diathermy or power-assisted debridement may have advantages over the standard method described above, chiefly in the reduction of peri-operative and post-operative haemorrhage. A Cochrane review of the evidence for these methods of adenoidectomy is currently underway (Poirier et al., 2018).

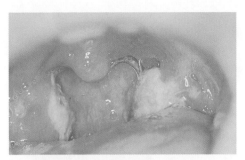

Fig. 38.11 Tonsillitis.

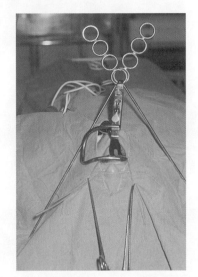

Fig. 38.12 Patient prepared for tonsillectomy.

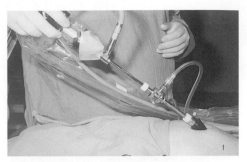

Fig. 38.13 Laparoscopic appendicectomy.

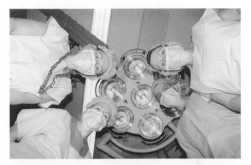

Fig. 38.14 A child's view from the operating table.

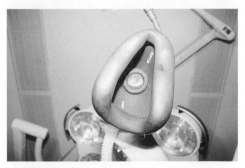

Fig. 38.15 A child's view of an anaesthetic mask.

Tonsillitis

Tonsillitis is a common illness of childhood, an infection that produces a purulent discharge which covers the inflamed tonsils (Fig. 38.11) and is accompanied by fever and often extreme discomfort. There is some controversy over the need for tonsillectomy (Fig. 38.12) and adenoidectomy, with ongoing debate about whether the relatively modest improvement in outcomes is worth the associated pain and risks (Burton et al., 2014). In children, adenotonsillectomy or adenoidectomy are performed to treat recurrent tonsillitis, obstruction of the nasopharynx and obstructive sleep apnoea (Nieminen et al., 2000). Traditionally, there have been two methods for tonsillectomy – using a tonsil snare (guillotine) which loops over the tonsil and cuts it off at its base (Homer et al., 2000), and more recently, by sharp or blunt dissection (Meeker and Rothrock, 1999). Despite newer technologies, tonsillectomy is still associated with a relatively high risk of post-operative morbidity such as pain and bleeding (Sargi and Younis, 2007). Although the majority of children undergoing a tonsillectomy will return to the ward post-operatively, some children may be transferred to the intensive care unit initially if complications are anticipated.

Laparoscopic Appendicectomy

Children presenting with acute appendicitis usually have a number of tell-tale signs and symptoms. The onset of acute appendicitis is usually over a period of 6–36 hours. The child complains of abdominal pain, which commences around the umbilical area but moves to the right upper quadrant of the abdomen. If the appendix is inflamed the child may be febrile. In appendicitis, vomiting usually begins after the onset of pain; if the child begins vomiting before the onset of pain then the prognosis is more likely to be gastritis (Ein, 2000). Diarrhoea does not usually commence unless the appendix has perforated, in which the case the sigmoid colon becomes involved and peritonitis may ensue.

Ultrasound is often performed to confirm a suspected appendicitis. Laparoscopic appendicectomy (Fig. 38.13) offers faster recovery times and a reduced rate of wound infection compared with open appendicectomy (Paterson, 2008), and is now

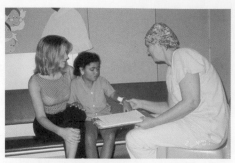

Fig. 38.16 A child coming into the operating room in their own pyjamas.

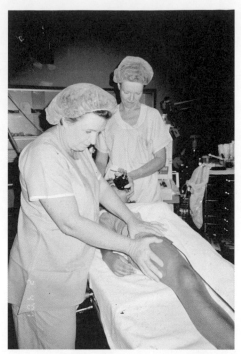

Fig. 38.18 Positioning an anaesthetised child and applying the diathermy plate.

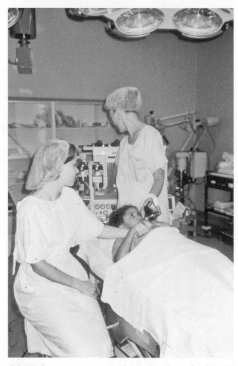

Fig. 38.17 A parent present for induction of anaesthetic.

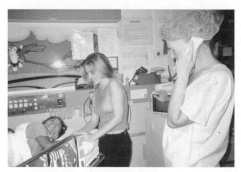

Fig. 38.19 A parent present in the post-anaesthetic care unit (PACU).

the preferred method. It involves the insertion of a large port or trocar for the camera at the umbilicus, and one to two other ports (usually 5 mm wide) for the grasping instruments. The appendix is ligated away from the appendiceal mesentery using diathermy. Once freed, the appendix is tied off, dissected from the bowel and removed via a 10-mm port (which is inserted to replace one of the 5-mm ports) and routinely sent for pathology.

REFERENCES

Australian and New Zealand College of Anaesthetists, 2020. PS26 Statement on Informed Consent for Anaesthesia and Sedation. Australian and New Zealand College of Anaesthetists, Melbourne. Online. Available from: https://www.anzca.edu.au/resources/professional-documents/standards-(1)/ps26-statement-on-informed-consent-for-anaesthesia.

Ayabe, T., Okumura, M., Itai, K., et al., 2017. Changes in safety attitude and improvement of multidisciplinary teamwork by implementation of the WHO surgical safety checklist in university hospital. Open J. Saf. Sci. Technol. 7, 22–41.

Baskin, L., Ebbers, M., 2006. Hypospadius: anatomy, aetiology and technique. J. Pediatr. Surg. 41, 463–472.

Bedford Russell, A.R., Passant, M., Kitt, H., 2014. Engaging children and parents in service design and delivery. Arch. Dis. Child. 99 (12), 1158–1162.

Bellew, M., Atkinson, K.R., Dixon, G., et al., 2002. The introduction of a paediatric anaesthesia information leaflet: an audit of its impact on parental anxiety and satisfaction. Paediatr. Anaesth. 12 (2), 124–130.

Bergendahl, H., Lönnqvist, P.A., Eksborg, S., 2006. Clonidine in paediatric anaesthesia: review of the literature and comparison with benzodiazepines for pre-medication. Acta Anaesthesiol Scand. 50, 135–143.

Binda, R., Mestad, P., 2000. Anaesthetic considerations. In: Ashcraft, K.W., Murphy, J.P., Sharp, R.J., et al. (Eds.), Pediatric Surgery, third ed. WB Saunders, Philadelphia, pp. 38–46.

Blom, G.E., 1958. The reactions of hospitalized children to illness. Pediatrics 22, 590–600.

Burton, M.J., Glasziou, P.P., Chong, L.Y., et al., 2014. Tonsillectomy or adenotonsillectomy versus non-surgical treatment for chronic/recurrent tonsillitis. Cochrane Database Syst. Rev. 11, CD001802. https://doi.org/10.1002/14651858.CD001802.pub3.

Chan, C., Molassiotis, A., 2002. The effects of an educational programme on the anxiety and satisfaction levels of parents having parent present induction and visitation in a post anaesthesia care unit. Paediatr. Anaesth. 12, 131–139.

Chiswell, C., Akram, Y., 2017. Impact of environmental tobacco smoke exposure on anaesthetic and surgical outcomes in children: a systematic review and meta-analysis. Arch. Dis. Child. 102 (2), 123–130.

Colville, G., Kerry, S., Pierce, C., 2008. Children's factual and delusional memories of intensive care. Am. J. Respir. Crit. Care Med. 177 (9), 976–982.

Daly, B., 2009. Patient consent, the anaesthetic nurse and the peri-operative environment: Irish law and informed consent. Br. J. Anaesth. Recovery Nurs. 10 (1), 3–10.

Davies, I.D.M., Sale, S.M., 2017. Anaesthesia for paediatric eye surgery. Anaesth. Intensive Care Med. 18 (1), 37–40.

De Oliveiria Pires, M.P., da Luz Goncalves Pedreira, M., Peterlini, M.A.S., 2013. Safe pediatric surgery: development and validation of preoperative interventions checklist. Rev. Latino-Am. Enferm. 21 (5). Available from: https://doi.org/10.1590/S0104-11692013000500010.

De Vries, E.N., Prins, H.A., Crolla, R.M., et al., 2010. SURPASS Collaborative Group. Effectiveness of a comprehensive surgical safety checklist on patient outcomes. N. Engl. J. Med. 363 (20), 1928–1937.

Ebrahim, A.F., 1995. Organ transplantation: contemporary Sunni Muslim legal and ethical perspectives. Bioethics 9, 291–302.

Ein, S., 2000. Appendectomy. In: Ashcraft, K.W., Murphy, J.P., Sharp, R.J., et al. (Eds.), Pediatric Surgery, third ed. WB Saunders, Philadelphia.

Erhaze, E.K., Dowling, M., Devane, D., 2016. Parental presence and anaesthesia induction: a systematic review. Int. J. Nurs. Pract. 22, 397–407.

Fallat, M.E., Caniano, D.A., Fecteau, AH., American Pediatric Surgical Association Ethics Advocacy Committee, 2007. Ethics and the pediatric surgeon. J. Pediatr. Surg. 42 (1), 129–136.

Gawande, A.A., Thomas, E.J., Zinner, M.J., et al., 1999. The incidence and nature of surgical adverse events in Colorado and Utah in 1992. Surgery 126 (1), 66–75.

Glasper, E.A., Charles-Edwards, I., 2002. The child first and always: the registered children's nurse over 150 years. Part one. Paediatr. Nurs. 14 (4), 38–42.

Goin, J.-P., Kiecolt-Glaser, J.K., 2011. The impact of psychological stress on wound healing: methods and mechanisms. Immunol. Allergy Clin. North Am. 31 (1), 81–93.

Haynes, A.B., Weiser, T.G., Berry, W.R., et al., 2009. A surgical safety checklist to reduce morbidity and mortality in a global population. N. Engl. J. Med. 360, 491–499.

Herron, A., Shields, L., Tanner, A., et al., 2002. In: Shields, L., Werder, H. (Eds.), Perioperative Nursing. Greenwich Medical Media, London.

Hines, S., Munday, J., Kynoch, K., 2015. Effectiveness of nurse-led preoperative assessment services for elective surgery: a systematic review update. JBI Database System Rev Implement Rep. 13 (6), 279–317.

Holm-Knudsen, R.J., Rasmussen, L.S., 2009. Paediatric airway management: basic aspects. Acta Anaesthesiol. 53 (1), 1–9.

Homer, J.J., Williams, B.T., Semple, P., et al., 2000. Tonsillectomy by guillotine is less painful than by dissection. Int. J. Pediatr. Otorhinolaryngol. 52, 25–29.

Ireland, D., 2006. Unique concerns of the pediatric surgical patient: pre-, intra-, and post-operatively. Nurs. Clin. North Am. 41 (2), 265–298.

Javid, P.J., Sanchez, S.E., Horslen, S.P., et al., 2013. Intestinal lengthening and nutritional outcomes in children with short bowel syndrome. Am. J. Surg. 205 (5), 576–580.

Jenkins, K.J., Castañeda, A.R., Cherian, K.M., et al., 2014. Reducing mortality and infections after congenital heart surgery in the developing world. Pediatrics 134 (5), e1422–e1430.

Jessner, L., Blom, G.E., Waldfogel, S., 1952. Emotional implications of tonsillectomy and adenoidectomy on children. Psychoanal Study Child 7, 126–169.

Jolley, J., Shields, L., 2008. The evolution of family centered care. J. Pediatr. Nurs. 24 (2), 164–170. https://doi.org/10.1016/j.pedn.2008.03.010.

Jonas, D., Worsley-Cox, K., 2000. Information giving can be painless. J. Child Health Care 4, 55–58.

Kable, A.K., Gibberd, R.W., Spiegelman, A.D., 2002. Adverse events in surgical patients in Australia. Int. J. Qual. Health Care 14 (4), 269–276.

Kain, Z.N., Caldwell-Andrews, A.A., Mayes, L.C., et al., 2007. Family-centered preparation for surgery improves perioperative outcomes in children: a randomized controlled trial. Anesthesiology 106 (1), 65–74.

Koinig, H., 2002. Preparing parents for their child's surgery: preoperative parental information and education. Paediatr. Anaesth. 12, 107–109.

Lagoo, J., Lopushinsky, S.R., Haynes, A.B., et al., 2017. Effectiveness and meaningful use of paediatric surgical safety checklists and their implementation strategies: a systematic review with narrative synthesis. BMJ Open 7, e016298. https://doi.org/10.1136/bmjopen-2017-016298.

Lambert, P., Cyna, A.M., Knight, N., et al., 2014. Clonidine premedication for postoperative analgesia in children. Cochrane Database. Syst. Rev. (1), CD009633. https://doi.org/10.1002/14651858.CD009633.pub2.

Lansdown, R., 1992. The psychological health status of children in hospital. J. R. Soc. Med. 85, 125–126.

Lundeberg, S., Lonnqvist, P.A., 2004. Update on systemic postoperative analgesia in children. Paediatr. Anaesth. 14, 394–397.

Manyande, A., Cyna, A.M., Yip, P., et al., 2015. Non-pharmacological interventions for assisting the induction of anaesthesia in children. Cochrane Database Syst. Rev. 14 (7), CD006447. https://doi.org/10.1002/14651858.CD006447.pub3.

Meeker, R.H., Rothrock, J.C., 1999. Alexander's Care of the Patient in Surgery, eleventh ed. Mosby, St Louis.

Mitchell, R., 2008. Sleep disordered breathing in children. Mo. Med. 105 (3), 267–269.

Mooney, K., 1997. Perioperative management of the pediatric patient. Plast. Surg. Nurs. 17, 69–73.

Mukherjee, S., Joshi, A., Carroll, D., et al., 2009. What is the effect of circumcision on risk of urinary tract infection in boys with posterior urethral valves? J. Pediatr. Surg. 44 (2), 17–421.

Nieminen, P., Tolonen, U., Copponen, H., 2000. Snoring and obstructive sleep apnea in children: a 6-month follow-up study. Arch. Otolaryngol. Surg. 126, 481–486.

Oremland, E.K., Oremland, J.D., 1973. The Effects of Hospitalization on Children: Models for Their Care. Charles C. Thomas, Springfield, MA.

Palabiyik, F., Cimilli, T., Kayhan, A., et al., 2009. Do the manipulations in paediatric inguinal hernia operations affect the vascularisation of the testes? J. Pediatr. Surg. 48, 788–790.

Paterson, H., Qadan, M., de Luca, S.M., et al., 2008. Changing trends in surgery for acute appendicitis. Br. J. Surg. 95 (3), 363–368.

Perera, A., 2008. Can I decide please? The state of children's consent in the UK. Eur. J. Health Law 15 (4), 411–420.

Poirier, J.F., Savage, J.R., Hilton, M.P., 2018. Curettage versus other methods of adenoidectomy in children. Cochrane Database Syst. Rev. 2018 (1). https://doi.org/10.1002/14651858.CD007642.pub4.

Price, S., 1994. The special needs of children. J. Adv. Nurs. 20, 227–232.

Prows, C.A., Zhang, X., Huth, M.M., et al., 2013. Codeine-related adverse drug reactions in children following tonsillectomy: a prospective study. Laryngoscope 124 (5), 1242–1250.

Raynor, S., 2000. Circumcision. In: Ashcraft, K.W., Murphy, J.P., Sharp, R.J., et al. (Eds.), Pediatric Surgery, third ed. WB Saunders, Philadelphia.

Royal College of Nursing (RCN), 2017. Standards for Assessing, Measuring, and Monitoring Vital Signs in Children and Young People. Royal College of Nursing, London.

Royal College of Surgeons (RCS), 2013. Standards for Children's Surgery. Available from: https://www.rcseng.ac.uk/-/media/files/rcs/library-and-publications/non-journal-publications/rcs_standards_for_childrens_surgery_2013.pdf.

Royal College of Surgeons (RCS), 2015. Standards for non-specialist emergency surgical care of children. Available from https://www.rcseng.ac.uk/-/media/files/rcs/library-and-publications/non-journal-publications/rcs_standards_for_childrens_surgery_2013.pdf.

Rullander, A.-C., Isberg, S., Karling, M., et al., 2013. Adolescents' experience with scoliosis surgery: a qualitative study. Pain Manag. Nurs. 14 (1), 50–59.

Sadhasivam, S., Cohen, L.L., Szabova, A., et al., 2009. Real-time assessment of perioperative behaviors and prediction of perioperative outcomes. Anesth. Analg. 108 (3), 822–826.

Sargi, Z., Younis, R., 2007. Tonsillectomy and adenoidectomy techniques: past, present and future. ORL J. Otorhinolaryngol. Relat. Spec. 69 (6), 331–335.

Shields, L., Waterman, L.A., 2002. Psychosocial care of children in the perioperative area. In: Shields, L., Werder, H. (Eds.), Perioperative Nursing. Greenwich Medical Media, London.

Shields, L., Werder, H., 2002. Perioperative Nursing. Greenwich Medical Media, London.

SickKids (nd) Preoperative Programme: Video tour. Available from: http://www.sickkids.ca/VisitingSickKids/Coming-for-surgery/Pre-Operative-Preparation-Program/video-tour/index.html.

Smith, J., Dearmun, A., 2006. Improving care for children requiring surgery and their families. Paediatr. Nurs. 18 (9), 30–33.

Spektor, Z., Saint-Victor, S., Kay, D.J., Mandell, D.L., 2016. Risk factors for pediatric post-tonsillectomy hemorrhage. Int. J. Pediatr. Otorhinolaryngol. 84, 151–155.

Steven, M., Broadis, E., Carachi, R., et al., 2008. Sign on the dotted line: parental consent. Pediatr. Surg. Int. 24 (7), 847–849.

Strachan, R.G., 1993. Emotional responses to paediatric hospitalization. Nurs. Times 89 (46), 45–49.

Turunen, E., Miettinen, M., Setälä, L., et al., 2017. An integrative review of a preoperative nursing care structure. J. Clin. Nurs. 26 (7–8), 915–930.

Vittinghoff, M., Lönnqvist, P.-A., Mossetti, V., et al., 2018. Postoperative pain management in children: guidance from the pain committee of the European Society for Paediatric Anaesthesiology (ESPA Pain Management Ladder Initiative). Pediatr. Anesth. 28 (6), 493–506.

Weber, T., Tracy, T., 2000. Groin hernias and hydroceles. In: Ashcraft, K.W., Murphy, J.P., Sharp, R.J., et al. (Eds.), Pediatric Surgery, third ed. WB Saunders, Philadelphia, pp. 654–662.

Winship, B., Ruston, H.G., Pohl, H.G., 2017. In pursuit of the perfect penis: hypospadias repair outcomes. J. Pediatr. Urol. 13 (3), 285–288.

Zeev, N., Kain, M., 2007. Family centred preparedness for surgery improves perioperative outcomes in children. Anaesthesiology 106, 65–74.

Zisk Rony, R.Y., Fortier, M.A., MacLaren Chorney, J., et al., 2010. Parental postoperative pain management: attitudes, assessment, and management. Pediatrics 125, e1372.

39

Caring for Children and Young People With Cancer

Wendy McInally, Lisa McCann

LEARNING OUTCOMES

- Explain what cancer is.
- Discuss the incidence of cancer in children and young people.
- Develop an understanding of how cancer is diagnosed and the treatments.
- Understand the common side effect from treatments.
- Discuss cancer care delivery models within the UK.
- Consider palliative and end of life care.

GLOSSARY

Some of the key terms listed here are used throughout the chapter. Others may not be used explicitly but are still relevant to the care of children and young people with cancer.

Biopsies are obtained in a number of different ways depending on the type of tissue required. For example, a biopsy of a skin cancer can be obtained by removing a small piece of tissue surgically, usually using local anaesthetic.

Blood tests are used in the diagnosis of cancers such as leukaemia and retinoblastoma. Blood is usually withdrawn from a peripheral vein, usually in the arm, and sent for pathological analysis.

Bone cancer can affect any bone, but most cases develop in the long bones of the legs or upper arms.

Bone marrow tests are used in the diagnosis of leukaemia and lymphoma. A sample of bone marrow is usually taken from either the hip bone or sternum (breast bone). The white blood cells within the bone marrow are then analysed under a microscope. The procedure usually involves a general anaesthetic.

CYP Children and young people.

Chemotherapy refers to the use of cytotoxic and cytostatic medication to destroy cancer cells.

Clinical trials are research studies carried out in people to evaluate medical, surgical or behavioural interventions. Clinical trials are the main way scientists and researchers find out if new drugs are safe and effective for people to use.

CT Computed Tomography (CT) scan is a special x-ray test that produces cross-sectional images of the body using x-rays and a computer.

Isotope bone scans are used in the diagnosis of primary bone tumours; involves injecting a small amount of a radioactive substance into a peripheral vein. Bones are a common site of metastases (secondary cancers). The radioactive substance migrates through the vascular system; therefore the whole skeleton can be reviewed rather than only the local site. The patient will then undergo x-ray scans of the whole of their skeleton.

Leukaemia is where white blood cells from the marrow are analysed to see if they are abnormal and will determine the type of leukaemia.

Lumbar puncture is a procedure to take a sample of fluid (known as cerebrospinal fluid [CSF]) to look for evidence of cancer cells, infection, and raised pressure in the central nervous system. A needle is inserted into the lower part of the spine. A lumbar puncture can also be used to inject chemotherapy into the cerebrospinal fluid, called intrathecal treatment. This can be done under general anaesthetic in very young children, as they need to lie very still. Young people may be able to tolerate the procedure using local anaesthetic to numb the skin.

Lymphoma is diagnosed through a bone marrow test to see if it contains any lymphoma cells.

Metastases are secondary cancers. They can develop in any area of the body, including bones, the brain and the liver.

MRI (magnetic resonance imaging) frequently used in the diagnosis and staging of cancer. This type of scan uses strong magnetic fields and radio waves to produce detailed images of the inside of the body. An MRI scanner is a large tube that contains powerful magnets.

PET scans are used in the diagnosis of brain tumours and lymphoma and involve injecting a glucose substance into the blood stream that has been labelled with radioactivity by a machine called a cyclotron. This substance is then able to show tissues that are either under-using or over-using glucose.

Retinoblastoma comes in either inherited or non-inherited form. A blood test can determine whether the retinoblastoma gene (Rb gene) is present. A needle is inserted through the skin and into the centre of the bone as this contains the marrow. Samples of the marrow cells are then aspirated into the syringe.

Staging of a cancer refers to how advanced the cancer is at the time it is diagnosed. This process is vital if the patient is to receive the treatment that is most appropriate for them.

TYA is the abbreviation used to refer to teenagers and young adults, typically those aged 15–24 years old.

INTRODUCTION

Cancer care across the United Kingdom (UK) has dramatically improved for children and young people (CYP) over the years (Department of Health, 2007; Scottish Government, 2016). Many CYP diagnosed with cancer survive into adulthood, but they may experience a range of acute and long-term health complications at different stages of this pathway. This chapter begins by providing a brief introduction to cancer, how many CYP are diagnosed with cancer (incidence rates) and an overview of different diagnoses and treatments relevant to CYP with cancer. This chapter focuses on the age range 0–24 years to encompass CYP. However, as some areas of cancer care provision are quite different and unique to the needs of children and young people, respectively, where relevant we discuss children (0–14 years old) and teenagers and young adults (TYA) (15–24 years old) separately. These age group separations are consistent with models of care and cancer service provision in the UK at this time. It is worth noting that there is no universal definition of a teenager or young person as the age parameters differ from within the literature around the world (Olsen and Smith, 2018). For the purposes of this chapter the authors will refer to CYP and TYA where appropriate. Although the care delivery is focused on nursing, many sections will include care delivery through the multi-disciplinary team (MDT).

WHAT IS CANCER?

The word 'cancer' originates from the Latin term for 'crab' and is said to have been first used by the Greek physician Hippocrates, also known as the 'Father of Medicine'. He is said to have applied the term because the finger-like spreading from a tumour reminded him of the shape of a crab burrowed in the sand with its legs spread in a circle. Cancer is not one disease but a collection of different pathologies affecting different parts of the body. The individuality of each person and the variety of pathologies are reflected in the varieties of treatments and outcomes (Cancer Research UK, 2018). Although the experiences and paths followed by individuals with cancer differ greatly, there are some similarities in the way cancer develops and spreads within the body. Cancer can be described as a group of diseases in which cells grow uncontrollably and have the ability to spread away from the site of origin (Children's Cancer and Leukaemia Group, 2018). Each type of cancer has its own characteristics, which means that different treatments will be required. Sometimes cancers can move from one area of the body to another and this is known as secondary cancer or metastases. When a cancer spreads to another part of the body it takes its own characteristics with it. So, for example, if a Wilms' tumour spreads to the lung, the tumour in the lung would both look and behave the same way as the original tumour. This is how primary tumours that have not been located can be found by examining the secondary tumour. Cancer cells develop as a result of damage to DNA, the controlling mechanism for all cell activities. This damage may be caused by a multitude of factors including environmental, dietary and genetic factors. Damaged DNA is normally repaired by the body, but in cancer cells this does not occur.

It is now believed that cancers originate from a single cell. This cell divides and eventually forms what is classed as a tumour. For a tumour to be recognised by either clinical or radiographic examination it is likely to contain about 1 billion cells (Cancer Research UK, 2018). Tumours can be either malignant or benign. Malignant tumours are usually cancerous and have a number of characteristics different to that of normal cells. The rate of reproduction in cancer cells is greater than the rate of cell death generally. This contrasts to normal cells where the number of cells produced equals those dying. Cancers do not always grow particularly fast. It is actually the lack of cell death in cancers that causes them to grow rather than the speed of reproduction being particularly fast.

Cancerous tumours can originate in any of the common tissue types in the body. For example, tumours that arise in the epithelium (tissue that lines the outer surfaces of organs and blood vessels throughout the body and the inner surfaces of cavities in many internal organs). These cancers which invade the bowel and oesophagus are termed 'carcinomas'. However, very few children are diagnosed with these particular kinds of carcinomas. The types of cancer that children are diagnosed with on the whole are different to those in young people and adults. The age at presentation varies with the different types of disease. Benign tumours are not classified as cancers. The main difference between benign and malignant (cancerous) tumours is that benign tumours do not attempt to spread away from the site of origin.

👤 ACTIVITY

Video link. Available from: https://youtu.be/Q6ucKWIIFmg. Explore cell cycle and division and why important to life.

Cancer Incidence

Worldwide cancer is a major concern. Over the past 40 years, the 5-year survival rates for CYP with cancer have risen dramatically in the UK. Recent statistics suggest that 7 in 10 children (70%) will survive cancer compared to 3 in 10 (30%) in the 1960's (see the Children with Cancer 2018 Cancer UK website: https://www.childrenwithcancer.org.uk). There are an estimated 1600 new cases of cancer diagnosed in children aged 0–14 years of age and, 2200 in TYA population aged 15–24 years annually in the UK (see the Cancer Research UK website: http://www.cancerresearchuk.org/). Cancer accounts for less than 1% of illnesses in children and young people; however, it is the leading cause of death for this age group in the developed world. The main types of cancer in children are leukaemia, brain tumours and lymphomas (Children with Cancer 2018), whereas in young people the main types of cancer are lymphoma, carcinomas and germ cell tumours (Cancer Research UK, 2013).

 ACTIVITY

What are the most common cancers seen in children and young people?
- https://www.childrenwithcancer.org.uk/childhood-cancer-info/types-of-cancer/

Five-year cancer survival for children and young people (0–24 years) varies between 50% and 95%, with survival in some cancers hardly having improved over the past two decades (Fern et al., 2013). Although cancer is one of the leading causes of death from disease in this age group, it is rare. Morbidity from both the treatment and disease is considerable, and interruptions to physical, emotional and social development are likely. Caring for a CYP with cancer can have an immense impact on family and friends (Taylor et al., 2013).

Reaching a Diagnosis

While cancer is relatively uncommon among CYP CCLG 2018a compared to adults, CYP will likely visit their general practitioner (GP) multiple times before referrals to haematology or oncology teams are made. Children will be taken by their families, but for the older child or young person, research has shown that there is often a reluctance to attend the GP often as they do not see their ailments as serious (Pinkerton et al., 2007). However, one-third of young people with cancer are diagnosed when their health deteriorates to the point of being admitted to Accident and Emergency (Teenage Cancer Trust, 2015). Recent data in the UK for the TYA population, for example, highlights that females were more likely than their male counterparts to have multiple GP consultation appointments prior to referral to specialists (Herbert et al., 2018) and before being referred to a child or adult haematologist/oncologist. Children and young people and their families report that receiving a cancer diagnosis is the most challenging part of the cancer pathway especially when they need to wait for an appointment or begin their treatment (Gibson and Soanes, 2008). A number of methods are used to confirm a cancer diagnosis. These methods are not exclusive and may be used in combination. For example, to diagnose a brain tumour, the patient will often undergo a Computed Tomography (CT) scan or magnetic resonance imaging (MRI) to find the position of the tumour and then a biopsy is taken by making a very fine hole in the skull and using a fine needle to remove a piece of tissue. Tests can be defined as invasive or non-invasive. Preparation of the child,

young person and their family will differ depending on the nature of the test and whether it is invasive or not (Gibson and Soanes, 2008). A common investigation will be a blood test to determine what is causing the bruising and/or bleeding if the child or young person for example has leukaemia. These clinical features are often associated with this type of cancer. At this time venous access may also be required if treatment is imminent. Most cancers are diagnosed with a blood test and/or biopsy. This applies to cancers where a tissue or cell sample can be obtained and includes all of the cancers described in this chapter (with the exception of retinoblastoma, which can be diagnosed using ophthalmological procedures).

Agreed treatment protocols available in the UK include the introduction of intensive multi-agent chemotherapy, immunotherapy, combined with radiotherapy, surgery and bone marrow transplant as required CCLG 2018. All treatments meet and comply with necessary national and international standards (Gibson and Soanes 2008; National Institute for Health and Care Excellence [NICE], 2005). A cancer may be suspected for a variety of reasons, but the definitive diagnosis of most malignancies must be confirmed by microscopic examination of the cancerous cells by a pathologist. The procedure of obtaining cells and/or pieces of tissue, and their examination, is referred to as a biopsy. The tissue diagnosis indicates the type of cell that is proliferating, its severity (degree of dysplasia) and its extent and size. Cytogenetic and immunohistochemistry tests may provide information about the future behaviour of the cancer and the best treatment.

 ACTIVITY

Jonathan, aged 6 years, was taken to his GP with a chest infection; he was treated with antibiotics for a week. As his chest infection did not improve after the course of antibiotics his mother returned to the GP with Jonathan. The GP requested a chest x-ray and a full blood count. Early evening, Jonathan's parents were telephoned by the GP, who explained to them that as Jonathan's blood count was abnormal, they needed to take him to their local hospital immediately. On arrival at the hospital, Jonathan's parents were advised that his blood results were indicative of leukaemia and the next morning, following a blood transfusion overnight, he would be transferred to a regional cancer unit where he would undergo investigations for leukaemia.

His blood results were haemoglobin 6.8 g/dL, platelets 48 $\times 10^9$, and total white cell count 25.4 $\times 10^9$. The differential showed 95% blast cells.
- What are the normal ranges for a full blood count?
- What do the terms anaemia, neutropenia, thrombocytopenia and pancytopenia mean?

CANCER TREATMENTS

This section of the chapter focuses on the main types of treatment for cancer in CYP, often termed 'treatment modalities'. The most appropriate treatment depends on the type of cancer a child or young person is diagnosed with, the anatomical position of the cancer and the stage and spread of the disease. Treatments for children and young people with cancer are highly complex. Treatments can involve chemotherapy regimens, multiple blood sampling and supportive care measures, all of which require reliable, safe and acceptable venous access to manage the child/young person through the cancer treatment experience. Among the most disturbing experiences for the younger child receiving cancer treatment is the trauma of venepuncture and associated needle phobia (Gibson and Soanes, 2008). Appropriate support is required for both the child/young person and family to remove or reduce these stressful experiences and is part of improving the quality of the patient's pathway in living with cancer (Gibson and Soanes, 2008).

Chemotherapy

The ultimate aim of chemotherapy as a treatment is to cure and ensure the person being treated maintains a good quality of life (Tomlinson and Kline, 2010). This will be delivered as adjuvant or neoadjuvant chemotherapy. Adjuvant chemotherapy means chemotherapy is delivered after another modality of treatment. For example, a child or young person may receive surgery to remove their tumour then may receive a course of adjuvant chemotherapy in the next stage of their treatment pathway. Neoadjuvant chemotherapy, on the other hand, means chemotherapy is delivered *before* another treatment modality. For example, a child or young person may need to undergo a course of chemotherapy to reduce the size of a tumour prior to surgical removal. Unfortunately, for some children and young people, the cancer is not curable and chemotherapy may be used to help control symptoms or discomfort. This is known as palliative chemotherapy.

Chemotherapy is administered in any of the following ways:
- Orally: by mouth.
- Intravenously: via a vein and often through a central venous access or percutaneous venous catheter.
- Subcutaneously: under the skin into subcutaneous tissue.
- Intrathecally: via the cerebral spinal fluid.
- Intramuscularly: directly into the muscle.
- Intracavity: into the bladder cavity (but this is rarely used with children and young people).

Chemotherapy treatment regimes (known as protocols) contain a combination of drugs to achieve the maximum damage and kill the cancer cells. The chemotherapy drug combinations are given in courses often called blocks of treatment and often over prolonged periods of time. It is not unusual for a child or young person to receive their chemotherapy drugs every 3 weeks, for a block of 5 days at a time for 6–9 months, or longer. In the breaks between each treatment block, the body is given time to recover from the damage caused by the previous treatment. This damage occurs as the chemotherapy cannot determine healthy cells from cancer cells and will destroy lots of healthy cells in the body (Gibson and Soanes, 2008; Tomlinson and Kline, 2010). It is this action on healthy cells that cause the side effects of the treatment, known as treatment toxicities. If the period of time between treatment blocks is too long then cancer cells may have the time to recover. For this reason, there are different treatment protocols for different cancers, with the type of individual drugs and the timing of treatments vitally important.

Radiotherapy

Radiotherapy is the use of ionising radiation to treat disease. It is essentially delivered in two forms – either electromagnetic (e.g. x-rays, gamma rays) or particulate (e.g. protons, neutrons). Radiotherapy is similar to chemotherapy in that it can lead to the destruction of cancer cells. Although normal cells are also damaged by radiotherapy, cancer cells are generally more sensitive (Children With Cancer UK, CCLG 2018). This means that a large enough dose to kill cancer cells can be given, while still allowing normal tissue to recover. This requires a careful balance between the radiation dose and an acceptable level of normal tissue damage – this is known as the therapeutic ratio. The effect that radiation has on normal tissue is variable and certain tissue types are particularly sensitive, for example, central nervous system tissue, eyes, lungs, bladder and bowel.

The aims of radiotherapy treatment are:
- To kill cancer cells.
- To cause minimum damage to healthy cells.

Uses of Radiotherapy

- Radiotherapy can be used as the sole treatment modality.
- Radiotherapy can be used in conjunction with chemotherapy or surgery.
- Radiotherapy can be used to control symptoms in an emergency situation. For example, if a tumour is compressing the spinal cord, radiotherapy can alleviate the pressure and prevent permanent damage.
- Radiotherapy may be palliative; for example, to help control symptoms or discomfort, such as bleeding or pain.

Prior to commencing treatment, consultation, planning and simulation is required to determine the most appropriate source and dose of radiotherapy. The following factors will influence the type of radiotherapy used:
- The overall treatment protocol.
- The cancer histology.
- Clinical assessment of the child and young person at the time of radiotherapy treatment planning.

To maintain accuracy of the radiotherapy beam, it is essential that the area of the body receiving the dose remains immobilised throughout each treatment. Often this will be achieved by providing the child and young person with a mould or mask, which will hold the area still and protect surrounding tissues. Furthermore, skin marking using ink is another method that ensures accurate delivery of radiotherapy to the correct site. The final stage of planning is a simulation using diagnostic x-rays to check the prescribed treatment plan. Published jointly on behalf of the Children's Cancer and Leukaemia Group, the Society and College of Radiographers and The Royal College of Radiologists, this guide will provide a framework for children and young people undergoing radiotherapy as part of their treatment (The Royal College of Radiologists (2018)).

Surgery

The improvements in treatments such as chemotherapy and radiotherapy mean that surgery is no longer the only treatment that offers a chance of cure for cancer. However, surgery remains the cornerstone of treatment for most solid cancers. It is used either alone or in combination with some of the other treatment modalities. The principles of surgery are that the primary tumour is removed along with a margin of normal tissue surrounding it (Tomlinson and Kline, 2010). This is to try and ensure that the cancer has been removed completely and that any microscopic malignant cells that are not visible are included within the tissue removed. Surgery is generally used in an attempt to cure the disease, but can also be used to reduce tumour bulk prior to other treatment or for symptom control. Surgery also has a role in the diagnosis and staging of some cancers.

Curative Surgery

If the primary tumour is localised to a particular area and can safely be removed, curative surgery can be attempted. The resected tumour is analysed under a microscope to make certain that the margins all contain normal tissue confirming that a complete resection has been performed. For more extensive cancers, it is becoming increasingly commonplace to use other treatment modalities, for example, chemotherapy, along with surgery in order to 'downstage' the cancer and thus increase the chance of a successful outcome. Surgery is not without risk, and dependent on the extent of the surgery, it may involve a long period of recovery. This stresses the importance of making certain that surgery is the correct treatment option as a failed attempt to resect a tumour can have a dramatic effect on quality of life.

Supportive Surgery

Surgery may be utilised in support of other treatments. For example, some chemotherapy regimens require insertion of a central venous catheter, which will remain in place for the duration of the treatment. This can be inserted surgically using either local or general anaesthesia and involves tunnelling the catheter under the skin and into a major vein, which provides a route for the administration of toxic drugs.

Bone Marrow Transplant (BMT) or Peripheral Blood Stem Cell Transplants (PBSCT)

Blood stem cells are the precursor cells for all the different cells present in blood. These precursor cells are able to develop into any of the cells that make up blood; for example, red blood cells, platelets or white blood cells. They are found in the bone marrow and in the umbilical cord blood of babies.

Indications for Blood Stem Cell Transplant

The primary goal of stem cell transplant is to cure life-threatening disease (either malignant or non-malignant) and restore normal bone marrow function by the reconstitution of both haematological and immune function. This can be achieved by three key treatment principles:

- Eliminate the patient's haemopoietic and immune system with high doses of chemotherapy and/or irradiation.
- Rescue with disease free stem cells, either from a donor (allograph) or the patient's own stem cells (autograph).
- Provide a graft versus leukaemia/tumour effect whereby donor immune cells recognise any residual disease and eradicate it.

Immunotherapy

Immunotherapy treatments, also known as targeted treatments or biological therapies, are a group of treatments that use the body's natural protective system to attack cancer cells (American Cancer Society, 2017; Cancer Research UK, 2018). Immunotherapy can be delivered on its own or alongside other cancer treatments. These treatments are still advancing and are only currently suitable to treat certain cancer diagnoses, but the hope is the use of these treatments will continue to grow once results of future clinical trials are known. The main types of immunotherapy are:

- Monoclonal antibodies (MABs)
- Cytokines
- Adoptive cell transfer
- Vaccines to treat cancer

  Read more about these different types of immunotherapy on the Cancer Research UK 2018 webpages via: https://www.cancerresearchuk.org/about-cancer/cancer-in-general/treatment/immunotherapy/what-is-immunotherapy.

Clinical Trials

Children and young people may be treated for their cancer on a clinical trial. Clinical trials are conducted in all areas of medicine, not just cancer, and are medical research studies with people. The Children's Cancer and Leukaemia Group (CCLG 2014) have produced information for children, young people and their families so they are informed about clinical trials; some of this is summarised below (see Activity for the weblink to access this information to review). Clinical trials are conducted to:

- test new treatments, including new chemotherapy drugs;
- look at new combinations of existing treatments;
- look at changing the way existing treatments are given to see if they are more effective or to help reduce side effects;
- find out how cancer treatments work;
- see which treatments have the least impact on patients' everyday lives;
- find supportive care treatments that help reduce side effects;

- look at the impact that cancer and its treatment have on quality of life.

Clinical trials are defined by phases – each phase has a different purpose and reason for being conducted:

- *Phase I.* New treatments are tested on a very small number of people for the first time.
- *Phase II.* Tested with a relatively small number of people to see if a particular treatment is likely to be effective for patients at given doses.
- *Phase III.* Large-scale trials with many participants from many different hospitals (and often countries) at the same time to confirm the benefits of the treatment. These studies are often known as randomised controlled trials and compare one group of participants who receive the new treatment compared to another who continue to receive the 'standard' treatment.

 ACTIVITY

Read the Fact Sheet on Clinical Trials produced by the Children's Cancer and Leukaemia Group (CCLG 2014) and identify possible benefits and disadvantages of participating in a clinical trial: Available from:

- https://www.cclg.org.uk/write/MediaUploads/Publications/PDFs/A_guide_to_clinical_trials_(Apr_14).pdf

Although many children are likely to be part of a clinical trial during their experience of cancer, this is not always the case for young people. The Teenage Cancer Trust has worked hard in recent years to increase opportunities and implement improvements for young people to participate in clinical trials.

 ACTIVITY

Read this report from the Teenage Cancer Trust (TCT 2014) and identify at least five challenges in provision of equitable access to clinical trials for young people: Available from:

- https://www.teenagecancertrust.org/sites/default/files/Clinical%20Trials%20Paper_JR_FINAL_April15.pdf

---

MODELS OF CARE DELIVERY

Across the UK, CYP with cancer usually begin their cancer journey within a children's service, teenage cancer unit or adult services. Children are normally managed in children's services from the age of 0–14 years. Young people 15–24 years are either nursed in Teenage Cancer Trust (TCT) units or adult services. The initial cancer diagnosis is normally made at the appropriate primary treatment centre (PTC). A PTC is a specialised centre for the provision of cancer treatment and recent recommendations suggest that all CYP are treated at such facilities (Pettit et al., 2016). Depending on the agreed treatment protocol and the needs of the patient and family, treatment is then delivered within the shared care centre (SCC) or home environment (Gibson and Soanes, 2008).

These links highlight the organisation of care for young people aged 13–24 years. There are 21 PTCs for 0–16 years. In addition, there are 28 TYA units ranging from the age of 13 or 16, up to the age of 24 cross the UK. These links provide in-depth knowledge around these centres.

- https://www.cclg.org.uk/CSOIR/Organisation-of-childrens-cancer-care-in-the-UK
- https://www.teenagecancertrust.org/about-us/what-we-do/cancer-units

Multi-disciplinary teams (MDTs) are central to the provision of effective care and treatment to improve outcomes for CYP diagnosed with cancer. MDTs facilitate the coming together of a wide range of health care professionals involved in care provision for children or young people diagnosed with cancer. The purpose of MDTs can vary – they may focus on confirming diagnoses, or they may be used to make treatment decisions for a patient or they may discuss how best the psychosocial needs of a patient can be met. In essence, the purpose of MDT working is to ensure each person diagnosed with cancer has the benefit of the best medical, nursing and allied health professional input when diagnosed and receiving treatments for cancer. Teenager and young adult-specific MDTs for those aged 16–24 years also consider the best place of care for the young person and what clinical trials are relevant to invite the young person to participate in (Pettit et al., 2016). For young people aged 19–24 years in England, there is more choice; they can choose to receive their treatment at a TYA designated hospital closer to their home or they can receive treatment at the PTC (Pettit et al., 2016).

For more information specifically relating to TYA cancer care and experiences of young people with cancer, read about the BRIGHTLIGHT study and complete the activity suggested in the information box below:

◎ **EVIDENCE-BASED PRACTICE**

The BRIGHTLIGHT study is a collection of research projects funded by the National Institute for Health Research (NIHR) in the UK to answer one overarching question: Do specialist services for teenagers and young adults add value? This large-scale programme of work was conducted between 2013 and 2019.

The main areas the research projects have focused on are:

- The environments in which care is delivered
- The competencies of health care professionals delivering care
- Young people's experience of care
- The cost of care (to the NHS, but also to young people and their families)
- Developing a metric to quantify specialist care

There have been lots of conference presentations and journal articles published on the BRIGHTLIGHT study. You can access these and read more about this programme of work via the study website: http://www.brightlightstudy.com .

Activity

Access the website and read two journal papers from the BRIGHTLIGHT resources page.

It is crucial that care is provided in an age appropriate setting. It is estimated that many young people are not treated within a setting appropriate for their age (NICE, 2005). The majority of these patients are not currently considered for entry into clinical trials (Chisholm et al., 2018), which ultimately impacts on the overall cancer survival and recovery from the disease. The experience of young people living with or beyond a cancer diagnosis is vital to the overall understanding of the cancer journey. Once a child or young person reaches a certain age, transition of care from a child to adult service should begin in an age appropriate, planned and seamless way. McCann et al. (2014) found that all health care professionals, young people and their families need to be too ready for transition. In order to achieve this, appropriate planning and preparation for the transition needs to be implemented. Currently some are transitioned to adult services at a well-defined and clearly communicated juncture, such as age or on completion of their treatment regime. Others remain within the children's oncology/haematology specialist service late into adulthood with no clear model of transition (McInally and Cruikshank, 2013). In addition, it is recommended that all patients are given the opportunity to decide when and where they would prefer to be treated. For example, the National Institute of Clinical Excellence (2005) suggests that young adults aged 19 years and above may make an informed choice regarding their place of care.

 ACTIVITY

Discover the number of Primary Treatment Centres across the UK.

Many families may well have to travel a significant distance away from home to their nearest centre.

Make a list of the advantages and disadvantages for the patient and family members when being transferred to a regional oncology centre.

Supportive Care

Meeting the supportive care needs of CYP living with and beyond a diagnosis of cancer is important to help ensure successful health and well-being outcomes. The treatment of a malignant disease attacks the body's normal defence mechanisms directly and indirectly. The direct effects are on the white cells and the immune system. The indirect effects are through the methods of administration, for example, via long lines that puncture the skin, other procedures such as venepunctures, bone marrow aspirates and lumbar punctures, which increase the risk of infection. The prevention and early detection of infection is therefore a priority.

As discussed previously, CYP undergoing treatment for cancer are likely to experience a prolonged treatment pathway. This means they may spend long periods of time as an inpatient in hospital or they may receive much of their treatment as outpatients. Either way, the effective symptom management of side effects they may experience is vital and so it is essential for nurses to have a good knowledge of both: (1) the disease

and its symptoms, and (2) treatments and their side effects. In addition, effective supportive care provision to address the psychological needs and well-being of the child or young person and their family members is essential. There are many acute/chronic side effects of treatment CYP may experience in addition to those discussed in detail in this chapter. Patients undergoing treatment for a malignancy are likely therefore, to receive a combination of therapies, which may last for months or, in the case of leukaemia, years. Some patients will undergo long periods of hospitalisation, others will receive much of their treatment as outpatients, attending both the regional centre and the shared care hospital. Therefore the effective management of side effects is vital. Effective management incorporates the physical and psychological care for the patient and the psychological care of family members. Symptom management for a patient undergoing treatment for a malignant disease requires nurses to have knowledge of the following:

- disease and its symptoms
- treatment and management of the side effects

Nurses and other members of the MDT must be able to prioritise their care and show flexibility in the way that the care is delivered (Gibson and Soanes, 2008). Many of the skills that nurses demonstrate will be carried out by the parents once the patient is discharged, and therefore negotiation and education are key aspects of care.

Febrile Neutropenia

Fever and neutropenia are common complications in CYP who receive chemotherapy for cancer and are the second most common reason for hospital admissions among this population (NICE, 2012). Regular observations of temperature, pulse, respirations and blood pressure and an accurate fluid balance are essential for the patient who is neutropenic. Nurses also need to be able to evaluate things like any changes such in skin colour, oral hygiene, skin integrity and nutritional intake (Gibson and Soanes, 2008). Neutropenia is responsible for significant morbidity in children and young people treated for cancer and accounts for a substantial use of resources and remains fatal in some instances. In the UK, specific NICE (2012) guidelines have been developed for neutropenic sepsis and management specifically focused on CYP with cancer (Bate et al., 2013).

Nausea and Vomiting

Nausea and vomiting are immediate side effects of chemotherapy, but they can persist for several days following administration of the drug, especially nausea. Children have identified nausea as being worse than vomiting, and assessment, which includes the patient and family, is therefore essential. Various rating scales have been developed (CCLG, 2018b). It is not unusual for some children and young people to experience anticipatory nausea and vomiting during their treatment. This is a complex reaction that triggers memories, thoughts and images from previous experiences. It could be a particular smell, such as disinfectant, food or a nurse's perfume, a particular room, generally something that the patient associates with nausea and/or vomiting. Pharmacological, non-pharmacological and complementary methods all have a role to play in establishing individualised approaches to managing nausea and vomiting for CYP.

Mucositis

The term 'mucositis' refers to inflammation of the oral mucosa, which relates to the mucous membranes of the digestive tract which begin at the mouth and end at the anus. Mucositis can be acute and chronic in nature and can reduce CYPs intake of fluids and solids, impacting negatively on general well-being and quality of life (Gibson and Soanes, 2008). For nurses, fluid balance charts need to be monitored extremely closely, as do output of stools, to ensure appropriate management. Mucositis is a prominent side effect of chemotherapy because oral epithelial cells have a lifespan of around 7 days and they continually renew. This makes these cells particularly vulnerable to attack by *cytotoxic drugs*, thus caring for the mouth throughout treatment is particularly important. This is even more so because chemotherapy treatment is likely to result in the patient's nutritional intake already being altered, through nausea (with or without vomiting), stomatitis, anorexia and taste alteration, or food restriction prior to procedures. Therefore working with dietitians, identifying at-risk patients, initiating flexible meal ordering, and provision of facilities for parents to cook or to bring food in for their child or young person are ways of preventing or minimising severe problems and helping to address people's nutritional needs.

Alopecia

Children and young people are concerned about their appearance, and it is important to be able to look and dress like their peers. Treatment, as already identified, can result in undesirable physical changes that make them look and feel different (Tomlinson and Kline, 2010). Although it is important to stress the temporary nature of side effects such as alopecia to CYP they and other family members will require help from the MDT to develop coping strategies to deal with these changes. Alopecia, or hair loss, is almost inevitable with most treatments for cancer for CYP. Often this is one of the most challenging aspects of the cancer experience, both for the person diagnosed and their family members. Chemotherapy-related hair loss is usually total (all body hair), although scalp hair is more severely affected as the hair follicles of the scalp are the most rapidly growing. Charities such as Clic Sargent, Macmillan Cancer Support and Teenage Cancer Trust all have website and written resources available to support children, young people and their families with side effects of treatment, including alopecia. As discussed previously, there are many more side effects of treatment such as pain, fatigue, constipation, anorexia and changes in skin condition and skin sensation.

🧑 ACTIVITY

Available from:
  https://www.youtube.com/watch?time_continue=28&v=FfeVcom5h-I
- Discuss why the patient with cancer, who is receiving treatment, is at risk of infection?
- What is febrile neutropenia?

PSYCHOLOGICAL WELL-BEING

Effective communication skills are a key aspect of the psychological care. In this section of the chapter, we draw on the example of a woman called Kate, a health professional diagnosed with cancer. Although diagnosed at 29 years old, which is slightly older than the focus of this chapter, the premise of her story is important for you in your roles as nurses when caring for people generally, but also CYP with cancer and their families. Sadly, Kate died in 2016; however, her work to improve the patient experience lives on. This is her story.

Kate, a Specialist Registrar in Geriatric Medicine, had incurable cancer. After five rounds of chemotherapy following her diagnosis with a rare and aggressive form of sarcoma in July 2011, Kate decided to stop receiving treatment and concentrate on enjoying a good quality of life.

Following that decision, Kate wrote two books, a series of blogs and tweeted extensively about living with cancer, and in particular, her experiences as a patient. She also launched the 'hello my name is' campaign after becoming frustrated by the number of health care professionals who failed to introduce themselves to her when she was being treated. This video is Kate's story which is useful when thinking about the communication skills required by health care professionals to reduce patient distress and improve patient centeredness.

🧑 ACTIVITY

Available from:
  https://www.hellomynameis.org.uk/
  After you have watched this video, write a few lines with your thoughts about her experiences and how it has possibly made you reflect on clinical practice.
- Why is communication important?
- What key skills do nurses require for effective communication?
- What are the core values from the work of the campaign?

The impact of a diagnosis of cancer in CYP is disruptive. The impact of these disruptions and the need for psychological support to ensure psychological well-being may be different depending on the age of the patient. Young people with cancer have identified their desire to use digital resources more to support their experiences of cancer (Abrol et al., 2017). This is especially important now, given that numerous digital technologies are available and present in society and influence many day-to-day activities, from internet banking to online shopping. Although the health care sector has been slower to adopt technology, gradually the sector is catching up, digital health and care strategic plans are developed and implemented (Scottish Government, 2016).

As CYP are now so often digital natives, a term used to reflect the population who have grown up in the digital age (Prenksy, 2001), researchers are increasingly developing and testing digital interventions to support children and young people diagnosed with cancer. These interventions include educational video games to involve young people in their own cancer treatment (Beale et al., 2007), apps to monitor treatment symptoms (Stinson et al., 2013), internet-based self-management solutions to support people post-treatment (Williamson et al., 2014; Winterling et al., 2016), and digital peer-support solutions, including social media (Lindberg et al., 2017).

TEENAGERS AND YOUNG ADULTS

As discussed at the beginning of this chapter there is no universal definition of teenager, adolescent, young person or young adult. The terminology and how we refer to this group of people differs across the globe. In the UK since the early 1990s teenagers and young adults have been referred to as TYA. When TYAs are diagnosed with cancer, their typical developmental pathways can be disrupted (Smith et al. 2016). Psychologically, physically, socially, educationally or vocationally, the impact of cancer can be wide-reaching. Relationships with peers and family members can be challenging and perhaps even compromised during a young person's experience of cancer. Therefore psychological and psychosocial assessments and support are essential to ensure young people's well-being. Often clinical psychologists are members of the MDT at PTCs and they can help support young people to adjust to their new circumstances, support them with their communication skills, particularly when discussing difficult topics, foster resilience and advise on coping strategies for young people to use throughout their experiences of cancer (Soanes and Gibson 2018).

👤 ACTIVITY

Imagine you are an 18-year-old female in your first year of University living away from home. You have been diagnosed with leukaemia and need to withdraw from your studies and move home to commence your treatment as the nearest PTC is there, not in your University town. How would you feel, what would you want to know, what would you do, and what emotions do you experience? Write a few lines to capture this.

LIVING BEYOND A CANCER DIAGNOSIS

Advancing treatments for cancer have had a significantly positive effect on survival rates for children, teenagers and young adults diagnosed with cancer over the decades. In the 1960s, for example, survivorship rates for children diagnosed with cancer were just 30% but now, more than 8 out of 10 (80%) children diagnosed will survive for at least 5 years beyond diagnosis (Cancer Research UK, 2018). For TYAs figures are similarly encouraging with more than 80% of young people in this age range surviving cancer for a least 5 years, with survival rate slightly higher in females (84%) than males (81%) (Cancer Research UK, 2018).

Remission

Treatment advances now mean many cancers can be cured, but the term more often used to describe this is remission (Cancer Research UK, 2017). Remission means there is no sign of cancer left in a person's body (Cancer Research UK, 2017).

For some diagnostic groups, such as acute lymphoblastic leukaemia, for example, once in remission children or young people will need to commence the treatment phase known as maintenance therapy. This treatment can last for many months and is to maintain the remission and minimise the chance of relapse (the disease returning).

Recurrence

It is possible, unfortunately, for some types of cancer to come back many years after they were first diagnosed and treated (Cancer Research UK, 2017). Relapse rates vary with individual diseases and depend on prognostic features and the stage of the disease at diagnosis. Relapse brings with it the need for information regarding confirmation and extent of the spread of recurrent disease and the possibility of further treatment.

Long-Term Late Effects

There are some long-term late effects and risks associated to surviving cancer in childhood or young adulthood and these are often related to diagnosis, treatment(s) and age at treatment of each individual young person. Long-term side effects are often related to the combination and dosage of drugs used, and multi-modal therapies can exacerbate toxicities further. The body systems that can be impacted by the toxicities are:

- lungs
- heart
- renal system
- liver
- gonads: fertility
- endocrine: growth and puberty
- hearing
- central nervous system
- skin
- skeletal
- eyes

SIGN (2013) (http://www.sign.ac.uk) and NICE (2005) (https://www.nice.org.uk) have developed specialist guidelines to inform the provision of appropriate care and support for survivors of childhood and young adult cancer. As more children, teenagers and young adults survive cancer, services have to be flexible and responsive given the varying experiences of those who have survived a diagnosis of cancer during childhood or young adulthood. Young people's transition through their developmental life-cycles naturally means their needs will vary so continued provision of age-appropriate care and support during these periods is particularly important. Increasingly, oncology and haematology services are implementing Late Effects Clinical Nurse Specialist roles as integral provision of multi-disciplinary, comprehensive and individualised patient-centred care for this population.

PALLIATIVE AND END-OF-LIFE CARE AND DEATH

Definitions

Palliative care should focus on the person, not the disease. It is defined as 'applying a holistic approach to meet physical, practical, functional, social, emotional and spiritual needs of the child or young person and their families facing progressive illness and bereavement (World Health Organization [WHO], 2018). End-of-life care is described as the child or young person's last remaining weeks, days or hours of life.

For many adults, hospice care is a large component of their palliative care and end of life care in the UK. However, this is not the case for children and young people. Throughout the UK now there is an extensive network of hospices for children and young people to now choose as an option (CCLG, 2019). Providing a choice for the majority of CYP with cancer and their family will involve choice; some families choose for the CYP to die at home in their familiar surroundings, though this may not always be possible. However, wherever the child/young person does spend their last few days or hours of their life, it is important that there is good communication and a holistic management of any symptoms. If the child/young person is able to die at home, then coordination of different community services, in order for the service to fit the family's needs, is required.

The Key to 'Good' Palliative and End-of-Life Care

- A named lead nurse and doctor to coordinate and oversee the child/young person's care.
- Early identification of the child and young person's palliative care needs. This allows more time around planning, and maximises the choice for child and family.
- The person delivering any 'bad news' has received training in 'breaking bad news'. In the palliative phase assessment of core needs and the development of a multi-agency plan is supportive. This should include, particularly, the child or young person reaching near the end of their life to have an 'anticipatory care plan' to aid the planning of the next steps for managing any symptoms they may have. This will also empower the parents if the child/young person is being cared for at home; the family do need access to 24-hour expert health care professional advice and support even if only via a phone.
- If a child/young person is being discharged from hospital to either their home or their local children's/young people's hospice, there is a requirement for good communication and planning between all professionals involved (Gibson and Soanes, 2008).
- Recognition of and planning for end-of-life, assuming there is time, which should include discussions and plans for resuscitation and management of symptoms and episodes of deterioration; making sure all organisations involved in the child/young person's care are informed of any plans. Another term for this type of planning is 'advance care planning'.
- Planning for care of the family after the child/young person's death – who will provide what/when. This can be discussed as part of the anticipatory care planning although it is important to understand that some CYP and the families may choose not to discuss such wishes prior to the death.

Within the time frame for palliative care a period where a young person may become of adult age, consideration of their transition between children and young people's services to adult services will need to be considered. There is also an important need for education and training in children/young people's palliative care of all health and social care practitioners who will care for this group of patients during this phase of their experience.

In addition to the above, any plans should also consider the psychological needs not only for the child/young person, but also any siblings and their parents. There may be a need to access additional financial assistance for the family; however, there are some families who find asking for help with any finances hard.

The child/young person should be able to continue attending school or college for as long as the child/young person feels well enough to attend and this may include taking school or national exams. Being at school/college will give the child/young person some 'normality' to their life during this phase of their cancer pathway, plus it enables them to continue with their friendship groups too, allowing their friends to build memories of them and provided their open honest discussions about the situation. Where the child/young person is being cared for at home there will be the need for assessment for what equipment they will require. This can be done through the Community Occupational Therapist or the Community Children's Nurse/District Nursing service as they may be able to provide aids to help with getting about like a wheelchair, bathing aids, specialist beds, equipment to assist the family/any health/social carer to move/transfer the child/young person safely. If the palliative care phase is continuing over a significant period of time there is an importance to protect the health needs of the child/young person's family members, as well as the needs of any siblings, ensuring these are met too. There may also be a need to access some short-term respite breaks for the CYP and the family.

👤 ACTIVITY

James is an 11-year-old who was diagnosed with an osteosarcoma in his pelvis. Initially James responded to his treatment despite presenting with a large tumour in his pelvis and metastases within his lung. However, as he nears the end of his chemotherapy, James started to complain of pins and needles/loss of feeling within one of his legs. He is also unable to pass urine. James required admission to hospital. On admission to hospital a urinary catheter was inserted to enable James to pass urine within his bladder. It was also discovered he had become incontinent of faeces. An MRI scan was undertaken and showed extensive tumour growth, which had started to erode through James' spinal cord which explained these new symptoms. James was also complaining of increased pain, especially when being helped to move. He is desperate to go home as previous experiences of hospital have been a challenge. James is also becoming very angry and uncooperative. He is also complaining of being unable to sleep while in hospital. Results from the MRI have been given to the parents, but not to James.

Using the scenario above answer the following questions below.

- Has James' cancer journey now become palliative or end-of-life rather than curative?
- How should this be communicated to James and his family?

SUMMARY

A national review of children's services has provided a real impetus for change with young people being a high priority area for the UK Government and national charities such as TCT, Macmillan and Children's Cancer and Leukaemia Group (CCLG). Research has shown that as young CYP survive, they are at significant risk of developing later complications following treatment for cancer including physical, emotional and psychological complications. As CYP grow and develop into independent and responsible individuals, they are encouraged to take responsibility for their own health care.

It is important to empower young people to make decisions regarding their own health care, yet there is currently a lack of clarity around which approach may impact on their ability to achieve this. Health care professionals must strive to ensure that the planning and preparation for individual patients is communicated well before the actual end of treatment arrives. It should be recognised that each individual may find this physically, emotionally and psychologically difficult. Further resources to support learning are available from: https://www.cclg.org.uk/elearning-for-health-professionals.

REFERENCES

Abrol, E., Groszmann, M., Pitman, A., et al., 2017. Exploring the digital technology preferences of Teenagers and Young Adults (TYA) with cancer and survivors: a cross-sectional service evaluation questionnaire. J. Cancer Surviv. 11 (6), 670–682. https://doi.org/10.1007/s11764-017-0618-z.

American Cancer Society, 2017. The current and future promise of immunotherapy for childhood cancers. Available from: https://www.cancer.org/latest-news/the-current-and-future-promise-of-immunotherapy-for-childhood-cancers.html.

Bate, J., Gibson, F., Johnson, E., et al., 2013. Neutropenic sepsis: prevention and management of neutropenic sepsis in cancer patients (NICE Clinical Guideline CG151). Arch. Dis. Child. Educ. Pract. Ed. 98, 73–75.

Beale, I.L., Kato, P.M., Marin Bowling, V.M., et al., 2007. Improvement in cancer related knowledge following use of a psycho-educational video game for adolescents and young adults with cancer. J. Adolesc. Health. 41 (3), 263–270.

BRIGHTLIGHT. 2018 BRIGHTLIGHT: do specialist services for teenage and young adults with cancer add value? Available from: http://www.brightlightstudy.com (accessed 14 June 2018).

Cancer Research UK, 2013. Young People's Cancers statistics. Available from: http://www.cancerresearchuk.org/health-professional/cancer-statistics/teenagers-and-young-adults-cancers#-heading-Six (accessed 14 June 2018).

Cancer Research UK, 2013. Teenagers and young adults cancer statistics. Available from: https://www.cancerresearchuk.org/health-professional/cancer-statistics/young-people-cancers/incidence#heading-Three (accessed 30 July 2018).

Cancer Research UK, 2017. Why some cancers come back. Available from: http://www.cancerresearchuk.org/about-cancer/what-is-cancer/why-some-cancers-come-back (accessed 13 June 2018).

Cancer Research UK, 2019. Children's cancers. Available from: https://www.cancerresearchuk.org/childrens-cancers (last accessed 25 April 19).

Children's Cancer and Leukaemia Group (CCLG), 2018. Childhood cancer. Available from: http://www.cclg.org.uk/ (accessed 25 July 2018).

Children with Cancer UK. Childhood cancer facts and figures. Available from: https://www.childrenwithcancer.org.uk/childhood-cancer-info/childhood-cancer-facts-figures/ (accessed 14 June 2018).

Children with Cancer UK. Childhood cancer info. Available from: https://www.childrenwithcancer.org.uk/childhood-cancer-info/types-of-cancer/ (accessed 30 July 2018).

Children's Cancer and Leukaemia Group (CCLG), 2014. A guide to clinical trials – for young people with cancer and their parents. Available from: https://www.cclg.org.uk/write/MediaUploads/Publications/PDFs/A_guide_to_clinical_trials_(Apr_14).pdf (accessed 30 July 2018).

Children's Cancer and Leukaemia Group (CCLG), 2018a. About childhood cancer. Available from: https://www.cclg.org.uk/About-Childhood-Cancer (accessed 25 April 2019).

Children's Cancer and Leukaemia Group (CCLG), 2018b. Chemotherapy induced nausea and vomiting. Available from: https://www.cclg.org.uk/CSOIR/Chemotherapy-induced-nausea-and-vomiting (accessed 31 July 2018).

Children's Cancer and Leukaemia Group (CCLG), 2019. Introduction to palliative care in children and young people with cancer. Available from: https://www.cclg.org.uk/CSOIR/Introduction-to-palliative-care-in-children-and-young-people-with-cancer.

Chisholm, J., Hough, R., Soanes, L., 2018. A Practical Approach to the Care of Adolescents and Young Adults With Cancer. Springer, London.

Department of Health, 2007. The Cancer Reform Strategy. The Stationery Office, London.

Fern, L.A., Birch, R., Whelan, J., Cooke, M., Sutton, S., Neal, R.D., Gerrand, C., Hubbard, G., Smith, S., Lethaby, C., Dommett, R., Gibson, F., 2013a. Why Can't We Improve the Timeliness of Cancer Diagnosis in Children, Teenagers, and Young Adults? BMJ, p. 6493. October.

Gibson, F., Soanes, L., 2008. Cancer in Children and Young People. Wiley, England.

Herbert, A., Lyratzopoulos, G., Whelan, J., et al., 2018. Diagnostic timeliness in adolescents and young adults with cancer: a cross-sectional analysis of the BRIGHTLIGHT cohort. The Lancet Child & Adolescent Health. Available from: https://doi.org/10.1016/S2352-4642(18)30004-X.

Lindberg, S., Svedberg, P., Berquist, M., et al., 2017. Evaluating digital peer support for children cured from cancer. International Journal Human Computer Interactive 33 (8), 664–676.

McCann, L., Kearney, N., Wengstrom, Y., 2014. It's just going to a new hospital…that's it. Or is it? An experiential perspective on moving from pediatric to adult cancer services. Cancer Nurs. 37 (5), E23–E31. https://doi.org/10.1097/NCC.0b013e3182a40f99.

McInally, W., Cruickshank, S., 2013. Transition from child to adult services for young people with cancer. Nurs. Child. Young People 25 (1), 14–18.

NICE, 2005. Accessed June 2018 https://www.nice.org.uk/guidance/csg7.

National Institute for Health and Care Excellence (NICE), 2012. Neutropenic sepsis: prevention and management in people with cancer, 2012. Available from: https://www.nice.org.uk/guidance/cg151accessed June 2018. National Institute for Health and Care Excellence (NICE), 2005. Guidance on Cancer Services: Improving Outcomes in Children and Young People With Cancer. NICE, London.

Olsen, P.R., Smith, S., 2018. Nursing Adolescents and Young Adults With Cancer, Developing Knowledge, Competence and Best Practice. Springer, London.

Pinkerton, R., Shankar, A., Matthay, K., 2007. Evidence-Based Paediatric Oncology, second ed. London. Blackwell.

SIGN 132, 2013. Long Term Follow up of Survivors of Childhood Cancer. Accessed June 2018 https://www.sign.ac.uk/media/1070/sign132.pdf.

Smith, S., Mooney, S., Cable, M., Taylor, R., 2016. The Blueprint of Care for Teenagers and Young Adults with Cancer, second ed. Teenage Cancer Trust, London.

Soanes, L., Gibson, F., 2018. Protecting an adult identity: a grounded theory of supportive care for young adults recently diagnosed with cancer. Int. J. Nurs. Stud. 40.

Stinson, J.N., Jibb, L.A., Nguyen, C., et al., 2013. Development and testing of a multidimensional iPhone pain assessment application for adolescents with cancer. J. Med. Internet Res. 15 (3), e51. https://doi.org/10.2196/jmir.2350.

Taylor, R., et al., 2013. Developing a conceptual model of teenager and young adult experiences of cancer through meta-synthesis. Int. J. Nurs. Stud. 50 (6), 832–846.

Teenage Cancer Trust, 2014. Giving more young people with cancer an opportunity to take part in clinical trials. Available from: https://www.teenagecancertrust.org/sites/default/files/Clinical%20Trials%20Paper_JR_FINAL_April15.pdf (accessed 30 July 2018).

Teenage Cancer Trust, 2015. A third of young people with cancer diagnosed in A&E. Available from: https://www.teenagecancertrust.org/about-us/news/third-young-people-cancer-diagnosed-ae.

The Royal College of Radiologists, 2018. Good Practice Guide for Paediatric Radiotherapy, second ed. Accessed June 2018. https://www.rcr.ac.uk/publication/good-practice-guide-paediatric-radiotherapy-second-edition.

The Scottish Government, 2016. Right Diagnosis, Right Treatment, Right Team, Right Place Cancer Plan for Children and Young People in Scotland 2016–19: Managed Service Network for Children and Young People with Cancer in Scotland. The Scottish Government, Edinburgh.

Tomlinson, D., Kline, N., 2010. Pediatric Oncology Nursing Advanced Clinical Handbook. Springer, London.

Williamson, R., Meacham, L., Cherven, B., et al., 2014. Predictors of successful use of a web-based healthcare document storage and sharing system for pediatric cancer survivors: cancer SurvivorLinkTM. J. Cancer Surviv. 8 (3), 355–363.

Winterling, J., Wiklander, M., Obol, C.M., et al., 2016. Development of a self-help web-based intervention targeting young cancer patients with sexual problems and fertility distress in collaboration with patient research partners. JMIR Research Protocols 5 (2), e60. https://doi.org/10.2196/resprot.5499.

World Health Organization (WHO), 2018. Palliative care. Available from: http://www.who.int/en/news-room/fact-sheets/detail/palliative-care (accessed 31 July 2018).

40

Children Living With Long-Term Conditions

Duncan C. Randall

LEARNING OUTCOMES

- Define long-term conditions, their dimension and duration.
- Set out the concepts of quality of life, the measures of health-related quality of life as applied to children's childhoods.
- Discuss children's self-care, children's agency in their self-care and the facilitation of self-care by children's carers and nurses.
- Discuss the use of technology, digital health monitoring and telemedicine to support children's self-care practices.

GLOSSARY

Categorical Approach to long-term conditions which considers the specific condition, e.g. diabetes.

Digital age The digital age or the information age is generally thought to have started in the 1970s with the introduction of personal computers. It can be defined as a period when health care became dominated by information retrieval, management, analysis and transition via electronic media and communication using computer technology.

Disease trajectory Observable pattern of a long-term condition over time. May include periods of exacerbation of the condition and incremental worsening or improvement in health status; may also include deterioration of health status leading to death.

Health-related quality of life Quality of life measures which relate to the health aspects of a person's life. This might include but not be limited to the effect of a condition and the required treatment or symptom management which affect a person's quality of life.

Key worker A worker who takes a lead role in coordinating a child's care often collaborating with others to ensure care is delivered. Also works with children and their carers to determine need and to articulate the views of child and their carers to other formal and informal carers/workers.

Long-term condition Various definitions have been put forward, but most recognise a person will live with the condition for more than 12 months, require some supervision or treatment with the expectation that they will experience symptoms and need support, and or treatment, for the foreseeable future, and possibly for life.

Non-categorical Approach to long-term conditions which considers the similarity between different conditions, rather than a specific condition, e.g. the stigma of having a long-term condition.

Patient reported outcome measures Outcome measures of health care as reported by a child.

Self-care Where a child accepts the responsibility for the management of their long-term condition themselves. Include the responses, interventions and actions of others, which facilitate a child managing their own health.

Stigma Concept described by Irving Goffman (1968) and expanded upon in relation to health by Eliot Freidson (1970). Stigma is a social phenomenon in which a person is disadvantaged because they are not accepted into the hegemonic or 'normal' group in a society. Here the hegemonic group would be well children and the families of well children.

Technological dependency Where a child relies on a medical device to compensate for the loss of a vital bodily function and where there is substantial and ongoing nursing care to avert death or further disability.

INTRODUCTION

In a way, long-term conditions are very simple to understand: they are health problems children live with for a prolonged period. However, this does not address a number of levels of complexity. To begin with living with a long-term condition may include acute care episodes. A child with sickle cell may have 'sickle cell crisis', an acute exacerbation which can be life threatening (Okpala, 2004; Dyson et al., 2010). Living with a long-term condition may also include palliative and end-of-life care needs. A child with a liver disease may need to

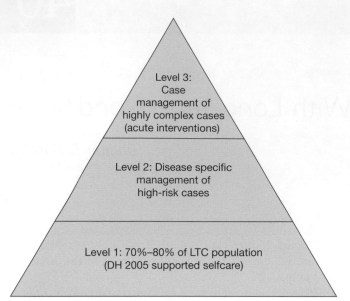

Fig. 40.1 Kaiser Permanente triangle *for Long Term Conditions*. (Adapted from Department of Health, 2005. Supporting People with Long-Term Conditions. An NHS and Social Care Model to Support Local Innovation and Integration. Department of Health, London.)

be helped to understand that their liver functioning is not improving and that they may die (Grinyer, 2012). There is also complexity in defining a long-term condition and a disability. While some conditions have pathological processes and disease processes, which arguably make them easier to identify as long-term conditions, perhaps a condition like cystic fibrosis and other conditions are less obvious to categorise. A condition such as cerebral palsy, for example, might well be seen more as a disability than having a long-term uncertain and variable pathological process (Kearney and Pryor, 2004). The boundaries then between long-term conditions and other aspects of children's health and nursing are often blurred. We will return to the challenges of defining long-term conditions later.

Despite these difficulties in deciding on the boundaries of what long-term conditions in childhood are, this aspect of children's nursing is important. Long-term conditions are an important aspect of children's health as they cost the most in terms of both financial cost and in the costs of caring emotionally, physically, in time resource and in the loss of opportunity for children and their carers. These 'costs' may be highly variable, dependent on the particular condition and on the child and their carers contexts or situations, but the long-term nature of the care means that the effects and cost accumulate over time. Thus while an acute illness may have a high cost, in terms of skilled resources, equipment costs as well as emotional aspects and disruption to a child's education and or childhood. These effects and costs are short term, and thus the effects and costs are limited. The Kaiser Permanente triangle based on insurance data from North America has been widely used to represent this cost breakdown for populations over time (see Fig 40.1). With the most complex cases requiring specialist (tertiary) care, often in regional centres costing the least overall, at

the top of the triangle. The middle section represents the cost of care for people who need active management of their condition; this might include periods of hospitalisation and/or community children's nursing service input. The bottom layer is the most costly and is the care of supporting people to undertake self-care. If this seems counterintuitive, consider the costs of an intensive care bed for a child per day (estimated at £1000–£2000 per day; Royal College of Paediatrics and Child Health [RCPCH], 2014), but which might be for 2–3 days, while the cost of, for example, diabetic blood testing and injection, is much less. However, a child will undertake blood glucose monitoring and injections up to perhaps six times each day, and every day for all of their childhood. Thus the cumulative costs of having a long-term condition far outweigh the short-term sporadic costs of intensive or acute care. Kaiser Permanente triangle graphic only accounts for financial costs to a provider, and it should be noted, to health care insurance companies in the USA. However, its widespread use and the logical arguments make it arguably relevant to children's nursing. We should remember that much of this financial cost is borne by parents and siblings in the child's family, and often the child's extended family and communities, rather than the health care system. Later we will consider some of the emotional and quality of life costs of a child living with a long-term condition.

In addition to the importance of being a child living with a long-term condition, we should consider the aspects of becoming an adult with a long-term condition. The nature of long-term conditions means that children will in the main grow up living with their condition. There are two aspects here: one is the transition into adult services (see Chapter 29) and secondly, the self-management styles and skills established in childhood which may affect a child's adult life of living with the condition. An example might be how a child with juvenile arthritis avoids physical exercise or intricate manual dexterity tasks in childhood. This may then affect their ability to participate in physical activities or certain occupations as an adult, which may have implications for mental health and social connection. A child who has never played football or any team game, as an adult may find joining local social groups based on these activities difficult, resulting in social isolation and potential depression. Thus in children's nursing we might need to consider what social activities a child with arthritis can undertake, encourage participation and support the management of pain to allow participation, with a view to their adult life, participation and social connection.

For children living with a long-term condition while some aspects for their nursing care might relate to the promotion, recovery and stability of the internal and external environments of health status, in the main our focus will be around the negotiation of care (see Chapter 2). In the triad relationship between child, their carer and nurse, our focus is on how we facilitate the child to take responsibility for their care. In other words, self-care for children is central to living with a long-term condition. As set out below self-care for children should be considered with the aspects of being a child and of becoming an adult living with the condition.

DEFINING LONG-TERM CONDITIONS

The defining of long-term conditions is not a simple matter. There are a number of terms which have been used over the years to describe these conditions and some concepts which continue to intersect and potentially overlap. Terms such as long-term conditions and disease, impairments, disability and life-limiting disease. Some of these terms have a negative association, such as chronic and disabled. The more recent shift to using the term long-term conditions reflects a desire to focus on the person's (the child's) experience of living with the condition and of how people can cooperate to find ways of living with conditions as active social participants.

There are some features of long-term conditions which appear across the definitions. These were brought together by the Office of National Statistics (2011). The definition they propose is that long-term conditions are physical or mental health conditions which are long lasting (12 months or more), and require some level of supervision and/or treatment over a long period of time, most likely for the rest of the person's life. While symptoms can be controlled with medication and/or other treatment, they are not curable and therefore relevant to the individual for the foreseeable future.

Caroline Eiser (1993) and Caroline Cooper (1999) were early nurse writers who set out much of the work on long-term conditions, or as they termed it, "chronic illness/disease". Eiser and Cooper outlined concepts and aspects which continue to be useful in considering long-term conditions, and these are summarised in Box 40.1.

☑ ACTIVITY

Make a list of the different long-term conditions that you have encountered in the last 12 months. Consider the particular needs and challenges of the children and their carers. Discuss in your study group those challenges/needs common to all, or many of the children and their carers and those which were condition specific.

Now reflect on the merits of grouping patients with the same condition as a useful way of predicting their needs, compared with the non-categorical approach of considering general issues of living with a long-term condition.

Dimensions of Long-Term Conditions: Incidence and Prevalence

Information about the incidence, the number of new cases of disease per unit of population in a defined period, and prevalence, the number of new and continuing cases of disease, is limited. And estimates of overall rates are problematic. The General Lifestyle Survey conducted by the Office for National Statistics (ONS) contains questions about long-term conditions in childhood, but is answered by adult carers (parents) who may over or under report symptoms (ONS, 2011). There are also problems in estimating mental health problems in children. Despite evidence from America that 50% of mental

health problems are established by age 14 years, and 75% by 26 years, there is a paucity of evidence about the extent of mental health issues in UK children. However, generally estimates are around 10% of children have mental health problems, with the incidence increasing in adolescents and higher rates in girls (Mental Health Foundation, 2015). A survey in England in 2017 found 12.8% of 5- to 19-year-olds had at least one mental health disorder (NHS digital, 2018). Of the mental health problems in 5- to 15-year-olds, emotional problems were most common (8.1% in 2017, having risen from 4.3% in 1999).

The way in which long-term conditions, palliative care and disability can overlap makes estimating the number of children living with a physical long-term condition difficult. However, the Children's Commissioner (2017) estimates that in England there are more than 1 million children living with disabilities (1,228,785) and almost 1.5 million with physical long-term conditions (1,478,487). There may also be some overlap with children living with a mental health problem (805, 950). Fraser et al. (2011) estimate that there are 40,042 children, 320 per 100,000 of the population, with life-threatening/limiting conditions, some of which will be considered long-term conditions such as cystic fibrosis, cerebral palsy, neuromuscular degenerative conditions and cancer.

It is advisable to access information about the incidence and prevalence of specific long-term conditions, for example, it is suggested that there are 1.1 million children being treated for asthma in the UK (Asthma UK, 2019). There has been an increase in the incidence of certain diseases such as asthma and diabetes and an increase in the life expectancy of children with other long-term conditions such as cystic fibrosis and cancer (Asthma UK, 2019; Norris and Wolfsdorf, 2005; Fraser et al., 2011).

Completely new categories of long-term conditions are emerging as technology develops and childhood mortality rates improve. Preterm babies are surviving at earlier gestation and increasingly low birth weights. Organ transplants are enabling children to survive longer with previously fatal diseases (Glendinning et al., 2001). Technology advances have given rise to many more children using various levels of respiratory support both in hospitals and the community (Walis et al., 2011). Understanding of the hereditary influences on the incidence of long-term conditions is constantly developing and nurses need a sound knowledge of genetics in order to deliver excellent care and advice to children and their carers and to participate in the ethical debates about treatment (Valentine and Hazell, 2007).

There is obviously a wide range in the severity of long-term conditions both within disease categories and between them. Some diseases, such as atopic eczema, may be common but not always perceived as an illness. This can bring further problems to children and their families as their experiences and needs may not be understood and even trivialised. A study of the prevalence of atopic symptoms in the UK found that almost half of the 12- to 14-year-olds surveyed reported one or more of the symptoms: itchy flexural rash, rhinoconjunctivitis or wheeze – and 4% reported all three (Austin et al., 1999).

BOX 40.1 Aspects of Long-Term Conditions

Aetiology	The aetiology of conditions which are long-term conditions are normally structural and functional problems. Type 1 diabetes being an example of a lack of insulin arising from the malfunction in the islets of Langerhans (Norris and Wolfsdorf, 2005). Thus long-term conditions tend to be caused, or be attributable to permanent changes to body systems or functions (consider sickle cell anaemia (Okpala, 2004).
	For mental health conditions this 'aetiology' approach is more problematic; however, long-term mental health issues tend to be associated with enduring relationship issues, environmental contexts, familial trends and personality issues (Thompson et al., 2012).
Onset	Onset or when a condition starts may vary in some conditions, but for others is well defined. Obviously for children's nurses to consider the consequences onset needs to be in childhood (not universally, but generally considered to be 0–18 years [WHO, 1989]). Some developmental conditions are particularly defined by their onset.
Stability, predictability and threat to life	Long-term conditions tend to be stable over time in that they endure over time; however the severity of the condition and the predictability of the condition can vary. Some conditions are highly unpredictable, for example, epilepsies. The pattern of the condition might include periods of stability and then sudden exacerbation (e.g. asthma), other conditions are more predictable in that they will result in gradual determination leading to death (e.g. Spinal muscular atrophy type 2). We should remember that 'professional' estimates of prognosis and predictability are often less than scientific or satisfactory (Brook and Hain, 2008). For children the fear of unpredictable exacerbation and even death may not be entirely rational based on the statistics, but is very real to the child and may also be real to their carers.
	Considering the stability of the condition and the degree to which exacerbations and prognosis can be predicted is useful in helping children and their carers to live with the condition and to cope with exacerbations and changes in health status, including preparing for death and bereavement.
Complexity and demandingness (impact of Rx)	Considering the variable degrees of complexity and the demands of treatment is also useful in helping children and their carers to understand the condition with which they are living. Some conditions have simple and less demanding treatment regimens or coping strategies. For a child with a nut allergy, avoiding the allergen and carrying an EpiPen might be seen as less demanding than the daily physiotherapy and the extensive medication that a child with cystic fibrosis might require.
	However, the interaction of stability, predictability, complexity and demands of living with a long-term condition are subjective and do interact. For some children and their families, living with a demanding and complex condition such as cystic fibrosis might have less effect than the child who lives in a difficult circumstance with challenging relationships and has an allergic condition.
	Rather than defining aspects of these phenomena (stability, predictability, complexity and demandingness) it is useful to consider each in the context of what we understand about the long-term condition and the child, their childhood and their social worlds.
Adaptations: physical, cognitive and social (parental)	The consideration of the stability, predictability, complexity and demandingness of living with a long-term condition can help us to understand the adaptations which the condition might place on a child and their carers, siblings and communities. These are aspects to which adaptations have to be made in order to facilitate a childhood for children living with the condition (see Chapter 2). Even if these adaptations are successful, they remain adaptations that other children would not have to make.
	It is useful to consider physical adaptions to a child's environment which may be required to facilitate free movement for a wheelchair user, but also, for example, the behavioural adaptation a child with a congenital heart condition might require to participate in school sports.
	Long-term conditions and exacerbations of the conditions may also affect cognitive functioning. This may be functional, when a condition itself affects cognitive abilities such as complex partial seizures (Collins, 2012), or social, such as repeated hospitalisation disrupting education and social development. This could also include more complex issues such as the effect on cognition of mood and/or behavioural aspects which we might see in diabetes, for example (Sorkin et al., 2015).
	For children, the physical and cognitive may combine to social adaptations. Children may experience the stigma of a long-term condition because of peer and/or adult reactions to their physical and/or cognitive problems arising from the long-term condition (Kyngas, 2004).
	Alongside the challenges for children, we might consider the challenges for carers such as parents. The expectations and social relationships associated with children are altered when a child has a long-term condition. This might affect a parent's work, their social life and their own self-esteem/efficacy. Caring for a child with a long-term condition can limit a parent's work opportunities, reduce their social life and therefore social connection, making them socially isolated, all of which can affect self-esteem giving rise to anxiety and depression (Gordon, 2009). The long-term nature of these conditions and the demands on carers when contrasted with a social expectation of children 'growing up' and becoming more independent, which might be less achievable for children living with a long-term condition, can result in despair and hopelessness. However, this 'tragic' picture of living with, and parenting a child with a long-term condition, should be considered alongside the reports in which that many people speak of the purpose and pleasure of caring for their child with a long-term condition and the social connectedness some parents get from communities of children and carers who also live with the condition (Kearney and Griffin, 2001; see Diabetes UK).

Continued

We can see both a non-categorical and categorical approach in the measure of the health-related quality of life discussed later.

BOX 40.1	Aspects of Long-Term Conditions—cont'd
Categorical versus non-categorical approaches	A categorical approach to long-term conditions is based upon the particular conditions; in effect such an approach states that living with diabetes is a unique experience. While a non-categorical approach seeks to unify all children living with long-term conditions; it might state that while diabetes is a unique condition, children living with diabetes share similar challenges such as stigma, reduced education opportunities and requirements for physical and cognitive adaptations to facilitate their experience of childhood, in common with children living with epilepsy, cystic fibrosis, etc.
	The attraction of a non-categorical approach is that it would provide a platform for children and their carers to demand more social support and consideration of long-term conditions. The numbers of children and the demand for resources would be combined, making long-term conditions in childhood a more significant social and therefore political issue. The challenge is that long-term conditions include such a disparate set of conditions with very different challenges for children and their carers. Making the case that the lived experience of a child with asthma is similar to that of a child with cerebral palsy is difficult, when both these conditions may themselves have very different effects on children and be reacted to by communities in very different ways. We can see both a non-categorical and categorical approach in the measure of the health-related quality of life discussed later.

Children with long-term conditions may not only have the symptoms of the disease and consequences of treatment to contend with, but they also have increased rates of mental health problems and psychological difficulties (Vessey, 1999). It has been suggested that an appropriate assessment tool to detect such problems should be added to routine paediatric outpatient assessments to aid detection and appropriate referral to child mental health services (Glazebrook et al., 2003). The importance of recognising and effectively managing psychological well-being is also supported by evidence that adults with persistent long-term conditions from childhood, which limit their daily life, suffer more depression and lower self-esteem than those with non-limiting conditions or healthy controls (Huurre and Aro, 2002).

LIVING WITH A LONG-TERM CONDITION: HEALTH-RELATED QUALITY OF LIFE

With the focus on medications and interventions for children there has been an increased interest in measuring quality of life associated with health interventions (Varni and Limbers 2009). Broadly, these are seen as *patient reported outcome measures* (or PROMs), which can be used to assess a child's health status, to compare lived experiences for different conditions (e.g. asthma vs diabetes), to measure quality of life issues over time, predict future outcomes and to monitor and improve clinical decisions on symptom management and interventions (Haverman et al., 2017).

These health-related quality of life (HRQOL) measures sit within a wider psychological concept and literature on quality of life more generally. These measures consist of various scales normally measured on some visual or numbered continuum. There are a number of both disease- or condition-specific measures (categorical) and generic (non-categorical) measures of children's perception of their health-related quality of life (Haverman et al., 2017).

Perhaps the most developed measure is Paediatric Quality of Life Inventory (PedsQL) 4.0 designed and tested by James

Varni and colleagues (www.pedsql.org). This has four items that relate to the child's perceptions of physical, emotional, social and school functioning. To administer the measure, 23 questions are rated 0–4 for the generic scale in relation to how much the statements have been a problem over the past month. Where 0 = never a problem and 4 = almost always a problem. Statements include for example 'it's hard for me to run' in the physical item list, or 'I feel afraid or scared' in the emotional item list.

The generic (non-categorical) measure is designed to be used with condition-specific measures or categorical measures as Eiser might term them. Varni and colleagues call these 'modules', and there are validated modules for diabetes, asthma, arthritis and brain tumour, among others (Varni and Limbers, 2009). Each contains a number of scales as in the generic measure. For example, the Arthritis module has scales on pain and hurt, daily activities, treatment, worry and communication.

The PedsQL inventory offers a set of measures that are validated in large scale trials and which address the generic or non-categorical aspects as well as condition-specific categorical issues of living with a long-term condition in childhood. However, it is one of many measures (Haverman et al., 2017).

There are challenges in using HRQOL measures with children. Some adults may still believe that children's reports of their experience of their own health cannot be reliable, despite the research evidence which demonstrates children as young as 5 years and certainly by 7 years can reliably report their own health (Haverman et al., 2017; Cremeens et al., 2006). Yet it is now well recognised that parent 'proxy' reports may differ from those of children (Cremeens et al., 2006; Scot, 2000). Some HRQOL-measure authors recognise this problem and suggest child self-report, for children of certain age ranges 5–18 (Varni and Limbers, 2009) alongside parental report 2–18. Children's self-report measures are normally tailored to various groups, for example, by referring to peers for teenage children rather than other kids, for younger children. The use of child self-report alongside parental report does not address issues of intergenerational power. A child's

BOX 40.2   Outcome Measures

3.3: Self-care	Nurses can demonstrate how they • assess and reassess children's capacity to self-care; • develop children's skills and understanding to facilitate self-care; • encourage and facilitate children to be active partners in their own care.
3.4: Negotiating care	The nurse has a negotiated plan of responsibilities for aspects of care where the child, their carer and the nurse all have defined and agreed responsibilities in the plan of care. This plan of responsibilities is regularly reviewed and revised.
3.5: Supporting children to live a childhood	Nursing care plan demonstrates understanding of the • child's position in their childhood; • parent's capacity to meet the child's needs and the skills or understanding that carers/parents need to develop to meet the child's needs; • illness process and how it may affect the child and their childhood. Where possible the child's main carer feels competent and confident to deliver care and care is delivered by the child's main carer to a proficient standard.

Randall, D., 2016. Pragmatic Children's Nursing: A Theory for Children and Their Childhoods. Routledge, Abingdon.

self-report may still be given less credence by nurses than the report of a parent. However, it does allow children to report their perceived view of their health and health care. It should be remembered that HRQOL measures are perceived quality of life, and parental views and a child's view can and do differ; neither is more or less 'correct', both are just the person's own perception. As Haverman et al. (2017) point out, children and or their carers living with the same long-term condition with similar health status, treatment burden and symptoms can and do have very different perceptions of their quality of life. Thus it may be legitimate to evaluate both a child and their carers' quality of life, but not to assume that a parent can answer for their child and give a valid 'proxy' view of how the child perceives their quality of life.

There are also challenges in the implementation of HRQOL measures which are of particular note in children's nursing. Children's abilities and interpretation of the questions asked in the measures may be variable by age, cognitive abilities and by cultural background. Care needs to be taken not just to translate HRQOL measures, but to adapt and interpret them in different cultural contexts. PedsQL has been adapted for more than 65 international contexts working in conjunction with the Mapi Research Institute in France (Varni and Limber, 2009). The challenge of variable cognitive states and interpretations of terms in such measures in clinical practice

is perhaps more complex, and nurses may need to think critically about a child and/or their carers' interpretation of the words and phrases used in an HRQOL measure (Haverman et al., 2017)

Health-related quality of life is an important concept and measure in long-term conditions. In childhood there are a number of challenges to using HRQOL measures, such as the use of parental proxy view and assumptions about the suitability of measures for children in certain age ranges, or from certain cultures. However, despite these challenges HRQOL measures have been shown to be valid and reliable in a number of long-term conditions, across the majority of childhood and in a number of cultural contexts.

Care of the Carers: Parenting a Child With a Long-Term Condition and Family Life

Long-term conditions in childhood occur in a social context in which a supportive relationship between parent and child is essential for successful management (see Chapter 2 and Box 40.2). The impact of childhood long-term conditions on the lives of parents, the adaptation processes required and their needs have been the focus of a considerable amount of research (e.g. Fisher, 2001; Hodgkinson and Lester, 2002; Lowes et al., 2005; Young et al., 2002a, b). There is an acceptance that parents are the main carers of children with long-term conditions and considerable effort has been made in trying to understand the impact of this role on their lives and how health care professionals can support them in their role and facilitate successful coping. Better understanding of the experience of parenting a child living with a long-term condition is thought to improve the relationship between health professionals and parents and ensure that care provided is appropriate and meaningful. Good relationships between health professionals and parents are considered to be beneficial both for children and parents. For example, a good relationship between doctors and mothers of children with atopic eczema was found to be the strongest predictor of adherence to skin-care treatment (Ohya et al., 2001).

The emphasis on the inevitable negative impact of childhood long-term conditions and disability has been criticised by some authors. It is not disputed that parenting a child with long-term conditions is stressful at times, but whether this causes distress in parents is questioned. The focus of research and nursing literature on the tragedy of childhood illness and disability, parental stress, the burden of care and need for successful coping mechanisms has shifted and the positive contributions to family life of children with disability has been recognised (Kearney and Griffin, 2001).

Treatment of long-term conditions may have a positive or negative impact on children's and carers' quality of life. Successful management of a disease may be at odds with children's and their carers' experience of the illness and it is important that treatment outcome measures include consideration of child and parent reported outcomes. International instruments to measure parents' experience of childhood long-term conditions, and which can be used to determine the acceptability and efficacy of pharmaceutical treatment, have been developed (Whalley et al., 2002).

In addition to influencing the child's carers' quality of life, the impact of long-term conditions on family units can be enormous. Efforts have been made to develop a scale to measure the impact of long-term conditions on parents and families (Stein and Reissman, 1980) and applied in specific diseases such as atopic eczema (Su et al., 1997). Bonner et al. (2006) developed and validated an instrument for measuring parents' experiences of child illness, which focuses on four critical domains of parental adjustment: guilt and worry, unresolved sorrow and anger, long-term uncertainty and emotional resources.

Within disease categories, parents' estimate of the severity of disease has been found to be the single strongest predictor of family impact of the disease (Balkrishnan et al., 2003). There may be differences in the perception of the impact of childhood illness between parents and paediatricians (Janse et al., 2005) and it is important to recognise that it is the assessment of severity by the parents, and not by the professionals, that predicts the impact on the family. Long-term conditions considered as relatively minor by health professionals may in fact have a greater impact on the family than other more serious diseases. For example, Powers et al. (2003) found that the quality of life of children suffering from migraines as assessed by the children themselves and their parents was similar to that of children with arthritis and cancer.

Emotional Responses

The emotional responses of parents to the diagnosis of long-term conditions in a child are frequently linked to loss and grief. Parents may experience multiple losses, loss of their healthy child, loss of freedom and lifestyle, loss of confidence and support systems and potential loss of their child's life (Lowes and Lyne, 2000). The grief reactions they may suffer have been studied in relation to many specific childhood diseases and are well documented in the nursing literature. For example, feelings of shock, anger, denial, sadness and frustration have been reported in parents of children newly diagnosed with diabetes (Hatton et al., 1995) and it is suggested that these reactions are a result of an awareness of the discrepancy between expectation and reality for their child's world (Lowes et al., 2005). Time-bound theories of grief have been applied to parents of children with long-term conditions, suggesting that they progress through a series of stages culminating in acceptance of their child's condition and resolution of their grief. Such theories have been challenged and an alternative model of 'chronic sorrow' has been suggested as representative of parents' experience of childhood long-term conditions. Teel (1991) describes chronic sorrow as a recurring sadness interwoven with periods of neutrality, satisfaction and happiness – suggesting that parents make a functional adaptation to childhood long-term conditions, but do not accept it.

It must be remembered that diagnosis may also result in feelings of relief and hope, particularly if the parents have been concerned for some time about their child's health.

Parents may also be falsely accused of being in denial when they are trying to remain positive and optimistic about their child's condition. Kearney and Griffin (2001) quote a mother of a child with significant health problems: 'I knew her condition was serious and her prognosis poor but to me she was my firstborn, beautiful child.'

SCENARIO

David is a third-year child branch student who is caring for a 6-month-old baby girl with cystic fibrosis. She has a chest infection but is otherwise well and her mother is delighted with her weight gain and achievement of normal development. David overhears the mother telling a friend that she doesn't think there is anything wrong with her baby and is considering stopping giving her medication because she is so well.

Consider how David might deal with this situation. How might he ensure that the mother recognises her baby's need for treatment, but maintain her positive approach and delight in her child's progress?

Parental Health

Parental health and well-being may suffer as a consequence of caring for a child with long-term conditions, and although not ill themselves, mothers in particular may suffer many of the consequences of long-term conditions (Young et al., 2002a). Mothers may experience stress in relation to caring for their child and coping with the demands of the illness. Stress may be experienced in relation to decision-making, the burden of care and accepting a change in identity (Hodgkinson and Lester, 2002). Many research studies throughout the 1970s and 1980s explored the stress experienced by parents (in particular mothers) and the coping strategies they developed when dealing with long-term conditions in a child (Faux, 1998).

Financial Consequences

Parents of children with long-term conditions may find it difficult to sustain full-time employment. Time off work to care for their child and attend hospital appointments, as well as the extra cost of childcare for a child with additional needs, may make paid employment impossible. In addition, there are costs involved in bringing up and caring for a child with long-term conditions that are extra to those for healthy children. In a study of families who care for a disabled child, Melnychuk et al. (2018) calculated that living with a disabled child cost families an extra £56–£79 per week; in part this may be compensated by state aid, but UK data suggests that 21% of children with disabilities live in poverty compared to 16% without (Melnychuk et al., 2018). In a study of parental coping with bereavement and living with a child with palliative care needs, Randall (2017) found that the financial picture for parents was complex as contextual factors interact to impact on the household. While the focus of research has been on monetary loss, little has been done to understand the interaction of factors. For example, Randall describes how families had retrained and relocated their work and homes to accommodate a child's long-term care needs. As access to health care and special education is better in more affluent areas, the families had moved to areas that were much more expensive to live in than where they originally lived. The picture then of the resource implications and costs to children's carers may be more complex and generally underestimated.

👤 ACTIVITY

Scenario

Laura is a 6-year-old girl with atopic eczema. She requires frequent application of ointment to keep her skin hydrated after a bath. This makes her clothes greasy and sticky and she requires several changes of clothes each day. She can only wear pure cotton clothes next to her skin as man-made fibres irritate her. Her bedding needs to be changed every morning as it is soiled with skin cells, exudate and ointment.

Laura's condition deteriorates if she eats certain foods. Her mother has to prepare special food for her meals, much of which is wasted if Laura does not like it.

It is thought that house-dust mites contribute to Laura's skin condition so her parents have replaced the carpet in her bedroom with laminate flooring and her curtains with wooden blinds.

List the additional financial costs to Laura's family involved in caring for her. What help with these additional costs might the family receive? What resources in your community could such a child and her carers access?

Social Consequences

The role of being a parent of a child with long-term conditions may compromise the ability to function adequately in other roles such as friend, professional, spouse or partner and parent of other children. Childhood long-term conditions may make parents reluctant to leave the child to pursue social and leisure activities. In addition, the disease may produce additional caring needs and treatment regimens for parents, such as regular injections or physiotherapy, which may reduce the time available to meet their own social needs.

There is evidence that the nature of normal childcare, such as bathing, feeding and entertaining, may be changed when a child has a long-term condition, and normally enjoyable tasks may become difficult and onerous. Parents of children with atopic eczema have described the constant struggle to keep their child entertained to distract them from scratching and the difficulties of bathing and nappy changing when skin is excoriated, itchy and sore (Elliott and Luker, 1996). There is evidence to suggest that parents can feel particularly stressed in relation to their parenting skills when a child has a long-term condition and may be less efficient in disciplining their affected child (Daud et al., 1993).

Restricted social activities may lead parents to perceive that they have less social support (Daud et al., 1993). This is a concern as ongoing social support is crucial for the successful adaptation of parents to their child's long-term conditions (Whyte, 1992). Perceived social support has been found to

be a predictor of family coping and a factor that influences the resilience of high-risk groups of families with a child with long-term conditions (Tak and McCubbin, 2002).

Marital Relationships

There is a belief that family dysfunction and marital problems frequently follow the diagnosis of long-term conditions in a child. However, there is conflicting empirical evidence in this area and much anecdotal evidence to suggest that caring for a child living with a long-term condition may bring a couple closer together. Gender differences between mothers and fathers in how they cope with long-term conditions in a child and from whom they receive their support have been reported (Katz, 2002), and conflict may arise from these differences.

There are conflicting reports in the literature of the effects of caring for a child living with a long-term condition on marital satisfaction and stability, with some studies showing a negative effect and others finding no differences. Most studies of parents of children with health problems report decreased marital satisfaction compared with parents of healthy children. A study by One plus One called *Growing Together or Drifting Apart* for Contact a Family (2012) found that couples face a number of challenges and that marital breakdown was common. However, support from nurses in coordinating care, offering emotional support and accessing financial support can be instrumental in helping couples to cope (Contact a Family, 2012). Childcare responsibilities and decision making are likely to cause conflict and are the most frequently cited stresses of parents of children with long-term conditions (Quittner et al., 1998). However, a study that compared 94 married parents caring for a child with long-term conditions with over 3000 married parents of well children found no differences in perceived marital quality or satisfaction between the two groups (Eddy and Walker, 1999). Similarly, Katz and Krulik (1999) found no difference in levels of marital satisfaction between fathers of healthy children and those of children with long-term conditions, although the latter group did experience a greater number of stressful life events and lower self-esteem.

Decreased marital satisfaction does not necessarily result in decreased marital stability. It is suggested that marital stability is a product of net outcomes (rewards minus costs), barriers to leaving the relationship and alternative attractions (Eddy and Walker, 1999). When parents have a child with long-term conditions there may be more strain on the relationship, resulting in fewer rewards and greater costs, but the barriers to leaving are increased and opportunities for alternative attractions reduced. All children, whether sick or healthy, constitute important marital capital in that they increase the barriers to leaving a relationship for the majority of parents.

Siblings

The family context in which children with long-term conditions live inevitably means that their well siblings are affected by the disease and its management. Within families, the relationship between siblings may be just as important as the parent–child relationship, if not more so. Brothers and sisters spend a considerable amount of time together and children can be very distressed by long-term conditions in a sibling. They may supply considerable emotional, social and physical support to the sick child, thus being a source of help to their parents. However, well siblings have their own unique needs and may themselves make additional demands at a time when their parents' attention is focused on the sick child.

However, the research literature in this area is contradictory as to the consequences of long-term conditions for well siblings (Bluebond-Langner, 1996; Eiser, 1993). There is a great deal of research literature reporting the negative effects of long-term conditions on well siblings. A whole range of problems have been reported including somatic and psychosomatic disorders, school problems, increased accidents, behaviour problems including hyperactivity and antisocial behaviour, emotional problems, aggressiveness, withdrawal and poor social adjustment. At the other end of the spectrum are studies that indicate that long-term conditions do not have a negative effect on well siblings, indeed there may be positive consequences. Empathy, compassion, coping and communication skills have been reported in well siblings, as well as an increased maturity, appreciation of their own health and increased family cohesion.

Explanations of why having a sibling with long-term conditions results in some children experiencing positive outcomes and others negative ones have been sought and it is apparent that factors other than the condition alone are influential. A number of factors have been considered by various researchers and summarised by Bluebond-Langner (1996). Factors such as age, birth order, gender, socioeconomic status of the family, parents' marital situation, prior family problems, character of the disease and relationship with the child, can all influence how a child copes with long-term conditions in a sibling. It should be noted that much of the research to date has relied on parental, usually the mother's, reporting of the behaviour and health of their children, which may be influenced by many factors including the parents' own health and adaptation to their child's illness and social presentation.

It is suggested that negative outcomes in well siblings should not be expected but that there should be an awareness of their unique relationship with the sick child and their individual needs. Childhood long-term conditions may be viewed as a stressor that combined with other factors, may result in an increased risk of psychological problems for some siblings of sick children. The factors that mediate the effects of long-term conditions on well siblings are poorly understood, but it is believed that the quality of family functioning and relationships has both direct and indirect effects on siblings (Drotar and Crawford, 1985).

CONTINUITY, RELATIONSHIPS AND MULTI-DISCIPLINARY/AGENCY TEAM WORKING

Nurses work with children with long-term conditions and their families in a variety of roles. Hospital nurses may care for the child and family around the time of diagnosis and during periods of acute exacerbation of their illness. Community children's nurses may support the child and family at home, helping them to incorporate care and treatment into their daily routine and manage the child's illness on a day-to-day basis. Health promotion and assessment of child development may be undertaken by Health Visitors. Many areas now employ nurses for specific diseases, such as cystic fibrosis and diabetes specialist nurses. These nurses use their specialist knowledge and expertise to support children and their families, and may also act in an advisory role for other nurses and other professionals involved in their care.

Looking back over the text above one can see that children living with long-term conditions sit in a nexus of care where health, education and social care interact. For many children, other professionals and non-professional with backgrounds in other disciplines can be vital to care, such as speech therapist, occupational therapists and physiotherapists, all of who's work might be assisted by voluntary workers such as organisers of a play group or children's social group, such as Scouts or a football team. A key worker will coordinate and ensure continuity of care. This might be a children's nurse who is assigned to this role and is dependent on the needs of the child. The key worker will provide information and advice, identify and address needs, access and coordinate services, provide emotional support and act as an advocate for the child and family (Mukherjee et al., 1999; Tait and Dejnega, 2001). The Department of Health (DoH, 2004, p 28) states that:

> … *studies of key workers consistently report positive effects on relationships with services, fewer unmet needs and greater family well-being.*

Key workers are an important aspect of care for children with long-term conditions and disabilities requiring complex health care provision and in recent years have received considerable interest in policy and research (Beecham et al., 2007; Children's Workforce Development Council, 2007; DoH, 2004; Greco et al., 2004, 2006; National Collaborating Centre for Cancer, 2005; Sloper et al., 2005).

Whether nurses are acting as key workers or simply involved in the care of a child with long-term conditions either in hospital or the community, they will be part of a team of health professionals. Multi-disciplinary and collaborative team-working skills and sound communication skills are fundamental to good nursing care of children and families.

Factors for Key Workers Consideration

The following six factors may be helpful when caring for children with long-term conditions and their families.

1. Finding out

Prior to caring for a child and family with a long-term condition, it is necessary to have some background knowledge and to be aware of previous medical, nursing, social and psychological issues and interventions. Information can be gained by reading case notes and contacting the health professionals and other support agencies involved in the care of the child and family. It can be cathartic for children and their carers to 'tell their story', and often people want to be assured that the nurse knows what has happened to them. However, many parents also point out the frustration of having to give the same information to many people involved in care, much of which is contained in easily accessible nursing and medical notes.

 ACTIVITY

During a clinical placement in the hospital or community, where you are involved in the care of children with long-term conditions, select three children and look at their case notes. What picture and knowledge do you gain about these children and their families from the case notes alone?

2. Building up relationships

Continuity of care is the main component in building up a relationship with children with long-term conditions and their families. It has been argued that parents with a child with a disability need a professional approach from nurses, which acknowledges hope, without labelling parents as unrealistic or in denial (Kearney and Griffin, 2001).

Visiting children and their families at home is less formal than the hospital setting and the home environment makes it easier for them to discuss issues openly. When undertaking nursing interventions in the busy home environment there can be many distractions but these can provide useful information about the ongoing care and relationships (see Chapter 33). It is important that nurses are mindful of the need to communicate effectively with children and their parents. The social position of children relative to adults means that communication between health professionals and children may be difficult and compromised by the influence of parents. Although parents have an important role in interpreting and facilitating communication between children and health professionals, they have been found to constrain communication and contribute to the marginalisation of children in encounters with health professionals (Young et al., 2003).

 ACTIVITY

Compare and contrast the picture and knowledge you gained from the case notes of the three children in the previous activity with the picture and knowledge you gained from caring for them either in hospital or on home visits.

Consider how information gained from different sources can be used to form a view of the child and family.

3. Preemptive advice and education

Long-term conditions are dynamic. The dynamic nature of the illness means that children and their families need to be prepared in advance for possible changes in their child's condition. The term 'disease trajectory' is frequently used to describe the course of a disease and the work involved in its management. The disease trajectory is the developmental process involved in learning to live with a chronic disease and is characterised by stages through which an individual progresses to achieve responsibility for his or her disease management. For nurses to

develop an understanding of long-term conditions, it may be useful to view the illness in terms of stages with key triggers, which move individuals from one stage to the next. There has been some questioning of the appropriateness of describing the development of childhood long-term conditions in such a manner when there are so many individual differences and factors affecting the course and severity of individual illness experiences. However, understanding of disease trajectories for particular illnesses can help nurses prepare children and their families for changes in their condition and factors likely to affect its progression trajectories have been suggested for a range of long-term conditions, for example, diabetes (Thorne and Paterson, 2001), juvenile rheumatoid arthritis (Pelaez-Ballestas et al., 2006) and leukaemia (Wills, 1999).

Carers need education about the usual minor illnesses that occur in childhood as these may have a greater significance to children with long-term conditions, for example, they may be more vulnerable to infection. Information about the expected growth and development of their child is also important. Preparing families for changes in their child's condition aids them in developing strategies to adapt.

 ACTIVITY

When on clinical placement, ask the senior nurse to identify an appropriate child with a long-term condition to whom you can talk (under supervision) about their knowledge of their disease and what care and treatment they undertake at home.

With the senior nurse's agreement and supervision, ask parents caring for a child with a long-term condition what they know about the disease and what care and treatment they undertake at home.

Discuss the information gained with your mentor or the senior nurse.

4. Advocacy

Advocacy means speaking out on behalf of a particular issue, idea or person (Waterston and Haroon, 2008). Nurses may have to act as advocates for children living with long-term conditions and their families who lack the assertiveness, confidence and eloquence to represent themselves (Ellis, 1995). Children living with a long-term condition may be particularly vulnerable because of the stigma of having a such a condition. We know that children with disabilities are more likely to be the victims of abuse and bullying (Balogh et al., 2000; Sullivan and Knutson, 2000). While advocacy may be required, nurses should aim to facilitate children and their cares to speak for themselves. This might include information on terms, providing assertiveness training and or access to expert patient groups and courses. Seeking permission and opportunities to link children and their carers to condition specific support groups such as Diabetes UK can be instrumental in encouraging the child and their carers' voice in health care. Advocacy is particularly important in the transition to adult services as the child enters and works their way through adolescence (see Chapter 29).

5. Support

Nurses need to work with children's existing support networks and help them to develop new ones to ensure that they and their families feel adequately supported. Family, friends, teachers, youth workers and others provide social support to all children. When a child has a long-term condition, these support systems may be reduced and new support networks may need to be developed in order to provide for the needs of the child and family. Ellerton et al. (1996) compared the social support networks of children with a range of long-term conditions with those of healthy children. Healthy children reported more support overall than children in the illness groups and children with spina bifida reported the smallest support networks and the fewest number of peers in their networks.

Families provide much practical support in managing children's long-term conditions and dimensions of family support have been studied in relation to specific diseases. For example, Siarkowski (1999) reviewed the literature on childhood adaptation to insulin-dependent diabetes mellitus and found that family guidance and control produced better glycaemic control, but that other dimensions of family support, such as warmth and caring, had no influence on glycaemic control.

School is an important source of support for children with long-term conditions. The school should be responsive to the emotional, social and educational needs of a child and should be a place of safety and normality for the child (Edwards and Davis, 1997) and it is important that children who live with a long-term condition are facilitated to integrate the management of their condition into school life, participating in sports/activities and achieving their full academic potential (Valentine and Mcnee, 2007). As interventions in managing children with long-term conditions are voluntary in many education settings, it is important that the school and staff feel supported, otherwise they may withdraw this voluntary care, which could restrict or deny such children an education in school (Watson et al., 2002). Approaches that facilitate good communication between health professionals and school staff have been explored and joint meetings, shared documentation and local policies have been found to be beneficial (Mukherjee et al.,

2002). Problems in communication arise when the parent is used as the conduit for information, there are practical difficulties in arranging meetings and there is a lack of knowledge about professional roles (Mukherjee et al., 2002).

The key worker or nurse together with the child and their carers should identify issues that require referring to other agencies and coordinate services required. Some support can be informally agreed, and in many communities (although not all) a network of informal carers can provide essential help such as babysitting siblings to allow the child and parents to attend clinic, and providing clothes and a listening ear. Formal and informal support as well as services need to be planned in advance, not on a crisis basis, because of the lengthy processes involved in recruiting and training carers (Kirk, 1999).

6. Outcomes

By attending to these aspects 1–5 (finding out, building up relationships, preemptive advice and education, advocacy and support) nurses can focus on three outcome measures described by Randall (2016). While all of the outcome measures set out in *Pragmatic Children's Nursing* are required for nursing children living with a long-term condition, arguably outcomes 3.3, 3.4 and 3.5 (see Box 40.2) provide a focus for measuring the outcomes of nursing care (Randall, 2016, p 109).

A principle of *Pragmatic* is that all aspects of care should be addressed (Randall, 2016). Although it is important to attend to promoting self-care, it is also required to acknowledge the limitations of self-care and the conditions in which the locus of control over care might move from the child to a carer and to the nurse. Outcome measures also need to address how well care and the plans of care attend to possible exacerbation of the condition, and to possible deterioration of health status (with the possibility of palliative and end of life care being considered). This might be included in the negotiation of care (3.4), and should clearly describe emergency measures a child and their carer might take, the circumstances in which nursing and medical assistance is sought and the communication strategy. In practical terms we might consider a child with epilepsy who has an aura, warning them that an episode is beginning. The care plan might identify that sensing the aura the child alerts a teacher or their parents. The carer (teacher or parents) agrees that they will monitor the child's episode and that they are aware of what action to take. For example, if the episode continues for more than 10 minutes or if the child has difficulty breathing, they will call an ambulance. Nursing staff might agree to monitor a child admitted for an episode, read their episode (or seizure) plan and when safe to do so contact the child's main carer.

There is a sense in which such planning for exacerbations and deterioration brings us full circle with these key worker factors. These plans allow us to find out how children and their carers want to deal with such events; this helps to build a trusting relationship where children and their carers are reassured that if they need extra nursing interventions it has been planned and resourced. The understanding of potential future events can be explored with children and their carers and it allows children to voice their concerns and state their needs and wishes. Finally, it should make clear the role of others who support the child such as teachers and other school workers.

> **ACTIVITY**

- Review the care plans you use in your placement area. Could you measure outcomes 3.3, 3.4 and 3.5 (Box 40.2) using these documents?
- What other information do you have access to which might allow you to evaluate how well your care meets outcomes 3.3–3.5?
- What plans do you have if the child experiences an exacerbation or deterioration in their health?

CHILDREN DOING IT FOR THEMSELVES! SELF-CARE IN CHILDHOOD

Self-management of long-term conditions has the potential:

> *… to allow people with chronic diseases to have access to opportunities to develop the confidence, knowledge and skills to manage their conditions better, and thereby gain a greater measure of control and independence to enhance their quality of life.*

> *DoH (2001)*

The more we focus on long-term conditions rather than chronic disease, the more essential it is to recognise the expertise of the people living with the condition. However, there are important issues to consider when applying these ideas in childhood long-term conditions. The first of these is who is the 'self' involved in self-management? Children cannot be seen in isolation because parents have legal and moral responsibilities for their care and protection. However, parents are proxies; their experience of the illness is different to their children's. Important differences emerge when children and their parents report symptoms or quality of life (QoL), and the impact of illness can differ between children and parents (Callery et al., 2003). To complicate matters further, the 'self' is not limited to one parent and one child. In addition to the adults in their family, children must deal with adult

carers in other settings, for example at school. A variety of adults can contribute to the care of children in the absence of their parents, adding further elements to the 'self' involved in self-management.

The range of people involved in self-management will have differing objectives. Parents of children with asthma can judge asthma by its observable effects on their children's behaviour and its impact on parents' own lives, so that they may be most concerned about avoiding acute attacks (Callery et al., 2003). They can accept a level of continuing symptoms and restriction of activity as 'tolerable' asthma. Children can be more concerned with the day-to-day effects of asthma and how these make them appear different to their peers (Callery et al., 2003). Again, this can lead to acceptance of restriction of activity, for example, to avoid appearing different by taking inhalers in public. These differences highlight the need to identify the objectives of children and of adult carers in planning self-management of long-term conditions.

Guidelines on asthma management stress the importance of individualisation of self-management plans (British Thoracic Society [BTS] and Scottish Intercollegiate Guidelines Network [SIGN], 2008). However, it appears that little attention has been paid to identification of children's objectives, concerns and experiences in self-management plans used in practice. In a survey of 47 UK centres using 30 self-management plans for school-aged children with asthma, only two plans had apparent space for inclusion of individualised objectives and 21 did not identify objectives even implicitly in the title (Milnes and Callery, 2003). Only three plans were clearly addressed to the child; the remainder were impersonal (six), addressed to an adult carer through the child (twelve), principally to an adult carer (four), ambiguous (four) or open ended (one). These findings suggest a lack of consensus about the role that children should take in self-management of asthma.

It is important to understand the meaning of long-term conditions to both child and parent, or other adult carer, because it influences the ways in which they respond to advice. Peak flow recording by children aged 5–16 years has been shown to be unreliable with the 'percentage of correct peak flow entries decreased from 56% to less than 50% from the first to the last study week ($P < 0.04$), mainly as a result of an increase in self-invented peak flow entries' (Kamps et al., 2001). One response to such findings is to describe the behaviours as 'non-compliant' and to obtain more control over the process, for example, by using electronic peak flow meters that would not record self-invented entries. However, an alternative approach is to seek to understand the perspectives of children and their adult carers to explain their reasons for behaving in this way in order to adapt advice to their needs. The differences between professional and family perspectives are highlighted by the different meanings attached even to apparently straightforward terms such as 'wheeze' by parents and professionals (Cane et al., 2000; Young et al., 2002b). Self-management education is effective in adults (Gibson et al., 2003). A review by Guevara et al. (2003) concluded that:

Educational programmes for the self-management of asthma in children and adolescents improve lung function and feelings of self-control, reduce absenteeism from school, number of days with restricted activity, number of visits to an emergency department, and possibly number of disturbed nights. Educational programmes should be considered a part of the routine care of young people with asthma. (pg1038)

The effect of education was most marked in children with severe asthma, when interventions were directed at individuals rather than groups and when interventions were based on peak flow recording. However, none of the studies included in this review assessed QoL, and other limitations in the study reports limited the conclusions that could be reached for various ages and other sub-groups of children. Further research is required to identify the best way to provide education for different groups of children. More child-centred approaches to self-management, which incorporate the objectives and perspectives of children as well as their adult carers, might be the most promising way to improve the effectiveness of self-management education.

 REFLECT ON YOUR PRACTICE

Think about a consultation between a child, parent and nurse or doctor that you have observed. How much of the time did each of those involved speak? What was the nature of the talk when each was speaking? Were the child's objectives for treatment discussed? Did the child have opportunities to influence decisions about treatment and/or care?

LONG-TERM CONDITIONS IN A DIGITAL AGE

The Topol review identified that we live in a unique time where technological advance has coincided with the creation of a digital infrastructure and revolutions in our understanding of health and medicine (Health Education England, 2019). Three aspects are now at the forefront of medical practice genomics, digital medicine and artificial intelligence with robotics. The Topol review panel argued that these will create opportunity to personalise health care and to augment the skills of health care workers such as nurses to enhance the interhuman relationships key to delivering personalised medicine. The review panel also highlight the group perhaps most affected by the new understanding of genomics; the capacity to create monitoring applications and to design robotics driven by artificial intelligence will be people living with long-term conditions. We can already see this potential in projects such as monitoring of blood glucose for children with diabetes (Clements and Staggs, 2017; Wong et al., 2018) and asthma apps (Hosseini et al., 2016). These combine monitoring technologies with the infrastructure to transmit, store and analyse large amounts of data via smart phone technologies. This allows children to input their data and receive feedback helping them to manage their long-term condition.

In addition to these more recent developments, there has been a trend of increasing technical capacity over a number of years (Glendinning et al., 2001; Toly et al., 2012). Increasing survival rates and the capacity through computerisation, to create more portable equipment such as Nippy ventilators and feeding pumps, have led to increasing numbers of children living with technologies, which help them to manage their long-term conditions. In 2001 Glendinning and colleagues estimated there were 6000 children living with some form of technology dependency, including: 2800 using artificial nutrition, 800 dependent on oxygen, 500 with tracheostomies and 156 having peritoneal dialysis at home. These were at the time thought to be underestimation of the numbers and are likely to have significantly increased due to changes in technology and in medical practices such as the use of continuous positive airway pressure (CPAP)/bilevel positive airway pressure (BiPAP) and other assisted respiratory technologies (Walis et al., 2011). Technological dependence has been defined as affecting children who live with a long-term condition and

who rely on … a medical device to compensate for the loss of a vital bodily function and substantial and ongoing nursing care to avert death or further disability.
Wagner et al. (1988, cited in Glendinning et al., 2001)

These children are then a group within the population of children with long-term conditions and or disabilities, possibly with palliative and end-of-life care needs who also require a medical technology or device and ongoing substantial nursing care. This definition might exclude children who use a communication aid, but would include those who have a sub-cut insulin pump.

Although we might welcome the improvements to life expectancy and quality of life technologies can bring, not all aspects of technology use in children's health care are positive. Some carers can come to feel that their home is being taken over with medical equipment and professional health care staff (Glendinning and Kirk, 2000). People can be fearful of technologies; this might take the form of automatonophobia. This is where a robot is very like a human, but as humans we can tell it is not human, but as the robot approaches more human form, anxiety in the person is increased. This is why some robotics experts purposefully design robots to look like robots, particularly in health care, to avoid this anxiety by clearly designing the robot not to look human. They might for example design a square head and body, rather than giving the robot a more human face and form. There is also a societal fear of artificial intelligence, centred on an anxiety that people will be replaced by robots or machines. There are already programmes to have robots react with children with autism, as robots can be programmed to always give the same answer, social cues which people not living with autism can find repetitive and frustrating (Robins et al., 2004; see https://robots4autism.com/milo/).

Wang and Barnard's (2008) study of 17 children dependent on home ventilation in Australia reported the following themes across the participants, but not shared by all participants:

- *'Hospital is another world to me'*. Routines and practice of hospital are not like home and the hospital environment places restrictions on carers, on 'family life', care of siblings, etc.
- *It's (home) a new world*. In this theme participants described how home and home-based practice familiar to the carer change when the child came home with the technology dependency. Issues included the possibility of medical emergencies, the ongoing relationships with health care professionals – an ambivalent relationship of needing nurses, but wanting to 'pass' as a 'normal' child in a 'normal family' (see Carnevale, 2007 on stigma and home ventilation).
- *Ambiguous social identity*. Conflicts of being medical carer and family relationship (mother and nurse? [see also Glendinning and Kirk, 2000]).
- *Medical machines frightening but necessary*. Carers appreciated the machines were needed but often also fearful. They comment on having to use the machinery with little training or support.
- *The difficulty is having the carers at home*. Here participants described the intrusion of professionals into the 'home' space. Where nurses and other professional carers were entering the home space and may be present for extended periods, making privacy and other 'normal' home practices difficult or socially awkward.
- *Social isolation*. Participants felt trapped at home and of low social status. They also discussed that when they went out they were stared at in public with one's child.
- *Changing as a person*. Participants suggested positive aspects of challenge and resilience. 'It wasn't all negative, like it was tiring for me physically and emotionally, but also I think I became stronger through it all.'

Technologies are changing many aspects of children's lives and their childhoods. In the coming few decades they will change children's nursing and in particular the management of long-term conditions. However, many warn against and debated technological determinism (Feenberg, 2004), the idea that we should be reliant on technology to solve human problems. There are anxieties and concerns over the use of technologies and these need to be respected and addressed. By working in partnership with children and their carers, we can harness the potential of technologies to transform children's lives who live with long-term conditions and allow them greater access to their childhood and opportunities in their communities.

SUMMARY

Children living with a long-term condition face significant challenges in attempting to live a childhood which is similar to their peers. By attempting to 'be like other children' (or their peers), these children are attempting to 'pass' to minimise or avoid stigma of a disease by appearing to be 'normal'. The child's carers, parents and siblings are also attempting to live their lives and meet the needs of the child, while not marking themselves as different from other families, brothers, sisters, etc. The demands of attempting to pass as ordinary and the demands a long-term condition placed on children and their carers can be overwhelming and often lead to significant relational, financial and mental health issues.

With the support of carers, teachers and communities many children live with their long-term condition and succeed in education, and in adulthood in employment and careers. There are many examples of high achieving actors, artists, sports people and even politicians who live with long-term conditions and have done so since childhood. With new technologies, and our improving understanding of managing long-term condition through self-care, children's nurses and nursing has the opportunity to help many more children to live their childhoods with a long-term condition.

REFERENCES

Asthma UK, 2019. Asthma data visualisations. Available from: https://www.asthma.org.uk/support-us/campaigns/data-visualisations/.

Austin, J.B., Kaur, B., Anderson, H.R., et al., 1999. Hay fever, eczema and wheeze: A nationwide UK study (ISAAC, international study of asthma and allergies in childhood). Arch. Dis. Child. 81 (3), 225–230.

Balkrishnan, R., et al., 2003. Disease severity and associated family impact in childhood atopic dermatitis. Arch. Dis. Child. 88 (5), 423–427. https://doi.org/10.1136/adc.88.5.423.

Balogh, R., Bretherton, K., Whibley, S., et al., 2001. Sexual abuse in children and adolescents with intellectual disability. J. Intellect. Disabil. Res. 45 (Pt 3), 194–201.

Beecham, J., Sloper, P., Greco, V., et al., 2007. The costs of key worker support for disabled children and their families. Child. Care Health Dev. 33 (5), 611–618.

Bluebond-Langner, M., 1996. The Shadow of Illness: Parents and Siblings of the Chronically Sick Child. Princeton University Press, Princeton, NJ.

Bonner, M.J., Hardy, K.K., Guill, A.B., et al., 2006. Development and validation of the parent experience of child illness. J. Pediatr. Psychol. 31 (3), 310–321.

British Thoracic Society and Scottish Intercollegiate Guidelines Network, 2008. British guideline on the management of asthma. Thorax 63 (suppl. 4), 1–121.

Brook, L., Hain, R., 2008. Predicting death in children. Arch. Dis. Child. 93 (12), 1067–1070.

Callery, P., Milnes, L., Couriel, J., et al., 2003. Qualitative study of children's and parents' beliefs about childhood asthma. Br. J. Gen. Pract. 53 (488), 185–190.

Cane, R.S., Ranganathan, S.C., McKenzie, S.A., 2000. What do parents of wheezy children understand by 'wheeze'? Arch. Dis. Child. 82, 327–332.

Carnevale, F.A., 2007. Revisiting Goffman's stigma: The social experience of families with children requiring mechanical ventilation at home. J. Child. Health Care. 11 (1), 7–18.

Children's Commissioner, 2017. On measuring the number of vulnerable children in England. Available from: https://www.childrenscommissioner.gov.uk/wp-content/uploads/2017/07/CCO-On-vulnerability-Overveiw.pdf.

Children's Workforce Development Council (CWDC), 2007. The Lead Professional Managers' Guide. Leeds Children's Workforce Development Council, UK.

Clements, M.A., Staggs, V.S., 2017. A mobile app for synchronizing glucometer data: impact on adherence and glycemic control among youths with type 1 diabetes in routine care. J. Diabetes Sci. Technol. 11 (3), 461–467. https://doi.org/10.1177/1932296817691302.

Collins, S., 2011. The psychosocial effect of epilepsy on adolescents and young adults. Nurs. Stand. 25 (43), 48–56.

Contact a Family, 2012. Relationships and caring for a disabled child. Available from: https://contact.org.uk/media/450037/relationshipscurrent_updated_march2012final.pdf.

Cooper, C., 1999. Continuing Care of Sick Children: Examining the Impact of Chronic Illness. Mark Allen, Salisbury.

Cremeens, J., Eiser, C., Blades, M., 2006. Characteristics of health-related self-report measures for children aged three to eight years: a review of the literature. Qual. Life Res. 15 (4), 739–754.

Daud, L.R., Garralda, M.E., David, T.J., 1993. Psychosocial adjustment in preschool children with atopic eczema. Arch. Dis. Child. 69, 670–676.

Department of Health (DoH), 2001. The Expert Patient a New Approach to Chronic Disease Management for the 21st Century. Department of Health, London.

Department of Health (DoH), 2004. National Service Framework for Children. In: Young People & Maternity Services. Department of Health, London.

Department of Health (DoH), 2005. Supporting People With Long-Term Conditions. An NHS and Social Care Model to Support Local Innovation and Integration. Department of Health, London.

Drotar, D., Crawford, P., 1985. Psychological adaptation of siblings of chronically ill children: research and practice implications. J. Dev. Behav. Paediatr. 6 (6), 355–362.

Dyson, S.M., Abuateya, H., Atkin, K., et al., 2010. Reported school experiences of young people living with sickle cell disorder in England. BERG 36 (1), 125e142.

Eddy, L.L., Walker, A.J., 1999. The impact of children With chronic health problems on marriage. J. Fam. Nurs. 5 (1), 10–31.

Edwards, M., Davis, H., 1997. Counselling Children with Chronic Medical Conditions. The British Psychological Society, Leicester.

Eiser, C., 1993. Growing up With a Chronic Disease: The Impact on Children and Their Families. Jessica Kingsley, London.

Ellerton, M., Stewart, M.J., Ritchie, J.A., et al., 1996. Social support in children with a chronic condition. Can. J. Nurs. Res. 28 (4), 15–36.

Elliott, B.E., Luker, K., 1996. The experiences of mothers caring for a child with severe atopic eczema. J. Clin. Nurs. 6 (3), 241–247.

Ellis, P.A., 1995. The role of the nurse as the patient's advocate. Prof. Nurs. 11 (3), 206–207.

Feenberg, A., 2004. Democratic rationalization. In: Kaplan, D.M. (Ed.), Readings in the Philosophy of Technology. Rowman & Littlefield, Oxford, pp. 209–225.

Fraser, L.K., Miller, M., Aldridge, J., et al., 2011. Life-Limiting and Life-Threatening Conditions in Children and Young People in the United Kingdom; National and Regional Prevalence in Relation to Socioeconomic Status and Ethnicity. Division of Epidemiology, University of Leeds and Together for Short Lives, Bristol.

Freidson, E., 1970. Profession of Medicine: A Study of the Sociology of Applied Knowledge. Dodd, Mead & Co, New York.

Faux, S.A., 1998. Historical overview of responses of children and their families to long-term conditions. In: Broome, M.E., Knafl, K., Pridham, K., Feetham, S. (Eds.), Children and Families in Health and Illness. Sage Knowledge, San Diego, pp. 179–195.

Fisher, H.R., 2001. The needs of parents with chronically sick children: A literature review. J. Adv. Nurs. 36 (4), 600–607.

Gibson, P., Powell, H., Coughlan, J., et al., 2003. Self-Management Education and Regular Practitioner Review for Adults with Asthma (Cochrane Review). The Cochrane Library, Oxford. https://doi.org/10.1002/14651858.CD001117.

Glazebrook, C., Hollis, C., Heussler, H., et al., 2003. Detecting emotional and behavioural problems in Paediatric clinics. Child. Care Health Dev. 29 (2), 141–150.

Glendinning, C., Kirk, S., Guliffrida, A., et al., 2001. Technology dependent children in the community definition, numbers and costs. Child. Care Health Dev. 27 (4), 321–334.

Glendinning, C., Kirk, S., 2000. High-tech care: high skilled parents. Paediatr. Nurs. 12 (6), 25–27.

Goffman, E., 1968. Stigma: Notes on the Management of Spoiled Identity. Penguin, Harmondsworth.

Gordon, J., 2009. An evidence-based approach for supporting parents experiencing chronic sorrow. Pediatr. Nurs. 35 (2), 115–119.

Greco, V., Sloper, P., Barton, K., 2004. Care Coordination and Key Worker Services for Disabled Children in the UK. Social Policy Research Unit University of York, York.

Greco, V., Sloper, P., Webb, R., et al., 2006. Key worker services for disabled children: the views of staff. Health Soc. Care Community 14 (6), 445–452.

Grinyer, A., 2012. Palliative and end of life care for children and young people: home, hospice and hospital. Wiley-Blackwell, Chichester.

Guevara, J.P., Wolf, F.M., Grum, C.M., et al., 2003. Effects of educational interventions for self management of asthma in children and adolescents: systematic review and meta-analysis. BMJ 326 (7402), 1308–1309.

Hatton, D.L., Canam, C., Thorne, S., et al., 1995. Parents' perceptions of caring for an infant or toddler with diabetes. J. Adv. Nurs. 22 (3), 569–577.

Haverman, L., Limperg, P.F., Young, N.L., et al., 2017. Paediatric health-related quality of life: what is it and why should we measure it? Arch. Dis. Child. 102 (5), 393–400.

Health Education England, 2019. The Topol Review: preparing the healthcare workforce to deliver the digital future. Available from: https://www.hee.nhs.uk/our-work/topol-review.

Hodgkinson, R., Lester, H., 2002. Stresses and coping strategies of mothers living with a child with cystic fibrosis: Implications for nursing professionals. J. Adv. Nurs. 39 (4), 377–383.

Hosseini, A., Buonocore, C.M., Hashemzadeh, S., et al., 2016. HIPAA Compliant Wireless Sensing Smartwatch Application for the Self-Management of Pediatric Asthma. International Conference on Wearable Implant Body Sens Netw. June 2016, 49–54. https://doi.org/10.1109/BSN.2016.7516231.

Huurre, T.M., Aro, H.M., 2002. Long-term psychosocial effects of persistent long-term conditions: a follow-up study of Finnish adolescents aged 16 to 32 years. Eur. Child. Adolescent. Psychiatry 12 (2), 85–91.

Janse, A.J., Sinnema, G., Uiterwaal, C.S.P.M., et al., 2005. Quality of life in long-term conditions: Perceptions of parents and paediatricians. Arch. Dis. Child. 90, 486–491.

Kamps, A.W., Roorda, R.J., Brand, P.L., 2001. Peak flow diaries in childhood asthma are unreliable. Thorax. 56, 180–182.

Katz, S., 2002. Gender differences in adapting to a child's long-term conditions: a causal model. J. Pediatr. Nurs. 17 (4), 257–269.

Katz, S., Krulik, T., 1999. Fathers of children with long-term conditions: do they differ from fathers of healthy children? J. Fam. Nurs. 5 (3), 292–315.

Kearney, P.M., Griffin, T., 2001. Between joy and sorrow: being a parent of a child with developmental disability. J. Adv. Nurs. 34 (5), 582–592.

Kearney, P.M., Pryor, J., 2004. The International Classification of Functioning, Disability and Health (ICF) and nursing. J. Adv. Nurs. 46 (2), 162–170.

Kirk, S., 1999. Caring for children with specialised health care needs in the community: the challenges for primary care. Health Soc Care Community 7 (5) 350–335.

Knutson, J., Tibbelin, A., Von Unge, M., 2006. Postoperative pain after paediatric adenoidectomy and differences between the pain scores made by the recovery room staff, the parent and the child. Acta Oto-Laryngologica. 126, 1079–1083. https://doi.org/10.1080/00016480600606715.

Kyngas, H., 2004. Support network of adolescents with chronic disease: adolescents' perspective. Nurs. Health Sci. 6, 287–293.

Lowes, L., Lyne, P., 2000. Chronic sorrow in parents of children with newly diagnosed diabetes: a review of the literature and discussion of the implications for nursing practice. J. Adv. Nurs. 32 (1), 41–48.

Lowes, L., Gregory, J.W., Lyne, P., 2005. Newly diagnosed childhood diabetes: A psychosocial transition for parents? J. Adv. Nurs. 50 (3), 253–261.

Melnychuk, M., Solmi, F., Morris, S., 2018. Using compensating variation to measure the costs of child disability in the UK. Eur. J. Health. Econ. 19, 419–433. https://doi.org/10.1007/s10198-017-0893-7.

Mental Health Foundation, 2015. Fundamental Facts About Mental Health. Mental Health Foundation, London.

Milnes, L.J., Callery, P., 2003. The adaptation of written self-management plans for children with asthma. J. Adv. Nurs. 41 (5), 444–453.

Mukherjee, S., Beresford, B., Sloper, P., 1999. Unlocking Key Working. Bristol Joseph Rowntree Foundation & The Policy Press, UK.

Mukherjee, S., Lightfoot, J., Sloper, P., 2002. Communicating about pupils in mainstream school with special health needs: The NHS perspective. Child. Care Health Dev. 28 (1), 21–27.

National Collaborating Centre for Cancer, 2005. Improving Outcomes in Children & Young People with Cancer: The Manual. National Institute for Health & Clinical Excellence, London.

NHS digital, 2018. Mental health of children and young people in England, 2017 [PAS]. Available from: https://digital.nhs.uk/data-and-information/publications/statistical/mental-health-of-children-and-young-people-in-england/2017/2017.

Norris, A.W., Wolfsdorf, J.I., 2005. Diabetes mellitus. In: Brook, C.G.D., Clayton, P.E., Brown, R.S., Savage, M.O. (Eds.), Clinical Pediatric Endocrinology, fifth ed. Blackwell, Malden.

Office of National Statistics, 2011. Harmonised Concepts and Questions for Social Data Sources Primary Standards Long-Lasting Health Conditions and Illnesses; Impairments and Disability. ONS, London. Available from: https://gss.civilservice.gov.uk/

wp-content/uploads/2016/03/P6-LLI-Impairments-and-Disability-June-16.pdf.

Ohya, Y., Williams, H., Steptoe, A., et al., 2001. Psychosocial factors and adherence to treatment advice in childhood atopic dermatitis. J. Invest. Dermatol. 117 (4), 852–857.

Okpala, I. (Ed.), 2004. The Practical Management of Haemoglobinopathies. Blackwell, Oxford.

Pelaez-Ballestas, I., Romero-Mendoxa, M., Ramos-Lira, L., et al., 2006. Illness trajectories in Mexican children with juvenile idiopathic arthritis and their parents. Rheumatology 45, 1399–1403.

Powers, S.W., Patton, S.R., Hommel, K.A., et al., 2003. Quality of life in childhood migraines: clinical impact and comparison to other long-term conditions. Pediatrics. 112 (1), e1–e5.

Quittner, A., et al., 1998. Role strain in couples with and without a long-term conditions: associations with marital satisfaction, intimacy and daily mood. Health Psychology 17 (2), 112–124.

Randall, D., 2016. Pragmatic Children's Nursing: A Theory for Children and Their Childhoods. Routledge, Abingdon.

Randall, D., 2017. Two futures: financial and practical realities for parents of living with a life limited child. Compr. Child. Adoles. Nurs. 40 (4), 257–267. https://doi.org/10.1080/24694193.2017.1376360.

Robins, B., Dautenhahn, K., te Boekhorst, R., et al., 2004. Robotic assistants in therapy and education of children with autism: can a small humanoid robot help encourage social interaction skills? Available from: https://uhra.herts.ac.uk/bitstream/handle/2299/1891/101152.pdf?sequence=1.

Royal College of Paediatrics and Child Health (RCPCH), 2014. High Dependency Care of Children- Time to Move on: A Focus on the Critically Ill Child Pathway Beyond the Paediatric Intensive Care Unit. RCPCH, London. Available from: http://rcpch.adlibhosting.com/files/High%20Dependency%20Care%20for%20Children%20-%20Time%20To%20Move%20On%202014-10.pdf.

Scot, J., 2000. Children as respondents: the challenge for quantitative methods. In: Christensen, P., James, A. (Eds.), Research With Children: Perspectives and Practices, second ed. Routledge, Abingdon.

Siarkowski, A.K., 1999. Children's adaptation to insulin dependent diabetes mellitus: A critical review of the literature. Pediatric. Nur. 5 (6), 627–639.

Sloper, P., Greco, V., Beecham, J., et al., 2005. Key worker services for disabled children: What characteristics of services lead to better outcomes for children and families? Child. Care Health Dev. 32 (2), 147–157.

Sorkin, D.H., Billimek, J., August, K.J., et al., 2015. Mental health symptoms and patient-reported diabetes symptom burden: Implications for medication regimen changes. Family. Pract. 32 (3), 317–322. https://doi.org/10.1093/fampra/cmv014.

Stein, R.E.K., Reissman, C.K., 1980. The development of an impact-on-family scale: preliminary findings. Medical. Care. 18, 465–472.

Su, J.C., Kemp, A.S., Varigos, G.A., et al., 1997. Atopic eczema: its impact on the family and financial cost. Arch. Dis. Child. 76, 159–162.

Sullivan, P.M., Knutson, J.F., 2000. Maltreatment and disabilities: A population based epidemiological study. Child. Abuse. Neglect. 24 (10), 1257–1273.

Tait, T., Dejnega, S., 2001. Coordinating Children's Services. Mary Seacole Research Unit. De Montfort University, Leicester.

Tak, Y.R., McCubbin, M., 2002. Family stress, perceived social support and coping following the diagnosis of a child's congenital heart disease. J. Adv. Nurs. 39 (2), 190–199.

Teel, C.S., 1991. Chronic sorrow: Analysis of the concept. J. Adv. Nurs. 16, 1311–1319.

Thorne, S.E., Paterson, B.L., 2001. Health care professional support for self-care management in long-term conditions: insights from diabetes research. Patient Educ. Couns. 42, 81–90.

Thompson, M., Hooper, C., Laver-Bradbury, C., et al., 2012. Child and Adolescent Mental Health: Theory and Practice, second ed. Hodder Arnold Taylor & Francis Group, Boca Raton, USA.

Toly, V.B., Musil, C.M., Carl, J.C., 2012. Families with children who are technology dependent: Normalization and family functioning. West. J. Nurs. Res. 34 (1), 52–71.

Valentine, F., Hazell, S., 2007. The definition and aetiology of long-term conditions. In: Valentine, F., Lowes, L. (Eds.), Nursing Care of Children & Young People with Long-Term Conditions. Blackwell Publishing, Oxford, pp. 1–28.

Valentine, F., Mcnee, P., 2007. Context of care & service delivery. In: Valentine, F., Lowes, L. (Eds.), Nursing Care of Children & Young People with Long-Term Conditions. Blackwell Publishing, Oxford, pp. 29–54.

Vessey, J., 1999. Psychological comorbidity in children with chronic conditions. Pediatr. Nurs. 25 (2), 211–214.

Varni, J.W., Limbers, C.A., 2009. The pediatric quality of life inventory: measuring pediatric health related quality of life from the perspective of children and their parents. Pediatric. Clin. North Am. 26, 843–863. https://doi.org/10.1016/j.pcl.2009.05.016.

Varni, J.W., 2020. The PedsQL Measurement Model for the Pediatric Quality of Life Inventory. Available from http://www.pedsql.org/index.html.

Walis, C., Paton, J.Y., Beaton, S., et al., 2011. Children on long-term ventilatory support: 10 years of progress. Arch. Dis. Child. 96, 998–1002. https://doi.org/10.1136/adc.2010.192864.

Wang, K.K., Barnard, A., 2008. Caregivers' experiences at home with a ventilator-dependent child. Qual. Health Res. 18, 501–508.

Waterston, T., Haroon, S., 2008. Advocacy and the paediatrician. Paediatr. Child Health. 18, 213–218.

Watson, D., Townsley, R., Abbott, D., 2002. Exploring multi-agency working in services to disabled children with complex healthcare needs and their families. J. Clin. Nurs. 11 (3), 367–375.

Whalley, D., Huels, J., McKenna, S.P., et al., 2002. The benefit of pimecrolimus on parents' quality of life in the treatment of pediatric atopic dermatitis. Pediatrics. 110 (6), 1133–1136.

Whyte, D.A., 1992. A family nursing approach to the care of a child with a chronic illness. J. Adv. Nurs. 17, 317–327.

Wills, B.S.H., 1999. The experiences of Hong Kong Chinese parents of children with acute lymphocytic leukemia. J. Pediatr. Nurs. 14 (4), 231–238.

Wong, J.C., Izadi, Z., Schroeder, S., et al., 2018. A pilot study of use of a software platform for the collection, integration, and visualization of diabetes device data by health care providers in a multidisciplinary pediatric setting. Diabetes Technol. Ther. 20 (12), 806–816. https://doi.org/10.1089/dia.2018.0251.

World Health Organization (WHO), 1989. Approaches to adolescents. WHO, Geneva.

Young, B., Dixon-Woods, M., Findlay, M., et al., 2002a. Parenting in crisis: Conceptualizing mothers of children with cancer. Soc. Sci. Med. 55 (10), 1835–1847.

Young, B., Fitch, G.E., Dixon-Woods, M., et al., 2002b. Parents' accounts of wheeze and asthma related symptoms: A qualitative study. Arch. Dis. Child. 87 (2), 131–134.

Young, B., Dixon-Woods, M., Windridge, K.C., et al., 2003. Managing communication with young people who have a potentially life threatening long-term conditions: Qualitative study of patients and parents. BMJ 326 (7384), 305–309.

41

Children Living With Long-Term Conditions: Child and Adolescent Mental Health: The Nursing Response

Celeste Foster

LEARNING OUTCOMES

- Understand the importance of attending to the emotional health and well-being needs of children and young people, and the policy frameworks that govern this element of work.
- Review the nature of adolescence.
- Consider the impact of the adolescent developmental tasks on health behaviours.
- Be able to locate the young person in terms of their developmental tasks.
- Understand the continuum of mental health and illness in relation to children and young people, and the risk

and resilience factors that can move children and young people along this continuum.
- Consider the impact of physical ill health on adolescent development and mental well-being.
- Review the interpersonal and communication skills required when working with young people.
- Explore the nature of the therapeutic relationship.
- Identify nursing responses to young people with emotional problems and/or mental health issues.
- Locate appropriate resources to inform best practice with young people.

INTRODUCTION – A CALL TO ACTION

It is estimated that in the UK one in five children and young people are experiencing emotional health or behavioural problems at any one time (Deighton et al., 2018). Since 1995, the prevalence of longstanding mental health conditions in children and young people (aged 4–24 years) has consistently increased (Pitchforth et al., 2018). Globally, depression causes the biggest burden of ill health in children and young people (Patton et al., 2016). Suicide is a leading cause of death for young people in the UK and has not declined in 30 years (Office for National Statistics [ONS], 2014). The impact of poor mental health on children and young people is profound, accounting for 45% of lost years due to disability in 10- to 24-year-olds (Gore et al., 2011). The case for intervening effectively to prevent mental ill health, maintain emotional well-being and to provide evidence-based treatment for mental illness, when it does occur in children and young people, cannot be overstated.

During adolescence, a young person acquires the physical, cognitive, emotional, social and economic resources or vulnerabilities that are the foundation for later life health and well-being or longer-term risk of illness. At an individual, family and population level the relative health capital that this balance of risk and resilience creates, influences the health and well-being of the next generation (Patton et al., 2016). It is estimated that up 75% of adult mental health conditions have their onset before the age of 24 (Kessler et al., 2005). Mental ill health in youth and beyond is associated with a wide range

of additional negative health and social outcomes such as sexually transmitted disease, road traffic accidents, domestic violence, physical fighting, crime, homicide and suicide and teenage pregnancy (Das et al., 2016).

Historically, and perhaps to some extent understandably, responding to the mental health needs of children and young people beyond making referrals to specialist Child and Adolescent Mental Health Services (CAMHS) services, has been seen by many children and young people's nurses as outside of their scope of practice. And yet children's nurses are more likely to meet young people experiencing acute mental distress than any other professional group within the children's work force.

The prevalence of mental health conditions in children with a long-term physical health condition is four times higher than the general population (Bennett et al., 2015). In national clinical guidelines, children's medical units are identified as essential components in the care pathway for children who self-harm, attempt suicide or have an eating disorder (National Institute for Health and Care Excellence [NICE], 2004, 2011, 2017). School nursing services play an important part in the government strategy for promoting mental health in school settings (Public Health England, 2015).

Children's nurses have a vital role to play, given the number of children with emotional health needs that children's nurses are likely to meet in their everyday practice, the high level of mortality associated with the mental health conditions that they will commonly encounter and the fact that it is estimated that up to 40% of children with a mental health disorder are not properly diagnosed and/or not receiving specialist treatment (Care Quality Commission [CQC], 2017). This is a role that includes safeguarding children and young people against experiences that can precipitate mental distress, identifying young people with a mental health need, providing advice, support and interventions for those young people and their families and acting as a bridge to more specialist mental health services when needed.

Lack of knowledge, the inappropriate nature of the paediatric units as a setting for meeting the needs of children in mental distress, fear of getting things wrong or making things worse, and negative assumptions about young people presenting with mental health problems have all been cited as reasons why children's nurses may struggle to meet the mental health needs of children in their care (Fisher and Foster, 2016).

Working with adolescents is a task many groups find challenging. Generally, adolescents are considered to have needs that differ from both adults and children, yet they are often nursed in environments that also contain either adults or children. If we add issues of emotional distress/mental health, things seem to move beyond the perceived areas of expertise or competence of many children's nurses (Fisher and Foster, 2016). The picture may be complicated further by the nurse having to move quickly from the parents of a child who is seriously physically ill, to an emotionally distressed, abusive, swearing adolescent, whose physical health may or may not appear to be seriously compromised (Foster, 2009). In addition, the legacy of successive governments underfunding adolescent mental health services, in spite of the knowledge that the burden of mental illness is higher in adolescence than at any other life stage (Singh et al., 2008), can mean that difficulties accessing tightly rationed specialist CAMHS services can leave children's nurses feeling frustrated and unsupported.

It is these dilemmas that this chapter wishes to address by providing information and educational resources, but more importantly some practical guidance on the interpersonal skills that might be helpful with this client group. It will set out the policy and legal frameworks in which children's nurses' responsibilities to the mental health and well-being of children are situated; explain the link between physical and emotional health issues; and outline how mental distress of children and young people can be understood in the context of their developmental and social history. Finally, how this knowledge can enable children's nurses to use elements of their core nursing skills and training to effectively contribute to meeting the mental health needs of children they meet in their everyday practice, will be demonstrated.

UNDERSTANDING THE POLICY FRAMEWORK AND LEGAL CONTEXT OF CARING FOR CHILDREN AND YOUNG PEOPLE WITH MENTAL HEALTH NEEDS

Since 2004, government policy in respect to child health and mental health has advocated child-centred services that consider the whole child, not simply the illness. Seeing the whole child also means recognising that health protection and promotion, and disease prevention are integral to the young person's care in any setting. All staff working with children need to recognise the contribution they can make to children's emotional well-being and that they understand their responsibilities for supporting children in difficulty (Department of Health [DoH], 2004). In exploring child-centred care, it is recognised that the child exists within the context of a family, school, friends and local community.

Further, children and young people have rights, and their treatment is a partnership. Children have rights to be consulted and involved in their care, for their needs to be paramount in all decision making, and depending on their age and stage of development, qualified rights of confidentiality and consent to treatment. These rights are afforded to them by *The Children Act (1989 & 2004)*, the United Nations Convention on the Rights of the Child (1990), *the Mental Health Act (1983)*, *the Mental Capacity Act (2005)* and specific case law, such as Fraser Guidelines for Gillick Competence. Parents also have rights and responsibilities outlined in *the Human Rights Act (1998)*, *the Family Law Act (1969)* and the *Children Act (1989 & 2004)*. Broadly speaking, as a child ages and matures the zone of parental control diminishes and the rights and autonomy of the child increases. Working to uphold young people's rights, whilst also respecting the role of parents is a significant part of providing services for children. It requires understanding of the legal framework that sets out each party's rights and responsibilities and the conflicts and dilemmas that application of the different legal frameworks can generate. (For a detailed explanation and case study exercise to help you understand the application of legal frameworks to different aspects of children's care, see: *The Legal Aspects of the Care and Treatment of Children and Young People with Mental Disorder: A Guide for Professionals.* London, NIMHE, 2009.)

In 2011, governmental strategy recognised the fact that most mental health problems in adulthood started in childhood and committed to improve access to early help for children and young people in mental distress as part of its 'No Health Without Mental Health' strategy (DoH, 2011).

The 2015 paper 'Future in Mind' (DoH, 2015) set out an ambition for improvements in mental health services for children and young people by 2020. These were also linked to the 'Five Year Forward View for Mental Health' (NHS, 2014) that included objectives for improving perinatal mental health services, access to psychological therapies for children and eating disorder treatment for children and young people. The key priorities for improving the mental health of our children can be summarised in Box 41.1.

Until 2017, children's mental health services were organised in a tiered model. All those who work with children (including children's nurses) were identified as part of universal mental health services at Tier 1, with increasing service specialism as the tiers progressed, ending at Tier 4 – specialist inpatient units for children with severe and complex mental health conditions. This approach has been criticised, due to the focus being on service organisation rather than being centred on children and their needs. As part of the governmental commitment to transform child and adolescent mental health services, a new model is now being implemented, known as the THRIVE model (Wolpert et al., 2014). The THRIVE model works by identifying where children are at in relation to level of help they need, and then matches this

to the kind of interventions that services provide (Fig. 41.1). This recognises that several different services may be contributing to meeting a child's needs. It also allows for the idea that children's level of need can change, and that this is not always based on the presence of a mental health condition – as many children have a diagnosis of a mental or a physical health condition, but with the right treatment and support can be thriving.

Within this model, children's nurses, in whatever context they work, have a responsibility to contribute to helping children thrive, cope, and when needed access appropriate information, guidance and help.

PROMOTING EMOTIONAL HEALTH AND WELL-BEING AND THE ROLE OF SCHOOLS

In line with the intention of the THRIVE model to provide services for children as early as possible in the places in which they usually live and learn. The most recent strategies for improving mental health services for children and young people (Public Health England, 2015; DoH, 2017) will re-organise services to make sure that access to mental health and well-being support is linked to schools and colleges. There is clear evidence that schools and colleges can, and do, play a vital role in identifying mental health needs at an early stage, referring young people to specialist support and working jointly with others to support young people experiencing problems. Over the coming years the government plan to strengthen this by making sure that there is a designated Senior Lead for Mental Health in each school to oversee the approach to mental health and well-being. An identified link person within the local specialist child and adolescent mental health service will provide rapid advice, consultation and signposting. There is also a plan to fund new Mental Health

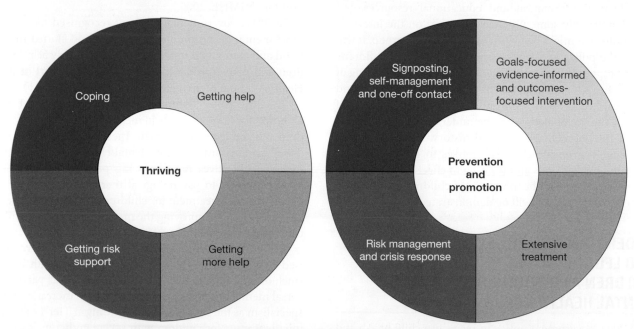

Fig. 41.1 The THRIVE Model: the place that young people are in and the input and help they need. (Wolpert, M., Harris, R., Jones, M., et al., 2014. THRIVE: The AFC-Tavistock Model for CAMHS. CAMHS Press, London.)

Support Teams, to provide specific extra capacity for early intervention and ongoing help to support those with mild to moderate needs. Their work will be managed jointly by schools, colleges and the NHS.

Schools are already responsible for making sure that mental health awareness training is provided for staff and for pupils, and that there are whole school approaches to well-being, tackling stigma and to addressing bullying and poor behaviour (Public Health England, 2015).

UNDERSTANDING THE LINK BETWEEN PHYSICAL AND PSYCHOLOGICAL HEALTH NEEDS IN CHILDREN AND YOUNG PEOPLE

A review of child and adolescent mental health (CAMH) services (DoH, 2008) highlighted the likelihood that children with a physical health problem, and particularly a long-term condition, will also have associated mental health needs. It is estimated that approximately 10% of adolescents are living with long-term conditions (Suris et al., 2004). Thus, emphasising the need for children's nurses to be sensitive to the needs of physically unwell children in relation to helping maintain their psychological well-being, not just addressing their immediate physical health needs.

This term 'psychological well-being' is thought to be the most useful description of mental health needs of children and adolescents, as too often we limit ourselves to viewing mental health problems as diagnosable, symptom-apparent mental illnesses. Contemporary understanding that mental distress in children and young people is most commonly a response to what is happening within the systems in which they live (Scott et al., 2010), requires a shift away from biomedical models of illness. The aim is to view the child or adolescent as a biopsychosocial being with interacting biological, psychological and social contributing factors to both their difficulties and the possible solutions. The term psychological well-being also incorporates emotional, cognitive and behavioural attributes of well-being (DoH, 2008).

Biological, psychological and social development of children and young people are interdependent: physical health conditions can affect psychological development and psychosocial adjustments to puberty and other facets of growing up can affect disease processes, treatment adherence and management. (For a comprehensive summary of the reciprocal impact of chronic conditions and psychosocial development upon each other see: Suris et al., 2004.)

Although the experience for each young person and their family is unique, broadly speaking chronic illness has the capacity to negatively affect identity development, self-esteem, self-efficacy, and hope for one's future. As well as creating psychological distress in themselves, such as feelings of loneliness, alienation and loss of developmental drive toward the achievement of adolescent tasks, these areas of development are all risk factors for reduced adherence with treatment and for development of mental illnesses such as clinical depression and anxiety disorders. The impact of the condition and associated treatment regimens also tend to disrupt ordinary social and occupational activities such as striving for independence and separation from families, school attendance and attainment, and peer/sexual relationships. Disruptions in these domains are all associated with wider health risk behaviours in adolescence and in later adulthood.

Children's nurses working have an important role to play in working to mitigate the risks factors associated with long-term conditions. Advocating for children's emerging independence to support self-management can be a vital part of helping young people move along the developmental continuum towards adulthood (Baltag and Sawyer, 2016). However, this is a careful balancing act that also involves supporting parents, as a result of the anxiety that this may understandably evoke in them, due to the risks associated with relinquishing control of their child's treatment. Providing accessible information about their condition and treatments supports young people to be informed stakeholders in their care, promoting a sense of control and protecting against feelings of hopelessness (World Health Organization [WHO], 2015). In addition, any activity that helps young people maintain connections with their peers and to continue with educational and leisure activities during periods of illness will help to foster positive identity formation, self-esteem and interpersonal skill development (Suris et al., 2004), as well as potentially buffer against the risk of depression (Collishaw et al., 2015). Central to all of these interventions is understanding the developmental and social context of the mental health and illness in young people.

THE DEVELOPMENTAL AND SOCIAL DETERMINANTS OF MENTAL HEALTH ISSUES IN CHILDREN AND YOUNG PEOPLE

Emergence of Mental Life and Resilience in Early Life

The perinatal periods and infancy are critical periods in development of the foundations for our mental functioning and resilience (i.e. ability to cope and adapt in response to the stresses and strains of everyday life), and the neurobiological structures that support these capacities. Research has significantly advanced our understanding of the way in which the physical and psychosocial environment affects gene expression (epigenetics), leaving lasting effects on neurological development (Bock et al., 2015). The hypothalamic-pituitary-adrenal axis, one of the brain's main system for regulating stress, is primed in utero and develops in the first few years of life. It is directly affected by the relative balance of stress and soothing/support available in the baby's environment, including the relative levels of prenatal stress experienced by the mother (Bock et al., 2015). The ability to name, understand and regulate changes in our emotions, to guess the feeling of others and to adapt to our surroundings all begin in infancy through the process of attachment (Bowlby, 1989). The carer–infant relationship is central within these growth processes because it acts on biological, emotional, cognitive and interpersonal aspects of the baby's development (Schore and Schore, 2014).

Attachment is the evolutionary mechanism by which we socially and physiologically connect with others to regulate our internal feeling states (Schore and Schore, 2010). It is easy to forget that being able to do this for ourselves is a not a developmental given that just comes with age and time, but rather it is a maturational achievement that requires certain conditions to foster it (Winnicott, 1984). These conditions come from provision of a relational environment that confers safety, belonging and legitimacy and that works to keep stress hormones at bay. In good enough circumstances we are held within a care relationship that sees everything we do as meaningful information to be decoded, in order to meet our needs, soothe our distress and creates an interactional environment in which we can learn to understand ourselves and others (Adshead, 2002).

Although attachment processes are often described in terms of the parent–infant relationship, they continue to operate throughout all stages of development and as the child moves into adolescence the task of containment becomes the function of its wider community and the adults who people the systems and organisations in which they live and learn (Waddell, 2002). For children who need to access health services this can include children's nurses.

Research is now beginning to show that the presence of multiple adverse childhood experiences increases the risk of an individual developing a range of health risk behaviours, illnesses such as diabetes and heart disease and mental health conditions by two- or three-fold (Hughes et al., 2017).

Positive attachment relationships can serve as protection against the impact of some adverse childhood experiences, helping children to feel safe, bounce back and to understand what has happened to them. However, if there is insufficient support and help for carers some forms of childhood adversity that affect children and their carers, can inhibit or disrupt the development of secure attachment bonds, which further adds to the risks the child may be facing. Chronic or severe insecurity, bereavement, disruption or maltreatment within key attachment relationships is an adverse childhood experience in itself, and can cause significant disturbances within the child's physiological systems that respond to stress. As the child gets older this can increase their vulnerability to further harm, particularly in adolescence, and increase the likelihood of them experimenting with ways of coping that are disease risk factors (Maunder and Hunter, 2008).

Adolescence

Adolescence is characterised by dynamic brain development in which the interaction with the social environment shapes the capabilities an individual takes forward into adult life. The only other period on the life course when our brains are subject to such a rapid and high level of neurological change is infancy (Patton et al., 2016). The emotional tone and sense of safety provided within the social contexts in which adolescents grow up are important facilitators or inhibitors of psychological, emotional, social and neurological maturation. For young people who are experiencing physical or mental ill-health to the extent that they are needing to spend time in hospital or other health care settings, means that we as nurses become important contributors to an individual child's social setting.

The Nature of Adolescence as a Life Stage

There are some dominant ideas about adolescence and young adulthood that are commonly accepted. It can be defined as a period in human development linked to biological markers, involving transitions (that can be seen as stages), in which the central task is establishing identity and independence from carers. It is suggested that universal definitions of adolescence should at best be restricted to describing adolescence as a 'period of transition' in which, although no longer seen as a child, the young person is not yet considered an adult. The World Health Organization's (WHO, 2014) definition of adolescence states that the stage is commonly associated with physiological changes occurring with the progression from the appearance of secondary sexual characteristics (puberty) to sexual and reproductive maturity. Pierce and Hardy (2012) suggest that these biological markers create problems because the falling age of onset of puberty attributed to improved health means there is now a widening gap between the age of sexual maturity, the age at which cognitive maturity (which develops with experience) catches up with the emotional and physical surges specific to puberty, and the age at which sexual relations become legitimate. A child experiencing early puberty can be overwhelmed by the experience of powerful emotions without the cognitive abilities to contain these strong feelings and impulses. Without the help and support of available and thoughtful adults, this can leave children who experience early puberty at risk of a range of psychosocial disorders and mental health conditions (Pierce & Hardy, 2012).

A central dilemma of the adolescent experience is that in some cultures, physical maturity comes well before legal definitions of adulthood in terms of legal sexual behaviour, the right to vote, join the military, etc.

The combination of young people's relative inexperience in sexual matters and the social stigma attached to them being sexually active creates vulnerability that is only now being recognised and addressed. However, adolescence is not characterised by just a sexual dilemma, there is also vulnerability in relationships with peers, with adults and with organisations. It seems that adults don't know how to take adolescents seriously because they do not find it easy to understand their experience. This leads to adolescents experiencing structural age-based discrimination in a range of contexts (Liebel, 2014). In addition, there is an acknowledged difficulty for adolescents in that health care workers can struggle to accept that they are not just older children or younger adults; therefore health care workers may have difficulty responding to adolescents' uniqueness regarding the ways in which they think, process and use information to make decisions (WHO, 2015).

There is, however, a view that the dilemma of adolescence has been overplayed, in terms of a life stage that by its very nature involves serious conflict and upheaval. More recent thinking suggests much less difficulty and much more continuity between the child that was, through adolescence to the adult that will be. It is considered that most adolescents negotiate this period of life transition with relatively little major disruption or sustained high-risk behaviour (Coleman, 2011).

Even if the more optimistic view of adolescence is taken, health care settings are likely to see more of those children involved in high-risk behaviours. These high-risk behaviours are also linked to the precursors of mental health problems, low self-esteem and dysfunctional families (British Medical Association [BMA], 2003).

The Psychological and Emotional Development Tasks of Adolescence

The period of transition from childhood to adulthood can be divided into early (10–14 years), late (15–19 years) and young adulthood (20–24 years) (Patton et al., 2016). Individuals will negotiate these stages in their own time, but as a general principle, it is helpful to view adolescence in this way.

It is helpful to see the key adolescent task as a search for identity, that is, a sense of separate self, but as always, the self in relation to others (Waddell, 2002). Adolescents are in search of an identity that will lead them to adulthood, they make a strong effort to answer the questions 'Who am I?' and 'Who am I in relation to you?' Developing a sense of a separate or independent sense of self and taking on the increased responsibilities that come with the move towards adulthood, also always involves an experience of loss and mourning of the child that the new adolescent once was (Polmear, 2004). This gradual process happens over time and can help us to understand the oscillation between more grown up and more childlike states of mind that can commonly be seen in young people who are working through the stage of adolescence.

Of the stage models, Erikson's psychosocial model is perhaps the best known. Erikson (1963) describes the adolescent task/crisis as identity versus confusion. He notes that the healthy resolution of earlier conflicts can now serve as a foundation for the search for an identity. If an individual has developed a sense of trust and a strong sense of industry in early life stages, then the search for identity will be easier. The adolescent must make a conscious search for identity. This is built on the outcome and resolution to conflict in earlier

stages. If the adolescent cannot make deliberate decisions and choices, especially about vocation, sexual orientation and life in general, role confusion becomes a threat.

Jacobs (1998) looks at adolescence in three stages:
- Early adolescence and sexuality
- Middle adolescence: authority and independence
- Later adolescence: faith and responsibility

In this model, early adolescence is linked to puberty and reinitiates issues of sexual identity and attitudes as part of the overall quest for personal identity. The young person may become very self-conscious and also very preoccupied with appearance and dress. The young person's changing physical appearance matters a great deal. This might evoke feelings of pleasure and confidence, or strangeness and shame. Rivalry and competition are often important elements at this time as part of the adjustments within peer groups. However, rivalry is not confined to peer groups: just at the time the children are finding their sexual identity, their parents are conscious of imminent or present changes in themselves.

Jacobs talks of how a mother may be entering her menopause at the same time as the daughter achieves her menarche or a father may be aware of his spreading midriff and lack of muscular tone just as his son is reaching his peak of physical fitness. Even if that is not the case, parents in the UK will be made aware of their changing life position in what is a very youth-oriented culture. These changes in life positions for all family members are the context in which the young person's ambivalence towards their parents is acted out. On the one hand, the parent is still needed as an object of love and a protector, but on the other hand there is a strong desire to push the parent away to find their own confidence and object of love. To both love and hate parents, who then may respond by being hurt or angry, can be a difficult conflict for the young person to contain and manage. It is important to consider the additional layer complexity that the onset of a long-term condition, for example diabetes, will add to this dynamic.

There is also the consideration of current cultural and technological changes to the adolescent landscape. One must consider that advances in technology and exposure via mobile technology, the internet and social media mean that our adolescent population is at risk of being bombarded with dialogue and imagery of both a volume and quality that may be far beyond their developmental capacity. Platforms for negative peer interactions and bullying now extend beyond the school day and playground, into the 24-hour cycle and the young person's home and bedroom. This can be one contributor to the high-octane mood swings and outbursts stereotypically attributed to adolescence, that are best understood as triggered by an increasing pressure to cope. This mismatch between cultural demand and emotional maturity means that sometimes adolescents can temporarily present with more toddler-like states and coping strategies and experience verbal and physical 'meltdowns'. This can be understood by proposing that the behaviour is symbolic to the return to a primitive manner of coping or regression in a time of increased stress and an inability to cope that leads the young person to be temporarily overwhelmed (Waddell, 2002). The lack of expressive ability inherent in the adolescent, at a time of emotional experience that is supremely complex means that their feelings can be expressed through acting-out behaviours like outbursts, rebellious dress sense and/or periods of withdrawal or refusal to communicate.

On the other hand, the internet and social media comes with increased access to information and advice regarding health and well-being, as well as new and diverse communities with which to engage and form strong social connections and peer relationships and opportunities for social activism and citizenship (Patton et al., 2016). A recent review found that the benefits of online communication and social media for young people included increased self-esteem, perceived social ort, increased social capital, safe identity experimentation and increased opportunity for self-disclosure. However, the negative effects included increased exposure to harm, social isolation, depression and cyber-bullying (Best et al., 2014).

Implications for the Health Care Professional

It is important to be mindful of the young person's need to assert themselves and of the adult response of meeting the challenge or setting the boundaries. This must be within a context of an acceptance of the young person and an understanding of what is motivating their behaviour. The limits must contain, but not crush, the young person's emotions and behaviour. It is important to recognise that although we (as nurses) may appear to be the target of their discontent, it is likely that bigger issues are being acted out. These issues relate to their main developmental task of trying to assert who they are, within the context of ill health. Their illness has the potential to undermine their sense of independence directly through their own thoughts and beliefs. This might also be done indirectly and unwittingly through the actions of anxious parents and/or the collusion of nursing and medical staff.

This natural process of adolescence – separating from the parents as a way of increasing independence – may happen without much drama or may be very dramatic. Separation can be made easier if the young person can achieve a degree of financial independence. This might be quite a challenge if the young person is in continuing education, unemployed or unable to work through ill health. In the last stage, Jacobs (1998) suggests the concern is for the wider issues of their place in the wider society and their own transition into adulthood. For some there is concern about what is wrong with society and optimism about their proposed solutions. It is at this stage that some of the compromises that underpin adult functioning are beginning to be made.

Coleman (2011) developed a 'focal theory' of adolescence, which suggests that at specific ages in adolescence different relationships come into focus, in the sense of being most prominent, or important. In early adolescence the concerns

about heterosexual relationships are to the fore. This is a time when normative uncertainties about sexual orientation and preferences are common but can also arouse much internal shame in the young person, due to anxieties of falling outside of the norm. It may be a period in which children and young people whose sexuality is developing in a non-heteronormative way, experience bullying or internal sense of anxiety and 'otherness'. In middle adolescence (15 years) the peer group becomes very important and in late adolescence (peaking at 17 years) conflicts with parents become central. Research has shown that adolescent decision-making processes differ from those of adults or children (Patton et al., 2016). The presence of peers affects the way in which they process social information, with heightened sensitivity to the perceived impact of decision making upon reputation, over and above other priorities (such as impact on health). Coleman (2011) added that there may well be overlap between the issues and that none of the issues are tied to a particular age or developmental level. A key idea that arises is that if the young person is able to deal with these issues one at a time, it is easier to cope with the complex issues of adolescence. This would be why only a minority of young people are overwhelmed by the transitions of adolescence and might also link with Erikson's assertion that successful transition is linked to the success, or not, of earlier life stages. Therefore the more difficulties there have been earlier in life, the more likely adolescence will be a difficult time. During this process of individuation (separating out one's own identity), adolescents increasingly transfer their emotional attachment from parents to peers. Close peer friendships have a positive influence on adolescents' social and personality development and adolescents who perceive their peer friends as supportive have fewer psychological problems, greater confidence and less loneliness (Hay and Ashman, 2003).

ACTIVITY

How might such knowledge about peer relationships influence our attempts to manage disruptive behaviour in a clinical setting?

In spite of the drive towards independence, parental relationships remain important in terms of self-worth, and facilitation of development of emotional processing skills and abilities to understand others, particularly for those adolescents whose transition is well adjusted. Those who are more troubled tend to disregard parents and teachers as sources of self-esteem, preferring alternative audiences such as peers, as a change to the negative feedback from parents and school (Hay and Ashman, 2003). This raises an important question about how therapeutic nursing relationships can be forged and used to provide positive or benign feedback to children who have become disaffected with adults, in order to try and re-engage them.

What is significant from a nursing point of view is that we should take as much account of the adolescent's developmental stage as we would of the developmental stage of the younger child. If we want to be helpful and respectful, we need to go to where they are. This is the starting point of any helping relationship. As nurses, we can begin to make progress in giving appropriate care only when we begin to understand how even the most undesirable of youthful behaviours usually represent:

- the attempts of adolescents to complete these developmental tasks;
- attempts to problem solve and to cope with the exacting demands of adolescence;
- ambivalence about whether they want to move on to adulthood;
- their perception that they may never complete the tasks successfully.

An understanding of the adolescent's developmental tasks will allow the nurse to focus caregiving in the most effective manner. For example, an important nursing intervention might be for the nurse to spend time with the young person's key friends, helping them accommodate the changed circumstances of the illness so that supportive peer relationships can be maintained. This in turn will enhance the young person's self-concept and self-esteem, which will be needed in facing the difficult adjustments ahead. This strategy will also serve as a protective factor against emotional distress and the risk of mental ill health. This would support the idea of moving beyond pure medical thinking and embrace the concept of adolescent health (WHO, 2015) in which:

- The developing person is seen as an active agent in his or her own development.
- Person and context are related: the individual must be seen within the context of their family, their peer group and their developmental stage.
- Developmental readiness: that is, adolescents will fare better if they are allowed more time to deal with important issues in their lives.
- 'Arena of comfort': this idea suggests that if adolescents feel comfortable in some environments then discomfort in other areas can be tolerated.

👤 ACTIVITY

- How might the young person's sense of agency be influenced by ill health?
- Do the assessment strategies consider the context of the person and their illness?
- Do the clinical procedures ensure space and the right information is being offered to help the young person accommodate the changes that are happening to them?
- How might the 'arena of comfort' concept be used in the planning of care?

When thinking of a holistic assessment process, it might be helpful to reflect on the interplay between the young person's illness and their transition through the adolescent developmental tasks. You might want to think of some questions you could ask during the assessment phase that might help you locate where the young person is in terms of their adolescent transition.

Supporting young people to be active agents in decision making about their care is an important component of the nurse's role. The more sense of power and control an adolescent perceives they have, the better they are able to balance short- and long-term risks and goals, which tends to lead to better health outcomes. Working to help young people manage high states of emotional arousal and facilitate decision making during periods of calm, will also enhance the likelihood of them making decisions in their own interests and foster maturation of their decision-making abilities.

There is a strong relationship between adolescent health and other aspects of adolescent life such as education, employment and housing. Interventions therefore should be multi-professional and involve cooperation between health, education and social services (BMA, 2003).

Issues of Sexuality, Gender Relationships and Physical Attractiveness

Sexuality might be seen as a taboo subject in that it is often an overlooked issue for those working with children and adolescents. Children and adolescents are aware of changes in their own bodies and those of their family and friends. There is a need to be sensitive to the young person's accommodation of their own sexuality in earlier adolescence, and their possible uneasiness with themselves in terms of sexuality. We need to be aware of issues of emerging primary sexual orientation, supporting young people to explore, find and inhabit their place along the continuum heterosexuality and homosexuality, without inadvertently reinforcing internalised stigma or assuming heteronormative development. Conversely, for a young person whose sexuality is not forming along heteronormative lines, it is equally important to avoid acting in ways that lead them to feeling pressure to 'fix' their sexuality absolutely as one thing or another and attribute a concrete label to it too quickly. The same principles need to be applied to gender identity development.

A key developmental achievement of middle adolescence is psychophysical integration, that is, assimilating changes in the body into the development of identity as a whole, including forming a relatively fixed body concept that reconciles the emergence of sexuality (Waddell, 2002). Part of this process drives the adolescent need for increased privacy and physical and psychological space from parents/carers. Contained within this task is a requirement to mourn. The childhood body and the passive nature of childhood object-relations must be given up in order to take active ownership of the new sexualised body that is now capable of enacting fantasies in reality (Polmear, 2004). The mourning component of the process can often be defended against through impulsive and provocative expressions of sexuality. During this period there is a need to keep the young person safe, and in some situations to keep staff safe as well. We need to be aware of how young people may be in a position to more readily relate to and engage with younger nurses, but that this may also come with the risk of being drawn by the young person into their peer network. They may want to see the nurse as a friend or identify with them, compete with them, or even reject them as a peer. The young person might develop intense feelings about individual nurses that may involve identification, love and/or sexual attraction. The issues and the careful boundary management needed to keep all parties safe are often underplayed, perhaps partly as an unconscious denial of the young person's sexuality.

Being ill can be a significant challenge to the individual's confidence about their sexuality, personal appearance and thus self-worth. Studies show that awareness of sexuality and physical attractiveness significantly influence females' and males' sense of self-worth (Hay and Ashman, 2003). Therefore developing skills and confidence to enter into dialogue with young people about changes in their body and body image in the context of ill health, and its impact upon expression of their sexuality, is essential.

THE CONTINUUM OF MENTAL HEALTH AND ILLNESS AND THE FACTORS THAT PROMOTE HEALTH AND INCREASE RISK FACTORS

In order to understand how to support children and young people in mental distress, we need to have a concept of mental wellness, in order to think about the state that we are hoping to support young people to return. Illness can be seen as easier to define than health and is often described in diagnostic manuals. However, the question needs to be asked: what is mental health? It is as difficult to define mental health as it is health in general, but it is widely agreed that in children, mental health is indicated by (NHS Health Advisory Service, 1995, p 15):

- A capacity to enter into and sustain mutually satisfying personal relationships.
- Continuing progression of psychological development.
- An ability to play and to learn so that attainments are appropriate for age and intellectual level.
- A developing moral sense of right and wrong.
- The degree of psychological distress and maladaptive behaviour being within normal limits for the child's age and context.

Young people themselves realistically do not view being mentally healthy as being happy all the time, but rather view it as being able to cope with the potential happiness that accompanies living (DoH, 2008). When assessing young people's mental health, their own views on their feelings and emotions are valuable indicators of their overall mental health and well-being, as well as their ability to participate in school, learn and socialise (Department of Health and Social Care [DHSC] and Department for Education [DE], 2017).

 ACTIVITY

Thinking About What Makes Us Mentally Healthy

It might be helpful to spend a little time thinking about how your mental health is maintained and what factors contribute to your maintenance of these attributes.

Risk and Resilience Factors

Mental health and ill health can be understood as a continuum upon which we all move up and down at different points of our life. Where children and young people find themselves on this continuum can be seen as a result of the interaction between risk factors (those things that serve to make us more vulnerable) and resilience factors (those things that can buffer against stress or strengths that can be used to help us manage the risks we are facing, and to bounce back from setbacks). Risk and resilience factors are summarised in Table 41.1 (Burton, 2014; Cabaj et al., 2014).

Mental ill health is much more likely to occur in the presence of three or more stressful events or risk factors (DoH, 2008). However, this is not a given, and the interaction between risk and resilience is also affected by the age and developmental stage of the child, the length of time to which they are exposed to the stressor, and the availability of helpful relationships with adults around them. It is also important to understand the difference between a statistical risk and an absolute inevitability that something will happen. For example, many parents experience mental ill health in their lifetime but remain very warm, loving and effective parents to their children. This is important to understand if we are to avoid labelling and stereotyping individuals. Equally, a young child can experience one risk factor of such severity that it is enough to cause mental ill health on its own. Similar to the presence of multiple stressors bringing about mental ill health, protection and recovery often requires the presence of multiple resilience factors. For example, supporting parents, providing opportunities for young people to have access to physical exercise, social relationships and activities that promote a sense of self efficacy, together have been found to provide mental health resilience in children whose parents are experiencing depression (Collishaw et al., 2015).

The extent of the negative impact of bullying, particularly if persistent or not responded to effectively by adults at the time, is only now really being understood. The effects of being both a victim and perpetrator of bullying have been shown to be directly associated with rates of depression, anxiety, self-harm and suicidality in childhood. The effects last well into early adulthood, affecting occupational, financial, health and social outcomes (Copeland et al., 2013).

There are also issues regarding equity of access for children who exist on the margins. Consequently, these children present as significantly at risk for developing mental health problems, due to lack of access to early help that may stop their difficulties developing. These children and young people may be vulnerable for a number of reasons, including the following (DHSC and DE, 2017):

- Their problems are hidden from or not understood by the system – for example, refugees, those seeking asylum, travelling communities, those who are homeless and young runaways.
- Their problems are not recognised or addressed due to discrimination or lack of awareness – for example, children from black and minority ethnic communities, children who identify as LGBTQ+.

TABLE 41.1 Summary of Statistically Significant Factors Known to Increase a Young Person's Risk and Resilience

Environmental/Contextual Risk Factors
Socioeconomic disadvantage
Homelessness
Disaster
Discrimination
Violence in the community
Being a refugee/asylum seeker
Other significant life event
Bullying

Family Risk Factors
Early attachment/nurturing problems
Parental conflict
Family breakdown
Inconsistent/unclear discipline
Hostile and/or rejecting relationships
Significant adults' failure to adapt to child's changing developmental needs
Physical, emotional, sexual abuse
Parental mental and/or physical illness
Parental criminal behaviour
Death and loss, bereavement issues relating to family members or friends

Child/Young Person Risk Factors
Genetic influences
Low IQ or learning difficulties
Specific developmental delay
Communication difficulties
Difficult temperament
Gender identity conflict
Chronic physical illness
Neurological disorder
Academic failure/poor school attendance
Low self-esteem

Resilience Factors
Secure attachments
Self-esteem
Social skills
Familial compassion and warmth
A stable family environment
Adequate quality time with parent/carers
Social support systems that encourage personal development and coping skills
Good academic performance
A skill or talent

- Of the presence of other serious conditions – as may be the case for children with learning difficulties or disabilities.
- Their mental health needs result in problems with their educational progress. Young people who are not in education, employment or training report particularly low levels of happiness and self-esteem.
- They are experiencing difficulties through abuse or neglect.
- They have needs in a number of areas and are at risk of falling between services – for example, children in care, teenage mothers and fathers, those in contact with the youth justice system, those with complex chronic illness.

There is an important distinction to be made here: it is the risk of marginalisation and inequitable access to services that brings with it an increased risk of mental ill health. Having a protected characteristic such as being gay, having a learning disability or being from a travelling or minority ethnic community, does not in itself cause mental ill health.

Prevalence of Mental Ill Health in Children and Young People

The problems of children accessing services in order to receive diagnosis and treatment, combined with the fact that many children in severe mental distress do not meet adult-focused diagnostic criteria, make accurately defining the rates of mental ill health in children and young people in the UK very difficult. The government recently estimated that 10% of children and young people of all ages have a diagnosable mental health condition of some kind (DHSC and DE, 2017). However, a review of child and adolescent mental health services by the Care Quality Commission (CQC, 2017) highlighted that up to 40% of children and young people are not getting access to the specialist services that they need, indicating that actual prevalence rates might be much higher.

In children under 10 years of age, the predominant difficulties tend to be school-related and behavioural difficulties, and the emotional and behavioural problems that can be secondary to neurodevelopmental or hyperkinetic disorders, such as attention deficit hyperactivity disorder (ADHD) and autistic spectrum characteristics. As children move into puberty, mood disorders such as anxiety, depression, obsessive compulsive disorders, eating disorders and psychotic disorders become more common. The highest burden of mental ill health falls upon the 16- to 24-year-old group. For this reason, people responsible for planning and designing mental health services are now being asked to think about services specifically for 14- to 25-year-olds. There is evidence to suggest that rates of self-harm are increasing in the UK (Morgan et al., 2017). Although self-harm is not a mental illness in itself, it is for some young people linked to suicidality, and can be an indicator of untreated anxiety or depression, or undisclosed safeguarding issues.

Not surprisingly, rates of mental ill-health are higher still in young people who belong to vulnerable groups. Young people involved in gangs face particularly high rates of mental illness. Up to 52% of children who witness domestic abuse experience behavioural problems and issues with social development and relationships. It is estimated that 45% of looked after children have a diagnosable mental disorder (compared to 10% of all children). This can be understood in terms of the impact that multiple or chronic adverse childhood experiences, including attachment and carer relationship problems have on mental well-being (DHSC and DE, 2017). These difficulties are sometimes referred to as developmental trauma or complex trauma, and there is an increasing understanding of the relationship between experiencing complex trauma in childhood and receiving a diagnosis of personality disorder in adulthood (Lamb et al., 2018).

Understanding What Children and Young People Want From Services

When asked what they want, each time the feedback is similar: young people want more say and more prominent involvement in decisions about their care and better explanations about procures, treatments, risks and benefits. To help with this there are a range of government approved resources you can access.

Young minds have developed a site to help young people understand common conditions and medical treatments available: https://www.headmeds.org.uk/.

Young minds general website has lots of resources for children, young people and parents to help them understand common mental health issues, how to access help and how to advocate for their needs when talking to professionals: https://youngminds.org.uk/.

The government has also funded a free to access training and education hub for parents and carers and all professionals working with children, to help them understand issues relating to child emotional health and well-being: https://www.minded.org.uk/.

Identified barriers to young people effectively using services include:
- lack of information;
- management of confidential issues;
- lack of expertise and continuity of care;
- failure to respect the validity of the young person's views;
- being cared for alongside younger children or with a population they regard as elderly;
- particular issues of access to services, disability, poverty, ethnicity, being looked after (in care) and sexual orientation (Royal College of Paediatrics and Child Health [RCPCH], 2003).

A consistent concern of young people is that they are not really listened to or taken seriously. There is a need for respect, a word that has strong currency with young people – particularly the idea of being disrespectful. Respect is related to the young person feeling empowered in the relationship, being listened to and what they say being acted upon if appropriate (Ahmad et al., 2003).

Although some of these studies were undertaken 10–15 years ago, more recent studies and surveys show that little has changed (Coyne et al., 2015).

As a starting point, we must be able to work with the young person within the context of their developmental stage, that is, in terms of their transition and what matters most to that individual right now: assessing the issues and the relationships that are in focus currently. A second important consideration might be the beliefs we bring to this relationship.

What are our thoughts and feelings about adolescents generally and this young person in particular? When we are thinking about the young person, we need to place them within the context of family and peers. Lastly, there is a need for an understanding of the nature of their condition and its unique interaction with their personhood.

Young people have identified certain key characteristics in adults who are approachable. The approachable adult:
- is welcoming, and so makes the young person feel comfortable;
- is interested in the young patient as a person, not just in the illness;
- explains things in a straightforward way;
- can help the young person express their opinions;
- will not patronise or judge the young person, but will take them seriously;
- will take forward issues raised, with the relevant staff;
- will mediate where there is conflict between patients and staff (Lightfoot and Slooper, 2003).

Young people can define their sense of well-being in terms of a continuum where feeling good and getting stressed are polarities of experience. Significant factors contributing to feelings of emotional well-being included: having people to talk to, personal achievement, being praised and generally feeling positive about oneself. Relationships with family or peers could contribute either positively or negatively to the sense of well-being (Ahmad, 2003).

Research into the experience of child and young people who use health services (Layard and Dunn, 2009) indicated that service users had the following expectations of staff who came in contact with them:
- A clear understanding of child development and mental health.
- An ability to actively promote mental health and psychological well-being.
- The use of language and communication that young people and their families understand.
- An ability to identify the mental health needs of young people early and direct them towards appropriate support services.

Some of the identified barriers to effective intervention included:
- The use of overcomplicated terminology and unclear interpretations.
- The presence of stigma around mental health problems and those seeking services.
- Mismatched expectations between young people and families and service providers.

Nurses often think they do not have the skills to work with young people with mental health problems or indeed any adolescents (Fisher and Foster, 2016). There is sometimes confusion about what the task is. Clearly it is not therapy or counselling – that is for skilled therapists. However, there is a duty to promote health (physical and mental) by enhancing protective factors and intervening to reduce health risk behaviours. The therapeutic relationship the nurse enacts with the young person is the key intervention strategy.

Furthermore, children's nurses are already well acquainted with developmental stages, so extending this concept into adolescence should not mean further extensive training. While it is totally appropriate for children's nurses to be supported by adolescent health/mental health specialists, it is also suggested that children's nurses can and should develop a therapeutic style that does allow meaningful engagement, but that is not specialist or a specific therapy.

THE ROLE OF CHILDREN'S NURSES IN HELPING SPECIFIC GROUPS OF YOUNG PEOPLE

Long-Term Conditions With Co-Existing Mental Health Needs
Why
* Contribution to reducing the number of youngsters who are not getting the specialist help they deserve.
* Mental distress actively disrupts recovery and self-management of asthma, diabetes, epilepsy, cystic fibrosis and cardiovascular problems in children.

Task
* Triage assessment, early identification and early help to avoid onset of more severe mental health problems, forging of therapeutic relationships and using these to help young people with positive self-management of their condition.

Self-Harm and Suicide
Why
* To provide a 24-hour cool down period in a safe place, to ensure accurate assessment of the young person's intent, needs and risks.
* To provide an essential place of safety in which safeguarding issues can be explored.
* To provide a non-harmful holding space while underlying function and causes of self-harm are established, in order to identify the correct care pathway for the young person (NICE, 2004, 2011).

Because it is a chance we may not get again – it is estimated that only about 13% of children who self-harm access health care services, and so every time we meet a young person in an acute setting it is a chance to intervene to try and ensure that they do not feel that they need to hurt themselves again.

Tasks
Know that:
* You never increase the risk of suicide by talking to children about it.
* Self-harm without suicidal intent is just as serious as with suicidal intent.
* The level of physical injury/risk is not a measure of severity of mental distress or risk, you can only find this out by talking to a young person.
* Children in distress are much less interested in seeking the attention of adults than you might think.

Express curiosity and a desire to understand the young person – it is known to reduce risk of repeated self-harm.

Be mindful that risk factors for young people may seem small to you, but are their whole world (e.g. bullying, relationships, school and family stress).

Be alert to potential for safeguarding concerns and understand your local safeguarding procedures.

Ensure issues of confidentiality, consent, and competence are included in your assessment/admission processes – young people need to feel in control and informed if they are going to confide in you about the underlying causes of their difficulties.

Triaging Children and Young People Who Present With Self-Harm and Suicidal Behaviours
The following questions have been devised to help non-mental health specialists undertake a screening assessment with young people, to help them think with the young person about next steps:
* **Meaning.** Can you help me understand the reasons or feelings that have led you to hurt yourself?
* **Intent to die.** Sometimes when people hurt themselves, they also have thoughts of wanting to end their life, have you ever experienced this? (don't be afraid to ask more detail about this if the person says yes).
* **Wider problems.** Are you having any problems in:
  - School life? Family life? With friends or other relationships?
* **Safeguarding.** Has/is anything unwanted, frightening or harmful been happening to you?
* **Mental health.** Look out for/ask about feelings of hopelessness, loss of enjoyment, repetitive, intrusive or disturbing worries – these can be indicators of anxiety and depression.
* **Internal triggers.** Be curious about the way the young person feels about themselves.
* **Resilience and self-help.** Ask questions about strengths and usual ways of coping.
* **Collaboration.** What do you think might help/we should do next? (Foster et al., 2016).

Disordered Eating
Why
* Low weight closes down thinking and the possibility of psychological treatment – physical risks must be addressed first.
* Raising a young person's body mass index (BMI) above 15 is essential for psychological shifts to occur in the young person's thinking that will enable recovery.
* Helping children start to eat again after a long period of calorie restriction or an acute period of fasting comes with significant physical risks, known as re-feeding syndrome, and they need to be in a place that can effectively monitor and address these risks.

Task
* Emotional containment and physical safety – enables positive risk-taking, safe re-feeding and engagement with other services, all of which are essential to recovery.

Remain in touch with realistic 'worry' for young person about their physical health status, at times when they are not able to, because restricting their diet feels essential to managing their emotional distress.

Maintain clear boundaries to keep children safe, but be open to limited negotiation, to help them maintain a sense of agency, dignity and hope.

Disentangle and separate the care challenges that the eating disorder symptoms bring from the child, so that the child is not subject to communication of our frustrations with the illness.

Maintenance of curiosity and hopefulness, to set the tone in which a young person can begin to think about the reasons why they might be struggling so much with maintaining a safe diet (Foster and Benson, 2016).

Medically Unexplained Symptoms
Why

- Because, if you were a parent who thought your child was physically unwell, where else would you go?
- Symptoms are often unconscious expression of undisclosed trauma, or unspeakable experiences and secrets.
- Feeling taken care of in the physical arena is an essential prerequisite to children and families making use of mental health services – they need to know that worries about physical ill health are not being dismissed.

Tasks

- Importance of accepting that all symptoms are real, even if you are sure that they are not due to an underlying pathophysiology (consider how often you have experienced a very painful headache that has not been due to any illness, but has needed rest and pain relief?).
- Never discount physical or psychological causes – 30% of unexplained symptoms have a physical cause.
- Using 'and' rather than 'either/or' explanations to avoid splitting body and mind. For example, 'I can hear that you are experiencing terrible pain and it is very worrying for you. Although we are confident that you are safe, we also know that to be in pain is very stressful, so we want to keep reviewing your physical health and also give you some help to understand and cope with the pain.'
- Promoting joined-up, working with other agencies, including mental health services. This includes *not* discharging patients as soon as they are offered a mental health service appointment. Families should not feel that they have to choose between good physical health care and good mental health care.

USING CORE INTERPERSONAL NURSING SKILLS TO SUPPORT CHILDREN AND YOUNG PEOPLE EXPERIENCING MENTAL DISTRESS

Observation Skills

Observation skills are a core component of all children nurse's skills. Within a paediatric medical setting, patients mainly attend with a problem/illness that has a clear presentation requiring specific tasks to be performed (Kraemer, 2010). A paediatric nursing approach will usually identify an illness and treatment based on patient presentation/symptoms, collected via physiological observation and history taking, more often than from interpersonal engagement. Frameworks such as the A–E framework are often used to help structure this process (Thim et al., 2012). When working with children whose primary problem is psychological, the answer is largely one from interpersonal engagement. This has been identified as potentially difficult for children's nurses who do not always possess the same level of confidence in their interpersonal engagement skills. One way of rethinking this concern is to understand that observation skills are just as key to assessing and understanding a young person's emotional health needs. However, instead of establishing physical proximity to take physiological observations, you are working to establish a relational proximity (Ranahan, 2014), in which you can observe and learn something about how the young person sees themselves, others and the world around them.

To illustrate this Table 41.2 outlines a possible alternative A–E framework to consider when caring for child or young person with emotional or mental health needs.

Using details and observation skills can also help to identify the underlying cause of a particularly challenging or risky behaviour, which in turn can help you to identify actions to help address the problem. Children and young people's behaviour always has a function, no matter how maladaptive or extreme it may appear, and even if seems to be doing the opposite of what the young person intended it to do.

Challenging behaviours can commonly be a way of defending against pain and vulnerability; distraction from unbearable feelings/states of mind; a concrete physical expression of something that cannot be said; an indirect way of communicating (e.g. giving us a 'taste' of what it feels like); an attempt to solve a problem; a way of gaining physical relief from emotional distress; or to regain a sense of control or to enlist our help.

TABLE 41.2	**Observe, Notice, Ask About and Record**	
	Standard A–E Framework for Top-to-Toe Assessment	**Framework for Observation of Emotional Health**
A	Airway	**Affect** (feelings) – the young person and yours
B	Breathing	**Behaviour** (what? why? consequences?)
C	Circulation	**Cognitions** (thoughts about self, other, world) **Context** (family, friends, school)
D	Disability	**Don't be afraid to ask** about unwanted frightening experiences
E	Exposure	**Exposure to life events** and risk factors

Therapeutic Style

Nurses need to find a way of interacting that is more than 'having a chat' or the collecting of information for assessment, but does not go as far as 'doing therapy'. Cooper and Glasper (2001, p 35) described this process as a 'therapeutic encounter', a dynamic and sensitive interaction between what is known (professional knowledge) and what is 'yet to be known' (the young person's story).

Two key elements to the therapeutic encounter are identified:

1. The nurse's ability to have an internal ongoing reflective conversation (reflection in action).
2. The interaction is influenced by the belief systems of the nurse and the 'tribal stories' present in their working environment.

The reflective conversation will be monitoring the potential impact of the nurse's personal beliefs and the collective 'tribal stories' on the relationship they are forming with the young person. In Cooper and Glasper's (2001) paper they gave an example of extracts from tribal stories related to young people who self-harm. Although this paper is 17 years old, a recent study investigating the perceptions of children's nurses regarding looking after children who self-harm, found evidence of exactly the same tribal stories being repeated (Fisher and Foster, 2016):

'Working with young people who self-harm often feels like it is a waste of time.' 'Our skills could be better used looking after someone who has a "real illness".' 'We are very busy here; there is not the time to give these people what they need.' 'They should be looked after somewhere else; this is not the place for them.'

'The kind of care required is not what we are trained in – we may say the wrong thing and trouble their mind further.' 'We came into nursing to look after people with real illnesses, these young people disrupt ward…upset other poorly children.' 'Anyway, even if we had the time what could we say? They are difficult to communicate with …. physically aggressive towards staff …'

An example of a reflective 'self-conversation' when confronted by a young person who is rejecting care, swearing and being abusive might be:

Initial thoughts: *I find adolescents difficult when they are like this. They are so self-centred. I am having a hard shift. I don't need this. What about the other children and parents? They don't deserve this either.***Initial formulation**: *This young person needs to be told what the limits are.*

This preliminary assessment is likely to be reinforced by the tribal story (collective staff belief) that this young person is disruptive and either needs 'sorting out' or shouldn't be there in the first place. There is a tendency to see adolescents as being disruptive in an environment aimed at younger children (Foster, 2009). These collective beliefs might reflect the difficulty nurses have in finding the appropriate way to relate to these young people. Further reinforcement for this formulation might come from other parents and children's disapproval of the young person's behaviour. Another thing that might support this initial position is that, as a principle, it is good to set boundaries. The issue here, however, is the timing of such an intervention and whether it will inflame or calm the situation. The nurse needs to hold back the response and ask:

Reflective question: What else should I be paying attention to in this situation?

The first internal conversation is focused primarily on the nurse. There is a need to re-focus on the young person and to try and assess what is motivating their behaviour by exploring the following issues:

- What is the young person's underlying emotional state?
- What do they need?
- Are they trying to assert themselves?
- Are they feeling vulnerable and dependent, not grown-up?
- Are they fearful for the future?
- How is the young person viewing me, my approach, and my non-verbal communication?

This should lead to a reformulation:

Reformulation – new hypothesis: This young person is scared. They are going for surgery tomorrow and want help but are fearful about appearing childlike. They are probably angry about being ill, being with little children, and are not sure if we can be trusted. This uncertainty might be influenced by their previous attachment history and how reliable adults have been in the past. Have they had a secure base in times of trouble? Other factors influencing their behaviour will be their level of self-esteem and feelings of self-efficacy.

Specific Core Communication Skills

Key communication skills make it more likely that the nurse will arrive at this more sensitive formulation. One of the key qualities central to all therapeutic communication is the ability to truly 'attend' to the other person. This is referred to as giving 'free attention'; it is the essential precursor of a second important quality 'active listening' (Egan, 2013).

Free Attention

Heron (2001) describes giving free attention as:

A subtle and intense activity of being present for the client; it involves gaze, posture, facial expression, maybe touch. It has the qualities of:

- being supportive: out there with the client
- being expectant: waiting for the human being to emerge in ways that are meaningful to them and their fulfilment
- being non-anxious: the practitioner is free of claims and demands, of any harrying attitude towards the client. It is always wider and deeper than the qualities of the client's speech, being attuned to his emerging potential, as well as his actual behaviour.

Egan (2013) identifies the following questions that nurses should ask when 'attending' a client:

- What are my attitudes towards this client?
- How would I rate the quality of my presence to the client?

- To what degree does my non-verbal behaviour indicate a willingness to work with the client?
- What attitudes am I expressing in my non-verbal behaviour?
- What attitudes am I expressing in my verbal behaviour?
- To what degree does my non-verbal behaviour reinforce my internal attitudes?
- In what ways am I distracted from giving my full attention to this client?
- What am I doing to handle these distractions?
- How might I be more effectively present for this person?

One of the tribal stories that have a basis in fact is that of the 'busy nurse'. It is certainly true that there are many demands on a nurse's time. Student nurses will often prefer to be busy because then they feel more 'nurse-like'. So 'attending' is a skill that requires some practice, and more significantly, a belief that it is an important thing to do. However, once the skill is acquired it takes up far less time than might be at first imagined.

Active Listening

The second core skill is active listening. Egan (2013) suggests that listening carefully to what the client has to say seems '… To be a concept so simple to grasp and so easy to do that one may wonder why it is given such explicit treatment here.'

He suggests that it is amazing how often people fail to listen to one another. Certainly young people often complain that they are not being listened to. Complete active listening involves four things:

1. Observing and reading the client's non-verbal behaviour: posture, facial expressions, movement, tone of voice, etc.
2. Listening to and understanding the client's verbal messages.
3. Listening to the whole person in the context of the social settings of life.
4. Tough-minded listening.

Points 1 and 2 can be understood from our life experience, but it might be helpful to enlarge on what Egan means by items 3 and 4.

He refers to a 'people in systems' framework, which is the need to understand each client not just in terms of a specific illness or problem, but also with careful attention to their life setting, personal values, and biological and sociopsychological characteristics.

Tough-minded listening is about accepting that the client's feelings and visions of themselves, others and the world are real and need to be understood. However, clients' perceptions of themselves and their worlds are sometimes distorted. This does not mean that helpers challenge clients as soon as they hear any kind of distortion. Rather, they note gaps and distortions and challenge them if and when it is appropriate to do so.

Egan (2013) identifies obstacles to listening and understanding clients:

- Inadequate listening: distracted, not giving our full attention.
- Evaluative listening: judging the merits of what is being said, comparing it to our own value system.

- Filtered listening: it is impossible to listen to others in an unbiased way; therefore the more self-knowledge we have the more we will recognise our particular filters.
- Knowledge as a filter, especially professional knowledge: we might be listening to validate a theory, maybe a diagnosis, rather than listening to the person. Children and young people are particularly at risk of being on the end of this as we tend to always view young people's experience through an adult lens (Liebel, 2014).
- Fact-centred rather than person-centred listening: some assessment strategies might put us into a fact-centred approach.

Attending and active listening are the key vehicles for conveying respect to others. Studies show that young people work best with professionals who convey respect for them (Ahmad et al., 2003).

The Importance of Listening to the Story

Narrative theory is based on the supposition that in large measure, people are the stories they tell themselves and that are told about them. Narratives can occur at different levels of social functioning. There are social and cultural narratives, interpersonal narratives and intrapersonal narratives. The narrative approach rests on the assumption that narratives are not representations of reflections of identities, lives and problems. Rather, narratives constitute or 'shape-up' identities, lives and problems. According to this position, the process of therapeutic re-authoring of personal narratives changes lives, problems and identities because personal narratives are constitutive of identity (Carr, 2016). In short, this approach suggests we are the stories we tell about ourselves and are told about us. Further, our stories are embedded in and influenced by a wider social and cultural context.

Such an approach can have a number of implications for nursing practice. Within the context of these ideas we can explore nursing in terms of dominant discourses or stories. A discourse is a dominant social and cultural story that can set the context in which an interaction takes place. Such discourse might relate to ideas as nursing, professionalism education, ethics and so on (Carr, 2016).

If the assessment process reflected narrative theory, the approach would first seek the meaning the young person and their family gives to the events, rather than a professional system that seeks to impose meaning and explain behaviour.

👤 ACTIVITY: REFLECT ON YOUR PRACTICE

How much is the nursing task to explain, to inform, to understand, or to help the young person, make sense of things?

Implications for the Health Care Professional

Nurses, when faced with the complex lives and backgrounds of young people with emotional disturbances, often feel powerless and think the situation is hopeless. Young people who come in with a history of repeated self-harm often provoke these feelings, accompanied sometimes by a degree of resentment. This may occur because the nurses fail to understand what the therapeutic task is. Clearly a life that has become so complex is hardly going to be turned around by an inpatient stay on a children's ward.

What we do know is that if the nurse can offer a secure, accepting base to the young person, this is a positive experience. The other main therapeutic strategy is to listen non-judgmentally and with care and compassion to the young person's unfolding story. This may not seem very active, but it could be life enhancing and possibly life saving for the young person.

One of the key ideas of narrative theory is the notion of 'repositioning', that is, taking up a different position in relation to the young person and or the problem. When we interact with young people and their families we are heavily influenced by a number of professional, personal and cultural discourses (tribal stories) (Glasper and Cooper, 2001). This can become problematic because instead of listening with a detached curiosity to what is being said – and through that process, really hearing the young person's story – their story can become 'entombed' with the professional narratives and belief systems. The client is then asked to enact a story told about them rather than their own story. To break out of our professional constructions and to reposition, it may be necessary to make an imaginative leap. We need to 'actively listen' in Egan's (2013) terms, repositioning ourselves so that we don't allow our professional knowledge and/or personal prejudices to interfere with the flow of the young person's story.

Helping the Story Unfold

Wilkes and Belsher (1994) offer some key principles for working with adolescents. Although they were considering the work in terms of cognitive therapy, the principles can translate as general principles for working with young people.

Acknowledge the adolescent's narcissism. Narcissism refers to the tendency of adolescent patients to be somewhat egocentric in their interests and goals. This tendency should be seen as developmentally appropriate and can be used to develop the therapeutic relationship. Rather than using statements, questions can often be a good way of demonstrating we are listening. For example, 'Would it be right to say you think …?' acknowledges the young person as the best judge of their own views and will reinforce the feeling that they are being listened to. Unless there is a specific need for them, avoid levelling comments such as 'I have heard that before' or 'You're not the only one that feels like that'. In short, the young person needs to feel at the centre of their world, so it makes sense to start the therapeutic process from where they actually are. Another way nurses can affirm the adolescent's self-importance is to offer choices every time it is possible to do so.

Collaborative empiricism. This is a central tenet of the cognitive therapy approach but again it can be adapted to general communication with adolescents.

To collaborate is to join with, to cooperate with in order to work something out together, and this is a particularly useful position to take up with the young person (Roberts et al., 2015). The nature of the nurse's specialist knowledge, life experience and health may lead the young person to feel in a one-down, less powerful position. Such a position would leave the young person very sensitive to the feeling of being patronised and more likely to want to assert themselves by being conflictual and oppositional, or through passivity and withdrawal. Another way that demonstrates collaboration is to be a voice for the young person; this links with young people's view that an approachable adult will take things forward on their behalf (Lightfoot and Slooper, 2003).

Empiricism means giving value to factual data and evidence. To excessively confront or challenge the evidence for the position the young person holds would be very unhelpful and lead to resistance and conflict; it would be an inappropriate form of Egan's tough listening. However, a genuine desire to see things from the young person's perspective by checking out the evidence they have for taking up their present position will demonstrate respect and help the young person's story become more coherent.

Adopt an objective stance. This means having the capacity of being able to be somewhat removed from the intricacies of the young person's situation. This is different from being disinterested or defensively detached from the situation. Objectivity is an important factor in all helping relationships, but it is – perhaps – sometimes harder to maintain with young people. Their high levels of emotionality and tendency to see things in black and white terms can draw nurses into a parental role or encourage them to over identify with the young person and into collusion. One of the ways to maintain a helpful objective stance is not to be drawn into the role of problem solver, but rather to act as a facilitator of the young person's problem-solving skills. Collaborative empiricism can help objectivity in that both parties are working together to find the evidence necessary to support whatever is being explored, therefore neither should need an emotional investment in a particular position or belief. These positions or beliefs stand or fall on the basis of the evidence there is to support them.

Include members of the social system. This links with Egan's (2013) reminder that active listening involves listening to the person within the context of his or her social system. Young people are rarely in a position to make important decisions without reference to their parents and other adults in positions of authority. Furthermore, their parents and peer group have a powerful effect on how they see themselves, and as such, can be helpful or unhelpful in terms of the young person's self-esteem (Patton et al., 2016).

Chase the affect. To chase the affect is to pay particular attention to expressions and changes in emotional state. This means being sensitive to the verbal and non-verbal cues the young person gives and following them up: 'You seem to be thinking about something that has made you sad'. Such attention to the emotional expression is likely to convey empathy and a more accurate assessment of the overall situation leading to the most therapeutic response.

Socratic questioning. This style of questioning and exploration aims to promote curiosity and support the young person to think about what he or she is saying and feeling, in order to develop self-knowledge. It is based on the understanding that learning is most effective when we are supported to come to arrive at our own conclusions, rather than being told (McLachlan et al., 2016). Again, any challenge to the young person's beliefs and assumptions must be made in a sensitive manner of genuine enquiry. The nurse must seek to understand the young person's world and thus help the young person become clearer about things. An example might be: 'When the doctor was talking to your parents about your illness what were you thinking?' or 'What did you feel like doing at that moment?'

Model for the adolescent. This should be a subtle process in the relationship whereby the nurse models aspects of the behaviour that will be helpful. For example, a nurse who wants to help the young person be more tolerant of younger children in the environment will model tolerance towards the young person. This can also include giving a commentary on one's own thinking, to help make it visible to the young person, so that they can see how problems can be solved and decisions arrived at, in a calm and logical way.

THE THERAPEUTIC RELATIONSHIP

The therapeutic relationship is grounded in an interpersonal process that occurs between the nurse and the young person. It is a purposeful, goal-directed relationship aimed at advancing the best interests of the client. The way we help (our style) seems to be at least if not more important than how we help (the model or theoretical approach we use). Research from nursing and psychotherapy suggests the therapeutic relationship to be the variable most highly correlated with positive outcome. The qualities of the therapeutic relationship include active listening, trust, respect, genuineness, empathy and responding to client concerns. The requisite capacities for establishing a therapeutic relationship with children and their families have been identified and defined as self-awareness, self-knowledge, empathy, the ability to collaborate and place families in the centre of decision making and awareness of boundaries and limits of the professional role (Roberts et al., 2015).

Requisite Capacities for Establishing Therapeutic Relationships

Self-Awareness

Self-awareness is the ability to reflect on one's subjective thoughts, feelings and actions. Thus, to be aware of any attitude being conveyed that could impede the therapeutic process and would react to counteract any potential negative effect on the client.

Self-Knowledge

With the development of self-knowledge, nurses are able to recognise that their own experience is shaped by nationality, race, culture, health, socioeconomic conditions, gender, education, early childhood experiences and development, as well as relationships, accomplishments, beliefs, issues and concerns. By gaining self-knowledge nurses are able to differentiate between their own experience and values and those of the client. In this way they are able to appreciate the unique perspective of the client (their story), are able to avoid burdening the client with their own issues and can prevent superimposing their own beliefs and preferred solutions on the client.

Empathy

Empathy is the ability of nurses to enter into the client's relational world, to see and feel the world as the client sees and feels it, and to explore the meaning it has for the client. Empathy involves nurses being able to attend to the subjective experience of the client and validate that their understanding is an accurate reflection of the client's experience. Understanding of the developmental tasks and experience of adolescence outlined earlier in the chapter is essential to this process.

Awareness of Boundaries and Limits of the Professional Role

Boundaries define the limits of the professional role. Nurses are obligated to place the client's needs before their own needs. Through self-awareness, nurses reflect on whether their actions are in the client's best interests. The supervision process should also be used to explore these issues. Sometimes our own conscious or unconscious wishes make it hard to recognise boundary violations. Indications that boundaries may have been crossed include having special patients, spending extra time with patients, keeping secrets with clients and doing activities with clients that you do not share with colleagues.

The Sequence of Events in the Relationship

For the sake of analysis, the therapeutic relationship can be seen in terms of a beginning, middle and end, although all three stages may occur in a single encounter. The beginning can be seen as the process of engagement, formulating the working alliance. The middle is the working phase during which how the work is structured is important. The end can be seen as the disengagement phase or letting go.

In her nursing model, Peplau (1952) describes three phases to the therapeutic relationship: orientation, working and resolution. In the beginning, both the nurse and the young person are strangers, each coming to the relationship with their own preconceptions of what to expect. These preconceptions will be based on their previous relationships, experiences, attitudes and beliefs. Peplau (1952) refers to the nurse and the client as being 'strangers' in this pre-orientation stage.

The Orientation Stage

In the orientation phase the parameters of the relationship are being established. The expectations of the young person and the nurse need to be explored and clarified. Consistency and listening are considered by clients to be critical at the beginning of a relationship. In this beginning stage, acceptance of the young person is important for the evolving relationship. Egan (2013) refers to this stage as 'The Present Scenario: helping the client identify, explore and clarify their problem situations and unused opportunities'. Egan suggests that people can neither manage problem situations nor develop opportunities unless they identify and understand them.

The Working Phase

As the name suggests, this is the active phase where problems are identified, and interventions decided on.

How this is structured will depend on the helping model used, although the nurse should be involved in some key communication strategies. One of the common mistakes when working with distressed young people who are expressing negative or aggressive thoughts is to try to move them on to a more positive frame or want to offer alternative more constructive positions. Although this aim is laudable in itself, the motivation is often to make the nurse feel more comfortable. Even if it is client focused, the timing is often wrong. One of the most important strategies, particularly with young people, is to validate the young person's thoughts, feelings and distress. This is not to collude with what in some cases might be a very distorted position (e.g. the anorexic stance), but to accept the young person's perspective and the distress caused by it. This working phase needs to be collaborative, led by the young person and facilitated by the nurse. The nurse needs to be the young person's advocate, ensuring that their views are considered in the overall care strategies. In Egan's model this is the preferred scenario (Stage 2): Helping clients develop goals, objectives, or agendas based on an action-oriented understanding of the problem situation. Once clients understand either their problem situations or opportunities for development more clearly, they may need help in determining what they would like to do differently. What things would look like if they were better than they are now? – The 'Getting there' stage (Egan, 2013).

The Resolution Phase

This final stage of the relationship is involved in completion of the relationship and endings. The process of ending is as important as the beginning but tends not to receive the same attention. It needs to be planned, talked about and should have been considered during the initial care planning: planning how and when the relationship should end. This is particularly important if the young person has a history of troubled or unreliable relationships. The nurse needs to be mindful of the experience of loss transition and change and the reactions of resistance, denial and ambivalence. While acknowledging the present, it may be helpful to be future orientated validating the young person's future plans.

 ACTIVITY

You might consider reading the chapter 'The overview of the model' in Egan (2013) 'The skilled helper' and judge how useful it could be for your nursing practice.

Integrating Understanding of Positive Characteristics of Attachment Relationships Into the Therapeutic Relationship

Earlier parts of this chapter have focused in detail on an understanding of child and adolescent development, and the role of primary carers and attachment figures in supporting the process of psychological development. This is because using the context of a therapeutic relationship to provide the characteristics of helpful attachment figures for the period in which the young person in our care, is a central part of how nurses can support the ongoing emotional health and well-being of children and young people. As the paediatrician Donald Winnicott (1971) observed, professional helping relationships of any kind are always a complex derivative of the primary carer's face.

The principle functions of any attachment figure are to provide a secure base and to modulate anxiety (Bowlby, 1988). In a professional helping situation both functions are simulated through active and reciprocal interactional process to which both the helper and the person help contribute. By providing information and consistent input anxiety can be contained and trust can be built. At a conscious level, empathic listening may be experienced as soothing and comforting. In ordinary circumstances of child development, attuned and empathic listening, in which the carer 'literally feels themselves in to the infant's place' is the foundation 'the holding environment'. The holding environment denotes not just the physical holding of the baby by the primary carer, but the entire psychophysiological system of protection, support, caring and containing that envelops the child, without which it would not survive physically or emotionally (Winnicott, 1971). In the context of acute physical and mental distress, the strength of parallel between this and the provision of good-enough nursing care within a paediatric environment, for both the child and the parent, cannot be overstated.

SUMMARY

- There is strong and growing evidence for the fundamental interrelationship between physical, mental and social health. Problems in adolescence in any of these areas indicate the likelihood of long-term adverse health and social consequences.
- Everyone in contact with young people should take the symptoms of emotional distress, behavioural difficulties and hyperactivity seriously, as they impair function and development and are unlikely to be transient, without help.
- It is imperative to the promotion of child and adolescent health that nurses develop the skills that will enable them to successfully engage with the young person and ensure a nursing interaction that is rewarding both for the young person and the nurse.
- An understanding of the adolescent's developmental tasks will allow you to focus caregiving in the most effective manner.
- Embrace the care of children in mental distress as a core part of your role.
- Know that in doing so you will probably save a young person's life.
- Remember that most mental distress, no matter how challenging, can be understood and is often related to adverse or stressful life events.

- See *all* behaviour as the fabulous gift of information that it is – just waiting for someone like you to decode it.
- Read up and skill up on triage assessment of mental distress in children, including understanding of risk factors.
- Find tools and resources to help you (make a note of the ones included in this chapter).
- Helping relationships are not just good for soothing the anxiety of children. Take time to build professional relationships with practitioners in local Children and Young People Mental Health Services.
- Be kind, brave, curious, observant, acceptant, and above all hopeful.
- Remember that small actions all add up to make a difference.

REFERENCES

Adshead, G., 2002. Three degrees of security: attachment and forensic institutions. Crim. Behav. Men. Health 12 (S2), S31–S45.

Ahmad, Y., Dalrymple, J., Daum, M., et al., 2003. Listening to Children and Young People. Faculty of Health and Social Care, University of the West of England, Bristol.

Baltag, V., Sawyer, S.M., 2016. Quality healthcare for adolescents. In: Cherry, A.L., Baltag, V., Dillon, M.E. (Eds.), International Handbook on Adolescent Health and Development. The Public Health Response. Springer International Publishing, Switzerland.

Bennett, S., Shafran, R., Coughtrey, A., et al., 2015. Psychological interventions for mental health disorders in children with chronic physical illness: a systematic review. Arch. Dis. Child. 100 (4), 308–316.

Best, P., Manktelow, R., Taylor, B., 2014. Online communication, social media and adolescent wellbeing: a systematic narrative review. Child. Youth. Ser. Rev. 41, 27–36.

Bock, J., Wainstock, T., Braun, K., et al., 2015. Stress in utero: prenatal programming of brain plasticity and cognition. Biol. Psychiatry 78 (5), 315–326.

Bowlby, J., 1988. A Secure Base: Clinical Applications of Attachment Theory. Routledge, London.

British Medical Association (BMA), 2003. Adolescent Health. BMA Publishing, London.

Burt, M.R., 2002. Reasons to invest in adolescents. J. Adolesc. Health 31 (Suppl. 6), 136–152. Online. Available from: http://www.sciencedirect.com.

Burton, M., 2014. Children and young people's mental health. In: Burton, M., Pavord, E., Williams, B. (Eds.), An Introduction to Child and Adolescent Mental Health. Sage Publishing. London.

Cabaj, J.L., McDonald, S.W., Tough, S.C., 2014. Early childhood risk and resilience factors for behavioural and emotional problems in middle childhood. BMC Pediatr. 14 (1), 166.

Care Quality Commission (CQC), 2017. Review of children and young people's mental health services: phase one report. Available from: https://www.cqc.org.uk/sites/default/files/20171103_cypmhphase1_report.pdf.

Carr, A., 2016. Narratives of hope. In: Vetere, A., Dowling, E. (Eds.), Narrative Therapies With Children and Their Families: A Practitioner's Guide to Concepts and Approaches, second ed. Taylor & Francis, London.

Children Act, 2004. UK https://www.legislation.gov.uk/ukpga/2004/31/contents.

Coleman, J., 2011. The Nature of Adolescence. Routledge.

Collishaw, S., Hammerton, G., Mahedy, L., et al., 2015. Mental health resilience in the adolescent offspring of parents with depression: a prospective longitudinal study. Lancet Psychiatry 3 (1), 49–57.

Cooper, M., Glasper, E., 2001. Deliberate self-harm in children: the nurse's therapeutic style. Br. J. Nurs. 10 (1), 34–40.

Copeland, W.E., Wolke, D., Angold, A., et al., 2013. Adult psychiatric outcomes of bullying and being bullied by peers in childhood and adolescence. JAMA Psychiatry 70 (4), 419–426.

Coyne, I., McNamara, N., Healy, M., et al., 2015. Adolescents' and parents' views of child and adolescent mental health services (CAMHS) in Ireland. J. Psychiatr. Ment. Health Nurs. 22 (8), 561–569.

Das, J.K., Salam, R.A., Lassi, Z.S., et al., 2016. Interventions for adolescent mental health: an overview of systematic reviews. J. Adolesc. Health 59 (4), S49–S60.

Deighton, J., Lereya, S.T., Patalay, P., et al., 2018. Mental Health Problems in Young People, Aged 11 to 14: Results from the First HeadStart Annual Survey of 30,000 Children. CAMHS Press, London.

Department of Health (DoH), 2004. National Service Framework for Children, Young People, and Maternity Services. HMSO, London.

Department of Health (DoH), 2008. Children and young people in mind: the final report of the CAMHS review. Available from: http://webarchive.nationalarchives.gov.uk/20120817174632/https://consumption.education.gov.uk/publications/standard/_arc_SOP/Page11/CAMHS-REPORT.

Department of Health (DoH), 2011. No health without mental health. Available from: https://www.gov.uk/government/publications/the-mental-health-strategy-for-england (accessed 31 October 2018).

Department of Health (DoH), 2015. Future in mind: promoting, protecting and improving our children and young people's mental health and well-being. Department for Education (DE) and NHS England. Available from: http://www.gov.uk/government/uploads/system/uploads/attachment_data/file/414024/Childrens_ Mental_Health.pdf.

Department of Health and Social Care (DHSC) and Department for Education (DE), 2017. Transforming children and young people's mental health provision: a green paper. Available from: https://www.gov.uk/government/consultations/transforming-children-and-young-peoples-mental-health-provision-a-green-paper.

Egan, G., 2013. The Skilled Helper: A Problem-Management and Opportunity-Development Approach to Helping. Cengage Learning. Belmont, CA. USA.

Erikson, E.H., 1963. Childhood and Society, second ed. Norton, New York.

Fisher, G., Foster, C., 2016. Examining the needs of paediatric nurses caring for children and young people presenting with self-harm/suicidal behaviour on general paediatric wards: findings from a small-scale study. Child. Care. Pract. 1–14. https://doi.org/10.1080/13575279.2015.1118013. Available from: http://usir.salford.ac.uk/id/eprint/36844.

Foster, C., 2009. Adolescents in acute mental distress on inpatient pediatric settings: reflections from a pediatric liaison practitioner. J. Child Adolesc. Psychiatr. Nurs. 22 (1), 16–22.

Foster, C., Benson, J., 2016. Emotional and mental health [part 6]. Case 2: a young woman with anorexia nervosa. In: Children's Nursing Case Book, Case Book Series. Open University Press, Berkshire.

Foster, C., Birch, L., Allen, S., et al., 2015. Enabling practitioners working with young people who self-harm. J. Men. Health Train. Edu. Pract. 10 (4), 268–280.

Gore, F.M., Bloem, P.J., Patton, G.C., et al., 2011. Global burden of disease in young people aged 10–24 years: a systematic analysis. Lancet 377 (9783), 2093–2102.

Hay, I., Ashman, A.F., 2003. The development of adolescents' emotional stability and general self-concept: the interplay of parent, peers, and gender. Int. J. Disabil. Develop. Educ. 50 (1), 77–91.

Heron, J., 2001. Helping the Client: A Creative Practical Guide, fifth ed. Sage Publications, London.

Hughes, K., Bellis, M.A., Hardcastle, K.A., et al., 2017. The effect of multiple adverse childhood experiences on health: a systematic review and meta-analysis. Lancet Public Health 2 (8), e356–e366.

Jacobs, M., 1998. The Presenting Past: The Core of Psychodynamic Counselling and Therapy. Open University Press. London.

Kessler, R.C., Berglund, P., Demler, O., et al., 2005. Lifetime prevalence and age-of-onset distributions of DSM-IV disorders in the national comorbidity survey replication. Arch. Gen. Psychiatry 62 (6), 593–602. https://doi.org/10.1001/archpsyc.62.6.593.

Kraemer, S., 2010. Liaison and cooperation between paediatrics and mental health. Paediatr. Child Health 20 (8), 382–387. https://doi.org/10.1111/j.1475-3588.2005.00373.x.

Lamb, N., Sibbald, S., Stirzaker, A., 2018. Shining lights in dark corners of people's lives: reaching consensus for people with complex mental health difficulties who are given a diagnosis of personality disorder. Crim. Behav. Ment. Health 28 (1), 1–4. https://doi.org/10.1002/cbm.2068.

Liebel, M., 2014. Adultism and age-based discrimination against children. In: Kutsar, D., Warming, H. (Eds.), Children and Non-Discrimination. Interdisciplinary Textbook. Children's Rights Erasmus Academic Network. University Press of Estonia, pp. 119–143.

Lightfoot, J., Slooper, P., 2003. Having a say in health: involving young people with a chronic illness or physical disability in local health services development. Child. Soc. 17 (4), 277–290.

Layard, R., Dunn, J., 2009. A Good Childhood: Searching for Values in a Competitive Age. The Children's Society, Penguin Books. London.

Maunder, R., Hunter, J., 2008. Attachment relationships as determinants of physical health. J. Am. Acad. Psychoanal. Dyn. Psychiatry 36, 11–32. Available from: https://doi.org/10.1521/jaap.2008.36.1.11.

McLachlan, N.H., Eastwood, L., Friedberg, R., 2016. Socratic questions with children: recommendations and cautionary tales. J. Cognitive Psychotherapy 30 (2), 105–119. https://doi.org/10.1891/0889-8391.30.2.105.

Morgan, C., Webb, R., Carr, M., et al., 2017. Incidence, clinical management, and mortality risk following self-harm among children and adolescents: cohort study in primary care. BMJ 359, 4351. Available from: http://www.bmj.com/content/359/bmj.j4351.

National Institute for Health and Care Excellence (NICE), 2004. The Short-Term Physical and Psychological Management and Secondary Prevention of Self-Harm in Primary and Secondary Care. NICE, London.

National Institute for Health and Care Excellence (NICE), 2011. Self Harm: Longer Term Management. NICE Clinical Guideline 133). NICE, London.

National Institute for Health and Care Excellence (NICE), 2017. Eating Disorders: Recognition and Treatment [NCG69]. NICE, London.

National Institute for Mental Health England (NIMHE), 2009. The Legal Aspects of the Care and Treatment of Children and Young People with Mental Disorder: A Guide for Professionals. NIMHE, London.

NHS, 2014. NHS five year forward view. Available from: https://www.england.nhs.uk/publication/nhs-five-year-forward-view/. (accessed 29 October 2018).

NHS Health Advisory Service, 1995. Together We Stand: The Commissioning, Role and Management of Child and Adolescent Mental Health Services. HMSO, London.

Office for National Statistics (ONS), 2014. Suicide in the United Kingdom, 2014 Registrations. Stat. Bullet. 2016, 1–33.

Patton, G.C., Sawyer, S.M., Santelli, J.S., et al., 2016. Our future: a Lancet commission on adolescent health and wellbeing. Lancet 387 (10036), 2423–2478.

Peplau, H.E., 1952. Interpersonal Relations in Nursing. Putnam, New York.

Pierce, M., Hardy, R., 2011. Commentary: the decreasing age of puberty–as much a psychosocial as biological problem? Int. J. Epidemiol. 41 (1), 300–302. Available from: https://doi.org/10.1093/ije/dyr227.

Pitchforth, J., Fahy, K., Ford, T., et al., 2018. Mental health and well-being trends among children and young people in the UK, 1995–2014: analysis of repeated cross-sectional national health surveys. Psychol. Med. 1–11.

Polmear, C., 2004. Dying to live: mourning, melancholia and the adolescent process. J. Child. Psychother. 30 (3), 263–274.

Public Health England, 2015. Promoting children and young people's emotional health and wellbeing – a whole school and college approach. Available from: https://www.gov.uk/government/uploads/system/uploads/attachment_data/file/414908/Final_EHWB_draft_20_03_15.pdf.

Ranahan, P., 2014. Watching in child and youth care suicide interventions: the potential for observation practices to be disengaging. Int. J. Child, Youth Family Stud. 5 (1), 4–23.

Roberts, J.F., Fenton, G., Barnard, M., 2015. Developing effective therapeutic relationships with children, young people and their families. Nurs. Child. Young People 27 (4), 30–35.

Royal College of Paediatrics and Child Health (RCPCH), 2003. Bridging the gaps: health care for adolescents. Council Report CR114. Available from: http://rcpch.adlibhosting.com/files/Bridging%20the%20Gaps%20%20Health%20Care%20for%20Adolescents%202003-06.pdf.

Schore, A., Schore, J., 2010. Clinical social work and regulation theory: implications of neurobiological models of attachment. In: Bennett, S., Nelson, T. (Eds.), Adult Attachment in Clinical Social Work. Essential Clinical Social Work Series. Springer Science. New York.

Schore, J., Schore, A., 2014. Regulation theory and affect regulation psychotherapy: a clinical primer. Smith Coll. Stud. Soc. Work 8 (2–3), 178–195.

Scott, D., Arney, F., Vimpani, G., 2010. Think Child, Think Family, Think Community (Doctoral dissertation). Cambridge University Press, Cambridge.

Singh, S.P., Paul, M., Ford, T., et al., 2008. Transitions of care from child and adolescent mental health services to adult mental health services (TRACK study): a study of protocols in Greater London. BMC. Health. Ser. Res. 8, 135.

Suris, J.C., Michaud, P.A., Viner, R., 2004. The adolescent with a chronic condition. Part 1: developmental issues. Arch. Dis. Child. 89 (10), 938–942.

The Children Act, 1989. UK https://www.legislation.gov.uk/ukpga/1989/41/contents.

The Family Law Reform Act, 1969. UK https://www.legislation.gov.uk/ukpga/1969/46.

The Human Rights Act, 1998. UK https://www.legislation.gov.uk/ukpga/1998/42/contents.

The Mental Capacity Act, 2005. https://www.legislation.gov.uk/ukpga/2005/9/pdfs/ukpga_20050009_en.pdf.

The Mental Health Act, 1983. England & Wales https://www.legislation.gov.uk/ukpga/1983/20/contents.

Thim, T., Krarup, N., Grove, E., et al., 2012. Initial assessment and treatment with the airway, breathing, circulation, disability, exposure (ABCDE) approach. Int. J. Gen. Med. 5, 117–121. https://doi.org/10.2147/IJGM.S28478.

UN Commission on Human Rights, 1990. Convention on the Rights of the Child. UN Commission on Human Rights, p. 7. March 1990, E/CN.4/RES/1990/74.

Waddell, M., 2002. Inside Lives: Psychoanalysis and the Growth of the Personality. Karnac Books, London.

Wilkes, T.C., Belsher, G., 1994. Ten key principles of adolescent cognitive therapy. In: Wilkes, T.C., Belsher, G., Rush, J., Frank, E. (Eds.), Cognitive Therapy for Depressed Adolescents. Guilford Press, New York.

Winnicott, D., 1971. Mirror-Role of Mother and Family in Child Development. Playing and Reality. Tavistock Publications, London.

Winnicott, D., 1984. The Maturational Processes and the Facilitating Environment Studies in the Theory of Emotional Development. Routledge, London.

Wolpert, M., Harris, R., Jones, M., et al., 2014. THRIVE: The AFC-Tavistock Model for CAMHS. CAMHS Press, London.

World Health Organization (WHO), 2014. Health for the world's adolescents: a second chance in the second decade.

World Health Organization (WHO), 2015. Building an adolescent-competent workforce: policy brief.

42

Children With a Learning Disability and/or Autistic Spectrum Conditions

Joann Kiernan

LEARNING OUTCOMES

- Be able to define the terms 'learning disability' and 'autistic spectrum conditions'.
- Develop an understanding of the importance of considering the individual holistic needs of a child/ young person with a learning disability and/or an autistic spectrum condition.

- Consider the nurse's role in supporting equality of access to health care for children and young people with a learning disability and/or an autistic spectrum conditions and their families through the provision of reasonable adjustments.

INTRODUCTION

This chapter has been written to support children's nurses to care for those children and young people with a learning disability and/or an autistic spectrum condition that they will meet throughout their nursing career. First and foremost, the chapter will advocate that these children should be supported as children first. Their needs and wishes will be similar to those of any child, whilst also being individual with bespoke requirements, as for all patients.

Currently, contemporary evidence highlights that people with a learning disability experience more difficulty than others in accessing appropriate health care. People with a learning disability and/or an autistic spectrum condition are more likely to use general hospital services, particularly paediatrics, psychiatry and dentistry (Public Health England, 2016). However, despite increased attendance and need for provision, it is clear that people with learning disabilities in England die much younger than the general population (Heslop et al., 2013).

The context of care for children and young people with a learning disability informs the content of this chapter. It stresses that children with a learning disability and/or an autistic spectrum condition are children and young people who have the same rights as any child. It further recognises the potential for additional needs that may require the provision of reasonable adjustments.

A range of additional needs will be considered with suggested ways in which children's nurses can work in partnership with the child, their family and other professionals to ensure these needs are identified and met. Ultimately, the need to adjust care (reasonable adjustments) to meet the needs of patients is a legal requirement *(Equality Act, 2010)*. As a profession, it is imperative we consider how to ensure that people are able to receive their care appropriately and in a timely person-centred way.

This chapter is written from the perspective of a social model of disability. In the past, society (which includes nurses and other members of the health care professions) tended to view disability and disabled people in terms of a medical or individual model of disability. This approach has meant that disabled people were viewed as not being able to do things because of their disability. In contrast, the social model of disability argues that whereas some people may have certain impairments (such as a visual, mobility or intellectual impairment) what hinders them most are a range of physical, social, psychological and economic barriers. It is these types of barriers that disable them. The removal of such barriers is everybody's business and will create accessible health care for all.

CONTEXT OF CARE

It is important for you to understand the context of care for children and young people with a learning disability and/or an autistic spectrum condition that you will nurse during your career. In 2010, the Royal College of Nursing (RCN) in consultation with people with a learning disability, published guidance to support dignity in health care for this group of potential patients. It defines dignity as '… being treated as a human being. It is about being treated as an individual and with respect.' (RCN, 2010, p. 3)

This does not seem to be unrealistic or unreasonable and may appear as obvious to the nurse.

However, achieving this aim for some people with a learning disability and/or an autistic spectrum condition has historically been difficult.

As a nurse, understanding the needs of this group of children and young people is paramount. It will support your ability to overcome barriers and empower you to ensure that you deliver the very best evidence-based care that realises dignity for all in health care.

THE PREVALENCE OF PEOPLE WITH A LEARNING DISABILITY AND/OR AN AUTISTIC SPECTRUM CONDITION

To consider how many children and young people with a learning disability and/or an autistic spectrum condition, you will, as a nurse, need to understand the prevalence of these conditions.

Through combining epidemiological research and numbers of people using services in England, Public Health England (PHE, 2016) estimated that 1,087,100 people were diagnosed with a learning disability, which includes 930,400 adults. 70,065 children were recorded as having a primary need associated with learning disabilities who also had an education health care plan (EHCP).

 ACTIVITY

Research the term 'educational health care plan'.

Consider the nurse's role in supporting the development of a plan for a child or young person.

Recent studies in the UK indicate a 1.1% prevalence in the population of people with an autistic spectrum condition. This has been estimated to mean that over 695,000 people in the UK may have autism (National Autistic Society, 2019).

Although difficulties remain in determining precisely who might be considered to have a learning disability or an autistic spectrum condition, it is clear that the number of people with a diagnosis is rising. This is attributed to a several factors that include:

- greater life expectancy;
- increasing numbers of children with complex and multiple disabilities surviving to adulthood;
- a significant rise in the number of children diagnosed with autistic spectrum disorders.

TERMINOLOGY

One of the key issues in meeting the needs of people with a learning disability and/or an autistic spectrum condition is the problem of terminology. There are multiple terms and descriptive labels used across services that can seem confusing to children, young people and their families as well as the myriad professionals with whom they may come into contact. Nurses may be involved with the child or young person before, during and after a diagnosis has been confirmed, so must always strive to ensure their care is child centred rather than diagnosis led.

It is important to understand that a learning disability and an autistic spectrum condition are not the same. An individual can have a learning disability or an autistic spectrum condition and may sometimes be diagnosed with both. The National Autistic Society (NAS, 2019) highlight that people with autism have a higher prevalence of learning disabilities or mental health issues with Autistica (2019) estimating that

four people in 10 with autism will also have a learning disability.

The term *disability* can be used in many ways, and this chapter will specifically consider the needs of children and young people described as having a learning/intellectual disability and/or an autistic spectrum condition. Intellectual impairment is currently termed in England as 'learning disability' or internationally as 'intellectual disability'. In virtually all areas of children's nursing there will be children and young people who will be described using these labels alongside many other terms, such as learning difficulties, global developmental delay, additional needs, special educational needs, and so on. Regardless of the language used to describe a person, such terminology indicates that as well as the usual health needs of children and young people this population may also experience additional health needs and comorbidities that may require the support of a range of professionals and agencies. Parents and carers may also require additional support to enable them to access appropriate care and support for their child in a coordinated and effective way.

Some groups of people who have been given the label 'learning disabilities' have indicated that, if they must have a label at all, 'people with learning difficulties' is the most acceptable or preferred term. They emphasise that people with a learning disability are people first and intellectually impaired second. Guidance from the Department of Health (DoH, 2009) considers this distinction and reinforces the use of the term 'learning disability' to refer to the same group of people. The term 'learning difficulty' is usually used in legislation to refer to a group of people with a wider range of educational needs. The term 'learning disability' is thus the current term that is used to refer to individuals and groups of people who would previously have been referred to as having a 'mental handicap' or being 'mentally subnormal'. Terminology, however, continues to evolve, with the term 'intellectual disability' currently favoured by some with variations across continents, for example, 'intellectual impairment' (Australasia) and 'mental retardation' (North America).

For people with autistic spectrum conditions, there are also multiple terms that can be used interchangeably. The NHS (2019) highlights current terminology including:

- autism spectrum disorder (ASD) – the medical name for autism
- autism spectrum condition (ASC) – used instead of ASD by some people
- Asperger's (or Asperger syndrome) – used by some people to describe autistic people with average or above average intelligence

DIAGNOSIS

Receiving or delivering the news that a child has a learning disability and/or an autistic spectrum condition can be extremely difficult. However, it can also be a point from which parents can begin to plan for the future. Crucial to this process is the manner in which concerns regarding the child's development are shared with the family, since problems occur when a carefully considered and planned approach is not taken. Unfortunately, there are many examples of parents and carers who have struggled to have their child's needs recognised, access appropriate services and gain adequate and timely support (Mencap, 2019b).

> **ACTIVITY**
>
> Read the range of family blogs on the Mencap website of how diagnosis and experiences can affect children and young people with a learning disability and their family or carers.
> - https://www.mencap.org.uk/

It must be highlighted that being diagnosed as having a learning disability and/or an autistic spectrum condition can have negative consequences for individuals because of prevailing social attitudes. People can view the person as being different, and difference in this context is viewed negatively. Low expectations, stereotyping and an emphasis on negative characteristics can have an impact on the opportunities and life experiences of an individual. Social attitudes can thus become one of the barriers that disable people who have impairments.

Having a label or a diagnosis can, however, also bring positive benefits. For many families and carers, a diagnosis can enable them to access appropriate service provision and support. An example of this might be access to additional educational support in the classroom or personalised health budgets.

> **ACTIVITY**
>
> - Reflect on the terminology and labels that you may have heard to describe children and young people with a learning disability and/or an autistic spectrum condition.
> - Consider the impact of labels and negative stereotypes on access to health care. What can you do to avoid this for the patients you will support?
> - Research personal health budgets for people with a learning disability and/or an autistic spectrum condition.

DEFINITIONS AND CAUSES OF LEARNING DISABILITY

Formal criteria have been developed to support the diagnosis of a learning disability. One of these is the cognitive functioning approach.

Despite there being a lot of disagreement about exactly what intelligence is, and whether we can establish fair and equal ways to measure it, intelligence has been used as a factor to determine if someone has a learning disability since the early 1900s.

The intelligence quotient (IQ) is a standardised figure that makes it possible to compare how an individual performs against other people in the population when taking a test of their cognitive ability. Historically such measures have been used to distinguish the degree of impairment experienced by

an individual. In this way a child's learning disability may be described as being:

- mild
- moderate
- severe
- profound (World Health Organization [WHO], 1993)

Although the cognitive approach is still currently in use for diagnostic purposes, the WHO's International Classification of Functioning, Disability and Health definition recognised the broader context of disability (WHO, 2001). It considers the effect a learning disability may have for an individual more holistically across multiple areas of their life; for example, how the person interacts with their environment. A Child and Youth Version of this International classification was published in 2007 (WHO, 2007) and placed further emphasis on the need to consider four key areas: the child in the context of the family, developmental delay, participation and the environment.

The WHO (1993) defines a learning disability as:

> ... *a state of arrested or incomplete development of mind, which is especially characterised by impairment of skills manifested during the developmental period* ...

In 2009 the Department of Health *Valuing People Now* White Paper (2009, p 14) stated that a learning disability included the presence of a significantly reduced ability to understand new or complex information and learn new skills (impaired intelligence) with a reduced ability to cope independently (impaired social functioning) that started before adulthood, with a lasting effect on development.

This definition is useful as it distinguishes a learning disability from other forms of impairment of social and cognitive functioning that may arise later in a person's life, such as brain injury or dementia.

When considering the causes of a learning disability, it is clear that it can result from a single factor or multiple interacting factors. To identify specific factors can be difficult, although advances in genetic testing and increased access to early diagnostic processes has increased the ability to highlight needs and provide early intervention for children and their families.

However, many children and young people with a learning disability may not receive a specific medical diagnosis or have labels applied to them while awaiting diagnosis. Terms such as global developmental delay, special educational needs, learning difficulties, etc. can cause some confusion when trying to meet the specific needs of an individual.

The British Institute of Learning Disabilities (BILD, 2019) groups possible causes of a learning disability into four broad stages:

Before birth (prenatal): this could include genetic or 'congenital' causes, such as Down's syndrome or fragile X syndrome. Maternal health behaviours may also be a factor, such as drug or alcohol use.

During birth (perinatal): damage to the brain during birth, such as oxygen deprivation or injury due to complications, and difficulties associated with premature birth.

After birth (postnatal): illnesses, injury or environmental conditions after birth, such as meningitis, brain injury or failure to receive appropriate care, such as deprivation of food, neglect or abuse.

Multiple causes: a combination of factors that can occur at any point stated above.

Although it may be possible to identify key factors to explain the presence of a learning disability in some children, it is often difficult to try and relate their level of cognitive or social functioning to one cause.

In addition, the link between the causative factor and the effects this has on the individual are often unclear. For example, in the case of children who have Down syndrome, the causative factor is known (i.e. trisomy 21), but exactly how this brings about the characteristic features of the syndrome is not so certain. The diagnosis itself cannot tell us the cognitive function of the child or what would be the best way to provide support. It does, however, tell us that because the child has Down syndrome, they have an increased risk of certain health conditions, such as cardiovascular problems, leukaemia, hypothyroidism and sensory impairments (National Institute of Child Health and Human Development, 2019). Ultimately the nurse must respond to the person as an individual and see their role as enabling accessible care based on child- and family-centred assessment.

ACTIVITY

Consider how you could meet the individual needs of a child or young person who may have a learning disability.

DEFINITIONS AND CAUSES OF AUTISM

Autism has been described as '… a lifelong, developmental disability that affects how a person communicates with and relates to other people, and how they experience the world around them' (National Autistic Society [NAS], 2019).

It is a developmental condition that can affect the way an individual receives and processes information. It is not considered to be a disease or illness and can have a variety of impacts on an individual's functioning.

Autism is viewed as a spectrum condition, with key characteristics that may include:

- difficulty in communicating and interacting with other people;
- difficulty in understanding how other people think or feel;
- heightened sensory issues that can mean finding everyday occurrences overwhelming, stressful or uncomfortable, e.g. noises, lighting;
- becoming anxious or upset in situations or social settings that are unfamiliar;
- needing additional time to understand information;
- doing or thinking about things repetitively.

The causes of autism remain unclear, with multiple theories still being researched. Currently there is not considered to be a single cause for the condition (NAS, 2019).

Current evidence suggests the following:

- Autism can be caused by a range of physical factors that can affect brain development.
- Autism is not related to the way a person is brought up.
- Genetic factors may have an influence on some types of autism.
- It is likely that multiple genes are involved rather than a single gene.
- There is difficulty associated with researching gene involvement because of the interaction of genes and potential environmental factors.

To ameliorate some of these difficulties and support the care of patients with autistic spectrum conditions Zanotti (2019) suggested the acronym 'SCRAMBLE'.

- **S**ensory management to reduce stimuli
- **C**ommunications that are kept simple and direct
- **R**educed or limited numbers of people
- **A**llowing extra time
- **M**edication reviews
- **B**ox of sensory toys – provision of appropriate distraction
- **L**istening actively to the child
- **E**xamination and treatment – child-centred modifications

ACTIVITY

Reflect on the children and young people you may have met with a learning disability and/or an autistic spectrum condition. Consider any specific conditions or syndromes that were related to their care. Access the Contact website to learn more about these and potential sources of support available for children's and families.

- http://www.cafamily.org.uk

THE HEALTH NEEDS OF CHILDREN WITH LEARNING DISABILITIES AND/OR AUTISTIC SPECTRUM CONDITIONS

As discussed, people with a learning disability and/or an autistic spectrum condition can experience multiple health needs. These can be exacerbated by issues with communication, access to health care and social and environmental factors. To evidence inequalities in health care the Confidential Inquiry into the Premature Deaths of People with a Learning Disability (Heslop et al., 2013) reviewed the deaths of 247 people. The findings of the inquiry highlighted a clear difference between the median age of death of men and women with a learning disability and the general population. For men the median age was 65 years (13 years younger than the general population), for women the median age was 63 years (20 years younger than the general population). The causes of these inequalities are currently being investigated and researched through a national review of deaths (Learning from Death Review [LEDER]) coordinated through Bristol University.

In response to the evidence associated with inequalities in health care, Mencap (2018) launched its 'Treat me well' campaign, which calls for adjustments in the way services are delivered for people with a learning disability. Key recommendations were associated with system-wide changes, such as training, resources and leadership, and also the application of reasonable adjustments associated with communication, time and information for people with a learning disability.

There is also increasing evidence that people with an autistic spectrum condition struggle to have their health needs met and experience significantly more chronic health conditions (Fortuna et al., 2016; Tyler et al., 2011).

Several research studies have highlighted potential barriers that can prevent people getting their needs met. These include:
- paucity of accessible transport links;
- patients not known to services;
- lack of staff knowledge and understanding;
- lack of recognition that a person with a learning disability is unwell;
- failure to make a correct diagnosis;
- lack of confidence or anxiety of staff;
- lack of joint working from different care providers;
- carers not being listened to;
- lack of aftercare or follow-up care.

(Allerton and Emerson, 2012; Heslop et al., 2013; Oulton et al., 2018; Tuffrey-Wijnes et al., 2013).

 ACTIVITY

Access the full findings from the CIPOLD 2013 inquiry (Heslop et al., 2013) about heath inequalities presented by people with a learning disability at:
- https://www.youtube.com/watch?v=hQXzcDbaVxc

THE IMPACT OF LEARNING DISABILITIES AND/OR AUTISTIC SPECTRUM CONDITIONS FOR THE CHILD AND THE FAMILY

When considering the impact of learning disability and/or autistic spectrum conditions on the child and their family, it is important to consider a number of different aspects, from initial diagnosis and growing up, through transition to adult services. An understanding of each of these aspects is important if children's nurses are to provide an effective service to children with learning disabilities and their families.

Beighton and Wills (2017) highlighted seven areas parents considered to be better in their lives due to their parenting experiences. These included the positive effects their child had on the community, an increase in their own strength and confidence, an enhanced appreciation of life, changes in priorities, pleasure in their child's achievements, increased faith and spirituality, and improvements in meaningful relationships.

 ACTIVITY

- Consider information provided for parents and families by Carers Trust at: https://carers.org/article/learning-disabilities.
- When reading the information consider the role that professionals can play in supporting children and young people and their families and carers.

Growing Up and Transitions

There are multiple transitions for children and young people as they develop and age. Usual transitions include such changes as moving through education into further education or employment, the move towards independent living, possibly away from their families, starting to make decisions about their own health care and attending adult service provision. For children and young people with a learning disability and/or an autistic spectrum condition, some of these usual life transitions can be more difficult.

It is known that the transition from child to adult services can be a particularly stressful time for individuals and their family/carers. Although it is a process that should be carefully planned, research suggests that it can be complex and uncoordinated. Barron et al. (2014) considered five areas that a person with a learning disability and/or an autistic spectrum condition may find difficult as they move into adulthood.

1. Leaving home – this can be later than their peers.
2. Staying at home – there is an increased risk that children and young people with a learning disability and/or an autistic spectrum condition may be already living away from home in residential or care environments.
3. Developing financial independence – individuals can have limited experience managing their own finances, and require support.
4. Reaching legal independence – some individuals with more severe learning disabilities may not have the mental capacity to be deemed legally competent to make their own decisions.
   - Moving towards social independence – difficulties are associated with access to transport, appropriate accessible activities and access to peers.
   - Gaining employment – young people with a learning disability and/or an autistic spectrum condition are less likely to be in paid employment.

Health transitions can be particularly difficult. There is clear national guidance available to support the transition from child to adult services for young people using health or social care services (NICE, 2016).

However, for children who have complex medical needs and comorbidities associated with their learning disability and/or autistic spectrum conditions, the Care Quality Commission (2014) states that:

> *In many cases, the health needs of these young people will have been met by the same people who have looked after them for as long as they can remember. However, one of the changes as they reach adulthood is the transfer to an adult environment where they may need to consult several different health teams, therapy teams, and adult social care services.*
>
> *CQC (2014, p 4)*

The complexity of provision and changes in access can add further difficulties in an individual's ability to meet their own health needs. Relationships and pathways of care will need to be established within adult services while leaving behind familiarity and often friendships that have been formed as the child or young person has developed.

Examples of best practice can be seen in relation to transition in health care, for example, the 'Ten Step Transition Toolkit' at Alder Hey Children's hospital.

 ACTIVITY

Access and read:
a. CQC (2014) report. 'From the pond into the sea. Children's transition to adult health services'. https://www.cqc.org.uk/sites/default/files/CQC_Transition%20Report.pdf.
b. 'Ten Step Transition Toolkit' – Alder Hey Children's hospital. https://www.entandaudiologynews.com/media/5451/ent-jf17-rogers_brook-new.pdf.

WORKING TOGETHER

Nurses can do many things to overcome the barriers described in this chapter that can affect children and young people's access to care. Some of these barriers may be removed or reduced by using child-centred strategies or 'reasonable adjustments' (Equality Act, 2010).

Such adjustments could include, for example:

- Practitioners being aware of the additional health needs that people with learning disabilities and autistic spectrum conditions may experience. Understanding these needs will support individuals to access appropriate care while alerting those involved to the possibility of diagnostic overshadowing.
- Enhancing practitioners' communication skills, including active listening to the patient as well as families and carers who know the person well.
- The development of practitioners' skills in augmented forms of communication, such as Makaton, is particularly useful for patients with a learning disability and helps to support and build therapeutic relationships.
- Provision of additional time for appointments or access to times that may be less busy for individuals with sensory impairments.

Access to reasonable adjustments is a right for any person who may require them. In health care it is particularly important that staff use their skills to gather the information that may enable effective and equal access for patients.

 ACTIVITY

a. Familiarise yourself with the 'Hello my name is' campaign.
 • https://www.hellomynameis.org.uk/
b. Teach yourself how to sign your name using Makaton, so you can effectively introduce yourself to another person.
 • https://www.youtube.com/watch?v=Zz711bmuUBw
c. Research Mencap's 'Treat me well' top 10 reasonable adjustments (Mencap, 2018).
 • https://www.mencap.org.uk/sites/default/files/2018-06/Treat%20me%20well%20top%2010%20reasonable%20adjustments.pdf

As well as children's nurses considering their own role in supporting patients with a learning disability and/or an autistic spectrum conditions, the development of new roles within health care has also started to improve provision. The importance of ensuring a skilled workforce that is able to make services accessible for all children has been recognised by the government (NHS England, 2017).

Examples of this include the employment of different fields of nursing and joint qualifications that can enhance the clinical skill mix and provide holistic care across multiple environments. These roles include, for example, integrated nurse/social work posts and acute liaison roles.

The Role of the Learning Disability Nurse

The learning disability nurse is one of the professionals who works specifically with people who have a learning disability and/or an autistic spectrum condition. Alongside mental health nurses the learning disability nurse works with people across the lifespan. Many learning disability nurses work across community, acute health and primary care environments. These roles include community posts as well as leading on community health facilitation and access to acute health care via liaison roles.

As with all nursing roles, the learning disability nurse's role has changed and evolved to meet the needs of a changing population.

Key roles of the learning disability nurse include:

- Health facilitation in the community to maximise health access through supporting appropriate provision through timely evidence-based interventions.
- Acute liaison roles to enable access to acute care through supporting the provision of reasonable adjustments.
- Encouraging and promoting an individual's meaningful access and presence within their local community.
- Supporting skills teaching for people with a learning disability and/or family/carers in the development of independence and good health.
- Accurate assessment and implementation of treatment and support to maximise health outcomes.
- Using accessible education and health promotion to support carers/families and people with a learning disability and/or autistic spectrum conditions to maintain good quality, healthy lifestyles.
- Multi-disciplinary working to liaise, train and model appropriate interventions to other professional groups.
- Supporting non-learning-disability specific trained staff in meeting the needs of people with a learning disability and/or an autistic spectrum condition.
- Coordination of care within the multi-disciplinary team.
- Challenging and reducing the incidence of inequality and discriminatory practice that affects health-care outcomes.
- Working alongside people with a learning disability and/or autistic spectrum conditions to promote independence.

Learning disability nurse roles differ, with wide variation across areas in relation to service provision for people with a learning disability and autistic spectrum conditions. As well as the generic skills that all nurses possess, a learning disability nurse may also have specialist skills, such as positive behaviour support, forensic skills, a specialist practitioner role, etc. As coordinators of care, and because of their experience of working with people with learning disabilities across the lifespan, learning disability nurses have much to offer in multiple contexts, so are often employed across all sectors, not just in health care.

It is important to note that not all acute hospitals have a learning disability acute liaison nurse, with different models of provision operating across trusts (Oulton et al., 2018). The importance of such roles has been emphasised via the publication of the Learning Disability Improvement Standards (NHSI, 2018). The value of such roles has been supported through the Oulton et al. (2018) study, where staff interviewed identified that they felt less confident in their ability to care for children with a learning disability, and often reported being unsure of what their service offered or what could or should be available.

ACTIVITY

What can you do in your role to support children and young people with a learning disability and/or an autistic spectrum condition?

- What can you do in your role to support children and young people with a learning disability and/or an autistic spectrum condition?
- If you nurse a child or young person with a learning disability and/or an autistic spectrum condition consider these simple points:
  - Who is with the child/young person? Encourage the patient and their family members/carers to share the child's preferred form of communication and their own assessment of the child's needs.
  - Consider this information and how you can obtain access to basic Makaton signs, pictures of your environment, a picture on your name badge if appropriate.
  - Has your clinical area got a resource file you can use? Has your clinical area got an acute liaison nurse or learning disability nurse that can support you in collecting resources?
  - Does the patient need information at a slower pace, in a story format, or through demonstration, as with any young person?
  - Does the young person have any sensory issues that may need to be considered, such as sensitivity to noises or lighting?
  - Are there any preferred methods/techniques that support the patient to access their care (early or prolonged appointment times, quiet areas, etc.)?
  - Discuss with the patient and their family/carers if their behaviour appears to have changed. Why might that be? What could this mean in relation to looking for effective interventions?
  - How is the patient best able to access their treatment, for instance taking medication, tolerating procedures, etc.

SCENARIOS

Consider the scenarios to follow. In the light of the points in the previous box, what could the nurses have put into place to support the child or young person in these examples to access effective and timely health care? What reasonable adjustments could have enhanced the care described?

JENNY

Jenny is a 12-year-old girl with severe learning disabilities. She lives at home with her parents and is a frequent visitor to her local children's ward as she has regular and severe epileptic seizures. She is currently on the ward for a review of her medication following a particularly severe seizure. She had the seizure at home and was found in the living room lying on the floor. When she recovered from the seizure she seemed very disorientated but did not appear to have otherwise injured herself as she got to her feet and started to walk around. While she was on the ward it was noticed that when she was assisted to bathe she would wince whenever her left hip was touched. She was x-rayed and found to have sustained a fracture during her seizure, which had not previously been detected.

SIMON

Simon is a 15-year-old boy with a mild learning and autistic spectrum condition. He is normally very active, but he does not enjoy being in close contact with other people. However, he does appear to have good understanding of what other people say to him and, when his mood allows, he is able to converse with others. He is currently in hospital following an appendectomy. When he was brought in to the ward he was very withdrawn and obviously in pain, but did not want anyone to go near him. His mother said that she had noticed him getting less active over the past couple of days and had tried to get him to tell her what was wrong. However, each time she did this he just got agitated and went to his room. Eventually, he had become so unwell that she had taken him to their general practitioner (GP). Their usual GP was away and so they saw a locum who appeared very hurried, did not take time to examine Simon because he was uncooperative and said that she thought that it was just to do with his condition (meaning his autism and learning disabilities). His mother then took him to the emergency department at the hospital where they (eventually) diagnosed him as having appendicitis.

He has now been on the ward for a couple of days following his operation, but the nurses are worried that he is not recovering as well as they would expect and they suspect that he is in pain. However, although he appears to understand what they say to him, they cannot get him to tell them what is wrong. He is also beginning to display what they feel is strange behaviour. Although most of the nurses are trying very hard to meet Simon's needs, one nurse on the ward says that children like Simon should not be on general wards – they should be looked after in specialist areas. In addition, another parent on the ward has complained to the ward staff about his behaviour, also believing that he should not be on the ward.

SUMMARY

This chapter has explored the care of children and young people with a learning disability and/or an autistic spectrum condition, its effect on the child and their family, and the ways in which nurses can work together with the child, their family, and other professionals to ensure that needs are identified and met in an appropriate and timely manner. Finally, when thinking about the key messages within this chapter, it may help to remember the following points:

- Children with a learning disability and/or an autistic spectrum condition are children first. They have the same needs as other children, but may also have additional needs.
- A learning disability and/or an autistic spectrum condition is a permanent condition. However, children and young people will continue to grow and develop into adults with their own wishes and aspirations, as would any other people.
- People with learning disabilities and/or an autistic spectrum condition have the same human rights as every other person.
- Some people are born with a learning disability, and some acquire a learning disability as the result of an injury or illness.
- An autistic spectrum condition is lifelong with multiple causal factors.
- Some people with learning disabilities and/or an autistic spectrum condition may also have a physical or sensory impairment, but many do not. Some are also at increased risk of certain health conditions.
- Children and young people with a learning disability and/or an autistic spectrum condition need to be seen in the context of their family and carers. Support may need to be provided to all family members.
- Professionals need to be aware of the significance of key stages in the life of a child with a learning disability and/or an autistic spectrum condition, such as initial diagnosis, commencing school and transition to adult services. These transitions can be more difficult because of the complexity of service provision.
- People with a learning disability and/or an autistic spectrum condition can achieve their life ambitions if they are included within their communities and able to access appropriate support.

As for all children, it is impossible to know what kind of a person a child with a learning disability and/or an autistic spectrum condition will be when they grow up. For this reason, it is of paramount importance to remember that they are children and young people first, with individual and additional needs second. They will continue to grow and develop throughout their lives. Owing to impairments, these stages may take longer. The failure to recognise this in the past has contributed to making the experience of a learning disability and/or an autistic spectrum condition more limiting than it might otherwise be. Nursing practitioners, as members of the multi-disciplinary team, can play a key role in minimising the negative impacts a learning disability may have on an individual and their family and in promoting quality of life for all.

Ensure that you will be a nurse who can enable this to happen for the children and young people you come across.

REFERENCES

Allerton, L., Emerson, E., 2012. British adults with chronic health conditions or impairments face significant barriers to accessing health services. Publ. Health 126, 920–927.

Autistica, 2019. https://www.autistica.org.uk/ (accessed 12 August 2019).

Barron, D., Coyle, D., Paliokosta, E., et al., 2014. Transition for Children With Intellectual Disabilities. Intellectual Disability and Health. University of Hertfordshire. Available from: http://www.intellectualdisability.info/life-stages/articles/transition-for-children-with-intellectual-disabilities (accessed 22 July 2019).

Beighton, C., Wills, J., 2017. Are parents identifying positive aspects to parenting their child with an intellectual disability or are they just coping? A qualitative exploration. J. Intellect. Disabil. 21 (4), 325–345. https://doi.org/10.1177/1744629516656073.

Care Quality Commission, 2014. From the pond into the sea. Children's transition to adult health services. Available from: https://www.cqc.org.uk/sites/default/files/CQC_Transition%20Report.pdf (accessed 23 July 2019).

Department of Health [DoH], 2009. Valuing People. A New Strategy for Learning Disability for the 21st Century. DoH, London.

Fortuna, R.J., Robinson, L., Smith, T.H., et al., 2016. Health conditions and functional status in adults with autism: a cross-sectional evaluation. J. Gen. Intern. Med. 31 (1), 77–84.

Heslop, P., Blair, P., Fleming, P., et al., 2013. Confidential inquiry into premature deaths of people with learning disabilities (CIPOLD) Final Report. http://www.bristol.ac.uk/cipold/fullfinalreport.pdf (accessed 4 August 2019).

Legislation.gov.uk, 2010. Equality Act 2010. [online] Available at: http://www.legislation.gov.uk/ukpga/2010/15/contents> [Accessed 11 January 2020].

Mencap, 2018. Treat me well. Available from: www.mencap.org.uk/treatmewell (accessed 4 August 2019).

Mencap, 2019a. https://www.mencap.org.uk/learning-disability-explained/research-and-statistics/children (accessed 14 July 2019).

Mencap, 2019b. https://www.mencap.org.uk/advice-and-support/diagnosis/dealing-diagnosis (accessed 23 July 2019).

National Autistic Society (NAS), 2019. www.autism.org.uk/ (accessed 10 August 2019).

NHS Digital, Health and care of people with learning disabilities: experimental statistics: 2016 to 2017. Available from: https://digital.nhs.uk/data-and-information/publications/statistical/health-and-care-of-people-with-learning-disabilities/health-and-care-of-people-with-learning-disabilities-experimental-statistics-2016-to-2017 (accessed 14 July 2019).

NHS England, 2017. Developing Support and Services for Children and Young People with a Learning Disability, Autism or Both. NHS England, Leeds.

NHS Improvement, 2018. The learning disability improvement standards for NHS trusts. Available from: https://improvement.

nhs.uk/resources/learning-disability-improvement-standards-nhs-trusts/ (accessed 21 July 2019).

NHS, 2019. Available from: https://www.nhs.uk/conditions/autism/what-is-autism/ Accessed 12 March 2019.

National Institute for Health and Care Excellence (NICE), 2016. Transition from children's to adults' services for young people using health or social care services. Available from: https://www.nice.org.uk/guidance/NG43 (accessed 23 July 2019).

National Institute of Child Health and Human Development, 2019. What conditions or disorders are commonly associated with Down syndrome? Available from: https://www.nichd.nih.gov/health/topics/down/conditioninfo/associated (accessed 21 July 2019).

Oulton, K., Gibson, F., Carr, L., et al., 2018. Mapping staff perspectives towards the delivery of hospital care for children and young people with and without learning disabilities in England: a mixed methods national study. BMC Health Serv. Res. 18 (1), 203.

Public Health England, 2016. Learning Disabilities Observatory People With Learning Disabilities in England 2015: Main Report. Available from: https://assets.publishing.service.gov.uk/government/uploads/system/uploads/attachment_data/file/613182/PWLDIE_2015_main_report_NB090517.pdf (accessed 19 July 2019).

Royal College of Nursing (RCN), 2010. *http://oxleas.nhs.uk/site-media/cms-downloads/RCN_Dignity_in_healthcare.pdf* (accessed 29 July 2019).

The Carers Trust, Learning disabilities. https://carers.org/article/learning-disabilities (accessed 22 July 2019).

Tuffrey-Wijne, I., Giatras, N., Goulding, L., Abraham, E., Fenwick, L., 2013. Identifying the factors affecting the implementation of strategies to promote a safer environment for patients with learning disabilities in NHS hospitals: a mixed-methods study. Health Serv. Deliv. Res. 1 (13).

Tyler, C.V., Schramm, S.C., Karafa, M., et al., 2011. Chronic disease risks in young adults with autism spectrum disorder: forewarned is forearmed. Am. J. Intellect. Dev. Disabil. 116 (5), 371–380. https://doi.org/10.1352/1944-7558-116.5.371.

World Health Organization, 1993. Describing Developmental Disability. Guidelines for a Multiaxial Scheme for Mental Retardation (Learning Disability). WHO, Geneva.

World Health Organization (WHO), 2001. International Classification of Functioning, Disability and Health, Geneva. Available from: http://www.who.int/classifications/icf/en (accessed 20 July 2019).

World Health Organization (WHO), 2007. International Classification of Functioning, Disability and Health: Children and Youth Version: ICF-CY. World Health Organization. Available from: https://apps.who.int/iris/handle/10665/43737 (accessed 20 July 2019).

Zanotti, J.M., 2019. Handle with care. Caring for children with autism spectrum disorder in the ED. Nursing 48 (2), 50–55.

USEFUL WEBSITES

http://www.nas.org/
http://www.cafamily.org.uk
https://www.nice.org.uk/
http://www.bild.org.uk
http://www.mencap.org.uk
https://www.makaton.org/
https://www.hellomynameis.org.uk/
https://www.rcn.org.uk/
https://www.mixitdays.com/

43

Care of the Child and Young Person Requiring Palliative and End-of-Life Care

Jayne Price, Marisa McFarlane

LEARNING OUTCOMES

- Examine the components that contribute to the philosophy of palliative care for children and families.
- Appreciate the importance of a family-centred and an interdisciplinary approach to care of a child with a life-limiting illness.

- Gain insight and understanding into the biopsychosocial and spiritual needs of the child with a life-limiting condition and their family.
- Understand the needs of the family in bereavement.

INTRODUCTION

Palliative care for children is about ensuring the child with a life-limiting condition and their family live as full a life as possible in the knowledge that early death is expected (Levetown, 2008; Together for Short Lives, 2018). The care of children with life-limiting illnesses has received increased attention over recent years, and as a result, children's palliative care has evolved as a small but distinct area of practice across the UK and internationally (Marston et al., 2018; Price and McNeilly, 2009). Evidence suggests that the numbers of children with life-limiting conditions in the UK are increasing (Fraser et al., 2014) due in part to advanced technology. A range of conditions require this type of care. Four broad groups of children, whose needs can change over time (TFsL), have been identified as likely to need this unique type of care. Within the four groups of children, many have complex chronic conditions and all the children have the possibility of an early death (Himelstein, 2006). These groups are listed on the companion PowerPoint.

Life-limiting conditions are those for which there is no reasonable hope of a cure and where death before adulthood is expected. It is also important to recognise that certain other conditions, for example cancer in childhood, are life threatening but may become life limiting if all treatment options are exhausted.

Government strategy and policy within the UK have placed children with palliative care needs and their families central to their agenda (Department of Health [DoH], 2005, 2007, 2008) and the National Institute for Health and Care Excellence (NICE, 2016) guideline outlines the importance of ensuring quality care for children with life-limiting conditions and their families specifically at the end of life. Knowing that a child is life limited poses a particular challenge for parents and professionals, resulting in much emotional and practical chaos as they juggle multiple, and often competing, demands while addressing the needs of the child in the context of the family (Price et al., 2013).

The subsequent death of the child is a devastating loss to families and communities, and in turn leads to one of the most profound and long-lasting of griefs. The death of a child defies the natural expected order of life events; no parent expects to outlive their child (Price and Jones, 2015; Sourkes et al., 2005).

Although it has been argued that the principles and ethics underpinning palliative care delivery are universal across age spans, caring for children within this and other specialist areas of health care bring different and unique challenges, issues and dilemmas. While some of the principles of caring for the adult patient may be useful in the care of children, it is essential to recognise and acknowledge the unique needs of the child requiring a palliative approach and of their family (Price et al., 2005). One of the most distinctive differences within children's palliative care is the broad diagnostic diversity, which results in the challenging uncertainty around prognosis experienced by children and families. Many of the disorders experienced by children are rare (Watterson and Hain, 2003). Others may be familial, and thus genetic counselling for the family is crucial. In addition, because of the degenerative nature of many of the life-limiting illnesses of childhood, palliative care services are traditionally involved with the child and family from an early stage, often over a long period of time. In fact, many children with life-limiting conditions do not have a diagnosis (Hoell et al., 2017). Thus palliative care for children is multi-faceted and complex. This chapter looks firstly at the historical development of palliative care for children and examines the different components of children's palliative care more than simply end-of-life care. It considers the impact of a diagnosis of a life-limiting condition on the child/family and ensuring ongoing quality of life including working in partnership through death into bereavement. Case studies, links and signposting evidence to underpin care are included.

PALLIATIVE CARE FOR CHILDREN

A Historical Perspective

Palliative care for children is about quality of living for both the child whose life is limited and their family (NICE, 2016). The development of this specialty can be attributed to the advent of the children's hospice movement and the further development of paediatric oncology outreach services. Born out of a desire to improve care for dying people, the hospice movement evolved as it had become accepted that the modern medical establishment was not fully addressing all the needs of dying people and their families. The need for an expansion of services was identified from simply providing care for adult cancer patients, and in 1982 the first children's hospice was opened in Oxford. Helen House developed from the special friendship between Sister Frances Dominica and a child called Helen, who had a life-limiting illness. Through this relationship, Sister Frances recognised the need for respite care and practical support for families in similar situations. Her vision was for a haven where this practical support and respite care could be delivered. Helen House provided a 'home from home' where families could share the caring, providing them with an environment where practical help, friendship and quality time were offered. This was to 'blaze a trail in the provision of hospice care for children and young people' (Worswick, 2000, p 160). Helen House remains an exemplar for the development of children's hospice services worldwide, and the number of children's hospices has grown in conjunction with the development of 'hospice-at-home' teams. The growth generated an appraisal into the care delivered to children with life-limiting illnesses and their families. In 1992 the ACT (Association for Children with Life-Threatening or Terminal Conditions and Their Families), since renamed the Association for Children's Palliative Care, was set up to influence and promote excellence and equity in care provision and support for children and young people with life-threatening or life-limiting conditions and their families.

ACT worked closely with other agencies, for example, Children's Hospices UK (formerly ACH), to promote excellence for all children requiring palliative care and their families (Price et al., 2005) and later merged to become Together for Short Lives. Together for Short Lives lobbies for the rights of children and families through raising awareness, advocating for change, and increasing funding for children's palliative care services. In addition, they have developed a range of resources for families and professionals. Other organisations, such as ICPCN (International Children's Palliative Care Network) and EAPC (European Association of Palliative Care) work around the needs of children requiring palliative care and their families.

🌐 **WWW**

- https://www.togetherforshortlives.org.uk/
Establish the current work of Together for Short Lives in the UK.
- http://www.icpcn.org/
Establish the current work internationally regarding care of children with palliative care needs.
- http://www.eapcnet.eu/
Establish the current work in Europe regarding palliative care for children.

Although this philosophy of care has developed largely from within the hospice movement, it has since permeated across a number of additional settings – namely hospital and home – to ensure seamless quality care. This being so, it is now referred to as *paediatric palliative care* or *palliative care for children and families*. The specialty has greatly developed in recent years through policy development and international networks. Despite the expansion and development of services in recent years, providing palliative care tailored to a child's individual needs has not been without its challenges. These challenges include difficulty recognising which children require palliative care, the variation in availability of services depending on geographical location, a lack of understanding by policy makers about what constitutes palliative care and the limited evidence base underpinning practice and transition to adult services. With regard to transition to adult services, a Teenager Cancer research project (Grinyer and Barbarachild, 2011) identified the gap in services for 16- to 18-year-olds and reported unsuitable hospice care in both paediatric and adult settings, and a lack of specialist paediatric palliative care services, as some of the challenges to providing appropriate support. Similar issues have been identified for young people with non-malignant conditions requiring transition (Kerr et al., 2018). In the last few years another specific group has received increased focus, this being babies both before or after birth, with the suggestions that perinatal and neonatal palliative care is the final frontier in the development of palliative (Wilkinson, 2013).

Palliative Care for Children – A Distinct Specialty

Although many of the terms within the specialty are used interchangeably, one of the most widely accepted definitions in the UK and further afield is from Together for Short Lives (2013, 2018).

> *Palliative care for children and young people with life-limiting conditions is an active and total approach to care, from the point of diagnosis or recognition, embracing physical, emotional, social and spiritual elements through to death and beyond. It focuses on enhancement of quality of life for the child/young person and support for the family and includes the management of distressing symptoms, provision of short breaks and care through death and bereavement.*
>
> ***Together for Short Lives (2018 p 9)***

Palliative care is not purely about dying or end of life, with the above definition highlighting the different attributes that contribute to the philosophy of palliative care for children. Palliative care for children requires an integrated approach, and it has become widely accepted that a mixed model of care is essential, commencing at diagnosis. Within this model, the principles of palliative care and cure-focused care are delivered concurrently, ensuring consistency throughout the child's illness (Michelson and Steinhorn, 2007) promoting long-term quality of life (Kreicbergs, 2018). So, for example, children with life-threatening conditions where treatment and cure is possible, such as a child with cancer, would have elements of palliative care philosophy applied throughout their active treatment. Quality of life, symptom management and psychological support are all inherent in active treatment for childhood cancer, and while some patients will become life limited and require end-of-life care, others will survive. This 'parallel planning' approach not only allows for a child's full potential to be achieved, but also informs and involves services and professionals where necessary. However, despite the recognition of an integrated approach, current attitudes within society and medicine continue to view palliative care as being restricted to the last few weeks of life (Kreicbergs, 2018).

 WWW

Together for Short Lives, 2013. A Core Care Pathway for Children with Life Limiting and Life Threatening Conditions, 3rd edition.
- https://www.togetherforshortlives.org.uk/resource/core-care-pathway/
  Consider how this could be used in your practice.

Reaction to a Life-Limiting Illness

The diagnosis of a life-limiting/life-threatening illness rocks the most stable of families (Chad, 2008). It is the start of a journey that can resemble a roller-coaster ride: the ups and downs along the uncertain road of the illness trajectory (Steele, 2005) and can lead to a long-term relationship with the health care team (Jordan et al., 2015; Nuutila and Salantera, 2006). For many families, their child may live for many years with periods of stability and then periods of deterioration. The way the news is broken can stay with a family for many years and a variety of models have been established to assist health care professionals in this complex and challenging task (Price et al., 2006). In addition, other factors affect the psychological impact of facing a life-limiting illness. These include the age and cognitive development of the child, the duration and type of treatment (if available), the prognosis, the degree of disruption to normal routine and education, the degree to which body image may be affected and the potential separation from siblings and main caregivers.

The overall reaction to the diagnosis of a child's life-limiting condition, or the birth of a baby with a life-limiting condition, is similar to that of bereavement as parents are grieving the loss of their 'well' child or the 'healthy baby' they wished for (Price et al., 2011). The child may also be grieving for the 'normal' life and the future they may feel they have lost (Maunder, 2004). Soricelli and Utech (1985) identify that grief symptoms are experienced from diagnosis and throughout the illness trajectory of a child with a life-limiting condition and highlighted four distinct phases of bereavement: firstly, bereavement at the time of diagnosis; secondly, bereavement during integration; thirdly, renewed bereavement if curative options have been available and are exhausted and death is approaching; with the fourth phase being post-death mourning.

Kubler-Ross (1970) identified five reactions to dying; these can equally be applied to a diagnosis of a life-limiting or life-threatening illness. These are denial, anger, bargaining, depression and acceptance. The child and the family may experience a multitude of different feelings at different times, and there is no set way for how the individual may feel at any particular time. Regardless of the type of feelings being experienced at any particular time, the child and family require cohesively planned care and support from an experienced team who are responsive to individual need. The family needs information and support at the time of diagnosis and afterwards (Royal College of Nursing [RCN], 2013). Planning palliative care for children must therefore be tailored to the individual and changing needs of that child and their families (Beardsmore and Fitzmaurice, 2002) and include a wide array of agencies and services within the NHS and outside to ensure holistic good quality care is provided (NICE, 2016).

The need for care can be unrelenting and can lead to social deprivation and extreme stress for the family. Short breaks are crucial, and hospices can provide essential breaks for families (Ling et al., 2015). In addition, burn-out and emotional distress in staff regularly caring for these children and families has also been noted (Forster and Hafiz, 2015; McCloskey and Taggart, 2010).

Psychological Care

Learning that a child has a life-limiting illness launches a family into what Steele (2005) describes as 'unchartered territory'. Emotional and practical chaos occurs as they navigate this unchartered territory (Price et al., 2011). Support is required as parents and the child can experience a range of emotions, including fear, anxiety, anger, guilt, uncertainty, blame and shock.

Hope has been identified as one of the greatest coping mechanisms for families (De Graves and Aranda, 2005). Hope is something that has been cited as important to parents throughout their child's illness trajectory and even up to the moment of their child's death (Lotz et al., 2017). Bereaved mothers who participated in a study by Laakso and Paunonen-Ilmonen (2002) identified that they expected nursing staff to maintain and provide hope as long as the child remained alive. However, hope for a cure may be replaced by the hope for a good death when parents have an awareness that death is imminent (Little & Sayers, 2004).

The emotional responses of the family impact on the care and support they give their child. Mothers appear to express their feelings more freely than fathers, and it is often assumed by health care professionals that fathers can cope. It is essential that the different members of the interdisciplinary team ensure that the needs of fathers are also addressed and that they are included in discussions and decision making.

Parents will have questions regarding their child and their child's care – examples of the questions that occur as the child is nearing the end of life are listed on the companion PowerPoint. Beardsmore and Fitzmaurice (2002) caution the use of timescales if parents ask: 'How long has my child got?' Parents can hold on to timescales, and if the child dies before or after the suggested time frame can feel cheated or frustrated.

Time should be permitted for parents to assimilate information before they decide how to approach it. Family members need to be empowered with information to enable them to make decisions about care. Jones (2006) suggests that in addition to information, families need control and advocacy for decisions they have to make. It is important to ensure that honest, accurate consistent responses and information are given. The family will have options but may require guidance when making decisions as parents are seen as the surrogate decision makers for their child (Hynson et al., 2003). There should be open communication where parents and the medical team discuss problems and hopes openly. These are important components in shared decision-making (Hill et al., 2015).

Being conscious of the needs of siblings in each stage of the process of dying can greatly benefit the surviving children (Fullerton et al., 2017).

EVIDENCE-BASED PRACTICE

Wallin et al. (2015) examined siblings' long-term psychological health in relation to their perception of communication with their family, friends and health care professionals during a brother or sister's last month of life. A nationwide questionnaire study was used to collect data from individuals whose brother or sister died from cancer. Of the 240 siblings contacted, 174 (73%) participated. Siblings who were not satisfied with the amount they talked about their feelings with others during their brother or sister's last month of life were more likely to report anxiety than those who were satisfied. Such feelings were similar for those who had been unable to talk to their family after bereavement. Siblings suggested that they avoided discussing their anxiety with health care professionals for fear of being in their way at follow-up. Long-term anxiety in bereaved siblings might be due to insufficient communication. Avoiding health care professionals, especially when the brother or sister is cared for at the hospital, may also increase the risk of anxiety.

Parents and health care professionals should ensure open, honest communication, inclusion and support for siblings as a child moves towards the end of life (Lovegren et al., 2016). Nurses can educate families on the importance of involving siblings and creating a supportive environment as soon as possible when it is clear that the child is going to die; this has been identified in the literature as anticipatory guidance (Giovanola, 2005).

SCENARIO

David is 8. His 11-year-old sister Clare was diagnosed with a brain tumour two years ago. After extensive treatment she is now approaching death. Clare is being cared for at home. Consider the changes David might be experiencing:
- in his family life;
- in his relationship with his sibling and parents;
- in his own feelings and emotions.

What strategies could David's mum and dad use to prepare David for Clare's imminent death?

An honest and truthful approach has been identified as one of the rights of the child and is viewed as an essential component of effective communication in quality palliative care. The understanding children have of death evolves gradually. Talking to children about illness and death is extremely difficult – the child's developmental stage must be given careful consideration when communicating effectively with life-limited children (Aldridge et al., 2017).

Children with life-limiting illness are suspected as having an awareness of their impending death (Bluebond-Langner, 1978). Bluebond-Langner's landmark study has shaped thinking on this issue and indicated that children as young as 3 years old were aware of their diagnosis and prognosis without having been told. It is understandable that parents want to protect their child from harm and distress. A situation of mutual pretence can arise where both the child and the parent pretend to be unaware of the situation to protect each other (Bluebond-Langner, 1978).

The nurse must accept that honesty can be extremely difficult and painful for families (van der Geest et al., 2015) and that sensitivity must be central to this. In certain situations, some parents may still wish to withhold the truth in an attempt to protect the child. This can be a difficult situation for the health care professional, who must respect the family's right. Swaffield (1985) identified that many of the children whose parents had chosen not to tell them of their impending death were aware of it anyway. The nurse must work in collaboration with the other members of the interdisciplinary team creating an atmosphere that fosters truthfulness and should ensure the family are fully informed as to the knowledge that exists around child awareness of death. (Helpful tips for talking to children about death can be found on the companion PowerPoint slide.)

Short Breaks

Short breaks, or respite care as it is sometimes called, are an instrumental part of palliative care for children and young people (Ling et al., 2015). Caring for a child with a life-limiting illness is both physically and emotionally draining for the family. The care may involve 24-hour devotion of the parent to the sick child. It is essential that the family is offered some time away from the physical and emotional exhaustion that the tasks of caring can cause.

Parents and families willingly undertake very complex care at home when their child has a life-limiting illness. Their ability to cope will decrease and their level of stress will increase unless they receive regular breaks. Judd (1994 p 218) defined respite care as:

> Complementary, flexible care in the home or home from home setting with appropriate medical and nursing support, offering parents or carers an interval of relief.

Contemporary children's palliative care has normally replaced the term 'respite' with 'short breaks' as the word 'respite' can impart the notion of burden, and understandably while still recognising the need for a break, families can reject the idea that caring for their child is a burden.

See the definition of short breaks on the companion CD and compare with the definition of Judd (1994).

As with all other aspects of palliative care for children and families, the need and type of respite care required should to be tailored to the individual family. The range of short break provision offered is limited in certain parts of the UK. However, with an increase in the profile of the needs of children with life-limiting illness and their families, new services continue to be developed in an attempt to meet the increasing demand.

Interprofessional/Interdisciplinary Approach Children's Palliative Care

The need for an interdisciplinary team approach to palliative care for children and their families is essential in the provision of a quality seamless service to children and their families (McNeilly and Price, 2008). Providing palliative care for children requires thorough planning and effective communication as well as coordination and cohesiveness within the interdisciplinary team (Hynson et al., 2003).

Clear, concise communication is a fundamental component of successful team working, with each team member having a role to play. Members of the interdisciplinary team must share identical goals of care and respect the individual roles of team members and also family needs and values. A cohesive package is required with clarity of roles in order that conflicting information is avoided. Team variance can create an environment where confusion is present. The health care professional must function effectively and efficiently on an individual basis and as part of the team. The palliative care package for the child and family should have an identified key worker (NICE, 2016). This worker will coordinate the care and ensure a seamless package is provided, that clarity of roles is established and good communication is maintained (NICE, 2016). The key worker could be a Community Children's Nurse (CCN), palliative care nurse, hospice nurse or paediatric oncology outreach nurse specialist (POONS). Vickers et al. (2007) purport that the POONS is in an ideal position to act as the key worker for a child with advanced cancer. The team will be made up of different professionals, depending on the individual child, family and their circumstances.

EVIDENCE-BASED PRACTICE

Khan et al. (2016) carried out a study exploring the role of pharmacists in providing palliative care to children in the UK. An online questionnaire was used to collect data from 114 pharmacists working in hospital and community. The response rate was 27% (114/430). Pharmacists reported supporting children receiving palliative care by supplying medicines, dealing with medication-related enquiries and providing advice to nursing and medical staff on the compatibility and stability of drugs. This is one of the first studies to outline the roles of pharmacists working in paediatric palliative care and has highlighted that pharmacists have an important input in the care of these patients.

Ensuring a robust family support network, including social support systems, is essential as a family face losing their child. Social isolation can be experienced when a child is ill; a study carried out by Steele (2005) gained insight into families' experiences of living with a child who has a neurodegenerative life-threatening illness. Families expressed that they often disengaged themselves from previous relationships outside the immediate family as the ill child was the focus of parental time and energy. This, in turn, could lead to them feeling isolated and alone, particularly at times of crisis. Parents and other family members should be encouraged to continue involvement in their child's care even as the child's condition deteriorates. Continual assessment of the needs of the parent and their coping is required, as is the necessary support.

A social worker will be able to advise, direct and assist the family in identifying and securing suitable resources to promote overall family functioning (Sourkes et al., 2005). Financial burdens can grip families who have to care for a child with life-limiting illnesses. The child's illness could necessitate one or both parents giving up work to care for the child. Families may be unaware of the help they are entitled to, which can include income support, care allowances and travel and other grants. Voluntary agencies may also provide help assistance with household chores. For example, Macmillan Cancer Support, in some areas, provides volunteer help with ironing, cleaning, etc., allowing parents to spend more time with the sick child and siblings.

Other organisations may be able to offer holidays for the complete family unit in purpose-built facilities. The interdisciplinary team should work together in ensuring that the family is aware of the availability of services and their entitlement. The child's education is an important part of maintaining a quality life for the child with a life-limiting illness. Its importance is two-fold. First, education is an essential way for the child continuing to develop to their potential. Second, it allows continuing socialisation and integration with peers. As the child's condition changes, their educational needs will need to be re-assessed to see how best they can be addressed. Hospitals and hospices have teachers as part of the interdisciplinary team, and home tutors can also be made available if the child is unable to attend their own school (DoH and DfES, 2004).

Examples of other members of the interdisciplinary team are listed on the companion CD-ROM.

The importance of good team working cannot be understated as the assessment, planning, implementing and evaluation of plans of care, including symptom control for children with a life-limiting illness, needs to be interdisciplinary (NICE, 2016).

Symptom Control for Children

Symptom management has been identified as a major component of palliative care (Michelson and Steinhorn, 2007). Parents have observed that children suffer multiple symptoms, particularly at the end of life (Wolfe et al., 2000). It is essential to recognise that the symptoms experienced by children are rarely simply physical events. Symptoms should more often be regarded as a complex experience with physical, psychological, social and emotional elements (Brady, 1996).

Reliable, valid and frequent assessment is central to successful symptom management. Assessment, regardless of the symptom, is an ongoing process that permits choice and flexibility when circumstances for the child and family change (Anghelescu et al., 2006). The child's stage of development must be central to the assessment and management of symptoms. A variety of assessment tools can be used in the extracting and assimilating of information with children. Many assessment tools offer a combination approach using verbal and non-verbal indicators (see Chapter 17). Paediatric pain profile (Hunt, 2003) is an example of an assessment tool for use with pre-verbal, unconscious and non-verbal children. Although a range of assessment tools exist, their underuse in practice with children with life-limiting conditions has been highlighted (McCluggage and Elborn, 2006).

Adequate symptom control is viewed as the ultimate aim of palliative care regardless of the setting in which care is provided. Negotiation with, and open lines of communication between, the child, family and nurse are essential in achieving optimum symptom control. Symptoms experienced vary depending on the child and specific diagnosis, and families have much to offer in the assessment and evaluation of symptom management. Symptom management plans should, in addition, be flexible, evidence based and include combinations of both pharmacological and non-pharmacological interventions (Anghelescu et al., 2006). Education of parents and their preparation regarding symptoms is crucial (Beardsmore and Fitzmaurice, 2002) so that they know what to expect. The nurse must consider the fact that symptoms that may not be disturbing to the child can be very distressing to parents.

Many symptoms are managed pharmacologically, which can be challenging given that many of the drugs used effectively for symptom management with adults are not licensed for use in children. A number of routes of administration can be used and the chosen route depends on the age, condition of the child and any access devices that the child may have in place.

The oral route is usually first choice for administration of medication in children and young people – many drugs are available in elixir form. The child and family should be involved in decisions about the preferred format. Intramuscular injections should be avoided in children where possible (Rainbows Children's Hospice, 2016). Many children at this stage in illness may have a central line in position, which provides a useful alternative route for administration. Some children may have a nasogastric tube in place and this can be utilised successfully for administration of medication. Infusions can be given subcutaneously via syringe drivers (McNeilly et al., 2004) or via an existing central venous access device. In recent years the transdermal route has become another option for the delivery of some drugs. Rectal preparations are available for many drugs, but they should not be used in children with a low platelet count. For many children or young people, using the rectal route can be a very distressing experience. The National Institute for Health and Care Excellence (NICE 2017) states that the rectal route should only be used in the treatment of constipation if oral laxatives do not work, and then only if the child/young person and family consent.

The focus of complementary therapies in palliative care is usually on symptom control. Buckle (2003) discusses the value of aromatherapy and massage in children's palliative care. These techniques can aid in promoting communication with children, reducing anxiety, enhancing relationships and enhancing quality of life in terms of symptom management. These therapies can be used in conjunction with conventional medicine. As with all interventions the child's welfare must be paramount and underpin all care delivered. There is little scientific evidence in this area of care.

◎ EVIDENCE-BASED PRACTICE

Thrane et al. (2017) carried out pre-post mixed-methods single group pilot study which focused on examining the feasibility, acceptability and outcomes on pain, anxiety and relaxation using reiki therapy with a convenience sample of 16 children (ages 7–16 years) receiving palliative care. Two 24-minute reiki sessions were carried out in the child's home. Results of this preliminary work indicated that reiki therapy did decrease pain, anxiety, heart and respiratory rates in children, but the small sample size prevented any specific statistical significance. Thus these findings would suggest that complementary therapies, such as reiki, may be beneficial in conjunction with traditional methods to manage anxiety and pain in children with palliative care needs.

Commonly occurring symptoms experienced by children and interventions to ameliorate them are identified in Table 43.1. Further details of symptoms and their management are listed in Rainbow Children's Hospice Guidelines (see box that follows). The Association of Paediatric Palliative Medicine Master Formulary (see box that follows) provides a detailed manual for symptom management for children.

TABLE 43.1   **Symptom Management in Children's Palliative Care**

Symptom	Possible Causes/ Exploration	Pharmacological Management	Non-Pharmacological Management	Comments/Special Notes
Pain. Pain is most feared by parents whose child is approaching death. Friedman et al. (2005) discuss that under-medication is a common issue relating to pain and other symptoms, particularly at the end of life.	Pain is multi-faceted, made up of physiological, emotional, spiritual and social aspects. Each of these elements requires consideration, as does the fact that the child continues to grow and develop.	Analgesia should be selected for the type of pain being experienced. Pain may be chronic, and a combination of drug types may be used (Friedman et al., 2005). Keep analgesia simple initially and gradually progress as necessitated by the specific need of the child. WHO (2012) guidance changed the analgesic ladder from a three-step to a two-step approach. (See CD-ROM.) A variety of routes can be used – oral, buccal, rectal, subcutaneous or IV infusion. Transdermal is a way of managing symptoms in children without needles and is increasingly being used (Hain and Wallace, 2008).	Non-pharmacological approaches to pain can include techniques such as guided imagery, relaxation, complementary therapies, distraction therapy, heat and cold (Anghelescu et al., 2006) and positioning of the child. Careful explanations to child and family, and parental presence, may have a positive effect in reducing fear and anxiety, and thus may reduce the intensity of the pain experienced.	Assessing and managing total pain is a priority when caring for the child and family. Refer to Chapter 17. Anticipation is critical in managing pain in children (Himelstein, 2006). Pain assessment must be developmentally and age appropriate (Himelstein, 2006). Parental support will be required regarding the use of opioids and associated fear (Beardsmore and Fitzmaurice, 2002).
Nausea and vomiting	This may be a result of constipation, raised intracranial pressure (ICP), intestinal obstruction, anorexia, cough, pain, or as a side-effect of opioid therapy.	A wide range of antiemetics are available. Antiemetics act on different sites, so it is essential to recognise the potential cause of the nausea and vomiting in order that the correct antiemetic is selected. If vomiting and nausea are not resolved treatments that work on different sites can be used in combination effectively. Dexamethasone can be added to first line to enhance efficacy.	Common sense measures include avoiding known stimuli to vomiting (McCluggage and Jassal, 2009). These can include: • avoiding strong odours; • offering small amounts of food; • good oral hygiene; • distraction techniques, including play.	These drugs can be given orally, often in elixir or tablet form. Certain antiemetics come in melt form that can provide a useful alternative for children. If the oral route is not suitable for a particular child, then rectal or subcutaneous routes can be used. Many antiemetic drugs are compatible with opiates and can be added to syringe drivers and administered with analgesia (McCluggage and Jassal, 2009). Nausea can contribute to weakness, inactivity and irritability. These non-specific signs can often be confused with pain (Himelstein, 2006).

TABLE 43.1   Symptom Management in Children's Palliative Care—cont'd

Symptom	Possible Causes/ Exploration	Pharmacological Management	Non-Pharmacological Management	Comments/Special Notes
Respiratory symptoms including cough, dyspnoea, congestion, respiratory distress, grunting	The cause of the respiratory symptom and the severity of the problem is dependent on the nature of the underlying disease. In children with malignancies, it may be due to pleural effusion, superior vena cava (SVC) obstruction, anaemia or ascites. Children with neurodegenerative disease and cystic fibrosis are most likely to experience problems related to the respiratory system in the terminal stage of illness.	Diazepam to reduce the anxiety associated with breathlessness, a simple linctus for an irritating cough and hyoscine can be used successfully for the management of excessive secretions. Laboured respiration and grunting may occur in the latter stages of illness when death is imminent; the child is normally in a deep unconscious state, this may be treated with diamorphine, subcutaneous midazolam or rectal diazepam. Parents require explanation and reassurance during this stage (Sourkes et al., 2005). Oxygen therapy and nebulised bronchodilators may be useful.	As anxiety can make breathlessness worse, calm reassurance for both child and family is important (McCluggage and Jassal, 2009). Appropriate positioning of the child may also ease this symptom, e.g. propping the child upright to permit optimal lung expansion. Physiotherapy, with or without suction, may help to settle the child. Use a fan to circulate air. Use relaxation and deep breathing exercises. Keep the room well ventilated.	Breathlessness can be increased by anxiety. Anxiety can exacerbate the physical symptoms. Anxiety of parents clearly affects the worries of the child.
Constipation	Constipation can result due to inactivity, dehydration, an obstruction (e.g. tumour involvement), nerve involvement or as a side-effect of medication (e.g. opioids).	Where possible, the aim of treatment should be to avoid it in the first place (Himelstein, 2006). If the child does develop constipation a variety of laxatives can be selected. Oral laxatives should be used in the first instance, and hopefully, if they are successful the use of rectal treatments can be avoided.	Encourage fluid intake. Enlist the help and support of the family, who will be able to give information to the nurse about the child's normal bowel movements. Encourage increased activity if appropriate given child's condition. Give attention to fluid intake and diet. Provide privacy and maintain dignity during defecation.	Prevention is key to management of constipation (Himelstein, 2006). A laxative should be prescribed and administered at the commencement of opioid therapy (McCluggage and Jassal, 2009).
Symptoms of central nervous system (seizures, agitation, twitching and restlessness)	Children with neurodegenerative conditions or brain tumour may suffer seizures. Twitching and agitation may be caused by electrolyte imbalance, hypoxia and opioids. Altered sleep pattern and depression can also lead to agitation.	Rectal diazepam is particularly useful and effective for children having a fit. Buccal midazolam is increasingly being used in older children or when the rectal route is difficult to access. Midazolam can be added into the syringe driver to address the agitation, which can be experienced in the late terminal stages of life in children.	Non-pharmacological interventions for agitation should include calm, reassuring, open communication with the child and the use of relaxation, guided imagery or massage.	If a child prone to a seizure is being cared for at home the families should have a supply of diazepam and be given practical advice on seizure management (Beardsmore and Fitzmaurice, 2002). The family should also be taught how to maintain their child's safety.

Continued

TABLE 43.1	Symptom Management in Children's Palliative Care—cont'd			
Symptom	**Possible Causes/ Exploration**	**Pharmacological Management**	**Non-Pharmacological Management**	**Comments/Special Notes**
Skin problems/pruritus	Children who are facing death are prone to this as a result of a decrease in oral intake, and medication such as opioids (Himelstein, 2006). Children who have biliary, renal or hepatic disease are also prone to skin irritation. Children who have been, or are on steroids may be predisposed to skin problems, as their skin can be thinned and papery in appearance. Skin breakdown can occur as a result of reduced mobility and a decrease in the child's nutritional intake.	Skin irritation can be managed by skin care products and antihistamines administered orally or intravenously. These may ease discomfort.	Avoid harsh soaps, which may dry the skin. Avoid the use of highly perfumed bath/shower products and moisturising products. Keep fingernails short and discourage scratching to prevent excoriation (Sourkes et al., 2005). Keep the child cool and dress them in cotton clothing. Distraction and relaxation may help (Sourkes et al., 2005).	Dry skin and pruritus are more common in children than breakdown of skin areas. Regular assessment of a child's skin condition should be carried out to establish if any change has taken place. Regular and accurate assessment of the child's skin integrity should be carried out and recorded. The parents or main caregivers should be educated as to how to carry this out. Mobility should be encouraged as the child's condition dictates. If the child is confined to bed then their position should be changed 2-hourly. Air mattresses can be obtained by nursing staff (either hospital or community).
Fatigue Most common symptom reported by families whose child died with malignant disease (Hechler et al., 2008; Wolfe et al., 2000)	Causes in children with malignancies include anaemia, poor nutrition, metabolic disturbances, medication and psychological factors. Signs can include low energy, weakness, altered sleep patterns or reduction in participation in usual activities (Himelstein, 2006).	Specific drug therapy does not currently exist (Himelstein, 2006).	Prioritise daily activities to conserve child's energy levels. Plan and pace activities throughout the day.	A thorough history should exclude other causes, such as depression or anaemia (Himelstein, 2006). Occupational therapists and physiotherapists may be able to assist with management programmes.
Anxiety	Anxiety usually takes the form of separation anxiety, loneliness, procedure-related anxiety, fear of abandonment and 'death anxiety'. Organic causes, such as pain, insomnia, breathlessness or weakness, may heighten anxiety (Twycross and Wilcock, 2018).	Midazolam and levomepromazine are the first two drugs of choice (although midazolam is known to cause paradoxical agitation). These can both be used via a syringe driver or midazolam can be given buccally or intranasally. Rectal diazepam or sublingual lorazepam are useful in acute cases of anxiety.	Provide the environment and opportunity for the child to raise their concerns or fears. Honesty, if offered gently, is helpful. Ensure the question being asked is being answered – listen to what is being asked. Consider complementary therapies, and input from a psychology or youth worker in the case of a young person.	The sedating effects of most of these drugs need to be discussed with parents – it may be a side-effect that parents will have difficulty with. Parents need to be aware and comfortable with health professionals discussing anxieties with their child.

This is only a selection of a few of the commonly experienced symptoms. Infections, bleeding, anorexia, muscle spasm, among others, are also symptoms that can be experienced by children. See Goldman et al. (2006a) Oxford Textbook of Palliative Care for Children, and Rainbows Children's Hospice Guidelines, 7th ed. (2008). The 9.5 edition (2016) gives a more exhaustive and detailed account of symptom management.

WWW

Refer to Rainbow Children's Hospice guidelines – basic symptom control in paediatric palliative care at:

- https://www.togetherforshortlives.org.uk/changing-lives/supporting-care-professionals/resources-and-research/
  Refer to The Association of Paediatric Palliative Medicine Master Formulary, 2017. Fourth Edition.
- https://www.togetherforshortlives.org.uk/resource/appm-master-formulary-2020-5th-edition/

A study by Pritchard et al. (2008) examined parents' perceptions of symptoms experienced by children with advanced cancer, including changes in their child's behaviour and appearance. Health care professionals should prepare and support parents regarding these two distressing symptoms.

Palliative care to children and families is developed around an ethos of holistic care delivery – that is care that embraces the interdependence between the physical, psychosocial and spiritual needs of the infant, child, young person, their family and those important to them (Goldman et al., 2006b).

Seldom are the issues and symptoms experienced by children and families simply in one category; much more often they are complex and multi-faceted. The child with palliative care needs must be viewed within the context of a family system (McNeilly et al., 2006). The philosophy of palliative care for children is thus premised on a holistic, individualised approach, which centres on the specific needs of each individual child and family during their limited life trajectory (Price et al., 2005). The care should be assessed, planned, implemented and evaluated using a collaborative partnership approach and should address the biological, psychological, social and spiritual needs of the child and family.

The collaborative partnership approach should be based on a trusting, therapeutic relationship with families (Monterosso and Kristjanson, 2008). Families should be welcomed as partners in all stages of the nursing process. Parents should feel they have a choice and be in control of the situation (Vickers and Carlisle, 2000).

END-OF-LIFE CARE

End-of-life care has been identified as:

> … care that helps all those with advanced, progressive, incurable illness to live as well as possible until they die. It focuses on preparing for an anticipated death and managing the end stage of a terminal medical condition. This includes care during and around the time of death and immediately afterwards. It enables the supportive and palliative care needs of both child/young person and family to be identified and met throughout the last phase of life and into bereavement. It includes management of pain and other symptoms and the provision of psychological, social, spiritual and practical support.
>
> ***Together for Short Lives (2018 p 33)***

However, identifying when a child enters the end-of-life phase is not easy and is dependent upon the child's condition,

with clinical patterns being variable (Finlay et al., 2008). For some families, there is little time to acknowledge that death is imminent; for others there is a clearer move to this phase – for example where a decision may have been made to stop treatment or where treatment options are exhausted.

ACTIVITY

Examine the resources available that you could use in your practice when caring for a child at the end-of-life developed by Together for Short Lives at the link below.

- https://www.togetherforshortlives.org.uk/resource/guide-end-life-care/

Families face many decisions throughout the whole palliative care journey but especially at the end-of-life stage (Popejoy, 2015). One of the choices is often the 'place of care' as the child approaches death. Improvements and developments within community services have led to many families choosing their own home as the place where they want their child to be nursed. Where appropriate, the child or young person should be included when the family considers the choice of where the child should be nursed. All their options should be outlined, and again, they may require time to discuss and make a decision. Parents often prefer the palliative care of their children to be carried out at home (Hynson and Sawyer, 2001; Vickers and Carlisle, 2000; Vickers et al., 2007).

ACTIVITY

Consider the advantages for the child and family if home is the place where the end-of-life care is delivered.

Children often prefer to be cared for at home in their own familiar environment, and home is also the place where the family may maintain greater control and a more normal family life can be managed (Friedman et al., 2005). Despite support from the interdisciplinary team, caring for the child at home can place a heavy responsibility on the parents. It is imperative to build a team around the child and family at home where good communication and coordination is essential. Anticipating symptoms, and having access to drugs and out of hours specialist advice, ensures that parents feel supported. Goldman et al. (1990) assert that the hospital environment can provide security, although the environment may not be comfortable and parental control may be lacking. It is important that parents who are not able to choose the home care option should not be made to feel guilty (Friedman et al., 2005). The hospice can provide a valuable alternative for families who cannot contemplate a home death (Watterson and Hain, 2003). Hospices can offer a homely, less clinical environment for families along with the security often desired by parents (Price et al., 2018).

The components of care already discussed in this chapter are also crucial at the end of life. End-of-life care should be based upon an individualised holistic approach to care centred on the changing needs of the child and family.

Communication, good team working, a therapeutic relationship with the child and family, good symptom management and a forum where family decisions are nurtured and facilitated are central aspects of quality end-of-life care. The stress and anxiety of families, often coupled with the reluctance to accept that death is imminent, can be particularly challenging. Changes in the child's behaviour and appearance were identified by parents as symptoms that caused them concern as they approached death (Pritchard et al., 2008). This finding has implications for health care professionals, as addressing the likelihood of these with families in advance is important.

Together for Short Lives (2013) Core Care Pathway gives an excellent framework to guide and structure end-of-life plans and ensures that all the child's and family's needs are considered. The end-of-life component of this pathway can be viewed on the companion CD-ROM.

The last days of a child's life, particularly, remain clear in the minds of parents (Postovsky and Ben Arush, 2004). Memories – negative and positive – that parents have of their child's end-of-life care can have an effect on parental adjustment, and theoretical perspectives on parental grief further support this (Davies, 2004). Therefore, the nurse has a professional responsibility to ensure that care is sensitively and carefully provided in response to the individual needs of both the child and family (Friedman et al., 2005). The family includes parents, siblings and the wider family circle.

Again, it is important to reiterate that individuality is the key in palliative care. However, the named nurse in this particular situation endeavoured to facilitate and support the parents in their decision. She sat down with John and, holding his hand, asked him if there was anything he wanted to talk about or if there were any questions he wanted to ask. He simply asked: 'Can you please make sure I am not in pain?' He did know that death was impending and did not wish to discuss it any further. Levetown and the Committee on Bioethics (2008) concede that children who do not ask should be given the opportunity to receive information; however, if they refuse it, this should not be forced upon them.

SCENARIO

John is an 11-year-old boy at the end stage of his illness. His parents want him to know the truth about his impending death. They think he probably already knows, but ask his named nurse to tell him. What would you do if you were that nurse?

It is widely recognised that managing end-of-life care for young people is challenging. Discussions around prognosis and decision-making are often delayed because of questions about the legal competence of the adolescent, staff feeling ill-equipped to engage in end-of-life discussions, and parental concern that discussing plans means the medical team wish to withdraw care. In recent years progress has been made in how health care professionals can approach advanced care planning with adolescents, involve their family and engage the entire health care team. Implementing a consistent approach at key points of the adolescence journey ensures preferences and goals are discussed. Ideally, these quality of life conversations should commence when treatment is started and can be revisited at progression of disease. It is important to assist parents to engage in end-of-life conversations with their child as lack of communication can lead to emotional isolation at a time when support is needed. It must be recognised that not every adolescent will be developmentally or cognitively able or wish to speak about their advancing disease.

Truth telling and talking to the dying child or young person can cause the nurse to face an ethical dilemma, especially if it contravenes the family's wishes. Other ethical dilemmas in palliative care include withdrawing treatment, decisions around 'Do Not Resuscitate', feeding and administering fluids to the child facing death, and more recently, parents using unlicensed/unprescribed medications such as cannabis, and in many cases not being transparent with the team caring for the child. These can also cause distress for families and raise ethical issues for staff. Go to Chapter xxx and identify the ethical principles and how they relate to children's palliative care.

Underpinning all decision-making must be the basic tenet of Article 3 of the UN Convention on the Rights of the Child (1989) – 'the best interests of children must be the primary concern in making decisions that may affect them'. When parental and professional interests are in conflict, good practice requires good communication between both parties to resolve disagreements.

Given the recent high profile cases with regard to the withdrawal of life-sustaining treatment (following court intervention), it is timely to mention how advances in medicine and technology have enabled previously fatal diseases to be managed, and ready access to information has led to more-informed parents with the expectation that their child will recover from the next episode in intensive care or that their child will be eligible for a clinical trial.

The Royal College of Paediatrics and Child Health document 'Making Decisions to Limit Treatment in Life Limiting and Life Threatening Conditions' (2015) offers a comprehensive framework for practice.

 POWERPOINT

Access the companion PowerPoint presentation and look at the case study.

A wide range of verbal and non-verbal communication strategies can be used when communicating with life-limited children. Touch, play, art and the therapeutic use of storytelling are important strategies in palliative care, aiding the child in expressing their concerns, fears and feelings (Done, 2001). These strategies are also useful in aiding siblings to express their feelings and are useful media for preparing them for the impending death. Play is widely recognised as the language of the child and, as such, play is an important communication medium for the child (see Chapter 10). Play specialists in both the hospital and community have expert training to enable them to fully implement play packages in order to maximise benefit to the child and family.

Charitable organisations have a role to play in the psychological well-being of children with life-limiting illnesses and their families, for example organisations such as Make-a-Wish, Dreams Come True and Dial a Dream. Wishes granted are wide-ranging and can give the family happy memories that can comfort them in bereavement.

> ### 🌐 WWW
>
> Visit the Make-a-Wish and Starlight Foundation websites and familiarise yourself with the mission statements of the charities and the ways in which they have in the past helped children and families. Read the personal stories of wishes that have been granted:
> - http://www.make-a-wish.org.uk
> - http://www.starlight.org.uk

Children and families can gain much psychological and social support from groups where they meet with other families whose children have the same condition. They also have experts and counsellors to assist the child and family in developing family and personal coping strategies. Examples of these groups are Contact, React and other local support groups.

The impact on the marital relationship, the interactions and communication between parents has also been examined. Evidence has indicated that a child's life-threatening illness can lead to strain on the relationship between parents as they focus on caring for the child and therefore can neglect their relationship (Steele, 2005). This provides a useful insight into the possible changes in the dynamics of relationships and endorses the importance of ensuring that within the 'family systems approach' to care, emotional support and communication is channelled to mothers, fathers, siblings and other family members.

SPIRITUAL CARE

Many families have established sources for spiritual support, and these will continue during their child's palliative journey and particularly at critical junctures – for example diagnosis, relapse or end of life. The nurse must ensure that the spiritual needs of the child and family are addressed and be cognizant of the fact that spiritual needs can occur independently of religious needs (Ferrell et al., 2016). Spiritual care should include the uniqueness of the child and family, and should address their needs, values and beliefs, encompassing moral aspects and value systems possessed by a parent and a child – for example insight and wisdom, reliance on values, and virtues such as hope, trust and love (Crisp, 2016). Evidence suggests that parents find issues around spirituality as a source of help as their child nears the end of life. Prayer, faith, access to clergy and the transcendent quality of the child–parent relationship that endures beyond death were identified as important by parents who had a child die in intensive care (Robinson et al., 2006).

Some families who have previously had little or no religious faith or belief may wish to have contact with a minister/chaplain as they face the death of their child – they should be facilitated in this as early as possible (Feudtner et al., 2003). The child, too, may wish to discuss ideas, views and fears from a spiritual stance. Some young people may want to talk, discuss and plan the arrangements for their funeral with the minister before their death. If this is their wish, it is important that they are given the opportunity to do so. Anger 'against God' can be common in some parents whose child is dying – the minister/chaplain may be a channel by which they can vent their anger with a professional who may help and facilitate them working through their feelings and emotions. For some families, to have their child baptised may be important at this time and should be facilitated. Children and families should be given the opportunity, time and privacy to perform any religious acts that may provide them comfort, for example lighting a candle (obviously safety must be paramount).

We are now living in a very wide and diverse cultural society. It is essential that all members of the team caring for the child recognise the individuality of the child and family and recognise, respect and accept any specific spiritual wishes, beliefs or rituals surrounding death.

CARE OF THE CHILD FOLLOWING DEATH

The need to support and advise parents is never greater than at the time when the death occurs (see Chapter 10 for an introduction to communication in bereavement). Even if the death has been expected, the parents' reactions at the time of death are unpredictable. Parents who have just lost their child will usually require guidance from the health care professional. Parental choice and control is essential (NICE, 2016). The health care professional must therefore be aware of the relevant issues and be knowledgeable and informed about the options facing the family at this sad time.

- Time and privacy should be given to parents when decisions have to be made.
- Death should be established by a medical officer/GP.
- Families should be able to stay with their child for as long as they wish and be encouraged to hold, cuddle, wash and dress their child if desired.
- Families should be prepared for how the child's appearance will change after death and the possible noises the body may make.
- Cultural and religious beliefs and practices should be respected.
- Families should be given the opportunity to talk through procedures and not merely be given the written information.
- Written booklets are useful to back up verbal information and guide parents to further support networks.
- The family might want a handprint or lock of hair to keep. Consent should be obtained from the family.
- Families should be given time to spend with their child; this may include siblings. They should never feel rushed or hurried.

- Parents should be informed of their choices regarding taking their child home following a planned death in hospice or hospital.
- All those professionals who have contact with the family must be immediately informed about the child's death so that appointments, etc., are not sent for the child. This can cause considerable distress to the family.
- Post-mortems are not usual if the death is expected. However, in some cases, a post-mortem may be useful if a diagnosis was not clear or to help gain insight into rare conditions. Parents will need support, reassurance and information to aid them to make decisions and choices.

 ACTIVITY

> In the Clinical Companion to this book, read McNeilly and Price (2008) Chapter 44 'Care of the child' in Kelsey and McEwing (Eds) 2008 Clinical Skills in Child Health.

BEREAVEMENT CARE

The death of a child is a uniquely traumatic experience for a parent (Brewis, 1995; Rando, 1986). The grieving process following such a loss is complex and multi-faceted. The definition of palliative care cited at the outset of this chapter includes bereavement support as one of the essential components of children's palliative care. This section therefore examines the needs of a family following the death of their child and the nurse's role in bereavement care. At this stage it seems appropriate to clarify the terms that are commonly used here. Hindmarch (2000) suggests that:

- bereavement is what happens;
- grief is what one feels in reaction to the bereavement;
- mourning is what one does to express grief.

 ACTIVITY

> Consider the factors that may affect an individual's grief.

The gendered differences in parental reaction to death of a child have been studied in a key work by Feeley and Gottlieb (1988). This study reported that mothers' grief reactions appeared angrier, despairing and much more isolating than that of fathers. Mothers were also more likely to talk about their feelings whereas fathers were more likely to keep busy. Duncombe and Marsden (1995) describe the 'tragedy of the inexpressive male' and in addition pointed out the more apparent willingness of mothers to 'recognise, label, express and disclose feelings'.

The devastation caused by a child's death is far reaching, affecting parents, siblings, grandparents, wider family circles, health care professionals and communities. Rando (1986) identifies that the loss of a child to a parent can seem like a physical loss (that is that they have lost a part of themselves), the loss of their role, loss of hopes, dreams and their identity as protector. Klass (1988) identifies two central features of parental grief following the death of their child. First, that

it represents to the parent a loss of self and, second, that it represents a loss of competence.

Worden (1991) describes the process of mourning as a series of tasks linked to stages. He identified four stages with inherent tasks, which the mourner must work through to resolve their grief:

- to accept the reality of loss
- to work through the pain of grief
- to adjust to an environment in which the deceased is missing
- to emotionally relocate the deceased and move on with life (the task of resolution)

However, this staged approach can be seen as providing a very rigid approach to grief work, although it does permit individuality, moving in and out of different stages, and overall provides a very prescriptive framework. It is important to recognise that Worden's grief work does not necessarily state that the stages are experienced sequentially or that any time limit can be applied. Uniformity is not part of the grieving process. There are no rules in grief and each parent is likely to respond in a different way.

Goldman (1999) states that the progress through phases of grief is not straightforward or only in one direction, and perspectives on parental grief would now indicate that bereaved parents negotiate the complexities of readjusted life with 'the dead child' and their continuing bonds with this child (Davies, 2004).

 ACTIVITY

> Consider some roles that may negatively affect fathers when dealing with their grief. See the text that follows.

William Schatz (1986) identified the following male roles as negatively affecting the way he dealt with his grief following the death of his son:

- The role of being strong, a macho man always in control of his emotions.
- The role of competing and winning in a crisis and being the best.
- The role of being protector of family and possessions.
- The role of being the family provider.
- The role of being problem solver, fixing things or finding someone who can.
- The role of controller.
- The role of self-sufficient standing on his own two feet.

The nurse who is coordinating the bereavement care of a family should be aware of these issues and patterns of grief.

Siblings require particular attention during the period leading up to the death of the child, as mentioned earlier, and following the death through bereavement. The period of time following the death, even though it may have been expected, is a time of great turmoil, interruption and uncertainty for the siblings. Their age and cognitive development will obviously affect their understanding. Children have very definite needs in bereavement. They require information, reassurance, time to express their feelings and the need to be involved. Children need also to have some type of routine maintained – this, coupled with support from the adults around them, may be difficult as the parents are struggling to deal with their own loss and feelings. Parents may need help from the health care professional in coordinating the bereavement care to gain an insight into patterns of childhood grief and suggestions as to how the child may be helped through the process.

Fox (1988) has outlined four tasks for grieving children:

- To understand or begin to make sense out of what is happening.
- To grieve and express emotional responses to loss.
- To commemorate in some formal or informal way the life of the person who has died.
- To learn how to integrate the loss into one's life to continue with everyday activities of living and loving.

Children can be helped in bereavement by having a memento of the person who has died. This way the child is provided with a tangible reminder of the person who is gone, is reminded of their existence and reassured that life does go on. This could be a favourite toy, photograph, another item of value to the child who has died, or even a selection of items in a designated memory box. A number of resources are available to help children experience a healthy grieving process (see the list of books available for children on the companion PowerPoint presentation).

Parents are often anxious about siblings attending the funeral. On the one hand, they want to protect them, and on the other the parents may feel unable to cope with their own feelings and the feelings of the child. Children should be involved in discussions about this, should be given information beforehand about what they should expect at the service, and their wishes and opinions should be listened to. If they do wish to attend, it may be appropriate for another adult to be assigned to look after them during the service. If they do not attend, they should be told as soon afterwards what happened and be given the chance to visit the grave.

It can be very helpful if children are involved in bereavement support groups, which enable the child to work through their grief and to see that they are not alone. Many children's hospices run groups such as these. With support and guidance from family and professionals, the child will learn to adapt to their loss and live their own life.

It is also important to remember the extended family circle and community that may be affected by the death of the child. Grandparents not only lose their grandchild, but also have the added burden of 'losing' their own child who is consumed with grief. Many grandparents may experience 'survivor guilt' asking 'Why am I still living when my grandchild is dead?'

🌐 WWW

Visit the Winston's Wish website and investigate ways in which this organisation helps support bereaved children.

- http://www.winstonswish.org.uk

  Examine some of the resources that could be used in practice.

The wider community is also affected by the death of a child, and it is important that the health care professional coordinating the bereavement follow-up ensures that contact is made with the child's school. Teachers may feel uncertain how to support the other pupils and staff at this time and usually welcome advice about how to manage the grief and commemorate the child who has died.

The bereavement component of palliative care may be coordinated and provided by a community children's nurse, Macmillan nurse, hospice nurse or other identified health care professional. The individual family should dictate the frequency of visits and type of support required. Contact should decrease as the family develops coping strategies, or the nurse may have to refer a parent to a psychologist or bereavement counsellor if they feel that the individual concerned needs further specialist bereavement support. Many hospitals and hospices hold annual remembrance services, which are important to families. Other ways organisations can assist with remembering the child are inclusion in the book of remembrance and sending cards and flowers on special dates, for example, the first anniversary of the child's death.

👤 ACTIVITY

List some organisations that help bereaved families. (Details of these can be found on the companion PowerPoint slide.)

THE NEEDS OF THE HEALTH CARE PROFESSIONAL

Care of children who are life limited can be a source of profound satisfaction for staff (Taylor and Aldridge, 2017). However, it can also be stressful for all those involved in providing care. The death of a child may lead to extreme guilt, anger, sadness and perhaps the feeling that the health care worker has failed the child and family (Michelson and Steinhorn, 2007).

Avoiding burn-out requires careful self-stress management strategies and awareness of the needs of oneself and others in the team (Baverstock and Finlay, 2006). All members of the team must be remembered: porters, domestic assistants and student nurses also can develop a bond with the child and family and can sometimes be overlooked when a death occurs. It is important to consider that you may be a health care professional but also that you are a human being with real feelings and emotions. Armstrong (2007) reported that the need to grieve often went unrecognised, and there was a lack of support to allow for the grieving process. Most nurses interviewed identified the need for formal mechanisms of support to be available, such as debriefing or counselling. It is essential to recognise our feelings and pain at a loss and deal with this. An 'ostrich approach' is dangerous, and ignoring one's own needs can have a detrimental effect in the long term. Organisations such as Child Bereavement UK offer support and training for health care workers in this area.

↩ REFLECT ON YOUR PRACTICE

Reflect on ways that you have seen, or consider may be useful strategies for, staff coping with death of a child.

Check out suggestions for staff coping management strategies on the companion PowerPoint slide.

SUMMARY

Palliative care and end-of-life care is an integrated approach to care that addresses holistic needs at different stages of the uncertain illness trajectory and focuses on quality of life for the child and family.

Quality palliative care for the child or young person requires a cohesive partnership approach, centred on the family with a collaborative interdisciplinary focus to care. Nurses play a key role within the team and are required to identify and address the needs, fears and anxieties of the child–family circle.

Although considerable development has occurred within children's palliative care over recent years, and policy has recognised the distinct needs of children with life-limiting conditions, future developments are required. The implementation of the recommendations of strategy and standards (NICE, 2017) is a good place to start while ensuring services for all children, regardless of where they live. In addition, further substantive research and further educational opportunities both nationally and internationally are required, as we move forward in the continual provision of care based on the best evidence (NICE, 2016).

Key Points

- Palliative care for children is an integrated philosophy of care provided in a variety of settings and has developed as a distinct specialty.
- The child and family should be central to decisions about the care delivered.
- Parallel planning in partnership with the family is crucial.
- The interdisciplinary team should address the holistic needs of the child.
- Parents and siblings need much support and information as death approaches.
- It is important to remember that for a parent who has lost a child bereavement is a long, complicated and very individual process.
- Nurses need to recognise that caring for children and families facing death is extremely stressful. They should be aware of the importance of developing their own personal management strategies.

REFERENCES

Aldridge, J., Shimmon, K., Miller, M., et al., 2017. 'I can't tell my child they are dying'. Helping parents have conversations with their child. Arch. Dis. Child. Educ. Pract. 102 (4), 182–187.

Anghelescu, D., Oakes, L., Hinds, P., 2006. Palliative care and pediatrics. Anesthesiol. Clin. North. Am. 24, 145–161.

Armstrong, D., 2007. Childhood Cancer: The Challenge of Providing Nursing Care in the Last Days of Life. Unpublished M.Sc. dissertation. University of Ulster.

Association of Paediatric Palliative Medicine Master Formulary, 2017, fourth ed. Available from: https://www.togetherforshortlives.org.uk/resource/appm-master-formulary-2017-4th-edition/.

Baverstock, A., Finlay, F., 2006. A study of staff support mechanisms within children's hospice. Int. J. Palliative Nurs. 12 (11), 506–508.

Beardsmore, S., Fitzmaurice, N., 2002. Palliative care in paediatric oncology. Eur. J. Can. 38, 1900–1907.

Bluebond-Langner, M., 1978. Mutual Pretence: Causes and Consequences. The Private Worlds of Dying Children. University Press, Princeton.

Brady, M., 1996. Symptom control in dying children. In: Hill, L. (Ed.), 1996. Caring for Dying Children and Families. Chapman Hall, London.

Brewis, E., 2004. Oncology Outreach: history in the making. Peadiatric Nursing 16 (9), 24–27.

Buckle, S., 2003. Aromatherapy and massage – the evidence. Paediatr. Nurs. 156, 24–27.

Chad, T., 2008. Losing a child to spinal muscular atrophy. Paediatr. Nurs. 203, 32–33.

Crisp, C.L., 2016. Supporting parents when their child has a life-limiting illness. J. Chris. Nur. 33 (1), 14–21.

Davies, R., 2004. New understandings of parental grief: literature review. J. Adv. Nurs. 46, 506–513.

De Graves, S., Aranda, S., 2005. When a child cannot be cured – reflections of health professionals. Eur. J. Cancer Care 14, 132–140.

Department of Health (DoH), 2005. National Service Framework for Children, Young People and Maternity Services – Commissioning Children's and Young People's Palliative Care Services. DoH, London.

Department of Health (DoH), 2007. Palliative Care Services for Children and Young People in England. An independent review for the Secretary of State for Health. DoH, London.

Department of Health (DoH), 2008. Better Lives: Better Care. Improving Outcomes and Experiences for Children, Young People and their Families Living with Life-Limiting and Life Threatening Conditions. DoH, London.

Department of Health (DoH) and Department for Education and Skills (DfES), 2004. National Service Framework for Children, Young People and Maternity Services. Disabled Children and Those with Complex Health Care Needs. DoH, London.

Done, A., 2001. The therapeutic use of story telling. Paediatr. Nurs. 133, 17–20.

Duncombe, J., Marsden, D., 1995. 'Workaholics' and 'whinging women': theorising intimacy and emotion work – the last frontier of gender inequality? Sociolog. Rev. 43, 150–170.

Feeley, N., Gottlieb, L.N., 1988. Parents' coping and communication following their infant's death. Omega 191, 51–67.

Feudtner, C., Haney, J., Dimmers, M.A., 2003. Spiritual care needs of hospitalized children and their families: a national survey of pastoral care providers' perceptions. Pediatrics 111, 67–72.

Finlay, F., Lewis, M., Lenton, S., et al., 2008. Planning for the end of children's lives--the lifetime framework. Child. Health Care Dev. 34 (4), 342–344.

Ferrell, B., Wittenberg, E., Battista, V., et al., 2016. Exploring the spiritual needs of families with seriously ill children. Int. J. Palliat. Nurs. 22 (8), 388–394.

Fox, S.S., 1988. Good grief: helping groups of children when a friend dies. Cited. In: Langton, H. (Ed.), The Child With Cancer – Family Centred Care, 2000. Baillière Tindall, London.

Forster, E., Hafiz, A., 2015. Paediatric death and dying: exploring coping strategies of health professionals and perceptions of support provision. Int. J. Palliat. Nurs. 21 (6), 294–301. https://doi.org/10.12968/ijpn.2015.21.6.294. PMID: 26126678.

Fraser, L., Lidstone, V., Miller, M., Aldridge, J., Norman, P., McKinney, P., Parslow, R., 2014. Patterns of diagnoses amongst children and young adults with life-limiting conditions: implications for service provision. BMJ Support. Palliat. Care 4 (Suppl. 1), A21. https://doi.org/10.1136/bmjspcare-2014-000654.58.

Friedman, D.L., Hilden, J.M., Powaski, K., 2005. Issues and challenges in palliative care for children with cancer. Curr. Pain Headache Rep. 9, 249–255.

Fullerton, J.M., Totsika, V., Hain, R., et al., 2017. Siblings of children with life-limiting conditions: psychological adjustment and sibling relationships. Child. Care Health Dev. 43 (3), 393–400.

Giovanola, J., 2005. Sibling involvement at the end of life. J. Pediatr. Oncol. Nurs. 22 (4), 222–226.

Goldman, A., 1999. Care of the Dying Child. Oxford University Press, Oxford.

Goldman, A., Beardsmore, S., Hunt, J., 1990. Palliative care for children: home hospital or hospice. Arch. Dis. Child. 65, 641–643.

Goldman, A., Hain, R., Liben, S. (Eds.), 2006a. Oxford Textbook of Palliative Care for Children. Oxford University Press, Oxford.

Goldman, A., Hewitt, M., Collins, G., Childs, M., Hain, R., 2006b. Symptoms in children/young people with progressive malignant disease. UKCCSG/Paediatric Oncology Nurses Forum Survey. Pediatrics 117, 1179–1186.

Grinyer, A., Barbarachild, Z., 2011. Teenage and Young Adult Palliative and End-of-life Care Service Evaluation; A Teenage Cancer Trust Project. Lancaster University.

Hain, R., Wallace, A., 2008. Progress in palliative care for children in the UK. Paediatr. Child Health 18 (3), 141–146.

Hechler, T., Blankenburg, M., Friedrichsdorf, S.J., Garske, D., Hubner, R., Menke, A., Wamsler, C., Wolfe, J., Zernikow, B., 2008. Parents' perspective on symptoms, quality of life, characteristics of death and end-of-life decisions for children dying from cancer. Klin Padiatric 220, 166–174.

Hill, D.L., Miller, V.A., Hexem, K.R., et al., 2015. Problems and hopes perceived by mothers, fathers and physicians of children receiving palliative care. Health Expect. 18 (5), 1052–1065.

Himelstein, B.P., 2006. Palliative care for infants, children, adolescents and their families. J. Palliat. Med. 9 (1), 163–180.

Hindmarch, C., 2000. On the Death of a Child, second ed. Radcliffe Medical Press, Oxford.

Hoell, J.I., Warfsmann, J., Gagnon, G., et al., 2017. Palliative care for children with a yet undiagnosed syndrome. Eur. J. Paediatr. 176 (10), 1319–1327.

Hunt, A., 2003. Paediatric pain profile. Available from: www.pppprofile.org.uk.

Hynson, J., Gillis, J., Collins, J., et al., 2003. The dying child: how is care different? Med. J. Aust. 179, S20–S22.

Hynson, J.L., Sawyer, S.M., 2001. Paediatric palliative care: distinctive needs and emerging issues. J. Paediatr. Child Health 37, 323–325.

Jones, B.L., 2006. Companionship, control, and compassion: a social work perspective on the needs of children with cancer and their families at the end of life. J. Palliat. Med. 9, 774–788.

Jordan, J., Price, J., Prior, L., 2015. Disorder and disconnection: parent experiences of liminality when caring for a dying child. Sociol. Health. Illness 37 (6), 839–855. https://doi.org/10.1111/1467-9566.12235.

Judd, D., 1994. Give Sorrow Words – Working with a Dying Child, second ed. Whurr Publishers, London.

Kerr, H., Price, J., Nicholl, H., et al., 2018. Facilitating transition from children's to adult services for young adults with life-limiting. conditions (TASYL). Programme theory developed from a mixed methods realist evaluation. Int. J. Nurs. Stud. 86, 126–138.

Khan, J., Gaze, S., Tomlin, S., 2016. The role of the pharmacist in paediatric palliative care. Arch. Dis. Child. 101 (9), e2.

Klass, D., 1988. Parental Grief, Solace and Resolution. Springer, New York.

Kreicbergs, U., 2018. Paediatric palliative care should focus on living as well as dying. Acta Paediatr. 107. https://doi.org/10.1111/apa.14319.

Kubler-Ross, E., 1970. On Death and Dying. Tavistock Press, London.

Laakso, H., Paunonen-Illmonen, M., 2002. Mother's experience of social support following the death of a child. J. Clin. Nurs. 11, 176–185.

Levetown, M., 2008. The Committee on Bioethics. Communicating with children and families; from everyday interactions to skill in conveying distressing symptoms. Pediatrics 121, e1441–e1460.

Ling, J., Payne, S., Connaire, K., et al., 2015. Parental decision-making on utilization of out-of-home respite in children's palliative care: findings of qualitative care study research – a proposed new model. Child. Care Health Dev. 42 (1), 51–59.

Little, M., Sayers, E., 2004. While there's life: hope and the experience of cancer. Soc. Sci. Med. 59, 1329–1337.

Lotz, J.D., Daxer, M., Jox, R.J., et al., 2017. "Hope for the best, prepare for the worst": a qualitative interview study on parents' needs and fears in pediatric advance care planning. Palliat. Med. 31 (8), 764–771.

Marston, J., Boucher, S., Downing, J., 2018. International Children's Palliative Care Network: a global action network for children with life-limiting conditions. J. Pain Symptom. Manage. 55 (2S), S104–s111.

Maunder, E.Z., 2004. The challenge of transitional care for young people with life-limiting illness. Br. J. Nurs. 13 (10), 594–596.

McCluggage, H.-L., Elborn, J.S., 2006. Symptoms suffered by life-limited children that cause anxiety to UK children's hospice staff. Int. J. Palliat. Nurs. 12, 254–258.

McCluggage, H.-L., Jassal, S.S., 2009. Symptom management. In: Price, J., McNeilly, P. (Eds.), Palliative Care for Children and Families: An Interdisciplinary Approach, 2009. Palgrave MacMillan, Basingstoke.

McCloskey, S., Taggart, L., 2010. How much compassion have I left? An exploration of occupational stress among children's palliative care nurses. Int. J. Palliat. Nurs. 16 (5), 233–240.

McNeilly, P., Price, J., McCloskey, S., 2004. The use of syringe drivers: a paediatric perspective. Int. J. Palliat. Nurs. 108, 399–402.

McNeilly, P., Price, J., McCloskey, S., 2006. Reflection in children's palliative care: a model. Eur. J. Palliat. Care 131, 31–34.

McNeilly, P., Price, J., 2008. Care of the child after death. In: Kelsey, J., McEwing, G. (Eds.), Clinical Skills in Child Health Practice, 2008. Elsevier, London.

Michelson, K.N., Steinhorn, D.M., 2007. Pediatric end-of-life issues and palliative care. Clin. Pediatr. Emerg. Med. 8, 212–219.

Monterosso, L., Kristjanson, G., 2008. Supportive and palliative care needs of families of children who die from cancer: an Australian study. Palliat. Med. 22, 59–69.

National Institute for Health and Care Excellence (NICE), 2016. End of life care for infants, children and young people with life limiting conditions. Planning and management (NG61). Available from: https://www.nice.org.uk/guidance/ng61.

National Institute for Health and Care Excellence (NICE), 2017. End of Life Care for Infants, Children and Young People – Quality Standard (QS160). Available from: https://www.nice.org.uk/guidance/qs160.

Nuutila, L., Salantera, S., 2006. Children with a long-term illness; parents' experiences of care. J. Pediatr. Nurs. 21, 153–160.

Popejoy, E., 2015. Parents' experiences of care decisions about children with life-limiting illnesses. Nurs. Child. Young People 27, 20–24.

Postovsky, G., Ben Arush, C., 2004. Care of a dying child of cancer – the role of the palliative care team in pediatric oncology. Pediatr. Hematol. Oncol. 21, 67–76.

Price, J., Jones, A.-M., 2015. Living through the life-altering loss of a child: a narrative review. Iss. Compre. Pediatric Nurs. 38 (3), 222–240 (IF 0.32).

Price, J., Jordan, J., Prior, L., 2013. A consensus for change: parent and professional perspectives on care for children at the end-of-life. Iss. Compre. Pediatric Nurs. 36 (1), 70–87.

Price, J., Jordan, J., Prior, L., et al., 2011. Living through the death of a child: a qualitative study of bereaved parents' experiences. Int. J. Nurs. Stud. 48 (11), 1384–1392.

Price, J., McCloskey, S., Brazil, K., 2018. The role of hospice in the transition from hospital to home for technology dependent children – a qualitative study. J. Clin. Nurs. 27 (1–2), 396–406.

Price, J., McNeilly, P., McFarlane, M., 2005. Paediatric palliative care in the UK: past, present and future. Int. J. Palliat. Nurs. 113, 124–126.

Price, J., McNeilly, P., Surgenor, M., 2006. Breaking bad news to parents – the children's nurse's role. Int. J. Palliat. Nurs. 12 (3), 115–120.

Price, J., McNeilly, P., 2009. Palliative Care for Children and Families. An Interdisciplinary Approach. Palgrave, London.

Pritchard, M., Burghen, E., Srivastava, D.K., et al., 2008. Cancer related symptoms most concerning to parents during the last week and last day of their child's life. Pediatrics 121, 1301–1309.

Rainbow Children's Hospice, 2016. (Edition 9.5) Guidelines – Basic Symptom Control. seventh ed. Available from: https://www.togetherforshortlives.org.uk/changing-lives/supporting-care-professionals/resources-and-research/.

Robinson, M., Thiel, M., Backus, M., et al., 2006. Matters of spirituality at the end of life in the paediatric intensive care unit. Pediatrics 118, 719–729.

Royal College of Nursing (RCN), 2013. Breaking Bad News: Supporting Parents When they are Told of their Child's Diagnosis. RCN Guidance for Nurses, Midwives and Health Visitors. Available from: https://www.rcn.org.uk/professional-development/publications/pub-004471.

Royal College of Paediatrics and Child Health (RCPCH), 2015. Making decisions to limit treatment in life-limiting and life threatening conditions in children: a framework for practice. Available from: https:// www.rcpch.ac.uk.

Schatz, W.H., 1986. Grief of fathers. In: Rando, A.T. (Ed.), Parental Loss of a Child. Research Press, Illinois.

Soricelli, B.A., Utech, C.L., 1985. Mourning the death of a child; the family and group process. Soc. Work. 30, 423–429.

Sourkes, B., Frankel, L., Brown, M., et al., 2005. Food, toys and love: pediatric palliative care. Curr. Prob. Pediatr. Adol. Health Care 35, 350–386.

Steele, R., 2005. Strategies used by families to navigate uncharted territory when a child is dying. J. Palliat. Care 21 (2), 103–110.

Swaffield, F., 1985. Protecting the parents? Nurs. Times 31, 51–52.

Taylor, J., Aldridge, J., 2017. Exploring the rewards and challenges of paediatric palliative care work – a qualitative study of a multi-disciplinary children's hospice care team. BMC Palliat. Care 73 (16), 73.

Thrane, S.E., Maurer, S.H., Ren, D., Danford, C.A., Cohen, S.M., 2017. Reiki Therapy for Symptom Management in children Receiving palliative care: a Pilot Study. Am J Hosp Palliat Care 34 (4), 373–379.

Together for Short Lives, 2013. A Core Care Pathway for Children with Life Limiting and Life Threatening Conditions, third ed. Bristol.

Together for Short Lives, 2018. A Guide to Children's Palliative Care. Supporting Babies, Children and Young People with Life Limiting and Life Threatening Conditions and Families, fourth ed. Bristol.

Tywcross, R., Wilcock, A., 2018. Introducing to Palliative Care, fifth ed.

United Nations Convention on the Rights of the Child, 1989. (20, xi, 1989; TS44; CM 1976) United Nations, New York. United Nations/human rights/CRC. http://www.unicef.org/crc/.

Vickers, J., Carlisle, C., 2000. Choices and control: parental experiences in pediatric terminal home care. J. Pediatr. Oncol. Nurs. 171, 12–20.

Vickers, J., Thompson, A., Collins, G.S., et al., 2007. Place and provision of palliative care for children with progressive cancer: a study by the Paediatric Oncology Nurses' Forum/United Kingdom Children's Cancer Study Group Palliative Care Working Group. J. Clin. Oncol. 25, 4472–4476.

Wallin, A.E., Steineck, G., Nyberg, T., et al., 2015. Insufficient communication and anxiety in cancer-bereaved siblings: a nation-wide long-term follow-up. Palliat. Support. Care 1–7.

Watterson, G., Hain, R., 2003. Palliative care; moving forward. Curr. Paediatr. 13, 221–225.

Wilkinson, D., 2013. We need palliative care for babies facing certain death. The Conversation. Available from: http://theconversation.com/we-need-palliative-care-for-babies-facing-certain-death-15932 (accessed 2 October 2018).

Wolfe, J., Grier, H.E., Klar, N., et al., 2000. Symptoms and suffering at the end of life in children with cancer. N. Engl. J. Med. 342, 326–333.

World Health Organization (WHO), 2012. Guidelines on the Pharmacological Treatment of Persisting Pain in Children with Medical Illnesses. World Health Organization, Geneva.

Worden, J.W., 1991. Grief Counselling and Grief Therapy. Tavistock Press, London.

Worswick, J., 2000. A House Called Helen – the Development of Hospice Care for Children. Oxford University Press, Oxford.

USEFUL WEBSITES

http://www.make-a-wish.org.uk – Make-a-Wish organization.
http://www.childhospice.org.uk – Children's Hospice UK
http://www.chionline.org – Children's Hospice International.
http://www.jessiesfund.org.uk – Jessie's Fund music therapy.
http://www.cafamily.org.uk – Contact.
http://dialadream-org.stackstaging.com/ – Dial a Dream.
http://www.reactcharity.org.
www.childbereavement.org.uk – Child Bereavement Charity
http://www.icpcn.org.uk/ – International Children's Palliative Care Network.

Page number followed by f indicate figures; t, tables; b, boxes.